Ebersole & Hess'
TOWARD HEALTHY AGING
Human Needs & Nursing Response

Theris A. Touhy, DNP, CNS, DPNAP

Emeritus Professor
Christine E. Lynn College of Nursing
Florida Atlantic University
Boca Raton, Florida

Kathleen Jett, PhD, GNP-BC

Gerontological Nurse Practitioner
Senior Care Clinic at Oak Hammock
Department of Aging and Geriatric Research
University of Florida
College of Medicine
Gainesville, Florida

NINTH EDITION

ELSEVIER

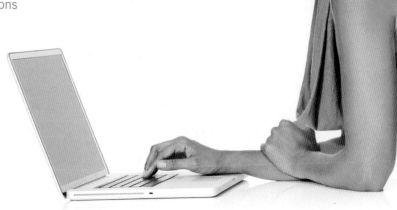

To my three sons and daughters-in-law, thanks for surrounding me with love and family. To my husband, just thanks for loving me for 47 years even though it's not always easy!

To my beautiful grandchildren, Colin, Molly, and Auden Touhy. Being your Grama TT makes growing older the best time of my life and I love you.

To all the students who read this book. I hope each of you will improve the journey toward healthy aging through your competence and compassion.

To all of my students who have embraced gerontological nursing as their specialty and are improving the lives of older people through their practice and teaching.

To the wise and wonderful older people whom I have been privileged to nurse, and to their caregivers. Thank you for making the words in this book a reality for the elders for whom you care, and for teaching me how to be a gerontological nurse.

Theris A. Touhy

To my patients and others who teach me every day about the highs and lows of the furthest reaches of age and what really matters the most in life.

To my husband Steve, for his patience during the year I worked on this edition, with little time for anything else.

To the staff at *The Diner* where I wrote and re-wrote for many hours in a place with no distractions and a sunny window. They always kept my iced tea glass full, knew what I wanted to eat, and how I liked it cooked!
I thank them.

And to Dr. Michael Johnson, who pushes me to grow and helps my soul seek peace.

Kathleen Jett

ELSEVIER

3251 Riverport Lane
St. Louis, Missouri 63043

EBERSOLE & HESS' TOWARD HEALTHY AGING, NINTH EDITION   ISBN: 978-0-323-32138-9

Notices

Knowledge and best practice in this field are constantly changing. As new research and experience broaden our understanding, changes in research methods, professional practices, or medical treatment may become necessary.

Practitioners and researchers must always rely on their own experience and knowledge in evaluating and using any information, methods, compounds, or experiments described herein. In using such information or methods they should be mindful of their own safety and the safety of others, including parties for whom they have a professional responsibility.

With respect to any drug or pharmaceutical products identified, readers are advised to check the most current information provided (i) on procedures featured or (ii) by the manufacturer of each product to be administered, to verify the recommended dose or formula, the method and duration of administration, and contraindications. It is the responsibility of practitioners, relying on their own experience and knowledge of their patients, to make diagnoses, to determine dosages and the best treatment for each individual patient, and to take all appropriate safety precautions.

To the fullest extent of the law, neither the Publisher nor the authors, contributors, or editors, assume any liability for any injury and/or damage to persons or property as a matter of products liability, negligence or otherwise, or from any use or operation of any methods, products, instructions, or ideas contained in the material herein.

Previous editions copyrighted 2012, 2008, 2004, 1998, 1994, 1990, 1985, and 1981.

Library of Congress Cataloging-in-Publication Data

Touhy, Theris A., author.
 Ebersole & Hess' toward healthy aging : human needs & nursing response/Theris A. Touhy, Kathleen F. Jett.—
Ninth edition.
   p.; cm.
 Ebersole and Hess' toward healthy aging
 Toward healthy aging
 Includes bibliographical references and index.
 ISBN 978-0-323-32138-9 (pbk. : alk. paper)
 I. Jett, Kathleen Freudenberger, author. II. Title. III. Title: Ebersole and Hess' toward healthy aging. IV. Title:
Toward healthy aging.
 [DNLM: 1. Geriatric Nursing.   2. Aged.   3. Aging.   4. Health Promotion. WY 152]
 RC954
 618.97'0231—dc23

                                                                            2015004733

Content Strategist: Sandra Clark
Content Development Manager: Laurie Gower
Senior Content Development Specialist: Karen C. Turner
Publishing Services Manager: Jeffrey Patterson
Senior Project Manager: Tracey Schriefer
Designer: Amy Buxton

Printed in China

Last digit is the print number: 9   8   7   6   5   4   3

ABOUT THE AUTHORS

Theris A. Touhy, DNP, CNS, DPNAP, has been a clinical specialist in gerontological nursing and a nurse practitioner for over 35 years. Her expertise is in the care of older adults in nursing homes and those with dementia. The majority of her practice as a clinical nurse specialist and nurse practitioner has been in the long-term care setting. She received her BSN degree from St. Xavier University in Chicago, a master's degree in care of the aged from Northern Illinois University, and a Doctor of Nursing Practice from Case Western Reserve University. Dr. Touhy is an emeritus professor in the Christine E. Lynn College of Nursing at Florida Atlantic University, where she has served as Assistant Dean of Undergraduate Programs and taught gerontological nursing and long-term, rehabilitation, and palliative care nursing in the undergraduate, graduate, and doctoral programs. Her research is focused on spirituality in aging and at the end of life, caring for persons with dementia, caring in nursing homes, and nursing leadership in long-term care. Dr. Touhy was the recipient of the Geriatric Faculty Member Award from the John A. Hartford Foundation Institute for Geriatric Nursing in 2003, is a two-time recipient of the Distinguished Teacher of the Year in the Christine E. Lynn College of Nursing at Florida Atlantic University, and was awarded the Marie Haug Award for Excellence in Aging Research from Case Western Reserve University. Dr. Touhy was inducted into the National Academies of Practice in 2007. She is co-author with Dr. Kathleen Jett of *Gerontological Nursing and Healthy Aging* and is co-author with Dr. Priscilla Ebersole of *Geriatric Nursing: Growth of a Specialty.*

Kathleen Jett, PhD, GNP-BC, has been actively engaged in gerontological nursing for over 30 years. Her clinical experience is broad, from her roots in public health to clinical leadership in long-term care, assisted living and hospice, researcher and teacher, and advanced practice as both a clinical nurse specialist and nurse practitioner. Dr. Jett received her bachelor's, master's, and doctoral degrees from the University of Florida, where she also holds a graduate certificate in gerontology. In 2000 she was selected as a Summer Scholar by the John A. Hartford Foundation—Institute for Geriatric Nursing. In 2004 she completed a Fellowship in Ethno-Geriatrics through the Stanford Geriatric Education Center. Dr. Jett has received several awards, including recognition as an *Inspirational Woman of Pacific Lutheran University* in 1998 and 2000 and for her excellence in undergraduate teaching in 2005 and Distinguished Teacher of the year within the Christine E. Lynn College of Nursing at Florida Atlantic University. A board-certified gerontological nurse practitioner, Dr. Jett was inducted into the National Academies of Practice in 2006. She has taught an array of courses including public health nursing, women's studies, advanced practice gerontological nursing, and undergraduate courses in gerontology. She has coordinated two gerontological nurse practitioner graduate programs and an undergraduate interdisciplinary gerontology certificate program. The majority of her research and practice funding has been in the area of reducing health disparities experienced by older adults. The thread that ties all of her work together has been a belief that nurses can make a difference in the lives of older adults. She is currently employed as a nurse practitioner at Oak Hammock, a life-care community associated with the University of Florida, and provides research consultation for the College of Nursing. In addition to her professional activities, Dr. Jett is actively engaged in the lives of her grandchildren in rural High Springs, Florida.

CONTRIBUTORS AND REVIEWERS

CONTRIBUTORS

Debra Hain, PhD, ARNP, ANP-BC, GNP-BC, FAANP
Associate Professor/Lead Faculty AGNP Program
Christine E. Lynn College of Nursing
Florida Atlantic University
Boca Raton, Florida
Nurse Practitioner
Department of Hypertension/Nephrology
Cleveland Clinic Florida
Weston, Florida

María de los Ángeles Ordóñez, DNP, ARNP/GNP-BC
Director, Louis and Anne Green Memory and Wellness Center
Memory Disorder Clinic Coordinator
Assistant Professor Christine E. Lynn College of Nursing
Assistant Professor of Clinical Biomedical Science (Secondary)
Charles E. Schmidt College of Medicine
Florida Atlantic University
Boca Raton, Florida

Lisa Burroughs Phipps, PharmD, PhD
Assistant Professor
Virginia Commonwealth University
Academic Learning Transformation Lab
Richmond, Virginia

Jo Lynne Robins, PhD, RN, ANP-BC, AHN-C, FAANP
Assistant Professor
Virginia Commonwealth University
School of Nursing
Department of Family and Community Health
Richmond, Virginia

REVIEWERS

Kathleen Koernig Blais, EdD, MSN, RN
Professor Emerita
Florida International University
College of Nursing and Health Sciences
Miami, Florida

Sherri Shinn Cozzens, MS, RN, GRN
Nursing Faculty
De Anza College Nursing Program
Cupertino, California

Gail Potter, RN, BScN, M. Div., MN, CGNC(C)
Nursing Faculty
Department of Health and Human Services
Selkirk College
Castlegar, British Columbia, Canada

P. Janine Ray, RN, CRRN, MSN, PhD(c)
Assistant Professor of Nursing
Department of Nursing
Angelo State University
Member, Texas Tech University System
San Angelo, Texas

Ann Christy Seckman, DNP, MSN-FNP, RN
Associate Professor
Goldfarb School of Nursing
Barnes-Jewish College
St. Louis, Missouri

JoAnn Swanson, MSN, RN-BC, ONC
Assistant Professor
BSN Program Director
Bellin College School of Nursing
Green Bay, Wisconsin

PREFACE

In 1981, Dr. Priscilla Ebersole and Dr. Patricia Hess published the first edition of *Toward Healthy Aging: Human Needs and Nursing Response,* which has been used in nursing schools around the globe. Their foresight in developing a textbook that focuses on health, wholeness, beauty, and potential in aging has made this book an enduring classic and the model for gerontological nursing textbooks. In 1981, few nurses chose this specialty, few schools of nursing included content related to the care of elders, and the focus of care was on illness and problems. Today, gerontological nursing is a strong and evolving specialty with a solid theoretical base and practice grounded in evidence-based research. Dr. Ebersole and Dr. Hess set the standards for the competencies required for gerontological nursing education and the promotion of healthy aging. Many nurses, including us, have been shaped by their words, their wisdom, and their passion for care of elders. We thank these two wonderful pioneers and mentors for the opportunity to build on such a solid foundation in the three editions of this book we have co-authored. We hope that we have kept the heart and spirit of their work, for that is truly what has inspired us, and so many others, to care with competence and compassion.

We believe that *Toward Healthy Aging* is the most comprehensive gerontological nursing text available. Within the covers, the reader will find the latest evidence-based gerontological nursing protocols to be used in providing the highest level of care to adults in settings across the continuum. The content is consistent with the Recommended Baccalaureate Competencies and Curricular Guidelines for the Nursing Care of Older Adults and the Hartford Institute for Geriatric Nursing Best Practices in Nursing Care to Older Adults. The text has been on the list of recommended reading for the ANCC Advanced Practice Exam for many years and is recommended as a core text by gerontological nursing experts. *Toward Healthy Aging* is an appropriate text for both undergraduate and graduate students and is an excellent reference for nurses' libraries. This edition makes an ideal supplement to health assessment, medical-surgical, community, and psychiatric and mental health textbooks in programs that do not have a freestanding gerontological nursing course.

Information about evidence-based practice is presented where available. A holistic approach, addressing body, mind, and spirit, along a continuum of wellness, and grounded in caring and respect for person, provides the framework for the text. The ninth edition has been totally revised to facilitate student learning. Several new chapters have been added to expand and update content areas from previous editions. We present aging within a cultural and global context in recognition of diversity of all kinds and health inequities which persist. We hope to encourage readers to develop a world view of aging challenges and possibilities and the significant role of nursing in promoting healthy aging.

ORGANIZATION OF THE TEXT

Toward Healthy Aging has 36 chapters, organized into 5 sections.

Section 1 introduces the theoretical model on which the text is based and discusses the concepts of health and wellness in aging and the roles and responsibilities of gerontological nurses to provide optimal and informed caring. It includes a discussion of the changing population dynamics around the globe as more and more persons live longer and longer.

Section 2 provides the reader with the basic information needed to perform the day-to-day activities of gerontological nursing such as assessment, communication, and interpretation of laboratory tests.

Section 3 explores concerns that may affect functional abilities in aging such as vision, hearing, elimination, sleep, physical activity, and safety and security. Nursing interventions to enhance wellness, maintain optimal function, and prevent unnecessary disability are presented.

Section 4 goes into more depth regarding the chronic disorders covered in just one chapter in previous editions. Among these are chapters on mental health and neurodegenerative disorders such as Alzheimer's and Parkinson's diseases.

Section 5 moves beyond illness and functional limitations that may occur in aging and focuses on psychosocial, legal, and ethical issues that affect elders and their families/significant others. Content ranges from the economics of health care to sexuality and palliative care. Aging is presented as a time of accomplishing life's tasks, developing and sharing unique gifts, and reflecting on the meaning of life. Wisdom, self-actualization, creativity, spirituality, transcendence, and legacies are discussed. The unique and important contributions of elders to society, and to each of us, calls for nurses to foster appreciation of each older person, no matter how frail.

KEY COMPONENTS OF THE TEXT

A Student Speaks/An Elder Speaks: Introduces every chapter to provide perspectives of older people and nursing students on chapter content

Learning Objectives: Presents important chapter content and student outcomes

Promoting Healthy Aging: Implications for Gerontological Nursing: Special headings detailing pertinent assessment and interventions for practice applications of chapter content

Key Concepts: Concise review of important chapter points

Nursing Studies: Practice examples designed to assist students in assessment, planning, interventions, and outcomes to promote healthy aging

Critical Thinking Questions and Activities: Assist students in developing critical thinking skills related to chapter and nursing study content and include suggestions for in-classroom activities to enhance learning

Research Highlights Box

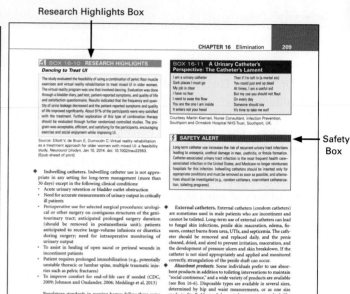

A Student Speaks

An Elder Speaks

Learning Objectives

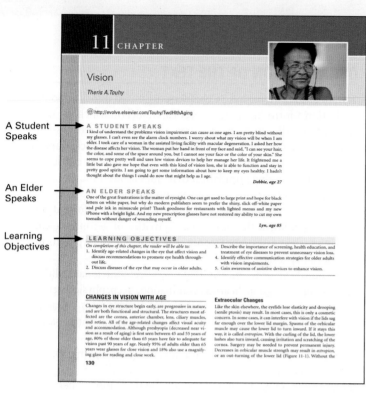

Safety Box

Key Concepts

Resources for Best Practice Box

Healthy People Box

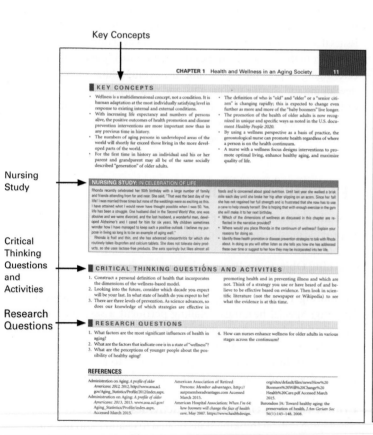

Nursing Study

Critical Thinking Questions and Activities

Research Questions

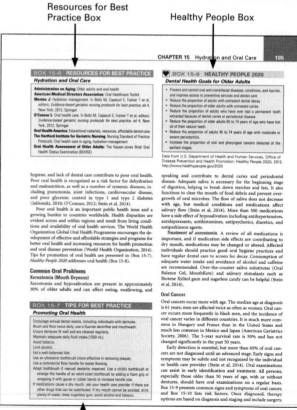

Tips for Best Practice Box

Research Questions: Suggestions to stimulate thinking about ideas for nursing research related to chapter topics

Boxes

Safety Alerts: QSEN competencies and safety issues related to care of older adults

Research Highlights: Summary of pertinent current research related to chapter topics

Resources for Best Practice (New to the ninth edition): Suggestions for further information for chapter topics and tools for practice

Tips for Best Practice (New to the ninth edition): Summary of evidence-based nursing interventions for practice

Healthy People: Reference to the goals cited in *Healthy People 2020*

EVOLVE ANCILLARIES

Instructors

Test Bank: Hundreds of questions with rationales to use in creating exams

PowerPoint: Lecture slides for each chapter, including integrated audience response questions

Teach for Nurses Lesson Plans: Detailed listing of resources available to instructors for their lesson planning, and including

unique case studies and class activities that can be shared with students

Students

Student Review Questions: Open-ended study questions covering nearly every element of each chapter

Case Studies: Accompanying select chapters, these provide short case studies with questions to help students see content put into practical use

ACKNOWLEDGEMENTS

This book would not have been possible without the support and guidance of the staff at Elsevier. Especially Karen C. Turner, who listened to all of our suggestions and concerns and understood how important this work was to us and to nursing students. Special thanks also to Sandra Clark, Content Strategist and Tracey Schriefer, Project Manager. We also acknowledge our reviewers and contributors, because without their efforts this edition would not have been possible. Finally, we acknowledge the past and future readers who, we hope, will provide us with enough feedback to keep us honest in any future writing.

Theris A. Touhy
Kathleen Jett

CONTENTS

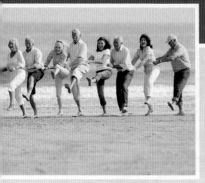

CHAPTER 1

Health and Wellness in an Aging Society

Kathleen Jett and Theris A. Touhy

http://evolve.elsevier.com/Touhy/TwdHlthAging

A STUDENT SPEAKS

I was so surprised when I went to the senior center and saw all those old folks doing tai chi! I feel a bit ashamed that I don't take better care of my own body.

Maggie, age 24

AN ELDER SPEAKS

Just a change in perspective! I can choose to be well or ill under all conditions. I think, too often we feel like victims of circumstance. I refuse to be a victim. It is my choice and I have control.

Maria, age 86

LEARNING OBJECTIVES

On completion of this chapter, the reader will be able to:

1. Compare and contrast the historical events influencing the health and wellness of those 60 and older.
2. Discuss the implications of the wide range of life expectancies of older adults in different parts of the world.
3. Describe a wellness-based model that can be used to promote the health of an aging, global community.
4. Describe the priorities of the National Prevention Council and suggest how these apply to the aging adult.
5. Discuss the multidimensional nature of wellness and its implications for healthy aging.
6. Define and describe the three levels of prevention.
7. Develop health-promoting strategies at each level of prevention that are consistent with the wellness-based model.
8. Describe the role of the nurse in promoting health in later life.

Herb is an 85-year-old man who considers himself "American." His great grandfather was born just after the American Civil War. Earlier in Herb's life he was a business executive but his passion was car racing. Today he works out in the gym and walks 8 miles a day. He no longer races but is active in teaching others to do so. He is talkative and enjoys interacting with those around him. He has mild hypertension and atrial fibrillation. For these conditions he takes a low dose of an antihypertensive and a blood thinner (warfarin), respectively. When asked why he is so healthy and active "at his age," he replies, "I never thought I would live to be this age, but I have lived life to the fullest. Mostly I think it is having the right genes, staying as active as possible and having a positive attitude."

From a perspective of Western medicine, health was long considered the absence of physical or psychiatric illness. It was measured in terms of the presence of accepted "norms," such as a specific range of blood pressure readings and results of laboratory testing, and the absence of established signs and symptoms of illness. When any of the parameters negatively affected the ability of the individual to function independently, debility was assumed. The measurement of a population's health status was usually inferred almost entirely from life expectancy, morbidity, and mortality statistics. The numbers provided information about illness but the health-related quality of life and wellness of the population could not be inferred. Measuring health in terms of illness does not reflect the life of persons with functional limitations, their ability to contribute to the community, or their movement toward self-actualization.

Although there had been efforts for many years to recognize that health meant more than the absence of disease, a national effort was not organized in the United States until 1979. At that time initial national goals were set and described in the document *The Surgeon General's Report on Health and Disease Prevention* (HealthyPeople, 2009). This has been updated every 10 years with the most current document *Healthy People 2020*. Many new topical foci have been added to the newest version, which are especially important to aging (HealthyPeople, 2013b). Among these are the dementias and a general area related to older adults. There is now a new area specific to health-related quality of life and wellness (HealthyPeople, 2013a). The importance of social well-being as a part of physical and mental health was recognized by the World Health Organization (WHO) in 1949, and the WHO recognized the importance of measuring social well-being in 2005 (WHO, 2005).

A wellness-based model, derived from a holistic paradigm, has reshaped how health is viewed and revolutionized the way health care and health are perceived. Instead of snapshots in time during a person's illness, a state of wellness can be uniquely defined anywhere along the continuum of health. Age and illness influence the ease at which one moves along the continuum but do not define the individual.

Aging is part of the life course. Caring for persons who are aging is a practice that touches nurses in all settings: from pediatrics involving grandparents and great-grandparents, to the residents of skilled nursing facilities and their spouses, partners, and children, to nurses providing relief support in countries outside of their own. Holroyd et al. (2009) have estimated that "by 2020, up to 75% of nurses' time will be spent with older adults" (p. 374). The core knowledge associated with gerontological nursing affects all of the profession and is not limited to any one subgroup of nurses (Young, 2003).

Gerontological nurses can help shape a world in which persons can thrive and grow old, not merely survive. They have unique opportunities to facilitate wellness in those who are recipients of care. As we move forward in the twenty-first century, the manner in which nurses respond to our aging society will determine our character because we are no greater than the health of the country and the world in which we live. This text is written using a wellness-based model to guide the reader in maximizing strengths, minimizing limitations, facilitating adaptation, and encouraging growth even in the presence of chronic illness or an acute health event. It is about helping persons move *Toward Healthy Aging*. In this ninth edition we appreciate your willingness to join us in this adventure.

THE YEARS AHEAD

As we look to the future, the world's population will soon include more persons older than 60 years than ever before. Although highly variable by country, in 2050 the number of persons older than 60 worldwide is expected to more than double from 2010— that is, the number will increase from 10% to 22%, the majority of whom are women (Figure 1-1). (United Nations, Department of Economic and Social Affairs, Population Division [UNDESAPD], 2005). Most of those older than 60 live in what is referred to as "less developed regions" and the percentage is expected to increase from 66% to 79% in this same time period (Figure 1-2) (United Nations [UN], 2012a). These elders are the most likely to be very poor and in need of support to an extent that is not seen in other parts of the world. For example, many grandparents are caring for the estimated 1.3 million Zimbabwean children orphaned by acquired immunodeficiency syndrome (AIDS). They have few, if any, organizations in place to help them (UNICEF, 2010).

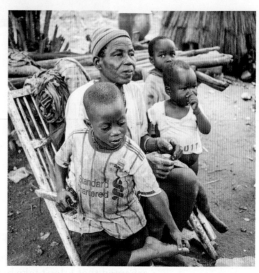

Many grandparents in Africa must care for their young grandchildren. (©iStock.com/Peeter Viisimaa.)

Population growth will change the face of aging as we know it and present many challenges today and in our future. Although healthy aging is now an achievable goal for many in developed and developing regions, it is still only a distant vision

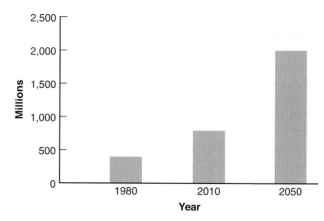

FIGURE 1-1 Growth in the Number of Persons at Least 60 Across the Globe. (Data from United Nations, Department of Economic and Social Affairs, Population Division: *World population prospects: the 2008 revision,* New York, 2009, United Nations.)

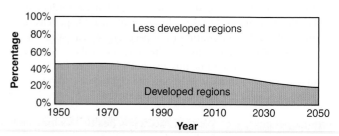

FIGURE 1-2 Distribution of World Population Aged 60 and Older by Development Region: 1950-2050. (From United Nations, Department of Economic and Social Affairs, Population Division: *World population ageing 2009,* New York, 2009, United Nations.)

for any of those living in less developed areas of the world, where lives are shortened by persistent communicable diseases, inadequate sanitation, and lack of both nutritious food and health care. It is essential that nurses across the globe have the knowledge and skills to help people of all ages achieve the highest level of wellness possible. Some of the questions that must be asked include the following: How can global conditions change for those who are struggling? How can the years of elderhood be maximized and enriched to the extent possible, regardless of the conditions in which one lives?

AGING

The term *geriatrics* was coined by American physician, Ignatz Nascher, around 1900 in recognition that the medical care of persons in later life differed from that of other population groups, such as pregnant women or children. Nascher authored the first medical textbook on treatment of the "old" in the United States (Nascher, 1914). Aging was reflected in his eyes as it was in society—a problem that must be reversed, eradicated, or held at bay as long as possible. From the early 1900s, the measurement of the incidence and prevalence of disease and associated morbidity or death was the focus. Although monitoring statistics is still important, the study of later life has been expanded to consideration of the nexus of time and human development, referred to as gerontology.

How Old Is Old?

Each culture has its own definition of when one is recognized as "old." A range of terms is used including elderly, senior citizens, elders, granny, older adult, or tribal elder. In some cultures elderhood is defined in functional terms—when one is no longer able to perform one's usual activities (Jett, 2003). Social aging is often determined by changes in roles, such as retirement from one's usual occupation, appointment as a wise woman/man of the community, or at the birth of a grandchild. Transitions may be marked by special rituals, such as birthday and retirement parties, invitations to join groups such as the American Association of Retired Persons (AARP, 2014), the qualification for "senior discounts" (Box 1-1), eligibility for age-related pensions, or recognition of special honor.

Biological aging is a complex and continuous process involving every cell in the body from birth to death (Chapter 3). The physical traits by which we identify one as "older" (e.g., gray hair, wrinkled skin) are referred to as the aging phenotype, that is, an outward expression of one's individual genetic makeup.

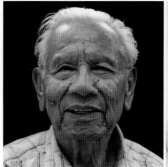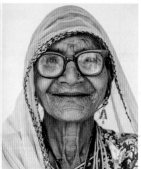

The aging phenotype. (©iStock.com/LPETTET; Mlenny.)

Chronological aging may be combined with any of the previously mentioned biological aging traits or used alone to define aging. In most developed and developing areas of the world, chronological late life is recognized as beginning sometime between the ages 50 and 65, with the World Health Organization using the age of 60 in their discussions (World Health Organization [WHO], 2013a). These arbitrary numbers have been defined with the expectation that persons are in the last decade or two of their lives. This is no longer applicable to men and women in some developed countries where life expectancies are rising. Japan is most notable. There, women have the longest potential life expectancy in the world—29 additional years at the age of 60 (UN, 2012b). In striking contrast are those living in many West African countries such as Mali, where both men and women can expect to live only 13 more years after 60 (Sanderson and Scherbov, 2008). Women at the age of 60 in the United States can expect to live another 25 years and men another 22 years (UN, 2012b). However, because the population in the United States is quite diverse, so is life expectancy. Although there has been a steady increase overall, this has been slower for those considered non-white when compared with those considered white (racial classification). For example, in 2010 the life expectancy at birth for black American men was 4.7 years less than that for white American men and 3.3 years less than that for black women (Kochanek et al, 2013) (Figure 1-3).

There is an ongoing controversy among demographers and gerontologists regarding the use and accuracy of chronological aging. In 1800 only 25% of men in Western Europe lived to the age of 60, yet today 90% of this same demographic live to the age of 90 (Sanderson and Scherbov, 2008, p. 3). So in 1800, was one "old" at 40? Is "old age" delayed until 70 today? How old is old and can there ever be a universal number?

As life expectancy increases how will we define aging? How will these definitions, as well as the meaning and the perception of aging, change as the health and wellness of individuals, communities, and nations improve? How will nursing roles and responsibilities change? How can we promote wellness in those who have a much greater chance of living into their 100s?

In the countries where the average life expectancies have expanded most rapidly, the following four generational subgroups have emerged: the super-centenarians, the centenarians,

---

BOX 1-1   The Aging Phenotype

A few years ago I stopped coloring my hair, which is almost completely silver now. It was quite a surprise to me the first time the very young clerk in the booth at the movie theater assumed I was 65 and automatically gave me the "senior discount." My husband's hair is only fading to a dull brown. When he goes alone they tentatively ask, "Do you have any discounts?"

Kathleen, at age 60

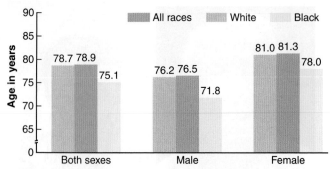

FIGURE 1-3 Life Expectancy at Birth, by Race and Sex: United States, 2010. (From Kochanek KD, Arias E, Anderson RN: *How did cause of death contribute to racial differences in life expectancy in the United States in 2010?* [NCHS data brief no. 125], Hyattsville, MD, 2013, National Center for Health Statistics. http://www.cdc.gov/nchs/data/databriefs/db125.htm. Accessed September 11, 2014.)

the baby boomers, and those in-between. Elderhood has the potential to span 40 years or more, attributable in a large part to increased access to quality health services and emphasis on improving the health of the public.

The Super-Centenarians

The super-centenarians are those who live until at least 110 years of age. As of 2015 they were born in 1905 or earlier (Box 1-2). This elite group emerged in the 1960s as those first documented to have lived so long. According to the New England Super-Centenarian Study at Boston University, there are about 200 to 300 of these exceptionally long-lived persons worldwide and about 60 in the United States (Schoenhofen et al, 2006).

Many of the fathers and older siblings of the oldest of this cohort fought and died in World War I (WWI) (1914 to 1918). Too old to fight in WWII, they saw their younger siblings repeat this service to their countries. There are no WWI veterans alive today. American Frank Buckles died at the age of 110 (1901 to 2011) (Duggan, 2011) and British veteran Florence Green died at the age of 111 (1901 to 2012) (Fox, 2012).

As teens or young adults the super-centenarians of today survived the influenza pandemic of 1918 to 1919, which killed an estimated 50 million people or one fifth of the world's population (National Archives, n.d.; U.S. Department of Health and Human Services [USDHHS], n.d.b). Referred to as the "Spanish Flu" or "Le Grippe," this outbreak began in the United States, Europe, and a small part of Asia. It spread worldwide almost overnight. The virulence was such that the period between exposure and death could be a matter of hours. In 1 year the life expectancy in the United States dropped by 10 to 12 years (National Archives, n.d.). Those alive today have also survived the three subsequent pandemics and three pandemic flu threats (Table 1-1).

In most developed countries, especially in nontropical areas, there were no new cases of yellow fever after 1905; however, cholera, typhoid, and polio still occurred. During the 1916 polio epidemic in New York City, many of the super-centenarians were toddlers. The sheer numbers affected by the communicable diseases of the 1800s and 1900s changed the view of science and the acceptance of governments' role in protecting the public's health.

A study of 32 super-centenarians in the United States found that "A surprisingly substantial portion of these individuals were still functionally independent or required minimal assistance (Schoenhofen et al, 2006, p. 1237)." Most functioned independently until after age 100, with no signs of frailty until about the age of 105. They were found to be remarkably homogeneous. None had Parkinson's disease, only 25% had ever had cancer, and stroke and cardiovascular disease were rare if they occurred at all. Few had been diagnosed with dementia. A study of super-centenarians in Japan corroborated these findings. It is theorized that these unusual persons have survived this long for "rare and unpredictable" reasons (Willcox et al, 2008). The unique phenotype is consistent, both biologically and socially. Scientists report that contributing factors include improvements in socio-political

---

BOX 1-2 A Remarkably Long Life: Truth or Fiction?

On August 4, 1997, Mme Calment of Arles, France, died a rich woman at reportedly the age of 122 years and 4½ months, a super-centenarian. In 1965, when she was 90 years old, her lawyer recognized the value of the apartment in which she lived and owned and made her, what turned out to be, the deal of a lifetime. In exchange for the deed to the apartment, he would pay her a monthly "pension" for life and she could live in the apartment the rest of her life. Over the next 32 years she was paid three times the apartment's value. She also outlived the lawyer, his son, her husband of 50 years, her daughter, and her only grandson. An active woman, she took up fencing at 85 and was still riding a bike at 100. She smoked until she was 117 and preferred a diet rich in olive oil.

Data from National Institute of Aging (NIA): *Aging under the microscope: a biological quest,* NIH Pub No. 02-2756, Bethesda, MD, 2003, U.S. Government Printing Office; Nemoto S, Finkel T: Aging and the mystery of Arles, *Science* 429:149, 2004.

TABLE 1-1   Pandemic Flu History Since 1918

YEAR(S)	HISTORICAL NAME
Pandemics	
1918	The Spanish flu; Le Grippe (H1N1)
1957-1960	Asian flu (H2N2)
1968-1969	Hong Kong flu (H3N2)
2009-2010	H1N1 (Swine flu)
Pandemic Flu Threats*	
1946-1947	Pseudopandemic
1976	Swine flu
1977	[Northern China] affecting mostly children
1997 and 1999	H5N1 (avian flu)
1997	Russian flu (Red flu), affecting only those <25 years old

*Those influenza outbreaks which were anticipated to spread worldwide but were controlled before this happened.
Data from the Centers for Disease Control and Prevention.

conditions, medical care, and quality of life (Vacante et al, 2012). While the number alive today is small, it is predicted to grow as the centenarians behind them live longer and healthier (Robine and Vaupel, 2001).

The Centenarians

Centenarians today are between 100 and 109 years of age, the majority of whom are between 100 and 104 years old (Meyer, 2012). Born between 1905 and 1914, they are primarily the younger siblings of the super-centenarians. Only the very youngest of these fought in WWII (1939 to 1946), when approximately 55 million people died, some of whom would have been centenarians today.

The Great Depression (approximately 1929 to 1940) was a global event with disastrous consequences for many. Jobs were scarce and poverty and malnutrition were rampant. Millions were unemployed. Young parents struggled to provide their children with even the barest necessities. American President Roosevelt implemented "New Deal" programs to provide some relief through the form of work programs. This included the Civilian Conservation Corp., which served as a source of a minimal amount of income for 3 million men but put great distances between family members. Nonetheless, entire families often had to work, and the skin color of the workforce shifted. African Americans lost the majority of jobs, with only 50% working in 1930 (Public Broadcasting Service [PBS], 1996-2013).

Smallpox has been a threat to centenarians until about 35 years ago when it was essentially eradicated globally (College of Philadelphia Physicians [CPP], 2013). Many centenarians had all or most of the "childhood" diseases, such as measles, mumps, chickenpox, and whooping cough; some survivors of today also had polio as children.

The percentage of those older than 100 years of age is rising more rapidly than the total population: an estimated increase of 93% between 1980 and 2012 or approximately 61,985 persons in the United States alone (Administration on Aging [AOA], 2013). However, several countries have a higher percentage of centenarians per 10,000 persons in their population (Figure 1-4). Based on the U.S. Census report of 2010, centenarians were overwhelmingly white (82.5%), women (82.8%), and living in urban areas of the Southern states (AOA, 2012). For the first time in history, parents and their children and grandchildren may all belong to this same "generation."

Along with the rapidly expanding numbers in this cohort, there is an exponential increase in genetics research to better understand exceptional longevity in humans and the underpinnings of morbidity that is compressed toward the end of their lives (Sebastiani et al, 2013). Although centenarians still carry genetic markers within their chromosomes for any number of health problems, for as yet unknown reasons, these are not "activated" until much later, if at all, when compared with other persons (Sebastiani and Perls, 2012).

Those In-Between

There is also a unique cohort born in the 30 years between 1915 and 1945, that is, between those referred to as the baby boomers and the centenarians; they are the 69- to 99-year-olds

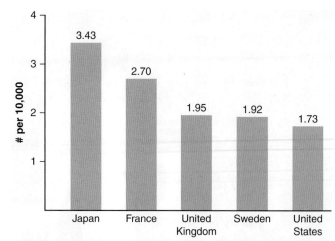

FIGURE 1-4 Number of Persons Older than 100 per 10,000 Persons in the Population (Select Countries). (Data from Meyer J: Centenarians: 2010, 2012. *2010 Census special reports,* C2010SR-03. https://www.census.gov/prod/cen2010/reports/c2010sr-03.pdf. Accessed October 1, 2014.)

of 2015. The oldest were born in the last year or two of WWI and the youngest at the very end of WWII. This age group includes some of the last survivors of the Holocaust. Many fought in WWII. It includes those considered "War Babies" conceived as a result of relationships between men in the military and local women and "left behind" in the countries of their births (Trucco, 1987).

This cohort in particular came of age during tumultuous times. Some witnessed or had personal experience with the American Civil Rights Movement (1955 to 1968) or the assassination of President John F. Kennedy (1963). Most were old enough to have been drafted or volunteered to serve in Vietnam (1959 to 1975). The "Cold War" was felt by many as the tensions between the United States and the former Soviet Union reached fever pitch. Others lost friends and family to the global AIDS epidemic before the human immunodeficiency virus (HIV) was isolated in France and the United States in 1983. If born between about 1929 and 1939, they were children during the Great Depression. Food was scarce, and for many, medical and dental care was not possible unless the care could be "bartered" (for example, a basket of eggs in exchange for a tooth extraction). In areas where the water lacked natural fluoride, children's teeth were soft and cavity prone. "Pigeon chest," a malformation of the developing rib cage caused by lack of vitamin D, was common. Goiter and myxedema were less common but were present regionally because of unrecognized iodine deficiencies. Those who were infants at this time have survived any number of childhood illnesses. Depending on the year they were born, they have also survived a number of communicable disease outbreaks and influenza pandemics (see Table 1-1).

Polio infection was a major fear for this cohort and for some, either they or their friends were affected. A vaccine was not available to children in the United States until 1955, providing the most benefits to the youngest of the "in-betweeners" (CPP, 2013). Penicillin, first discovered in 1928 by Alexander

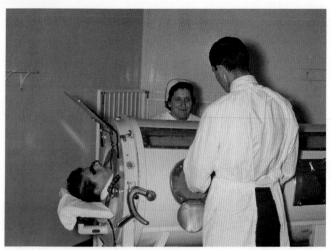

Hospital staff examining a patient in an iron lung during the Rhode Island polio epidemic, 1960. (From the Centers for Disease Control and Prevention Public Health Image Library.)

Fleming, became usable in humans in 1936 and likely prevented many infection-related mortalities from then to the present time (Markel, 2013).

The number of persons between the ages of 70 and 99 is growing at an exponential rate as the boomers begin to join their ranks. At this time the population in the United States of those 85+ years of age is expected to triple between 2011 and 2040—from 5.7 million to 14.1 million. There is slowly growing racial and ethnic heterogeneity—88.5% of persons in their 90s self-identified as white alone, 87.6% in their 80s, and 84% in their 70s. The group growing older at an increased rate is those who self-identify as Hispanic (AOA, 2012) (Figure 1-5).

The "Baby Boomers"

The youngest of the "older generation" are referred to as "baby boomers" or "boomers." They were born somewhere between approximately 1946 and 1964 depending on how they have been defined by any one country. In the United States the first to become baby boomers turned 64 in 2010; the last will do so

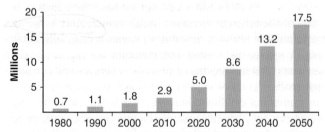

FIGURE 1-5 Projected Increase in Number of Persons Considered Hispanic in the United States. (From U.S. Administration on Aging, U.S. Department of Health and Human Services: *A statistical profile of Hispanic older Americans aged 65+*. http://www.aoa.gov/Aging_Statistics/minority_aging/Facts-on-Hispanic-Elderly.aspx. Accessed September 11, 2014.)

21 years later in 2031. More babies were born in the United States in 1946, the year after the end of WWII, than any other year—3.4 million or 20% more than in 1945. These numbers increased every year until they tapered off in 1964. In just 18 years, 76.4 million babies had been born (History, 1996-2013). Each day another 11,000 "boomers" turn 50 years old (American Hospital Association [AHA], 2007).

The differences in the life experiences between those born in the late 1940s and early 1960s are quite significant. For example, the eldest had mothers and fathers who had served in WWII and as young adults they may have been drafted into the Vietnam War, obtained a "college deferment," or volunteered to serve in the military. The youngest in this cohort may have had only a childhood recollection, if any, of that period of time.

The baby boomers of today have better access to medication and other treatment regimens than previous cohorts but will nevertheless live longer with chronic disease than any of their predecessors (see Chapter 21). Of particular concern are obesity, diabetes, arthritis, congestive heart failure, and dementia, all of which we discuss in this text. Some of this increased rate is related to a lack of importance placed on what we now consider healthful living as they were growing up. For example, in the 1950s and 1960s smoking was not only condoned, but also considered a sign of status. Candy in the shape and appearance of cigarettes was popular with children. Work and public places and homes were filled with smoke, affecting both the smokers themselves and those who were exposed to second-hand smoke. In the 1950s, 50% of the men and 33% of the women in the United States smoked cigarettes. By 2005 this had decreased to 23% and 19%, respectively (AHA, 2007). Although there has been improvement in some areas and some parts of the world, the damage done to the cardiovascular system has already occurred. Cardiovascular disease is the overall number one cause of noncommunicable death worldwide, killing almost 17 million in 2011 (Figure 1-6) (WHO, 2014b).

The "boomers" in developed countries have had the benefit of the ongoing development of immunizations against communicable diseases. Although the super-centenarians and centenarians may not have received these immunizations, they became a standard of care from 1960 on, when the eldest boomer was 13 years of age. The ability to produce the potent antibiotic penicillin and those to follow has been significantly influential in the survival of this cohort into 2015. The social emphasis today on healthier lifestyles will go far to help persons reach higher levels of wellness, but for this group, the challenges are many.

A WELLNESS-BASED MODEL

The burgeoning population of persons entering the last 20 to 40 years of life presents the nurse with opportunities to make a difference in promoting wellness and stemming the tide of prolonged life accompanied by chronic disease and disability, especially for the baby boomers. While we provide the implications for nursing practice for the most common health challenges in aging, we do this from the perspective that a state of relative

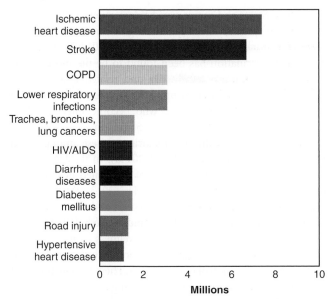

FIGURE 1-6 Ten Leading Causes of Noncommunicable Causes of Death Worldwide, 2012. (From World Health Organization: *The top 10 causes of death* [Fact sheet no. 310]. http://www.who.int/mediacentre/factsheets/fs310/en/index.html. Accessed September 11, 2014.)

wellness can be an ongoing goal for both nursing practice and individuals themselves. This includes how we approach those to whom we provide care and how we foster health-promoting behaviors.

In this text we use a broad view of wellness to provide nurses with a framework for addressing the needs of our aging population on a global scale. A wellness-based model encompasses the idea that health is composed of multiple dimensions. Wellness is expressed in functional, environmental, intellectual, psychological, spiritual, social, and biological dimensions of the human experience within the context of culture (Figure 1-7). These dimensions are juxtaposed on a myriad of other factors, including normal changes of aging, income, education, gender, race, ethnicity and country of origin, place of residence, life

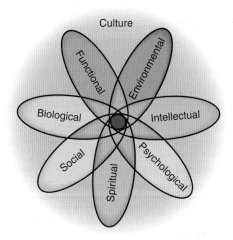

FIGURE 1-7 Flower model.

opportunities, and access to health care. The challenge to both living and dying in wellness is to balance each of these dimensions to the extent possible. The dimensions are like overlapping petals on a flower, anchored together at the center. Wellness involves each of these singularly and in interaction making a fully, richer whole.

A wellness-based model is one in which health is viewed on a continuum. At one end there is either an absence of disease as we know it or the presence of chronic diseases that are controlled to the point where their damaging effects are minimized (e.g., a person's blood pressure reading or blood glucose level is within normal limits). At the other end of the continuum is the point when an acute episode or multiple concurrent conditions result in approaching death but one in which suffering of all kind is minimized to the extent possible. The gerontological nurse has the opportunity and the responsibility when working with persons all along the continuum, including at the time of death, to promote wholeness and wellness as defined by the individual at any point in time.

The Wellness-Based Model for Healthy Aging

Healthy aging can no longer be viewed by looking only at later life. Reaching for wellness begins in the prenatal period and continues to death. "To a substantial degree, the health of the emergent adult is in the hands of the pediatrician" (Barondess, 2008, p. 147). Exciting research in the field of epigenetics is leading to new understanding of the effect of environmental factors and lifestyle habits such as diet, stress, smoking, and prenatal nutrition on life expectancy and healthy aging.

The concept of healthy aging from a wellness perspective is uniquely defined by each individual and likely to change over time. The subcomponents within the wellness model particularly applicable to healthy aging are functional independence, self-care management of chronic illness and disability, positive outlook, personal growth, social contribution, and activities that promote one's health.

The exponential increase in the number of persons older than the age 65 across the globe is a driving force behind the social and political pressure to develop, test, and implement strategies to promote wellness and healthful living across the continuum of life and country (WHO, 2013b). Some of these strategies have been found to be effective based on empirical evidence, others are no longer supported, and many others are believed to be helpful but we do not yet have the evidence. Because of the inherent increased health vulnerability as we age, the efficacy of health-promoting strategies is especially important in helping us achieve and maintain the highest level of wellness possible along the continuum. There are still considerable challenges to implement evidence-based practices as a result of the paucity of research specific to health promotion and aging, especially when applied to those from historically underrepresented groups. Although this may change as the "baby boomers" enter the stage of elderhood, the numbers of those who participate in preventive services at this time are low—only 25% of those between 40 and 64 years of age and less than 40% of those 65 years and older utilize the preventive services available to them (Centers for Disease Control [CDC], 2014).

DISEASE PREVENTION AND HEALTH PROMOTION FOR OLDER ADULTS

In an effort to move forward, a provision of the Affordable Care Act in the United States called for creation of the National Prevention Council. Chaired by Surgeon General Dr. Regina Benjamin, the charges were to partner community and governmental agencies and establish an action plan for the specific purpose of accelerating prevention in six priority areas (USDHHS, n.d.a) (Box 1-3). The overarching goals are to implement evidence-based prevention strategies at the community level (Box 1-4). These strategies are consistent with both our wellness-based model and the goals and objectives established by *Healthy People 2020* (see www.healthypeople.gov) with a new emphasis on the needs of the older adult (Box 1-5) (USDHHS, 2012) (http://www.healthypeople.gov/2020/topics-objectives/topic/older-adults).

Primary Prevention

Primary prevention refers to strategies that can and are used to prevent an illness before it occurs. For example, through a collaboration of the Centers for Disease Control and Prevention in the United States and many worldwide partners, wellness is promoted at the primary level by reducing the incidence and prevalence of annual influenza infections (CDC, 2013; WHO, 2013c). An annual vaccination has been found to be the most safe and effective way to prevent influenza and related illness globally; complications are reduced by up to 60% in the elderly and deaths reduced by 80% among those who become infected (WHO, 2014a). Worldwide there are 3 to 5 million cases a year and 250,000 to 500,000 deaths, the majority of these among persons more than 65 years of age (WHO, 2014a). In the United States 90% of flu-related death and 60% of flu-related hospitalization occur in persons 65+ years of age (CDC, 2013). Yet the rates for influenza vaccinations for persons 65 years and older vary by age, economic status, place of residence, and race/ethnicity (Box 1-6).

Moving toward and maintaining wellness along the continuum in the context of primary prevention includes many choices that are under the control of the person. These may include never starting or stopping smoking, maintaining an ideal body weight, exercising regularly, eating a well-balanced diet, and using select age-appropriate dietary supplements such as vitamin D and calcium (see Chapters 14, 18, & 19). Among other strategies at the primary level are stress management, social engagement, intellectual stimulation, and restful sleep, all of which are essential but too often not emphasized in gerontological nursing practice.

BOX 1-3   National Prevention Council's Six Priority Areas

Tobacco-free living
Preventing drug abuse and excessive alcohol use
Healthy eating
Injury and violence free living
Reproductive and sexual health
Mental and emotional well-being

BOX 1-4   Goals of the National Prevention Council

Empowered people
Healthy and safe community environments
Clinical and community preventive services
Elimination of health disparities

 ### BOX 1-5   HEALTHY PEOPLE 2020

Regarding the Health of Older Adults

Goal
Improve the health, function, and quality of life of older persons.

Emerging Issues
Coordination of care
Helping older adults manage their own care
Establishing quality of care measures
Identifying the minimum levels of training for people who care for older adults
Promoting research and analysis of appropriate training to equip providers with the tools they need to meet the needs of older adults

Data from U.S. Department of Health and Human Services, Office of Disease Prevention and Health Promotion: Healthy People 2020, 2012. http://www.healthypeople.gov/2020

BOX 1-6   Comparison of Influenza and Pneumococcal Immunizations by Ethnic and Racial Groups*

Non-Hispanic Black People
- In 2009 non-Hispanic blacks at least 65 years old were 30% less likely (50.8%) to have received the influenza vaccination than their non-Hispanic white counterparts (68.6%).
- In 2010 non-Hispanic blacks were 30% less likely (46.2%) to have ever received a pneumonia vaccination than their non-Hispanic white counterparts (63.5%).

American Indian/Native Alaskan People
- Between 2010 and 2011 American Indians/Native Alaskans at least 65 years of age were slightly more likely (68.7%) to have received an influenza vaccination than their non-Hispanic white counterparts (67.7%).[†]

Asian People
- In 2011 Asians at least 65 years of age were only 20% less likely (48%) to have received the pneumococcal vaccination than their white counterparts (63.5%).
- In 2011 Asians were only 20% less likely (48%) to have received the pneumococcal vaccination than their white counterparts (63.5%).

Hispanic People
- In 2010 Hispanics at least 65 years of age were only 40% less likely (39%) to have received the pneumococcal vaccination than their white counterparts (63.5%).
- In 2010 Hispanics were only 30% less likely (50.6%) to have received the influenza vaccination than their white counterparts (68.6%).

*Only U.S. statistics are available. Data from the U.S. Department of Health and Human Services, Office of Minority Health. http://minorityhealth.hhs.gov.
[†]Data for the specific age group not available.

Secondary Prevention

Secondary prevention is the early detection of a disease or health problem that has already developed. The goal of early detection is to increase the likelihood that the problem can be adequately and effectively addressed and therefore the person may return to the prior level of wellness or as close to it as possible (CDC, 2014). The majority of the strategies considered secondary prevention are in the form of health screenings of some type and are particularly important in promoting healthy aging in those whose life expectancy increases with each year and are active and engaged. Secondary prevention occurs in community and senior centers, health fairs, and in health care providers' offices. Nurses and nurse practitioners are usually advocates and organizers of these strategies. While one cannot entirely compensate for a lifetime of lifestyle choices that were detrimental to one's health, many small health-promoting changes can ameliorate their impact in later life.

Although primary prevention is extremely important and has demonstrated efficacy, secondary and tertiary prevention (see following section) take on new meaning for older adults. For example, determining who should undergo health screening depends on several key factors, especially relevant as we age or develop comorbid conditions: if *knowing* one has a disease or condition will change the course along the continuum and projected timing of death or if aggressive treatment such as radiation or surgery is a reasonable option for any one person (Box 1-7).

Tertiary Prevention

A wellness-based model is most salient in facilitating tertiary prevention for persons living with chronic diseases or subsequent to an acute health event. Tertiary prevention addresses the needs of persons who have their day-to-day wellness challenged, either by slowing a disease process (e.g., chemotherapy) or by limiting complications from a previous event (e.g., rehabilitation following a stroke) (Box 1-8). The goals of tertiary prevention are to promote wellness to the extent possible in the presence of an active health challenge. Tertiary prevention may be as "simple" as diabetic meal planning or as complex as combining speech, swallowing, and occupational and physical therapy for the person who has had a stroke. With aggressive

---

BOX 1-7 When Is Secondary Prevention in Question?

A breast mass was noted in a patient in a skilled nursing facility. The nurse was adamant that the patient should have a mammogram. Although the 85-year-old woman was still quite mobile and cheerful, she also had very advanced dementia. My inclination was to not pursue this screening. In conversation with her only living child, we decided that a screening (the mammogram) would be a hardship for her mother because she would not understand what was being done to her and the screening itself was not innocuous. If cancer was found (which was very likely), questions about radiation, chemotherapy, and so on would need to be addressed. It was agreed that the patient could neither understand her screening procedure nor withstand any treatment, both of which would negatively affect her current quality of life. The woman did not receive the mammogram and died of an acute myocardial event about 3 months later.

BOX 1-8 Tertiary Prevention in Action

About 9 months ago Helen suffered a stroke that left her partially paralyzed on the right side. With extensive rehabilitation she was able to regain independent ambulation with the help of a cane (declining a walker) and functional use of her affected hand with a brace. The left shoulder had become quite tender because of a combination of chronic arthritis and overuse, the latter occurring because she relied on it to a great extent to remain mobile. She came to the wellness clinic requesting a referral for physical therapy for stretching, heat therapy, and massage therapy, all of which she was readily given. She has now returned to her usual activities, until she needs another "dose" of tertiary prevention.

---

tertiary prevention the person may reach a new level of wellness in the face of health challenges.

◆ Promoting Healthy Aging: Implications for Gerontological Nursing

The gerontological nurse can use the wellness-based model to promote healthy aging across the continuum of wellness and care settings. The model builds on the goals described in the strategies of the National Prevention Council (Box 1-9) and *Healthy People 2020,* expanded now to recognize emerging issues relevant to healthy aging (see Box 1-4). Gerontological nurses are active in promoting wellness at the primary level through participating in and facilitating even the simplest of activities, such as when the bedside nurse ensures that the patient is served a meal that is nutritious but also culturally appropriate. Nurses in the community promote wellness as health educators, advocates, and case managers, making sure people know the services to which they are entitled and recommended. Advanced practice nurses are becoming champions of the Annual Health Promotion visit for Medicare recipients (see Chapter 30).

Yet both the goals and the objectives and interventions for healthy older adults will differ from those for very frail older adults or those with limited life expectancies. When select preventive approaches are questionable, the nurse can inform those involved in health care conversations, leading to the best decision for any one person. Secondary prevention such as health screening for the most impaired or those with very short life expectancies is generally not recommended, but primary and tertiary prevention is always appropriate. It is the responsibility of the skilled gerontological nurse to design interventions all along the continuum—from the very active person, like

---

BOX 1-9 Examples of Strategies of the National Prevention Council

Active Living
   Encourage community design and development that support physical activity.
Healthy Eating
   Improve nutritional quality of food supply (e.g., that provided to residents in nursing facilities).
Mental and Emotional Well-Being
   Promote the early identification of mental health needs and access to quality services.

Herb in the opening paragraph, to those with advanced cognitive impairments, to those who are nearing death.

The nurse promotes *biological wellness* by promoting regular physical activity such as playing tennis, participating in wheelchair bowling, or sitting upright for intervals throughout the day. Healthy lifestyles can also be encouraged by promoting healthy eating and adequate and restful sleep, taking control of acquired health problems such as hypertension or diabetes, and avoiding tobacco or tobacco products. Fostering maximal biological wellness also means advocating for the person to secure the highest quality of medical care when it is needed. The implementation of evidence-based care and cutting-edge research is no longer an option (Box 1-10). At all times the wellness-based model requires that the lifestyle recommendations be balanced between burden and benefit.

The nurse promotes *social wellness* by facilitating activities in which interactions with others, pets, or both are possible, as desired. Ongoing social interactions have been found to have a significant effect on cognition, memory, and mood (Chapters 28 and 29). Through social interaction, persons can be recognized with inherent value not only in the neutral "person" but also as sexual beings, as men and women, regardless of sexual orientation, age, or functional ability (Box 1-11).

Nurses promote *functional wellness* across the continuum of care and roles. The bedside nurse ensures that the physical environment is one that promotes healing and encourages the person to remain active and engaged at the highest level possible. For example, it is not appropriate to help someone out of a chair who is able to do so, albeit slower. This type of "help" negatively affects both muscle tone and self-esteem.

Addressing the *environmental* dimension of the wellness model is individual to the person but often includes political activism. Those living in the inner city may be facing increased crime and victimization, exposure to pollution, reduced access to fresh fruits and vegetables, and greater dependence on dwindling public transportation. It may be necessary for the nurse to become involved in creating healthy living spaces by advocating for adequate funding for a wide range of resources from street lighting to funding of local agencies that provide aging-related services, such as the American Aging Association (http://www.americanagingassociation.org), the National Society for American Indian Elderly (http://nsaie.org), or EUROFAMCARE (Family Care of Older Adults in Europe). The gerontological nurse helps to create living spaces and practices that respect and support an environment that supports healthy aging.

Addressing the *psychological dimension* of the wellness model most often calls for identifying potential threats to this aspect of the person. Psychological health includes being aware of and accepting one's feelings. The nurse is often the one to observe and assess this dimension and challenge the view held by both persons themselves and health care providers—that declines in mental and cognitive health are "normal changes with aging." In many cases the signs and symptoms of dementia may actually be the misdiagnosis of depression (Chapter 28). The nurse can take the lead in addressing these misconceptions and helping persons who are wrestling with new or life-long psychological challenges as they age.

The *spiritual dimension* of the wellness-based model may be described as that which gives one's life meaning, be this a relationship with a greater source (e.g., God, Allah, The Great Spirit, Wakan Tanka, Gitche Manitou) or a relationship with others or the sense of the community or world. The nurse fosters the spiritual dimension of the person through awareness or at least openness to how others view and express their own spirituality. This may be ensuring that the person's spiritual rituals are taken into account when scheduling medical appointments or procedures or even when taking vital signs in the hospital setting. It also means that the nurse and the rest of the health care team respect and account for dying and death rituals as appropriate (Chapter 35).

When nurses address the person's needs along the continuum within his or her personal perspective, they are respecting the patient's culture regardless of what it is and the form it takes. It may be ensuring the appropriate food is provided, such as a serving of pasta or rice with each meal, or facilitating the inclusion of an indigenous healer in the care team.

The nurse promotes wellness in all dimensions within the context of the person's culture. By listening closely, nurses can hear what is most important to persons and what can be done to promote their wellness. The nurse's role across the globe is to facilitate the creation of economic, social, and physical environments that enhance the opportunity for persons to move toward wellness through the promotion of healthy lifestyles, timely health screening, and the ability to participate in tertiary prevention at every stage of life. The wellness-based approach is perhaps the most equitable in supporting the individual's potential for maximal health and functioning at all ages.

BOX 1-10 **RESEARCH HIGHLIGHTS**

Promoting Health

Norwegian researchers recruited 30 persons at least 75 years old to participate in a study to test the effectiveness of a series of telephone support calls on a number of factors, including mental health, sense of coherence, self-care, and a sense of ability to perform self-care activities. A significant difference was found between those who received the calls and those who did not. Those who received the calls improved especially in the indicators of mental health, thought to be precursors of the use of health-promoting activities.

Data from Sudsli K, Söderhamn U, Espner GA, et al: Self-care telephone talks as a health promotion intervention in urban home-living 75+ years of age: a randomized controlled study, *Clin Interv Aging* 9:95–103, 2014.

BOX 1-11 **The Social Dimension**

There was a long-term care facility in which the staff was consistently friendly to the residents, regardless of their functional or cognitive status. For many of the residents the staff was all of the family they had left. One of the residents had been there a long time and would likely spend the rest of his life there because of brain damage from uncontrollable seizures. Although communication was difficult, he got much pleasure in "flirting" with the staff. One day a nurse was observed stopping by his chair and commenting on a new baseball cap he had been given. She said "you're smokin' in that cap there!" His smile could not be broader and they each went about their different directions.

KEY CONCEPTS

- Wellness is a multidimensional concept, not a condition. It is human adaptation at the most individually satisfying level in response to existing internal and external conditions.
- With increasing life expectancy and numbers of persons alive, the positive outcomes of health promotion and disease prevention interventions are more important now than in any previous time in history.
- The numbers of aging persons in undeveloped areas of the world will shortly far exceed those living in the more developed parts of the world.
- For the first time in history an individual and his or her parent and grandparent may all be of the same socially described "generation" of older adults.

- The definition of who is "old" and "elder" or a "senior citizen" is changing rapidly; this is expected to change even further as more and more of the "baby boomers" live longer.
- The promotion of the health of older adults is now recognized in unique and specific ways as noted in the U.S. document *Healthy People 2020*.
- By using a wellness perspective as a basis of practice, the gerontological nurse can promote health regardless of where a person is on the health continuum.
- A nurse with a wellness focus designs interventions to promote optimal living, enhance healthy aging, and maximize quality of life.

NURSING STUDY: IN CELEBRATION OF LIFE

Rhonda recently celebrated her 90th birthday with a large number of family and friends attending from far and near. She said, "That was the best day of my life! I was married three times but none of the weddings were as exciting as this. I have attained what I would never have thought possible when I was 50. Yes, life has been a struggle. One husband died in the Second World War, one was abusive and we were divorced, and the last husband, a wonderful man, developed Alzheimer's and I cared for him for six years. My children sometimes wonder how I have managed to keep such a positive outlook. I believe my purpose in living so long is to be an example of aging well."

Rhonda is frail and thin, and she has advanced osteoarthritis for which she routinely takes ibuprofen and calcium tablets. She does not tolerate dairy products, so she uses lactose-free products. She eats sparingly but likes almost all foods and is concerned about good nutrition. Until last year she walked a brisk mile each day until she broke her hip after slipping on an acorn. Since her fall she has not regained her full strength and is frustrated that she now has to use a cane to help steady herself. She is hoping that with enough exercise in the gym she will make it to her next birthday.

- Which of the dimensions of wellness as discussed in this chapter are reflected in the narrative provided?
- Where would you place Rhonda in the continuum of wellness? Explain your reasons for doing so.
- Identify three health promotion or disease prevention strategies to talk with Rhoda about. In doing so you will either listen as she tells you how she has addressed these over time or suggest to her how they may be incorporated into her life.

CRITICAL THINKING QUESTIONS AND ACTIVITIES

1. Construct a personal definition of health that incorporates the dimensions of the wellness-based model.
2. Looking into the future, consider which decade you expect will be your last. In what state of health do you expect to be?
3. There are three levels of prevention. As science advances, so does our knowledge of which strategies are effective in promoting health and in preventing illness and which are not. Think of a strategy you use or have heard of and believe to be effective based on evidence. Then look in scientific literature (not the newspaper or Wikipedia) to see what the evidence is at this time.

RESEARCH QUESTIONS

1. What factors are the most significant influences of health in aging?
2. What are the factors that indicate one is in a state of "wellness"?
3. What are the perceptions of younger people about the possibility of healthy aging?

4. How can nurses enhance wellness for older adults in various stages across the continuum?

REFERENCES

Administration on Aging: *A profile of older Americans: 2012*, 2012. http://www.aoa.acl. gov/Aging_Statistics/Profile/2012/index.aspx.

Administration on Aging: *A profile of older Americans: 2013*, 2013. www.aoa.acl.gov/ Aging_Statistics/Profile/index.aspx. Accessed March 2015.

American Association of Retired Persons: *Member advantages*. http:// aarpmemberadvantages.com Accessed March 2015.

American Hospital Association: *When I'm 64: how boomers will change the face of health care*, May 2007. https://www.healthdesign. org/sites/default/files/news/How%20 Boomers%20Will%20Change%20 Health%20Care.pdf Accessed March 2015.

Barondess JA: Toward healthy aging: the preservation of health, *J Am Geriatr Soc* 56(1):145–148, 2008.

Centers for Disease Control: *Clinical preventive services*, 2014. http://www.cdc.gov/aging/services/. Accessed December 1, 2013.

Centers for Disease Control: *Influenza update for geriatricians and other clinicians caring for people 65 and older*, 2013. http://www.cdc.gov/flu/professionals/2012-2013-guidance-geriatricians.htm. Accessed December 1, 2013.

College of Philadelphia Physicians: *The history of vaccines*, 2013. http://www.historyofvaccines.org. Accessed December 1, 2013.

Duggan P: *Last U.S. World War I veteran Frank W. Buckles dies at 110*, The Washington Post, Feb 28, 2011.

Fox M: *Florence Green, last World War I veteran, dies at 110*, The New York Times, Feb 7, 2012.

HealthyPeople: *History and development of healthy people*, 2011. http://healthypeople.gov/2020/about/history.aspx. Accessed March 2014.

HealthyPeople: *Health-related quality of life and well-being*, 2013a. http://healthypeople.gov/2020/topicsobjectives2020/overview.aspx?topicid=19. Accessed March 2014.

HealthyPeople: *2020 Topics & objectives*, 2013b. http://healthypeople.gov/2020/topicsobjectives2020/default.aspx. Accessed March 2014.

History: *Baby boomers*, 1996-2013. http://www.history.com/topics/baby-boomers. Accessed December 1, 2013.

Holroyd A, Dahlke S, Fehr C, et al: Attitudes toward aging: implications for a caring profession, *J Nurs Educ* 48(7):374–380, 2009.

Jett KF: The meaning of aging and the celebration of years, *Geriatr Nurs* 24(4):290–293, 2003.

Kochanek KD, Arias E, Anderson RN: *How did cause of death contribute to racial differences in life expectancy in the United States in 2010?* (NCHS data brief no. 125), Hyattsville, MD, 2013, National Center for Health Statistics. http://www.cdc.gov/nchs/data/databriefs/db125.htm. Accessed December 1, 2013.

Markel H: *The real story behind penicillin*, PBS NewsHour, Sept 27, 2013. http://www.pbs.org/newshour/rundown/2013/09/the-real-story-behind-the-worlds-first-antibiotic.html. Accessed December 1, 2013.

Meyer J: Centenarians: 2010, *2010 Census Special Reports* (Report no. C2010SR-03), 2012.

Nascher I: *Geriatrics*, Philadelphia, 1914, P. Blakiston's Sons & Co.

National Archives: *The deadly virus: the influenza epidemic of 1918*. http://www.archives.gov/exhibits/influenza-epidemic/index.html. Accessed December 1, 2013.

Public Broadcasting Service: *The Great Depression*, 1996–2013. http://www.pbs.org/wgbh/americanexperience/features/general-article/dustbowl-great-depression. Accessed December 1, 2013.

Robine J, Vaupel JW: Supercentenarians: slower ageing individuals or senile elderly? *Exp Gerontol* 36(4–6):915–930, 2001.

Sebastiani P, Bae H, Sun FX, et al: Meta-analysis of genetics variants associated with human exceptional longevity, *Aging* 5(9):653–661, 2013.

Sebastiani P, Perls TT: The genetics of extreme longevity: lessons from the New England centenarian study, *Front Genet* 3(277):1–7, 2012.

Sanderson W, Scherbov S: Rethinking age and aging, Population Bulletin: *A Publication of the Population Reference Bureau* 63(4), 2008.

Schoenhofen EA, Wyszynski DF, Andersen S, et al: Characteristics of 32 supercentenarians, *J Am Geriatr Soc* 54:1237–1240, 2006.

Trucco T: *English war babies search for American fathers*, The New York Times, Apr 9, 1987. http://www.nytimes.com/1987/04/09/garden/english-war-babies-search-for-american-fathers.html?pagewanted=all&src=pm. Accessed December 1, 2013.

UNICEF: *Humanitarian action report 2010: Partnering for children in emergencies*, Feb 2010. http://www.unicef.org/har2010/index_zimbabwe_feature.html. Accessed November 1, 2013.

United Nations: *Linking population, poverty and development*, 2012a. http://www.unfpa.org/pds/trends.htm. Accessed November 1, 2013.

United Nations: *Social indicators: Health: Life expectancy*, 2012b. http://unstats.un.org/unsd/demographic/products/socind/. Accessed December 1, 2013.

United Nations, Department of Economic and Social Affairs, Population Division: *Population challenges and development goals*, 2005. http://www.un.org/esa/population/publications/pop_challenges/Population_Challenges.pdf. Accessed November 1, 2013.

U.S. Department of Health and Human Services: *National Prevention Council*, n.d.a. http://www.surgeongeneral.gov/initiatives/prevention/about/index.html. Accessed December 1, 2013.

U.S. Department of Health and Human Services: *Pandemic flu history*, n.d.b. http://www.flu.gov/pandemic/history. Accessed December 1, 2013.

U.S. Department of Health and Human Services: *HealthyPeople: Older adults*, 2012. http://www.healthypeople.gov/2020/topicsobjectives2020/overview.aspx?topicid=31. Accessed December 1, 2013.

Vacante M, D'Agata V, Motta M, et al: Centenarians and supercentenarians: a black swan. Emerging social, medical and surgical problems, *BMC Surg* 12(Suppl 1):S36, 2012.

Willcox DC, Willcox BJ, Wang NC, et al: Life at the extreme limit: phenotypic characteristics of supercentenarians in Okinawa, *J Gerontol A Biol Sci Med Sci* 63(11):1201–1208, 2008.

World Health Organization: The World Health Organization Quality of Life Assessment (WHOQOL: position paper from the World Health Organization), *Soc Sci Med* 41(10):1403–1409, 2005.

World Health Organization: *Influenza (seasonal)*, 2014a. http://www.who.int/mediacentre/factsheets/fs211/en/index.html. Accessed October 31, 2014.

World Health Organization: *Definition of and older or elderly person*, 2013a. http://www.who.int/healthinfo/survey/ageingdefnolder/en/. Accessed December 1, 2013.

World Health Organization: *The 8th global conference on health promotion – the Helsinki Statement on Health in all policies*, 2013b. http://www.who.int/healthpromotion/conferences/8gchp/en/index.html. Accessed December 1, 2013.

World Health Organization: *Influenza: Surveillance and monitoring*, 2013c. http://www.who.int/influenza/surveillance_monitoring/en/. Accessed December 1, 2013.

World Health Organization: *The top 10 causes of death*, 2014b. http://www.who.int/mediacentre/factsheets/fs310/en/index.html. Accessed December 2013.

Young H: Challenges and solutions for an aging society, *Online J Issues Nurs* 8:1, 2003.

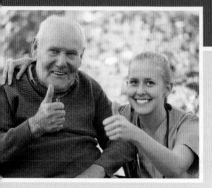

CHAPTER 2

Gerontological Nursing: Past, Present, and Future

Theris A. Touhy

e http://evolve.elsevier.com//Touhy/TwdHlthAging

A YOUTH SPEAKS

Until my grandmother became ill and needed our help, I really didn't know her well. Now I can look at her in an entirely different light. She is frail and tough, fearful and courageous, demanding and delightful, bitter and humorous, needy and needed. I'm beginning to think that old age is the culmination of all the aspects of living a long life.

Jenine, 28 years old

A PERSON AT MID-LIFE SPEAKS

Gerontological nursing brings one in touch with the most basic and profound questions of human existence: the meanings of life and death; sources of strength and survival skills; beginnings, endings, and reasons for being. It is a commitment to discovery of the self—and of the self I am becoming as I age.

Stephanie, 46 years old

AN ELDER SPEAKS

I'm 95 years old and have no family or friends that still survive. I wonder if anyone will be there for me when I leave the planet, which will be very soon I am sure. Mothers deliver, but who will deliver me into the hand of God?

Helen, 87 years old

LEARNING OBJECTIVES

On completion of this chapter, the reader will be able to:
1. Discuss strategies to prepare an adequate and competent eldercare workforce to meet the needs of the growing numbers of older people across the globe.
2. Identify several factors that have influenced the development of gerontological nursing as a specialty practice.
3. Discuss several formal geriatric organizations and describe their significance to nurses.
4. Discuss the role of gerontological nurses in research related to aging
5. Compare various gerontological nursing roles and requirements across the health-wellness continuum.
6. Discuss interventions to improve outcomes for older adults during transitions between health care settings.

CARE OF OLDER ADULTS: A NURSING IMPERATIVE

Healthy aging is now an achievable goal for many. It is essential that nurses have the knowledge and skills to help people of all ages, races, and cultures to achieve this goal. The developmental period of elderhood is an essential part of a healthy society and as important as childhood or adulthood (Thomas, 2004). We can expect to spend 40 or more years as older adults. Enhancing health in aging requires attention to health throughout life, as well as expert care from nurses.

How do nurses maximize the experience of aging and enrich the years of elderhood for all individuals regardless of the physical and psychological changes that commonly occur? Nurses have a great responsibility to help shape a world in which older people can thrive and grow, not merely survive. Most nurses care for older people during the course of their careers. Estimates are "that by 2020, up to 75% of nurses' time will be spent with older adults" (Holroyd et al, 2009, p. 374). In addition, the public will look to nurses to have the knowledge and skills to assist people to age in health. Every older person should expect care provided by nurses with competence in gerontological nursing.

Who Will Care for an Aging Society?

By 2040, the number of older people in the world will be at least 1.3 billion (Tolson et al, 2011) (Chapter 1). It is a critical health and societal concern that gerontological nurses, other health professionals, and direct care workers are prepared to deliver care in all settings across the globe. The aging workforce is in shortage in most of the developed world, and the increased aging population is posing challenges for many countries to meet the expanding need for care services for older people (European Economic and Social Committee, 2012). The developing countries are experiencing the most rapid growth in numbers of older people and lack systems of care and services.

In the United States, eldercare is projected to be the fastest growing employment sector in health care. In spite of demand, the number of health care workers who are interested and prepared to care for older people remains low (Institute of Medicine, 2008). Less than 1% of registered nurses and less than 3% of advanced practice nurses (APNs) are certified in geriatrics (Cortes, 2012; Institute of Medicine, 2008; Robert Wood Johnson Foundation, 2012). "We do not have anywhere close to the number of nurses we need who are prepared in geriatrics, whether in the field of primary care, acute care, nursing home care, or in-home care" (Christine Kovner, RN, PhD, FAAN, as cited in Robert Wood Johnson Foundation, 2012).

Geriatric medicine faces similar challenges with about 7000 prepared geriatricians, 1 for every 2546 older Americans; and this number is falling with the trend predicted to be less than 5000 by 2040 (Cortes, 2012; Institute of Medicine, 2008). Other professions such as social work, physical therapy, and psychiatry have similar shortages. It is estimated that by 2030 nearly 3 million additional health care professionals and direct care workers will be needed to meet the care needs of a growing older adult population (Eldercare Workforce Alliance, 2014).

The geriatric workforce shortage also presents a looming crisis for the 43.5 million unpaid family caregivers providing care for someone 55 years or older. Without improvement in the eldercare workforce, even more stress will be placed on family and other informal caregivers. With smaller family sizes, the rising divorce rate, and the increase in geographical relocation, the next generation of older adults may be less able to rely on families for caregiving (Eldercare Workforce Alliance, 2014) (Chapter 34). Will there be care workers to assist families in care of loved ones?

The Eldercare Workforce Alliance, a group of 28 national organizations representing older adults and the eldercare workforce, including family caregivers, health care professionals, direct care workers, and consumers, has begun to address these concerns. Immediate goals of the Alliance are as follows:

- strengthen the direct care workforce through better training, supervision, and improved compensation; address clinician and faculty shortages through incentives such as loan forgiveness; increase public funding for training; and provide better compensation
- ensure a competent workforce by encouraging agencies and organizations that certify and regulate the eldercare workforce to require demonstrated and continued competence
- redesign the health care delivery by adopting cost-effective care coordination models

The Patient Protection and Affordable Care Act (2010) provides many initiatives that will have a direct impact on

BOX 2-1   HEALTHY PEOPLE 2020

Objective 7-A

Increase the proportion of the health care workforce with geriatric certification (physicians, geriatric psychiatrists, registered nurses, dentists, physical therapists, registered dieticians).

Data from U.S. Department of Health and Human Services, Office of Disease Prevention and Health Promotion: Healthy People 2020, 2012. http://www.healthypeople.gov/2020

gerontological nursing with regard to workforce, education, and practice. Funding to support advanced education in gerontological nursing, education of faculty, and advanced training for direct care workers employed in long-term care settings is included in the provisions of the law.

Improving the competency and adequacy of the eldercare workforce is essential to meet the needs and demands of a burgeoning aging population (Bardach and Rowles, 2012). "The consequences of inaction will be profound" (Besdine et al, 2005, p. S246). See Box 2-1 for a *Healthy People 2020* objective related to the workforce crisis.

DEVELOPMENT OF GERONTOLOGICAL NURSING

Historically, nurses have always been in the frontlines of caring for persons as they age. They have provided hands-on care, supervision, administration, program development, teaching, and research and are, to a great extent, responsible for the rapid advance of gerontology as a profession. Nurses have been, and continue to be, the mainstay of care of older adults (Mezey and Fulmer, 2002). Gerontological nurses have made significant contributions to the body of knowledge guiding best practice care of older people.

Efforts to determine the appropriate term for nurses caring for older people have included gerontic nurses, gerontological nurses, and geriatric nurses. We prefer the term gerontological nurse because it reflects a more holistic approach encompassing both health and illness. *Gerontological* nursing has emerged as a circumscribed area of practice only within the past 6 decades. Before 1950, gerontological nursing was seen as the application

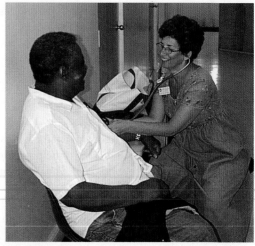

Nurses provide care in a number of settings. (Courtesy Kathleen Jett.)

of general principles of nursing to the older adult client with little recognition of this area of nursing as a specialty similar to obstetric, pediatric, or surgical nursing. Whereas most specialties in nursing developed from those identified in medicine, this was not the case with gerontological nursing because health care of the older adult was traditionally considered within the domain of general nursing (Davis, 1985). In examining the history of gerontological nursing, one must marvel at the advocacy and perseverance of nurses who have remained deeply committed to the care of older adults despite struggling against insurmountable odds over the years.

The foundation of gerontological nursing as we know it today was built largely by a small cadre of nurse pioneers, many of whom are now deceased. The specialty was defined and shaped by these innovative nurses who saw, early on, that older individuals had special needs and required the most subtle, holistic, and complex nursing care. These pioneers challenged the current thinking and investigated new ideas related to the care of older people; refuted mythical tales and fantasies about aging; and found realities through investigation, clinical observation, practice, and documentation, setting in motion activities that markedly influenced the course of the aging experience. They saw new possibilities and a better future for those in the later stages of life. The wisdom the pioneers shared is still relevant today, and we owe them a debt of gratitude for their commitment, compassion, and persistence in establishing the specialty practice. Box 2-2 presents the views of some of the geriatric nursing pioneers, as well as those of current leaders, on the practice of gerontological

---

BOX 2-2 Reflections on Gerontological Nursing from Gerontological Nursing Pioneers and Current Leaders in the Field

Doris Schwartz, Gerontological Nursing Pioneer

"We need to remind ourselves constantly that the purpose of gerontic nursing is to prevent untimely death and needless suffering, always with the focus of doing with as well as doing for, and in every instance to attempt to preserve personhood as long as life continues."

(From interview data collected by Priscilla Ebersole between 1990 and 2001.)

Mary Opal Wolanin, Gerontological Nursing Pioneer

"I believe that one of the most valuable lessons I have learned from those who are older is that I must start with looking inside at my own thinking. I was very guilty of ageism. I believed every myth in the book, was sure that I would never live past my seventieth birthday, and made no plan for my seventies. Probably the most productive years of my career have been since that dreaded birthday and I now realize that it is very difficult, if not impossible, to think of our own aging."

(From interview data collected by Priscilla Ebersole between 1990 and 2001.)

Bernita Steffl, Gerontological Nursing Pioneer

"There is always an interesting person there, sometimes locked in the cage of age. I think I have helped at least a few of my students with this approach, 'You see me as I am now, but I see myself as I've always been and all the things I've been—not just an old lady.'"

(Ebersole P, Touhy T: Geriatric nursing: growth of a specialty, New York, 2006, Springer, p. 52.)

Terry Fulmer, Dean, College of Nursing, New York University, and Co-Director, John A. Hartford Institute for Geriatric Nursing

"I soon realized that in the arena of caring for the aged, I could have an autonomous nursing practice that would make a real difference in medical outcomes. I could practice the full scope of nursing. It gave me a sense of freedom and accomplishment. With older patients, the most important component of care, by far, is nursing care. It's very motivating."

(Ebersole P, Touhy T: Geriatric nursing: growth of a specialty, New York, 2006, Springer, p. 129.)

Neville Strumpf, Edith Clememer Steinbright Professor in Gerontology, University of Pennsylvania, Director of the Hartford Center of Geriatric Nursing Excellence and Center for Gerontological Nursing Science

"My philosophy remains deeply rooted in individual choice, comfort and dignity, especially for frail, older adults. I fervently hope that the future will be characterized by a health care system capable of supporting these values throughout a person's life, and that we shall someday see the routine application of evidence-based practice to the care of all older adults, whether they are in the community, a hospital, or the nursing home. We have not yet achieved that dream."

(Ebersole P, Touhy T: Geriatric nursing: growth of a specialty, New York, 2006, Springer, p. 145.)

Mathy Mezey, Professor Emerita and Retired Founding Director, The Hartford Institute for Geriatric Nursing, New York University College of Nursing

"Because geriatric nursing especially offers nurses the unique opportunity to dramatically impact people's lives for the better and for the worst, it demands the best that you have to offer. I am very optimistic about the future of geriatric nursing. Increasing numbers of older adults are interested in marching into old age as healthy and involved. Geriatric nursing offers a unique opportunity to help older adults meet these aspirations while at the same time maintaining a commitment to the oldest and frailest in our society."

(Ebersole P, Touhy T: Geriatric nursing: growth of a specialty, New York, 2006, Springer, p. 142.)

Jennifer Lingler, PhD, CRNP, Assistant Professor, School of Nursing, University of Pittsburgh

"When I was in high school, a nurse I knew helped me find a nursing assistant position at the residential care facility where she worked. That experience sparked my interest in older adults that continues today. I realized that caring for frail elders could be incredibly gratifying, and I felt privileged to play a role, however small, in people's lives. At the same time, I became increasingly curious about what it means to age successfully. I questioned why some people seemed to age so gracefully, while others succumbed to physical illness, mental decline, or both. As a Building Academic Geriatric Nursing Capacity (BAGNC) alumnus, I now divide my time serving as a nurse practitioner at a memory disorders clinic, teaching an ethics course in a gerontology program, and conducting research on family caregiving. I am encouraged by the realization that as current students contemplate the array of opportunities before them, seek counsel from trusted mentors, and gain exposure to various clinical populations, the next generation of geriatric nurses will emerge. And, I am confident that in doing so, they will set their own course for affecting change in the lives of society's most vulnerable members."

(As cited in Fagin C, Franklin P: Why choose geriatric nursing? Six nursing scholars tell their stories, Imprint Sep-Oct, 2005, p. 74.)

nursing and what draws them to the specialty. For a comprehensive review of the history of the specialty, including Dr. Ebersole's interviews with geriatric nursing pioneers, the reader is referred to *Geriatric Nursing: Growth of a Specialty* (Ebersole and Touhy, 2006). Nurses are proud to be the standard bearers of excellence in the care of older people (Table 2-1).

Early History

The origins of gerontological nursing are rooted in England and began with Florence Nightingale as she accepted a position in the Institution for the Care of Sick Gentlewomen in Distressed Circumstances. Nightingale's concern for the frail and sick elderly was continued by Agnes Jones, a wealthy Nightingale-trained

TABLE 2-1	**Professionalization of Gerontological Nursing**
1906	First article is published in *American Journal of Nursing* (AJN) on care of the elderly.
1925	AJN considers geriatric nursing as a possible specialty in nursing.
1950	Newton and Anderson publish first geriatric nursing textbook.
	Geriatrics becomes a specialization in nursing.
1962	American Nurses Association (ANA) forms a national geriatric nursing group.
1966	ANA creates the Division of Geriatric Nursing.
	First master's program for clinical nurse specialists in geriatric nursing developed by Virginia Stone at Duke University.
1970	ANA establishes *Standards of Practice for Geriatric Nursing.*
1974	Certification in geriatric nursing practice offered through ANA; process implemented by Laurie Gunter and Virginia Stone.
1975	*Journal of Gerontological Nursing* published by Slack; first editor, Edna Stilwell.
1976	ANA renames Geriatric Division "Gerontological" to reflect a health promotion emphasis.
	ANA publishes *Standards for Gerontological Nursing Practice;* committee chaired by Barbara Allen Davis.
	ANA begins certifying geriatric nurse practitioners.
	Nursing and the Aged edited by Burnside and published by McGraw-Hill.
1977	First gerontological nursing track funded by Division of Nursing and established by Sr. Rose Therese Bahr at University of Kansas School of Nursing.
1979	*Education for Gerontic Nursing* written by Gunter and Estes; suggested curricula for all levels of nursing education.
1980	*Geriatric Nursing* first published by AJN; Cynthia Kelly, editor.
1983	Florence Cellar Endowed Gerontological Nursing Chair established at Case Western Reserve University, first in the nation; Doreen Norton, first scholar to occupy chair.
	National Conference of Gerontological Nurse Practitioners is established.
1984	National Gerontological Nurses Association is established.
	Division of Gerontological Nursing Practice becomes Council on Gerontological Nursing (councils established for all practice specialties).
1989	ANA certifies gerontological clinical nurse specialists.
1992	John A. Hartford Foundation funds a major initiative to improve care of hospitalized older patients: Nurses Improving Care for Healthsystem Elders (NICHE).
1996	John A. Hartford Foundation establishes the Institute for Geriatric Nursing at New York University under the direction of Mathy Mezey.
2000	Recommended baccalaureate competencies and curricular guidelines for geriatric nursing care published by the American Association of Colleges of Nursing and the John A. Hartford Foundation Institute for Geriatric Nursing (2010).
	The American Academy of Nursing established Building Academic Geriatric Nursing Capacity (BAGNC) in 2000 with support from the John A. Hartford Foundation.
2001	Hartford Coalition of Geriatric Nursing Associations formed.
2002	Nurse Competence in Aging (funded by the Atlantic Philanthropies Inc.) initiative to improve the quality of health care to older adults by enhancing the geriatric competence of nurses who are members of specialty nursing.
2004	Nurse Practitioner and Clinical Nurse Specialist Competencies for Older Adult Care published by the American Association of Colleges of Nursing and the Hartford Institute for Geriatric Nursing.
	Atlantic Philanthropies committed its resources to postdoctoral fellowships in gerontology nursing.
2007	Atlantic Philanthropies provides a grant to the American Academy of Nursing of $500,000 to improve care of older adults in nursing homes by improving the clinical skills of professional nurses (Nursing Home Collaborative).
	American Association for Long-Term Care Nurses formed.
2008	Four new Centers of Geriatric Nursing Excellence (CGNE) are funded by the John A. Hartford Foundation, bringing the total number of Centers to nine. Existing Centers are at the University of Iowa, University of California San Francisco, Oregon Health Sciences University, University of Arkansas, University of Pennsylvania, Arizona State University, Pennsylvania State University, University of Minnesota, and University of Utah.
	Research in Gerontological Nursing launched by Slack Inc; Dr. Kitty Buckwalter, Editor.
	Geriatric Nursing Leadership Academy established by Sigma Theta Tau International with funding from the John A. Hartford Foundation.
	John A. Hartford Foundation funds the Geropsychiatric Nursing Collaborative (Universities of Iowa, Arkansas, Pennsylvania, American Academy of Nursing).
	Institute of Medicine publishes *Retooling for an aging America: building the health care workforce* report and addresses the need for enhanced geriatric competencies for the health care workforce.
	Consensus Model for APRN Regulation:
	Licensure, Accreditation, Certification & Education designates adult-gerontology as one of six population foci for APRNs
2009	*Sigma Theta Tau's Center for Nursing Excellence in Long-Term Care launched*
	John A. Hartford Foundation funds Phase 2 of the Fostering Geriatrics in Pre-Licensure Nursing Education, a partnership between the Community College of Philadelphia and the National League for Nursing.

TABLE 2-1	**Professionalization of Gerontological Nursing—cont'd**
2010	Adult-gerontology primary care nurse practitioner competencies published by the John A. Hartford Foundation Institute for Geriatric Nursing, the AACN, and NONPF.
	Sigma Theta Tau's Center for Nursing Excellence established.
	ANCC Pathways to Excellence—Long-Term Care Program established.
	ANA Gerontological Nursing Scope and Standards of Practice published.
2012	The Gerontological Society of America is now home to the Coordinating Center for the National Hartford Centers of Gerontological Nursing Excellence (HCGNE), also known as the Building Academic Geriatric Nursing Capacity Initiative.
	U.S. Department of Health and Human Services provides funding to five designated medical center hospitals for clinical training to newly enrolled APRNs to deliver primary care, preventive care, transitional care, chronic case management, and other services appropriate for Medicare recipients.
2013	Adult-Gerontology Acute Care Nurse Practitioner and Adult-Gerontology Primary Care Nurse Practitioner certifications through ANCC begin.
	Hartford Institute of Geriatric Nursing (HIGI) receives a $1.5 million Nurse Education, Practice, Quality, and Retention (NEPQR) Grant from HRSA to enhance interprofessional education, leadership, and team-building skills for practitioners and students to help address the complexity of medication management for frail older adults in the community. The grant is a practice/education partnership between HIGI, New York University (NYU) College of Nursing, NYU Silver School of Social Work, Touro College of Pharmacy, and Visiting Nurse Service of New York.
	Primary Care for Older Adults Initiative e-learning clinical training modules released; supported by funds from DHHS, HRSA, Bureau of Health Professions (BHPr), and Division of Public Health and Interdisciplinary Education (DPHIE). Modules available on GenerationNP.com.
	Post-master's certificate in Interprofessional Primary Care for Older Adults with Multiple Chronic Conditions: Hartford Institute of Geriatric Nursing and New York University College of Nursing.

nurse, who in 1864 was sent to the Liverpool Infirmary, a large Poor Law institution. The care in the institution had been poor, the diet meager, and the "nurses" often drunk. Under the tutelage of Nightingale, Miss Jones was able to dramatically improve the care and reduce the costs.

In the United States, almshouses were the destination of destitute older people and were insufferable places with "deplorable conditions, neglect, preventable suffering, contagion, and death from lack of proper medical and nursing care" (Crane, 1907, p. 873). As early as 1906, Lavinia Dock and other early leaders in nursing addressed the needs of the elderly chronically ill in almshouses and published their work in the *American Journal of Nursing* (AJN). Dock and her colleagues cited the immediate need for trained nurses and pupil education in almshouses, "so that these evils, all of which lie strictly in the sphere of housekeeping and nursing—two spheres which have always been lauded as women's own—might not occur" (Dock, 1908, p. 523). In 1912, the Board of Directors of the American Nurses Association (ANA) appointed an Almshouse Committee to continue to oversee nursing in these institutions. World War I distracted them from attention to these needs. But in 1925, the ANA advanced the idea of a specialty in the nursing care of the aged.

With the passage of the Social Security Act of 1935, federal monies were provided for old-age insurance and public assistance for needy older people not covered by insurance. To combat the public's fear of almshouse placement, Congress stipulated that the Social Security funds could not be used to pay for care in almshouses or other public institutions. This move is thought to have been the genesis of commercial nursing homes. During the next 10 years, many almshouses closed and the number of private boarding homes providing care to elders increased. Because retired and widowed nurses often converted their homes into such living quarters and gave care when their boarders became ill, they can be considered the first geriatric nurses in the community and their homes the first nursing homes.

In the 1940s, two nursing journals described centers of excellence for geriatric care: the Cuyahoga County Nursing Home in Ohio and the Hebrew Home for the Aged in New York. An article in the *American Journal of Nursing* (AJN) by Sarah Gelbach (1943) recommended that nurses should have not only an aptitude for working with the elderly but also specific geriatric education. The first textbook on nursing care of the elderly, *Geriatric Nursing*, was published by Newton and Anderson in 1950, and the first published nursing research on chronic disease and the elderly (Mack, 1952) appeared in the premier issue of *Nursing Research* in 1952.

In 1962 a focus group was formed to discuss geriatric nursing, and in 1966 a geriatric practice group was convened. Also in 1966 the ANA formed a Division of Geriatric Nursing. The first geriatric standards were published by the ANA in 1968, and soon after, geriatric nursing certification was offered. Geriatric nursing was the first specialty to establish standards of practice within the ANA and the first to provide a certification mechanism to ensure specific professional expertise through credentialing (Ebersole and Touhy, 2006). In 1976 the Division of Geriatric Nursing changed its name to the Gerontological Nursing Division to reflect the broad role nurses play in the care of older people. In 1984 the Council on Gerontological Nursing was formed and certification for geriatric nurse practitioners (GNPs) and gerontological clinical nurse specialists (GCNSs) became available. The most recent edition of *Scope and Standards of Gerontological Nursing Practice* was published in 2010 and identifies levels of gerontological nursing practice (basic and advanced) and standards of clinical gerontological nursing care and gerontological nursing performance.

Current Initiatives

The most significant influence in enhancing the specialty of gerontological nursing has been the work of the Hartford Institute for Geriatric Nursing, established in 1996 and funded by the John A. Hartford Foundation. It is the only nurse-led organization in the country seeking to shape the quality of the nation's health care for older Americans by promoting geriatric nursing excellence to both the nursing profession and the larger health care community. Initiatives in nursing education, nursing practice, nursing research, and nursing policy include enhancement of geriatrics in nursing education programs through curricular reform and faculty development and development of the National Hartford Centers of Gerontological Nursing Excellence, predoctoral and postdoctoral scholarships for study and research in geriatric nursing, and clinical practice improvement projects to enhance care for older adults (www. hartfordign.org).

Another significant influence on improving care for older adults was the Nurse Competence in Aging (NCA) project. This initiative addressed the need to ensure competence in geriatrics among nursing specialty organizations. The initiative provided grant and technical assistance to more than 50 specialty nursing organizations, developed a free web-based comprehensive gerontological nursing resource center (ConsultGeriRN.org) where nurses can access evidence-based information on topics related to the care of older adults, and conducted a national gerontological nursing certification outreach (Stierle et al, 2006). There is also a new mobile app (http://consultgerirn.org/resources/apps/) that can be purchased for $1.99 and gives access to information and tools to treat common problems encountered in the care of older adults. The Resourcefully Enhancing Aging in Specialty Nursing (REASN) project extended this work and focused on building intensive collaborations with 13 hospital-based specialty associations to create geriatric educational products and resources to ensure the geriatric competencies of their members.

Sigma Theta Tau's Center for Nursing Excellence in Long-Term Care was launched in 2009. The Center sponsors the Geriatric Nursing Leadership Academy (GNLA) and offers a range of products and services to support the professional development and leadership growth of nurses who provide care to older adults in long-term care. In 2013, The Hartford Institute for Geriatric Nursing, in collaboration with several other organizations, began several initiatives focusing on interprofessional education, leadership, and team building skills, as well as improving the knowledge and skill sets of primary care providers caring for older adults (Table 2-1).

GERONTOLOGICAL NURSING EDUCATION

According to the ANA's *Gerontological Nursing: Scope and Standards of Practice* (2010), "Nurses require the knowledge and skills to assist older adults in a broad range of nursing care issues, from maintaining health and preventing illnesses, to managing complex, overlapping chronic conditions and progressive/protracted frailty in physical and mental functions, to palliative care" (pp. 12, 13).

Essential educational competencies and academic standards for care of older adults have been developed by national organizations such as the American Association of Colleges of Nursing (AACN) for both basic and advanced nursing education (ANA, 2010). *The Essentials of Baccalaureate Education for*

Professional Nursing Practice (AACN, 2008) specifically address the importance of geriatric content and structured clinical experiences with older adults across the continuum in the education of students. In 2010, AACN and the Hartford Institute for Geriatric Nursing, New York University, published the *Recommended Baccalaureate Competencies and Curricular Guidelines for the Nursing Care of Older Adults,* a supplement to the *Essentials* document (Appendix 2-A). In addition, gerontological nursing competencies for advanced practice graduate programs have also been developed. All of these documents can be accessed from the AACN website. "Despite these lists of competencies, however, there remains a lack of consistency among nursing schools in helping students gain needed gerontological nursing information and skills" (ANA, 2010, p. 12).

There has been some improvement in the amount of geriatrics-related content in nursing school curricula, but it is still uneven across schools and hampered by lack of faculty expertise in the subject (IOM, 2011; Robert Wood Johnson Foundation, 2012). Faculty with expertise in gerontological nursing are scarce and there is a critical need for nurses with master's and doctoral preparation and expertise in care of older adults to assume faculty roles. Most schools still do not have freestanding courses in the specialty similar to courses in maternal/child or psychiatric nursing. AACN's 2007 report on the education and role of the clinical nurse leader stated: "In the past, nursing education has been dogged about assuring that every student has the opportunity to attend a birth, but has never insisted that every student have the opportunity to manage a death, even though the vast majority of nurses are more likely to practice with clients who are at the end of life" (p. 7). Best practice recommendations for nursing education include provision of a stand-alone course, as well as integration of content throughout the curriculum "so that gerontology is valued and viewed as an integral part of nursing care" (Miller et al, 2009, p. 198).

It is important to provide students with nursing practice experiences caring for elders across the health-wellness continuum. For clinical practice sites, one is not limited to the acute care setting or the nursing home. Experiences with well elders in the community and opportunities to focus on health promotion should be the first experience for students. This will assist them to develop more positive attitudes, understand the full scope of nursing practice with older adults, and learn nursing responses to enhance health and wellness. Rehabilitation centers, subacute and skilled nursing facilities, and hospice settings provide opportunities for leadership experience, nursing management of complex problems, interprofessional teamwork, and research application for more advanced students (Fox, 2013; Neville et al, 2014).

ORGANIZATIONS DEVOTED TO GERONTOLOGY RESEARCH AND PRACTICE

The Gerontological Society of America (GSA) demonstrates the need for interdisciplinary collaboration in research and practice. The divisions of Biological Sciences, Health Sciences, Behavioral and Social Sciences, Social Research, Policy and Practice, and Emerging Scholar and Professional Organization include individuals from myriad backgrounds and disciplines who affiliate with a section based on their particular function rather than their educational or professional credentials. Nurses can be found in all sections and occupy important positions as officers and committee chairs in the GSA.

This mingling of the disciplines based on practice interests is also characteristic of the American Society on Aging (ASA). Other interdisciplinary organizations have joined forces to strengthen the field. The Association for Gerontology in Higher Education (AGHE) has partnered with the GSA, and the National Council on Aging (NCOA) is affiliated with the ASA. These organizations and others have encouraged the blending of ideas and functions, furthering the understanding of aging and the interprofessional collaboration necessary for optimal care. International gerontology associations, such as the International Federation on Aging and the International Association of Gerontology and Geriatrics, also have interdisciplinary membership and offer the opportunity to study aging internationally.

Organizations specific to gerontological nursing include the National Gerontological Nursing Association (NGNA), the Gerontological Advanced Practice Nurses Association (GAPNA), the National Association Directors of Nursing Administration in Long Term Care (NADONA/LTC) (also includes assisted-living RNs and LPNs/LVNs as associate members), the American Association for Long-Term Care Nursing (AALTCN), and the Canadian Gerontological Nursing Association (CGNA).

The CGNA, founded in 1985, addresses the health needs of older Canadians and the nurses who care for them. In 2003, the CGNA formed an alliance with the NGNA to exchange information and share mutual goals and opportunities for the advancement of both groups. NGNA and CGNA published *Prescriptions for Excellence in Gerontological Nursing Education* (2008). In 2001, the Coalition of Geriatric Nursing Organizations (CGNO) was established to improve the health care of older adults across care settings. The CGNO represents more than 28,500 geriatric nurses from 8 national organizations and is supported by the Hartford Institute for Geriatric Nursing and located at New York University College of Nursing (New York, NY).

RESEARCH ON AGING

Inquiry into and curiosity about aging is as old as curiosity about life and death itself. Gerontology began as an inquiry into the characteristics of long-lived people, and we are still intrigued by them. Anecdotal evidence was used in the past to illustrate issues assumed to be universal. Only in the past 60 years have serious and carefully controlled research studies flourished.

The impact of disease morbidity and impending death on the quality of life and the experience of aging have provided the impetus for much of the study by gerontologists. Much that has been thought about aging has been found to be erroneous, and early research was conducted with older people who were ill. As a result, aging has been inevitably seen through the distorted lens of disease. However, we are finally recognizing that aging and disease are separate entities although frequent companions.

Aging has been seen as a biomedical problem that must be reversed, eradicated, or controlled for as long as possible. The trend toward the medicalization of aging has influenced the general public as well. The biomedical view of the "problem" of aging is reinforced on all sides. A shift in the view of aging to one that centers on the potential for health, wholeness, and quality of life, and the significant contributions of older people to society, is increasingly the focus in the research, popular literature, the public portrayal of older people, and the theme of this text.

The National Institute on Aging (NIA), the National Institute of Nursing Research (NINR), the National Institute of Mental Health (NIMH), and the Agency for Healthcare Research and Quality (AHRQ) continue to make significant research contributions to our understanding of older people. Research and knowledge about aging are strongly influenced by federal bulletins that are distributed nationwide to indicate the type of research most likely to receive federal funding. These are published in requests for proposals (RFPs). Ongoing and projected budget cuts are of concern in the adequate funding of aging research and services in the United States.

Theoreticians and researchers most commonly interested in the study of aging are sociologists, psychologists, and biologists. Their conceptual bases underlie their perspectives regarding survival issues. Nursing research draws from its own body of knowledge, as well as from all of these disciplines, to describe, monitor, protect, and evaluate the quality of life while aging and the services more commonly provided to the aging population, such as hospice care.

Nursing Research

Gerontological nursing research and practice have evolved to such a point that the best practice standards are being published and distributed widely. Nurses have generated significant research on the care of older adults and have established a solid foundation for the practice of gerontological nursing. Research with older adults receives considerable funding from the National Institute of Nursing Research (NINR), and their website (www.nih.gov/ninr) provides information about results of studies and funding opportunities. A current initiative is The Palliative Research Cooperative (PCRC): Enhancing Sustainability and Building the Science of Palliative Care. This opportunity will encourage cutting-edge studies focused on biobehavioral research and the impact of transitions along the palliative care spectrum, as well as caregiving issues. Gerontological nurse researchers publish in many nursing journals and journals devoted to gerontology such as *The Gerontologist* and *Journal of Gerontology* (GSA), and there are several gerontological nursing journals including *Journal of Gerontological Nursing*, *Research in Gerontological Nursing*, *Geriatric Nursing*, and the *International Journal of Older People Nursing*.

Nursing research has significantly affected the quality of life of older people and gains more prominence each decade. Federal funding for gerontological nursing research is increasing, and more nurse scholars are studying nursing issues related to older people. Many nursing research studies and evidence-based protocols are featured in this text. Some of the most important nursing studies have investigated methods of caring for individuals with dementia, reducing falls and the use of restraints, pain management, delirium, care transitions, and end-of-life care.

Knowledge about aging and the lived experience of aging has changed considerably and will continue to change in the future. Past ideas and current practices will not be acceptable to a generation of healthier and better educated individuals who expect a much higher quality of life than did their elders. Nursing research will continue to examine the best practices for care of older people who are ill and living in institutions but increasing emphasis will be placed on strategies to maintain and improve health while aging, especially in light of the increasing numbers of older individuals across the globe.

Current research priorities include a focus on community and home-care resources for older adults, family caregiving issues, and a shift from the emphasis on illness and disease to the expectation of wellness, even in the presence of chronic illness and functional impairment. Translational research and continued attention to interprofessional studies are increasingly important. Future research directions from prominent gerontological nurse researchers are presented in Box 2-3. Brendan McCormack, editor of the *International Journal of Older People Nursing*, provides suggestions for a global research agenda in Box 2-4.

GERONTOLOGICAL NURSING ROLES

Gerontological nursing roles encompass every imaginable venue and circumstance. The opportunities are limitless because we are a rapidly aging society. "Nurses have the potential to improve elder care across settings through effective screening and comprehensive assessment, facilitating access to programs and services, educating and empowering older adults and their families to improve their health and manage chronic conditions, leading and coordinating the efforts of members of the health care team, conducting and applying research, and influencing policy" (Young, 2003, p. 9).

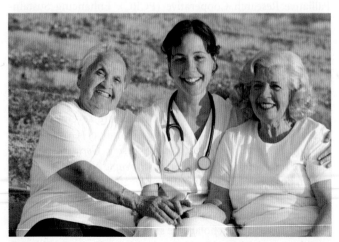
Gerontological nursing is important in this rapidly aging society. (©iStock.com/DianaHirsch.)

BOX 2-3   Future Directions for Gerontological Nursing Research

- Staffing patterns and the most appropriate mix to improve care outcomes in long-term care settings; role of the registered nurse in residential long-term care settings
- Strategies to increase preparation in gerontological nursing and increased recruitment into the specialty
- Influence of culture, diversity, and ethnicity on aging and preparation of nurses to work with older adults
- Gay, lesbian, bisexual, transgender couples/families/relationships
- Factors contributing to successful aging, health promotion, and wellness, including resilience and spirituality
- Retirement decisions of current and future older people, how they are made and how they are changing
- Dementia as a chronic illness and staying well with the disease
- Developing the science behind other pain management devices such as TENS, acupuncture, distraction, and various skin stimulation techniques
- Adaptation of electronic medical records (EMRs) to capture the complexity of older adults with multiple comorbid conditions and provide person-centered care
- Increasing the sophistication of physical, psychosocial, and environmental assessments for older adults
- Nonpharmacological treatments nurses can use to help older people including counseling and teaching skills
- Caregiving, particularly intergenerational and cross-cultural
- Interventions for drug and alcohol abuse and mental health problems of current and future generations of older adults
- Integration of current best practice protocols into settings across the continuum in cost-effective and care-efficient models
- Models of acute care designed to prevent negative outcomes in elders
- Nursing interventions for individuals with dementia in acute care settings
- Delirium—prevention, management, and care
- Interprofessional care: what is it, how to do it, and what impact does it have on quality of care and quality of life of older adults?
- Health promotion and illness management interventions in the assisted living setting; role of professional nurses and advanced practice nurses in this setting; aging in place
- Development of models for end-of-life care in the home and nursing home

From Resnick B, Kovach C, McCormack B: Personal communication, December 18, 2013; and Wykle ML, Tappen RM as cited in Ebersole P, Touhy T: *Geriatric nursing: growth of a specialty*, New York, 2006, Springer.

BOX 2-4   Suggestions for Global Gerontological Nursing Research

Aging in low- and middle-income nations
Ethnic elders in Western societies
Homeless older people
Older people in rural isolated communities
Older people as caregivers
Aging in war-torn societies
Older people in the context of natural disaster management

From personal communication: Brendan McCormack, December 20, 2013.

A gerontological nurse may be a generalist or a specialist. The generalist functions in a variety of settings (primary care, acute care, home care, subacute and long-term care, and the community), providing nursing care to individuals and their families. National certification as a gerontological nurse is a way to demonstrate one's special knowledge in care for older adults and should be encouraged (http://www.nursecredentialing.org/GerontologicalNursing).

The gerontological nursing specialist has advanced preparation at the master's level and performs all of the functions of a generalist but has developed advanced clinical expertise, as well as an understanding of health and social policy and proficiency in planning, implementing, and evaluating health programs.

Specialist Roles

Under the Consensus Model for APRN Regulation: *Licensure, Accreditation, Certification and Education* (2008), advanced practice registered nurses (APRNs) must be educated, certified, and licensed to practice in a role and a population. APRNs may specialize but they may not be licensed solely within a specialty area. APRNs are educated in one of four roles, one of which is adult-gerontology. This population focus encompasses the young adult to the older adult, including the frail elder.

Today, there are only about 5700 geriatric nurse practitioners but there are 25,000 adult nurse practitioners (ANPs) and 52,000 family nurse practitioners (FNPs) (Cortes, 2012, 2013). The number of APRNs with gerontological certification and interest in the specialty practice has historically been low. It is hoped that this new focus in role and population, combining ANP and gerontological nurse practitioner (GNP) specialty education, will assist in meeting the critical need for APRNs so that more are well prepared to care for the aging population.

Family and adult nurse practitioner programs often attract more students, and many of these graduates go on to practices that include a large number of older adults. Some have had intensive attention in their curricula to gerontological nursing care, but many have not and must "learn on the job." The lack of faculty with expertise in gerontological nursing and limited knowledge of the scope of gerontological nursing have led to less than ideal preparation of FNP and ANP students in care of older adults and those with the complex medical conditions often seen in aging. Further, the faculty may have little to no experience or negative attitudes of care provided in long-term care settings, discouraging advanced practice nursing (APN) students from practicing in these settings. The routing of federal grants for education in medicine and nursing to family practice is an additional reason for the low numbers of nurses choosing specialty preparation in gerontological nursing.

Titles of APRNs educated and certified across both areas of practice will include the following: Adult-Gerontology Acute Care Nurse Practitioner, Adult-Gerontology Primary Care Nurse Practitioner, and Adult-Gerontology Clinical Nurse Specialist. Certification is available for all of these levels of advanced practice; in most states this is a requirement for licensure.

Advanced practice nurses with certification in adult-gerontology will find a full range of opportunities for collaborative and independent practice both now and in the future. Direct care sites include geriatric and family practice clinics, long-term care, acute and subacute care facilities, home health care agencies, hospice agencies, continuing care retirement communities, assisted living facilities, managed care organizations, and specialty care clinics (e.g., Alzheimer's, heart failure, diabetes). Specialty gerontological nurses are also involved with community agencies such as local Area Agencies on Aging, public health departments, and national and worldwide organizations such as the Centers for Disease Control and the World Health Organization. They function as care managers, eldercare consultants, educators, and clinicians.

One of the most important advanced practice nursing roles that emerged over the last 40 years is that of the gerontological nurse practitioner (GNP) and the gerontological clinical nurse specialist (GCNS) in skilled nursing facilities. The education and training programs arose from evident need, particularly in the long-term care (LTC) setting (Ploeg et al, 2013). Nurse practitioners have been providing care in nursing homes in the United States since the 1970s, in Canada since 2000, and only recently in the United Kingdom. Numbers remain small and there is a need for continued attention at the policy and funding level for increased use of nurse practitioners in LTC. Recommendations from expert groups in the United States and Canada have called for a nurse practitioner in every nursing home (Harrington et al, 2000; Ploeg et al, 2013). This role is well established and there is strong research to support the impact of advanced practice nurses working in LTC settings (Bakerjian, 2008; Oliver et al, 2014; Ploeg et al, 2013) (Box 2-5).

The Evercare Care Model, a federally funded Medicare demonstration project, originally designed by two nurse practitioners, is a very successful innovative model with a long history of positive outcomes. This model utilizes APRNs, either certified in gerontology or specially trained by Evercare, for care of long-term nursing home residents and individuals with severe or disabling conditions (see www.innovativecaremodels.com). Box 2-6 presents research highlights from a study examining resident and family perceptions of the nurse practitioner role in long-term care settings.

Generalist Roles
Acute Care

Older adults often enter the health care system with admissions to acute care settings. Older adults comprise 60% of the

---

BOX 2-5   Outcomes of APNs Working in LTC Settings

Improvement in or reduced rate of decline in incontinence, pressure ulcers, aggressive behavior, and loss of affect in cognitively impaired residents

Lower use of restraints with no increase in staffing, psychoactive drug use, or serious fall-related injuries

Improved or slower decline in some health status indicators including depression

Improvements in meeting personal goals

Lower hospitalization rates and costs

Fewer ED visits and costs

Improved satisfaction with care

Data from Ploeg J, Kaaslainen S, McAiney C, et al: Resident and family perceptions of the nurse practitioner role in long term care settings, *BMC Nurs* 12:24, 2013.

BOX 2-6 RESEARCH HIGHLIGHTS

In-depth and focus group interviews were conducted with residents and family members in four Canadian nursing homes to explore their perceptions of the nurse practitioner role. The major themes that emerged were as follows:

NPs were seen as providing resident and family-centered care and providing enhanced quality of care. Residents and families perceived the NP as improving availability and timeliness of care and helping to prevent unnecessary hospitalization. Participants spoke eloquently about the NP role as "catalyst," "light switch," and "bridge" in shaping the culture and working relationships in long-term care (LTC). "She (NP) helps me and my sister a lot just by listening and providing suggestions . . . not just communicating but she is also listening. It's almost like having a midwife or doula or something like that, from an emotional point of view" (p. 7).

Residents and families valued the caring relationship with the NP and this was a central means through which enhanced quality of care occurs. Increased use of NPs in LTC settings can enhance outcomes and satisfaction. Including the concepts of caring relationships and person-centered care in NP education is important.

Data from Ploeg J, Kaaslainen S, McAiney C, et al: Resident and family perceptions of the nurse practitioner role in long term care settings, *BMC Nurs* 12:24, 2013.

BOX 2-7 Guiding Principles for the Elder-Friendly Hospital/Facility

For the Patient
- Each patient is a unique individual and should be evaluated as such.
- Measures are taken to accommodate the patient's and family's special needs.

For the Staff
- Nurses demonstrate clinical competence in geriatric nursing.
- Nurses provide therapeutic response, patience, and presence when caring for geriatric patients.
- Nurses and staff who provide direct care identify and address the patient's individual needs and preferences; staff creates a positive experience for the patient and family.
- Nurses coordinate care across the continuum and "Manage the Journey" of the patient and family.
- Excellent communication, tailored to meet the needs of the geriatric patient, results in a "Climate of Confidence" for the patient and the nurse.
- The organization provides appropriate resources and systems that support best practice in geriatric nursing care.

For the Environment
- The physical environment supports the needs of the geriatric patient and family and the staff who care for them.
- An elder-friendly environment, as defined by the patient and family, also enhances the practice environment for the staff.
- The elder-friendly environment is embraced hospital wide.

From American Association of Nurse Executives: *The guiding principles for creating elder-friendly hospitals*. Copyright 2010 by the American Organization Nurse Executives (AONE). All Rights Reserved.

medical-surgical patients and 46% of the critical care patients. Acutely ill older adults frequently have multiple chronic conditions and comorbidities and present many challenges. Even though most nurses working in acute care are caring for older patients, many have not had gerontological nursing content in their basic nursing education programs and few are certified in the specialty. "Only a small number of the country's 6000 hospitals have institutional practice guidelines, educational resources, and administrative practices that support best practice care of older adults" (Boltz et al, 2008, p. 176).

Kagan (2008) reminds us that "older adults are the work of hospitals but most nurses practicing in hospitals do not say they specialize in geriatrics . . . We, as a profession and a force in an aging society, must make the transformation to understanding care of older adults is acute care nursing . . . Care of older adults would be the rule instead of the exception" (2008, p. 103). Kagan goes on to suggest that such a transformation would mean that acute care nurses would proudly describe themselves as geriatric nurses with subspecialties (geriatric vascular nurses, geriatric emergency nurses) and, along with geriatric nurse generalists, would populate hospital nursing services across the country.

Nurses caring for older adults in hospitals may function in the direct care provider role; or as care managers, discharge planners, care coordinators, or transitional care nurses; or in leadership and management positions. Many acute care hospitals are adopting new models of geriatric and chronic care to meet the needs of older adults. These include geriatric emergency rooms and specialized units such as acute care for the elderly (ACE), geriatric evaluation and management units (GEM), and transitional care programs. This will increase the need for well-prepared geriatric professionals working in interprofessional teams to deliver needed services. Box 2-7 presents guiding principles for the elder-friendly hospital.

NICHE. The Nurses Improving Care for Health System Elders (NICHE), a program developed by the Hartford Geriatric Nursing Institute in 1992, was designed to improve outcomes for hospitalized older adults and offers many opportunities for new roles for acute care nurses such as the geriatric resource nurse (GRN). The GRN role emphasizes the pivotal role of the bedside nurse in influencing outcomes of care and coordination of interprofessional activities (Resnick, 2008). "All geriatric models of care include a high level of nursing input but only NICHE stresses nurse involvement in hospital decision-making regarding care of older adults. This professional nursing practice perspective supports nurse competencies related to the complex interdisciplinary care management of older adults and the resources they need to improve the safety and outcomes of hospitalized older adults" (Capezuti et al, 2012, p.3117).

NICHE especially targets the prevention of iatrogenic complications, which occur in as many as 29% to 38% of hospitalized older adults, a rate three to five times higher than that seen in younger patients (Inouye et al, 2000). Common iatrogenic complications include functional decline, pneumonia, delirium, new-onset incontinence, malnutrition, pressure ulcers, medication reactions, and falls. Recognizing the impact of iatrogenesis, both on patient outcomes and on the cost of care, the Centers for Medicare and Medicaid Services (CMS) has instituted changes that will reduce payment to hospitals relative to these often preventable outcomes. The changes target conditions that are high cost or high volume, result in a higher payment when present as a secondary diagnosis, are not present on admission, and could have reasonably been prevented through the use of evidence-based guidelines. Targeted conditions include catheter-associated urinary tract infection (CAUTI), pressure ulcers, and falls (Chapters 13, 16, 19). Expertise in gerontological nursing is essential in prevention of these conditions.

NICHE has been the most successful acute care geriatric model in recruiting hospital membership and contributing to the depth of geriatric hospital programming. More than 500 hospitals in more than 40 states, as well as parts of Canada, are involved in NICHE projects (www.nicheprogram.org).

Community- and Home-Based Care

Nurses will care for older adults in hospitals and long-term care facilities, but the majority of older adults live in the community. Community-based care occurs through home and hospice care, provided in persons' homes, independent senior housing complexes, retirement communities, residential care facilities such as assisted living facilities, and adult day health centers. It also takes place in primary care clinics and public health departments. Care will continue to move out of hospitals and long-term care institutions into the community because of rapidly escalating health care costs and the person's preference to "age in place." Gerontological nurses will find opportunities to create practices in community-based settings with a focus on not only care for those who are ill but also health promotion and community wellness.

Nurses in the home setting provide comprehensive assessments including physical, functional, psychosocial, family, home, environmental, and community. Care management and working with interprofessional teams are integral components of the home health nursing role. Nurses may provide and supervise care for elders with a variety of care needs (including chronic wounds, intravenous therapy, tube feedings, unstable medical conditions, and complex medication regimens) and for those receiving rehabilitation and palliative and hospice services. Schools of nursing must increase education and practice experiences for nursing students in home- and community-based care.

New roles for registered nurses in the community may emerge with the implementation of the Patient Protection and Affordable Care Act (2010). The California Institute for Nursing and Health Care *Nurse Role Exploration Project* (2013) discusses the following emerging roles: care coordinator (including population health management and tiered coordination); nurse/family cooperative facilitator (bringing virtual and in-person health care to people where they live and work); and primary care provider (performing intake screening, education, coaching, and support for people with complex illnesses, as well as preventative information and support for wellness in collaboration with physicians and nurse practitioners). Nurse practitioners are now Medicare-accepted providers of the annual wellness visits for beneficiaries. Advances in technology for remote monitoring of health status and safety and the development of point-of-care testing devices show promise in improving outcomes for elders who

want to age in place (see Chapter 20). These technologies present exciting opportunities for nurses in the management and evaluation of care.

Certified Nursing Facilities (Nursing Homes)

Certified nursing facilities, commonly called nursing homes, have evolved into a significant location where health care is provided across the continuum, part of a range of long-term post–acute care (LTPAC) services. Estimates are that 37% of all acute hospitalizations require post–acute care services and older adults now enter nursing homes with increasingly acute health conditions. The old image of nursing homes caring for older adults in a custodial manner is no longer valid. Today, most facilities have subacute care units that more closely resemble the general medical-surgical hospital units of the past. Most people enter nursing homes for short stays that last no more than 1 week to 3 months (Toles et al, 2013). "Nursing homes are no longer just a destination but rather a stage in the recovery process" (Thaler, 2014). Subacute care in nursing facilities will continue to grow with health care reform, and there are many new roles and opportunities for professional nursing in the setting.

Roles for professional nursing include nursing administrator, manager, supervisor, charge nurse, educator, infection control nurse, Minimum Data Set (MDS) coordinator, case manager, transitional care nurse, quality improvement coordinator, and direct care provider. Professional nurses in nursing facilities must be highly skilled in the complex care concerns of older people, ranging from subacute care to end-of-life care. Excellent assessment skills; ability to work with interprofessional teams in partnership with residents and families; skills in acute, rehabilitative, and palliative care; and leadership, management, supervision, and delegation skills are essential.

Practice in this setting calls for independent decision-making and is guided by a nursing model of care because there are fewer physicians and other professionals on site at all times. In addition, stringent federal regulations governing care practices and greater use of licensed practical nurses and nursing assistants influence the role of professional nursing in this setting. Many new graduates will be entering this setting upon graduation so it is essential to provide education and practice experiences to prepare them to function competently in this setting, particularly leadership and management skills. Box 2-8 presents research highlights of a study of quality geriatric care in long-term and acute care settings. Chapter 32 provides comprehensive information about long-term care.

TRANSITIONS ACROSS THE CONTINUUM: ROLE OF NURSING

Care transition refers to the movement of patients from one health care practitioner or setting to another as their condition and care needs change. Older people have complex health care needs and often require care in multiple settings across the health-wellness continuum. This makes them and their family and/or caregivers vulnerable to poor outcomes during

BOX 2-8   RESEARCH HIGHLIGHTS

Quality Geriatric Care as Perceived by Nurses in Long-Term and Acute Care Settings

The study examined differences in nurses' satisfaction with the quality of care of older people and with organizational characteristics and work environment in acute care and long-term care (LTC) settings. Nursing staff in LTC facilities were significantly more satisfied with the quality of geriatric care provided at their facilities than nursing staff in acute care settings. Obstacles to providing geriatric care (inadequate staffing, lack of time, inadequate educational opportunities, lack of resources) were identified by both acute and LTC nursing staff, but acute care staff perceived significantly more obstacles. Dissatisfaction with the continuity of care for older adults across settings was a source of dissatisfaction for both acute and LTC nursing staff.

Implications include the need to improve knowledge of best practices in geriatric care and enhance organizational resources. Programs such as NICHE can contribute to enhanced quality of geriatric care in hospitals. Adequate staffing and resources are essential in all settings so that nurses have time to deliver quality care to the complex older adult patient.

Data from Barba B, Hu J, Efird J: Quality geriatric care as perceived by nurses in long-term and acute care settings, *J Clin Nurs* 21(5–6): 833–840, 2012.

transitions (Naylor, 2012). An older person may be treated by a family practitioner or internist in the community and by a hospitalist and specialists in the hospital; discharged to a nursing home and followed by another practitioner; and then discharged home or to a less care-intensive setting (e.g., assisted living facilities/residential care settings) where their original providers may or may not resume care. Most health care providers practice in only one setting and are not familiar with the specific requirements of other settings. Each setting is seen as a distinct provider of services and little collaboration exists. This is changing with health care reform initiatives such as accountable care organizations, health homes, and bundled care payments (Chapters 30 and 32).

Readmissions: The Revolving Door

One in five older patients is readmitted to the hospital within 30 days of discharge. Some readmissions may be predictable but many can and should be prevented. Ninety percent of these readmissions for Medicare patients are unplanned, resulting in annual costs of more than $17 billion, paying for return trips that need not happen if patients received the right care. These statistics do not consider emergency department "treat-and-release" visits within 30 days of discharge, which have been found to account for nearly 40% of all hospital post–acute care use for Medicare recipients (Vashi et al, 2013). Place of residence and the health care system providing care also influence readmission rates. Many patients are readmitted because they live in an area where the hospital is used more frequently as a site for illness care or there are limited resources for community-based care (Robert Wood Johnson Foundation, 2013).

Additionally, one in four Medicare patients admitted to skilled nursing facilities from hospitals is readmitted to the hospital within 30 days. Up to two thirds of these hospital transfers

are rated as potentially avoidable by expert long-term care health professionals (http://interact2.net/). These rehospitalizations are costly, potentially harmful, and often preventable (Chapter 32). Older adults who are discharged home after nursing home stays also have a high use of acute care services. This is an area that has received little attention and there is a need for transitional care interventions in this population as well (Toles et al, 2014).

The Centers for Medicare & Medicaid Services (CMS) has identified avoidable readmissions as one of the leading problems facing the U.S. health care system and penalizes hospitals (with fines) that have high readmission rates for patients with heart failure, heart attack, and pneumonia (Robert Wood Johnson Foundation, 2013). There are several CMS demonstration projects, funded by the Patient Protection and Affordable Care Act (2010), designed to address avoidable readmissions and care transitions (Lind, 2013). Many hospitals and nursing homes have begun programs to address the issue with transitional care programs and there has been some improvement (Chapter 32). The average hospital was fined less in the second year of the penalty program but ongoing efforts are needed (Ness, 2013).

Factors Contributing to Poor Transitional Care Outcomes

Multiple factors contribute to poor outcomes during transitions: patient, provider, and system. Many are the result of a fragmented system of care that too often leaves discharged patients to their own devices, unable to follow instructions they did not understand, and not taking medications or getting the necessary follow-up care (Box 2-9).

Patient characteristics such as language, literacy, and cultural and socioeconomic factors are contributing factors to hospital readmissions. The nursing role in discharge planning and patient and family education is critical. Teaching must be based on a complete assessment of the unique needs of the individual and family and adapted to ensure understanding (Chapters 5 and 7).

Engaging patients and families in learning about care required after discharge contributes to improved outcomes. Patients who lack the knowledge, skills, and confidence to manage their own care after discharge have nearly twice the rate of readmissions as patients with the highest level of engagement (Kangovi et al, 2014; Schneidermann and Critchfield, 2012-2013). The nursing role in discharge planning and patient and family education is critical. Teaching must be based on a complete assessment of the unique needs of the individual and adapted to ensure understanding (Chapter 5).

SAFETY ALERT

Medication discrepancies are the most prevalent adverse event following hospital discharge and the most challenging component of a successful hospital-to-home transition (Foust et al, 2012; Hain et al, 2012; Pincus, 2013). Nurses' attention to an accurate prehospital medication list; medication reconciliation during hospitalization, at discharge, and after discharge; and patient and family education about medications are required to enhance safety.

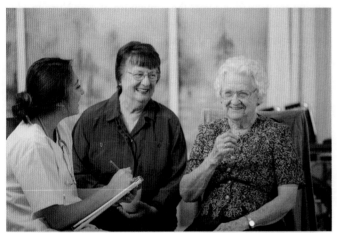

Working with the patient and the caregiver to provide education to enhance self-care abilities and to facilitate linkages to resources is important for the consideration of promoting safe discharges and transitions to home and other care settings. (©iStock.com/Pamela Moore.)

Improving Transitional Care

Transitional care "refers to a broad range of time limited services to ensure health care continuity, avoid preventable poor outcomes among at-risk populations, and promote the safe and timely transfer of these patient groups from one level of care (e.g., acute to subacute) or setting (e.g., hospital to home) to another" (Naylor, 2012, p. 116). National attention to improving patient safety during transfers is increasing, and a growing body of evidence-based research provides data for design of care to improve transition outcomes.

Nurses play a very important role in ensuring the adequacy of transitional care, and many of the successful models involve the use of advanced practice nurses and registered nurses in roles such as transition coaches, care coordinators, and care managers (Chalmers and Coleman, 2008; Naylor, 2012). Nurse researchers Dorothy Brooten and Mary Naylor, along with their colleagues, have significantly contributed to knowledge in the area of transitional care and the critical role of nurses in transitional care improvement. One of the most rigorously studied acute care approaches, the Transitional Care Model (TCM), has demonstrated reductions in preventable hospital readmissions,

improvements in health outcomes, enhancement in patient satisfaction, and reductions in total health care costs (Naylor, 2012)

In addition to roles as care managers and transition coaches, nurses play a key role in many of the elements of successful transitional care models, such as medication management, patient and family caregiver education, comprehensive discharge planning, and adequate and timely communication between providers and sites of service. Box 2-10 presents Resources for Best Practice and Box 2-11 gives Tips for Best Practice for

BOX 2-12   Suggested Elements of Transitional Care Models

- Multidisciplinary communication, collaboration, and coordination from admission to transition
- Clinician involvement and shared accountability during all points of transition
- Evaluation of transitional interventions
- Information systems (electronic medical records) that span traditional settings; well-designed and structured patient transfer records
- Comprehensive planning and risk assessment throughout hospital stay including targeting of high-risk patients and high-risk families
- Improved communication among patients, family caregivers, and providers
- Improved communication and collaboration between sending and receiving clinicians
- Medication reconciliation on admission, discharge, post discharge; simplify posthospital medication regimen
- Education to improve patient/family knowledge of medications before discharge
- Adapt educational materials for language and health literacy
- Discuss warning signs that require reporting and medical evaluation and explain how to access assistance
- Schedule follow-up care appointments before discharge
- Timely follow-up, support, and coordination after the patient leaves a care setting; follow-up discharge with home visits/telephone calls.
- Care coordination by advanced nurse practitioners
- Coach patients, teach self-care skills, and encourage active involvement in their own care
- Assessment of informal support
- Involvement, education, and support of family caregivers
- Share community resources and make appropriate referrals to resources and sources of financial assistance
- Interventions to enhance discussions of palliative and end-of-life care and communication of advance directives

transitional care nursing. Further research is needed to evaluate which transitional care models are most effective in various settings and for which group of patients, particularly those who are most frail or cognitively impaired and medically underserved populations (Golden and Shier, 2012-2013). Box 2-12 presents suggested elements of transitional care models. Chapter 32 discusses transitional care in the nursing home setting.

◆ PROMOTING HEALTHY AGING: IMPLICATIONS FOR GERONTOLOGICAL NURSING

The rapid growth of the older population brings forth opportunities and challenges for the world now and in the future. With the promise of a healthier old age, health care professionals, particularly nurses, will play a significant role in creating systems of care and services that enhance the possibility of healthy aging for an increasingly diverse population. Nurses have the skills needed to create a more person-centered, coordinated health care system and improve outcomes in health and illness. Continued attention must be paid to the recruitment and education of health professionals and direct care staff prepared to care for older people to meet critical shortages that threaten health and safety.

Exciting roles for nurses with preparation in gerontological nursing are increasing across the continuum of care. Nursing education is called upon to prepare graduates to assume positions across the continuum of care, with increasing emphasis on community-based and long-term care settings. Of particular importance is improving outcomes during transitions of care for older people. Dare we say that gerontological nursing will be the most needed specialty in nursing as the number of older people continues to increase and the need for our specialized knowledge becomes even more critical in every specialty and every health care setting?

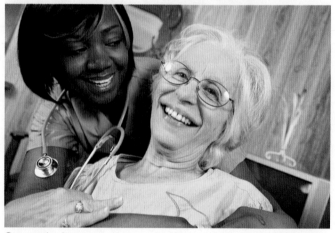

Gerontologic nurses have a significant role in the healthy aging of older adults. (©iStock.com/Pamela Moore.)

▮ KEY CONCEPTS

- The eldercare workforce is dangerously understaffed and unprepared to care for the growing numbers of older adults.
- Nursing has led the field in gerontology, and nurses were the first professionals in the nation to be certified as geriatric specialists.
- Certification assures the public of nurses' commitment to specialized education and qualification for the care of older people.
- Research in gerontological nursing has provided the foundation for improved care of older people.

- Health care reform initiatives and a growing older adult population offer many exciting opportunities for nurses with competence in care of older adults.
- Advanced practice role opportunities for nurses are numerous and are seen as potentially cost-effective in health care delivery while facilitating more holistic health care.
- Professional nursing involvement is an essential component in models to improve transitions of care across the continuum.

CRITICAL THINKING QUESTIONS AND ACTIVITIES

1. What content and clinical experiences on care of older adults is included in your nursing program?
2. Reflect on the Recommended Baccalaureate Competencies for Care of Older Adults (Appendix 2-A). Which have you had the opportunity to meet in your nursing program?
3. Review one of the gerontological nursing journals (*Geriatric Nursing, Journal of Gerontological Nursing, Research in Gerontological Nursing*) and choose a research study of interest to you. How could you use the findings of the study in your clinical practice with older adults?
4. What programs to improve transitional care are being implemented in the acute care setting where you are studying?
5. What settings for care of older adults are of interest to you as you consider a nursing practice area after graduation?

RESEARCH QUESTIONS

1. What aspects of gerontological nursing roles do practicing nurses find most rewarding and which do they find most challenging?
2. Why do so few students choose gerontological nursing as an area of practice? What factors might encourage more interest in the specialty?
3. What is the actual time in the curriculum of baccalaureate nursing schools spent on content and practice experiences related to the care of older people?
4. What is the phenomenon of interest in nursing research? How does it differ from other disciplines?
5. What roles in gerontological nursing and which settings of practice are of most interest to new graduates?

REFERENCES

American Association of Colleges of Nursing: *White paper on the education and role of the clinical nurse leader,* Feb 2007. http://www.nursing.vanderbilt.edu/msn/pdf/cm_AACN_CNL.pdf. Accessed September 16, 2014.

American Association of Colleges of Nursing: *The essentials of baccalaureate education for professional nursing practice,* Oct 2008. http://www.aacn.nche.edu//education-resources/baccessentials08.pdf. Accessed February 12, 2014.

American Association of Colleges of Nursing: *Adult-gerontology primary care nurse practitioner competencies,* Mar 2010. http://www.aacn.nche.edu/geriatric-nursing/adultgeroprimcareNPcomp.pdf. Accessed February 10, 2014.

American Association of Colleges of Nursing. *Recommended baccalaureate competencies and curricular guidelines for the nursing care of older adults.* A supplement to The Essentials of Baccalaureate Education for Professional Nursing Practice, Sept 2010. http://www.aacn.nche.edu/education/pdf/AACN_Gerocompetencies.pdf. Accessed February 12, 2014.

American Nurses Association: *Gerontological nursing: scope and standards of practice,* ed 3, Silver Spring, MD, 2010, American Nurses Association.

APRN Consensus Work Group & National Council of State Boards of Nursing APRN Advisory Committee: *Consensus model for APRN regulation: licensure, accreditation, certification & education,* March 2008. http://www.nursingworld.org/EspeciallyForYou/AdvancedPracticeNurses/Consensus-Model-Toolkit. Accessed December 2014.

Bakerjian D: Care of nursing home residents by advanced practice nurses: a review of the literature, *Res Gerontol Nurs* 1:177–185, 2008.

Bardach S, Rowles G: Geriatric education in the health professions: are we making progress? *Gerontologist* 52(5):607–618, 2012.

Besdine R, Boult C, Brangman S, et al: Caring for older Americans: the future of geriatric medicine, *J Am Geriatr Soc* 53(Suppl 6):S245–S256, 2005.

Boltz M, Capezuti E, Bower-Ferris S, et al: Changes in the geriatric care environment associated with NICHE, *Geriatr Nurs* 29:176–185, 2008.

California Institute for Nursing and Health Care: *Nurse role exploration project: the Affordable Care Act and new nursing roles,* Sept 25, 2013. http://www.calhospital.org/sites/main/files/file-attachments/cinhc_whitepapernurseroles.pdf. Accessed December 17, 2013.

Capezuti E, Boltz M, Cline D, et al: Nurses improving care for health system elders – a model for optimizing the geriatric nurse practice environment, *J Clin Nurs* 21(21–22):3117–3125, 2012.

Chalmers S, Coleman E: Transitional care. In Capezuti E, Swicker D, Mezey M, et al, editors: *The encyclopedia of elder care,* ed 2, New York, 2008, Springer, pp 740–743.

Cortes T: Out of the ashes, *Hot Issues in Geriatrics Now: HIGN blog,* May 30, 2012. http://hartfordinstitute.wordpress.com/?s=Out+of+the+Ashes. http://hartfordinstitute.wordpress.com/page/3/Accessed February 9, 2014.

Cortes T: NPs bridging the gap in primary care, *Hot Issues in Geriatrics Now: HIGN blog,* April 8, 2013. http://hartfordinstitute.wordpress.com/2013/04. Accessed February 9, 2013.

Crane C: Almshouse nursing: the human need, *Am J Nurs* 7:872, 1907.

Davis B: Nursing care of the aged: historical evolution, *Bull Am Assoc Hist Nurs* 47, 1985.

Dock L: The crusade for almshouse nursing, *Am J Nurs* 8:520, 1908.

Ebersole P, Touhy T: *Geriatric nursing: growth of a specialty,* New York, 2006, Springer.

Eldercare Workforce Alliance: *Geriatrics workforce shortage: a looming crisis for our families* (Issue brief). http://www.eldercareworkforce.org/files/Issue_Brief_PDFs/EWA_Issue.Supplydemand.final-3.pdf. Accessed February 5, 2014.

European Economic and Social Committee: *Active ageing and solidarity between generations,* 2012. http://www.eesc.europa.eu/resources/docs/eesc-12-16-en.pdf. Accessed September 12, 2014.

Foust J, Naylor M, Bixby B, et al: Medication problems occurring at hospital discharge among older adults with heart failure, *Res Gerontol Nurs* 5(1):25–33, 2012.

Fox J: Educational strategies to promote professional nursing in long-term care: an integrative review, *J Gerontol Nurs* 39(1):52–60, 2013.

Gelbach S: Nursing care of the aged, *Am J Nurs* 43:1112–1114, 1943.

Golden R, Shier G: What does "care transitions" really mean? *Generations* 36(4): 6–12, 2012–2013.

Hain D, Tappen R, Diaz S, et al: Characteristics of older adults rehospitalized within 7 days and 30 days of discharge, *J Gerontol Nurs* 38(8):32–44, 2012.

Harrington C, Kovner C, Mezey M, et al: Experts recommend minimum nurse staffing for nursing facilities in the United States, *Gerontologist* 40(1):5–16, 2000.

Holroyd A, Dahlke S, Fehr C, et al: Attitudes towards aging: implications for a caring profession, *J Nurs Educ* 48(7):374–380, 2009.

Inouye S, Bogardus S, Baker D, et al: The Hospital Elder Life Program: a model of care to prevent cognitive and functional decline in older hospitalized patients, *J Am Geriatr Soc* 48:1657–1706, 2000.

Institute of Medicine, National Academies: *Retooling for an aging America: building the health care workforce,* 2008. http://www.iom.edu/Reports/2008/Retooling-for-an-Aging-America-Building-the-Health-Care-Workforce.aspx. Accessed November 2010.

Institute of Medicine, National Academies: *The future of nursing: leading change, advancing health,* 2011. http://www.iom.edu/Reports/2010/The-future-of-nursing-leading-change-advancing-health.aspx. Accessed February 4, 2014.

Kagan S: Moving from achievement to transformation, *Geriatr Nurs* 29: 102–104, 2008.

Kangovi S, Barg F, Carter T, et al: Challenges faced by patients with low socioeconomic status during the post-hospital transition, *J Gen Intern Med* 29(2):283–289, 2014.

Lind K: *Recent Medicare initiatives to improve care coordination and transitional care for chronic conditions,* Mar 2013. http://www.aarp.org/health/medicare-insurance/info-03-2013/recent-medicare-initiatives-to-improve-care-coordination-AARP-ppi-health.html. Accessed February 10, 2014.

Mack M: Personal adjustment of chronically ill old people under home care, *Nurs Res* 1:9–30, 1952.

Mezey M, Fulmer T: The future history of gerontological nursing, *J Gerontol A Biol Sci Med Sci* 57:M438–M441, 2002.

Miller J, Coke L, Moss A, et al: Reluctant gerontologists: integrating gerontological nursing content into a prelicensure program, *Nurs Educ* 34:198–203, 2009.

Naylor M: Advancing high value transitional care: the central role of nursing and its leadership, *Nurs Admin Q* 36(2):115–126, 2012.

National Gerontological Nurses Association and Canadian Gerontological Nursing Association: *Prescriptions for excellence in gerontological nursing education: a joint position statement,* May 2008. http://www.ngna.org/_resources/documentation/position_papers/CGNANGNAJointPositionStatement.pdf. Accessed February 9, 2014.

Ness D: Reducing hospital readmissions: it's about improving patient care, *Health Affairs Blog,* Aug 16, 2013.http://healthaffairs.org/blog. Accessed February 10, 2014.

Neville C, Dickie R, Goetz S: What's stopping a career in gerontological nursing? Literature review, *J Gerontol Nurs* 40(1):18–27, 2014.

Newton K, Anderson H: *Geriatric nursing,* St. Louis, 1950, Mosby.

Oliver G, Pennington L, Revelle S, et al: Impact of nurse practitioners on health outcomes of Medicare and Medicaid patients, *Nurs Outlook,* Aug 1, 2014. doi: 10.1016/j.outlook.201407.004. [Epub ahead of print].

Patient Protection and Affordable Care Act, 42 U.S.C. § 18001 (2010).

Pincus K: Transitional care management services, *J Gerontol Nurs* 39(10):10–15, 2013.

Ploeg J, Kaasalainen S, McAiney C, et al: Resident and family perceptions of the nurse practitioner role in long term care settings: a qualitative descriptive study, *BMC Nurs* 12(1):24, 2013. http://www.biomedcentral.com/content/pdf/1472-6955-12-24.pdf. Accessed September 16, 2014.

Resnick B: Hospitalization of older adults: are we doing a good job? *Geriatric Nursing* 29(3):153–154, 2008.

Robert Wood Johnson Foundation: *United States in search of nurses with geriatrics training,* 2012. http://www.rwjf.org/en/about-rwjf/newsroom/newsroom-content/2012/02/united-states-in-search-of-nurses-with-geriatrics-training.html. Accessed February 5, 2014.

Robert Wood Johnson Foundation: *The revolving door: a report on U.S. hospital readmission,* 2013. http://www.rwjf.org/content/dam/farm/reports/reports/2013/rwjf404178. Accessed January 21, 2014.

Schneidermann M, Critchfield J: Customizing the "teachable moment": ways to address hospital transitions in a culturally conscious manner, *Generations* 36(4): 94–97, 2012–2013.

Stierle L, Mezey M, Schumann M, et al: The Nurse Competence in Aging initiative: encouraging expertise in the care of older adults, *Am J Nurs* 106:93–96, 2006.

Thaler M: The need for SNFs for baby boomers. *McKnight's Long-Term Care News and Assisted Living,* 2014. http://www.mcknights.com/the-need-for-snfs-for-baby-boomers/article/327724/. Accessed February 5, 2014.

Thomas W: *What are old people for? How elders will save the world,* Acton, MA, 2004, VanderWyk & Burnham.

Toles M, Anderson R, Massing M, et al: Restarting the cycle: incidence and predictors of first acute care use after nursing home discharge, *J Am Geriatr Soc* 62(1): 79–85, 2014.

Tolson D, Rolland Y, Andrieu S, et al: International Association of Gerontology and Geriatrics: a global agenda for clinical research and quality of care in nursing homes, *J Am Med Dir Assoc* 12:184–189, 2011.

Toles M, Young H, Ouslander J: Improving care transitions to nursing homes, *Generations* 36(4):78–85, 2013.

Vashi A, Fox J, Carr B, et al: Use of hospital-based acute care among patients recently discharged from the hospital, *JAMA* 309(4):364–371, 2013.

Young H: Challenges and solutions for care of frail older adults, *Online J Issues Nurs* 8:1, 2003.

Recommended Baccalaureate Competencies and Curricular Guidelines for the Nursing Care of Older Adults

Gerontological Nursing Competency Statements

1. Incorporate professional attitudes, values, and expectations about physical and mental aging in the provision of patient-centered care for older adults and their families.

Corresponding to Essential VIII

2. Assess barriers for older adults in receiving, understanding, and giving of information.

Corresponding to Essentials IV and IX

3. Use valid and reliable assessment tools to guide nursing practice for older adults.

Corresponding to Essential IX

4. Assess the living environment as it relates to functional, physical, cognitive, psychological, and social needs of older adults.

Corresponding to Essential IX

5. Intervene to assist older adults and their support network to achieve personal goals, based on the analysis of the living environment and availability of community resources.

Corresponding to Essential VII

6. Identify actual or potential mistreatment (physical, mental, or financial abuse, and/or self-neglect) in older adults and refer appropriately.

Corresponding to Essential V

7. Implement strategies and use online guidelines to prevent and/or identify and manage geriatric syndromes.

Corresponding to Essentials IV and IX

8. Recognize and respect the variations of care, the increased complexity, and the increased use of health care resources inherent in caring for older adults.

Corresponding to Essentials IV and IX

9. Recognize the complex interaction of acute and chronic comorbid physical and mental conditions and associated treatments common to older adults.

Corresponding to Essential IX

10. Compare models of care that promote safe, quality physical and mental health care for older adults such as PACE, NICHE, Guided Care, Culture Change, and Transitional Care Models.

Corresponding to Essential II

11. Facilitate ethical, noncoercive decision-making by older adults and/or families/caregivers for maintaining everyday living, receiving treatment, initiating advance directives, and implementing end-of-life care.

Corresponding to Essential VIII

12. Promote adherence to the evidence-based practice of providing restraint-free care (both physical and chemical restraints).

Corresponding to Essential II

13. Integrate leadership and communication techniques that foster discussion and reflection on the extent to which diversity (among nurses, nurse assistive personnel, therapists, physicians, and patients) has the potential to impact the care of older adults.

Corresponding to Essential VI

14. Facilitate safe and effective transitions across levels of care, including acute, community-based, and long-term care (e.g., home, assisted living, hospice, nursing homes), for older adults and their families.

Corresponding to Essentials IV and IX

15. Plan patient-centered care with consideration for mental and physical health and well-being of informal and formal caregivers of older adults.

Corresponding to Essential IX

16. Advocate for timely and appropriate palliative and hospice care for older adults with physical and cognitive impairments.

Corresponding to Essential IX

17. Implement and monitor strategies to prevent risk and promote quality and safety (e.g., falls, medication mismanagement, pressure ulcers) in the nursing care of older adults with physical and cognitive needs.

Corresponding to Essentials II and IV

18. Use resources/programs to promote functional, physical, and mental wellness in older adults.

Corresponding to Essential VII

19. Integrate relevant theories and concepts included in a liberal education into the delivery of patient-centered care for older adults.

Corresponding to Essential I

From American Association of Colleges of Nursing, Hartford Institute for Geriatric Nursing, New York University College of Nursing: *Recommended baccalaureate competencies and curricular guidelines for the nursing care of older adults* [supplement to *The essentials of baccalaureate education for professional nursing practice*], Sept 2010. http://www.aacn.nche.edu/education/pdf/AACN_Gerocompetencies.pdf. Accessed September 12, 2014.

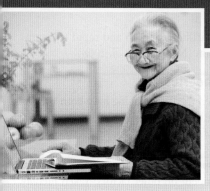

Theories of Aging

Kathleen Jett

http://evolve.elsevier.com/Touhy/TwdHlthAging

A STUDENT SPEAKS

Until I started learning about the science of the aging process I had no idea how complicated it could be. We seem to have learned so much but still have so much more to learn.

Helena, age 23

AN ELDER SPEAKS

When I was a young girl Einstein was proposing the molecular theory of matter, and we had never heard of DNA or RNA. We only knew of genes in the most rudimentary theoretical sense. Now I hear that scientists believe there is a gene that is controlling my life span. I really hope they find it before I die.

Beatrice, age 72

LEARNING OBJECTIVES

On completion of this chapter, the reader will be able to:
1. Describe the interrelationships among the various biological theories of aging.
2. Compare and contrast the major psychosocial theories of aging.
3. Describe the cultural and economic limitations of the current psychosocial theories associated with aging.
4. Use at least one psychosocial theory of aging to support or refute commonly provided social services for older adults living in the community.
5. Create theory-based strategies to foster the highest level of wellness while aging.

Theories are attempts to explain phenomena, to give a sense of order and to provide a framework from which one can interpret and simplify the world (Einstein, 1920). The theories of aging have been broadly drawn, from biological to psychosocial. To a great extent, the current theories are no longer thought to be in competition with each other. Instead, each offers different but often overlapping views of the process of aging.

This chapter provides the reader with an overview of several prominent biological and psychosocial theories and frameworks of aging. The nurse can use the biological theories to help understand the physical changes of aging and the genetic underpinnings of some of the most common disorders. Although they are more subjective and ethnocentric, psychosocial theories and models can provide potential context for aging and social behavior. Taken together, the nuances of the bio-psychosocial being can be better understood.

BIOLOGICAL THEORIES OF AGING

Biological aging, referred to as *senescence*, is an exceedingly complex interactive process of change (Ostojifá et al, 2009). It is accepted that changes occur in the most basic structures of the cells, especially the mitochondria (Lagouge and Larsson, 2013). These changes in turn affect the functioning and longevity of the organism, be it a yeast cell, a mouse, or a human. It may be from unchecked damage from atoms or clusters of atoms called "free radicals" or from genetic mutation (Lagouge and Larsson, 2013). These changes are made visible in what is referred to as the aging phenotype.

While there is a growing body of knowledge about the genomics of aging, complex questions remain. What triggers the changes at the cellular or organ level? Are the changes orderly and predictable or random and chaotic? What are the roles of cellular mutation and epigenetics, that is, the effect of the environment on the RNA? What are the effects of lifestyle choices and how do they influence the aging phenotype? Can we extend life (Box 3-1)? It is the causes and patterns of effect at the cellular level that are in debate and subject to further discovery.

Cellular Functioning and Aging

Survival of an organism depends on successful cellular reproduction, or mitosis. The genetic components of each cell

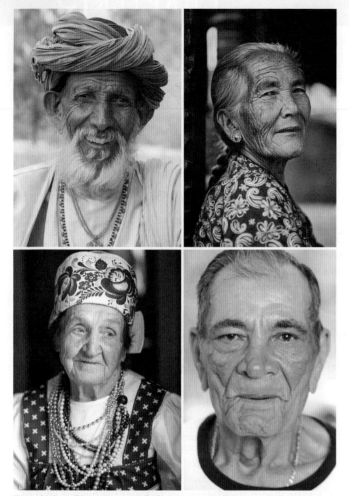

The Aging Phenotype. (©iStock.com/kailash soni; Bartosz Hadyniak; De Visu; ProArtWork.)

BOX 3-1 **Theories Postulated to Prolong Life**

The *neuroendocrine theory* is built on the observation that some organs (and the cells within them) appear to have somewhat of a programmed decline, such as the ovary and the immune system. The foci of research in this area have been on the effect of DHEA and melatonin and the ability to delay senescence of the reproductive organs.

The *caloric restriction theory* has garnered interest for many years. A significant amount of bench research has been conducted with non-humans. The results have been conflicting. In a recent report published by the National Institutes of Health, a diet composed of 30% fewer calories than the standard diet in rhesus monkeys did not extend their lives. A restriction to this level would be intolerable to most humans.

From National Institutes of Health: *Can we prevent aging?* 2014. http://www.nia.nih.gov/health/publication/can-we-prevent-aging#calorie. Accessed April 2014.

(deoxyribonucleic acid [DNA] and ribonucleic acid [RNA]) serve as templates for ensuring that, theoretically, mitosis results in new cells that are exactly the same as the old cells in form and function. If reproduction was always perfect, the organism would never age. Instead, cells become increasingly complex over time. For example, an infant does not learn to walk or talk until the neurons have adequate myelination—until the myelin

sheath is thick enough to facilitate smooth and rapid transmission of messages to the brain (Nomellini et al, 2008).

Programmed Aging Theories

For many years programmed theories of aging have been the foci of bench research (Goldsmith, 2013). They were notably advanced in 1981 through the work of Hayflick and Moorhead, who coined the term "biological clock" (1981). They purported that each cell had a preprogrammed life span; that is, the number of replications were limited and not dependent on other factors. Taken literally, programmed aging means that the age at which cells die in any one person is predetermined and inevitable. It may be inferred that the preventive strategies we now believe enhance health-related quality of life or extend the life span may be ineffective (e.g., smoking cessation) (see Chapter 1). Although programmed theories of aging still have many proponents (Goldsmith, 2013), they are being eclipsed by those made possible by advances in cellular research.

Error Theories

In contrast to programmed aging, error theories propose that the changes at the cellular level are random and unpredictable. These have matured from the very simplistic wear-and-tear theory to the highly complex theories relating to the effect of telomere shortening.

Wear-and-Tear Theory

Wear-and-tear theory proposed that cellular errors were the result of "wearing out" over time because of continued use. The associated damage was accelerated by the harmful effects of internal and external stressors, which include pollutants and injurious metabolic by-products we now refer to as *free radicals* (see section titled Free Radical Theory of Aging). It was thought that the damage caused either progressive decline in function or death of an increasing number of cells.

Oxidative Stress Theories

While the wear-and-tear theory provided building blocks for later work (e.g., identification of free radicals), advances in scientific methods have increased our ability to better understand more changes at the molecular level, particularly the activity and effect of the reactive oxygen species (ROS). As natural products in the metabolism of oxygen, they have an important role in homeostasis. The number of ROS is increased by several external factors (such as pollution and cigarette smoke) and by internal factors (such as inflammation) (Dato et al, 2013). If there is a dramatic rise in the level of ROS, significant damage to the cell results; this is referred to as oxidative stress (Harman, 1956; Murphy, 2009). For the most part, the damage from oxidative stress appears to be random and unpredictable, varying from one cell to another, from one person to another. While still not unequivocal, oxidative stress theories and their associated mitochondrial theories of aging are among those most studied and most widely accepted at this time (Shi et al, 2010).

Free Radical Theory of Aging

Among the end products of cellular reproduction are atoms, molecules, or ions referred to as "free radicals." From a physiological perspective they are quite unstable and their presence alone causes damage to cell functioning (Figure 3-1) (Dato et al, 2013; Gruber et al, 2008). In youth, naturally occurring vitamins, hormones, enzymes, and antioxidants are able to neutralize an adequate number of free radicals to minimize this damage (Valko et al, 2005). The changes we associate with normal aging and vulnerability to many of the diseases common in later life have been suggested to be a result of the point when the accumulation of damage occurs faster than the cells can repair themselves (Dato et al, 2013; Grune et al, 2001; Hornsby, 2010).

For many years it was thought that the consumption of supplemental antioxidants, such as vitamins C and E, could delay or minimize the effects of aging by counteracting the oxidative stress caused by free radicals (Box 3-2). However, it is now known that the intake of supplemental antioxidants is deleterious to one's health (National Center for Complementary and Alternative Medicine [NCCAM], 2013). At the same time, diets inclusive of natural antioxidants, such as those high in fruits and vegetables or a Mediterranean diet rich with red wine and olive oil, have been found to be healthful (Dato et al, 2013).

As evidence has accumulated, *oxidative stress theories of aging* have garnered strong support (Goldsmith, 2013; Jang and Van Remmen, 2009; Lagouge and Larsson, 2013).

Mutations

The rapidly growing field of genomics has allowed scientists to go within the cells and examine the DNA itself. There is

growing evidence suggesting that the presence of ROS and free radicals alone does not trigger the aging process itself but instead results in mutations in cellular DNA and resultant replicative errors, with the number of mutations increasing with age (Lagouge and Larsson, 2013; Wang et al, 2013). Although supported by early research, the findings are not yet conclusive.

Telomeres and Aging

Studies of the human genome have also led to those related to the interaction between aging and telomeres—small pieces of DNA located at the tip of each strand (Figure 3-2). The presence of the enzyme telomerase ensures the reproductive ability of the telomeres, which in turn ensures the life of the DNA and that of the cell (Cefalu, 2011). The length of the telomere may affect longevity, immunity, and overall health (Box 3-3) (Dehbi et al, 2013). Each telomere appears to have a maximum length before it begins to undergo senescence. Consistent with the

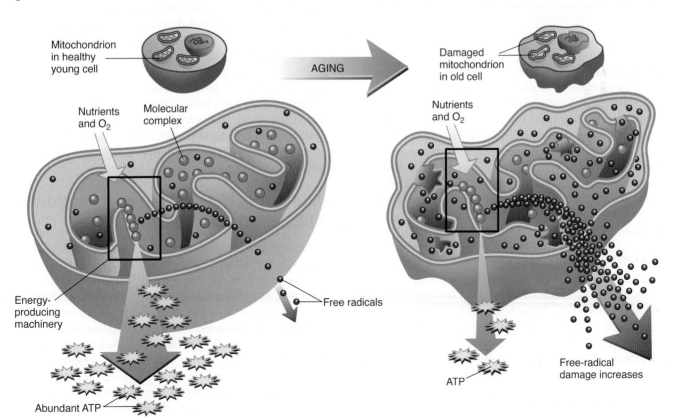

FIGURE 3-1 Mitochondria in Young and Old Cells. *ATP,* Adenosine triphosphate. (From McCance KL, Huether SE: *Pathophysiology: the biologic basis for disease in adults and children,* ed 6, St Louis, 2010, Mosby.)

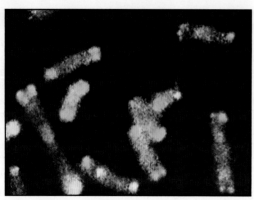

FIGURE 3-2 Chromosomes with Telomere Caps. (Modified from Jerry Shay and the University of Texas Southwestern Medical Center at Dallas, Office of News and Publications, 5323 Harry Hines Blvd, Dallas, TX 75235.)

BOX 3-3   Telomeres, Aging, and Longevity

Telomere length decreases at a rate of 24.8 to 27.7 base pairs per year. A number of lifestyle factors can increase the rate of shortening (Box 3-3). Daily smoking of 1 pack of cigarettes a day for 40 years is associated with the loss of 5 additional base pairs or 7.4 years of life. Obesity also causes accelerated telomere shortening, resulting in 8.8 years of life lost. Excessive emotional stress results in the release of glucocorticoids by the adrenal glands. They have been shown to reduce antioxidants and thereby increase oxidative and premature shortening of telomeres. Shorter telomeres are suggested as greatly increasing one's vulnerability to early onset of age-related health problems such as heart disease.

From Shammas MA: Telomeres, lifestyle, cancer and aging, *Curr Opin Clin Nutr Metab Care* 14(1):28–34, 2011.

BOX 3-4   Factors That Appear to Accelerate Telomere Shortening

Environmental exposure to pollutants
Low social and economic status
Lack of exercise
Obesity
Smoking
Increased age
Unhealthy diet
Excessive dietary protein
Low intake of omega-3 fatty acids

From Shammas MA: Telomeres, lifestyle, cancer and aging, *Curr Opin Clin Nutr Metab Care* 14(1):28–34, 2011.

---

findings of Hayflick and Moorhead (1981), the telomere may have its own "biological clock." At the same time, the shortening is the result of and influenced by oxidative stress. Premature shortening can occur, increasing the individual's risk for any number of disease states and a decreased life span (Shammas, 2011). A recent study indicated that telomere shortening is influenced by a number of factors, especially lifestyle choices (Box 3-4). Research related to aging and the reproductive ability of telomeres has become an intriguing area of inquiry, showing great promise to untangling the mysteries of the aging process (Lin et al, 2012; Shammas, 2011).

Autoimmune Theory

The immune system in the human body is a complex network of cells, tissues, and organs that function separately. The body maintains homeostasis through the actions of this protective, self-regulatory system, controlled by B lymphocytes (humoral immunity) and T lymphocytes (De la Fuente, 2008). Together they protect the body from invasion by exogenous substances, such as exposure to toxins, and endogenous conditions, such as emotional stress, inflammation, and infection.

The *autoimmune theory* suggests that aging is a result of an accumulation of damage as a result of changes in the activities and function of the immune system, or immunosenescence. According to the autoimmune theory, the decreased ability of lymphocytes to withstand oxidative stress appears to be a key factor in the aging process (Swain and Nikolich-Zugich, 2009). Cellular errors in the immune system have been found to lead to an auto-aggressive phenomenon in which normal cells are misidentified as alien and are destroyed by the body's own immune system. The T cells in particular are thought to be responsible for hastening age-related changes caused by auto-immune reactions as the body battles itself.

Although the current biological theories provide possible clues to aging, they also raise many questions and stimulate continuing research. A unifying theory does not yet exist that explains the mechanics and causes underlying biological aging (Viña et al, 2013). It is apparent that the theories are no longer distinct. The science of the biology of aging continues to advance at a rapid pace, fueled in large part by the success of the human genome project. Other related areas of intense inquiry are the relationship between oxidative stress and the development of diseases, and the science of *epigenetics*, or how the genes are influenced by environment, lifestyle, and other factors (Borghini et al, 2013; Brooks-Wilson, 2013; Cefalu, 2011). It is hoped that more research will lead to the discovery of other pathways and key changes in gene expression seen as the aging phenotype and perhaps more importantly, their association to preventable and treatable illnesses.

◆ PROMOTING HEALTHY AGING: IMPLICATIONS FOR GERONTOLOGICAL NURSING

In the application of our growing knowledge of biological aging, it appears reasonable to expect that slowing or reducing cellular damage may have the potential for promoting healthy aging (Box 3-5). Although we do not know if this will lead to increased longevity, it may be a way to ultimately reduce or delay those diseases commonly associated with or acquired by many as they age (Dato et al, 2013). Helping persons reduce external factors (e.g., pollutants in the environment such as second-hand smoke) that are known to increase the development of ROS is one important approach. Facilitating improved nutrition for all persons has been found to reduce the speed of telomere shortening, but this is far from possible in many parts of the world where food is scarce (Box 3-6). Levels of *naturally* occurring antioxidants can be increased through regular exercise, but supplements

BOX 3-5 Promoting Healthy Aging Consistent with the Biological Theories of Aging

What Can Be Done to Reduce Cellular Damage?

- Avoid environmental pollutants and unnecessary radiation. (Oxidative stress)
- Watch for research on the use and presence of antioxidants. (Oxidative stress)
- Avoid stress. (Oxidative stress, Immune)
- Minimize the potential for infection: wash hands frequently, undergo immunizations, and avoid those who are ill. (Immune)

BOX 3-6 TIPS FOR BEST PRACTICE

Finding ways for all persons to have access to nutritious food is an important nursing intervention.

can cause damage. Because we have realized the deleterious effects of antioxidants, the gerontological nurse can use this knowledge to encourage persons to abandon long-held habits and beliefs and replace these with the healthiest diets and judicious use of herbs and dietary supplements (see Chapters 10 and 25).

Of significant importance in the clinical setting is the auto-immune theory and indications of increased susceptibility to infections, autoimmune disorders, and cancers (Cefalu, 2011; Gomez et al, 2008). Observing for early signs and symptoms of infections in older adults is a particular contribution nurses can make to facilitate a return to wellness (see Chapter 1).

With an understanding of these potential changes in immunity, the conscientious nurse can take an active role in promoting specific preventive strategies such as the use of immunizations (especially influenza and pneumococcal) and the avoidance of exposure to others with infections. It is nurses' responsibility to not only promote healthy lifestyles but also serve as role models.

PSYCHOSOCIAL THEORIES OF AGING

A person is not just a biological being but a multidimensional whole (see Chapter 1, Figure 1-7). Only when life is considered in its totality can we begin to truly understand aging. Here we discuss the psychosocial theories of aging and acknowledge that most are more accurately conceptual models or approaches to understanding. Because they are most often referred to as theories in the gerontological literature, we will do so here for the ease of discussion. They can be classified as first-, second-, and third-generation theories (Hooyman and Kiyak, 2011).

First Generation

Early psychosocial theories of aging were an attempt to explain and predict the changes in middle and late life with an emphasis on adjustment. Adjustment was seen as an indication of success, at least by the academic theoreticians who developed them. The majority of these theories began appearing in the

gerontological literature in the 1940s and 1950s. They were based on little research and primarily on "face validity," that is, emerging from the personal and professional experience of both scientists and clinicians and appearing to be reasonable explanations of aging. This set of theories has varied very little since they were first proposed. The major theories in the first generation were those of *role* and *activity*.

Role Theory

Role theory was one of the earliest explanations of how one adjusts to aging (Cottrell, 1942). Self-identity is believed to be defined by one's role in society (e.g., nurse, teacher, banker). As individuals evolve through the various stages in life, so do their roles. Successful aging means that as one role is completed it is replaced by another one of comparative value to the individual and society. For example, the wage-earning work role is replaced by that of a volunteer, or a parent becomes a grandparent. The ability of an individual to adapt to changing roles is a predictor of adjustment to aging. Resistance to change is seen as a harbinger of difficulty at the end of life.

Role theory is operationalized in the phenomenon of *age norms*. They are culturally constructed expectations of what is deemed acceptable behavior in society and are internalized by the individual. Age norms are based on the assumption that chronological age and gender, in and of themselves, imply roles; for example, one may hear, "If only they would act their age," or "You are too old to do/say/behave like that," or "That is unbecoming to a woman of your age." Although beliefs in age- and gender-segregated roles are still present, challenges began with the socially controversial but popular television show of the 1970s *Maude* (1972-1978), later in *The Golden Girls* (1985-1993), and more recently Betty White's role in *Hot in Cleveland* (2010-2014). In each of these, the characters behaved in ways that challenged long-established age norms for white middle- and late-aged women. While older men have long served as role models (albeit unrealistic ones) in movies and television, they are now becoming available to women such as those performed by Dame Judi Dench and Maggie Smith (both born in 1934), Dame Helen Mirren (born in 1945), and American Meryl Streep, born in 1949. With the aging of the "baby boomers" (Chapter 1), popular culture is challenging age norms; for example, "older persons" are now depicted as still sexually active; from advertisements for genital lubricants featuring actors with graying hair to news of the availability of medications to treat erectile dysfunction. These images replace the historical view that persons become asexual as they age (or so their grandchildren hope!). Both men and women are assuming roles and engaging in behaviors in 2014 that were unimaginable when role theory was first proposed.

Activity Theory

In 1953 Havinghurst and Albrecht proposed that continued activity and the ability to "stay young" were indicators of successful aging. Based on data from the Kansas City Studies of Adult Life, successful aging was based on the individual's ability to maintain an *active lifestyle*. It is expected that the productivity and activities of middle life are replaced with equally engaging pursuits in later life (Maddox, 1963). The theory was based on the assumption that it is better to be active (and young) than inactive (Havinghurst, 1972). *Activity theory* is consistent with Western society's emphasis on work, wealth, and productivity and therefore continues to influence the perception of unsuccessful aging (Wadensten, 2006).

The first generation theories of aging have been criticized because of their limited applicability. Problems of intersubjectivity of meaning, testability, and empirical adequacy have persisted. Consistent with the historical period of their development, they failed to consider social class, education, health, and economic and cultural diversity as influencing factors (Hooyman and Kiyak, 2011; Marshall, 1994).

Second Generation

Second generation theories were also referred to as those in the first transformation and "alternative theoretical perspectives" (Hooyman and Kiyak, 2011). They expanded or questioned those of the first generation. These include the *disengagement, continuity, age-stratification, social exchange, modernization,* and *gerotranscendence theories.*

Disengagement Theory

Disengagement theory is in contrast to both role and activity theories. In 1961, Cumming and Henry proposed that in the natural course of aging the individual does, and should, slowly withdraw from society to allow the transfer of power to the younger generations. The transfer is viewed as necessary for the maintenance of social equilibrium (Wadensten, 2006). A belief in the appropriateness of disengagement provided the basis of age discrimination for many years when an older employee was replaced by a younger one. Although this practice was overtly accepted in the past, it is still present more covertly but is now being challenged socially and legally. An elder's withdrawal is no longer an indicator of successful aging, is not *necessarily* a good thing for society, and does not take into account the needs of the individual or culture in which one lives.

Continuity Theory

Also in contrast with role theory but similar to activity theory is *continuity theory.* Havinghurst and colleagues (1968) proposed that individuals develop and maintain a consistent pattern of behavior over a lifetime. Aging, as an extension of earlier life, reflects a *continuation of the patterns* of roles, responsibilities, and activities. Personality influences the roles and activities chosen and the level of satisfaction drawn from these. Successful aging is associated with one's ability to maintain and continue previous behaviors and roles or to find suitable replacements (Wadensten, 2006) (Box 3-7).

BOX 3-7   **TIPS FOR BEST PRACTICE**

If you followed continuity theory in the design of a special living facility for persons with dementia, using their own furniture may be very helpful. "Shadowboxes" are also sometimes used. This is a protected area on the person's door or nearby wall that holds memorabilia with special meaning to these persons earlier in their lives.

Age-Stratification Theory

Age-stratification theory is based on the belief that aging can be best understood by considering the experiences of individuals as members of cohorts with similarities to others in the same group (Riley, 1971). The importance of the similarities exceeds that of the differences. Age stratification can take a number of different forms, such as the historical perspective described in Chapter 1, the traditional conceptualization of "young-old," "middle-old," and "old-old" (Neugarten, 1968), and the view of Thomas (2004) that "childhood" and "adulthood" are followed by "elderhood."

The cohort of baby boomers born between approximately 1947 and 1964 are presenting a significant challenge to this theory in the developed world. As described in Chapter 1, the range of experiences and when they occurred to individuals within the cohort have resulted in substratifications within baby boomers themselves. The wide range of socioeconomic and education levels furthers this diversity (Chapter 4).

Social Exchange Theory

Social exchange theory is conceptualized from an economic perspective. The presumption is that as one ages, one has fewer and fewer economic resources to contribute to society. This paucity results in loss of social status, self-esteem, and political power (Hooyman and Kiyak, 2011). Only those who are able to maintain control of their financial resources have the potential to remain fully participating members of society and anticipate successful aging. Although this may have some applicability in the communities in the world that have been able to develop a stable economy for its citizens, this theory marginalizes those in communities and underdeveloped countries who struggle for the barest necessities now and into the foreseeable future (World Health Organization [WHO], 2014).

Modernization Theory

Although not usually associated with social exchange theory, *modernization theory* can be used to consider nonmaterial aspects of exchange. This theory is an attempt to explain the social changes that have resulted in devaluing the contributions of elders. In the United States before about 1900, material and political resources were controlled by the older members of a society (Achenbaum, 1978). The resources included their knowledge, skills, experience, and wisdom (Fung, 2013). In agricultural cultures and communities, the oldest members held power through property ownership and the right to make decisions related to food distribution. Older men and women often held valuable religious and cultural roles of instructing youth and controlling ceremony (Sokolovsky, 1997).

According to modernization theory, the status and value of elders are lost when their labors are no longer considered useful, kinship networks are dispersed, their knowledge is no longer pertinent to the society in which they live, and they are no longer revered simply because of their age (Hendricks and Hendricks, 1986). Modernization has had a notable effect on cultures such as those in China and Japan where filial duty predominated as an underlying construct of eldercare (Fung, 2013). As more and more adult children enter the marketplace or emigrate for social or economic reasons, conflicts between traditional values mount (see *The Bonesetter's Daughter* by Amy Tan). It is proposed that these changes are the result of advancing technology, urbanization, and mass education (Cowgill, 1974). In some cultures or family structures and in underdeveloped areas of the world, "modernization" as described may not yet be applicable.

Gerotranscendence Theory

This theory is similar to that of disengagement yet the reason for the withdrawal is not for societal needs but to give the person time for self-reflection, exploration of the inner self, contemplation of the meaning of life, and movement away from the material world (Chapter 36) (Maslow, 1954; Moody, 2004; Tornstam, 1989, 2000, 2005; Wadensten, 2007). Aging is viewed as movement from birth to death and maturation toward wisdom, an ever-evolving process that alters one's view of reality, sense of spirituality, and meaning beyond the self. Inasmuch, gerotranscendence implies achieving wisdom through personal transformation. Tornstam (2005), Erikson (1993), and Peck (1968) describe the necessity of transcending individual identity (Table 3-1). With aging, time becomes less important, as do superficial relationships. Transcendence is viewed as a universal goal, the highest goal any person can achieve and a marker of successful aging. This theory is based on a highly egocentric approach to aging. It is less likely to be applicable in cultures based on the quality of interpersonal relationships (see Chapter 4). It also does not account for differences in economic resources, which may or may not provide the individual the "luxury" of time for introspection.

Third Generation

The third generation of theoretical development related to aging is also referred to as the "second transformation" occurring since the 1980s. The goal is "understanding the human meanings of social life in the context of everyday life rather than the explanation of facts" (Hooyman and Kiyak, 2011, p. 326). This may or may not rise to the level of a theory.

A phenomenological approach is used to achieve a qualitative understanding of the individual as an aging person. Aging is considered a personal interpretation rather than one that is

socially or culturally constructed. A number of methods are used in this approach to understand aging, including critical theory, feminism, and postmodernism (Box 3-8).

This level is particularly useful in the application of nursing care and the incorporation of recognition of the aging person as unique and valuable in any circumstance and within the context of any culture. It can be used to promote healthy aging as the person is supported on the wellness continuum.

◆ PROMOTING HEALTHY AGING: IMPLICATIONS FOR GERONTOLOGICAL NURSING

Psychosocial theories and perspectives of aging provide the gerontological nurse with useful information to serve as a backdrop for the development of one's philosophy of care. Although they have been neither proved nor disproved, some of the first two generations have stood the test of time but may have limited applicability to privileged persons wherever they live. They have been used as the rationale for many things, from the creation of senior activity centers to laws regulating employment. They do not, per se, address "crucial issues regarding the attitudes and structure of good nursing" (Wadensten, 2006, p. 347).

BOX 3-8 Third Generation of Theoretical Development Related to Psychosocial Aging

Critical Theory
Inclusion of an understanding of the individual rather than limiting examination to "how things are." In aging, this means that an understanding of the person telling the story is as important as the story of aging being told.

Feminist Theory
A theory proposing that the stories and lives of women have not been adequately told and that to understand the whole experience of aging their voices must be heard as clearly as those of men. This may assume special meaning in aging because of the significant gender shift that occurs in later life.

Postmodernist Theory
Life and meaning are socially constructed. Presumption is not possible. This supports the notion against stereotyping and ageism.

TABLE 3-1 Comparison of Theoretical Proposals of the Developmental Tasks Associated with Aging

ERIKSON		PECK	
THEORY	**DESCRIPTION**	**THEORY**	**DESCRIPTION**
Generativity	Establishes oneself and contributes to society in meaningful ways	Ego differentiation	Begins to define self as separate from work role
v. Stagnation (midlife)	Self is restricted to identification with one's major role (e.g., nurse)	v. Work role preoccupation	Inability to identify as someone outside of a work role
Ego integrity	Attaining a sense of completeness and cohesion of the self	Body transcendence and ego transcendence	Body changes accepted as part of life. Sees oneself as part of a greater whole
v. Despair	A sense that one's self no longer has purpose in life, physically or mentally	v. Body preoccupation and ego preoccupation	Body changes as a source of focus. Sees oneself as an individual needing special attention

Nurses have a unique opportunity to work with multiple approaches to understanding aging. In doing so, they can have an important voice in testing, modifying, and discussing psychosocial theories and frameworks and how they apply to worldwide diversity.

Many questions about late life development remain unanswered. Do biological differences exist between persons of different races and ethnicities, and how does this influence the aging of the human body? How do people change in the later years? What are the effects of epigenetics and are these limited to biology? What is the reason for and purpose of aging? What is the meaning of aging and can this ever be generalized? These are not new questions but they still beg an answer. The answers may be the essence of maturity in later life.

KEY CONCEPTS

- What is meant by the phrase that later life is culturally and socially determined.
- The timing of when one begins to have features that are identified as "old" is significantly affected by one's genetic make-up and environmental stressors experienced over a lifetime.
- There is no longer one exclusive explanation for aging or for adaptation to aging.
- Regardless of the theory, biological aging results in damage within the cell itself, resulting in a decrease in its ability to function or reproduce.
- The increased incidence of many chronic diseases in later life can be explained by biological theories of aging.

- A commonality of the biological theories of aging is the effect of oxidative stress occurring at the cellular level.
- While the psychosocial theories in use today apply to some populations, this applicability is limited by socioeconomic, educational, and cultural factors.
- The third generation of theoretical development related to psychosocial aging, still in the early stages, uses a phenomenological viewpoint to better understand aging regardless of setting or circumstances.

CRITICAL THINKING QUESTIONS AND ACTIVITIES

1. Consider the psychosocial theories of aging and discuss how each would or would not apply to the oldest person with whom you most commonly interact.
2. Identify at least two "older persons" among your family or friends and ask them their own theories of how the body ages. In a classroom discussion, compare their responses to the current state of the science of biological aging.
3. Discuss the meanings and the thoughts triggered by the student's and elder's viewpoints as expressed at the beginning of the chapter. How do these vary from your own experience?
4. Imagine yourself at 90 years old and describe the lifestyle you will have and the factors that you believe account for your long life.
5. Organize a debate in which each individual attempts to convince others of the logic of one particular generation of the psychosocial theories of aging.

RESEARCH QUESTIONS

1. What physical changes can be attributed strictly to the aging of an organism?
2. What environmental factors have the potential to affect longevity?
3. What factors in relationships have the potential to contribute to survival?
4. What are the identifiable factors in extreme longevity?

REFERENCES

Achenbaum WA: *Old age in a new land*, Baltimore, 1978, Johns Hopkins Press.

Borghini A, Cervelli T, Galli A, et al: DNA modifications in atherosclerosis: from the past to the future, *Atherosclerosis* 230(2):202–209, 2013.

Brooks-Wilson AR: Genetics of healthy aging and longevity, *Hum Genet* 132(12): 1323–1338, 2013.

Cefalu CA: Theories and mechanisms of aging, *Clin Geriatr Med* 27:491–506, 2011.

Cottrell L: The adjustment of the individual to his age and sex roles, *Am Sociol Rev* 7:617–620, 1942.

Cowgill D: Aging and modernization: a revision of the theory. In Gubrium J, editor: *Late life communities and environmental policy*, Springfield, IL, 1974, Charles C Thomas.

Cumming E, Henry W: *Growing old*, New York, 1961, Basic Books.

Dato S, Crocco P, D'Aquila P, et al: Exploring the role of genetic variability and lifestyle in oxidative stress response for healthy aging and longevity, *Int J Mol Sci* 14: 16443–16472, 2013.

Dehbi AZ, Radstake TR, Broen JC: Accelerated telomere shortening in rheumatic disease: cause or consequence? *Expert Rev Clin Immunol* 9(12):1193–1204, 2013.

De la Fuente M: Role of neuroimmunomodulation in aging, *Neuroimmunomodulation* 15:213–233, 2008.

Einstein A: *Relativity: the special and the general theory*, New York, 1920, Henry Holt.

Erikson E: *Childhood and society*, 1950. Reprint, New York, 1993, Norton.

Fung HH: Aging in culture, *Gerontologist* 53(3):369–377, 2013.

Goldsmith TC: Arguments against non-programmed theories of aging, *Biochemistry (Mosc)* 78(9):971–978, 2013.

Gomez CR, Nomellini V, Faunce DE, et al: Innate immunity and aging, *Exp Gerontol* 43:718–728, 2008.

Gruber J, Schaffer S, Halliwell B: The mitochondrial free radical theory on ageing—where do we stand? *Front Biosci* 13:6554–6579, 2008.

Grune T, Shringarpure R, Sitte N, et al: Age-related changes in protein oxidation and proteolysis in mammalian cells, *J Gerontol A Biol Sci Med Sci* 56:B459–B467, 2001.

Harman D: Aging: a theory based on free radical and radiation chemistry, *J Gerontol* 11:298–300, 1956.

Havinghurst RJ: *Developmental tasks and education*, New York, 1972, David McKay.

Havinghurst RJ, Albrecht R: *Older people*, New York, 1953, Longmans, Green.

Havinghurst RJ, Neugarten BL, Tobin SS: Disengagement and patterns of aging. In Neugarten BL, editor: *Middle age and aging*, Chicago, 1968, University of Chicago Press.

Hayflick L, Moorhead PS: The serial cultivation of human diploid cell strains, *Exp Cell Res* 25:585–621, 1981.

Hendricks J, Hendricks CD: *Aging in mass society: myths and realities*, Boston, 1986, Little, Brown.

Hooyman NR, Kiyak HA: *Social gerontology: a multidisciplinary approach*, New York, 2011, Allyn & Bacon.

Hornsby PJ: Senescence and life span, *Pflügers Arch* 459:291–299, 2010.

Jang Y, Van Remmen H: The mitochondrial theory of aging: insight from transgenic and knockout mouse models, *Exp Geront* 44:256–260, 2009.

Lagouge M, Larsson NG: The role of mitochondrial DNA mutations and free radicals in disease and aging, *J Int Med* 273:529–543, 2013.

Lin J, Epel E, Blackburn E: Telomeres and lifestyle factors: roles of cellular aging, *Muta Res/Found and Molec Mechanisms Mutagenesis* 730(1–2): 85–91, 2012.

Maddox G: Activity and morale: a longitudinal study of selected elderly subjects, *Soc Forces* 42:195–204, 1963.

Marshall VW: Sociology, psychological and the theoretical legacy of the Kansas City studies, *Gerontologist* 34(4):768–774, 1994.

Maslow A: *Motivation and personality*, New York, 1954, Harper & Row.

Moody HR: From successful aging to conscious aging. In Wykle M, Whitehouse P, Morris D, editors: *Successful aging through the life span*, New York, 2004, Springer, pp 55–68.

Murphy MP: How mitochondria produce reactive oxygen species, *Biochem J* 417: 1–13, 2009.

National Center for Complementary and Alternative Medicine (NCCAM): *Antioxidants and health: an introduction*, 2013. http://nccam.nih.gov/health/antioxidants/introduction.htm. Accessed February 2014.

Neugarten BL: *Middle age and aging*, Chicago, 1968, University of Chicago Press.

Nomellini V, Gomez CR, Kovacs EJ: Aging and impairment of innate immunity, *Contrib Microbiol* 15:188–205, 2008.

Ostojić S, Pereza N, Kapović M: A current genetic and epigenetic view on human aging mechanisms, *Coll Antropol* 33: 687–699, 2009.

Peck R: Psychological developments in the second half of life. In Neugarten B, editor: *Middle age and aging*, Chicago, 1968, University of Chicago Press.

Riley MW: Social gerontology and the age of stratification of society, *Gerontologist* 11:79–87, 1971.

Shammas MA: Telomers, lifestyle, cancer and aging, *Curr Opin Clin Nutr Metab Care* 14(1):28–34, 2011.

Shi Y, Buffenstein R, Pulliam DA, et al: Comparative studies of oxidative stress and mitochondrial function in aging, *Integr Comp Biol* 50(5):869–879, 2010.

Sokolovsky F, editor: *The cultural context of aging: worldwide perspectives*, ed 2, Westpoint, CT, 1997, Plenum Press.

Swain SL, Nikolich-Zugich J: Key research opportunities in immune system aging, *J Gerontol A Biol Sci Med Sci* 64:183–186, 2009.

Tan A: *The Bonesetter's daughter*, New York, 2001, Random House.

Thomas WH: *What are old people for? How elders will save the world*, New York, 2004, VanderWyk & Burnham.

Tornstam L: Gerotranscendence: a meta-theoretical reformulation of the disengagement theory, *Aging: Clin Exper Res* 1:55–64, 1989.

Tornstam L: Transcendence in later life, *Generations* 23:1014, 2000.

Tornstam L: *Gerotranscendence: a developmental theory of positive aging*, New York, 2005, Springer.

Valko W, Morris H, Cronin MT: Metals, toxicity and oxidative stress, *Curr Med Chem* 12:1161–1208, 2005.

Viña J, Borras C, Abdelaziz KM, Garcia-Valles R, et al: The free radical theory of aging revisited, *Antioxid Redox Signal* 19(8): 779–787, 2013.

Wadensten B: An analysis of the psychosocial theories of ageing and their relevance to practical gerontological nursing in Sweden, *Scand J Caring Sci* 20:347–354, 2006.

Wadensten B: The theory of gerotranscendence as applied to gerontological nursing—part 1, *Int J Older People Nurs* 2:289–294, 2007.

Wang CH, Wu SB, Wu YT, et al: Oxidative stress response elicited by mitochondrial dysfunction: implication in the pathophysiology of aging, *Exp Biol Med* 238:450–460, 2013.

World Health Organization: *Global financial crisis and the health of older people*. http://www.who.int/ageing/economic_issues/en/. Accessed February 2014.

4 CHAPTER

Cross-Cultural Caring and Aging

Kathleen Jett

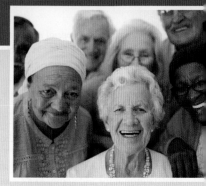

ⓔ http://evolve.elsevier.com/Touhy/TwdHlthAging

A STUDENT SPEAKS

We are trying to do our work with the patient but her daughter keeps getting in the way and keeps saying that it "is not the way we do things." I don't understand, we are just trying to do what we were taught to do.

Sandy, age 20

AN ELDER SPEAKS

It seems like I don't fit in anywhere anymore. My children do their best, but they have to work and my grandchildren don't have the same respect for me that I had for my grandparents. I know they love me but it is just not the same.

Yi Liu, age 87

LEARNING OBJECTIVES

On completion of this chapter, the reader will be able to:
1. Describe the global changes in the aging population.
2. Compare the major paradigms of health and illness.
3. Identify strategies one might take to move toward cultural proficiency in the delivery of cross-cultural care.
4. Accurately identify situations in which expert interpretation is essential.
5. Be prepared to work with interpreters effectively.
6. Formulate a care plan incorporating culturally sensitive interventions.
7. Develop gerontological nursing interventions geared toward reducing health disparities.

CULTURE AND HEALTH CARE

Culture is most often referred to in terms of the shared and learned values, beliefs, expectations, and behaviors of a group of people. Culture guides thinking, decision-making, and beliefs about aging, health and health-seeking, illness, treatment, and prevention (Jett, 2003; Spector, 2012). Cultural values extend into health care delivery any time the "seeker" and "giver" meet. The giver determines the problems that are recognized, the treatments that are appropriate, and the way seekers are expected to respond. In turn, seekers decide if they agree with the problems identified, if they will accept the "prescription," and if they will act on it.

Culture provides directions for individuals as they interact with family and friends within the same group and outside of their group, such as during health care encounters. Culture allows members of the group to predict each other's behavior and respond in ways that are considered appropriate. Cultural beliefs are passed down from one generation to another through *enculturation* and involve the family, the community, and even the political and structural aspects of an environment, such as where they live.

In contrast, *acculturation* is the process by which persons from one culture adapt to another. There has been much concern about aging immigrants and the adjustments needed to find late life satisfaction in their adopted countries. Fung (2013) and Spector (2012) wrote that some aspects of acculturation were more critical to functional adaptation than others. For example, outward adaptations that incorporate language and dress are expressions of cultural identity, but many have less importance than those enculturated at a young age (Fung, 2013). These include attitudes toward aging, health, illness and treatment; use of time; and interactions with others.

This chapter provides an overview of cross-cultural health care and the aging adult. Strategies are provided to help the gerontological nurse respond to the changing face of elders, regardless of their backgrounds, but particularly those with beliefs and values that differ from those of the nurse. The goal of

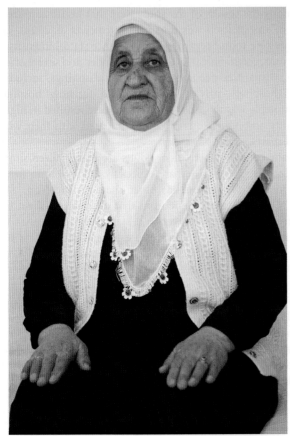

Common attire of Muslim women as expressions of culturally expected modesty. (©iStock.com/Reddiplomat.)

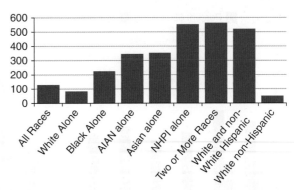

FIGURE 4-1 Projected Percent Increase in Total Number of Persons at Least 65 Years of Age from 2012 to 2060 by Race and Ethnicity. *AIAN*, American Indian/Alaska Native; *NHPI*, Native Hawaiian/Pacific Islander. (Data from U.S. Census: *2012 National population projections*, 2013. http://www.census. gov/population/projections/data/national/2012.html. Accessed March 2014.)

DIVERSITY

Extending the idea of culture is that of *cultural diversity* or simply the existence of more than one group with differing values and perspectives. Morin (2013) describes the extent of diversity in the world, identifying those countries with the least amount of cultural diversity to those with the most. In Argentina, 97% of the citizens are white (of European descent), Roman Catholic, and Spanish is their primary language.

At the other end of the spectrum are many of the countries on the African continent. The 37 different tribal groups in Togo speak 39 different languages and share little in common other than geography. Canada is the only "Western" country in the top 20 in terms of diversity. The United States ranks near the middle, but with considerable changes anticipated in the years to come (Morin, 2013).

Diversity in the United Stated usually refers to the six major ethnoracial groups: African American, Asian American, Native Hawaiian/Pacific Islander, American Indian/Alaskan Native, White (of European descent), and the ethnic group who self-identify as "Hispanic" (regardless of race) (Office of Minority Health [OMH], 2013). Of note: The most accurate use of the term "African American" includes the more than 4 million people who were transported to the United States against their

will between 1619 and 1860 (Spector, 2012). With the exception of those classified as "White," the number of persons who identify with one of these groups is growing rapidly (U.S. Census, 2013). The majority of this growth will occur through immigration, especially among those at 30 years of age in 2010 (U.S. Census, 2014) (Figures 4-1 and 4-2).

In 2010 the United States added experimental questions to its census forms, allowing persons to self-identify with subethnoracial groups such as mixed race, Puerto Rican (Hispanic), or Samoan (Pacific Islanders) (Krogstad and Cohn, 2014; Perez and Hirschman, 2009). This may prove to be very empowering to older adults who are recent immigrants or who still strongly identify with their country of origin.

It is important to note that within any one group, culturally similar or disparate, there is diversity of other kinds, most notably that of gender, power, and status. These factors, in particular, greatly influence the delivery and receipt of health care in many, if not all, places in the world.

HEALTH INEQUITIES AND DISPARITIES

The terms *health inequities* and *health disparities* are often used interchangeably. Although they are somewhat different, both have implications for health care outcomes. Health inequities most often relate to differences as a result of distribution of wealth. One of the most dramatic examples is the 37-year discrepancy in life expectancy between the impoverished nation of Malawi and the high-income country of Japan. It is always important to note that health inequities are not limited to those between countries. In London the life expectancy of men ranges from 88 years of age to 71 years of age, depending on neighborhood, from the most affluent to the least, respectively (World Health Organization [WHO], 2011).

The term *health disparity* refers to differences in health outcomes between groups. It is usually discussed in terms of the excess burden of illness in one group compared with another. Most often the latter hold the majority of the power and influence in a culture including control of the resources, such as health care.

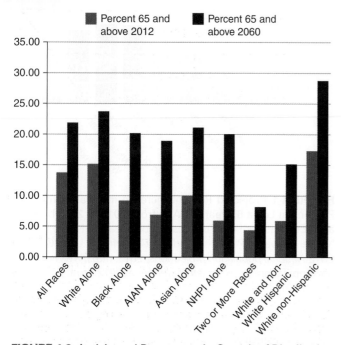

FIGURE 4-2 Anticipated Percentage in Growth of Distribution of Race and Ethnic Groups of Persons 65 and Older in the United States, 2012 to 2060. *AIAN,* American Indian/Alaska Native; *NHPI,* Native Hawaiian/Pacific Islander. (Data from U.S. Census: *2012 National population projections,* 2013. http://www.census.gov/population/projections/data/national/2012.html. Accessed March 2014.)

In 2002 the Institute of Medicine published the landmark report of the state of the science of health disparities in the United States, aptly entitled *Unequal Treatment* (Smedley et al, 2002). Previous research had demonstrated an irrefutable differential in access to health care between white Americans and all others (Box 4-1). Hence, the analysis began with this and researchers were charged with determining the state of care in light of this disparity.

BOX 4-1   The Tuskegee Experiment

Among some older African Americans today there remains mistrust of receiving care from white health care providers, especially those conducting research. This distrust will continue at some level until the memory of the infamous "Tuskegee Experiment" fades. In an effort to study the "natural history of syphilis," nearly 600 black men from Macon County, Mississippi, were recruited in 1932 to participate in a study conducted jointly by the Public Health Service and the Tuskegee Institute. About half of the men had documented syphilis and were told they were being treated for "bad blood," a phrase with several meanings in the U.S. Southern dialect. The men were never treated, even when penicillin became the evidenced-based practice in 1947. While concerns were raised in 1968, the study was not discontinued until 1972 when it was deemed to be unethical for being misleading and failing to inform the subjects of the risks of participation. In 1973 a class action suit was filed, and in 1974 $10 million dollars was provided to the survivors and their surviving families. In 1997 President Clinton apologized on behalf of the nation, and not long afterward strict rules on the conduct of research were created. The last participant died on January 16, 2004. The last widow died on January 27, 2009.

Source: Centers for Disease Control and Prevention. *The Tuskegee timeline,* 2013. http://www.cdc.gov/tuskegee/timeline.htm. Accessed November 2013.

Among the results of the study were that health care treatment in and of itself was unequal (Smedley et al, 2002). The barriers were found regardless of insurance status, intensity of symptoms, geographical location, age, gender, and sexual orientation. Disparities occurred in all clinical settings, including public hospitals, private hospitals, and teaching hospitals. Most notable was that the disparities in care resulted in higher mortality among persons of color compared with their white counterparts.

In any country where older adults are marginalized simply because of their age, they are especially vulnerable to health disparities. If the person has other characteristics (e.g., skin color, religion, sexual orientation) that differentiate them further from those with power and status, the disparities are amplified (Agency for Healthcare Research and Quality [AHRQ], 2013; CDC, 2014; Gushulak and MacPherson, 2006; PAHO/WHO, 2013; WHO, 2008).

In the years since *Unequal Treatment* was published, the U.S. Agency for Healthcare Research and Quality has produced an annual report, the *National Healthcare Quality and National Healthcare Disparities* to track the prevailing trends in health care quality and access for vulnerable populations, including the elderly and those from statistically minority populations. In the past, the comparisons were limited to those primarily between black and white Americans (see Chapter 1). The World Health Organization contributes to this knowledge base by monitoring special needs groups such as migrants, migrant workers, and asylum seekers (Gushulak and MacPherson, 2006).

OBSTACLES TO CROSS-CULTURAL CARING

Providing cross-cultural care does not always mean addressing disparities or inequities, but it does mean overcoming common obstacles. Both overt and covert barriers to care include ethnocentrism and stereotyping, both of which can lead to significant conflict and decreased quality of care. Conflict can occur in the nursing situation any time one person interacts with another whose beliefs, values, customs, languages, and behavior patterns differ from their own (Box 4-2). Gerontological nurses will have to find ways to overcome these obstacles themselves and in their workplaces in order to promote healthy aging.

Ethnocentrism

Both nurses in Box 4-2 denigrated the other's nationality as a proxy for culture. These are examples of what is known as *ethnocentrism,* or the belief that one ethnic/cultural group is superior to that of another. This belief may be acquired through enculturation learned at an early age or acculturation later in life. In Western health care it is expected that seekers adapt to the rules of the givers: to be on time for appointments; to listen and follow the directions that are relayed by their caregivers. In an institutional setting, acculturated elders will accept the type, frequency, and timing of such things as bathing and personal grooming and sleep and rest schedules. The more acculturated an elder is to the culture of the institution and nurse, the less

BOX 4-2 Intercultural Conflicts in Nursing Care

A newly immigrated Korean nurse is instructed to ambulate an 80-year-old male patient. He says that he is tired and wants to remain in bed. The nurse does not insist. The nurse manager reprimands the nurse for not getting the patient out of bed. The Korean nurse says to another Korean nurse: "Those Americans do not respect their elders; they treat them as if they were children." The nurse manager complains to another nurse, "Those Asian nurses allow patients to run all over them." In the traditional Korean culture, elders are revered.

From McHale JP, Dinh KT, Rao N: Understanding co-parenting and family systems among East and Southeast Asian–heritage families. In Selin H, editor: Parenting across cultures: childrearing, motherhood and fatherhood in non-western cultures, Dordrecht, Netherlands, 2014, Springer, pp 163–173.

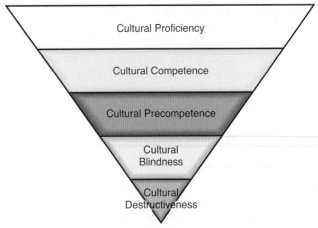

FIGURE 4-3 A Model for Cross-Cultural Caring. (Adapted from Cross T, Bazron B, Dennis K, et al: *Toward a culturally competent system of care*, vol 1, Washington, DC, 1989, CASSP Technical Assistance Center, Center for Child Health and Mental Health Policy, Georgetown University Child Development Center; Goode TD: *Cultural competence continuum*, Washington, DC, revised 2004, National Center for Cultural Competence, Georgetown University Center for Child and Human Development, University Center for Excellence in Developmental Disabilities; and Lindsey R, Robins K, Terrell R: *Cultural proficiency: a manual for school leaders*, Thousand Oaks, CA, 2003, Corwin Press.)

the potential for conflict. The elder will eat the meals provided, even if the food does not look or taste like what he/she is accustomed to eating. A "compliant" non–English-speaking resident will accommodate the staff, with or without the help of an interpreter.

Stereotyping

Stereotyping is the application of limited knowledge of a race, ethnicity, age, or culture to an individual. The nurse may hear or say something about what "old people are like" without getting to know the person as a unique individual and member of a tribe, clan, or family, for example. When stereotypes are used, the identification of the heterogeneity within the group is not recognized. However, the use of some stereotypes can be a helpful starting point in the provision of the fast-paced health care expected today. For example, a common stereotype about Hispanic elders is that they live with a child and grandchildren and that a male in the family is the decision-maker. If the nurse simply assumes this to be true, it could have a negative outcome, such as fewer referrals for support (e.g., home-delivered meals). On the other hand, this stereotype can be used to shortcut the assessment. In discussing discharge plans, the nurse may say, "Are any members of your family available to help you when you get home?" This must be done with utmost tact to avoid the patient from embarrassment if this is not the case.

PROVIDING CROSS-CULTURAL HEALTH CARE

Providing cross-cultural care in a way that challenges ethnocentrism and negative stereotyping is no longer an option; it is an expectation and a necessity as we move to a world community (Bearskin, 2011; The Joint Commission, 2010). It is also a means to an end—of reducing health disparities and inequities experienced by vulnerable populations, among them, many older adults (Kirmayer, 2012). Gerontological nurses can learn to do this more expertly as they move along a continuum from cultural destructiveness to cultural proficiency (Figure 4-3). This requires a willingness to become more self-aware, to learn to know others from their perspectives (i.e., "where they are coming from"), and finally by applying new skills to more effectively work with individuals to support rather than hinder their cultural strengths (Box 4-3).

Cultural Destructiveness

Cultural destructiveness is the systematic elimination of the recognized culture of another. There are many well-known examples of this: the genocide of the Jews in Eastern Europe, of the Hutu in Rwanda, and of many American Indians and African Americans in the United States. In both Australia (WHO, 2008) and the United States cultural destructiveness occurred with the removal of children to boarding schools where the

BOX 4-3 Moving Toward Cultural Proficiency and Healthy Aging

- Become familiar with your own cultural perspectives, including beliefs about disease etiology, treatments, and factors leading to outcomes.
- Examine your personal and professional behavior for signs of bias and the use of negative stereotypes.
- Remain open to viewpoints and behaviors that are different from your expectations.
- Appreciate the inherent worth of all persons from all groups.
- Develop the skill of attending to both nonverbal and verbal communication.
- Develop sensitivity to the clues given by others, indicating the paradigm from which they face health, illness, and aging.
- Learn to negotiate, rather than impose, strategies to promote healthy aging consistent with the beliefs of the persons to whom we provide care.

language, dress, and food of their origins were forbidden (Lewis, 2013). American Indian healing ceremonies, performed by tribal elders, were forbidden. Practices referred to as "traditional" or "folk" healing were and continue to be discounted. Suspiciousness of Western medicine is still present among many African American and American Indians, especially those in their 80s and 90s who may have first- or second-hand knowledge of the cultural destruction to which they and others were subjected (Grandbois et al, 2012).

Cultural Blindness

It is hoped by this point the reader has begun to understand that there are multiple cultures coexisting in countries and continents and that such things as skin color, socioeconomic, political, and educational power affect the health care experience. Yet some people, including health care providers, voice that they see the outward differences such as skin color but that "everyone is the same" and "all old people are grumpy" but are blind to the fact that life experiences such as prejudice and historical trauma may influence both the pursuit and the receipt of health care. It is not possible to provide cross-cultural care or reduce health disparities in the context of cultural destructiveness or cultural blindness unless individual and community health belief paradigms, factors such as poverty and racism, are considered (Feagin and Bennefield, 2014; Williams and Mohammed, 2009). Cultural blindness prevents the nurse from providing sensitive and, more importantly, effective care.

Cultural Precompetence

The development of precompetence begins in the cross-cultural setting with self-awareness of one's personal biases, prejudices, attitudes, and behaviors toward persons different from oneself in age, gender, sexual orientation, social class, economic situations, religious beliefs, and many other factors. For persons whose culture or status places them in a position of power, cultural awareness is realizing that this alone often means special privilege and freedoms (White Privilege Conference, 2014) (Box 4-4). Achieving cultural precompetence requires a willingness to learn how health is

viewed by others. It means playing an active role to combat ageism in society.

Cultural Competence

The nurse who moves beyond precompetence is able to step outside of one's biases and accept that others bring a different set of values, choices, and even priorities to the health care setting. The nurse who is able to provide competent cross-cultural care accepts that all persons are deserving of respect. The nurse has some knowledge of other cultures, particularly those she or he is most likely to encounter in the health care setting. This is especially important when the nurse and the elder are of different ages or have different values, backgrounds, and cultures. The acquisition of cross-cultural knowledge takes place in the classroom, at the bedside, and in the community. Cultural knowledge is both what the nurse brings to the caring situation and what the nurse learns from others (Fung, 2013).

Cultural Knowledge

Cross-cultural knowledge has the potential to optimize health care and minimize frustration and conflict between older patients and other health care providers (Kirmayer, 2012). It is expected that knowledge will allow the nurse to more appropriately and effectively improve health outcomes (Campinha-Bacote, 2011; Kirmayer, 2012). Some nurses prefer to use what can be called an "encyclopedic" approach in learning the details of a *particular* culture group, such as proper name usage, greeting, eye contact, gender roles, foods, and attitudes toward aging.

Although this information is important, it can be combined with conceptual knowledge by coming to know others as whole persons. Instead, basic knowledge of what is *more likely* to be important to someone from a specific culture, such as dietary preference or patterns of interaction, starts the conversation. Providing for choices and then assuring these are met are factors that allow the delivery of competent cross-cultural nursing care (Fung, 2013).

Definitions of terms. Cultural knowledge includes the appropriate use of terms, especially race and ethnicity. Often used interchangeably, each actually has a separate meaning. *Race* is a phenotype as expressed in observable traits, such as eye color, facial structure, hair texture, and especially skin tones. However, at this time it is best used as a proxy for geographical origins and lineage such as Africa, Central Europe, or the Pacific Rim (Gelfand, 2003).

Ethnicity refers to the culture group with which one self-identifies. Persons may share a common nationality, migratory status, language or dialect, religion, or even geographical location (e.g., rural versus urban). Traditions, symbols, literature, folklore, food preferences, and dress are often expressions of ethnicity. Persons from a specific ethnic group may not share a common race. For example, persons who identify themselves as "Hispanic" may be from any race and from a number of countries. However, most Hispanic persons share the Catholic religion and the Spanish language. It is more accurate to ask an elder to self-identify ethnicity rather than make assumptions (Box 4-5).

BOX 4-4 Unrecognized Privilege and Ethnocentrism

A gerontological nurse responded to a call from an older patient's room. While she was with him, he repeatedly, and without comment, dropped his watch on the floor. She calmly picked it up, handed it back to him, and continued talking. One time an aide walked in the room when the patient dropped the watch. The aide picked it up and handed it back to him just as the nurse had done. The patient immediately started yelling and cursing at the aide for attempting to steal his watch. When telling this story, the nurse thought the whole situation odd, but not too remarkable.

The patient and nurse were white and the aide was black. The nurse did not realize that the behavior of the patient was both ethnocentric and culturally destructive until the nurse learned of the concepts while taking a formal class on cross-cultural health care.

Orientation to family and self. A useful concept in cross-cultural health care is orientation to self and family. Many North Americans, especially those of northern European descent, place great value on independence, that is, personal autonomy and individuality (Fung, 2013). Identity is closely bound to oneself. In the classic study, Rathbone-McCune (1982) found that a large group of American elders living in a segregated ("white") senior apartment building went to great lengths and lived with significant discomforts rather than ask for help. To seek or receive help was considered a sign of weakness and dependence, something to be avoided at all costs.

In the United States the cultural expression of autonomy was institutionalized in the passing of the Patient Self-Determination Act of 1990 wherein individuals were recognized as the sole decision-makers regarding their health. Health care providers are now legally bound to restrict access to health care information only to the patient, without the person's explicit permission.

This orientation is in sharp contrast to that of a collectivist or interdependent culture, a norm in many parts of the world. In the Latino culture this is referred to as "Familism" (Lukwago et al, 2001; Scharlach et al, 2006). Self-identity is drawn from family ties (broadly defined) rather than the individual. The "family" (e.g., extended, tribe, clan) is of primary importance; decisions are made by the group or designee based on the needs and beliefs of the group rather than those of the individual (Box 4-6). Within families, the exchange of help and resources is both expected and commonplace. The cultural belief of families is particularly significant for healthy aging because it relates to eldercare and health-related decision-making. When a nurse from a culture in which independent decision-making is expected cares for an elder whose dominant value is interdependence or vice versa, the potential for cultural conflict and poor outcomes is great.

Orientation to time. Orientation to time is often overlooked as a culturally constructed factor influencing the use of health care and the attitudes toward preventive practices (Lukwago et al, 2001). Time orientations are culturally described as future, past, or present (Box 4-7).

Conflicts between the future-oriented Westernized medical care and those with past or present orientations are many. Patients are likely to be labeled as *noncompliant* for failing to keep an appointment or for failing to participate in preventive measures, such as a "turning schedule" for a bed-bound patient to prevent pressure ulcers or immunizations to prevent future infections. Members of present-oriented cultures are often accused by the media of overusing hospital emergency departments in the United States, when in fact it may be considered the only reasonable option available for today's treatment of today's problems.

Regardless of the health and illness orientation of an individual or members of a culture, community, poverty, geography, and a country's infrastructure have significantly confound-

Dress as an expression of ethnicity. (©iStock.com/Bartosz Hadyniak.)

BOX 4-7   Cultural Orientations to Time as Applied to Health Care

A *past orientation* to health and health problems views both as dependent on the actions in the past (such as a past life or earlier in this life) or on events or circumstances of one's ancestors. For example, dishonoring ancestors by failure to perform certain rituals or having poor interactions with others earlier in one's life may result in illness today. Illness today may be considered punishment for past deeds, and it may be prevented by living an honorable life.

A *present orientation* means that when a health care problem occurs, immediate treatment is needed. Future treatment is considered potentially too late for a positive outcome. The success of freestanding "immediate care centers" or those associated with pharmacy chains in the United States may be a reflection of a present orientation. In general, preventive actions for future health are not consistent with a present orientation toward illness and need for treatment.

Future time orientation is consistent with a belief that when one is ill today, a health care appointment can be made for the future (e.g., the "next available" opening). In other words, the health problem and its treatment can "wait." The problem will still be there and the delay will not necessarily affect the outcome. Prevention is important because of its effect on future health days, years, and even decades later, such as weight control.

---

ing effects. In many developing countries, health care may only be available when provided by outside organizations such as Doctors without Borders (www.doctorswithoutboarders.com).

Obtaining health care may mean a walk of many days, and once at the clinic the waiting time to be seen may be hours to days. Such a walk may be impossible for a frail or ill elder. Those living in remote areas, such as those in the state of Montana or the Inuit living near the Arctic, have to wait until the public health nurse and midwife make their next rounds by helicopter. For elders living with chronic diseases this infrequency of contact may be inadequate for even near-optimal outcomes. In such circumstances, older adults are much more dependent on their own resources to deal with illness. Increasing use of technology, such as telemedicine, may decrease some of the disparities between those near health care services and those far away.

In providing cross-cultural care, the nurse can listen closely, determine which orientation has the *most* value to the individual, and find ways to work with it rather than expecting conformity to the cultural model in which the health care is provided. In this way we are reaching out beyond our own perspectives and ethnocentrism to improve the quality of gerontological nursing care.

Beliefs about health, illness, and treatment. The diversity of the population has brought the strong potential for a clash of health belief systems, languages, and attitudes about health and illness in the delivery of care. Aging itself further increases the diversity of beliefs because of the life-long experiences with illness of self, family, and others. The major health belief paradigms are the biomedical, magico-religious, and naturalistic/holistic. The biomedical paradigm is consistent with what is referred to as "Western" medicine (allopathic). The magico-religious paradigm is often referred to as "folk" medicine. Many naturalistic/holistic practices are referred to as "Eastern Medicine" when contrasted to the biomedical model.

Biomedical. The biomedical health paradigm espouses that disease is the result of abnormalities in structure and function of body organs or illness/disease caused by the intrusion of pathogens (e.g., bacteria or a virus) into the body. Clinicians use what is referred to as the *scientific method*, such as quantitative laboratory tests and other procedures, to make a diagnosis. Treatment involves repairing the abnormality, destroying the pathogen, or at least ameliorating the damage caused by its presence. Surgery, medications, and rehabilitation programs are typical treatments. Health is viewed as the absence of illness or abnormalities. Biomedical care is considered highly impersonal because the focus is on the abnormality and disease rather than on the person. Preventive strategies are those in which pathogens, chemicals, activities, and dietary agents known to cause malfunction are avoided. Screenings, as described in Chapters 1 and 30, are those activities that identify the disease in an early stage and are consistent with this paradigm.

Magico-religious. In the magico-religious health belief paradigm, illness is believed to be caused by the actions of a higher power, a supernatural force such as God, ghosts, ancestors, or evil spirits (Winkelman, 1990). This belief system can be traced back thousands of years to ancient Egypt and persists in whole or in part in many groups. Health is viewed as a blessing or reward and illness as a punishment for breaking a rule or taboo or displeasing or failing to please the source of power. Beliefs that illness and disease are attributed to the

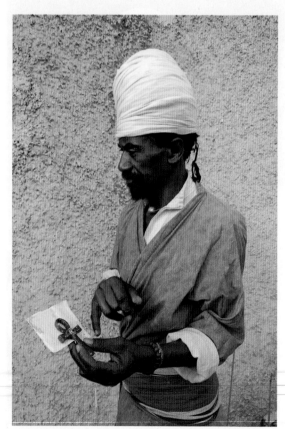

The "ankh" is sometimes used in healing practices. (©iStock.com/tapuzina.)

wrath of the higher power are prevalent among members of many groups, including the Holiness, Pentecostal, and Fundamentalist Baptist churches in the United States. Examples of magical causes of illness are voodoo, especially among persons from the Caribbean; root work among southern African Americans; hexing among Mexican Americans and African Americans; and Gaba among Filipino Americans. Magico-religious healing is often in the form of rituals lead by culturally trained and appointed persons such as Faith Healers, Shaman, or Curanderos.

Treatments may consist of, or include, religious practices such as meditating, fasting, wearing amulets, burning candles, "laying of hands" and prayer circles, or establishing family altars. Such practices may be used both curatively and preventively. Another preventive strategy is to ensure that one maintains good relationships with others (Samovar et al, 2010).

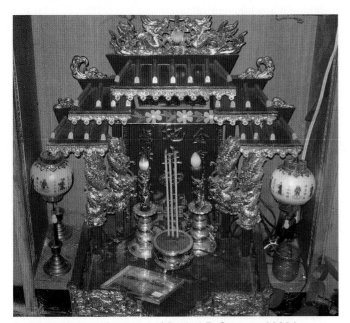

Buddhist shrine. (Courtesy of Rachel E. Spector, 2006.)

Significant conflict with Western-trained nurses can occur when a patient refuses biomedical treatments because to do so is viewed as a sign of disrespecting ancestors or challenging "God's will." Most of us adhere to magico-religious practices to some extent. How many nurses and their patients have prayed to a higher power that health be restored or maintained? It is not uncommon to hear an older adult pray for a cure or to lament "What did I do to cause this?" or "God please help me."

Naturalistic or holistic. The naturalistic or holistic health belief system is based on the concept of balance. Many people throughout the world view health as a sign of balance—of the right amount of exercise, food, sleep, evacuation, interpersonal relationships, or geophysical and metaphysical forces in the universe, such as Qi in the Chinese culture.

The ancient health practice based on the concept of Yin-Yang stems from the ancient civilizations of China, India, and Greece (Young and Koopsen, 2005). Health is viewed as a state of balance. The balance is between the Yin and the Yang, dark and light, male and female. Disturbances in this balance result in disharmony and subsequent illness. Diagnosis requires the determination of the type of imbalance and treatment requires a specific strategy to restore balance. Treatments include the use of herbs, acupuncture, acupressure, controlled deep-breathing exercises, and lifestyle changes as appropriate. When one is in balance there is the serenity of inner and outer peace.

Another naturalistic approach is based on a balance between hot and cold. It is a common paradigm throughout the world, especially in the Latino culture. Illness is classified as either hot or cold and believed to be the result of an imbalance between the two. Diagnosis is the determination of the cause of the imbalance (e.g., too much cold) and treatment is usually through countering this with a substance with the opposite properties (e.g., something hot) (Ortiz et al, 2007).

Ayurveda is the oldest known medical paradigm in the naturalistic system, practiced in India and many other countries. Like others in this category, health is in terms of balance of key elements. In this case the major foci are earth, wind, water, and air. Illness is the result of imbalance. However, both diagnosis and selection of appropriate treatments are very complex. Health promotion and disease prevention are key aspects in the lives of those who practice Ayurveda; other strategies to maintain health and live a long life include good hygiene, yoga, and meditation (National Center for Complementary and Alternative Medicine [NCCAM], 2013).

Cultural Proficiency

In order to provide the best care to all persons regardless of race, ethnicity, or culture, it is now expected that the nurse not only demonstrate cultural competence but also strive for cultural proficiency—which is at a higher level of expertise (Figure 4-3). The culturally proficient nurse is able to move smoothly between two worlds for the promotion of health and the care of persons. Culturally proficient health care is that which is respectful, compassionate, and relevant. Cultural proficiency includes putting cultural knowledge to use in assessment, communication, negotiation, and intervention.

It includes the recognition of factors beyond culture, such as the effect of past and current trauma, social status, and poverty leading to health disparities and inequities. The nurse providing proficient cross-cultural health care is able to work with, and build relationships with, members from a variety of cultural groups as a natural part of daily practice. The relationship building results in the ability to communicate effectively, sensitively assess the individual's state of health, formulate mutually acceptable goals, and support interventions that are culturally acceptable and empowering.

Cultural Skills: Communication

Communication and language are foundational skills and intimately tied to the concept of the self. The self is continuously constructed and inextricably intertwined with the linguistic categories available in a given culture (Berman, 1991). We can conceive of ourselves only within the language we know. Promoting healthy aging and providing the highest quality of cross-cultural care for elders require not only awareness and knowledge but also the ability to communicate in new and expert ways. In doing so, the self-esteem of the elder is enhanced and health-related quality of life is increased to the extent possible (Kirmayer, 2012).

Communication means listening carefully to the person, especially for his or her perception of the situation, and attending not just to the words but also to nonverbal expressions and the meaning behind both of these. It includes attention to idiom, style, jargon, voice tone, inflection, and body language to make each contact meaningful. Communication begins long before a word is spoken. In many cultures the unspoken message may be as, or more important than, what is said.

The application of cross-cultural communication skills plays an essential part in assessment, in relationship and trust building, and in the development of the plan of care. In caring in the cross-cultural setting the gerontological nurse must have expert communication skills, and without these, only less than optimal outcomes can be achieved.

The handshake. A handshake is the customary and expected greeting in most of North America. A firm handshake is thought to be a sign of good character and strength. Yet this is not always the case and the types of acceptable physical contact vary widely. In a number of East Asian cultures the handshake is used in the business setting, but it is expected to be slight and accompanied by a bow (eDiplomat, 2014). Traditional American Indian elders may interpret firm or vigorous handshakes as signs of aggression. Their handshake may instead be more of a passing of the hand with a light touch as a sign of respect rather than of weakness. In the Muslim culture, cross-gender physical contact (including handshakes) may be considered highly inappropriate or even forbidden. Before the nurse makes physical contact with an elder of any culture, he or she should ask the person's permission or follow his or her lead, such as an outstretched hand.

Eye contact. Eye contact is another highly culturally constructed behavior. In some cultures direct eye contact is believed to be a sign of honesty and trustworthiness. Nursing students in the United States are taught to establish and maintain eye contact when interacting with patients, but this behavior may be misinterpreted by persons from elsewhere. Some persons avoid eye contact, not as a sign of deceit, but as a sign of respect. A more traditional American Indian elder may not allow the nurse to make eye contact, moving his or her eyes slowly from the floor to the ceiling and around the room. During a health care encounter, in most Asian cultures, direct eye contact is considered disrespectful (eDiplomat, 2014). Looking one directly in the eye implies equality. Older adults may avoid eye contact with physicians and nurses if health professionals are viewed as authority figures. In other cultures, direct eye contact between men and women is considered a sexual advance. The gerontological nurse can follow the lead of the elder by being open to eye contact but neither forcing it nor assigning it any inherent value.

The use of silence. The value, use, and interpretation of silence also vary markedly from one culture to another. In many Eastern cultures, especially those in which the Confucian philosophy is embraced, silence is highly valued. It is expected of young family members and family members with less authority. Silence may be considered a sign of respect for the wisdom of an elder. In traditional Japanese and Chinese families, silence during a conversation may indicate the speaker is giving the listener time to ponder what has been said before moving on to another idea. In traditional American Indian cultures, it is believed that one learns self-control, courage, patience, and dignity from remaining silent. Silence during a conversation may signify that the listener is reflecting on what the speaker has just verbalized. In contrast, Western cultures place much importance on verbal communication. French, Spanish, and older adult immigrants from the former Soviet Union may interpret silence as a sign of agreement (Purnell and Paulanka, 2003; Tripp-Reimer and Lauer, 1987).

Spoken communication. If the nurse and the elder share the same spoken language, communication is facilitated, although attention to cross-cultural factors is not precluded, such as the appropriate use of specific words and phrases. In health care, recognition of this is especially important such as in the appropriateness of directions (e.g., related to assessment techniques), requests, and instructions (Box 4-8).

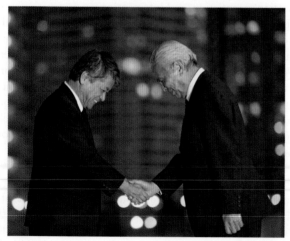

The bow is a gesture of respect in many East Asian cultures and religions. (©iStock.com/stockstudioX.)

BOX 4-8   When a Professional Interpreter Is Needed

An interpreter is needed any time the nurse and the elder speak different languages, when the elder has limited proficiency in the language used in the health care setting, or when cultural tradition prevents the elder from speaking directly to the nurse. The more complex the decision-making, the more important are the interpreter and his or her skills. These circumstances are many, such as when discussions are needed about the treatment plan for a new condition, the options for treatment, advanced care planning, or even preparation for care after discharge from a health care institution. The use of a specially trained interpreter is essential in the setting of lowered levels of health literacy.

Interpretation and translation are needed when different languages are spoken. *Interpretation* is the processing of one **spoken** language into another in a manner that preserves the meaning and tone of the original language without adding or deleting anything. The job of the interpreter is to work with two different linguistic codes in a way that will produce equivalent messages, that is, without adding meaning or opinion (Haffner, 1992).

It is ideal to engage those who are trained in medical interpretation who are adults and of the same culture and gender (Box 4-9). Unfortunately, too often children or even grandchildren are called on to fulfill this role. When they are not available, secretaries or housekeepers may be asked to interpret. When depending on these interpreters, the nurse must realize that either the interpreter or the elder may "edit" his or her comments because of cultural restrictions about the content, that is, what is or is not appropriate to speak about to, or in front of, a parent, child, or stranger. Regardless of who is available to assist, there are guidelines available to maximize the quality and acceptability of the communication (Box 4-10). When there are no other reasonable options, "interpreter lines" via the phone or computer are used. Again, the nurse must expect that the information obtained is limited at best and that misunderstandings are likely.

Translation is the exchange of one **written** language for another, such as in the translation of patient education materials.

BOX 4-9 Cross-Cultural Health Care

A Haitian woman about 70 years old came to the clinic where I was working, complaining of vaginal itching. I explained that I needed to examine her before I would be able to treat her correctly. When I started to step out of the room after the examination so that she could re-dress, she smiled and said (through and interpreter), "No need for that, you just saw where only my mother and God ever saw, you might as well stay."

Kathleen

BOX 4-10 Guidelines for Working with Interpreters

- Before an interview or session with a client, meet with the interpreter to:
  - Explain the purpose of the session.
  - Instruct the interpreter to use the person's own words and avoid paraphrasing.
  - Instruct the interpreter to avoid inserting his or her own ideas or omitting any information.
- Look and speak directly to the client, not the interpreter.
- Be patient. Interpreted interviews take more time because of the need for three-way communication.
- Use short units of speech. Long, involved sentences or complex discussions create confusion.
- Use simple language. Avoid technical terms, professional jargon, slang, abbreviations, abstractions, metaphors, and idiomatic expressions.
- Listen to the client and watch nonverbal communication (facial expression, voice intonation, body movement) to learn about emotions regarding a specific topic.
- Clarify the client's understanding and the accuracy of the interpretation by asking the client to tell you in his or her own words what he or she understands, facilitated by the interpreter.

Modified from Lipson JG, Dibble SL, Minarik PA, editors: Culture and nursing care: a pocket guide, San Francisco, 1996, UCSF School of Nursing Press.

It is recommended that a "back translation" is done for accuracy. This is to first translate the material into the language needed and then translate it back to the original language in which it was written to ensure accuracy. There are many patient education materials in multiple languages available on the websites www.cdc.gov and www.ahrq.gov.

◆ PROMOTING HEALTHY AGING: IMPLICATIONS FOR GERONTOLOGICAL NURSING

To provide proficient cross-cultural care, one must enter into an unknown conceptual world in which time, space, religion, tradition, and wellness are expressed through a unique language that conveys the perceived nature of the health, illness, and humanity. It requires sensitive and effective assessment, mutual goal setting, and acceptable interventions that are possible within the limitations of available resources.

◆ Assessment

A number of "cultural assessment" tools have been created to detail an individual's beliefs and practices in very specific and comprehensive ways, especially that of Leininger's Sunshine Model (Reynolds and Leininger, 1993), Giger and Davidhizer's Transcultural Assessment Model (2002), and Spector's Heritage Assessment Tool (Spector, 2012). However, adding one of the larger tools, such as that of Leininger, to the already inherently complex and lengthy assessments required in working with aging adults may be too burdensome for all involved. The Explanatory Model can serve as a guide to assessment questions that have helped nurses and other health care professionals obtain relevant assessment information in a culturally sensitive manner (Kleinman et al, 1978; Pfeifferling, 1981) (see Chapter 7, Box 7-3).

The assessment should include a discussion of which of the overall health belief paradigms are most meaningful to the individual. Some ascribe to only one, but many find parts of them or some of the practices of one or the other to have meaning to them.

◆ Interventions
◆ The On Lok Program

The most well-known model for the provision of gerontological cross-cultural care in the United States is the On Lok Program of All-inclusive Care for the Elderly (PACE) in San Francisco. It has long been recognized for its cultural relativism. Originally designed to meet the home care needs of Chinese and Italian immigrants, it is now structured to meet the needs of seniors at every level of care from senior housing to long-term care (www.onlok.org). Services are provided in the language of the elder and in a manner that optimizes each person's cultural heritage (Lehning and Austin, 2011). Nurses can learn from the work of On Lok and other programs to promote wellness and healthy aging and to help reduce health disparities and inequities. It is suggested that modifications of existing long-term care services that enhance the well-being of aging persons regardless of their race, ethnicity, or culture should include the following:

1. Ensure that the individual has access to a professional interpreter if needed.

2. Develop programs that reflect the diversity of the participants or residents.
3. Consider monocultural facilities or units when population demographics warrant this.
4. Employ staff who reflect the diversity of residents/clients/patients.

◆ The LEARN Model

Regardless of the assessment model chosen, this information must be operationalized into a plan of care that addresses the special needs of the person and is realistic and consistent with the person's cultural patterns and beliefs. The LEARN model (Berlin and Fowkes, 1983) is a simple and highly effective model and can be used not only in the cross-cultural encounter but also any time the nurse wants to increase the probability that the highest level of wellness is achieved.

The LEARN Model is a negotiated plan of care and includes the identification of the availability of culturally appropriate and sensitive community resources (Box 4-11). It is likely to include the identification of others who will be part of the care team, such as indigenous healers, priests, monks, rabbis, or ministers, if their presence is desired or believed to be helpful.

Through the skilled use of this simple model gerontological nurses can provide culturally sensitive care regardless of setting. When caring for persons from marginalized groups, including many older adults, using the model has the potential to reduce health disparities and increase health equity.

INTEGRATING CONCEPTS

Promoting cross-cultural healthy aging provides the gerontological nurse with new challenges and the opportunity to learn from new perspectives. Unfortunately, poverty is very common in many households of persons who are not of the dominant culture in a country. Meeting basic needs, especially food and health care, may be difficult. Some elders immigrated to the United States or other adopted countries much earlier in their lives and their moves were not traumatic. Others have experienced horrific events in their home country or during their immigration process and hold a

unique concern for safety and security. The nurse must be sensitive to this possibility without making assumptions or stereotyping. The nurse can assess the components of biological integrity and, if necessary, facilitate the elder or family obtaining support services (e.g., food stamps, home-delivered meals) that are possible and appropriate.

Cultural identity is one of the major elements of self-concept and a key to self-esteem, increasingly so as a person ages or becomes more mentally or physically frail (Fung, 2013). Older adults may be closely tied to family and community and, in some cases, religious beliefs. Estrangement from their country of origin may be ameliorated if they live in homogeneous communities and may be exacerbated if they live in social isolation or away from persons with similar backgrounds. The monoethnic community (e.g., barrio, Nihonmachi, Chinatown) serves as a buffer and a means of strengthening cohesiveness for elders from similar cultural groups. Within the community, elders are protected from discrimination and the language and customs of the society outside.

Familial supports are variable among groups, social classes, and subcultures, yet the nuclear or extended family is the chief avenue of transmitting cultural values, beliefs, customs, and practices. The family may provide stability and sanctuary. Making the broadest of generalizations, we may say that persons from Asian cultures value familial piety and respect for elders (McHale et al, 2014); Hispanics treasure large, extended networks (*compadres* translates to *co-parents*, usually the appointed godparents) and church affiliations; African Americans embrace extended families or fictive kin supports; and American Indians value a system of kinship and line of descent. Independent decision-making and self-care is a common characteristic of those of northern European descent.

Spirituality or religiosity plays a major role in defining many cultures. Religion may function as a consistent experience that affords psychic support in the individual's life. The *Issei* seek religious tradition in the face of aging and death (Kitano, 1969). Padilla and Ruiz (1976) noted that Hispanics sought Spanish-speaking clergy rather than mental health professionals when they had emotional problems.

Changes are threatening the historical role of aging in families across the globe. Different degrees of assimilation between generations create a communication gap between the young and older immigrants, as they join their families in new countries where the language and customs may be unknown to them. This may cause isolation and estrangement between the oldest and youngest generations. Enculturated and acculturated expectations may clash (see any of the books by author Amy Tan). In marginalized groups of elders, illness, poverty, and migration are destroying the insulation previously afforded by the family and community (Jett, 2006) (Box 4-12). Members of minorities in any community are extremely vulnerable as they age. They may experience triple jeopardy when devalued because of age, race, and ethnicity.

The study of aging is one of the most complex and intriguing opportunities of our day. Realistically, it will be almost impossible to become familiar with the whole range of clinically relevant cultural differences of older adults one may encounter.

BOX 4-11 LEARN Model

L Listen carefully to what the person is saying. Attend not just to the words but to the nonverbal communication and the meaning behind them. Listen to the perception of the person's situation, desired goals, and ideas for treatment.

E Explain your perception of the situation and the problems.

A Acknowledge and discuss both the similarities and the differences between your perceptions and goals and those of the elder and their significant other/decision-makers as appropriate.

R Recommend a plan of action that takes both perspectives into account.

N Negotiate a plan that is mutually acceptable and possible.

Adapted from Berlin E, Fowkes W: A teaching framework for cross-cultural health care: application in family practice, *West J Med* 139: 934–938, 1983.

From Jett KF: Mind-loss in the African American community: dementia as a normal part of aging, *J Aging Studies* 20(1):1–10, 2006.

BOX 4-13   A Cross-Cultural Caring Encounter

Determine the following about the elder:
- Preferred cultural, ethnic, and racial identity
- Expectations concerning formality of the encounter
- Expectations concerning use of names, titles, addressing the patient and the nurse
- Preferred language
- Level of health and reading literacy and availability of assistance if needed
- Past personal experience with the Western health care model
- Level of acculturation, adherence to traditional approaches, openness to new approaches
- Factors influencing decision-making: who, how, when, what

 BOX 4-14   HEALTHY PEOPLE 2020

Key Overarching Goals

- Achieve health equity, eliminate disparities, and improve the health of all groups.
- Create social and physical environments that promote good health for all.

Data from U.S. Department of Health and Human Services: *Healthy People 2020*. http://healthypeople.gov/2020/about/default.aspx. Accessed May 2014.

Attempting to provide care holistically and sensitively is the most challenging opportunity leading to personal growth for both the nurse and the person receiving care.

Today's nurse is expected to provide culturally proficient care to persons regardless of their age, health beliefs, experiences, values, and styles of communication (Box 4-13). Cross-cultural communication is especially important because of the inherent complexity of health while aging and the combination of generational and cultural differences between the person and the nurse. The nurse will need to communicate effectively with persons regardless of the languages spoken. In doing so, the nurse may depend on limited verbal exchanges and attend more to facial and body expressions, postures, and gestures and know how to work with the many aspects of communication. Effective gerontological nurses provide cross-cultural care through the application of cultural knowledge and skills needed to optimize intercultural communication.

To skillfully assess and intervene, nurses must develop cultural proficiency through awareness of their own ethnocentricities. They must be acutely sensitive to the cues suggested (e.g., eye contact) to know how best to respond. Promoting healthy aging in cross-cultural settings includes the ability to develop a plan of action that considers the perspective of both the elder/family and the nurse/health care system to negotiate an outcome that is mutually acceptable. Skillful cross-cultural nursing means developing a sense of mutual respect between the nurse and the elder. A sense of caring is conveyed in gestures of personal recognition. It is working "with" the person rather than "on" the person; and in doing so, health disparities and inequities, if they exist, can begin to be reduced and movement toward healthy aging can be facilitated (Box 4-14). Unbiased caring can surmount cultural differences.

█ KEY CONCEPTS

- Global population diversity is rapidly increasing and will continue to do so for many years. This suggests that nurses will be caring for a greater number of elders from a broader number of cultural backgrounds than they have in the past.
- Recent research has shown that significant disparities and inequities in the outcomes of health care persist. Those who bear the greatest burden of morbidity and mortality are those who are the most marginalized from those in control of health care resources.
- Nurses can contribute to the reduction of health disparities and the promotion of social justice by increasing their own cultural awareness, knowledge, and skills.
- Cultural proficiency and sensitivity require awareness of issues related to culture, race, social class, and economic situations.
- Ethnicity is a complex phenomenon of self-identity expressed as language, dress, traditions, symbols, and folklore.

- Stereotyping can negate the fact that significant heterogeneity exists within cultural groups.
- Health beliefs of various groups emerge from three general belief systems: biomedical (allopathic), magico-religious, and naturalistic. Elders may adhere to one or more of these systems.
- Effective cross-cultural care to elders includes skills related to both verbal and nonverbal communication.
- The more complex the decision-making, the more important the quality of communication. For those with limited English proficiency, expert interpretation is needed whenever serious decisions are needed (e.g., end-of-life care or treatment changes).
- The use of family, children, or support staff as interpreters is not recommended and may result in censored interpretation because of rules of cultural etiquette that may be unknown to the nurse.
- The LEARN model provides a useful framework for working to reach mutually agreeable and possible health care goals.

NURSING STUDY: WHERE DO I BELONG? WHO AM I?

Georgia thought she was a misfit. She had always thought this. She was born in China in 1920 where her parents had built and managed a school for orphaned children in Shanghai. When she was 15 the family returned to the United States and moved to an Appalachian mining village to manage a small school and clinic. Having grown to adolescence in China, she felt more Chinese than English. She had a difficult adjustment in the poverty-stricken rural mining village in Appalachia, so different from Shanghai. In a few years, her parents sent her to a private religious college, attended mainly by the children of the affluent elders of her church. She married a young army officer, and they were immediately sent to France. Her life from then on seemed to consist of nothing but moves as she followed her husband. She was grateful that she had never had children, as she said, "My life has always seemed so unsettled, I don't think I could have provided any stability for children." When she was widowed at 80, she almost immediately entered a nursing home. There, she found that most of the staff were Filipino and talked among themselves in Tagalog. Again, she felt disconnected with the prevailing culture in which she found herself. She became very difficult to get along with, and the staff members were at their wits' end trying to please her. You recently went to work as director of nursing in the facility. How will you help her and the staff maximize life satisfaction?

On the basis of this nursing study, propose:

- How best to reach out to Georgia and attempt to understand the story behind her current behavior.
- A method to work with Georgia to develop a plan of care that meets both her physical and her psychological needs.
- A means of working with the staff to facilitate optimizing Georgia's life satisfaction while minimizing the demands on their already heavy workload.

CRITICAL THINKING QUESTIONS AND ACTIVITIES

1. Define the terms *culture, ethnicity, ethnocentricity,* and *cultural proficiency.*
2. Identify several personal values or beliefs that are derived from your ethnic roots.
3. Relate major historical events that have affected you and your birth cohort, and explain in what way your cohort has been affected.
4. Privately list your stereotypes and "ethnocentrisms" for various ethnoracial cultural groups, and explore the basis of these beliefs (e.g., taught, fear, experience, lack of knowledge). Then consider what you can do to address these stereotypes.
5. Select a food or particular behavior and examine differences in custom that arise from ethnic/cultural interpretations.
6. Describe the advocacy role of nurses to reduce health disparities.
7. What are the primary difficulties in providing nursing care for individuals from a different background from one's own?

RESEARCH QUESTIONS

1. What are the factors that identify a group as an ethnic minority?
2. What are the enduring cohort differences that are unlikely to change throughout life?
3. What are the outcomes of an integrated cultural approach versus a separate-course approach in a curriculum?
4. What effect will the baby boomers have on gender parity or disparity?

REFERENCES

Agency for Healthcare Research Quality (AHRQ): *2012 National healthcare disparities report*, 2013. http://www.ahrq.gov/research/findings/nhqrdr/nhdr12/chap10.html. Accessed May 2014.

Bearskin RLB: A critical lens on culture in nursing practice, *Nurs Ethics* 18(4): 548–559, 2011.

Berlin E, Fowkes W: A teaching framework for cross-cultural health care: application in family practice, *West J Med* 139:934–938, 1983.

Berman HJ: From the pages of my life, *Generations* 15:33–40, 1991.

Campinha-Bacote J: Delivering patient-centered care in the midst of a cultural conflict: the role of cultural competence, *Online J Nurs Issues* 16(2):5, 2011.

Centers for Disease Control and Prevention (CDC): *Minority health*, 2014. http://www.cdc.gov/minorityhealth/. Accessed May 2014.

eDiplomat: *Japan*, 2014. http://www.ediplomat.com/np/cultural_etiquette/ce_jp.htm. Accessed April 2014.

Feagin J, Bennefield Z: Systematic racism in U.S. healthcare, *Soc Sci Med* 103:7–14, 2014.

Fung HH: Aging in culture, *Gerontologist* 53(3):369–377, 2013.

Gelfand D: *Aging and ethnicity: knowledge and service*, ed 2, New York, 2003, Springer.

Giger JN, Davidhizer R: The Giger and Davidzar transcultural assessment model, *J Transcult Nurs* 13(3):185–188, 2002.

Grandbois DM, Warne D, Eschiti V: The impact of history and culture on nursing care of Native American elders, *J Geron Nurs* 38(10):3–5, 2012.

Gushulak BD, MacPherson DW: The basic principles of migration health: population mobility and gaps in disease prevalence, *Emerg Themes Epidemiol* 3:1–11, 2006.

Haffner L: Translation is not enough. Interpreting in a medical setting, *West J Med* 157:255–259, 1992.

Jett KF: Making the connection: seeking and receiving help by elderly African Americans, *Qual Health Res* 12:373–387, 2002.

Jett KF: The meaning of aging and the celebration of years among rural African American women, *Geriatr Nurs* 24:290–293, 2003.

Kirmayer LJ: Rethinking cultural competence, *Transcult Psychiatry* 49(2):149–164, 2012.

Kitano H: *Japanese Americans*, Englewood Cliffs, NJ, 1969, Prentice-Hall.

Kleinman A, Eisenberg L, Good B: Culture, illness, and care: clinical lessons from anthropologic and cross-cultural research, *Ann Intern Med* 88:251–258, 1978.

Krogstad JM, Cohn D'V: *U.S. census looking at big changes in how it asks about race and ethnicity*, Pew Research Center, Mar 14, 2014. http://www.pewresearch. org/fact-tank/2014/03/14/u-s-census-looking-at-big-changes-in-how-it-asks-about-race-and-ethnicity. Accessed March 2014.

Lehning AJ, Austin MJ: On Lok: a pioneering long-term care organization for the elderly (1971-2008), *J Evid Based Soc Work* 8(1–2):218–234, 2011.

Lewis JP: The importance of optimism in maintaining healthy aging in rural Alaska, *Qual Health Res* 23(11):1521–1527, 2013.

Lukwago S, Kreuter MW, Bucholtz DC, et al: Development and validation of brief scales to measure collectivism, religiosity, racial pride, and time orientation in urban African American women, *Fam Community Health* 24:63–71, 2001.

McHale JP, Dinh KT, Rao N: Understanding co-parenting and family systems among East and Southeast Asian–heritage families, In Selin H, editor: *Parenting across cultures: childrearing, motherhood and fatherhood in non-western cultures*, Dordrecht, Netherlands, 2014, Springer, pp 163–173.

Morin R: *The most (and least) culturally diverse countries in the world*, Pew Research Center, July 18, 2013. http://www. pewresearch.org/fact-tank/2013/07/18/the-most-and-least-culturally-diverse-countries-in-the-world/. Accessed March 2014.

National Center for Complementary and Alternative Medicine (NCCAM): *Ayurvedic medicine: Get the facts*, 2013. http://nccam.nih.gov/health/ayurveda/introduction.htm. Accessed April 2014.

Office of Minority Health (OMH): *About OMH*, 2013. http://minorityhealth.hhs. gov/. Accessed May 2014.

Ortiz BI, Shields KM, Clauson KA, et al: Complementary and alternative medicine use among Hispanics in the United States, *Ann Pharmacol* 41(6):994–1004, 2007.

Padilla A, Ruiz R: Prejudice and discrimination. In Hernandez CA, Haug MJ, Wagner NN, editors: *Chicanos: social and psychological perspectives*, ed 2, St. Louis, 1976, Mosby.

Pam American Health Organization (PAHO)/World Health Organization (WHO): *Addressing the causes of disparities in health service and utilization for lesbian, gay, bisexual and trans (LGBT) persons* (WHO ref. no. CD52/18), 2013. http://www.who.int/hiv/pub/populations/lgbt_paper/en. Accessed April 2014.

Perez AD, Hirschman C: The changing racial and ethnic composition of the US population: emerging American identities, *Popul Dev Rev* 35(1):1–51, 2009.

Pfeifferling JH: A cultural prescription for mediocentrism. In Eisenberg L, Kleinman A, editors: *The relevance of social science for medicine*, Boston, 1981, Reidel.

Purnell LD, Paulanka BJ: *Transcultural health care: a culturally competent approach*, ed 2, Philadelphia, 2003, F.A. Davis.

Rathbone-McCune E: *Isolated elders: health and social intervention*, Rockville, MD, 1982, Aspen.

Reynolds CL, Leininger MM: *Madeleine Leininger: cultural care diversity and universality theory*, Newbury Park, CA, 1993, Sage.

Samovar LA, Porter RE, McDaniel ER: *Communicating between cultures*, Boston, 2010, Wadsworth.

Scharlach AE, Kellam R, Ong N, et al: Cultural attitudes and caregiver service use: lessons from focus groups with racially and ethnically diverse family caregivers, *J Gerontol Soc Work* 47:133–156, 2006.

Smedley B, Stith AY, Nelson AR, editors: *Unequal treatment: confronting racial and ethnic disparities in health care*, Washington, DC, 2002, National Academy Press.

Spector RE: *Cultural diversity in health and illness*, ed 8, Upper Saddle River, NJ, 2012, Prentice-Hall Health.

The Joint Commission: *Advancing effective communication, cultural competence and patient and family centered care: a roadmap for hospitals*, Oakbrook, IL, 2010, The Joint Commission. http://www. jointcommission.org. Accessed May 2014.

Tripp-Reimer T, Lauer GM: Ethnicity and families with chronic illness. In Wright LM, Leahy M, editors: *Families and chronic illness*, Springhouse, PA, 1987, Springhouse.

U.S. Census: *2012 National population projections*, 2014. http://www.census.gov/population/projections/data/national/2012.html. Accessed March 2014.

White Privilege Conference: *What is white privilege?* 2014. http://www.whiteprivilegeconference.com/white_privilege. html. Accessed May 2014.

Williams DR, Mohammed SA: Discrimination and racial disparities in health: evidence and needed research, *J Behavioral Med* 32(1):20–47, 2009.

Winkelman MJ: Shaman and other "magicoreligious" healers: a cross-cultural study of their origins, nature and social transformations, *Ethos* 18:308–352, 1990.

World Health Organization (WHO): Australia's disturbing health disparities set Aboriginals apart, *Bull World Health Org* 86(4):241–320, 2008.

World Health Organization (WHO): *10 facts on health inequities and their causes*, 2011. http://www.who.int/features/factfiles/health_inequities/en/. Accessed April 2014.

Young C, Koopsen C: *Spirituality, health and healing*, Sudbury, MA, 2005, Jones & Bartlett.

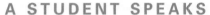
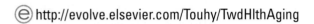

Cognition and Learning

Theris A. Touhy

ⓔ http://evolve.elsevier.com/Touhy/TwdHlthAging

A STUDENT SPEAKS

I was shocked the other day when I got a message on my Facebook page from my grandmother. I had no idea that older people even knew about Facebook but my Gram says she has 30 friends and has reconnected with some of her classmates from high school. She's been pretty lonely since Grandpa died and I wouldn't be surprised if she finds her old boyfriend next. Older people can be pretty cool.

Kate, age 19

AN ELDER SPEAKS

Imagine, they tell us now that our brain continues to develop even though we are older. I thought it was all downhill to dementia when I turned 70. My nurse practitioner advised me to get involved in some activities for stimulating my brain and improving my memory. I found a free class at the high school where I could learn French, something I have always wanted to do. I am having such fun and am already looking at brochures for river cruises through France.

Marie, age 74

LEARNING OBJECTIVES

On completion of this chapter, the reader will be able to:

1. Explain cognitive changes with age and strategies to enhance cognitive health.
2. Identify nursing responses to assist older adults to maintain or improve cognitive abilities.
3. Discuss factors influencing learning in late life, including health literacy, and appropriate teaching and learning strategies.

The processes of normal cognition and learning in late life and strategies to enhance cognitive health and effective teaching-learning are discussed in this chapter. Assessment of cognition is discussed in Chapters 7 and 23, and care of older adults with mild and major neurocognitive disorders is discussed in Chapter 29.

ADULT COGNITION

Cognition is the process of acquiring, storing, sharing, and using information. Components of cognitive function include language, thought, memory, executive function, judgment, attention, and perception (Desai et al, 2010). The determination of intellectual capacity and performance has been the focus of a major portion of gerontological research. Developing knowledge today suggests that cognitive function and intellectual capacity is a complex interplay of age-related changes in the brain and nervous system and many other factors such as education, environment, nutrition, life experiences, physical function, emotions, biomedical and physiological factors, and genetics (Glahn et al, 2013; National Institutes of Health, 2004).

Before the development of sophisticated neuroimaging techniques, conclusions about brain function as we age were based on autopsy results (often on diseased brains) or results of cross-sectional studies conducted with older adults who were institutionalized or had coexisting illnesses. Changes seen were considered unavoidable and the result of the biological aging process rather than disease. As a result, the bulk of research has focused on the inevitable cognitive declines rather than on cognitive capacities. There are many old myths about aging and the brain that may be believed by both health professionals and older adults. It is important to understand cognition and memory in late life and dispel the myths that can have a negative effect on wellness and may, in fact, contribute to unnecessary cognitive decline (Box 5-1).

BOX 5-1   Myths About Aging and the Brain

MYTH: People lose brain cells every day and eventually just run out.

FACT: Most areas of the brain do not lose brain cells. Although you may lose some nerve connections, it can be part of the reshaping of the brain that comes with experience.

MYTH: You cannot change your brain.

FACT: The brain is constantly changing in response to experiences and learning, and it retains this "plasticity" well into aging. Changing our way of thinking causes corresponding changes in the brain systems involved; that is, your brain believes what you tell it.

MYTH: The brain does not make new brain cells.

FACT: Certain areas of the brain, including the hippocampus (where new memories are created) and the olfactory bulb (scent-processing center), regularly generate new brain cells.

MYTH: Memory decline is inevitable as we age.

FACT: Many people reach old age and have no memory problems. Participation in physical exercise, stimulating mental activity, socialization, healthy diet, and stress management helps maintain brain health. The incidence of dementia does increase with age, but when there are changes in memory, older people need to be evaluated for possible causes and receive treatment.

MYTH: There is no point in trying to teach older adults anything because "you can't teach an old dog new tricks."

FACT: Basic intelligence remains unchanged with age, and older adults should be provided with opportunities for continued learning. Minimizing barriers to learning such as hearing and vision loss and applying principles of geragogy enhance learning ability.

Modified from American Association of Retired Persons: *Myths about aging and the brain*, April 10, 2006. http://www.aarp.org/health/brain-health/info-2006/myths_about_aging_and_the_brain.htm. Accessed October 31, 2014.

Changes in the aging nervous system (Box 5-2) cause a general slowing of many neural processes, but they are not consistent with deteriorating mental function, nor do they interfere with daily routines. Age-related changes in brain structure, function, and cognition are also not uniform across the whole brain or across individuals. Recent research suggests that the reason older brains slow down is because they take longer to process constantly increasing amounts of information (Ramscar et al, 2014).

Cognitive functions may remain stable or decline with increasing age. The cognitive functions that remain stable include attention span, language skills, communication skills, comprehension and discourse, and visual perception. The cognitive skills that decline are verbal fluency, logical analysis, selective attention, object naming, and complex visuospatial skills. Overall cognitive abilities remain intact, and it is important to remember that if

BOX 5-2   Changes in the Central Nervous System

Neurons

- Shrinkage in neuron size and gradual decrease in neuron numbers
- Structural changes in dendrites
- Deposit of lipofuscin granules, neuritic plaque, and neurofibrillary bodies within the cytoplasm and neurons
- Loss of myelin and decreased conduction in some nerves, especially peripheral nerves (PNs)

Neurotransmitters

- Changes in the precursors necessary for neurotransmitter synthesis
- Changes in receptor sites
- Alteration in the enzymes that synthesize and degrade neurotransmitters
- Significant decreases in neurotransmitters, including acetylcholine (ACh), glutamate, serotonin, dopamine, and γ-aminobutyric acid

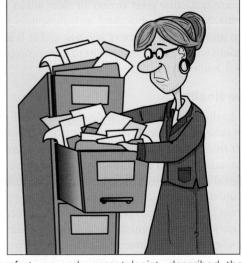

Alex Comfort, an early gerontologist, described the slowed response time of an older adult: By the time you are 80, you have a lot of files in the file cabinet. Your secretary is 80 so it also takes her a lot longer to locate the files, go through them, find the one you want, and bring it to you.

brain function becomes impaired in old age, it is the result of disease, not aging (Crowley, 1996).

Neuroplasticity

It is very important to know that the aging brain maintains resiliency or the ability to compensate for age-related changes. Developing knowledge refutes the myth that the adult brain is less plastic than the child's brain and less able to strengthen and increase neuronal connections (Petrus et al, 2014). The old adage "use it or lose it" applies to cognitive and physical health. Stimulating the brain increases brain tissue formation, enhances synaptic regulation of messages, and enhances the development of cognitive reserve (CR). CR is based on the concept of neuroplasticity and refers to the strength and complexity of neuronal/dendrite connections from which information is transmitted and cognition/mentation emerges. The greater the strength and complexity of these connections, the more the brain can absorb damage before cognitive functioning is compromised. "CR can be increased or decreased due to two complex, overarching processes—positive or negative neuroplasticity. Positive neuroplasticity is the brain's ability to make more and stronger connections between neurons in response to novel situations. Negative neuroplasticity refers to the atrophy of such connections in response to low stimulation or physiological insults" (Vance, 2012, p. 28).

To maximize brain plasticity and CR, it is important to engage in challenging cognitive, sensory, and motor activities, as well as meaningful social interactions, on a regular basis throughout life. People vary in the CR they have, and this variability may be because of differences in genetics, overall health, education, occupation, lifestyle, leisure activities, or other life experiences. Brain diseases and injuries may be less apparent in those with greater CR because they are able to tolerate lost neurons and synapses. For example, people who have attained more years of education may have high levels of Alzheimer's pathology, but few, if any, clinical symptoms (Desai et al, 2010).

Recent research seems to suggest that cognitive ability may be improving in the cohort of the oldest-old when compared with those born a decade earlier as a result of better nutrition, improved health care, healthier environment, enhanced intellectual stimulation, and better general living conditions (Christensen et al, 2013). Centenarians and supercentenarians also have a lower prevalence of dementia than those younger than 100 years (Vacante et al, 2012). Additionally, results of several recent studies report a decline in the incidence of cognitive impairment and dementia in Europe and the United States. Further research is needed to confirm the decline and explore the underlying mechanisms, but increasing efforts to promote cognitive health throughout life are important (Rocca et al, 2011; Qiu et al, 2013).

Changes in the brain with aging, once seen only as compensation for declining skills, are now thought to indicate the development of new capacities. These changes include using both hemispheres more equally than younger adults, greater density of synapses, and more use of the frontal lobes, which are thought to be important in abstract reasoning, problem solving, and concept formation (Grossman et al, 2010; Hooyman and Kiyak, 2011). The scaffolding theory of aging and cognition suggests that the increased frontal lobe activation with age is a marker of an adaptive brain that engages in compensatory scaffolding in response to the challenges of declining neural structures and function (Park and Reuter-Lorenz, 2009).

Later adulthood is no longer seen as a period when growth has ceased and cognitive development halted; rather, it is seen as a life stage programmed for plasticity and the development of unique capacities. The renewed emphasis on the development of cognitive capabilities that can develop with age provides a view of aging that reflects the history of many cultures and provides a much more hopeful view of both aging and human development.

Fluid and Crystallized Intelligence

Fluid intelligence and crystallized intelligence are factors of general intelligence and can be measured in standardized IQ tests. Fluid intelligence (often called *native intelligence*) consists of skills that are biologically determined, independent of experience or learning. It involves the capacity to think logically and solve problems in novel situations, independent of acquired knowledge. Fluid intelligence has been likened to "street smarts." Crystallized intelligence is composed of knowledge and abilities that the person acquires through education and life ("book

smarts") and is demonstrated largely through one's vocabulary and general knowledge. Crystallized intelligence is long-lasting and improves with experience.

Older people perform more poorly on performance scales (fluid intelligence), but scores on verbal scales (crystallized intelligence) remain stable. This is known as the classic aging pattern. The tendency to do poorly on performance tasks may be related to age-related changes in sensory and perceptual abilities, as well as psychomotor skills. Speed of cognitive processing, slower reaction time, and testing methods also affect performance.

Memory

Memory is defined as the ability to retain or store information and retrieve it when needed. Memory is a complex set of processes and storage systems. Three components characterize memory: immediate recall; short-term memory (which may range from minutes to days); and remote or long-term memory. Biological, functional, environmental, and psychosocial influences affect memory development throughout adulthood. Recall of newly encountered information seems to decrease with age, and memory declines are noted in connection with complex tasks and strategies. Even though some older adults show decrements in the ability to process information, reaction time, perception, and capacity for attentional tasks, the majority of functioning remains intact and sufficient.

Familiarity, previous learning, and life experience compensate for the minor loss of efficiency in the basic neurological processes. In unfamiliar, stressful, or demanding situations, however, these changes may be more marked (e.g., hospitalization). Healthy older adults may complain of memory problems, but their symptoms do not meet the criteria for mild or major neurocognitive impairment (Chapter 23). The term *age-associated memory impairment* (AAMI) has been used to describe memory loss that is considered normal in light of a person's age and educational level. This may include a general slowness in processing, storing, and recalling new information, as well as difficulty remembering names and words. However, these concerns can cause great anxiety in older adults who may fear dementia. Many medical or psychiatric difficulties (delirium, depression) also influence memory abilities, and it is important for older adults with memory complaints to have a comprehensive evaluation (Chapters 7, 23, 29).

Cognitive Health

Cognitive health is defined as "the development and preservation of the multidimensional cognitive structure that allows the older adult to maintain social connectedness, an ongoing sense of purpose, and the abilities to function independently, to permit functional recovery from illness or injury, and to cope with residual functional deficits" (Hendrie et al, 2006, p. 12). A healthy brain is "one that can perform all mental processes that are collectively known as cognition, including the ability to learn new things, intuition, judgment, language, and remembering" (CDC, 2014). Cognitive health is influenced by many of the factors that comprise the multiple dimensions of wellness discussed in Chapter 1. Attention to cognitive health, beginning at conception and continuing throughout life, is just as important as attention to physical and emotional health. Many of the behaviors influencing physical and emotional health also promote cognitive health. Findings from a large, long-term, randomized controlled trial suggest that a healthy diet, physical activity, and brain exercises can help slow mental decline in older people at risk for dementia (Ngandu et al, 2015).

This view of healthy cognitive aging (healthy brain aging) is comprehensive and proactive; it implies that cognitive health is much more than simply a lack of decline with aging (Desai et al, 2010). The National Center for Creative Aging campaign, *Beautiful Minds: Finding Your Lifelong Potential,* describes four steps to a beautiful mind (Box 5-3). The Centers for Disease Control and Prevention and the National Institute on Aging have large-scale programs focused on healthy brain aging and provide resources nurses can use in health promotion education (Box 5-4).

PROMOTING HEALTHY AGING: IMPLICATIONS FOR GERONTOLOGICAL NURSING

Nurses need to educate people of all ages about effective strategies to enhance cognitive health and vitality and to promote cognitive reserve and brain plasticity. Barnett et al. (2013) suggest that despite considerable fatalism among both health professionals and patients about the extent to which risk factors for dementia can be modified, there is growing evidence that good health promotion practices, from conception throughout life, affect cognitive function as you age (Figure 5-1). Although it is important to continue research examining strategies to enhance the cognitive health of older people, larger longitudinal studies

BOX 5-3   Four Steps to a Beautiful Mind

The Nourished Mind: A diet low in saturated fats and cholesterol, rich in good fats like polyunsaturated fats and omega-3 fatty acids, and packed with protective foods with nutrients such as vitamin E and lutein may protect brain cells and promote brain health.

The Mentally Engaged Mind: Brain cells, like muscle cells, can grow bigger and stronger with cognitive challenges and stimulation. Continued learning and new activities, skills, and interests help build connections in the brain and enhance function.

The Socially Connected Mind: Social connectedness is vital to health, wellness, and longevity. A rich social network supports brain health and provides individuals with better resources and stimulation.

The Physically Active Mind: Physical activity is important and is associated with improved cognitive skills or reduced cognitive decline.

Data from National Center for Creative Aging: *Four steps to a beautiful mind,* 2014. http://www.beautiful-minds.com/four-dimensions-of-brain-health. Accessed March 19, 2014.

BOX 5-4   RESOURCES FOR BEST PRACTICE

Cognitive Health

- National Institutes of Health: *Cognitive and Emotional Health Project: The Healthy Brain*
- Centers for Disease Control and Prevention: *The Healthy Brain Initiative: A National Public Health Road Map to Maintaining Cognitive Health*
- National Institute on Aging: *Alzheimer's Disease Education and Referral Center: Understanding Memory Loss: What to Do When You Have Trouble Remembering*
- National Center for Creative Aging: *Beautiful Minds: Finding Your Lifelong Potential; 2014, America's Brain Health Index*

of younger people need to be conducted so that health promotion efforts can begin earlier. Figure 5-2 presents a checklist to promote healthy brain aging that can be used by clinicians.

Education provided about health promotion activities should be tailored to specific communities and cultural subgroups because there are differences in perceptions about cognitive health among racial/ethnic groups. Results of a study examining perceptions about aging well in the context of cognitive health among a large and diverse group of older adults suggest that there are common themes about aging well among groups but also differences (Laditka et al, 2009) (Box 5-5).

There is a great deal of interest and some positive research findings about the role of cognitive (brain) training in enhancing memory and stimulating cognitive function, both in cognitively intact individuals and in those with cognitive impairment (Rebok et al, 2014; Tappen and Hain, 2014). Further research is needed on the effect of cognitive stimulation activities on cognitive function but recent studies have reported improved reasoning, increased speed of processing skills, improved activities of daily living (ADL) performance, greater brain volumes, and higher cognitive scores. Physical activity is also important and interesting new findings suggest that dancing improved reaction time and working memory as well as posture and balance while providing socialization (Kattenstroth et al, 2013). Findings from a recent large, long-term, randomized controlled trial suggest that a healthy diet, physical activity, and brain exercises can help slow mental decline in older people at risk for dementia (Ngandu et al, 2015).

Nurses can share research findings with older people and encourage the use of cognitive stimulation activities. Older adults, whether they have normal memory or mild memory problems, should engage in some type of memory training or brain fitness program a couple of times a week for at least 25 minutes. These may include computer-based programs and games or memory training techniques (Table 15-1), but can also be game playing (Scrabble, Trivial Pursuit, cards), puzzles, learning a new language, developing a new hobby, reading books, and engaging in interesting conversations. Among the various types of cognitive stimulating activities, games such as cards or puzzles seem to be particularly useful (Jeffrey, 2014; Rebok et al, 2014). There are many classes, games, computer programs, and phone and tablet applications available and these have captured the public imagination.

The brain exercising activity chosen should meet the following criteria: 1) it is new, unfamiliar, and out of your comfort zone; 2) it is challenging and takes some mental effort; and 3) it is fun and stimulates your interest and enjoyment. Tips for Best Practice are presented in Box 5-6.

LEARNING IN LATER LIFE

Basic intelligence remains unchanged with increasing years, and older adults should be provided with opportunities for continued learning. Adapting communication and teaching to enhance understanding requires knowledge of learning in late life and effective teaching-learning strategies with older adults. *Geragogy* is the application of the principles of adult learning theory to teaching interventions for older adults.

The older adult demands that teaching situations be relevant; new learning must relate to what the person already

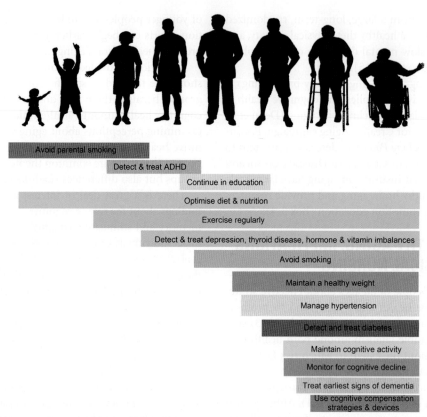

FIGURE 5-1 Factors Affecting Cognitive Health across the Life Span. (From Barnett J, Hachinski V, Blackwell A: Cognitive health begins at conception: addressing dementia as a lifelong and preventable condition, *BMC Med* 11:246, 2013.)

knows and should emphasize concrete and practical information. Aging may present barriers to learning, such as hearing and vision losses and cognitive impairment. Pain and discomfort can also interfere with learning. Moreover, the process of aging may accentuate other challenges that had already been factors in a person's life, such as cultural and cohort variations and education. Many older adults may have special learning needs based on educational deprivation in their early years and consequent anxiety about formalized learning.

Attention to literacy level and cultural variations is important to enhance learning and the usefulness of what is learned. Mood is extremely important in terms of what individuals (both young and old) will recall. In other words, when we attempt to measure recall of events that may have occurred in a crisis situation or an anxiety state, recall will be impaired. This is significant for health care professionals who give information to older adults who are ill or upset, particularly at times of crisis such as hospital discharge. Box 5-7 presents Tips for Best Practice in guiding older learners.

Learning Opportunities

Opportunities for older adults to learn are available in many formal and informal modes: self-teaching, college attendance, participation in seminars and conferences, public television programs, CDs, Internet courses, and countless others. In most colleges and universities, older people are taking classes of all types. Fees are usually lower for individuals older than 60 years of age, and elders may choose to work toward a degree or audit classes for enrichment and enjoyment. Senior centers and local

school districts often provide a wide array of adult education courses as well. The Road Scholar (formerly Elderhostel) program is an example of a program designed for older people that combines continued learning with travel. The program offers trips to 90 countries and presents learning programs in the United States and Canada. Road Scholar offers intergenerational programs for grandparents and grandchildren ages 4 and older.

Information Technology and Older Adults

Older adults comprise the fastest growing population using computers and the Internet. According to data from the Pew Research Center's Internet and American Life Project, 56% of American adults ages 65 and older use the Internet or email as compared with 82% of overall Americans. After age 75, Internet usage is less prevalent (36%). Older American women comprise the fastest growing group using social networking sites such as Facebook, Twitter, and Myspace (Madden, 2010; Zickuhr and Madden, 2012). More than any other age group, older adults perceive the Internet as a valuable resource to help them more easily obtain information and connect to loved ones. This could range from using a cell phone to set medication reminders to using Skype and FaceTime to interact with long-distance grandchildren. Many individuals are also using email to communicate with their health care providers. Organizations such as CyberSeniors and AARP provide basic computer and Internet training for older people.

With the aging of the baby boomers and the young tech-savvy adults, the future of technology in care and services for older adults can only be imagined. Technology has the potential

1	Counseled regarding smoking cessation	☐
	Comments:	
2	Advised to follow guidelines proposed jointly by the American Heart Association and the American College of Sports Medicine regarding daily physical activity	☐
	Comments:	
3	Counseled regarding healthy nutrition (e.g., Mediterranean diet, DASH [Dietary Approaches to Stop Hypertension] diet)	☐
	Comments:	
4	Counseled regarding the importance of intellectually challenging and creative leisure activities	☐
	Comments:	
5	Counseled regarding strategies to promote emotional resilience and reduce psychological distress and depression (e.g., relaxation exercises, mindfulness-meditation practices)	☐
	Comments:	
6	Advised to maintain an active, socially integrated lifestyle	☐
	Comments:	
7	Discussed strategies to achieve and maintain optimal daily sleep	☐
	Comments:	
8	Provided education about strategies to reduce risk of serious head injury (e.g., wearing seat belts, wearing helmets during contact sports, bicycling, skiing, skateboarding)	☐
	Comments:	
9	Provided education about strategies to reduce exposure to hazardous substances (e.g., wearing protective clothing during the administration of pesticides, fumigants, fertilizers, and defoliants)	☐
	Comments:	
10	Provided education and counseling regarding negative health effects of alcohol consumption more than recommended as safe by the National Institute of Alcoholism and Alcohol Abuse	☐
	Comments:	
11	Provided education about importance of achieving and maintaining healthy weight to promote overall health	☐
	Comments:	
12	Discussed and implemented strategies to achieve optimal blood pressure control	☐
	Comments:	
13	Discussed and implemented strategies to achieve optimal control of dyslipidemia (e.g., high cholesterol)	☐
	Comments:	
14	Discussed and implemented strategies to achieve optimal control of blood sugar/diabetes	☐
	Comments:	
15	Discussed risks and benefits of medications, supplements, herbal remedies, and vitamins to promote brain health	☐
	Comments:	
16	Discussed and implemented secondary prevention of stroke strategies (e.g., daily baby aspirin)	☐
	Comments:	

FIGURE 5-2 Promoting Healthy Aging: Cognitive Health. (Courtesy Center for Healthy Brain Aging, St Louis University School of Medicine, St Louis, MO. From Desai A, Grossberg G, Chibnall J: Healthy brain aging: a road map, *Clin Geriatr Med* 26:1–16, 2010.)

to improve the quality of life for older adults across settings by enhancing access to health information and resources, making communication with family and friends easier, providing cognitive stimulation and enjoyable activities, and alleviating isolation among community-dwelling older adults and those in nursing homes (Culley et al, 2013; Tak et al, 2007) (Box 5-8).

◆ PROMOTING HEALTHY AGING: IMPLICATIONS FOR GERONTOLOGICAL NURSING

Traditional ways of providing health information and services are changing, and both public and private institutions are increasingly using the Internet and other technologies.

This presents challenges for people with limited experience using computers and for those with limited literacy.

Nurses can share resources available for older adults who want to learn computer skills and adaptations that can be made to make computers as user-friendly as possible (e.g., touch screens, voice systems) for those who may have limitations (Choi and Dinitto, 2013). Nurses and other health professionals need to develop skills in the understanding and use of consumer health information and teach clients how to evaluate the reliability and validity of health information on the Internet (Box 5-9). Using social media as a platform for health promotion and health education presents exciting possibilities (Kolanowski et al, 2013). Continued attention to access to technology, especially among disadvantaged

From Laditka S, Corwin S, Laditka J, et al: Attitudes about aging well among a diverse group of older Americans: implications for promoting cognitive health, *Gerontologist* 49(51):S30–S39, 2009.

BOX 5-5   RESEARCH HIGHLIGHTS

Focus groups were conducted with a large and diverse group of older adults to explore perceptions of aging within the context of cognitive health. All groups perceived aging well as living to an advanced age, having good physical health, being mobile, having a positive mental outlook, being cognitively alert, having a good memory, and being socially involved. There were differences among the groups with Asian participants emphasizing the relationship between mental outlook and physical abilities; American Indians did not relate aging well to diet or physical activity; and African American and Vietnamese participants rarely mentioned cognitive stimulation techniques (game playing, puzzles, learning new things) as contributing to cognitive health. Not all groups have the same beliefs about aging and cognitive health. In designing education, it is important to understand the views of the intended audience and the individualize approaches based on perceptions about cognitive health and what is important to the group.

groups, and also efforts to enhance culturally and language-appropriate materials are important (Culley et al, 2013).

HEALTH LITERACY

Health literacy is defined as the degree to which individuals have the capacity to obtain, process, and understand basic health information and services needed to make appropriate health decisions (Kobylarz et al, 2010; National Research Council, 2004). Limited health literacy has been linked to increased health disparities, poor health outcomes, inadequate preventive care, increased use of health care services, higher health care costs, higher risk of mortality for older adults, and several health care safety issues, including medical and medication errors.

Health literacy plays a major role in improving health and health care quality for all Americans. In the past, health literacy has been viewed in terms of individual patient deficits (lack of knowledge regarding health issues) but is now recognized as a complex issue that involves the patient, the health care professional, and the health care system.

Health care literacy has been identified as 1 of the 20 necessary actions to improve health care quality on a national scale, and there are many national and local efforts addressing health literacy. Three major initiatives on the national level are the Affordable Care Act, the Department of Health and Human Services (HHS) National Action Plan to Improve Health Literacy, and the Plain Writing Act of 2010, requiring all new federal publications, forms, and publicly distributed documents to be written in a clear, concise, and well-organized manner (Koh et al, 2012). *Healthy People 2020* includes goals and objectives to improve health literacy and use of information technology (Box 5-10).

Nearly 9 of 10 adults do not have the level of proficiency in health literacy skills necessary to successfully navigate the health care system. Health literacy skills involve more than the basic reading and writing skills, although reading ability and education influence

TABLE 5-1   Tips for Improving Your Memory

TECHNIQUE	EXAMPLE
Pay attention to the task at hand; minimize distractions, avoid multitasking.	When listening to someone giving you directions while you are driving, do not keep the radio on.
Involve your senses.	To help remember the names of people you are meeting, look them in the eye, shake their hand, and repeat their name. Use auditory cues such as timers, alarm clocks, cell phone reminders.
Use repetition.	Say what you are trying to remember several times. Say things aloud ("I am putting my car keys on the hall table"). Review new learning at the end of the day.
Chunk it and organize it.	When trying to remember a telephone number, chunk it into 3 pieces of information (area code, 3-digit prefix, and a 4-digit number). Write things down, organize routine tasks, try to prepare things in advance when you have time to concentrate.
Use mneumonic devices (clues to help you remember) (visual images, acronyms, rhymes and alliterations).	Use the word HOMES to remember the names of the Great Lakes: Huron, Ontario, Michigan, Erie, and Superior. Remember the months of the year with 30 days using the rhyme "Thirty days has September…." Search the alphabet when trying to remember something. Do an Internet search for what you are trying to remember.
Relate information to what you already know.	Remember a new address by thinking of someone you know who lives on the same street.
Get adequate sleep; use stress-relieving techniques; and engage in physical activity.	Sleep is necessary for memory consolidation, and the key memory-enhancing activity occurs during the deepest stages of sleep. Cognitive training and memory training exercises may improve sleep. Mindfulness meditation encourages more connections between brain cells and increases mental acuity and memory ability. Exercise increases oxygen to the brain, reduces the risk of illness, enhances helpful brain chemicals, and protects brain cells.

Adapted from Grobol J: *8 tips for improving your memory,* Psych Central, 2010. http://psychcentral.com/blog/archives/2010/09/03/8-tips-for-improving-your-memory. Accessed February 17, 2014; Smith M, Robinson L: *How to improve your memory.* http://www.helpguide.org/articles/memory/how-to-improve-your-memory.htm. Accessed February 17, 2014.

BOX 5-6   TIPS FOR BEST PRACTICE

Cognitive Health

- Dispel myths about brain aging and teach about cognition and aging.
- Educate people of all ages about factors that influence cognitive health.
- Be aware of cultural differences in perceptions of cognitive health and adapt education accordingly.
- Advise older adults to have comprehensive assessment if they are experiencing cognitive decline.
- Encourage socialization and participation in intellectual stimulating activities, exercise, healthy diets (e.g., Mediterranean, DASH diet).
- Teach chronic illness prevention strategies and ensure good management of chronic illnesses.
- Share resources for cognitive training (memory enhancing techniques, computer games, puzzles, card games).

BOX 5-7   TIPS FOR BEST PRACTICE

Guiding Older Adult Learners

- Make sure the person is ready to learn before trying to teach. Watch for cues that would indicate that the person is preoccupied, fatigued, or too anxious to comprehend the material.
- Ensure that the person is comfortable (appropriate seating, room temperature); pain and discomfort can interfere with learning. Provide pain medication if needed before teaching.
- Be sensitive to cultural, language, health literacy level, and other differences among the older adults you serve. Some suggestions may not be appropriate for everyone and materials need to be individualized.
- Provide adequate time for learning, and use self-pacing techniques.
- Create a shame-free environment where older adults feel free to ask questions.
- Provide regular positive feedback.
- Avoid distractions, and present one idea at a time.
- Present pertinent, specific, practical, and individualized information. Emphasize concrete rather than abstract material.
- Use past experience; connect new learning to what has already been learned.
- Use plain language, use large readable font (e.g., Arial, 14 to 16 points), and use both uppercase and lowercase letters.
- Use high contrast on visuals and handout materials (dark colors for text and lighter for background; black print on white, dark blue on pale yellow).
- Pay attention to reading ability; use tools other than printed material such as pictures, videos, discussion, demonstrations.
- Use bullets or lists to highlight pertinent information. Use only two to three main concepts.
- Sit facing the client so that he or she can watch your lip movements and facial expressions.
- Speak slowly, keeping the pitch of your voice low; low sounds are heard better than high-frequency sounds.
- Encourage the learner to develop various mediators or mnemonic devices (e.g., visual images, rhymes, acronyms, self-designed coding schemes).
- Use shorter, more frequent sessions with appropriate breaks; pay attention to fatigue and physical discomfort.
- If using computers, adapt as needed for physical limitations (large icons and font, voice systems, touch screens, volume adjustments).
- Use "teach-back" methods to ensure understanding.

BOX 5-8   This Is What 90 Looks Like

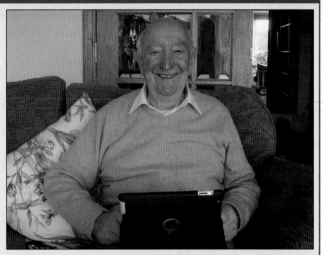

When Britain entered the war in Europe I decided that further attendance at formal schooling was out and as soon as I was old enough I volunteered for aircrew duties in the Royal Air Force and was accepted and trained as a pilot. Following an injury, I left the RAF in 1951 and soon found that entering the industrial market was not easy. Soon after my return to civilian status I married a nurse whom I had met while I was at the RAF rehabilitation unit, and over the 50 years of our marriage we raised 6 children.

I eventually found employment in the new plastics industry and was surprised to find how short of background knowledge the new factories and their management were; therefore, having gained some knowledge in processing I joined an engineering group that intended to manufacture processing machinery. Fortunately I had received good background training in hydraulics and electrics in the services. I was able to take an active part in improving their equipment.

During my employment the Rubber and Plastics Institute elected me a fellow for my service to the industry. When I retired I was the director of development and technical training. After retirement I worked for a further 17 years as a consultant specializing in processing and training.

Losing my wife while we were both in our mid-80s was a double blow. Living alone after more than 50 years of shared companionship was difficult but the restriction of advancing years in my new solitary state made the years ahead look very bleak. My children all helped me at this difficult period and I learned to live with what I had and modify my life to suit. Now that I am 90 years of age I no longer fly my own plane but I still feel confident driving, so I do have a degree of mobility that I feel is helping me deal with life's problems. I find learning to recognize what is possible and what is hazardous and to realize that these factors do change is an important lesson when growing old.

Victor T. Gardner

information, operate a computer, search the Internet and evaluate websites, calculate or reason numerically, and interact with health professionals (National Network of Libraries of Medicine, 2013).

Health Literacy and Older Adults

Some older adults may be disproportionately affected by inadequate health literacy. Chronic illness and sensory impairments further contribute to challenges related to communication and understanding (Warren, 2013). Older adults have lower health literacy scores than all other age groups. Today, more than half of individuals older than 65 years of age are at the below-basic level (CDC, 2009; Kobylarz et al, 2010; USDHHS, n.d.). Older adults are a heterogeneous group in their characteristics and literacy skills, so strategies to enhance their understanding of health

health literacy. Anyone can have low health literacy, including people with good literacy skills. Most people will have trouble understanding health information at some point in their lives (USDHHS, n.d.). In today's complex health care system health literacy may include the ability to obtain and apply relevant information, understand visual

BOX 5-9 Evaluating Internet Health Information

- **SPONSORSHIP**: Consider the source: use only recognized authorities. Government agencies have .gov in the address; educational institutions or medical schools have .edu in the address; professional organizations will be identified as .org. These are usually the best websites to use to obtain health information. MedlinePlus, NIH Senior Health, Centers for Disease Control and Prevention, and Healthfinder provide credible information and can get you started by pointing to other credible sites.
- The site should clearly identify the sponsor of the site, including the identities of commercial and noncommercial organizations that have contributed to funding, service, or material on the site. Some commercial websites (.com) have valuable or credible information (e.g., www.mayoclinic.com), but others may represent a specific company using the web for commercial reasons—to sell products. Advertisements should be labeled.
- **PURPOSE**: Is the purpose of the site to inform? Is it to sell a product? Is it to raise money? Be cautious about sites trying to sell a product or service. If it sounds too good to be true, it probably is.
- **CURRENCY**: The site should be updated frequently and be consistently available, with the date of the latest revision clearly posted (usually at the bottom of the page).
- **FACTUAL INFORMATION**: Information should be presented in a clear manner capable of being verified. Information presented as opinion should be clearly stated and the source should be identified as a qualified professional or organization.
- **AUDIENCE**: The website should state if information is intended for the consumer or health professional.
- **OTHER**: Reliable websites have a policy about how they establish links to other sites. Look for the site's linking policy, often found in a section titled "About This Web Site."
- Check the Privacy Policy and be cautious about providing personal information until you determine what is done with your information.
- Check with your health care provider before using information found on web searches.

Adapted from Medline Plus: *Medline Plus guide to healthy Web surfing,* 2012. http://www.nlm.nih.gov/medlineplus/healthywebsurfing.htm.; Medical Library Association: *Find and evaluate health information on the Web,* 2014. https://www.mlanet.org/resources/userguide.html. Accessed March 23, 2014.

♥ BOX 5-10 HEALTHY PEOPLE 2020
Information Technology, Health Literacy

Goal

Use health communication strategies and health information technology (IT) to improve population health outcomes and health care quality, as well as to achieve health equity.

Objectives

- Improve the health literacy of the population.
- Increase the proportion of persons with access to the Internet.
- Increase the proportion of persons with broadband access to the Internet.
- Increase the proportion of persons who use mobile devices.
- Increase the proportion of persons who use the Internet to keep track of personal health information, such as care received, test results, or upcoming medical appointments.
- Increase the proportion of persons who use the Internet to communicate with their health provider.
- Increase the proportion of health-related websites that meet three or more evaluation criteria disclosing information that can be used to assess information reliability.
- Increase the proportion of online health information seekers who report easily accessing health information.

Data from U.S. Department of Health and Human Services, Office of Disease Prevention and Health Promotion: Healthy People 2020, 2012. http://www.healthypeople.gov/2020

cultural competence, and knowledge of what matters most to the person are essential.

◆ Assessment

There are many widely available resources (Box 5-11) that nurses can use to assess health literacy and design effective teaching programs (brochures, one to one or group teaching, web resources). Identifying high-risk older adults (non-English speakers, less than high school education) can assist in targeting interventions (Chapter 4). There are several validated easy-to-administer health literacy screening tools readily available (Rapid Estimate of Adult Literacy in Medicine, Test of Functional Health Literacy in Adults, and Newest Vital Signs assessment). The *Health Literacy Universal Precautions Toolkit* (AHRQ, 2013) was developed to help structure the delivery of care as if every patient may have limited health literacy. This strategy may benefit everyone, regardless of health literacy levels, because it improves understanding.

◆ Interventions

Patient education materials should use plain language and provide information at no higher than a sixth grade level in the person's language (may vary depending on person's abilities), be culturally appropriate, and use varying methods to communicate information (pictures, videos) (Box 5-12). The Centers for Medicare and Medicaid Services (CMS) describes written material as clear and effective when it meets the following criteria: (1) attracts the intended reader's attention; (2) holds the reader's attention; (3) makes the reader feel respected and understood; (4) helps the reader understand the messages in the material; and (5) moves the reader to take action. Translation of materials should be done by certified medical interpreters or a native speaker of the target language rather than by the literal

information need to be individualized. However, as the major consumers of health care in this country, many are at risk for poor outcomes related to understanding of health care information and navigating the health care system.

◆ PROMOTING HEALTHY AGING: IMPLICATIONS FOR GERONTOLOGICAL NURSING

An integral part of the nursing role across the continuum is provision of health information. Older adults are the major users of health care, so nurses will have many opportunities to provide health education to this age group. Knowledge of health literacy and its relationship to health status in older adults is a growing area of concern (Zamora and Clingerman, 2011). In addition to poorer health literacy skills, some older adults may also have multiple risk factors that affect their ability to understand and use health information (sensory changes, cognitive changes, complex medical regimens). Knowledge of the principles of geragogy, an understanding of health literacy, excellent communication skills, creativity,

BOX 5-11 RESOURCES FOR BEST PRACTICE

Health Literacy/Teaching Older Adults

AHRQ: Health literacy universal precautions toolkit

CDC: Improving health literacy for older adults; Simply Put: a guide for creating easy-to-understand materials

USDHHS, Office of Disease Prevention and Health Promotion: A guide to writing and designing easy-to-use health websites; Quick guide to health literacy and older adults; Plain language: a promising strategy for clearly communicating health information and improving health literacy

NIH Senior Health: Helping older adults search for health information online: a toolkit for trainers

HRSA: Effective communication for healthcare professionals (free online course)

BOX 5-12 RESEARCH HIGHLIGHTS

Discharge instructions for low-literate diverse older adults following hip replacement surgery were designed using pictographs (simple line drawings with stick figures showing explicit care actions). The pictographs were evaluated for acceptability and comprehension. All were well received by all participants of various races/ethnicities and they felt the pictograph instructions helped them understand the health care messages, particularly for step-by-step procedures and post-discharge care. Pictographs are culturally and language neutral, making them appropriate for different ethnicities, ages, languages, and genders. The pictograph approach is an effective strategy for discharge instructions for patients with low literacy levels and also for immigrants with significant communication challenges. Using pictographs may also be appropriate as a supplement to written instructions.

Further research is needed to evaluate this approach and compare it with text-based instructions on adherence to instructions and health outcomes.

From Choi J: Older adults' perceptions of pictograph-based discharge instructions after hip replacement surgery, *J Gerontol Nurs* 39(7): 48–54, 2013.

translation of English to another language because many concepts cannot be translated (Pearce and Clark, 2013).

Individuals should be able to both understand and use the information presented. Using the "teach-back" (also known as "show-me" or "closing the loop") method involves having people explain back to you or demonstrate what you have told them. For example, you might say "I want to be sure you understand your medication correctly. Can you tell me how you are going to take this medicine?"

Because medication management is a high-risk activity for older adults, attention to improving older adults' ability to understand their medications and take them correctly is essential.

In addition to effective teaching, simplified drug regimens, and use of assistive medication management devices, pharmaceutical companies should be encouraged to develop educational materials at lower literacy levels to ensure comprehension (Ingram and Ivanov, 2013; Zamora and Clingerman, 2011). Nurses should also be advocates for continued development and research on the most effective age-specific, culturally appropriate health literacy materials and interventions for older adults.

KEY CONCEPTS

- Although there are changes in the aging brain, cognitive function, in the absence of disease, remains adequate. Any changes in cognitive function require adequate assessment.
- The aging brain maintains resiliency or the ability to compensate for age-related changes. Developing knowledge refutes the myth that the adult brain is less plastic than the child's brain and can strengthen and increase neuronal connections.
- Late adulthood is no longer seen as a period when growth has ceased and cognitive development halted; rather, it is seen as a life stage programmed for plasticity and the development of unique capacities.
- Cognitive stimulation and attention to brain health are just as important as attention to physical health.
- Learning in late life can be enhanced by utilizing principles of geragogy and adapting teaching strategies to minimize barriers such as hearing and vision impairment and low literacy.
- Older adults are disproportionally affected by inadequate health literacy, and nurses must ensure that health information is provided in an appropriate manner to ensure understanding.

CRITICAL THINKING QUESTIONS AND ACTIVITIES

1. Review the myths about aging and the brain (Box 5-1). Were any of the facts surprising to you?
2. Partner with another student and use the checklist of promoting cognitive health (Figure 5-2). Discuss what areas may need improvement to enhance cognitive health in aging.
3. What types of health teaching would you provide to a young adult to enhance cognitive health in aging?
4. Work with another student and design a brochure to teach older adults about interventions to enhance cognitive health. What adaptations would you incorporate to ensure understanding for individuals with low health literacy?

RESEARCH QUESTIONS

1. What do older adults of different cultures believe about aging and brain function?
2. What types of cognitive stimulating activities do older adults report engaging in on a daily basis?
3. What strategies to improve the understanding of health information are most effective for older adults?
4. What are the learning needs of older adults related to the use of computers?
5. What do older adults perceive as the benefits of participation in social networking sites such as Facebook?

REFERENCES

Agency for Healthcare Research and Quality: *Health literacy universal precautions toolkit*, 2013. www.ahrq.gov/professionals/quality-patient-safety/quality-resources/tools/literacy-toolkit/index.html. Accessed February 20, 2014.

Barnett J, Hachinski V, Blackwell A: Cognitive health begins at conception: addressing dementia as a lifelong and preventable condition, *BMC Med* 11:246, 2013.

Centers for Disease Control and Prevention (CDC): *Improving health literacy for older adults: expert panel report* 2009. Atlanta, 2009, U.S. Department of Health and Human Services.

Centers for Disease Control and Prevention (CDC): *Healthy Brain Initiative*, 2014. http://www.cdc.gov/aging/healthybrain/index.htm. Accessed October 2014.

Choi N, Dinitto DM: The digital divide among low-income homebound older adults: Internet use patterns, eHealth literacy, and attitudes toward computer/Internet use, *J Med Internet Res* 15(5):e93, 2013.

Christensen K, Thinggaard M, Oksuzyan A, et al: Physical and cognitive functioning of people older than 90 years: a comparison of two Danish cohorts born 10 years apart, *Lancet* 382(9903):1507–1513, 2013.

Crowley SL: Aging brain's staying power, *AARP Bulletin* 37:1, 1996.

Culley J, Herman J, Smith D, et al: Effects of technology and connectedness on community-dwelling older adults, *Online J Nurs Inform* 17(3), 2013.

Desai A, Grossberg G, Chibnall J: Healthy brain aging: a road map, *Clin Geriatr Med* 26:1–16, 2010.

Glahn D, Kent J Jr, Sprooten E, et al: Genetic basis of neurocognitive decline and reduced white-matter integrity in normal human brain aging, *Proc Natl Acad Sci U S A* 110(47):19006–19011, 2013. http://www.pnas.org/content/early/2013/10/30/1313735110.abstract. Accessed February 13, 2014.

Grossman I, Na J, Varnum M, et al: Reasoning about social conflicts improves into old age, *Proc Natl Acad Sci U S A* 107(16):7246–7250, 2010.

Hendrie H, Albert M, Butters M, et al: The NIH Cognitive and Emotional Health Project: report of the Critical Evaluation Study Committee, *Alzheimers Dement* 2:12–32, 2006.

Hooyman NR, Kiyak HA: *Social gerontology: a multidisciplinary perspective*, ed 9, Boston, 2011, Pearson.

Ingram R, Ivanov L: Examining the association of health literacy and health behaviors in African American older adults: does health literacy affect adherence to antihypertensive regimens? *J Gerontol Nurs* 39(3):22–32, 2013.

Jeffrey S: More evidence brain games boost cognitive health, *Medscape Medical News from the Alzheimer's Association International Conference*, 2014. http://www.medscape.com/viewarticle/828285#3. Accessed July 2014.

Kattenstroth J, Kalisch T, Holt S, et al: Six months of dance intervention enhances postural, sensorimotor, and cognitive performance in elderly without affecting cardiorespiratory functions, *Front Aging Neurosci* 5:5, 2013.

Kobylarz F, Pomidor A, Pleasant A: Health literacy as a tool to improve the public understanding of Alzheimer's disease, *Ann Longterm Care* 18:34–40, 2010.

Koh H, Berwick D, Clancy C, et al: New federal policy initiatives to boost health literacy can help the nation move beyond the cycle of costly "crisis care," *Health Affairs* 31(2):434–443, 2012.

Kolanowski A, Resnick B, Beck C, et al: Advances in nonpharmacological interventions 2011-2012, *Res Gerontol Nurs* 6(1):5–8, 2013.

Laditka S, Corwin S, Laditka J, et al: Attitudes about aging well among a diverse group of older Americans: implications for promoting cognitive health, *Gerontologist* 49(51):S30–S39, 2009.

Madden M: *Older adults and social media*, Pew Research Center, Aug 27, 2010. http://www.pewinternet.org/2010/08/27/older-adults-and-social-media. Accessed February 17, 2014.

National Institutes of Health: *Cognitive and emotional health project: the healthy brain*, 2004. http://trans.nih.gov/CEHP. Accessed February 14, 2014.

National Network of Libraries of Medicine: *Health literacy*, 2013. http://nnlm.gov/outreach/consumer/hlthlit.html. Accessed February 17, 2014.

National Research Council: *Health literacy: a prescription to end confusion*, Washington, DC, 2004, National Academies Press.

Ngandu T, Lehtisaio J, Solomon A, et al: A 2 year multidomain intervention of diet, exercise, cognitive training, and vascular risk monitoring versus control to prevent cognitive decline in at-risk elderly people (FINGER): a randomised controlled trial, The Lancet, published on line March 11, 2015, DOI:http://dx.doi.org/10.1016/S0140-6736(15)60461-5.

Park D, Reuter-Lorenz P: The adaptive brain: aging and neurocognitive scaffolding, *Ann Rev Psychol* 60(1):173–196, 2009.

Pearce T, Clark D: Strategies to address low health literacy in the older adult, *Top Geriatr Rehabil* 29(2):98–106, 2013.

Petrus E, Isaiah A, Jones A, et al: Crossmodal induction of thalamocortical potentiation leads to enhanced information processing in the auditory cortex, *Neuron* 51(3):664–673, 2014.

Qiu C, von Strauss E, Bäckman L, et al: Twenty-year changes in dementia occurrence suggest decreasing incidence in central Stockholm, Sweden, *Neurology* 80(20):1888–1894, 2013.

Ramscar M, Hendrix P, Shaoul C, et al: The myth of cognitive decline: non-linear dynamics of lifelong learning, *Top Cogn Sci* 6(1):5–422, 2014.

Rebok G, Ball K, Guey L, et al: Ten-year effects of the advanced cognitive training for independent and vital elderly cognitive training trial on cognition and everyday functioning in older adults, *J Am Geriatr Soc* 62:16–24, 2014.

Rocca W, Petersen R, Knopman D, et al: Trends in the incidence and prevalence of Alzheimer's disease, dementia, and cognitive impairment in the United States, *Alzheimers Dement* 7(1):80–93, 2011.

Tak S, Beck C, McMahon E: Computer and Internet access for long-term care residents, *J Gerontol Nurs* 33:32–40, 2007.

Tappen R, Hain D: The effect of in-home cognitive training on functional performance of individuals with mild cognitive impairment and early-stage Alzheimer's disease, *Res Gerontol Nurs* 7(1):15–24, 2014.

U.S. Department of Health and Human Services (USDHHS): *Quick guide to health literacy and older adults* (n.d.). Accessed February 17, 2014.

Vacante M, D'Agata V, Motta M, et al: Centenarians and supercentenarians: a black swan. Emerging social, medical and surgical problems, *BMC Surg* 12(Suppl 1):S36, 2012.

Vance D: Potential factors that may promote successful cognitive aging, *Nursing (Auckl)* 2:27–32, 2012.

Warren M: Promoting health literacy in older adults with low vision, *Top Geriatr Rehabil* 29(2):107–115, 2013.

Zamora H, Clingerman E: Health literacy among older adults: a systematic literature review, *J Gerontol Nurs* 37(10):41–51, 2011.

Zickuhr K, Madden M: *Older adults and Internet use*, Pew Research Center, June 2012. http://www.pewtrusts.org/our_work_report_detail.aspx?id=85899396673. Accessed February 17, 2014.

CHAPTER 6

Communicating with Older Adults

Theris A. Touhy

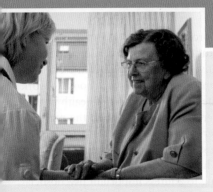

http://evolve.elsevier.com/Touhy/TwdHlthAging

A STUDENT SPEAKS

When they told us we were going to a senior center to interview an older person about their life, I was really nervous. My grandparents are no longer living and I really wasn't close to them when they were alive. I have little contact with older people and to tell you the truth, I find them a little boring. Seems to me they are always complaining and criticizing and talking about the good old days. I am just not sure what I am going to learn from this assignment. I plan to go into pediatrics, so it isn't very relevant to me.

James, age 22

AN ELDER SPEAKS

I love living in my retirement community but I tell you I miss being around younger people. My grand-children live far away and I don't see them often. I would enjoy being around the young folks more. They really bring a new perspective on things and have a lot of enthusiasm and energy. It's good to keep up on the new things they are involved in. I think older people and younger people could learn a lot from each other.

Frances, age 82

LEARNING OBJECTIVES

On completion of this chapter, the reader will be able to:

1. Describe the importance of communication to the lives of older adults.
2. Discuss how ageist attitudes affect communication with older adults.
3. Understand the significance of the life story in coming to know older adults.
4. Discuss the modalities of reminiscence and life review.
5. Identify effective methods to facilitate communication with older adults individually and in groups.

Communication is the single most important capacity of human beings, the ability that gives us a special place in the animal kingdom. Few things are more dehumanizing than the inability to communicate effectively and engage in social interaction with others. The need to communicate, to be listened to, and to be heard does not change with age or impairment. Meaningful communication and active engagement with society contributes to healthy aging and improves an older adult's chances of living longer, responding better to health care interventions, and maintaining optimal function (Herman and Williams, 2009; Levy, 2009; Levy et al, 2009; Levy and Leifheit-Limson, 2009; Rowe and Kahn, 1998; Van Leuven, 2010; Williams, 2006; Williams et al, 2008).

For some elders, opportunities for social interaction may be more limited as a result of loss of family and friends, illnesses, and sensory and cognitive losses. The ageist attitudes of the public, as well as health professionals, also present barriers to communicating effectively with older people. Good communication skills are the basis for accurate assessment, care planning, and the development of therapeutic relationships between the nurse and the older person.

This chapter discusses the effect of health professionals' attitudes toward aging on their communication with older people and communication skills essential to therapeutic interaction with older adults. The significance of the life story, reminiscence, life review, and communication with groups of elders are also included in this chapter. Communication with individuals with hearing and vision loss is discussed in Chapters 11 and 12, and communicating with individuals with cognitive impairment is discussed in Chapter 29.

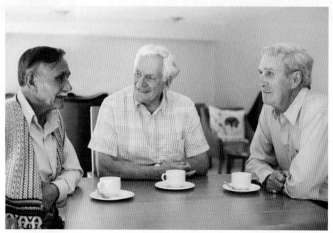

Group of older men talking over coffee. (©iStock.com/ Squaredpixels.)

AGEISM AND COMMUNICATION

Beliefs in myths and stereotypes about aging and ageist attitudes on the part of health professionals and older people themselves can interfere with the ability to communicate effectively. For example, if the nurse believes that all persons he or she perceives as old have memory problems or are unable to learn or process information, he or she will be less likely to engage in conversation, provide appropriate health information, or treat the person with respect and dignity. If an older person believes that illness is inevitable with increased age, he or she may fail to report changes in health or adopt health promotion strategies.

Ageism, a term coined by Robert Butler (1969), the first director of the National Institute on Aging (Bethesda, MD), is the systematic stereotyping of and discrimination against people because they are old, in the way that racism and sexism discriminate against color and gender. Ageism will affect us all if we live long enough. Although ageism is found cross-culturally, it is more prevalent in the United States, where aging is viewed with sadness, fear, and anxiety (International Longevity Center, 2006). Some research indicates that individuals in many non-Western cultures are more tolerant toward their elders, perceive older adults as significantly more important to their society, and engage in less avoiding behaviors toward older people (Bergman et al, 2013).

Ageist attitudes, as well as myths and stereotypes about aging, can be detrimental to older people. A recent study (Rogers et al., 2015) reported that one out of five adults over the age of 50 years experiences discrimination in healthcare settings. Discrimination contributes to substandard experiences with the healthcare system, increasing the burden of poor health in older adults. On the other hand, holding a positive self-perception of aging can contribute to a longer life span (Levy et al, 2002). While older people, collectively, have often been seen in negative terms, a most striking change in attitudes toward aging has occurred in the past 30 years. Undoubtedly, this will continue to change with the influence of the baby boomers and beyond. The impact of media presentation is enormous, and it is gratifying to see robust images of aging; fewer older people are portrayed as victims or as those to be pitied, shunned, or ridiculed by virtue of achieving old age.

Ageism affects health professionals as well and, with few exceptions, studies of attitudes of health professional students toward aging reflect negative views. Examples of the effect of ageism include the few number of students who choose to work in the field of aging and the lack of education of health professionals in the care of older people, even though the majority of their patients are older adults (Kydd et al, 2014). Other effects include spending less time with older patients, taking a more authoritarian role, having less patience, providing less information, and neglecting to address important psychosocial and preventive factors (Gerontological Society of America, 2012). It is important for nurses who care for older people to be aware of their own attitudes and beliefs about aging and the effect of these attitudes on communication and care provision. Enhancing one's interpersonal communication skills is the foundation for therapeutic interactions with older adults.

Elderspeak

An example of ageism is the use of elderspeak. It is especially common in communication between health care professionals and older adults in hospitals and nursing homes but occurs in non–health care settings as well (Herman and Williams, 2009; Williams et al, 2003, 2004, 2008; Williams, 2006; Williams and Tappen, 2008). Elderspeak is a form of patronizing speech, similar to "baby talk," which is often used to talk to very young children (Box 6-1).

Nurses may not be aware that they are using elderspeak and may view it as an effective way to communicate with elders, especially those with cognitive impairment. However, research has shown that use of this form of speech conveys messages of dependence, incompetence, and control (Williams, 2006; Williams et al, 2008). Elderspeak may also increase the likelihood of resistance to care among cognitively impaired nursing home residents (Lombardi et al, 2014). Some features of elderspeak (speaking more slowly, repeating, or paraphrasing) may be beneficial in communication with older people with dementia, and further research is needed. Other examples of communication that conveys ageist attitudes are ignoring the older person and talking to family and friends as if the person was not present, and limiting interaction to task-focused communication only (Touhy and Williams, 2008) (Box 6-2).

BOX 6-1 Characteristics of Elderspeak

- Using a singsong voice, changing pitch and tone, and exaggerating words
- Using short and simple sentences
- Speaking more slowly
- Using limited vocabulary
- Repeating or paraphrasing what has just been said
- Using pet names (diminutives) such as "honey" or "sweetie" or "grandma"
- Using collective pronouns such as "we"—for instance, "Would we like to take a bath now?"
- Using statements that sound like questions

Modified from Williams K, Kemper S, Hummert L: Enhancing communication with older adults: overcoming elderspeak, *J Gerontol Nurs* 30:17–25, 2004; Williams K: Improving outcomes of nursing home interactions, *Res Nurs Health* 29:121–133, 2006.

BOX 6-2   RESEARCH HIGHLIGHTS

This study explored the experiences of people with disabilities in their interactions with nurses and unlicensed assistive personnel and their perceptions of care they received during hospital stays. A total of 35 people with cognitive and physical disabilities participated in focus groups and semistructured interviews. There were some individuals older than 65 among the participants, but the mean age was 50 years. Poor communication by nursing staff was identified by every participant and included failing to listen to patients, talking to family members rather than the individual with the disability, not respecting the individual's knowledge of his or her care regimen, and being talked to like a child. Other studies have reported similar findings. There is a need to educate nurses and other health care personnel about effective communication strategies to enhance person-centered respectful care for individuals with disabilities.

Source: Smeltzer S, Avery C, Haynor P: Interactions of people with disabilities and nursing staff during hospitalization, *Am J Nurs* 112(4): 30–37, 2012.

THERAPEUTIC COMMUNICATION WITH OLDER ADULTS

Basic communication strategies that apply to all situations in nursing, such as attentive listening, authentic presence, non-judgmental attitude, clarifying, giving information, seeking validation of understanding, keeping focus, and using open-ended questions, are all applicable in communicating with older adults. Basically, elders may need more time to give information or answer questions simply because they have a larger life experience from which to draw information. Sorting thoughts requires intervals of silence, and therefore listening carefully without rushing the elder is important. Word retrieval may be slower, particularly for nouns and names (Chapter 5).

Open-ended questions are useful but can also be difficult. Those who wish to please, especially when feeling vulnerable or somewhat dependent, may wonder what it is you want to hear rather than what it is they would like to say. Communication that is most productive will initially focus on the issue of major concern to the individual, regardless of the priority of the nursing assessment.

When using closed questioning to obtain specific information, be aware that the individual may feel on the spot, and thus the appropriate information may not be immediately forthcoming. This is especially true when asking questions to determine mental status. The elder may develop a mental block because of anxiety or feel threatened if questions are asked in a quizzing or demeaning manner.

Older people may also be reluctant to disclose information for fear of the consequences. For example, if they are having problems remembering things or are experiencing frequent falls, sharing this information may mean that they might have to relinquish desired activities or even leave their home and move to a more protective setting.

When communicating with individuals in a bed or wheelchair, position yourself at their level rather than talking over a side rail or standing above them. Pay attention to their gaze, gestures, and body language, as well as the pitch, volume, and tone of their voice, to help you understand what they are trying to communicate. Thoughts unstated are often as important as those that are verbalized. You may ask, "What are you thinking about right now?" Clarification is essential to ensure that you and the elder have the same framework of understanding. Many generational, cultural, and regional differences in speech patterns and idioms exist. Frequently seek validation of what you hear. If you tend to speak quickly, particularly if your accent is different from that of the patient, try to speak more slowly and give the person time to process what you are saying.

THE LIFE STORY

As we age, we accumulate complex stories from the long years lived. In caring for older adults, listening to life stories is an important component of communication. The life story can tell us a great deal about the person and is an important part of the assessment process. Stories provide important information about etiology, diagnosis, treatment, prognosis, and experience of living with an illness from the patient's point of view. Listening to stories is also a way of demonstrating cultural competence (Chapter 4).

Listening to memories and life stories requires time and patience and a belief that the story and the person are valuable and meaningful. A memory is an incredible gift given to the nurse, a sharing of a part of oneself when one may have little else to give. The more personal memories are saved for persons who will patiently wait for their unveiling and who will treasure them. Stories are important. "The people who come to see us bring us their stories. They hope they tell them well enough so that we understand the truth in their lives. They hope we know how to interpret their stories correctly" (Coles, 1989, p. 7).

The life story as constructed through reminiscing, journaling, life review, or guided autobiography has held great fascination for gerontologists in the last 25 years. The universal appeal of the life story as a vehicle of culture, a demonstration of caring and generational continuity, and an easily stimulated activity has held allure for many professionals. "One of the few universals is that humans in all known cultures use language to tell stories" (Ramírez-Esparza and Pennebaker, 2006, p. 216).

The most exciting aspect of working with older adults is being a part of the emergence of the life story: the shifting and blending patterns. When we are young, it is important for our emotional health and growth to look forward and plan for the future. As one ages, it becomes more important to look back, talk about experiences, review and make sense of it all, and end with a feeling of satisfaction with the life lived. This is important work and the major developmental task of older adulthood that Erik Erikson called *ego integrity versus despair*. Ego integrity is achieved when the person has accepted both the triumphs and the disappointments of life and is at peace and satisfied with the life lived (Erikson, 1963) (Chapter 3).

Storytelling is a complementary and alternative therapy nurses can use with older adults to enhance communication (Moss, 2014). The nurse can learn much about an older adult's history, communication style, relationships, coping mechanisms, strengths, fears, affect, and adaptive capacity by listening thoughtfully as the life story is constructed.

Reminiscing

Reminiscing is an umbrella term that can include any recall of the past. Reminiscing occurs from childhood onward, particularly at life's junctures and transitions. Reminiscing cultivates a sense of security through recounting of comforting memories, belonging through sharing, and promotion of self-esteem through confirmation of uniqueness. Robert Butler (2002) emphasized that in the past, reminiscing was thought to be a sign of senility or what we now call Alzheimer's disease. Older people who talked about the past and told the same stories again and again were said to be boring and living in the past. From Butler's landmark research (1963), we now know that reminiscence is the most important psychological task of older people. The emerging model of reminiscence and well-being has been evaluated with Eastern and Western cultures, but further research is needed about ways of reminiscing among other cultures (Bergman et al, 2013; Cappeliez, 2013; O'Rourke et al, 2012).

For the nurse, reminiscing is a therapeutic intervention important in assessment and understanding. The work of several gerontological nursing leaders, including Irene Burnside, Priscilla Ebersole, and Barbara Haight, has contributed to the body of knowledge about reminiscence and its importance in nursing. The International Institute for Reminiscence and Life Review (University of Wisconsin, Superior, WI), an interdisciplinary organization uniting participants to study reminiscence and life review, is another valuable resource for nurses and members of other disciplines involved in research or practice. This group also publishes a journal, the *International Journal of Reminiscence and Life Review.*

Reminiscence can have many goals. It not only provides a pleasurable experience that improves quality of life but also increases socialization and connectedness with others, provides cognitive stimulation, improves communication, facilitates personal growth, and can decrease depression scores (Bohlmejier et al, 2003; Grabowski et al, 2010; Haight and Burnside, 1993; Pinquart and Forstmeier, 2012; Stinson, 2009). The process of reminiscence can occur in individual conversations with older people, be structured as in a nursing history, or can occur in a group where each person shares his or her memories and listens to others sharing their memories. Intergenerational reminiscence activities could have benefits for both older and younger individuals. Reminiscence can also be used by caregivers to enhance communication with family members experiencing cognitive impairment (Latha et al, 2014). Box 6-3 provides some suggestions for encouraging reminiscence, and group work is discussed later in this chapter.

Stinson (2009) offers a protocol for structured reminiscence based on research from earlier studies and the Nursing Interventions Classifications (NIC) recommendations. Mudiwa (2010) reports on an innovative use of "You Tube" reminiscence therapy in Ireland and proposes that this medium can be easily used in reminiscence interventions. "In-the-Moment" recording of reminiscence episodes via new mobile devices also hold promise, and results of life review therapy for depression in older adults in a face-to-face setting with additional computer use are promising (Cappeliez, 2013; Preschl et al, 2012). Although further research on the effectiveness of reminiscence and the development of evidence-based protocols is needed, nurses can have confidence in using this technique in work with older people (Latha et al, 2014; Stinson, 2009).

Reminiscence and life story have entered the computer age through the use of digital storytelling. Digital storytelling is another medium that can be used with older people to record their stories and memories in a format that can be shared with others. The digital story is a first-person narrative created by combining personal narration, video, animation, artifacts, and music or other sounds. Digital storytelling brings the ancient

---

BOX 6-3   Suggestions for Encouraging Reminiscence

- Listen without correction or criticism. Older adults are presenting their version of their reality; our version belongs to another generation.
- Encourage older adults to discuss various ages and stages of their lives. Use questions such as, "What was it like growing up on that farm?", "What did teenagers do for fun when you were young?", or "What was WWII like for you?"
- Be patient with repetition. Sometimes people need to tell the same story often to come to terms with the experience, especially if it was meaningful to them. If they have a memory loss, it may be the only story they can remember, and it is important for them to be able to share it with others.
- Be attuned to signs of depression in conversation (dwelling on sad topics) or changes in physical status or behavior, and provide appropriate assessment and intervention.
- If a topic arises that the person does not want to discuss, change to another topic.
- If individuals are reluctant to share because they do not feel their life was interesting, reassure them that everyone's life is valuable and interesting and tell them how important their memories are to you and others.
- Keep in mind that reminiscing is not an orderly process. One memory triggers another in a way that may not seem related; it is not important to keep things in order or verify accuracy.
- Keep the conversation focused on the person reminiscing, but do not hesitate to share some of your own memories that relate to the situation being discussed. Participate as equals, and enjoy each other's contributions.

- Listen actively, maintain eye contact, and do not interrupt.
- Respond positively and give feedback by making caring, appropriate comments that encourage the person to continue.
- Use props and triggers such as photographs, memorabilia (e.g., a childhood toy or antique, short stories or poems about the past, favorite foods, YouTube videos, old songs).
- Use open-ended questions to encourage reminiscing. If working with a group, you can prepare questions ahead of time, or you can ask the group members to pick a topic that interests them. One question or topic may be enough for an entire group session.
- Consider using questions such as the following:
  How did your parents meet?
  What do you remember most about your mother? Father? Grandmother? Grandfather?
  What are some of your favorite memories from childhood?
  What was the first house you remember?
  What were your favorite foods as a child?
  Did you have a pet as a child?
  What do you remember about your first job?
  How did you celebrate birthdays or other holidays?
  If you were married, what are your memories of your wedding day?
  What was your greatest accomplishment or joy in your life?

art of telling stories to life using technology to promote a deeper level of understanding and meaning of the story for the storyteller, listener, and audience (Flottemesch, 2013).

Digital storytelling is an excellent tool for intergenerational connection that can help nursing students begin to know and value older people and their life journeys. A study producing personalized multimedia biographies for individuals with cognitive impairment reported that the biography stimulated reminiscence, brought mostly joy but occasionally moments of sadness, aided family members in remembering and better understanding their loved ones, and stimulated social interactions with family members and formal caregivers (Damianakis et al, 2010). Buron (2010) presents a lovely format for person-centered life history collages for use in a nursing home. There are many resources available for those interested in digital storytelling, and community centers and educational institutions, as well as the Internet, provide instruction on this medium.

Reminiscing and Storytelling with Individuals Experiencing Cognitive Impairment

Cognitive impairment does not necessarily preclude older adults from participating in reminiscence or storytelling groups. Opportunities for telling the life story, enjoying memories, and achieving ego integrity should not be denied to individuals on the basis of their cognitive status. Modifications must be made according to the cognitive abilities of the person, and although individual life review from a psychotherapeutic approach is not an appropriate modality, individuals with mild to moderate memory impairment can enjoy and benefit from group work focused on reminiscence and storytelling.

Research suggests that communication skills' training that involves memory book and life review activities with those who have dementia and their families can (1) increase the quantity and quality of communication between care recipients and caregivers, (2) lower caregiver stress and burden, and (3) reduce behavioral problems (Damianakis et al, 2010).

When the nurse is working with a group of persons who are cognitively impaired, the emphasis in reminiscence groups is on sharing memories, however they may be expressed, rather than specific recall of events. There should be no pressure to answer questions such as "Where were you born?" or "What was your first job?" Rather, discussions may center on jobs people had and places they have lived. Displaying additional props, such as music, pictures, familiar objects (e.g., an American flag, an old coffee grinder), and doing familiar activities that trigger past memories (e.g., having a tea party, folding linens) can prompt many recollections and sharing. The leader of a group with participants who have memory problems must assume a more active approach.

The TimeSlips program (Bastings, 2003, 2006; Fritsch et al, 2009) is an evidence-based innovation, cited by the Agency for Healthcare Research and Quality (AHRQ, 2014), that uses storytelling to enhance the lives of people with cognitive impairment. Positive outcomes associated with the program include enhanced verbal skills and provider reports of positive behavioral changes, increased communication, increased sociability, and less confusion. TimeSlips is a beneficial and cost-effective therapeutic intervention that can be used in many settings.

Using the TimeSlips format, group members looking at a picture are encouraged to create a story about the picture. The pictures can be fantastical and funny, such as from greeting cards, or more nostalgic, such as Norman Rockwell paintings. All contributions are encouraged and welcomed, there are no right or wrong answers, and everything that the individuals say is included in the story and written down by the scribe. Stories are read back to the participants during the session, using their names to identify their contributions. At the beginning of each session, the story from the last session is read to the participants. Care is taken to compliment each member for his or her contribution to the wonderful story. The stories that emerge are full of humor and creativity and often include discussions of memories and reminiscing.

One of the authors of this text (T. Touhy) has used the storytelling modality extensively with mild to moderately impaired older people with great success as part of a research study on the effect of therapeutic activities for persons with memory loss. Qualitative responses from group participants and families indicated their enjoyment with the process. At the end of the 16-week group, the stories were bound into a book and given to the participants with a picture of the group and each member's name listed. Many of the participants and their families have commented on the pride they feel at their "book" and have even shared them with grandchildren and great-grandchildren. In work by Bastings (2003), some of the stories were presented as a play.

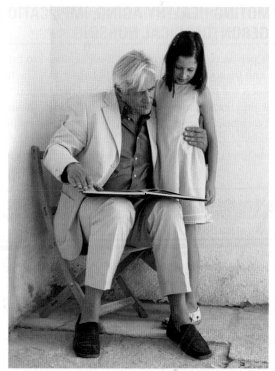

Grandfather sharing stories with his granddaughter. (©iStock. com/IS_ImageSource.)

Life Review

Robert Butler (1963) first noted and brought to public attention the review process that normally occurs in the older person as the realization of his or her approaching death creates a resurgence of unresolved conflicts. Butler called this process *life review*. Life review occurs quite naturally for many persons during periods of crisis and transition. However, Butler (2002) noted that in old age, the process of putting one's life in order increases in intensity and emphasis. Life review occurs most frequently as an internal review of memories, an intensely private, soul-searching activity.

Life review is considered more of a formal therapy technique than reminiscence and takes a person through his or her life in a structured and chronological order. Life review therapy (Butler and Lewis, 1983), guided autobiography (Birren and Deutchman, 1991), and structured life review (Haight and Webster, 2002) are psychotherapeutic techniques based on the concept of life review. Gerontological nurses participate with older adults in both reminiscence and life review, and it is important to acquire the skills to be effective in achieving the purposes of both of these techniques. Life review may be especially important for older people experiencing depressive symptoms and those facing death (Chan et al, 2014; Pot et al, 2010).

Life review should occur not only when we are old or facing death but also frequently throughout our lives. This process can assist us to examine where we are in life and change our course or set new goals. Butler (2002) commented that ongoing life review by an individual may help avoid the overwhelming feelings of despair that may surface for some individuals at the end of life when there may not be time to make changes. Resources for best practice in communication with older adults and reminiscence are presented in Box 6-4.

◆ PROMOTING HEALTHY AGING: IMPLICATIONS FOR GERONTOLOGICAL NURSING

As each person confronts mortality, there is a need to integrate events and then to transcend the self (Chapter 36). The human experience, the person's contributions, and the poignant anecdotes within the life story bind generations, validate the uniqueness of each brief journey in this level of awareness, and provide the assurance that one will not be forgotten. When the nurse takes the time to listen to an older person share memories and life stories, it communicates respect and valuing of the individual and provides important data for assessment and coming to know the person. What more can one ask at the end of life than to know that who one is and what one has accomplished hold personal meaning and meaning for others as well?

COMMUNICATING WITH GROUPS OF OLDER ADULTS

Group work with older adults has been used extensively in institutional settings to meet a myriad of needs in an economical manner. Nurses have led groups of older people for a variety of therapeutic reasons. Expert gerontological nurses, such as Irene Burnside and Priscilla Ebersole, have extensively discussed advantages of group work both for older people and for group leaders and have provided in-depth guidelines for conducting groups. Box 6-5 presents some of the benefits of group work.

Many groups can be managed effectively by staff with clear goals and guidance and training. Volunteers, nursing assistants, students, and recreational staff can be taught to conduct many types of groups, but groups with a psychotherapy focus require a trained and skilled leader. Perese et al. (2008) and Heliker (2009) provide excellent suggestions for group reminiscence therapy and story-sharing interventions. Some basic considerations for group work are presented in this chapter, but nurses interested in working with groups of older people should consult a text on group work for more in-depth information.

Groups can be implemented in many settings, including adult day health programs, retirement communities, assisted living facilities, nutrition sites, and nursing homes. Examples of groups include reminiscence groups, psychoeducational groups, caregiver support groups, and groups for people with memory impairment or other conditions such as Parkinson's disease or stroke. Groups can be organized to meet any level of human need; some meet multiple needs.

BOX 6-4   RESOURCES FOR BEST PRACTICE

Communication

Center for Digital Storytelling, Berkeley, CA

Gerontological Society of America: *Communicating with older adults: an evidence-based review of what really works,* Washington, DC, 2012, Author

International Institute for Reminiscence and Life Review, University of Wisconsin, Superior, WI

Laurenhue K: *Getting to know the life stories of older adults: activities for building relationships,* Baltimore, MD, 2007, Health Professions Press

Roberts B: *I remember when: activity ideas to help people reminisce,* Herefordshire, U.K., 2000, Elder Books

---

BOX 6-5   Benefits of Group Work with Elders

- Group experiences provide older adults with an opportunity to try new roles—those of teacher, expert, storyteller, or even clown.
- Groups may improve communication skills for lonely, shy, or withdrawn older people, as well as those with communication disorders or memory impairment.
- Groups provide peer support and opportunities to share common experiences, and they may foster the development of warm friendships that endure long after the group has ended.
- The group may be of interest to other residents, staff, and relatives and may improve satisfaction and morale. Staff, in particular, may come to see their patients in a different light—not just as persons needing care but as persons.
- Active listening and interest in what older people have to say may improve self-esteem and help them feel like worthwhile persons whose wisdom is valued.
- Group work offers the opportunity for leaders to be creative and use many modalities, such as music, art, dance, poetry, exercise, and current events.
- Groups provide an opportunity for the leader to assess the person's mood, cognitive abilities, and functional level on a weekly basis.

Adapted from Burnside IM: Group work with older persons, *J Gerontol Nurs* 20:43, 1994.

BOX 6-6 Special Considerations in Group Work with Elders

- The leader must pay special attention to sensory losses and compensate for vision and hearing loss.
- Pacing is different, and group leaders must slow down in both physical and psychological actions depending on the group's abilities.
- Group members often need assistance or transportation to the group, and adequate time must be allowed for assembling the members and assisting them to return to their homes or rooms.
- Time of day a group is scheduled is important. Meeting time should not conflict with bathing and eating schedules, and evening groups may not be good for older people, who may be tired by then. For community-based older people, transportation logistics may become complicated in the evening.
- Having a warm and friendly climate of acceptance of each member and showing appreciation and enjoyment of the group and each member's contribution are all important.
- Groups generally should include people with similar levels of cognitive ability. Mixing very intact elders with those who have memory and communication impairments calls for special skills. Burnside (1994) suggests that in groups of people with varying abilities, alert persons tend to ask, "Will I become like them?" whereas the people with memory and communication impairments may become anxious when they are aware that they cannot perform as well as the other members.
- Many older people likely to be in need of groups may be depressed or have experienced a number of losses (health, friends, spouse). Discussion of losses and sad feelings can be difficult for group leaders. A leader prone to depression would not be appropriate.

- Remind members of the termination date for the group so that they can prepare and not experience another loss.
- Leaders must be prepared for some members to become ill, deteriorate, and die. Plans regarding recognition of missing members will need to be clear. The following, which occurred during a reminiscence group conducted by one of the authors (T.T.), illustrates this: "As I arrived at the nursing home for the weekly reminiscence group meeting, I was told by the nursing home staff that one of our members had died. One of the members had been a priest, so we asked him to say a prayer for our deceased group member. He did so beautifully, and the group was grateful. The next week, to our surprise, the supposedly deceased member showed up for the group (she had been in the hospital). We didn't know how to handle the situation, but the other members came to our rescue by saying, 'Father's prayers really worked this time.'" Older people's wisdom and humor can teach us a lot.
- Leaders are continually confronted with their own aging and attitudes toward it. Co-leaders are ideal and can support each other. If leading the group alone, locate someone with expertise in group work with elders who can discuss the group experiences with you and provide support and direction. Students generally should work in pairs and will need supervision. Skills in developing and implementing groups for older adults improve with experience. Burnside (1994) reminds us that "all new group leaders should have guidance from an experienced leader to help them weather the difficult times" (p. 43).
- Evaluate each group session and the total group experience. Involve the group members in the evaluation.

Source: Burnside IM: Group work with older persons, *J Gerontol Nurs* 20:43, 1994; Stinson C: Structured group reminiscence: an intervention for older adults, *J Contin Educ Nurs* 40(11):521–528, 2009.

Group Structure and Special Considerations

Implementing a group intervention follows a thorough assessment of environment, needs, and the potential for various group strategies. Major decisions regarding goals will influence the strategy selected. For instance, individuals with diabetes in an acute care setting may need health care teaching regarding diabetes. The nurse sees the major goal as education and restoring order (or control) in each individual's lifestyle. The strategy best suited for that would be motivational or educational. A group of people experiencing mild neurocognitive impairment (dementia) may benefit from a support group to express feelings or a group that teaches memory-enhancing strategies. Successful group work depends on organization, attention to details, agency support, assessment and consideration of the older person's needs and status, and caring, sensitive, and skillful leadership.

Group work with older people is different from that with younger age groups; and there are some unique aspects that require special skills and training and an extraordinary commitment on the part of the leader. Although these unique aspects may not apply to all types of groups of older adults, some strategies are presented in Box 6-6.

◆ PROMOTING HEALTHY AGING: IMPLICATIONS FOR GERONTOLOGICAL NURSING

Throughout this chapter we have tried to convey the potential for honest and hopeful communication with individuals as they age. Communicating with older people requires special skills, patience, and respect. We must break through the barriers and continue to reach toward the humanity of the individual with the belief that communication is the most vital service we offer. This is the heart of nursing. Skilled, sensitive, and caring individual and group communication strategies with older adults are essential to meeting needs and are the basis for therapeutic nursing relationships. Just as all people have the need to communicate and have their basic needs met, they also have the right to experiences that are meaningful and fulfilling. Age, language impairment, or mental status does not change these needs.

▮ KEY CONCEPTS

- Communication is a basic need regardless of age or impairment.
- The life history of an individual is a story to be developed and treasured. This is particularly important toward the end of life.
- Storytelling is a complementary and alternative therapy that nurses can use to come to know older adults and enhance communication.

- In a rapidly changing society, the shared life histories of elders provide a sense of continuity among the generations.
- Group work can meet many needs and is satisfying and rewarding for both the older adult and the group leader.

CRITICAL THINKING QUESTIONS AND ACTIVITIES

1. Observe communication styles of people talking to older people, e.g., in restaurants, stores, and in the health care setting. Do you see examples of elderspeak?
2. Watch some commercials on television that feature older people. What image do they portray?
3. Ask an elder whom you know to tell you their life story. Reflect on whether or not you learned anything surprising.
4. If you were going to create a digital life story of your own life, what kinds of music, pictures, and artifacts would you include to help people know about your life?
5. Sit with another student and share your life stories. Reflect on what this exercise meant to you and to the other person.

RESEARCH QUESTIONS

1. Are there particular care settings and activities in which elderspeak is more prevalent?
2. What benefits do older people experience in sharing their life stories?
3. Can digital storytelling be used to promote more positive attitudes toward older people among nursing students?
4. Does the use of reminiscence and storytelling lead to more holistic assessment of older people?

REFERENCES

Agency for Healthcare Research and Quality: *Weekly group storytelling enhances verbal skills*, encourages positive behavior change, and reduces confusion in patients with Alzheimer's and related dementias, AHRQ Innovations Exchange, 2014. https://innovations.ahrq.gov/profiles/weekly-group-storytelling-enhances-verbal-skills-encourages-positive-behavior-change and https://innovations.ahrq.gov/. Accessed October 2014.

Bastings A: Reading the story behind the story: context and content in stories by people with dementia, *Generations* 27:25–29, 2003.

Bastings A: Arts in dementia care: "This is not the end…it's the end of this chapter," *Generations* 30:16–20, 2006.

Bergman Y, Bodner E, Cohen-Fridel S: Cross-cultural ageism: ageism and attitudes toward aging among Jews and Arabs in Israel, *Int Psychogeriatr* 25(1): 6–15, 2013.

Birren JE, Deutchman DE: *Guiding autobiography groups for older adults: exploring the fabric of life*, Baltimore, 1991, Johns Hopkins University Press.

Bohlmeijer E, Smit F, Cuijpers P: Effects of reminiscence and life review on late-life depression: a meta-analysis, *Int J Geriatr Psychiatry* 18:1088–1094, 2003.

Burnside IM: Group work with older persons, *J Gerontol Nurs* 20:43, 1994.

Buron B: Life history collages: effects on nursing home staff caring for residents with dementia, *J Gerontol Nurs* 36(12): 38–48, 2010.

Butler R: The life review: an interpretation of reminiscence in the aged, *Psychiatry* 26:65–76, 1963.

Butler R: Age-ism: another form of bigotry, *Gerontologist* 9:243–246, 1969.

Butler R: Age, death and life review. In Doka K, editor: *Living with grief: loss in later life*, Washington, DC, 2003, Hospice Foundation.

Butler R, Lewis M: *Aging and mental health: positive psychosocial approaches*, ed 3, St. Louis, MO, 1983, Mosby.

Cappeliez P: Neglected issue and new orientations for research and practice in reminiscence and life review, *Int J Reminiscence Life Rev* 1(1):19–25, 2013.

Chan M, Leong K, Heng B, et al: Reducing depression among community-dwelling older adults using life-story review: a pilot study, *Geriatr Nurs* 35:105–110, 2014.

Coles R: *The call of stories*, Boston, 1989, Houghton Mifflin.

Damianakis T, Crete-Nishihata M, Smith K, et al: The psychosocial impacts of multimedia biographies on persons with cognitive impairments, *Gerontologist* 50:23–35, 2010.

Erikson EH: *Childhood and society*, ed 2, New York, 1963, Norton.

Flottemesch K: Learning through narratives: the impact of digital storytelling on intergenerational relationships, *Acad Educ Leadership* 17(3):53–60, 2013.

Fritsch T, Kwak J, Grant S, et al: Impact of TimeSlips, a creative expression intervention program, on nursing home staff and residents with dementia and their caregivers, *The Gerontologist* 49:117–127, 2009.

Gerontological Society of America: *Communicating with older adults: an evidence-based review of what really works*, Washington, DC, 2012, Gerontological Society of America.http://www.agingresources.com/cms/wp-content/uploads/2012/10/GSA_Communicating-with-Older-Adults-low-Final.pdf. Accessed October 31, 2014.

Grabowski D, Aschbrenner K, Tome V, et al: Quality of mental health care for nursing home residents: a literature review, *Med Care Res Rev* 67:627–656, 2010.

Haight B, Burnside IM: Reminiscence and life review: explaining the differences, *Arch Psychiatr Nurs* 7:91–98, 1993.

Haight B, Webster J: *Critical advances in reminiscence work: from theory to application*, New York, 2002, Springer.

Heliker D: Enhancing relationships in long-term care through story-sharing, *J Gerontol Nurs* 35(6):43–49, 2009.

Herman R, Williams K: Elderspeak's influence on resistiveness to care: focus on behavioral events, *Am J Alzheimers Dis Other Demen* 24:417–423, 2009.

International Longevity Center, Anti-ageism Task Force: *Ageism in America*. New York, 2006, International Longevity Center.

Kydd T, Touhy T, Newman D, et al: Attitudes toward caring for older people in Scotland, Sweden and the United States, *Nurs Older People* 26(2):33–40, 2014.

Latha K, Bhandury P, Tejaswini S, et al: Reminiscence therapy: an overview, *Middle East J Age Ageing* 11(1):18–22, 2014.

Levy B, Slade M, Kunkel S, et al: Longevity increased by positive perceptions of aging, *J Pers Soc Psych* 83:261–270, 2002.

Levy BR, Leifheit-Limson E: The stereotype-matching effect: greater influence on functioning when age stereotypes correspond to outcomes, *Psychol Aging* 24:230–233, 2009.

Lombardi N, Buchanan J, Afflerbach S, et al: Is elderspeak appropriate? A survey of certified nursing assistants, *J Gerontol Nurs* Apr 14:1–8, 2014. doi: 10.3928/00989134-20140407-02. [Epub ahead of print].

Levy BR, Zonderman A, Slade M, et al: Age stereotypes held earlier in life predict cardiovascular events in later life, *Psychol Sci* 20:296–298, 2009.

Moss M: Storytelling. In Lindquist R, Snyder M, Tracy M, editors: *Complementary and alternative therapies in nursing*, ed 7, New York, 2014, Springer, pp 215–228.

Mudiwa L: *The online future of reminiscence therapy*, Nov 24, 2010, Irish Medical Times. http://www.imt.ie/features-opinion/2010/11/the-online-future-of-reminiscence-therapy.html

O'Rourke N, Carmel S, Chaudhury H, et al: A cross-national comparison of reminiscence functions between Canadian and Israeli older adults, *J Gerontol B Psychol Sci Soc Sci* 68(2):184–192, 2012.

Perese E, Simon M, Ryan E: Promoting positive student clinical experiences with older adults through the use of group reminiscence therapy, *J Gerontol Nurs* 34(12):46–51, 2008.

Pinquart M, Forstmeier S: Effects of reminiscence on psychosocial outcomes: a meta-analysis, *Aging Ment Health* 16:1–18, 2012.

Pot A, Bahlmeijer E, Onrust S, et al: The impact of life review on depression in older adults: a randomized controlled trial, *Int Psychogeriatr* 22:572–585, 2010.

Preschl B, Maercker A, Wagner B, et al: Life-review therapy with computer supplements for depression in the elderly: a randomized control trial, *Aging Ment Health* 16:964–974, 2012.

Ramírez-Esparza N, Pennebaker J: Do good stories produce good health? Exploring words, language and culture, *Narrat Inq* 16(11):211–219, 2006.

Rogers S, Thrasher A, Miao Y, et al: Discrimination in healthcare settings is associated with disability in older adults: Health and Retirement Study, 2009-2012, *Jour General Internal Medicine:* published onine March 13, 2015, 10.1007/s11606-015-3233-6.

Rowe JW, Kahn RL: *Successful aging*, New York, 1998, Pantheon Books.

Stinson C: Structured group reminiscence: an intervention for older adults, *J Contin Educ Nurs* 40(11):521–528, 2009.

Touhy T, Williams C: Communicating with older adults. In Williams C, editor: *Therapeutic interaction in nursing*, ed 2, Boston, 2008, Jones & Bartlett.

Van Leuven KA: Health practices of older adults in good health: engagement is the key, *J Gerontol Nurs* 36:38–46, 2010.

Williams K: Improving outcomes of nursing home interactions, *Res Nurs Health* 29:121–133, 2006.

Williams K, Herman R, Gajewski B, et al: Elderspeak communication: impact on dementia care, *Am J Alzheimers Dis Other Demen* 24:11–20, 2008.

Williams K, Kemper S, Hummert L: Enhancing communication with older adults: overcoming elderspeak, *J Gerontol Nurs* 30:17–25, 2004.

Williams K, Kemper S, Hummert L: Improving nursing home communication: an intervention to reduce elderspeak, *Gerontologist* 43:242–247, 2003.

Williams C, Tappen R: Communicating with cognitively impaired persons. In Williams C, editor: *Therapeutic interaction in nursing*, ed 2, Boston, 2008, Jones & Bartlett.

Health Assessment

Kathleen Jett

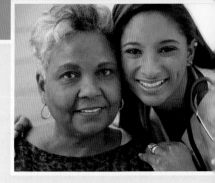

e http://evolve.elsevier.com/Touhy/TwdHlthAging

A STUDENT SPEAKS

It takes so long to get a health history from an older person—they have so many stories. I now know to listen carefully, and I will find out what I need to know to give good nursing care. After all, most of them have had their health problems longer than I have been alive!

Michelle, age 20

AN ELDER SPEAKS

Whenever I go to one of my doctors I feel like they are rushing through and never really give me a good examination. Then I had an appointment with a nurse practitioner who specializes in us older folks. I couldn't believe the difference. I not only felt listened to, but I also felt like I got the best exam I have had in a long time. I am sure she will help me get better!

Henry at age 76

LEARNING OBJECTIVES

On completion of this chapter, the reader will be able to:

1. Identify the findings of the physical assessment of older adults that differ in meaning from those for younger adults.
2. List the essential components of a comprehensive health assessment of an older adult.
3. Discuss the advantages and disadvantages of the use of standardized assessment instruments.
4. Describe the purpose of the functional assessment when caring for an older adult.

In the promotion of healthy aging, gerontological nurses conduct skilled and detailed assessments of, and with, the persons who entrust themselves to their care. The process is strikingly different from that of younger adults in that it is more complex, even when it is limited to a particular problem. A comprehensive assessment may be performed by a team of professionals for several reasons, such as when a person is being admitted to a health care facility for a specific reason, or enrolling in an insurance plan (e.g., Medicare), or being seen by a provider for the first time.

Assessment of the older adult requires the following special skills—to listen patiently, to allow for pauses, to ask questions that are not often asked, to observe minute details, to obtain data from all available sources, and to recognize the normal changes associated with late life that might be considered abnormal in one who is younger. In gerontological nursing, assessment takes more time than it does with younger adults because of the increased medical, functional, and social complexities of having lived longer. When it is necessary to use a medical interpreter, approximately double the amount of time

will be needed for the assessment (see Chapter 4). The quality and speed of the assessment are arts born of experience. Novice nurses should neither be expected to nor expect themselves to do this quickly, but should expect to see their skills and efficiency increase over time.

According to Benner (1984), assessment is a task for the expert. However, an expert is not always available. Nurses at all skill levels can learn to conduct health assessments that promote healthy aging when using a high degree of compassion, being aware of the normal changes with aging, and knowing how and when to use reliable instruments.

The assessment provides information critical to goal setting and leads to the development of a plan of care that enhances healthy aging, decreases the potential for complications related to chronic conditions, and increases elders' self-efficacy and self-care empowerment. The nurse uses the results of the initial assessment as a baseline, in other words, a snapshot of the person's health status at that point in time. Subsequent assessments are used for comparison and modification of goals as the person moves along the wellness trajectory. Health assessment is a complex process that requires entire textbooks to address in detail. Specialized aspects of the assessment can be found in chapters in this text specific to the issue, such as falls, continence, caregiver burden, and safety. In this chapter we provide an overview of key aspects of the geriatric assessment and a discussion of instruments that are unique to, or helpful in, caring for the older adult.

THE HEALTH HISTORY

The health history marks the beginning of the nurse-patient relationship in the assessment process. It is the subjective report of health and is collected through the completion of a form by the patient in advance of the health care contact, through a face-to-face interview, or, most often, in a combination of the two (Box 7-1). The data needed for the health history include demographic information, a past medical history, current medications and dietary supplements (prescribed, over-the-counter, "home remedies," and herbals), social and functional histories, and finally the review of systems. The health history in an older adult will take longer because of both the high number of concurrent illnesses and the unknown etiologies of some of these.

The social component of the health history is often a part of the functional history and assessment. Several of the instruments discussed later in this chapter address the collection of data for the social health history. It is very important that the social history includes information about those who are involved in health care decision-making, such as health care proxies or surrogates, and the presence or absence of living wills (Chapters 31 and 35).

A discussion of functional status may be one of the more difficult parts of the health history because it deals with the person's ability to manage independently or to need assistance. This must be discussed with the utmost tact to avoid embarrassing the person who has developed limitations, such as the inability to hold a spoon without spilling its contents because of tremors. In some Asian countries such an admission runs counter to the cultural concept of "saving face," where it is necessary to preserve dignity, or at least its appearance, at all costs (Kim et al, 2004). Most often, the history of functional status is in the form of a screening tool, several of which are discussed later in this chapter.

Review of Systems (ROS)

The review of systems (ROS) is often conducted immediately before or during a physical exam. In a younger adult it is likely to be quick and limited to the system involved with the symptom at hand. However, as one ages and collects health problems, this review becomes more complex and time consuming because one system affects another. The ROS may be more aptly referred to as a "review of symptoms," which becomes the focus of the assessment. When there are no particular presenting symptoms, the ROS begins with the areas where problems are most likely to be problematic simply attributable to the normal changes with aging (Box 7-2) or the health problems most often encountered in the country, race, ethnicity, or socioeconomic class of the patient.

It is ideal to obtain the history from the elder himself or herself. This allows the gerontological nurse to better understand the person's priorities. If this is not possible, it is necessary to obtain the information from a proxy, that is, someone who knows the person well and has permission to speak on the patient's behalf. In some cases, the person with a cognitive impairment can still be part of the process when simple language is used, such as "Are you having any pain today?" or "Where are you hurting?"

The explanatory model provides questions to supplement the usual data collected in the health history and is particularly helpful. It will better enable the nurse to understand the older adult and plan individually designed and effective interventions (Box 7-3) (Kleinman, 1980).

PHYSICAL ASSESSMENT

The physical assessment is followed by, or at the same time as, the review of systems, depending on the stamina of the patient or other time constraints. When a comprehensive exam is needed, this is often done in two visits or more contacts, depending on the level of complexity of the current health problems and functional status.

Many of the manual techniques of the physical examination, such as the use of the otoscope, do not differ from those used with younger adults; however, it is always necessary to consider the normal changes with aging and their effect on both the exam and the findings (Box 7-4). When either physical or cognitive limitations are present (Box 7-5), it is not always possible to perform these tests as precisely as is ideal in all settings. For example, in the outpatient setting, a thorough abdominal exam may not be possible if the person cannot get to a lying position because of arthritis, kyphosis, or other skeletal deformity. Instead, the best that can be done is for the person to lean as far back in the chair as possible and then for the examiner to auscultate, percuss, and palpate as usual. (This is documented as a "limited abdominal exam.") It is highly unlikely that a complete "head-to-toe" exam is done, except under special circumstances (Box 7-6) (Zambas, 2010). It is always best that the exam begin with the presenting problem(s), the associated systems, and the problems/symptoms that place the person at most risk, such as evidence of any of the geriatric syndromes (Box 7-7). In many cases, the aspects of the exam that require special attention are determined by the setting and purpose of the assessment. It is

---

BOX 7-1   Factors Affecting the Collection of Information for the Health History
Visual and auditory acuity
Manual dexterity
Language and health fluency
Adequacy of translation of materials
Availability of a trained interpreter
Cognitive ability and reading level

BOX 7-2   TIPS FOR BEST PRACTICE

Areas of Emphasis When Conducting a Review of Systems with an Older Adult

Constitutional
- Changes in the level of energy

Senses
- Changes in vision, in hearing acuity, and in the situations or complaints of others related to these
- Increase in dental caries; changes in taste, bleeding gums, or level of current dental care
- Changes in smell

Respiratory
- Shortness of breath and, if so, under what circumstances
- Frequency of respiratory problems
- Need to sleep in chair or elevated on pillows

Cardiac
- Chest, shoulder, or jaw pain and under what circumstances
- If already taking antianginal medication such as nitroglycerin, whether there is a need for more than usual dosage
- Sense of heart palpitations
- If using anticoagulants, and evidence of bruising or bleeding

Vascular
- Cramping of extremities, decreased sensation (see also neurological), edema, what time of the day and how much
- Change of color to the skin, especially increased pigment to the lower extremities, cyanosis, or any other change in color

Urinary
- Changes in urine stream and for how long; difficulty starting stream
- Incontinence and, if so, under what circumstances and degree

Sexual
- Desire and ability to continue physical sexual activity
- Ability to express other forms of intimacy
- Changes with aging that may affect sexuality (e.g., vaginal dryness, erectile dysfunction)

Musculoskeletal
- Pain in joints, back, or muscles
- Changes in gait and sense of safety in ambulation
- If stiffness is present, when is it the worst and is it relieved by activity?
- If limited, effect on day-to-day life

Neurological
- Changes in sensation, especially in extremities
- Changes in memory other than very minimal
- Ability to continue usual cognitive activities
- Changes in sense of balance or episodes of dizziness
- History of falls, trips, slips

Gastrointestinal
- Continence, constipation, bloating, anorexia

Integument
- Dryness, frequency of injury, and speed of healing
- Itching, dryness, history of skin cancer

BOX 7-3   The Explanatory Model for Culturally Sensitive Assessment

1. How would you describe the problem that has brought you here? (What do you call your problem; does it have a name?)
   a. Who is involved in your decision-making processes about health concerns?
2. How long have you had this problem?
   a. When do you think it started?
   b. What do you think started it?
   c. Do you know anyone else with it?
   d. Tell me what happened to that person when dealing with this problem.
3. What do you think is wrong with you?
   a. How severe is it?
   b. How long do you think it will last?
4. Why do you think this happened to you?
   a. Why has it happened to the involved part?
   b. What do you fear most about your sickness?
5. What are the chief problems your sickness has caused you?
6. What do you think will help this problem? (What treatment should you receive and what are the most important results you hope to receive?)
   a. If specific tests, medications are listed, ask what they are and do.
7. Apart from me, who else do you think can make you feel better?
   a. Are there therapies that make you feel better that I do not know? (Maybe in another discipline?)

Modified from Kleinman A: *Patient and healers in the context of culture: an exploration of the borderland between anthropology, medicine, and psychiatry,* Berkeley, 1980, University of California Press.

always necessary to be aware of cultural rules of etiquette and taboos that influence the physical examination (Box 7-8).

Instruments for Use When Conducting a Physical Assessment

To address the complex interrelationship between parts of the physical assessment, standardized, evidence-based instruments have proven helpful. The websites of the Hartford Institute for Geriatric Nursing (http://hartfordign.org) and the Iowa Geriatric Research Center (http://www.nursing.uiowa.edu/hartfor.) provide a compilation of key tools for individual use. In some cases, videos demonstrating their use are included. These sites are portals of a wealth of information, especially for assessing specific conditions or situations.

Two early instruments include mnemonics to assist gerontological nurses to remember the parts of the exam and therefore serve as useful guides. These are *SPICES* and *FANCAPES*. The resultant findings will indicate the domain where more detailed assessments are needed, many of which are discussed in subsequent chapters.

FANCAPES

The mnemonic *FANCAPES* stands for Fluids, Aeration, Nutrition, Communication, Activity, Pain, Elimination, and Socialization. The guide was developed by Barbara Bent (2005) in her work as a geriatric resource nurse at Missouri Hospital in Ashville, North Carolina. It has broad applicability in any setting.

BOX 7-4   TIPS FOR BEST PRACTICE

Considerations of Common Changes Specific to Late Life during the Physical Assessment

Height and Weight
- Monitor for changes in weight.
- Weight gain: especially important if the person has any heart disease; be alert for early signs of heart failure.
- Weight loss: be alert for indications of malnutrition from dental problems, depression, or cancer. Check for mouth lesions from ill-fitting dentures. There is an increased rate of mortality for rapid weight loss in persons with dementia.

Temperature
- Even a low-grade fever could be an indication of a serious illness. Temperatures as low as 100° C may indicate pending sepsis.

Blood Pressure
- Positional blood pressure readings should be obtained because of the high occurrence of orthostatic hypotension (drop of 20/10 mm Hg or more when changing from sitting to standing). Isolated systolic hypertension is common. Common auscultatory gap heard due to high rate of hypertension.

Skin
- Check for indications of solar damage, especially among persons who worked outdoors or live in sunny climates. Due to thinning, "tenting" is not a good indicator of hydration status. Examine bruises.

Ears
- As a result of drying cerumen, impactions are common. These must be removed before hearing can be adequately assessed.

Hearing
- High-frequency hearing loss (presbycusis) is common. Whisper test of little utility. The person often complains that he or she can hear but not understand because some, but not all, sounds are lost, such as consonants. The person with severe but unrecognized hearing loss may be incorrectly thought to have dementia.

Eyes
- Reduced pupillary responsiveness (miosis). Normal if equal bilaterally. Gray ring around the iris (arcus senilis). Sagging of lids. Position of lids.

Vision
- Increased glare sensitivity, decreased contrast sensitivity, and need for more light to see and read. Ensure that waiting rooms, hallways, and exam rooms are adequately lit.
- Decreased color discrimination may affect ability to self-administer medications safely.

Mouth
- Excessive dryness common and exacerbated by many medications. Cannot use mouth moisture to estimate hydration status. Periodontal disease common. Decreased sense of taste. Tooth surface abraded.

Neck
- Because of loss of subcutaneous fat it may appear that carotid arteries are enlarged when they are not.

Chest
- Any kyphosis will alter the location of the lobes, making careful assessment more important. Crackles in lower lobes may clear with cough.
- Risk for aspiration pneumonia increased and therefore the importance of the lateral exam and measurement of oxygen saturation.

Heart
- Listen carefully for third and fourth heart sounds. Fourth heart sounds common. Determine if this has been found to be present in the past or is new. Up to 50% of persons have heart murmur.

Extremities
- Dorsalis pedis and posterior tibial pulses very difficult or impossible to palpate. Must look for other indications of vascular integrity. Edema common.

Abdomen
- Because of deposition of fat in the abdomen, auscultation of bowel tones may be difficult.

Musculoskeletal
- Osteoarthritis very common and pain often undertreated. Ask about pain and function in joints. Conduct very gentle passive range-of-motion exercises if active range-of-motion exercises not possible. Do not push past comfort level. Observe for gait disorders. Observe the person get in and out of chair in order to assess independent function and fall risk.

Neurological
- Although there is a gradual decrease in muscle strength, it still should remain equal bilaterally. Greatly diminished or absent ankle jerk (Achilles) tendon reflex is common and normal. Decreased or absent vibratory sense of the lower extremities, testing unnecessary. Slowed reflexes. Coherence, memory. Verbal fluency should be intact.

Genitourinary: Male
- Pendulous scrotum with less rugae; smaller penis; thin and graying pubic hair.

Genitourinary: Female
- Small to nonpalpable ovaries; short, dryer vagina; decreased size of labia and clitoris; sparse pubic hair. Use utmost care with exam to avoid trauma to the tissues.

BOX 7-5   An Abbreviated Exam

Alice has severe dementia. She spends most of her time walking around the unit where she lives. When she gets tired she lays down in whatever bed she is near, occupied or not. When an exam in the outpatient clinic was needed, the only way we could exam her was to very quietly and gently "follow her around" as she wandered. An aide was with her and knew exactly how to redirect her back to the clinic hallway.

F: Fluids. An assessment of a person's state of hydration (fluids) includes those physiological, situational, functional, and mental factors that contribute to the maintenance of its adequacy. Attention is directed to the ability of the person to obtain adequate fluids independently, to express thirst, and to swallow effectively. Medications are reviewed to identify those with the potential to affect intake. This is especially important when working with older adults who are not able to independently access fluids because of functional

BOX 7-6   Select Components of the Welcome to Medicare Exam*

Comprehensive review of medical and social history
Assessment of risk for depression
Assessment of functional ability and safety
Brief education related to the identified risk factors and the development of a plan to address these factors

*These are often conducted by advanced practice gerontological nurse practitioners. There is no charge to the patient. See Chapter 30 for more detail.
For more information see: www.cms.gov/Outreach-and-Education/Medicare-Learning-Network-MLN/MLNProducts/downloads/AWV_Chart_ICN905706.pdf.

BOX 7-7   Geriatric Syndromes*

Falls and gait abnormalities
Frailty
Delirium
Urinary incontinence
Sleep disorders
Pressure ulcers

*Note that there is considerable discussion about the exact "conditions" that are considered "geriatric syndrome." There is agreement that a syndrome is something that does not neatly fit into another disease category. From Brown-O'Hara T: Geriatric syndromes and their implications for nursing, *Nursing* 43(1):1–3, 2013.

BOX 7-8   Key Points to Consider in Observing Cultural Rules and Etiquette

- Be aware of past experiences in the health care setting.
- Ask if there are persons (e.g., males in the family) who need to be present or involved in some way with the exam.
- Respect the communication style used, especially in the health care setting.
- Do not intrude into personal space without permission.
- Determine general health orientation related to time (past, present, future).
- Inquire as to appropriate wording reference to the person; presume use of last name unless otherwise welcomed.
- Inquiry as to acceptable level of touch and gender of provider.

limitations, or for anyone with the reduced sense of thirst, a common change with aging (Chapters 14 and 15).

A: Aeration. Because of the close relationship between pulmonary function (aeration) and cardiovascular function, these are assessed simultaneously. Careful pulmonary auscultation in the older adult should include the lateral aspects of the lower lobes, which are part of every exam but are particularly important in assessing the older adult. The measurement of the oxygen saturation rate is a part of this exam and easily done in any setting with a small, inexpensive fingertip device. Those with any amount of chronic peripheral cyanosis will have artificially low readings. Assessment of the respiratory rate and depth at rest and with activity should be done any time respiratory or cardiac compromise is suspected (Chapter 24). Assessment of the cardiovascular system is addressed in Chapter 22.

N: Nutrition. Protein-calorie malnutrition is common among the frail and those who live alone or are socially isolated. Nutritional assessment is a complex process but especially important in frail elders or those with dementia. For the frail elder who is losing weight, even with an adequate intake, the risk for mortality escalates considerably. Assessment of nutritional status and gerontological nurses' responses to alterations in nutrition are addressed in Chapter 14.

C: Communication. While the assessment of communication in the healthy older adult may be the same as that of a younger adult, many of those who are aging today have the potential to have, or already have, some level of communication impairment such as those associated with dysarthria (motor speech disorder affecting muscles of mouth and face and therefore speech). Assessment includes the physical capacity to communicate effectively, with visual and auditory acuity that is adequate enough to negotiate the environment and meet self-care needs. The impoverished childhoods of some and racist educational practices for others, even in developed countries, have resulted in very low literacy levels, and communicating health information cannot take the usual route of written materials. Inadequate assessment of communication by the nurse will lead to erroneous conclusions and significantly reduce the quality of care and health outcomes. Assessment of communication is discussed in detail in Chapter 6.

A: Activity. The ability to continue to ambulate safely and the capacity to participate in enjoyable physical activities are important parts of healthy aging. However, activity assessment is exceedingly complex because of the range of abilities among those referred to as "older adults." As more baby boomers join this group, the complexity of assessment increases. It ranges from the risk for falling; to the need for, and correct use of, assistive devices; to the degree to which one can participate in aerobic exercises. Assessment of activity abilities may be accomplished by the combined efforts of nurses, physical therapists, and personal trainers (Chapters 18 to 19).

P: Pain. The assessment of pain includes that which is physical, psychological, and spiritual. One rarely occurs in isolation. Many nurses hear their patients implore, "What did I do to deserve this [pain]?" A number of evidence-based instruments have been developed for the assessment of physical pain in persons with and without cognitive difficulties. Because of the increasing amount of pain common with each decade of life (e.g., progression of arthritis or number of losses), this deserves particular attention by gerontological nurses (Chapter 27).

E: Elimination. Although difficulties with bowel and bladder functioning are not normal parts of aging, they are more common than they are in younger adults and can be triggered by such things as immobility attributable to physical limitations (e.g., post-stroke) or medications (e.g., diuretics). Incontinence can result from cognitive changes that may cause a reduced, or even nonexistent, sensation indicating a need to void or defecate. There are many elimination problems for older adults living in institutional settings where they are dependent on others for assistance to maintain continence (e.g., getting to the toilet in time). If the person is having a problem with bowel or bladder functioning, including

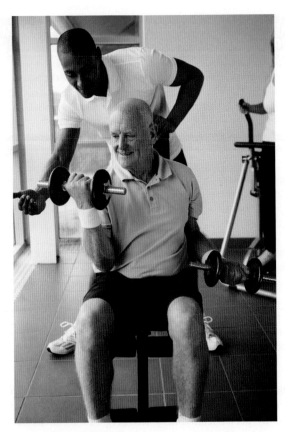

©iStock.com/Dean Mitchell.

FANCAPES, anything that indicates a problem in one of the categories warns the nurse that more in-depth assessment is needed. It is a system for alerting the nurse about problems that are interfering with the person's health and well-being, particularly those who have one or more unstable medical conditions or are at risk for further physical and functional decline.

FUNCTIONAL ASSESSMENT

Whereas FANCAPES and SPICES address primarily physical parameters, a functional assessment is the evaluation of a person's ability to carry out the tasks needed for self-care and those needed to support independent living. Other aspects of the functional assessment include the individual's ability to negotiate physical and social environments. The functional assessment helps the gerontological nurse work with the individual to move toward healthy aging by accomplishing the following:

- Identifying the specific areas in which help is needed or not needed
- Identifying changes in abilities from one time to another
- Providing information that may be useful in assessing the safety of a particular living situation.

Evidence-based instruments are available to screen, describe, monitor, and predict an individual's ability to perform the activities or tasks needed for daily living. On most tools the activities are considered mutually exclusive and the scoring is arbitrary. For example, eating is not broken down into its component parts, such as picking up a cup or swallowing water. It is seen as a total task, when in reality, a person may be able to perform one part and not the other. In several of the tools, ability is rated and scored as (1) is able to do the task alone, (2) needs assistance, or (3) is not able to perform the task at all. The ratings are done by self-report, proxy, or observation. This type of scoring is not sensitive to small changes and can only be used as part of a holistic assessment. It should be noted that some research has found that self-reports overestimate functional ability and differ from that of proxy report (Sakurai et al, 2013; Stratford et al, 2010). While all of the ADL tasks are universal human needs, the way they are met are socially and culturally constructed. However, the tools are beneficial in that they provide caregivers with a common nomenclature and therefore have the potential to increase the quality of care. When deficits are found in any aspect of functional status, a more detailed assessment is expected of the gerontological nurse or care team.

incontinence and constipation, and it has not been discussed, the assessment begins by "opening the door" to communication about problems that may be embarrassing to admit, much less discuss. The observant nurse may notice the upper edge of an incontinence brief when examining the chest or the advanced practice nurse may notice perigenital irritation when conducting a gynecological exam. Providing a safe and nonjudgmental avenue of communication and finding mutually acceptable and understandable language are ways to approach this difficult topic (Chapter 6). Sensitivity is required to determine if such conversations are even culturally acceptable at all.

S: Social skills. Socialization and social skills include the individual's ability to negotiate in society, to give and receive love and friendship, and to feel self-worth. The type of persons included in one's social network is highly culturally influenced (Box 7-9). Assessment focuses on the individual's ability to deal with loss and to interact with other people in give-and-take situations. Assessment of social skills can be quite complex. It is addressed in more detail in Chapters 33 and 34.

SPICES

As with FANCAPES, the mnemonic "*SPICES*" helps the nurse remember key aspects of the assessment (Fulmer and Wallace, 2012; Montgomery et al., 2008). *SPICES* refers to six common and very serious geriatric syndromes that require nursing interventions: Sleep disorders, Problems with eating, Incontinence, Confusion, Evidence of falls, and Skin breakdown. As with

- Bathing
- Dressing
- Toileting
- Transferring
- Continence
- Feeding/eating

Table 7-1	**Functional Assessment Staging Tool (FAST)**
Stage 1—Normal adult	Shows no functional decline.
Stage 2—Normal older adult	Shows personal awareness of some functional decline.
Stage 3—Early Alzheimer's disease	Demonstrates noticeable deficits in demanding job situations.
Stage 4—Mild Alzheimer's disease	Requires assistance in complicated tasks such as handling finances or planning parties.
Stage 5—Moderate Alzheimer's disease	Requires assistance in choosing proper attire.
Stage 6—Moderately severe Alzheimer's disease	Requires assistance dressing, bathing, and toileting. Experiences urinary and fecal incontinence.
Stage 7—Severe Alzheimer's disease	Speech ability declines to about a half-dozen intelligible words. Demonstrates progressive loss of abilities to walk, sit up, smile, and hold up head.

From Reisberg B: Functional Assessment Staging (FAST), *Psychopharmacol Bull* 24:653–659, 1998. Copyright ©1984 by Barry Reisberg, MD. Reproduced with permission.

Activities of Daily Living

The day-to-day functions related to personal needs are referred to as the *activities of daily living* or *ADLs* (Box 7-10). Two of these tasks (dressing [including grooming] and bathing) require higher cognitive function than the others. The ability to feed oneself, in at least some rudimentary manner, remains intact until late in dementia, assuming other health problems do not interfere, such as a dominant-side stroke.

Katz index. Activities of daily living (ADLs) were first classified as such by Sidney Katz and colleagues in 1963 (Katz et al, 1963). The *Katz index* has served as a basic framework for most of the subsequent measures. On the Katz index the ADLs are considered only in dichotomous terms: the ability to complete the task independently (1 point) or the complete inability to do so (0 points). With equal weight on all activities, this index cannot be used to identify the particular areas of need and cannot show change in any one task. Over the years this instrument has been refined to afford more sensitivity to the nuances of, and changes in, functional status (Nikula et al, 2003).

Barthel index (BI). The *Barthel index* (BI) (Mahoney and Barthel, 1965; Wade and Collin, 1988) is a quick and reliable instrument for the assessment of both mobility and the ability to perform ADLs. It can be completed in 2 to 3 minutes using self-report or in about 20 minutes when direct observation is necessary. The items are rated in various ways, depending on the item. The BI has been found to be sensitive enough to identify when a person first needs help and to measure progress or decline, especially following a stroke (Quinn et al, 2011).

Functional independence measure (FIM). The *functional independence measure* (FIM) was designed to assess a person's need for assistance with ADLs during inpatient stays and for discharge planning, especially following a stroke (Cournan, 2011). In some studies the BI and FIM were found to be comparable (Sangha et al, 2005). In others the FIM was deemed preferable (Kidd et al, 1995). The FIM is a highly sensitive functional assessment tool and includes measures of ADLs, mobility, cognition, and social functioning. The tasks are rated using a seven-point scale from totally independent to totally dependent. Although it is commonly used in acute rehabilitation and veterans administration hospitals in the United States and several other countries (Lundgren-Nilsson et al, 2005; Ottenbacher et al, 1996). Information about this tool is easily found on the web. For related software and training in its use, see http://www.udsmr.org/WebModules/FIM/Fim_About.asp.

FAST. FAST (functional assessment staging tool) is unique in that it is descriptive in nature and specific to the functional changes seen and anticipated in persons with a progressive dementia such as Alzheimer's disease (Table 7-1). It was designed by geriatrician Barry Reisberg (1988) to assist clinicians to identify the level (stage) of ability and, in doing so, help the family know what to expect and how to prepare for the changes ahead. It uses an ordinal scale from stage 1 (no functional impairment associated with any cognitive impairment) to 7 (unable to perform any ADLs associated with very severe [late stage] cognitive impairment). It has been found to be a reliable and valid instrument for the evaluation and staging of functional decline in persons with Alzheimer's disease (Sclan and Reisberg, 1992).

Instrumental Activities of Daily Living

Those activities considered necessary for independent living in many cultures are referred to as *instrumental activities of daily living* or *IADLs* (Box 7-11). This does not mean that the person performs the tasks, just that he or she could perform them if called upon to do so (Box 7-12). It is generally agreed that the ability to perform IADLs requires higher cognitive and physical functioning than do the ADLs.

The Lawton IADL scale. The original *Lawton IADL scale* rated the IADLs from zero (lowest functioning) to eight (highest functioning) (Lawton and Brody, 1969). The level of functioning is determined by a summary score. It may be useful as a screening tool to establish an overall baseline of general functioning, but like the Katz index, it is not sensitive to changes in any one area. The original tool and the subsequent iterations take about 15 minutes to administer using self-report, proxy, or observation. Persons with dementia will progressively lose the ability to perform IADLs beginning with those associated with the highest neuropsychological functioning, such as handling finances and shopping. There are English, Chinese, and

BOX 7-12 Evelyn: Moving from Dependence to Independence

When I first met Evelyn she was 65 and recently widowed. She had married young, moving from her parents' home into that of her husband's. During their entire marriage she had never driven, pumped gas, shopped alone, or taken care of anything but personal and child care, cooking, and house cleaning. She knew nothing about their finances. She had significant IADL deficits but had no choice but to learn how to take care of herself independently after her husband died. She never did learn how to drive very well!

Japanese versions of the tool (APA, 2014). Unfortunately, it may be biased by age and culture (LaPlante, 2010). Fieo and colleagues (2011) have suggested that if some of the IADLs and ADLs were to be combined into a new instrument, it may be more sensitive to change.

FUNCTION AND COGNITION

When conducting health screenings of both function and cognition simultaneously, a slightly different tool is necessary. *The Blessed Dementia Scale* is a 22-item instrument that incorporates aspects of ADLs, IADLs, memory, recall, and finding one's way outdoors (Blessed et al, 1968). If it is administered using self-report, it takes about 10 to 15 minutes. The higher the score, the greater the degree of suspected dementia-related impairment (Chapter 29).

Cognition

Cognition is easily threatened by any disturbance in health or homeostasis. Altered mental status, including reduced cognitive abilities, may be the first sign of anything from a heart attack to a reversible condition such as a urinary tract infection. In a comprehensive assessment, baseline measures of cognition are obtained. However, the gerontological nurse should have the skills to conduct a "quick" assessment when symptoms are reported, expressed, or observed so that the person can be referred or treated promptly. For those with potential problems, any screening or testing is often particularly stressful to the person and significant others. An environment and relationship of trust leads to the most accurate assessment possible with the least amount of embarrassment. Techniques may be honestly described as similar to auscultation of the heart, to "see how the brain is doing." Like most other assessments, these are best administered when the person is comfortable, rested, and free of pain. Gerontological nursing requires the sensitivity to note subtle changes that may indicate a reversible health problem or the need for a more in-depth assessment (see Chapter 29).

Mini-Mental State Examination (MMSE)

For many years the MMSE has been the mainstay for the gross screening of cognitive status (Folstein et al, 1975; Mitchell, 2009). It is a 30-item instrument that is used to screen for and monitor orientation, short-term memory and attention, calculation ability, language, and construction (Wattmo et al, 2011). It has now been revised into a briefer 16-item instrument, the *MMSE-2: BF*, and takes between 10 and 15 minutes to administer. There is also a slightly longer *Expanded Version*. Both are reported to be equivalent to the original instrument and are available in multiple languages. To ensure reliability, the advanced practice nurse must be able to administer them correctly each time they are used. The instruments, permission for use, and instructions can be purchased from the PAR (Psychological Assessments Resources) Company (www.parinc.com).

Clock Drawing Test

The *Clock Drawing Test*, in use since 1992, is reported to be used second most often as the MMSE across the world (Aprahamian et al, 2010; Ehreke et al, 2010). It is not appropriate for use with those who are blind or who have limiting conditions such as tremors, or a stroke that affects their dominant hand. While reading fluency is not necessary, completion of the Clock Test requires number fluency, the ability to hear and see, manual dexterity adequate to hold a pencil, and experience with analog clocks (Box 7-13). Scoring is based on the position of both the numbers and the hands. This tool cannot be used as the sole measure for dementia, but it does test for constructional apraxia, an early indicator (Shulman, 2000) (Figure 7-1). The Clock Test is an evidence-based instrument that has been found to be useful across cultures and languages (Borson et al, 1999).

Mini-Cog

In some settings the use of the *Mini-Cog* has replaced the MMSE as a screening tool for cognitive impairment (Borson et al, 2000). It has been found to be as accurate and reliable as the MMSE but less biased, easier to administer, and possibly more sensitive to dementia (Mitchell and Malladi, 2010). The Mini-Cog combines the test of short-term memory in the original MMSE with the Clock Test (Box 7-14). It has been found to be equally reliable with English-speaking and non–English-speaking individuals (Borson et al, 2003). It takes 3 to 5 minutes to administer and like the other screening tools discussed in this chapter, only serves as an indicator of the need for more detailed assessments leading to diagnosis. It requires number fluency and the ability to hear and see, hold a pencil, and have experience with analog clocks. For more information about this useful tool see The Hartford Institute for Geriatric Nursing, *Try This* series.

Global Deterioration Scale

This scale is very similar to Reisberg's FAST and widely used to "stage" dementia (Reisberg et al, 1982). It uses an ordinal scale

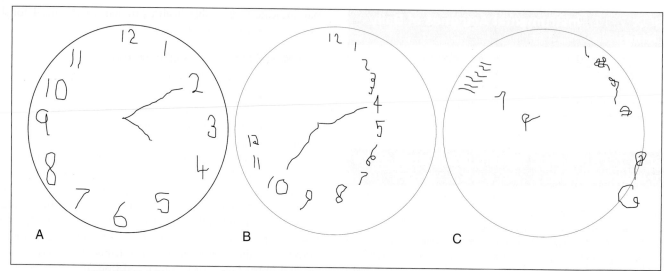

FIGURE 7-1 Examples of Results of a Clock Drawing Test. **A,** Unimpaired; **B** and **C,** impaired. (From Stern TA, Rosenbaum JF, Fava M, et al: *Massachusetts General Hospital comprehensive clinical psychiatry,* St Louis, MO, 2008, Mosby.)

BOX 7-13   Instructions for the Administration of the Mini-Cog and Clock Drawing Tests

1. State three unrelated words, such as "chair," "coin," "tree"; state each word clearly and slowly, about 1 second for each.
2. Ask the person to repeat these words; if the person is unable to do so, you may repeat the words up to 3 times to give the person three attempts to say them back to you correctly.
3. The person is asked to draw a clock as in the Clock Drawing Test.
   a. Provide the person with a piece of plain white paper with a circle drawn on it.
   b. Ask the person to draw numbers in the circle so that it looks like a clock, and then to put the hands in the circle to read "10 after 4."
4. The person is asked to recall the three words from step 1.

BOX 7-14   Scoring of the Mini-Cog and Clock Drawing Tests

Scoring

Points are awarded for recalled words first. The following scoring system is used: none remembered, dementia likely; all three words remembered, dementia unlikely; recall of one or two words upon consideration of the results of the clock drawing, normal (all numbers and hands correct) or abnormal (any errors).

There are several suggestions by psychologists about how the clocks are scored. All consider (1) the symmetry of the numbers (able to plan ahead): if all the numbers are included, repeated, or missed; whether they are inside or outside of the circle; if they appear as numbers; and (2) the hands of the clock: whether the numbers appear at all and if they are in the correct place relative to the numbers (abstract thinking).

---

from stage 1 (no cognitive decline; i.e., no dementia) to 7 (late-state, very severe cognitive decline) that is sensitive enough to show therapeutic changes (e.g., those related to medication adjustments) (Reisberg, 2007). It is used in the United States, including veterans administration hospitals, in Canada, and in many other countries (Alzheimer Society Toronto, 2014).

Nurses can use the scale to help individuals with dementia and their families recognize and prepare for the cognitive changes that are likely (Table 7-2).

ASSESSMENT OF MOOD

Assessment of mood is especially important because of the high rate of depression in late life, either as a side effect of a medication or in association with several health conditions including stroke and Parkinson's disease (Bowker et al, 2012). Older adults with untreated or undertreated depression are more functionally impaired and will have prolonged hospitalizations and nursing home stays, lowered quality of life, and overall increased morbidity and mortality. Persons with depression may appear to have dementia and many persons with dementia are also depressed (Bowker et al, 2012). The interconnection between the two, calls for skill and sensitivity on the part of the nurse to ensure that elders receive the most appropriate, effective, and timely care possible. Although several tools have been used, the most common one is the Geriatric Depression Scale. The Cornell Scale is an observational tool specifically for persons with dementia (Chapter 28).

Geriatric Depression Scale

The Geriatric Depression Scale was developed as a 30-item tool specifically for screening older adults (Brink, 1982; Yesavage et al, 1983). It has been tested extensively with translations in multiple languages (Ortiz and Romero, 2008). A shortened 15-item version is now used (Table 7-3). With the free resources provided by Drs. Yesavage and Brink, the instrument can be completed on an iPhone or Android with an automatic calculation of the results that can be downloaded to a computer. A score of 5 or greater indicates the potential of a major depressive disorder and indicates the need for a more detailed clinical

TABLE 7-2 The Global Deterioration Scale

Diagnosis	Stage	Signs and Symptoms
No dementia	Stage 1: no cognitive decline	In this stage the person functions normally, has no memory loss, and is mentally healthy. People with no dementia would be considered to be in Stage 1.
No dementia	Stage 2: very mild cognitive decline	This stage is used to describe normal forgetfulness associated with aging; for example, forgetfulness of names and where familiar objects were left. Symptoms are not evident to loved ones or the physician.
No dementia	Stage 3: mild cognitive decline	This stage includes increased forgetfulness, slight difficulty concentrating, decreased work performance. People may get lost more often or have difficulty finding the right words. At this stage, a person's loved ones will begin to notice a cognitive decline. Average duration: 7 years before onset of dementia.
Early stage	Stage 4: moderate cognitive decline	This stage includes difficulty concentrating, decreased memory of recent events, and difficulties managing finances or traveling alone to new locations. People have trouble completing complex tasks efficiently or accurately and may be in denial about their symptoms. They may also start withdrawing from family or friends because socialization becomes difficult. At this stage a physician can detect clear cognitive problems during a patient interview and exam. Average duration: 2 years.
Midstage	Stage 5: moderately severe cognitive decline	People in this stage have major memory deficiencies and need some assistance to complete their daily activities (e.g., dressing, bathing, preparing meals). Memory loss is more prominent and may include major relevant aspects of current lives; for example, people may not remember their address or phone number and may not know the time or day or where they are. Average duration: 1.5 years.
Midstage	Stage 6: severe cognitive decline (middle dementia)	People in stage 6 require extensive assistance to carry out daily activities. They start to forget names of close family members and have little memory of recent events. Many people can remember only some details of earlier life. They also have difficulty counting down from 10 and finishing tasks. Incontinence (loss of bladder or bowel control) is a problem in this stage. Ability to speak declines. Personality changes, such as delusions (believing something to be true that is not), compulsions (repeating a simple behavior, such as cleaning), or anxiety and agitation may occur. Average duration: 2.5 years.
Late stage	Stage 7: very severe cognitive decline (late dementia)	People in this stage have essentially no ability to speak or communicate. They require assistance with most activities (e.g., using the toilet, eating). They often lose psychomotor skills, for example, the ability to walk. Average duration: 2.5 years.

From Reisberg B, Ferris SH, de Leon MJ, et al: The Global Deterioration Scale for assessment of primary degenerative dementia, *Am J Psychiatry* 139:1136–1139, 1982. Copyright ©1983 Barry Reisberg, MD. Reproduced with permission.

TABLE 7-3 Geriatric Depression Scale (Short Form)

Are you basically satisfied with your life?	Yes	No*
Have you dropped many of your activities and interests?	Yes*	No
Do you feel that your life is empty?	Yes*	No
Do you often get bored?	Yes*	No
Are you in good spirits most of the time?	Yes	No*
Are you afraid that something bad is going to happen to you?	Yes*	No
Do you feel happy most of the time?	Yes	No*
Do you often feel helpless?	Yes*	No
Do you prefer to stay at home, rather than going out and doing new things?	Yes*	No
Do you feel you have more problems with memory than most?	Yes*	No
Do you think it is wonderful to be alive?	Yes	No*
Do you feel pretty worthless about the way you are now?	Yes*	No
Do you feel full of energy?	Yes	No*
Do you feel that your situation is hopeless?	Yes*	No
Do you think that most people are better off than you?	Yes*	No

*Each answer indicated by an asterisk counts as 1 point. Scores greater than 5 indicate need for further evaluation. Contact Dr. Yesavage directly at Stanford University in Palo Alto, Calif, or see http://www.stanford.edu/~yesavage/GDS.html.
From Yesavage J, Brink TL, Rose TL, et al: Development and validation of a Geriatric Depression Screening Scale: a preliminary report, Journal of Psychiatric Research 17:37, 1982-1983.

assessment by a psychiatrist or a mental health advanced practice nurse. However, when some of the items are "missed," prorating of scores is possible. It has also been suggested that the 15-item version can be used by some who are aphasic but are able to use a point-board. The Geriatric Depression Scale has been extremely successful in identifying depression because it deemphasizes physical complaints, libido, and appetite (Lach et al, 2010). Dr. Yesavage may be contacted directly at Stanford University in the United States for more information and the products he has available. See also http://www.stanford.edu/~yesavage/GDS.html.

Cornell Scale for Depression in Dementia

The Cornell Scale for Depression in Dementia (CSD-D) was designed to identify major depressive disorders in persons who may have dementia (Alexopoulos et al, 1988; Lim et al, 2012). The first person to be interviewed is a proxy followed by an attempted interview with the patient. If he or she is unable to respond to the questions, many of these can be completed through observation. The questions are related to the signs and symptoms of depression in the *week* before the interview. The CSD-D takes about 20 minutes to administer. Each item is assessed for severity: 0 = absent, 1 = mild or intermittent, 2 = severe. The instrument is introduced with "I am going to ask you questions about how you/your relative has been feeling during the past week. I am interested in changes you have noticed and the duration of these changes." For a downloadable document, see www.health.vic.gov.au.

COMPREHENSIVE GERIATRIC ASSESSMENT

In some cases an integrated approach is used rather than an individual or collection of separate instruments, that is, one that combines physical, functional, and psychosocial components. The most well-known comprehensive tools are the OARS Multidimensional Functional Assessment Questionnaire (OMFAQ), the Resident Assessment Instrument (RAI), and the Outcomes and Assessment Information Set (OASIS). All are quite comprehensive and therefore lengthy but, once completed, can serve as a basis for a detailed plan of care. They are all very labor intensive and therefore expensive to administer.

The OARS Multidimensional Functional Assessment Questionnaire (OMFAQ)

The classic instrument, the *Older Americans Resources and Services* (OARS), was developed at the Center for the Study of Aging and Human Development at Duke University (Pfeiffer, 1976). It was later updated as the OMFAQ (Duke University Center for the Study of Aging and Human Development, 2014). The updated instrument includes (1) an evaluation of the ability, disability, and capacity level at which the person is able to function and (2) the determination of the extent and intensity of utilization of resources. In the first section, the assessment is divided into five subscales that may be used separately or alone. The person's functional capacity in each area is rated on a scale of 1 (excellent functioning) to 6 (totally impaired functioning). At the conclusion of the assessment a cumulative impairment score (CIS) is calculated ranging from the most capable (6) to total disability (30). It takes approximately 45 minutes to administer and does not require training. The subscales are described in the following sections.

Social Resources

Social resources is a measurement of social skills and the ability to negotiate and make friends. Is the person able to ask for things from friends, family, and strangers? Are caregivers available if needed? Who are the caregivers and how long are they available? Does the person belong to any social network or group, such as a church, synagogue, ashram, temple, or other support system?

Economic Resources

Information about monthly income and sources is needed to determine the adequacy of income compared with needs. This will provide insight into the elder's relative standard of living and highlight areas of need that might be alleviated by the use of additional resources.

Mental Health

Consideration is given to intellectual function in the presence or absence of psychiatric symptoms and the amount of enjoyment the person gets from life (Chapter 28).

Physical Health

The physical health subscale includes the current diagnoses, the type of prescribed and over-the-counter medications used, and the person's perception of his or her health status. Excellent physical health includes participation in vigorous activities, such as walking, dancing, or biking at least twice each week. Seriously impaired physical health is determined by the presence of one or more illnesses or disabilities that are very painful or life-threatening, or that require extensive care.

ADLs and IADLs

The ADLs included in this instrument are the ability to walk, get into and out of bed, bathe and groom oneself (e.g., combing hair, shaving), dress, eat, and get to the bathroom on time. The IADLs include tasks such as dialing the telephone, driving a car, hanging up clothes, obtaining groceries, taking medications, and having the correct knowledge of medication dosages.

The OMFAQ and training materials can be purchased for a nominal fee from the Center for the Study of Aging and Human Development at Duke University http://centerforaging.duke.edu/services/141. Information can also be found through the website for the University of Western Ontario.

Resident Assessment Instrument (RAI)

In 1986 the Institute of Medicine (IOM) completed a study indicating that although there was considerable variation, residents in skilled nursing facilities in the United States were receiving an unacceptably low quality of care. As a result, nursing home reform was legislated as part of the Omnibus Budget Reconciliation Act (OBRA) of 1987. The creators of OBRA recognized the challenging work of caring for sicker and sicker persons discharged from acute care settings to nursing homes and, along with this, the need for comprehensive assessments, complex decision-making, and documentation regarding the care that was needed, planned, implemented, and evaluated.

In 1990 a Resident Assessment Instrument (RAI) was created and mandated for use in all skilled nursing facilities that receive compensation from either Medicare or Medicaid (Chapter 30). In March 2014 Quality Indicators were updated to provide a standardized measure of the quality of care provided (Box 7-15) (CMS, 2014).

The Quality Indicators along with the RAI are used in several countries outside of the United States, including provinces in Canada, and have been found to provide a foundation for quality care (Touhy et al, 2012). Now in its third version, the 450-item *Minimum Data Set* (MDS 3.0) is the basis for the assessment. As the MDS is analyzed, specific areas of need are identified and guide the development of the plan of care (Care Area Assessments) (Box 7-16) (CMS, 2014). The most recent revision has been found to be more reliable, efficient, and clinically relevant than previous versions; evidence-based assessment tools are included whenever possible (Saliba and Buchanan, 2008). In a significant change from the MDS 2.0, care recipient interviews are included.

The RAI provides a comprehensive health, social, and functional profile of persons as they enter skilled nursing facilities and at designated times thereafter. The initial assessment serves as the framework for the initial goals and outcomes for the individual. As reassessments are done, the nurse and other members of the care team have the opportunity to track the progress toward the resolution of identified problems and make changes to the plan of care as appropriate. As goals are met and resources are available, the assessment leads to discharge to a lower level of care, such as returning home or to an assisted living facility. For a person whose condition is one of progressive decline, the RAI

BOX 7-15 Quality Indicators: Factors Considered in the Measurement of Quality of Care Provided in a Skilled Nursing Facility

Short-Term Stay Residents	Long-Term Stay Residents
Self-report severe pain	All of the indicators for short stays **plus:**
Pressure ulcers: new or worsened	Developed urinary tract infection(s)
One or more falls with major injury	Developed incontinence
Assessed for/given seasonal influenza vaccination	Had catheter inserted into bladder
Assessed for/given pneumococcal vaccine	Was physically restrained
Newly received antipsychotic medication	Demonstrated increased need for assistance with ADLs
	Showed excessive weight loss
	Showed depressive symptoms
	Received an antipsychotic medication

From Centers for Medicare and Medicaid Services: *Quality measures,* 2014. Available at http://www.cms.gov/Medicare/Quality-Initiatives-Patient-Assessment-Instruments/NursingHomeQualityInits/NHQIQualityMeasures.html Accessed June 2014.

BOX 7-16 Examples of Care Area Assessments

Delirium	Feeding tubes
Vision	Dental care
ADL/rehabilitation potential	Psychotropic medication use
Well-being	Pain
Behavioral symptoms	Mood
Falls	Nutritional status

From Centers for Medicare and Medicaid Services (CMS): *MDS 3.0 RAI manual,* 2014. Available at http://www.cms.gov/Medicare/Quality-Initiatives-Patient-Assessment-Instruments/NursingHomeQualityInits/MDS30RAIManual.html. Accessed June 2014.

leads to a plan of care focused on comfort. The RAI process is dynamic and solution oriented. It is used to gather definitive information and promote healthy aging in a specific care setting and in a holistic manner. The RAI is coordinated by a nurse and requires his or her signature attesting to its accuracy.

OASIS C1

The plan for the nursing care provided in the home is based on, and documented in, the Outcomes and Assessment Information Set (OASIS). Now in its third revision (OASIS-C), further modifications were effective October 1, 2014 (OASIS C1). The assessment is very comprehensive and focuses on the development of nursing interventions to prevent rehospitalization and ensure safety in the home setting. Among the items on the instrument are those that identify the person's risk for hospitalization (Box 7-17). The majority of the documentation takes place in the patient's home and is entered into a laptop or tablet for transmission to the agency database and ultimately the Centers for Medicare and Medicaid Services. Completion is required for all care that is compensated by Medicare or

BOX 7-17 Risk for Hospitalization from the OASIS Assessment

- ☐ 1: History of falls (2 or more falls—or any fall with an injury—in the past 12 months)
- ☐ 2: Unintentional weight loss of a total of 10 pounds or more in the past 12 months
- ☐ 3: Multiple hospitalizations (2 or more) in the past 6 months
- ☐ 4: Multiple emergency department visits (2 or more) in the past 6 months
- ☐ 5: Decline in mental, emotional, or behavioral status in the past 3 months
- ☐ 6: Reported or observed history of difficulty complying with any medical instructions (e.g., medications, diet, exercise) in the past 3 months
- ☐ 7: Currently taking 5 or more medications
- ☐ 8: Currently reports exhaustion
- ☐ 9: Other risk(s) not listed in 1-8
- ☐ 10: None of the above

Medicare and forms the basis for the level of reimbursement. As with other instruments, the assessment is completed at the time the care is begun and at intervals thereafter. Nurses supplement the OASIS data to include information necessary to personalize the care provided. It is exceedingly complex and training is required. For more information see www.cms.gov or search OASIS-C.

◆ PROMOTING HEALTHY AGING: IMPLICATIONS FOR GERONTOLOGICAL NURSING

Whether the nurse is working with a standardized instrument or creating a new one, the goal is always to assist the person to move along the wellness trajectory toward healthy aging, regardless of the care setting or health status. The nurse is expected to collect data that are the most accurate, and to do so in the most efficient yet caring manner possible. The use of assessment instruments serves as a way to organize the data and be able to compare it at various points in time. Each tool has strengths and weaknesses, as does each completed assessment. A number of factors complicate assessment of the older adult: differentiating the effects of aging from those originating from disease, determining the presence of comorbidities, underreporting of symptoms by older adults, manifesting atypical presentations or nonspecific presentations of illnesses, and increasing numbers of iatrogenic illnesses.

Overdiagnosis and underdiagnosis occur when the normal age changes are not considered and assessments are inadequate. Assessing the person in later life with multiple chronic conditions is a complex task at the least. Many symptoms or complaints are ascribed to normal aging rather than to a disease entity that may be developing, necessitating careful and often problem-oriented assessments. Symptoms of one condition can exacerbate or mask symptoms of another. The gerontological nurse is challenged to provide the highest level of excellence in the assessment of the elderly without burdening the person in the process.

KEY CONCEPTS

- Assessment of the physical, cognitive, psychosocial, functional, and environmental status is essential to identifying specific needs, leading to implementation of appropriate interventions designed to enhance quality of life while aging.
- The quality and quantity of the data are affected by the source of collection, whether by self-report, report-by-proxy, or through nurse observation.
- Evidence-based instruments are available for most aspects of the assessment of the older adult.
- Knowledge of, and sometimes training in, the use of a particular assessment instrument is needed to accurately administer it.
- Multiple factors complicate obtaining and interpreting assessment data and providing the highest quality of care.

NURSING STUDY: IS A COMPREHENSIVE ASSESSMENT NEEDED?

Eighty-year-old Señora Hernandez is newly admitted to your acute care hospital unit. She is there for observation and testing after a witnessed syncopal episode. She lives with her 90-year-old husband, who has mild dementia, and her 60-year-old daughter. Her daughter admits to you that neither of her parents have been doing well and that the doctors "just haven't been able to figure it out." You know that Señora Hernandez will be receiving both neurological and cardiac testing. However, as a gerontological resource nurse you also know that she and her family may benefit from a comprehensive evaluation. The decision of which aspects of the assessment to complete is within your scope of practice at your facility.

- Of the assessment instruments available to you, which do you think is most important in determining the immediate needs of Señora Hernandez?
- In order to prepare Señora Hernandez for discharge, which one or which selection of instruments will you use to collect the data needed to promote her well-being and safety?
- What information will you collect to supplement the information that you obtain through the use of standardized instruments?

CRITICAL THINKING QUESTIONS AND ACTIVITIES

1. Of the assessment tools that are available to you, which are the most reasonable to perform within the limitations of an acute care setting?
2. How would any of your answers to the preceding questions change in a skilled nursing facility? In an assisted living facility? In the home setting?
3. If you cannot do a complete head-to-toe examination and detailed history, list the parts you will do when assessing an older adult, in order of priority.
4. Review the literature and present to your class two instruments that are applicable for use in cultures or languages other than the ones for which they were created.
5. Select the instrument or the portion of an instrument you are the least comfortable with and role-play with a classmate in conducting the assessment until you become comfortable.

RESEARCH QUESTIONS

1. What is the importance of measuring ADLs and IADLs in older adults?
2. What makes an assessment tool effective?
3. What tool or tools would be most appropriate for assessing an elder in the community, in the hospital, in long-term care, or in day care? Give your rationale for the choices.

REFERENCES

Alexopoulos GS, Abrams RC, Young RC, et al: Cornell Scale for Depression in Dementia, *Biol Psychiatry* 23:271–284, 1988.

Alzheimer Society Toronto: *The progression of Alzheimer's disease*, 2014.http://www.alzheimertoronto.org/ad_ProgressionAD.htm. Accessed May 2014.

American Psychological Association (APA): *Instrumental Activities of Daily Living Scale: Construct: assessment of complex activities of daily living*, 2014.http://www.apa.org/pi/about/publications/caregivers/

practice-settings/assessment/tools/daily-activities.aspx. Accessed May 2014.

Aprahamian I, Martinelli JE, Neri AL, et al: The accuracy of the Clock Drawing Test compared to that of standard screening tests for Alzheimer's disease: results from a study of Brazilian elderly with heterogeneous educational backgrounds, *Int Psychogeriatr* 22:64–71, 2010.

Benner P: *From novice to expert*, Menlo Park, CA, 1984, Addison-Wesley.

Bent B: FANCAPES Assessment: Increases in longevity lead to need for expertise in

geriatric care, *Advance Healthcare Network for Nurses* 7(14):10, 2005.

Blessed G, Tomlinson BE, Roth M: The association between qualitative measures of dementia and of senile change in the cerebral grey matter of elderly subjects, *Br J Psychiatry* 114:797–811, 1968.

Borson S, Brush M, Gil E, et al: The Clock Drawing Test: utility for dementia detection in multiethnic elders, *J Gerontol A Biol Sci Med Sci* 54(11):M534–M540, 1999.

Borson S, Scanlan J, Brush M, et al: The Mini-Cog: a cognitive "vital signs" measure for dementia screening in multi-lingual elderly, *Int J Geriatr Psychiatry* 15(11): 1021–1207, 2000.

Borson S, Scanlan JM, Chen P, et al: The Mini-Cog as a screen for dementia: validation in a population-based sample, *J Am Geriatr Soc* 51(10):1451–1454, 2003.

Bowker LK, Price JD, Smith SC, editors: *Oxford handbook of geriatric medicine,* ed 2, Oxford, 2012, Oxford University Press.

Brink TL, Yesavage JA, Lum O, et al: Screening tests for geriatric depression, *Clin Gerontol* 1:37–44, 1982.

Centers for Medicare & Medicaid Services (CMS): *MDS 3.0 RAI manual,* 2014. http://www.cms.gov/Medicare/Quality-Initiatives-Patient-Assessment-Instruments/NursingHomeQualityInits/MDS30RAIManual.html. Accessed June 2014.

Cournan M: Use of the Functional Independence Measure for outcomes measurement in acute inpatient rehabilitation, *Rehabil Nurs* 36(3):111–117, 2011

Duke University Center for the Study of Aging and Human Development: *Older Americans Resources and Services,* 2013. http://centerforaging.duke.edu/services/141. Accessed May 2014.

Ehreke L, Luppa M, König HH, et al: The Clock Drawing Test a screening tool for the diagnosis of mild cognitive impairment? A systematic review, *Int Psychogeriatr* 22:56–63, 2010.

Fieo RA, Austin EJ, Starr JM, et al: Calibrating ADL-IALD scales to improve measurement and accuracy and to extend the disability construct into the pre-clinical range: a systematic review, *BMC Geriar* 11:42, 2011. http://www.biomedcentral.com/1471-2318/11/42.

Folstein MF, Folstein SE, McHugh PR: Mini-mental state: a practical method for grading the cognitive state of patients for the clinician, *J Psychiatr Res* 12:189–198, 1975.

Fulmer T, Wallace M: *Fulmer SPICES: an overall assessment tool for older adults,* New York, 2012, Hartford Institute for Geriatric Nursing.http://consultgerirn.org/uploads/File/trythis/try_this_1.pdf. Accessed October 31, 2014.

Katz S, Ford AB, Moskowitz RW, et al: Studies of illness in the aged: the index of ADL: a standardized measure of biological and psychosocial function, *JAMA* 185:914–919, 1963.

Kidd D, Stewart G, Baldry J, et al: The Functional Independence Measure: a comparative validity and reliability study, *Disabil Rehabil* 17:10–14, 1995.

Kim EY, Bean RA, Harper JM: Do general treatment guidelines for Asian American families have applications to specific ethnic

groups? The case of culturally-competent therapy with Korean American, *J Marital Fam Ther* 30(3):359–372, 2004.

Kleinman A: *Patient and healers in the context of culture: an exploration of the borderland between anthropology, medicine, and psychiatry,* Berkeley, CA, 1980, University of California Press.

Lach H, Chang Y, Edwards D: Can older adults accurately report depression using brief forms? *J Gerontol Nurs* 36:30–37, 2010.

LaPlante MP: The classic measure of disability of activities of daily living is biased by age but an expanded IADL/ADL measure is not, *J Gerontol B Psychol Sci Soc* 656: 720–732, 2010.

Lawton MP, Brody EM: Assessment of older people: self-maintaining and instrumental activities of daily living, *Gerontologist* 9:179–186, 1969.

Lim HK, Hong SC, Won WY, et al: Reliability and validity of the Korean version of the Cornell Scale for Depression in Dementia, *Psychiatry Invest* 9(4):332–338, 2012.

Lundgren-Nilsson A, Grimby G, Ring, H, et al: Cross-cultural validity of Functional Independence Measure items in stroke: a study using Rasch analysis, *J Rehabil Med* 37:23–31, 2005.

Mahoney FI, Barthel DW: Functional evaluation: the Barthel Index, *Md State Med J* 14:61–65, 1965.

Mitchell AJ: A meta-analysis of the accuracy of the Mini-Mental Status Examination in the detection of dementia and mild cognitive impairment, *J Psychiatr Res* 43:411–431, 2009.

Mitchell AJ, Malladi S: Screening and case finding tools for the detection of dementia. Part 1. Evidence-based meta-analysis of multidomain tests, *Am J Geriatr Psychiatry* 18:759–782, 2010.

Montgomery J, Mitty E, Flores S: Resident condition change: should I call 911? *Geriatr Nurs* 29:15–26, 2008.

Nikula S, Jylhä M, Bardage C, et al: Are ADLs comparable across countries? Sociodemographic associates of harmonized IADL measures, *Aging Clin Exp Res* 15(6): 451–459, 2003.

Ortiz I, Romero L: Cultural implications for assessment and treatment of depression in Hispanic elderly individuals, *Ann Longterm Care* 16:45, 2008.

Ottenbacher KJ, Hsu Y, Granger CV, Fielder RC: The reliability of the functional independence measure: a quantitative review, *Ach Phys Med Rehabil* 77(12):1226–1232, 1996.

Pfeiffer E: *Physical and mental assessment—OARS,* Durham, NC, 1976, Duke University, Center for the Study of Aging and Human Development.

Quinn TJ, Langhorne P, Stott DJ: Barthel Index for stroke trials: development, properties and application, *Stroke* 42: 1146–1151, 2011.

Reisberg B: Functional Assessment Staging (FAST), *Psychopharmacol Bull* 24:653, 1988.

Reisberg B: Global measures: utility in defining and measuring treatment response in dementia, *Int Psychogeriatr* 19:421–456, 2007.

Reisberg B, Ferris SH, de Leon MJ, et al: The Global Deterioration Scale for assessment of primary progressive dementia, *Am J Psychiatry* 139:1136–1139, 1982.

Sakurai R, Fujiwara Y, Ishihara M, et al: Age-related self-overestimation of step-over ability in the healthy older adults and its relationship to fall risk, *BMC Geriatr* 13:14–23, 2013.

Saliba D, Buchanan J: *Development and validation of a revised nursing home assessment tool: MDS 3.0,* Santa Monica, CA, Apr 2008, RAND Corporation.

Sangha H, Lipson D, Foley N, et al: A comparison of the Barthel Index and the Functional Independence Measure as outcome measures in stroke rehabilitation: patterns of disability scale usage in clinical trials, *Int J Rehabil Res* 28:135–139, 2005.

Sclan SG, Reisberg B: Functional Assessment Staging (FAST) in Alzheimer's disease: reliability, validity, and ordinality, *Int Psychogeriatr* 4:55–69, 1992.

Shulman KI: Clock drawing: is it the ideal cognitive screening test? *Int J Geriatr Psychiatry* 15:545–561, 2000.

Stratford PW, Kennedy DM, Maly MR, et al: Quantifying self-report measures' overestimation of mobility scores postarthroplasty, *Phys Ther* 90(9):1288–1296, 2010.

Touhy TA, Jett KF, Boscart V, et al: *Ebersole and Hess' Gerontological nursing and healthy aging,* Toronto, ON, 2012, Elsevier Canada.

Wade C, Collin C: The Barthel ADL Index: a standard measure of physical disability, *Int Disabil Stud* 10(2):64–67, 1988.

Wattmo C, Wallin ÅK, Londos E, et al: Long-term outcome and prediction models of activity of daily living in Alzheimer disease with cholinesterase inhibitor treatment, *Alzheimer Dis Assoc Disord* 25(1):63–72, 2011.

Yesavage JA, Brink TL, Rose TL, et al: Development and validation of a geriatric depression screening scale: a preliminary report, *J Psychiatr Res* 17:37–49, 1983.

Zambas SI: Purpose of the systematic physical assessment in everyday practice: critique of a "sacred cow," *J Nurs Educ* 49(6):305–311, 2010.

Laboratory Values and Diagnostics

Kathleen Jett

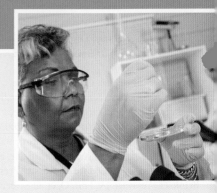

http://evolve.elsevier.com/Touhy/TwdHlthAging

A STUDENT SPEAKS

I always thought that as people got older, their blood sugars went up a little and that was OK. Now I realize that an elevation in fasting glucose means a problem regardless of one's age.

Susan, age 20

AN ELDER SPEAKS

Every time I turn around somebody wants my blood. They say that they need to "watch me closely" but I am not sure what that has to do with my blood. What if they take too much and it causes me to get sick?

Sung Ye, age 92

LEARNING OBJECTIVES

On completion of this chapter, the reader will be able to:

1. Discuss the key laboratory tests used to monitor common health problems.
2. Understand the implications of deviations in key abnormal diagnostic laboratory values that can occur in the older adult.
3. Define precautions the nurse should take when interpreting laboratory values for the older adult.

The nurse's knowledge related to laboratory values and diagnostic tests assumes special meaning when working with older adults. The older the person is, the more difficult the interpretation of findings. The bedside or home health nurse is expected to have skills in basic interpretation, knowledge of the appropriate timing of the testing, and awareness of factors that could affect the results. For nurses working in long-term care settings, knowledge of interpretation is especially important to ensure that when abnormalities are identified, the person is treated promptly and appropriately. Advanced practice nurses are responsible for knowing when and what testing to order and to use the results for prescriptive responses to promote healthy aging.

Laboratory findings are often reported in relationship to a range of normalized values or reference ranges referred to as "within normal limits (WNL)." Special diligence is needed to interpret the results within the context of the person's overall health and normal changes with aging (Box 8-1).

HEMATOLOGICAL TESTING

Hematological testing refers to testing associated with the blood and lymph and their component parts: red blood cells (RBCs),

white blood cells (WBCs), and cell fragments called *platelets*. Together the cells float in a fluid matrix called *plasma*. A basic complete blood count (CBC) provides a measure of the number of RBCs, WBCs, platelets, and the hematocrit and hemoglobin indices. A CBC with a "differential" refers to the inclusion of the subtypes of the WBCs: granulocytes (neutrophils, basophils, and eosinophils) and agranulocytes (lymphocytes and monocytes).

Hematological laboratory tests are used to monitor illnesses such as anemia, check for the presence of potential side effects of treatment such as chemotherapeutic agents, or evaluate symptoms such as fatigue or indications of an infection. A number of disorders commonly seen in later life are diagnosed or monitored through hematological testing. Several conditions affect the interpretation of the results, such as dehydration, inadequate nutrition, infections, and inflammation.

Red Blood Cell Count

The primary function of the RBCs (erythrocytes) is to transport molecules of hemoglobin. Because the erythrocytes have no nucleus of their own, they cannot reproduce. With an average life span of 120 days, the RBCs are constantly being replenished.

BOX 8-1 Few Changes with Aging

While there are no differences in what is a normal result in a laboratory finding in an older compared with a younger adult, deviations are more likely to occur and put the older person at greater risk of poor outcomes.

They are produced primarily by the bone marrow of the long bones.

Hemoglobin and Hematocrit

Hemoglobin, a conjugated protein, is the main component of the red blood cell. It contains iron and the red pigment porphyrin. The iron is part of protein synthesis in the mitochondria, essential for generating cellular energy, and serves as the transport medium for oxygen from the lungs to the tissues and for carbon dioxide from the tissues to the lungs. Each saturated gram of hemoglobin carries 1.39 mL of oxygen. A hemoglobin level equal to or less than 5 g/dL, or more than 20 g/dL, is considered a "critical value" for the average adult and requires urgent intervention (Box 8-2). Older adults may begin to show signs of physiological distress well before these values are reached.

The term *hematocrit* means "to separate blood." It is the *relative percentage* of packed RBCs to the plasma in blood, after the two have been separated (often referred to as "spun down"). Although they measure different aspects of the RBCs, the hematocrit and hemoglobin values are comparative numbers, with the hemoglobin level approximately one third of the hematocrit value. For example, a person with a hemoglobin level of 12 g/dL will have a hematocrit of approximately 36% (Chernecky and Berger, 2013).

There is no indication that there is a change in RBCs in healthy aging; however, the speed at which new blood cells can be produced in late life is reduced (*decreased marrow reserve*). This becomes a potential problem with a loss of blood such as after phlebotomy or frank bleeding. Recovery from the loss takes much longer, increasing the risk of falling, delirium, and other geriatric syndromes.

Iron. The primary source of iron is through the consumption of iron-containing foods such as dark-green leafy vegetables and red meats. Iron is transported into bone marrow by the plasma protein *transferrin* for storage and later use. The serum concentration of iron is determined by a combination of its absorption and storage and the breakdown and synthesis of hemoglobin. Iron studies include measurements of iron, ferritin, total iron binding capacity, and transferrin levels.

BOX 8-2 Caution with the Interpretation of Hematocrit and Hemoglobin Levels

Elevations in hematocrit and hemoglobin levels may be the result of a pathological process but are more often an early sign of hypovolemia from malnutrition, dehydration, or severe diarrhea. The volume depletion must be corrected before an accurate interpretation can be done.

Serum iron (Fe) level is reported as micrograms per deciliter (mcg/dL). The total iron binding capacity (TIBC) is a measure of the combination of the amount of iron already in the blood and the amount of transferrin available in the blood serum. *Ferritin* is a complex molecule made up of ferric hydroxide and a protein; its measurement reflects body iron stores. If the person has adequate iron, the body is able to respond quickly to the demand for increased oxygen and energy and to replenish iron lost through bleeding.

Anemia. Anemia is a condition in which there is a reduced number of red blood cells and consequentially a reduced capacity for the transport of oxygen and carbon dioxide and a reduced ability to synthesize the protein needed for cell energy. Although not a normal part of aging, it is a common finding, especially in those who are frail or who have had a chronic disease for an extended period of time. Anemia of some type has been found in 10% of those more than 65 years of age, increasing to 50% of those older than age 80 (Berliner, 2013) (Box 8-3).

Diagnostic testing for anemia includes a CBC with differential, iron studies, and the measurement of several vitamins, especially the levels of folic acid and B_{12}. The most common types of anemia in late life are associated with blood loss, especially in the postoperative period (e.g., post fracture or hip replacement surgery), and chronic inflammation, such as with diabetes (Balducci, 2014) (Box 8-4). Anemia of chronic inflammation is the second most common type of anemia worldwide (Lichtin, 2013). The hemoglobin value is more important than the RBC measurement as a diagnostic indicator of anemia.

The World Health Organization (WHO, 1968) defines anemia as hemoglobin concentrations <13.5 g/dL for men and <12.0 g/dL for women. Using this definition the prevalence of anemia is higher in black men than in any other group after the age of 65 (Balducci, 2014). Several studies, including the Women's Health and Aging Study in Baltimore, found that a hemoglobin level <13.0 g/dL was a risk factor for mortality and that a level <13.4 g/dL was a risk factor for functional decline in older adults (Chavez, 2008; Semba et al, 2007). In another study,

BOX 8-3 Implications for Aging: Misinterpretation of Potential Signs of Anemia

In older adults the signs and symptoms of anemia are easily confused with other disorders, making diagnosis difficult or delayed. For example, one of the first signs of anemia is fatigue. This could also be a side effect of a medication or falsely attributed to normal aging.

BOX 8-4 Types of Anemia Found in Older Adults

Anemia of chronic inflammation (33.6%)
Unknown causes (24%)
Iron deficiency (16%)
Vitamin B_{12} and/or folate deficiency (14.3%)
Renal insufficiencies (12%)

Source: NHANES: National Health and Nutrition Examination Survey.

a hemoglobin level below 12.6 g/dL was an independent risk factor for death among women 65 and older (Zakai et al, 2005). It is reasonable to consider 12.5 to 13.0 g/dL to be the lowest range for older women (Balducci, 2014). Anemia that is progressive untreated or not responsive to treatment will result in the person's death. The advanced practice gerontological nurse must be able to recognize the need to consider anemia as a causative factor in complaints of weakness, fatigue, or a number of other symptoms, including altered mental status. The nurse should be able to recognize the potential for anemia and to monitor its treatment.

White Blood Cells

White blood cells (leukocytes) are the cells of the immune system that primarily function to protect the body from infection and other foreign invaders. They are produced by the bone marrow and thymus and are stored in the lymph nodes, spleen, and tonsils. They are found mainly in the interstitial fluid until they are needed and then travel to the site of invasion or infection. The number of WBCs and the type of WBC are regulated largely by the endocrine system and by the need for a particular type of cell (Table 8-1). Each cell has a life span of 13 to 20 days, after which it is destroyed in the lymphatic system and excreted in feces. An excess is referred to as leukocytosis and a deficiency is leukopenia. Either of these conditions is more common in the older adult, especially because of adverse side effects of medications. Leukopenia can be caused by common medical conditions and commonly prescribed medications, such as some antibiotics, anticonvulsants, antihistamines, analgesics, sulfonamides, or diuretics. On the other hand, leukocytosis may be a side effect of other drugs including allopurinol, aspirin, heparin, or steroids (Dugdale, 2013).

The average adult has 5000 to 10,000 WBCs/mm^3. A major concern in the elderly is WBC elevations. A WBC count greater than 10,000/mm^3 in conjunction with an increase in the number of immature neutrophils (referred to as *bandemia* or a *left shift*) in an older adult is an indicator of infection. Rather than an increase in the total number of lymphocytes, only immature neutrophils are found (Chernecky and Berger, 2013). Due to age-related decreases or delayed responses in the immune system, the traditional indication of infection is not immediately apparent. This change has significant implications for the gerontological nurse.

TABLE 8-1	Functions of the Types of White Blood Cells
CELL TYPE	**CELL FUNCTION**
Neutrophils	Stimulated by pyogenic infections, to fight bacteria
Eosinophils	Stimulated by allergic responses, to fight antigens and parasites
Basophils	Stimulated by the presence of allergens; transport histamine
Lymphocytes	Stimulated by the presence of viral infections
Monocytes	Stimulated by severe infections including viral, parasitic, and rickettsial

Data from Chernecky CC, Berger BJ: *Laboratory tests and diagnostic procedures*, ed 6, St Louis, MO, 2013, Elsevier.

SAFETY ALERT

Due to the decreased immune function in the older adult, laboratory indicators of infection may be delayed. Waiting for the "usual signs" of infection in an older adult may result in his or her death. Instead, the nurse must be alert for more subtle signs of illness such as new-onset or increased confusion, falling, or incontinence, and respond to these changes earlier rather than later.

Granulocytes

Neutrophils. Neutrophils are produced in 7 to 14 days in the bone marrow and are in circulation for about 6 hours. They fight illness by phagocytizing bacteria and other products perceived to be foreign (Chapter 25). *Neutrophilia,* or increased numbers of neutrophils, is a nonspecific finding. It may be an indicator of a number of conditions more common in late life, including infections and connective tissue diseases, such as rheumatoid arthritis; a side effect of medications, such as corticosteroids; or a result of trauma such as a fall (Chernecky and Berger, 2013).

Eosinophils and basophils. Eosinophils ingest antigen-antibody complexes induced by IgE-mediated reactions to attack allergens and parasites. High eosinophil counts are found in people with type I allergies such as hay fever and asthma. Eosinophils are involved in the mucosal immune response, which is known to diminish in late life (Liesveld and Reagan, 2014). Basophils transport histamine, a factor in immune and antiinflammatory responses. Like eosinophils, they play a role in allergic reactions but are not involved in bacterial or viral infections (Chernecky and Berger, 2013).

Agranulocytes

Lymphocytes. Lymphocytes are divided into two types: T cells and B cells. T cells are produced by the thymus and are active in cell-mediated immunity; B cells are produced in the bone marrow and are involved in the production of antibodies (humoral immunity). In adulthood, 80% of lymphocytes are T cells, with a slight decrease in T cells and an increase in B cells with aging. T-cell activity is especially important in late life, due in part to the naturally occurring immunosenescence, especially depressed T-cell responses and T-cell–macrophage interactions (Chapter 3) (Inal et al, 2014). Measurement of the number of T cells is included in the monitoring of the health status and treatment response of persons who are immunocompromised such as those who are receiving chemotherapeutic agents, are infected with human immunodeficiency virus (HIV), or have acquired immunodeficiency syndrome (AIDS). Together with neutrophils, lymphocytes make up 75% to 90% of all white blood cells (Chernecky and Berger, 2013).

Monocytes. Monocytes are the largest of the leukocytes. When matured they become macrophages and help defend the body against foreign substances or, more importantly, what the body believes are foreign substances. The macrophages migrate to a site in the body where they can remove microorganisms, dead RBCs, and foreign debris through the physiological process of phagocytosis. If the number of monocytes is low, the person has reduced physiological capacity to fight infection. This value must be watched carefully, especially in frail elders.

Platelets

Platelets are small, irregular particles known as thrombocytes, an essential ingredient in clotting. They are formed in the bone marrow, lungs, and spleen and are released when a blood vessel is injured. As they arrive at the site of injury, they become "sticky," forming a plug at the site to stop the bleeding and to help trigger what is known as the *clotting cascade* (Schwartz and Rote, 2014; Thibodeau and Patton, 2003). Although the platelet count does not change with aging, there is an increase in the concentrations of a large number of coagulation enzymes (factors VII and VIII and fibrinogen). This and other developments indicate a greater possibility of hypercoagulability. At the same time, older adults are more likely to have blood diatheses, resulting in unexplained bruising, nosebleeds, and excessive bleeding with surgery, for example. If any of these signs are present, platelet counts and coagulation studies are done. Counts of 150,000 to 400,000/mm^3 are considered normal. Counts less than 100,000/mm^3 are a cause for concern and considered thrombocytopenia; spontaneous hemorrhage may occur when the count falls below 20,000/mm^3; at 40,000/mm^3 spontaneous bleeding is uncommon but prolonged bleeding can occur with trauma or surgery, and there is a significantly exacerbated risk of excessive bleeding when anticoagulants are used at the same time (Schwartz and Rote, 2014). *Thrombocythemia* indicates a platelet count greater than 1 million/mm^3; bleeding still may occur as a result of abnormal functioning.

The gerontological nurse caring for older adults, especially those who are frail or who have vague symptoms of fatigue, is expected to monitor patients at risk for bleeding. A basic understanding of the meaning of the patient's hematological laboratory findings is expected. For frail elders, such as those in long-term care facilities, thrombocytopenia can quickly lead to death should bleeding occur, such as from nonsteroidal antiinflammatory drug (NSAID)–related gastric bleeding or from an unrecognized subdural hematoma following a fall.

MEASURES OF INFLAMMATION

Erythrocyte Sedimentation Rate

The *erythrocyte sedimentation rate* (ESR), also referred to as the "sed rate," is the rate at which an RBC falls to the bottom of a saline solution or plasma in a set period of time. It is a proxy measure for the degree of inflammation, infection, necrosis, infarction, or advanced neoplasm. It may be slightly elevated (10 to 20 mm/hour) in many normal, healthy older adults, most likely attributable to the prevalence of long-standing chronic disease. In a large number of older adults unexplainable elevations may be found (Cankurtaran et al, 2010). A more than minimal elevation indicates elevated levels of serum proteins and inflammatory activity. The ESR may be useful for monitoring several inflammatory diseases and their treatments, such as polymyalgia rheumatica, temporal arteritis, or rheumatoid arthritis (Chapter 26). However, the ESR is a nonspecific test and this must be always taken under consideration when evaluating the results (Kreiner et al, 2010). Slight elevations in the ESR in older adults are to be expected in the presence of long-standing chronic diseases.

C-reactive Protein

C-reactive protein (CRP) is produced by the liver during the acute phase of inflammation or in the course of various diseases. Although originally used to determine cardiac events, it has been found a useful indicator for other forms of inflammation, such as after an injury, following surgery, or in the presence of infection. Tests of both CRP and ESR together are currently used, especially for the evaluation of an acute myocardial infarction (AMI). However, in a study of 5777 patients, Colombet and colleagues (2010) concluded that the joint measurement was not necessary and the results of the ESR could be misleading. The authors recommended that priority be given to the CRP measurement when inflammation is suspected. In another study of 163 persons, the CRP measurement was found to be helpful in diagnosing septic joints, whereas the ESR value was not (Ernst et al, 2010). The CRP value was also found useful for predicting the risk for coronary heart disease among intermediate-risk subjects (Helfand et al, 2009). There is now a high-sensitivity assay for CRP (hs-CRP), which has increased the accuracy of the measurement even at low levels.

VITAMINS

Vitamin deficiencies are common in later life and should be considered any time the person complains of vague symptoms (especially fatigue), cognitive impairment is present, wound healing is delayed, or anemia is suspected. Those at highest risk are persons with protein-calorie malnutrition. Vitamin B and C deficiencies are more likely in persons undernourished for long periods of time such as many of those living in low-income countries (Mathew and Jacobs, 2014). Vitamin D deficiencies are now being found in both apparently healthy and ill adults. When vitamin supplementation is used, it should be carefully tailored to the individual.

B Vitamins

The two B vitamins that are especially important are folic acid and B$_{12}$, two of the eight B vitamins found in the B complex.

Folic Acid

Folic acid is formed by bacteria in the intestines; it is necessary for the normal functioning of both RBCs and WBCs, as well as for deoxyribonucleic acid (DNA) synthesis (CDC, 2009). It is stored in the liver and can be found in eggs, milk, leafy vegetables, yeast, liver, and fruit. Decreases in folic acid may indicate protein-energy malnutrition, several types of anemia, and liver and renal disease. It is more common among persons with chronic alcohol abuse. Due to the number of foods that are enhanced with folic acid in the United States, associated anemias are rare. Nonetheless, the nurse must be alert for potential folic acid deficiencies when the person has significant nutritional deficits, such as those who are very frail.

Vitamin B$_{12}$

Vitamin B$_{12}$ (cyanocobalamin) is a water-soluble vitamin required for the normal development of RBCs, for a number of neurological functions, and also for DNA synthesis. It cannot be synthesized in the human body and thus must be provided by the diet. Conditions that lead to folate and B_{12} deficiency can result in megaloblastic anemia. B_{12} deficiency is common in older adults and is estimated to affect about 3.2% of those older than age 51 (Box 8-5). Tests of B_{12} and folate levels are now part of the standard workup for dementia (CDC, 2009). Testing for a B_{12} deficiency is indicated when there is unexplained neurological or functional decline.

Vitamin B_{12} is found in the proteins of foods such as eggs, fish, shellfish, and meat; typically only half of the B_{12} ingested by healthy adults with normal gastric function is absorbed. It is primarily extracted from proteins in the stomach in the presence of gastric acid and a number of other compounds including intrinsic factor (IF). Pernicious anemia is a type of anemia characterized by lowered intrinsic factor production by gastric cells. The normal age-related decreases in the acidity of the stomach, combined with any loss of IF, can lead to this condition, the average age of diagnosis of which is 60 years of age (Antony, 2012).

While the ability to absorb B_{12} from food declines with aging, the body is still able to absorb synthetic formulations. Adequate amounts should be obtained from a combination of eating foods high in B_{12} and supplementation.

Vitamin D

Vitamin D deficiencies have been found to be common among all ages. Vitamin D is produced in the skin when exposed to ultraviolet light through the conversion of 7-dehydrocholesterol to vitamin D_3 (cholecalciferol) (NHLBI, 2011). Levels are measured in the blood, using 25-hydroxyvitamin D_2 and 25-hydroxyvitamin D_3 to determine total 25-hydroxyvitamin D levels. A level of 20 ng/mL indicates a deficiency, 20 to 30 ng/mL an insufficiency, and greater than 30 ng/mL a sufficiency (optimal).

Those with decreased exposure to ultraviolet (UV) light, such as many who live in institutional settings or at the extremes of the hemispheres (e.g., the Inuit living near the Arctic Circle), are at higher than usual risk for vitamin D deficiencies. The normal changes in the aging skin exacerbate the risk. Vitamin D deficiencies reduce the absorption of calcium into bone.

It has been demonstrated that in response to the lowered levels of calcium, the secretion of parathyroid hormone increases, triggering increased bone resorption. Ensuring adequate intake of calcium and vitamin D is essential for healthy aging.

There is a considerable amount of research currently under way examining the effect and implications of the wide-scale deficiencies of vitamin D that have been observed (NCCAM, 2013).

BLOOD CHEMISTRY STUDIES

Blood chemistry studies include an assortment of laboratory tests used to identify and measure circulating elements and particles in the plasma and blood including thyroxin-stimulating hormone, glucose, proteins, amino acids, nutritive materials, excretion products, hormones, enzymes, vitamins, and minerals. Due to the most common chronic diseases in older adults, typical tests include lipid, vitamin D, and hepatic function panels; basic chemistry; comprehensive chemistry; and thyroid panels. Some of these are used for screening and others for monitoring specific health problems or treatments. All tests are individually selected and must be justified by a current diagnosis for reimbursement (Table 8-2). The nurse must become familiar with the names and test components used by the laboratory that provides services to her or his patients. The advanced practice nurse is expected to know when urgent and disease-monitoring blood chemistry studies are needed.

Electrolytes

Electrolytes are inorganic substances that maintain a complex balance between the intracellular and extracellular environments. They regulate hydration and blood pH and are critical for nerve and muscle function. For example, if there is an imbalance of calcium, sodium, and potassium levels, muscle weakness or contractions may occur. The blood levels of these electrolytes are reported as solitary measurements or as a part of panels, such as a basic or comprehensive metabolic panel.

Because older adults are more sensitive to electrolyte imbalances, these should be checked anytime there is a sudden mental status change, an adjustment or addition of a medication (e.g., potassium), an increase or decrease in fluid intake, or a transfer of the patient from one setting to another (e.g., home to hospital, nursing home to hospital, general unit to intensive care unit). Excessive diuresis, medication interactions (such as

---

BOX 8-5   Laboratory Testing and Vitamin B_{12}

Laboratory testing with the following findings indicate a vitamin B_{12} deficiency:
Serum cobalamin level <200 pg/mL
- With clinical signs or symptoms and/or related hematological abnormalities

OR

Serum cobalamin level <200 pg/mL
- On two different occasions

OR

Serum cobalamin level <200 pg/mL
- With total serum homocysteine level >13 μmol/L in the absence of renal failure or deficiencies in folate or B_6

OR

Low serum holotranscobalamin levels, <35 pmol/L

Adapted from Cadogan MP: Functional implications of vitamin B_{12} deficiency, *J Gerontol Nurs* 36:16–21, 2010.

TABLE 8-2   Examples of Laboratory Testing and Associated Diagnoses

DIAGNOSIS	EXAMPLES OF JUSTIFIED LABORATORY TEST
Hypertension	Basic metabolic panel (monitoring renal function and electrolytes related to treatment)
Altered mental status	Comprehensive metabolic panel, vitamin D, vitamin B_{12}, thyroid-stimulating panel
Dyslipidemia	Lipid panel, liver function (usually part of the comprehensive metabolic panel)

the use of both potassium and a potassium-sparing medication), and dehydration are probably the most common causes of electrolyte imbalances in older adults. Those who are frail, residing in long-term care facilities, or taking multiple medications are at especially high risk (Mentes, 2006). The most common electrolytes of concern in gerontological care include sodium and chloride, potassium, and glucose.

> ## ⚡ SAFETY ALERT
>
> A minor electrolyte imbalance may have little effect in a younger adult but may have significantly deleterious results in an older adult, especially one who is medically or cognitively fragile.
> The signs and symptoms of an imbalance in the older adult include weakness, fatigue, immobility, or delirium.

Sodium and Chloride

The test for sodium (Na^+) concentration, measured in circulating blood, is a proxy index of hydration. Sodium is necessary for the maintenance of blood pressure, the transmission of nerve impulses, and the regulation of body fluids into and out of the cells (Cho, 2013) (Table 8-3). The movement of fluids affects blood volume and is related to thirst, yet a reduced sense of thirst is a common change with aging (Mathew and Jacobs, 2014). Sodium balance is influenced by renal filtration and blood flow, cardiac output, and glomerular filtration rate (see Chapter 9). Laboratory sodium levels indicate the balance between ingested sodium and that which is excreted by the kidneys. Changes in sodium (Na^+) levels are always accompanied by changes in chloride (Cl^-) levels because they are predominantly found in combinations as sodium chloride.

Hyponatremia. A high prevalence of hyponatremia (≤ 130 mmol/L) has been found in long-term care facilities (Cho, 2013). Hyponatremia can be divided into three types: decreased extracellular fluid (ECF) volume (e.g., diarrhea, renal salt–losing circumstances); increased ECF volume (e.g., heart failure); or normal ECF from syndrome of inappropriate antidiuretic hormone secretion (SIADH)—with the latter more common in older adults compared with younger adults (Cho, 2013). Hyponatremia is usually asymptomatic as the plasma sodium concentration drops slightly below 130 mEq/L

and is usually accompanied by decreased osmolality (<280 mOsm/kg) (Cho, 2013). However, with further loss, central nervous system (CNS) symptoms appear and can become quickly significant, leading to seizures and coma secondary to cerebral edema. Mental status changes and other CNS effects can be seen with levels ≤ 125 to 130 mEq/L. Hypovolemic hyponatremia is always accompanied by a significant drop in postural blood pressure and tachycardia as the body attempts to compensate. In the most severe cases, hyponatremia can result in a high rate of morbidity and mortality. *Slow replacement is necessary*. Hyponatremia is one of the more common causes of delirium in older adults.

Hypernatremia. Hypernatremia, or an elevation of plasma sodium concentration (>145 mEq/L), is accompanied by hyperosmolality. It is most often caused by free water loss (e.g., vomiting or diarrhea, or dehydration), which is common among ill older adults in hospitals and long-term care facilities. The prevalence in this age group is up to 30% with a death rate of 42% (Cho, 2013). Low body weight is a risk factor. The death rate for hypernatremia is 40% in hospitalized elders, especially if it occurs quickly and is severe (>158 mEq/L). When sodium levels are >155 mEq/L, mental status changes should be expected, which indicates a poor prognosis in older adults. Signs include lethargy, irritability, and weakness. Severe hypernatremia (>158 mEq/L) is associated with delirium, coma, and seizures (Cho, 2013).

Potassium

Potassium (K^+) is an electrolyte found primarily within the cells themselves. It is essential in maintaining cell osmolality, ensuring muscle functioning, and transmitting nerve impulses and is a key component in the maintenance of the acid-base balance. Serum potassium levels decrease as lean body mass decreases, a normal part of aging. When the person is taking any K^+-sparing or wasting medication, as is common in later life, potassium level must be closely monitored.

Hypokalemia. Hypokalemia (K^+ <3.5 mEq/L) is associated with cardiac arrhythmias and may cause glucose intolerance and renal tubular dysfunction. Mild hypokalemia is asymptomatic. Potassium levels less than 2.5 mEq/L are critical and produce muscle weakness, cramping, confusion, fatigue, paralytic ileus, atrial and ventricular ectopy and tachycardia, fibrillation, and sudden death (Chernecky and Berger, 2013). Chronic low levels of potassium may lead to significant renal tubular dysfunction.

Hyperkalemia. Hyperkalemia (K^+ >5 mEq/L) usually occurs only in persons with advanced kidney disease. However, it is also found in those with acidosis, inadequate monitoring of potassium-sparing medications such as angiotensin-converting enzyme (ACE) inhibitors, or excessive potassium supplementation, all highly relevant to older adults. The signs and symptoms of a disturbance in potassium levels may not be evident until cardiac toxicity occurs (Box 8-6) (Cho, 2013).

Glucose

Glucose—a substance made from a combination of starch, cellulose, and glycogen—is the main source of energy used by the body. For optimal functioning, the levels of fasting glucose in the body must be maintained between about 70 and 110 mg/dL

TABLE 8-3   Signs and Symptoms of Disturbances in Sodium Levels

	HYPONATREMIA	HYPERNATREMIA
Signs	Plasma Na^+ ≤ 130 mmol/L (approximately)	Plasma Na^+ ≥ 150 mmol/L (approximately)
	Drop in BP (in hypovolemia)	Poor skin turgor
	Tachycardia (in hypovolemia)	Dry mucous membranes
Symptoms	Mental status changes	Mental status changes

BP, Blood pressure.
Data from Doig AK, Huether SE: The cellular environment fluids and electrolytes, acids and bases. In McCance KL, Huether SE, Brashers VL, et al, editors: *Pathophysiology: the biological basis for disease in adults and children,* ed 7, St. Louis, MO, 2014, Elsevier.

BOX 8-6   Signs and Symptoms of Disturbances in Potassium Levels

HYPOKALEMIA	HYPERKALEMIA
Generalized muscle weakness	Impaired muscle activity
Fatigue	Weakness
Muscle cramps	Muscle pain/cramps
Constipation	Increased GI motility
Ileus	Bradycardia
Flaccid paralysis	Cardiac arrest
Hyporeflexia	ECG changes:
Hypercapnia	P wave flattened
Tetany	T wave large, peaked
ECG changes:	QRS broad
Q-T interval prolonged	Biphasic QRS-T complex
T wave flattened or depressed	
ST segment depressed	

ECG, Electrocardiogram; *GI,* gastrointestinal.
For additional information, see Cho KC: Fluid and electrolyte disorders. In McPhee SJ, Papadakis MA, editors: *Current medical diagnosis and treatment 2010,* New York, 2010, McGraw-Hill.

(depending on the laboratory). Although the required levels do not change with aging, the signs and symptoms of persons with elevations or reductions may change. The fasting blood glucose levels are in the high range and it takes longer to return to normal levels after eating. These changes appear to be most likely related to a decrease in the insulin sensitivity of the tissues. For many older adults, even slight hypoglycemia can result in confused and depressed CNS activity. Elevations may not be evident until the person is in a hyperosmolar hyperglycemic nonketotic coma (now called hyperosmolar hyperglycemic state, or HHS). Interpretation of findings and related nursing interventions must always be done within the context of time since the person has ingested meals or snacks.

Glycosylated Hemoglobin A_{1C}

Laboratory testing of blood glucose or plasma glucose level provides "snapshot" information about the glucose level at any one time. For more accurate measurement and monitoring of glucose concentration, as is done in persons with diabetes, the glycosylated hemoglobin A_{1C} (Hb A_{1C}) measurement is used. About 7% of the hemoglobin in the RBCs can combine with glucose through the process of glycosylation. The glucose attachment is not easily reversible and therefore stays for the life of the RBC, approximately 120 days, and provides a good estimate of the overall average blood glucose level. In non-diabetics 4% to 5.9% is the normal range regardless of one's age; <7% indicates good diabetic control, 8% to 9% fair control, and >9% poor control (Chernecky and Berger, 2013).

URIC ACID

Uric acid is a naturally occurring end product of purine metabolism. It is usually measured in serum chemistry studies but is also found in the urine. Two thirds of the amount normally produced is excreted by the kidneys and the rest via the stool.

Elevations in uric acid levels (>7.5 mg/dL) are found when there is either *overproduction* or *underexcretion.* Measurement of uric acid levels is indicated in the evaluation of renal failure or leukemia, or, most often, in the diagnosis or treatment of gout or kidney stones. Hyperuricemia (>13 mg/dL) indicates a high risk for kidney stones or gout. While all persons with gout have an elevated uric acid level, others with elevated uric acid levels do not have gout (Nakasato and Christensen, 2014). A number of conditions and situations can result in increased uric acid levels, including binge alcohol drinking; medications, especially thiazide diuretics; surgery; or acute medical illness. The use of thiazide diuretics in the person with preexisting higher than usual uric acid levels may trigger an episode or recurrence of gout. The levels also increase slightly with age and vary between men and women (Chernecky and Berger, 2013).

PROSTATE-SPECIFIC ANTIGEN

One of the primary screening tools for prostate cancer has been a measure of the prostate-specific antigen (PSA). However, it can be elevated by a number of conditions; and the relative use of it as a screen for prostate cancer has been seriously questioned. As of May 2012 the U.S. Preventive Services Task Force (USPSTF) concluded that many men are harmed as a result of this screening test and few have any benefit from being tested (USPSTF, 2012). It does continue to be useful as a gross monitor of men's responsiveness to *treatment* of prostate cancer.

LABORATORY TESTING FOR CARDIAC HEALTH

Heart disease remains the primary cause of death for all persons. As a result, the gerontological nurse must be knowledgeable about the most common laboratory testing related to cardiac function. These include measures performed after acute cardiac events and those used in the determination of cardiac health and health risk.

Acute Cardiac Events

Older adults who appear to have acute and unexpected changes that may be related to an ischemic event need immediate transportation to an emergency department for evaluation. At the emergency department, initial testing for an acute cardiac event or acute myocardial infarction (AMI) will include at least an ECG and measurement of cardiac enzymes or tissue markers (creatinine kinase and troponin measurements), measurement of hs-CRP, and determination of ESR as discussed earlier.

Creatinine Kinase

The cardiac enzyme creatinine kinase (CK) is present in various parts of the body and in several forms (called isoenzymes). The isoenzyme CK-MB is associated with cardiac tissue, and laboratory values for CK-MB are used in the diagnosis of AMI, myocardial muscle injury, unstable angina, shock, malignant hyperthermia, myopathies, and myocarditis (Bashore et al, 2013). The CK-MB level rises 3 to 6 hours after an AMI occurs. It peaks at 12 to 24 hours (unless the infarction extends) and returns to normal after 12 to 48 hours; therefore it is not a useful measure after that period of time. A number of medications used to manage chronic diseases can cause false CK-MB testing results (Box 8-7). For the best diagnosis, CK-MB is used as a comparative measure with troponin measurement.

Troponin

Troponin I and troponin T are specific biomarkers for cardiac disease and have become the "gold standard" for diagnosis of heart injury. Their levels become elevated as early as 3 hours after an acute event and troponin I concentration remains elevated for 7 to 10 days; troponin T concentration remains elevated for 10 to 14 days. The normal level of troponin I is <0.03 ng/mL and that for troponin T is <0.2 ng/mL for persons at any age (Bashore et al, 2013).

Monitoring Cardiovascular Risk and Health

Increasing attention has been given to three biochemical markers that are believed to have value in the detection of heart disease or in the assessment for risk of cardiovascular disease. These are high-sensitivity C-reactive protein (hs-CRP), homocysteine, and brain natriuretic peptide (BNP). Detection and monitoring of dyslipidemia and elevated triglyceride levels are important for determining both health and health risk, at least in those younger than about age 80 (Takata et al, 2014).

Homocysteine

Homocysteine is a naturally occurring amino acid produced in the metabolism of proteins such as meat. When elevated (about >10 μmol/L) it may be associated with atherosclerosis and increase the risk for strokes, AMI, and peripheral vascular disease (AHA, 2014). It is now thought that there may be some association to neurocognitive impairments as well (Faux et al, 2011). Adequate amounts of vitamin B_{12} and folate appear to facilitate the breakdown of homocysteine, and therefore it is recommended that any deficiencies be treated and monitored (see Box 8-5).

B-type Natriuretic Peptide (BNP)

B-type natriuretic peptide (BNP) is an amino acid secreted by the ventricles in response to excessive stretching, such as in heart failure. It is secreted at the same time as a similar but inactive fragment, NT-proBNT. BNP levels are determined to identify and stratify persons in acute heart failure and possibly to monitor the effectiveness of treatment. The BNP level may also be a predictor of mortality from heart disease and diabetes (Sanchez et al, 2014). Serum levels >100 pg/mL indicate a poor prognosis (Jensen et al, 2012).

BOX 8-7 Medications that can Cause False CK-MB Results	
Anticoagulants	Alcohol
Aspirin	Lovastatin
Dexamethasone	Lidocaine
Furosemide	Propranolol
Captopril	Morphine
Colchicine	

Lipid Panels

Dyslipidemia and elevated levels of triglycerides have been found to be health risks regardless of one's age and are major predictors of coronary heart disease. Laboratory testing is usually done as a "lipid panel" and includes both cholesterol and triglyceride levels. It is done both as a health screen for persons at high risk and as a means of monitoring the response to treatment, usually for those taking lipid-lowering medications and/or altering their diet. For the most accurate results, the person should have fasted 12 to 15 hours before the test.

Cholesterol. Cholesterol is a sterol compound used by the body to stabilize cell membranes. It is metabolized in the liver, where it is combined with low-density lipoprotein (LDL), high-density lipoprotein (HDL), and very-low-density lipoprotein (VLDL). Men's cholesterol levels slowly increase from puberty until about age 60 years. They appear to stabilize, only to rise again after age 80 years; however, the elevations after the age of 80 may be an indication of increased longevity (Freitas et al, 2014). While this renewed increase in LDL levels may increase the risk again for atherosclerosis, an elevated HDL level may have the opposite effect (Freitas et al, 2014). The cholesterol levels of women are relatively stable until menopause, at which time they begin to rise.

Although lipid panels are usually conducted for the management of statin therapy, according to the most recent guidelines of the American Heart Association there is no longer a "one size fits all" in the consideration of the component parts of lipids. Instead, they recommend that multiple factors be taken into account when the "numbers" are reviewed. These include family history, other risk factors for heart disease, and long-term risk/benefit ratios (Stone et al, 2014).

An unexplained low serum cholesterol level (≤200 mg/dL) is indicative of several conditions including malnutrition—a common problem for those with difficulty swallowing, trouble feeding themselves, or finding themselves in an environment where the foods they are served are different from those to which they are accustomed (e.g., a long-term care facility).

A total cholesterol level less than 160 mg/dL in a frail elder is a risk factor for increased mortality. A total cholesterol level ≥200 mg/dL has also been suggested to increase neuropsychiatric symptoms in Alzheimer's disease, especially in men (Hall et al, 2014). Triglycerides are the primary lipids found in the blood and are bound to a protein. They are produced in the liver and circulated in the blood. Excess blood levels are deposited into fatty tissue. Triglycerides peak at midlife. Abnormally low triglyceride levels are suggestive of malnutrition or hyperthyroidism. Reasons for elevated levels include chronic renal failure and poorly controlled diabetes. Severely elevated triglyceride levels (>2000 mg/dL) are a strong risk factor for pancreatitis (Mathew and Jacobs, 2014).

TESTING FOR BODY PROTEINS

Body proteins are measured by determining the amount of albumin and globulin in the serum. Serum albumin is a measure of nutritional status. Globulins are important in the functioning of antibodies and in the maintenance of osmotic pressure. The measurement and knowledge of the protein status of frail elders will help determine when additional consultation (e.g., dietitian or speech therapist) or dietary supplements are needed.

Serum Albumin

Serum albumin and globulin levels are used most often as measures of nutritional status but are also used to diagnose and monitor cancer, protein-wasting states, immune disorders, and liver function (Chernecky and Berger, 2013). Although serum protein measurements are commonly ordered, they are neither sensitive nor specific for nutritional health and are often in the low range of normal in older adults. Medications such as corticosteroids, insulin, and progesterone increase protein stores but are not recommended. Dehydration will show a deceptive increase in albumin levels at the same time albumin levels appear to decrease with overhydration, liver and renal disease, malabsorption, and changes from an upright position to a supine position during the blood draw (Chernecky and Berger, 2013). The half-life of albumin is about 3 weeks, so changes are not quickly apparent except in sudden and acutely severe conditions. However, albumin levels are most useful as an indicator of the severity of illness and the risk of mortality. Prealbumin (transthyretin) has a half-life of only 2 to 3 days and is therefore a more sensitive marker for change. A low prealbumin level can confirm poor nutritional status and serve as a monitor for active treatment.

LABORATORY TESTS OF RENAL HEALTH

Renal function decreases substantially with age, but in most cases the body is able to compensate adequately and there are only slight changes so that laboratory findings are still "within normal limits." However, laboratory findings may be *unreliable* in those with reduced lean body mass (a normal change with aging), excessive dietary intake of protein, alterations in metabolism, and strenuous physical activity before measurement. Because of the frequency of health problems and medications that further affect renal health, measuring and monitoring renal functioning are particularly important to the older adult and the gerontological nurse. Laboratory indices particularly diagnostic of renal disease are elevated blood urea nitrogen and creatinine levels. They are included in a basic metabolic panel.

Blood Urea Nitrogen

Urea is the end product of protein metabolism. The serum chemistry test for blood urea nitrogen (BUN) is used as a gross measurement for renal functioning and level of hydration. Blood levels are often in the high-normal range because of the age-related changes to the liver and kidney. Changes over time in the BUN level may be more important than any one laboratory result, especially in the assessment of dehydration, renal insufficiency, or renal failure. *Azotemia* is an elevation of BUN level. Prerenal azotemia refers to elevations before blood reaches the kidneys; causes include shock, severe dehydration, congestive heart failure, and excessive protein catabolism such as in starvation. Normal BUN findings for adults are 10 to 20 mg/dL (Chernecky and Berger, 2013).

Creatinine

Creatinine is a by-product of the breakdown of muscle creatinine phosphate that is normally produced in energy metabolism; its level is highly dependent on muscle mass. As long as muscle mass remains the same, the serum creatinine level should be constant. The reduced lean muscle mass of normal aging will result in a decreased creatinine level. The creatinine level is a key aspect of the determination of the glomerular filtration rate (GFR)—that is, the ability of the kidneys to handle the fluids and products passing through them. The creatinine level has been specifically used to diagnose and monitor impaired renal function. Although the measurement of creatinine is a more accurate reflection of renal health than BUN, it can also overestimate renal function in the elderly. Consideration of both the creatinine level and the BUN level must be considered in the dosing of a number of medications excreted through the kidneys.

However, because of the number of factors that can alter the BUN/creatinine level (and therefore the measurement of creatinine clearance), another test—cystatin C—is a more sensitive marker for estimating the GFR (Inker et al, 2012). Cystatin C is a very small molecule biomarker associated with detecting early breakdown in a number of muscles, including the kidney. It is less dependent on age, sex, race, and muscle mass than creatinine and therefore more appropriate to use in older adults. When used together with creatinine measurements, it has been found to more accurately predict GFR-related death for those with end-stage renal disease (Shlipak et al, 2013).

MONITORING FOR THERAPEUTIC BLOOD LEVELS

The monitoring of physiological levels of certain medications is especially important at any time but more so in later life. Medications are in need of monitoring not only because they are given more often but also because inappropriate dosing can have a more dramatic effect. At levels too low, the effects of medications may be negligible, and at levels too high they may easily result in adverse or even life-threatening drug events (Chapter 9).

Anticoagulants

Anticoagulation therapy has become the mainstay of stroke prevention for persons with atrial fibrillation (Chapter 22) and in the prevention of deep vein thrombosis and pulmonary embolus following surgery, such as a hip repair. When the blood is excessively anticoagulated, the person is at risk for life-threatening bleeding. When the levels of anticoagulants in the blood are too low, the protective qualities are lost.

At the present time there are six anticoagulants available in the United States, but only the levels of warfarin and heparin and of heparin's variation enoxaparin (low-molecular-weight heparin) can be monitored (Fogerty and Minichiello, 2013). Anyone who is taking warfarin or heparin must have their coagulation time monitored because of the narrow therapeutic windows. Prothrombin, produced by the liver, is a key component in blood clotting. For the body to produce prothrombin, it must have adequate intake and absorption of vitamin K. During clotting, prothrombin is converted to thrombin as the first part of the coagulation cascade. The prothrombin time (PT) is the most sensitive measure of deficiencies in vitamin K–dependent clotting factors II, VII, IX, and X affected by warfarin use. The PT is not sensitive to fibrinogen deficiencies and heparin, and instead the combination of PT with a partial prothrombin time (PT/PTT) is used to monitor coagulation status and determine the drug dose needed to provide the desired effect, especially in the acute care setting. The results are important for prompt adjustment of an individual's dosage for the anticoagulants.

In the past, precise monitoring of the anticoagulation effects of warfarin was difficult because of the amount of variation in test results between laboratories. An international normalized ratio (INR) is now used to overcome these difficulties. The INR can be measured by a laboratory or at the "point of care" (POC) such as in a clinic or a care facility, using a device similar to a blood glucose monitor. Because there are standard ranges for the INR (Table 8-4), some persons self-monitor, with their cardiologists receiving the results and adjusting the dose of the warfarin as needed. Nurses often perform the POC INR test.

Antiarrhythmics: Digoxin

Digoxin (Lanoxin) is a drug that is commonly used to control ventricular response to chronic atrial fibrillation. It is initiated slowly and carefully to prevent too rapid a reduction in heart rate. Once the patient's dose is stabilized, the nurse monitors the effect of the medication by measuring the heart rate before drug administration and by observing for signs of adverse effects. Monitoring includes periodic determination of blood levels. The normal therapeutic range is 0.9 to 2.0 ng/mL with toxicity occurring at levels greater than 3.0 ng/mL. However, because of the normal changes with aging that affect pharmacokinetics, toxicity may be evident at levels well below 3.0 ng/mL. Observing for signs of toxicity, regardless of laboratory results, is probably more meaningful; this is especially important for an older adult who is receiving a dose >0.125 mg/day. The nurse can use the blood level only as a general guide, and it must be combined with the clinical presentation (including heart rate) of the person being treated.

Thyroid Panels

Thyroid panels are used to both diagnose and monitor thyroid disorders and their treatment (Chapter 25). The panel includes measurement of the level of thyroid-stimulating hormone (TSH), free T_3 (triiodothyronine), and free T_4 (thyroxin). The levels of each of these, considered relative to each other, are used to make a diagnosis (see Chapter 25). If the person has a goiter, a thyroid scan with technetium may be necessary (Brashers et al, 2014). In most cases, treatment (especially thyroid replacement) can be monitored easily on the basis of TSH levels alone. Testing is repeated initially at 6- to 8-week intervals until a euthyroid state is reached and confirmed. After that, only annual reevaluations are necessary unless there is a change in the person's condition. The nurse is in a key position to monitor the thyroid function of the patient by ensuring timely and appropriate laboratory testing of TSH level.

URINE STUDIES

Urine is the end-product of metabolism and contains products that have exceeded the body's threshold of usefulness. If the kidneys are working well and the urine level of a compound is elevated, there should be a corresponding elevation in the blood. However, if the kidney is diseased, urine levels may be deceptively low. The most common urine test in the everyday care of older adults is a urinalysis.

A macroscopic urinalysis may be performed in the outpatient primary care setting, but more often is done by a diagnostic laboratory. In healthy aging, the findings do not differ by age, but abnormalities are frequently found because of the high rate of diabetes, renal insufficiency, subclinical bacteriuria, and proteinuria.

> ### ⚡ SAFETY ALERT
> A finding of hematuria, even in outpatient macroscopy, always requires further evaluation.

A urine specimen is collected either by using the clean-catch method or via catheterization. In the outpatient setting, it is best that the specimen be collected at the laboratory or sent to the lab immediately. If this is not possible, it may be collected and refrigerated for up to 2 hours if absolutely necessary. Any specimen that has not been properly stored or tested promptly should be disposed of and a new one obtained. The cleaner and fresher the specimen, the more accurate the analysis will be. There is a long history of conflicting evidence of the accuracy and reliability of urine testing using a "dip stick" method in the outpatient setting. Both laboratory and outpatient office analyses will yield results for urine specific gravity, pH, and the presence of urine protein, glucose, ketones, blood, bilirubin, nitrates, and leukocytes.

The specific gravity is a measure of the adequacy of the renal concentrative mechanism; it measures hydration and therefore is a useful measure when caring for frail elders. Specific gravity in the adult is normally between 1.005 and 1.030. These values decrease with aging because of the 33% to 50% decline in the number of nephrons, which impairs the ability of the kidney to

INDICATION	PREFERRED INR
Deep vein thrombosis management and prevention of emboli	2.0-3.0
For those with mitral or aortic tissue valves	
Post–myocardial infarction (with aspirin)	
Potential range for post–myocardial infarction	3.0-4.0 (target 3.5)
Prophylaxis for high-risk surgery (e.g., orthopedic)	2.5-3.5
Stroke prevention for those older than age 75 with atrial fibrillation	2.0-3.0

TABLE 8-4 Preferred International Normalized Ratio According to Indication for Anticoagulation

INR, International normalized ratio.
From Chernecky CC, Berger BJ: *Laboratory tests and diagnostic procedures*, ed 6, St Louis, MO, 2013, Elsevier.

concentrate urine. The urine pH indicates its acid-base balance. An alkaline pH is usually caused by bacteria (which may indicate a urinary tract infection), a diet high in citrus fruits and vegetables, or the intake of sodium bicarbonates. Acidic urine occurs with starvation, dehydration, and diets high in meats and cranberries. A urine albumin level of almost 30 mg/dL translates into a considerably high rate of proteinuria and always indicates a need for further evaluation of renal function. Ascorbic acid and aspirin can cause false-negative results for glucose. Ketones may be positive in high-protein diets, "crash" diets, or starvation.

Nitrates and/or leukocytes are often found in the presence of infection. A urinalysis suggestive of the presence of bacteria usually results in further testing, most often a culture of the urine and a subsequent testing of sensitivity of the bacteria to select antibiotics. This is often ordered as a "U/A (urine analysis) C & S (culture and sensitivity) as indicated." However, because of the potential lethality of any infection in ill older adults, empirical clinical evidence of a potential infection may require treatment before the 3 or 4 days needed to obtain culture results.

◆ PROMOTING HEALTHY AGING: IMPLICATIONS FOR GERONTOLOGICAL NURSING

Laboratory tests and regular screening tests are commonly employed when caring for a resident of a nursing home. Protocols for establishing routine laboratory testing procedures for long-term care vary widely from one institution to the next and from one laboratory to the next. Gerontological nurses advocate good resident care by requesting laboratory tests and developing protocols to comply with recommended minimal standards for screening and monitoring for both long-term and short-term residents in residential settings.

Knowledge about the use of, frequency of, and basic interpretations of laboratory findings is important to the quality of care provided. These skills are especially important in gerontological nursing practice—not because of the expected normal changes in laboratory results but because of the potential influence of commonly prescribed medications in the presence of chronic diseases often prevalent in the older adult.

Laboratory values are helpful tools in understanding clinical signs and symptoms, although clinical decisions based on laboratory values alone are not enough for treatment of the whole person. Abnormal laboratory results trigger comprehensive patient assessments, obtaining information about clinical signs and symptoms, patient history, and psychosocial and physical examination. The nurse combines this information with the interpretation of laboratory values to establish the most appropriate care in collaboration with the person's nurse practitioner or physician. The nurse practitioner quickly and accurately interprets the findings and translates these into the overall plan of care.

▎KEY CONCEPTS

- The normal range of diagnostic laboratory results does not differ by age.
- Because of more limited reserves, the older adult is often more sensitive to slight variations in biological parameters.
- The nurse is often responsible for the initial interpretation of laboratory results. The nurse cannot depend entirely on laboratory values when considering the possibility of medication toxicity.
- The interactions between medications and chronic disorders complicate the interpretation of laboratory values in older adults.

▎NURSING STUDY: EVALUATING LABORATORY RESULTS

An 84-year-old white male, Mr. Jones, is being admitted to the nursing home where you work. He has a history of heart disease, hypertension, diabetes, constipation, and anemia of chronic inflammation. You find that he denies any fever, chest pain, numbness or tingling, leg swelling, or palpitations. His diabetes has been under fairly good control while at home, but he has difficulty telling you how much insulin he has been taking. His skin is slightly warm to the touch. He is lethargic, but you notice that he also has some muscle twitching. He has an order to have blood tests done today, including a CBC and a complete metabolic panel. You request it and get the following results later in the evening. Medications include lisinopril, 20 mg/day; Lasix, 40 mg/day; potassium, 5 mEq/day; Lantus insulin, 12 units every morning; laxative as needed; multivitamin daily. Blood sugar before supper is 243.

	RESULT	NORMAL RANGE
Sodium	135 mEq/L	136-148 mEq/L
Potassium	5.8 mEq/L	3.5-5.3 mEq/L
Chloride	110 mEq/L	97-108 mEq/L
Glucose	60 mg/dL	70-110 mg/dL
BUN	25 mg/dL	10-20 mg/dL

	RESULT	NORMAL RANGE
Creatinine	1.8 mg/dL	0.6-1.2 mg/dL
Albumin	2.4 g/dL	3.5-5.8 g/dL
WBCs	7000/mm³	5000-10,000/mm³
RBCs	$4.0 \times 10^6/\mu L$	4.4-$5.8 \times 10^6/\mu L$
Hb	10.2 g/dL	14-18 g/dL
Hct	30.6%	39-48%

- Considering Mr. Jones and his current health status, which of the preceding lab results concerns you most?
- Are there any deviations in the results that are consistent with normal aging?
- Which of these deviations from normal are potentially the most dangerous for Mr. Jones at this time? If so, why?
- Could any of the abnormal blood tests be related to his medications?
- Are there any results that need prompt referral to the primary care provider for Mr. Jones? If so, which one(s)?

CRITICAL THINKING QUESTIONS AND ACTIVITIES

1. The next time you are working with an older adult either as his or her nurse/nurse practitioner or as a student nurse, review the most recent laboratory report and determine which variations are more likely a reflection of the person's disease state rather than age.

2. In a classroom discussion, consider a 90 year old with increasing dyspnea (shortness of breath) and fatigue. If you were ordering laboratory tests for this person, which ones would you choose in order of priority?

3. Summarize laboratory values that are considered the most "critical" in older adults and require some type of immediate response.

RESEARCH QUESTIONS

1. In what way does food and alcohol intake affect the accuracy of laboratory test results?

2. If someone has had a number of chronic diseases for an extended period of time and yet the person is active and "healthy," what laboratory finding(s) may still be outside of the normal limits?

REFERENCES

American Heart Association (AHA): *Homocysteine, folic acid and cardiovascular health*, 2014. http://www.heart.org/HEARTORG/GettingHealthy/NutritionCenter/Homocysteine-Folic-Acid-and-Cardiovascular-Disease_UCM_305997_Article.jsp. Accessed August 2014.

Antony AC: Megaloblastic anemias. In Hoffman R, Benz EJ Jr, Silberstein LE, et al, editors: *Hematology: basic principles and practice*, ed 6, Philadelphia, 2012, Elsevier Saunders, chap 37.

Balducci L: Anemia. In Ham RJ, Sloane PD, Warshaw GA, et al, editors: *Primary care geriatrics: a case-based approach*, ed 6, Philadelphia, 2014, Elsevier, pp 491–496.

Bashore TM, Granger CB, Hranitzky PK, et al: Heart disease. In Papadakis MA, McPhee SJ, editors: *Current medical diagnosis and treatment 2013*, New York, 2013, McGraw-Hill, pp 324–432.

Berliner N: Anemia in the elderly, *Trans Am Clin Climatol Assoc* 124:230–237, 2013.

Brashers VL, Jones RE, Huether SE: Mechanisms of hormonal regulation. In McCance KL, Huether SE, Brashers VL, et al, editors: *Pathophysiology: the biological basis for disease in adults and children*, ed 7, St. Louis, 2014, Mosby, pp 689–716.

Cankurtaran M, Ulger Z, Halil M, et al: How to assess high erythrocyte sedimentation rate (ESR) in elderly? *Arch Gerontol Geriatr* 50(3):323–326, 2010.

Centers for Disease Control and Prevention (CDC): Vitamin B$_{12}$ deficiency, 2009. http://www.cdc.gov/ncbddd/b12/intro.html. Accessed August 2014.

Chavez PH: Functional outcomes of anemia in older adults, *Semin Hematol* 45: 255–260, 2008.

Chernecky CC, Berger BJ: *Laboratory tests and diagnostic procedures*, ed 6, St. Louis, MO, 2013, Elsevier.

Cho KC: Fluid and electrolyte disorders. In Papadakis MA, McPhee SJ, editors: *Current medical diagnosis and treatment 2013*, New York, 2013, McGraw-Hill, pp 870–897.

Colombet I, Pouchot J, Kronz V, et al: Agreement between erythrocyte sedimentation rate and C-reactive protein in hospital practice, *Am J Med* 123:863.e7–e13, 2010.

Dugdale DC: *Blood differential*, Medline Plus, 2013.http://www.nlm.nih.gov/medlineplus/ency/article/003657.htm. Accessed August 2014.

Ernst AA, Weiss SJ, Tracy LA, et al: Usefulness of CRP and ESR in predicting septic joints, *South Med J* 103:522–526, 2010.

Faux NG, Ellis KA, Porter L, et al: Homocysteine, vitamin B$_{12}$, and folic acid in Alzheimer's disease, mild cognitive impairment, and health elderly: baseline characteristic in subjects of the Australian Imaging Biomarker Lifestyle Study, *J Alzheimers Dis* 27(4):909–922, 2011.

Fogerty PF, Minichiello T: Disorders of hemostasis, thrombosis, and antithrombotic therapy. In Papadakis MA, McPhee SJ, editors: *Current medical diagnosis and treatment 2013*, New York, 2013, McGraw-Hill, pp 538–563.

Freitas WM, Quaglia LA, Santos SN, et al: Low HDL cholesterol but not high LDL cholesterol is independently associated with subclinical atherosclerosis in healthy octogenarians, *Aging Clin Res*, June 7, 2014. [Epub ahead of print].

Hall JR, Weichmann AR, Johnson LA, et al: Total cholesterol and neuropsychiatric symptoms in Alzheimer's disease: the impact of total cholesterol level and gender, *Dement Geriatr Cogn Disord* 38 (5–6):300–309, 2014.

Hefland M, Buckley D, Freeman M, et al: Emerging risk factors for coronary heart disease: a summary of a systematic reviews for the U.S. Prevention Services Task Force, *Ann Intern Med* 151(7): 496–507.

Inal A, Koc B, Bircan HY, et al: The effects of aging on lymphocyte subgroups in males and females, *Med Sci Monit Basic Res* 20:93–96, 2014.

Inker LA, Schmid CH, Tighiouart H, et al: Estimating glomerular filtration rate from serum creatinine and cystatin C, *N Engl J Med* 367:20–29, 2012.

Jensen J, Ma LP, Bjurman C, et al: Prognostic values of NTpro BNP/BNP ration in comparison with NTproBNP or BNP alone in elderly patients with chronic heart failure in a 2-year follow up, *Int J Cardiol* 55(1):1–5, 2012.

Kreiner F, Langberg H, Galbo H: Increased muscle interstitial levels of inflammatory cytokines in polymyalgia rheumatica, *Arthritis Rheum* 62:3768–3775, 2010.

Lichtin AE: Anemia of chronic disease (iron-reutilization anemia). *Merck manual: Professional edition*, 2013. http://www.merckmanuals.com/professional/hematology_and_oncology/anemias_caused_by_deficient_erythropoiesis/anemia_of_chronic_disease.html. Accessed August 2014.

Liesveld J, Reagan P: Eosinophilia. In *Merck manual: Professional edition*, 2014. http://www.merckmanuals.com/professional/hematology_and_oncology/eosinophilic

_disorders/eosinophilia.html. Accessed August 2014.

Mathew MK, Jacobs MS: Malnutrition and feeding problems. In Ham RJ, Sloane PD, Warshaw GA, et al, editors: *Primary care geriatrics: a case-based approach*, ed 6, Philadelphia, 2014, Elsevier, pp 315–322.

Mentes J: A typology of caps and oral rehydration: problems exhibited by frail nursing home residents, *J Gerontol Nurs* 32:13–19, 2006.

Nakasato Y, Christensen M: Arthritis and related disorders. In Ham RJ, Sloane PD, Warshaw GA, et al, editors: *Primary care geriatrics: a case-based approach*, ed 6, Philadelphia, 2014, Elsevier, pp 456–465.

National Center for Complementary and Alternative Medicine (NCCAM): *Got (enough vitamin D? "Current Controversies in Medicine" STEP event series*, 2013. http://nccam.nih.gov/node/4816. Accessed August 2014.

National Heart, Lung, and Blood Institute (NHLBI): *Pernicious anemia*, 2011. http://www.nhlbi.nih.gov/health/health-topics/topics/prnanmia. Accessed August 2014.

Sanchez I, Santana S, Escobar C, et al: Clinical implications of different biomarkers in elderly patients with heart failure, *Biomark Med* 8(4):535–541, 2014.

Schwartz A, Rote NS: Alterations of leukocyte, lymphoid, and hemostatic function. In McCance KL, Huether SE, Brashers VL, et al, editors: *Pathophysiology: the biological basis for disease in adults and children*, ed 7, St. Louis, MO, 2014, Mosby, pp 1008–1054.

Semba RD, Ricks MO, Ferrucci L, et al: Types of anemia and mortality among elderly women living in the community: the Women's Health and Aging Study I, *Aging Clin Exp Res* 19:259–264, 2007.

Shlipak MG, Matsushita K, Ärmlöv J, et al: Cystatin C versus creatinine in determining risk based on kidney function, *N Engl J Med* 369:932–943, 2013.

Stone NJ, Robinson JG, Lichtenstein AH, et al: ACC/AHA Prevention guideline on the treatment of blood cholesterol to reduce atherosclerotic cardiovascular risk in adults, *Circulation* 129:S1–S45, 2014.

Takata Y, Ansai T, Soh I, et al: Serum total cholesterol concentration and 10-year mortality in an 85-year-old population, *Clin Interventions Aging* 9:293–300, 2014.

Thibodeau GA, Patton KT: *Structure and function of the body*, ed 12, St. Louis, MO, 2003, Mosby.

U.S. Preventive Services Task Force: *Prostate cancer: screening*, 2012. http://www.uspreventiveservicestaskforce.org/Page/Topic/recommendation-summary/prostate-cancer-screening. Accessed August 2014.

World Health Organization (WHO): *World Health Organization definition of anemia: reports of a WHO scientific group*, Geneva, Switzerland, 1968, World Health Organization.

Zakai NH, Katz R, Hirsch C, et al: A prospective study of anemia status, hemoglobin concentrations, and mortality in an elderly cohort: the Cardiovascular Health Study, *Arch Intern Med* 165:2214–2220, 2005.

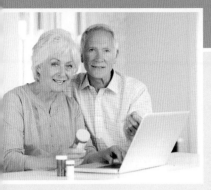

CHAPTER 9

Geropharmacology

Kathleen Jett

http://evolve.elsevier.com/Touhy/TwdHlthAging

A STUDENT SPEAKS

Whenever I see patients in the clinic I try to think very carefully before adding any medications, but since most of them have so many things going on with them, I sometimes wonder where I can start!

Helen, age 32, gerontological nurse practitioner student

AN ELDER SPEAKS

Every time I go to the clinic I get another prescription. It just doesn't seem like I should need to take so many, so sometimes I don't.

Annie, age 72

LEARNING OBJECTIVES

On completion of this chapter, the reader will be able to:

1. Describe the pharmacokinetic and pharmacodynamic changes that occur as a result of normal changes with aging.
2. Describe potential problems associated with medication therapy in late life.
3. Identify medications that are more commonly used in late life.
4. Identify inappropriate medication use and explain its application in gerontological nursing.
5. Identify the early signs of adverse medication reactions and develop strategies to prevent these.
6. Discuss barriers to medication adherence in older adults.
7. Develop a nursing plan to promote safe medication practices and prevent medication toxicity.

In the United States, persons 65 years of age and older are prescribed more medications than any other age group. Although the exact statistics vary from study to study, all findings indicate that as one ages, the number of prescribed medications, dietary supplements, and herbal products taken increases. When used appropriately, pharmacological interventions can enhance the quality of life and promote healthy aging. When used inappropriately, they contribute to both morbidity and mortality at any age. Unfortunately, even when medications are prescribed, administered, and taken appropriately, adverse medication reactions and events can and do occur, especially to older adults. The reasons for this are many and include reduced organ function and physiological reserve, as well as varying levels of skills of health care providers (Ajemigbitse et al, 2013).

This chapter reviews the effect of aging on pharmacokinetics and pharmacodynamics. Issues in medications are discussed including polypharmacy, medication interactions, adverse medication reaction and events, and the uses of psychoactive agents relative to the aging adult.

PHARMACOKINETICS

Pharmacokinetics is the study of the movement and action of a medication in the body. Pharmacokinetic processes determine the concentration of medications in the body, which in turn determines the effect. The concentration of the medication at different times depends on how the medication is taken into the body (absorption), where the medication is dispersed (distribution), how the medication is broken down (metabolism), and how the body gets rid of the medication (excretion) (Figure 9-1). Although there are important age-related changes in absorption, distribution, and elimination, there are few such changes in metabolism.

Absorption

There does not seem to be conclusive evidence that absorption in older adults is appreciably different from that in younger adults. There are, however, several normal age-related changes that have the potential to affect absorption and therefore the amount of the medication that is available for use and the potential to cause unintended effects. Most medications are

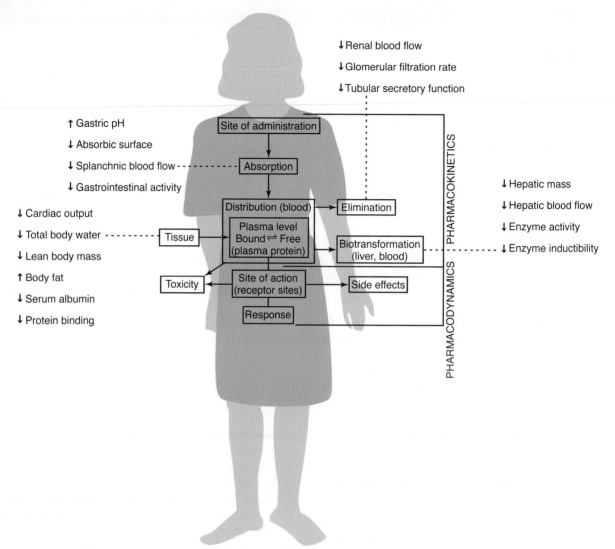

FIGURE 9-1 Physiological Age Changes and the Pharmacokinetics and Pharmacodynamics of Medication Use. (Data from Kane RL, Abrass ID, Ouslander JG: *Essentials of clinical geriatrics*, New York, 1984, McGraw-Hill; Lamy PP: Hazards of medication use in the elderly: common sense measures to reduce them, *Postgrad Med* 76:50, 1984; Montamat SC, Cusack BJ, Vestal RE: Management of medication therapy in the elderly, *N Engl J Med* 321: 303, 1989; Roberts J, Tumer N: Pharmacodynamic basis for altered medication action in the elderly, *Clin Geriatr Med* 4:127, 1988; Vestal RE, Dawson GW: Pharmacology and aging. In Finch CE, Schneider EL, editors: *Handbook of biology and aging*, New York, 1985, Van Nostrand Reinhold.)

administered orally, and many of those more often taken by older adults lead to a dry mouth and decreased salivation, especially those with anticholinergic effects (Box 9-1). With sublingual administration, medication is absorbed directly into the systemic circulation through the mucous membrane, but a dry mouth will reduce or delay buccal absorption. Normal age-related decreases in esophageal motility can lead to swallowing difficulties and tissue erosions. One possible alternative, rectal administration, may be useful when the patient cannot tolerate oral or sublingual medications, especially for those nearing the end of life.

BOX 9-1 Use of Medications with Strong Anticholinergic Properties

Examples of Medications	Select Potential Effects of Any of the Medications
Antihistamines	
Some antidepressants	Constipation
Most antipsychotics	Dry mouth
Antimuscarinics (for urinary incontinence)	Blurred vision
	Dizziness
Antispasmodics	Urinary retention
	Altered mental status

Age-related changes in the stomach have several potential effects. Decreases in the amount of gastric acid may retard the action of acid-dependent medications. Delayed stomach emptying may diminish or negate the effectiveness of short-lived medications that could become inactivated before reaching the small intestine. Some enteric-coated formulations of medications, such as aspirin, which are specifically meant to bypass stomach acidity, may be delayed so long that their action begins in the stomach and may cause gastric irritation or nausea.

Once a medication has been administered orally (or enterally), it may be absorbed directly into the bloodstream from the stomach (e.g., alcohol), but usually absorption begins in the duodenum of the small intestine and continues in the large intestine. Slowed intestinal motility, while not a normal change of aging, is frequently encountered in older patients. This additional time for contact of the medication with the intestinal walls increases the risk for adverse reactions and unpredictable effects.

Nurses working with older adults are usually familiar with the transdermal medication delivery system (TDDS). Designed for the slow absorption of fat-soluble medications, it has been found to be extremely useful for those who require very small doses of a medication over a longer period of time (usually over 72 hours). This route overcomes any first-pass problems (through an aging liver) and is more convenient, acceptable, and potentially more reliable than other routes, especially for persons with cognitive disorders. Ideally the TDDS provides for a more constant rate of medication administration and eliminates concern about gastrointestinal absorption variation, gastrointestinal intolerance, and medication interaction. However, the use of these patches requires manual dexterity that is not always possible, especially for persons with orthopedic deformities such as osteoarthritis. Additionally, for the person who is underweight or overweight, absorption may be unreliable. The characteristic thinning, dryness, and roughness of older skin also may affect absorption of the intended dose. An increased risk for an allergic reaction to a transdermal patch is due to age-related changes in the immune system, especially in the skin and mucous membranes (Saxon et al, 2010).

Distribution

The systemic circulation transports a medication throughout the body to receptors on the cells of the target organ where a therapeutic effect is initiated. The organs of high blood flow (e.g., brain, kidneys, lungs, and liver) rapidly receive the highest concentrations. Distribution to organs of lower blood flow (e.g., skin, muscles, fat) occurs more slowly and results in lower concentrations of the medication in these tissues. Circulatory diseases common in late life, such as peripheral vascular disease, can negatively affect medication distribution.

Normal changes with aging include lower total body water and higher body fat (as fat replaces lean tissue). Adipose tissue nearly doubles in healthy older men and increases by one half in older women. Lipophilic (fat-soluble) medications concentrate in adipose tissue to a greater extent than in other tissues. If the medication accumulates to an excess in the adipose tissue, it may increase medication effect and can even result in a potentially fatal overdose (Hughes and Beizer, 2014). In contrast, the decreased amount of body water found in normal aging leads to higher serum concentrations of water-soluble medications such as digoxin, ethanol, and aminoglycosides.

Distribution also depends on the availability of plasma protein in the form of lipoproteins, globulins, and especially albumin. Some medications are bound to protein for distribution. In healthy adults of any age, a predictable percentage of an absorbed medication is inactivated as it is bound to the protein. The remaining free medication is available in the bloodstream for therapeutic effect when an effective concentration is reached in the plasma.

Serum albumin level may be significantly reduced in those with malnutrition, acute illness, or a long-standing chronic condition. This reduction is common among those who are frail and in need of skilled care at home or in long-term care settings (Chapter 32). This decrease in serum albumin level can increase the amount of free medication available in an unpredictable manner. This effect can also occur when a person who had been well, with controlled medication responses, becomes ill (Hughes and Beizer, 2014). Signs of medication toxicity can occur quickly; this is especially dangerous in medications with narrow therapeutic windows (Box 9-2).

Excretion

Medications are excreted either unchanged or as metabolites (Box 9-3). A few medications are eliminated through the lungs, in bile and feces, or in breast milk. Very small amounts of medications and metabolites can also be found in hair, sweat, saliva, tears, and semen. The renal system, however, is the primary site of medication excretion. Excretion occurs when a medication passes through the kidneys and into the bladder and depends on the mechanisms of glomerular filtration, active tubular secretion, and passive tubular reabsorption (Chapter 16). The glomerular filtration rate (GFR) in turn depends on both the rate and extent

---

BOX 9-2 Medications Commonly Used by Older Adults with Narrow Therapeutic Windows

Unpredictable concentrations of drug are especially dangerous in those with narrow therapeutic windows such as salicylates, lorazepam, diazepam, chlorpromazine, phenobarbital, or haloperidol.

BOX 9-3 What is a Metabolite?

A metabolite is a substance that results from the breaking down of a medication in the body (metabolism). It may continue to work in a way in which the original medication did or it becomes inactivated in the process.

of protein binding of the medication; only unbound medications are filtered.

Age-related changes in renal function have the most significant effect on pharmacokinetics in the aging body. A decline in kidney function is a normal change with aging, especially a decrease in the GFR, which reduces the body's ability to excrete or eliminate medications in a timely manner. The significantly decreased GFR leads to prolongation of the half-life of medications eliminated through the renal system, that is, the amount of time it takes for the body to lose half of a medication's pharmacological effect. This results in more opportunities for accumulation and can lead to potential toxicity or other adverse events.

Creatinine, a by-product of muscle metabolism, can be measured in the serum. Because it is excreted unchanged by the kidneys, it is often used as a reflection of renal health. The GFR, or the body's ability to excrete medications, can be approximated by calculating a creatinine clearance rate. For someone with any measurable renal impairment, a urine albumin level must be measured (Chapter 8) and a creatinine clearance rate must be calculated before a dosing decision is made. The creatinine clearance value will provide an estimated GFR. Although there are several normograms and algorithms available to estimate GFR, the most reliable for those at the extremes of age or active diseases may be the Cockcroft-Gault equation (Hughes and Beizer, 2014). A number of free automatic calculators are available online (see http://nephron.com/cgi-bin/CGSI.cgi).

PHARMACODYNAMICS

Pharmacodynamics refers to the physiological interactions between a medication and the body, specifically the chemical compounds introduced into the body and the receptors on the cell membrane. These receptors are cellular proteins with unique shapes and ionic charges that bind to medications very specifically. The molecule (medication) fits into the receptor protein like a glove to a hand, with complementary ionic charges. When this binding occurs, a structural change in the receptor protein is initiated, which in turn leads to a biochemical cascade and resultant therapeutic effect (e.g., nerve conduction, enzyme inhibition).

The older a person becomes, the more likely he or she will have altered and unreliable pharmacodynamics. Although it is not always possible to explain or predict all of these alterations, several are well-known. Those of special note in aging are the side effects associated with anticholinergic medications. These side effects can significantly increase the rate of functional decline and the risk for accidental injury in older patients (Peron et al, 2011). Baroreceptor reflex responses decrease with age, causing increased susceptibility to positional changes (orthostatic hypotension) and volume changes (dehydration). A decreased responsiveness of the α-adrenergic system results in decreased sensitivity to β-agonist and β-antagonist medications (e.g., beta-blockers).

ISSUES IN MEDICATION USE

Polypharmacy

Polypharmacy has been defined in many ways: the use of approximately five or more medications or the use of multiple medications for the same problem. Either way, it is extremely common among older adults and a source of potential morbidity and mortality. Gnjidic and colleagues (Gnjidic et al, 2012) concluded that when five or more medications are taken, for each additional medication there was a significant increased risk for the development of frailty, disability, death, and falls. If the patient has multiple chronic conditions, simple polypharmacy may be necessary, even if the prescribing provider is following evidence-based guidelines. It may occur unintentionally, especially if an existing medication regimen is not considered when new prescriptions are given, or any number of the hundreds of over-the-counter (OTC) preparations, supplements, and herbs are added to those prescribed (Table 9-1).

Polypharmacy is exacerbated by the combination of a high use of health care specialists and a reluctance of prescribers to discontinue potentially unnecessary medications that have been prescribed by someone else. This can lead to the continued use of medications that may be no longer necessary (Rochon, 2014). When communication among patients, nurses, other health care providers, and caregivers becomes fragmented, the risk for duplicative medications, inappropriate medications, potentially unsafe dosages, and potentially preventable interactions is heightened. The two major concerns with polypharmacy are the increased risk for medication interactions and the increased risk for adverse events.

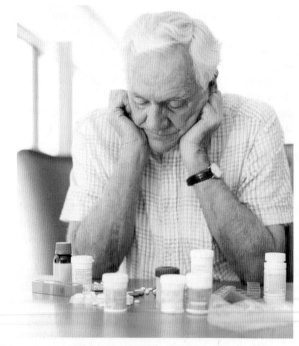

Older man with many prescriptions. (From ©iStock.com/Squaredpixels.)

TABLE 9-1 Select Herb-Medication Interactions*

HERB	MEDICATION	COMPLICATION	NURSING ACTION
Echinacea	**Any anticoagulant drug** such as warfarin sodium; digoxin	Risk of bleeding may increase; therapeutic digoxin level may be altered	Advise person not to take without provider approval
Garlic	**Any anticoagulant or antiplatelet drug** such as warfarin sodium, streptokinase, aspirin, other NSAIDs	Risk of bleeding may increase	Advise person not to take without provider approval
	Antihypertensives	Increased hypotensive effect	Advise provider approval with use
	Antivirals, such as ritonavir	Altered drug effect	Advise against use
	Antimetabolites such as cyclosporine	Risk of less effective response	Advise against use
	Insulin or oral hypoglycemic agent such as pioglitazone or tolbutamide	Serum glucose control may improve; less antidiabetic drug needed	Monitor blood glucose levels
Ginkgo	Aspirin, other NSAIDs, heparin sodium, warfarin sodium, **any anticoagulant**	Risk of bleeding may occur	Teach person not to take without approval of provider
	Antiplatelet drugs such as ticlopidine		
	Antidiabetic drugs: insulin, oral DMT2 drugs such as metformin	May alter blood glucose levels	Monitor blood glucose level closely
	Antidepressants, MAOIs, SSRIs	May cause abnormal response or decrease effectiveness	Advise not to take with these drugs
	Antihypertensives	May cause increased effect	Monitor blood pressure
	Antiseizure drugs	Risk for seizure if history of seizure	Advise against use
Ginseng	Insulin and oral antidiabetic drugs	Blood glucose levels may be altered	Monitor blood glucose levels closely
	Anticoagulant and antiplatelet drugs	May increase bleeding	Advise use with caution and provider oversight
	Aspirin and other NSAIDs		
	MAOIs such as isocarboxazid	Headaches, tremors, mania	Advise against use
	Antihypertensives, cardiac drugs such as calcium channel blockers	May alter effects of drug	Advise against use unless provider monitors closely
	Immunosuppressants	May interfere with action	Advise against use
	Stimulants	May cause additive effect	Advise against use
	Fenugreek	Decreased blood glucose	Monitor closely
Green tea	**Warfarin sodium**	May alter anticoagulant effects	Advise against use
	Stimulants	May cause additive effect	Advise to use with care
Hawthorn	Digoxin	May cause a loss of potassium, leading to drug toxicity	Monitor blood levels
	Beta-blockers and other drugs lowering blood pressure and improving blood flow	May be additive in effects	Monitor blood pressure meticulously; advise that this concern holds true for erectile dysfunction drugs also
Red yeast rice	Fibrate drugs; other cholesterol drugs	May cause additive effects	Avoid concomitant use
	Drugs for diabetes management	May alter blood sugar levels	Monitor blood sugar carefully
	Anticoagulants, antiplatelet drugs, NSAIDs	May increase risk of bleeding	Warn patient and monitor carefully
St. John's wort	Triptans such as sumatriptan, zolmitriptan	May increase risks of serotonergic adverse effects, serotonin syndrome, cerebral vasoconstriction	Advise against use
	HMG-CoA reductase inhibitors	May decrease plasma concentrations of these drugs	Monitor levels of lipids
	MAOIs	May cause similar effects as with use with any SSRI	Advise against use
	Digoxin	Decreases the effects of the drug	Advise against use
	Alprazolam	May decrease effect of drug	Advise against use
	Ketoprofen	Photosensitivity	Advise sun block use
	Tramadol and some SSRIs	May increase risk of serotonin syndrome	Advise against use
	Olanzapine	May cause serotonin syndrome	Advise against use
	Paroxetine	Sedative-hypnotic intoxication	Advise against use
	Theophylline	Increases metabolism; decreases drug blood level	Monitor drug effects
	Albuterol		
	Warfarin	May decrease anticoagulant effect	Advise against use
	Amlodipine	Lowers efficacy of calcium channel	Advise against use
	Estrogen or progesterone	May decrease effect of hormones	Advise that this effect may occur
	Protease inhibitors or nonnucleoside reverse transcriptase inhibitors in HIV/AIDS treatment; antivirals	May alter drug effects	FDA advises avoidance of this herb for patients taking these drugs

*The interactions listed represent only a few of the possible herb-drug interactions. Use of herbs that interfere with metabolism of drugs by the liver's cytochrome P450 enzyme system should be avoided or monitored closely by the provider.

AIDS, Acquired immunodeficiency syndrome; *DMT2,* diabetes mellitus type 2; *FDA,* U.S. Food and Drug Administration; *HIV,* human immunodeficiency virus; *HMG-CoA,* 3-hydroxy-3-methylglutaryl coenzyme-A; *MAOIs,* monoamine oxidase inhibitors; *NSAIDs,* nonsteroidal antiinflammatory drugs; *SSRIs,* selective serotonin reuptake inhibitors.

Data from Natural Standard: *The Authority on Integrative Medicine.* Available at http://www.naturalstandard.com Accessed May 2014; Wilson BA, Shannon MT, Stang CL: *Nurse's drug guide,* Upper Saddle River, NJ, 2004, Pearson Prentice Hall; Yoon SL, Schaffer SD: Herbal, prescribed, and over-the-counter drug use in older women: prevalence of drug interactions, *Geriatr Nurs* 27:118–129, 2006.

Medication Interactions

The more prescribed medications or other substances (e.g., herbs, dietary supplements) a person takes, the greater the possibility one or more will interact with another. At the same time, the more chronic conditions one has, the more likely it is that a medication for one condition will affect the body in such a way as to influence another condition (e.g., a person takes ibuprofen for arthritis pain and subsequently has an increase in his or her already high blood pressure). When two or more medications (or products of any kind, including food) are given at the same time or closely together, one substance may potentiate another (i.e., cause it to have stronger effects than when given alone) or may antagonize (lower the potency) the other, even to the point that the medication is inactivated.

Medication–Herb/Supplement Interactions

As the popularity of medicinal herbs and other dietary supplements rises, so does the risk for interactions with prescribed medications. Although much remains unknown, new knowledge is added almost daily upon which the gerontological nurse may base her or his practice. For example, a number of herbs have a direct effect on coagulability. When these herbs are taken with warfarin, the risk of bleeding may significantly increase (see Table 9-1). If the herb influences the results of the international normalized ratio (INR) or other measure of coagulation, adjustments to the warfarin dose will lead to inappropriate and potentially dangerous consequences. The interactions presented in Table 9-1 represent only a small fraction of the many real and potential problems in prescribing medications and caring for persons who take an herb or a dietary supplement in addition to prescribed medications.

Medication-Food Interactions

Many foods interact with medications, producing increased, decreased, or variable effects. They may also bind to medications, affecting their absorption. For example, calcium in dairy products will bind to levothyroxine, tetracycline, and ciprofloxacin, greatly decreasing their absorption; lovastatin absorption is increased by a high-fat, low-fiber meal. All of these are medications frequently prescribed to older adults. Grapefruit juice contains substances that inhibit CYP3A4-mediated metabolism in the gut and bind with the statins used for cholesterol-lowering medications, clopidogrel, and many other medications (Table 9-2).

Spironolactone, prescribed for end-stage heart failure, increases potassium (K^+) reabsorption by the renal tubule. If a patient ingests a diet high in potassium (e.g., KCl salt substitute, molasses, oranges, bananas) or other potassium-sparing agents (e.g., Lisinopril) at the same time, K^+ levels can rise significantly and quickly reach toxic levels. The vitamin K in leafy green vegetables antagonizes (decreases) the anticoagulant effects of warfarin and may have a significant effect on the coagulability of the blood (Burchum, 2011). It is recommended that patients taking warfarin ingest a consistent amount of greens to avoid variations in their warfarin levels (Box 9-4).

TABLE 9-2 Common Drug-Food Interactions

FOOD	DRUG	POTENTIAL EFFECT
Fiber	Digoxin	Absorption of drug into fiber, reducing drug action
Foods with vitamin K	Warfarin	Decreased effect of drug
Food	Many antibiotics	Reduced absorption rate of drug
Vitamin B_6 supplements	Levodopa-carbidopa	Reverses antiparkinsonian effect
Grapefruit juice	Multiple medications	Altered metabolism and elimination can increase concentration of drug
Citrus juice	Calcium channel blockers	Gastric reflux exacerbated

BOX 9-4   Top 10 Foods to Avoid When Taking Warfarin

Kale	Turnip greens
Spinach	Parsley
Collards	Broccoli
Swiss chard	Brussels sprouts
Mustard greens	

See for expanded list and for patient information: http://www.cc.nih.gov/ccc/patient_education/drug_nutrient/coumadin1.pdf

Medication-Medication Interactions

The polypharmacy that may be a necessary part of health care in later life significantly increases both the risk for and the frequency of medication-medication interactions. These may occur at any time from preparation to excretion. For example, persons who cannot swallow after a stroke may receive all feedings and medications enterally. Medications intended for oral administration must be converted to a soluble form for passage through the tube without clogging and yet also remain in their original form. When several medications are crushed, mixed together, and then dissolved in water for administration, a new product is created and medication-medication interactions may have already begun (Box 9-5).

⚡ SAFETY ALERT

Safe Administration of Medications through Enteral Feeding Tubes

Persons who receive their medications via the enteral route are at high risk for medication errors. Safe administration of such drugs is a time-consuming process that requires detailed knowledge of the medications (and their formulation) and the skill to prepare them appropriately. Most often this preparation occurs at the bedside, further increasing the risk for errors. The possible outcomes of such errors may include the following: occluded tube, reduced medication effect, medication toxicity, patient harm, and patient death. The three most common errors are incompatible route, improper preparation, and improper administration.

BOX 9-5 TIPS FOR BEST PRACTICE

Factors to Consider When Giving Medications via the Enteral Route

Drugs given enterally (via tube) are intended for an oral administration route but mechanically bypass the mouth and potentially the stomach or duodenum. Many factors affect the rate at which a medication is dissolved. These factors include the amount of liquid in the stomach, the type of coating on the tablet, the extent of tablet compression used in making the tablet, the presence of expanders in the tablet, the solubility of the drug in the acidic environment of the stomach, and the rate of peristalsis. The most common errors are (1) incompatible route (cannot use sustained-release formulations), (2) improper preparation (must be liquid or semiliquid; oral suspensions and tinctures will partially adhere to the tubing and affect the dose), and (3) improper administration: Can it be given with food? Should it go to the stomach or duodenum and is the tube in the proper anatomical location?

BOX 9-6 TIPS FOR BEST PRACTICE

Examples of Medication Interaction Potential for Adverse Reactions

- ACE inhibitors and potassium-sparing diuretics
- ACE inhibitors or ARBs and Septra (Bactrim)
- Macrolide antibiotics (e.g., Cipro) and either calcium channel blockers or digoxin
- Warfarin and any of the antibiotics or NSAIDs

ACE, Angiotensin-converting enzyme; *ARB*, α-receptor blocker.
From Hines LE, Murphy JE: Potentially harmful drug-drug interactions in the elderly: a review, *Am J Geriatr Pharmacother* 9(6):364–377, 2011.

effect on everyday prescribing, administration, and monitoring of effects of medications taken by older adults (Box 9-6).

Adverse Drug Reactions and Events

Adverse drug reactions (ADRs) or *adverse drug events* (ADEs) occur when there is a noxious response to a medication. The effects of such reactions may range from a minor annoyance to death and are a common cause of hospitalization. Between 2004 and 2008 there was a 52% increase in the number of ADEs in inpatient settings. More than half of these were related to corticosteroids, anticoagulants, and sedative-hypnotics. While only 18.5% of persons treated for adverse drug reactions in the emergency department (ED) and released were older than 65 years of age, 53% of patients hospitalized for ADRs were at least age 65 (Lucado et al, 2011).

Altered absorption can occur when one medication binds another medication in the small intestine to form a nonabsorbable compound. For example, ciprofloxacin and iron compounds are both taken frequently by older adults; however, when these drugs bind, both are inactivated. Other medications may compete to simultaneously bind and occupy the same receptor site, creating varied bioavailability of one or both drugs. Interference with enzyme activity may alter metabolism and cause deficiencies or toxicities. Antispasmodic medications, which are commonly prescribed, slow gastric and intestinal motility even further than that present in normal aging. In some instances this may be useful if a prolonged effect is beneficial but may prove harmful when it leads to an accumulation and potential medication intoxication.

Altered distribution may be caused by displacement of one medication from its receptor site by another medication or by binding of the drug to plasma albumin or α_1-acid glycoprotein. Altered distribution is a common cause of adverse medication reactions in older adults and is an especially important issue in patients with lowered albumin levels. Thus it is common among chronically ill, frail elders, such as many of those residing in long-term care facilities (Beyth and Shorr, 2007).

Altered excretion coupled with age-related decreases in renal function can occur when one medication changes the urinary pH such that another medication is either reabsorbed or excreted to a greater extent than is desired. Another mechanism may involve one medication increasing or decreasing active transport in the renal tubules (e.g., probenecid decreases the active transport of penicillin, thereby prolonging its half-life) (Hughes and Beizer, 2014).

In pharmacodynamic interactions, one medication alters the patient's response to another medication without changing the pharmacokinetic properties. Pharmacodynamic medication interactions can be especially dangerous for older adults, including the additive pharmacological effects of two or more similar medications; that is, together they are more potent than they are separately (e.g., central nervous system [CNS] effects of sedative-hypnotic medications and anticholinergic medications) (Hughes and Beizer, 2014). Due to the frequency of polypharmacy, medication-medication interactions can have a significant

Sometimes an ADR can be predicted from the pharmacological action of the medication, such as bone marrow suppression from chemotherapeutic agents or bleeding from anticoagulants. At other times they are unpredictable, such as in an allergic reaction to antibiotics. Allergic reactions become more common in older adults as the immune system decreases in function (Chapter 25). It is reasonable to assume that many ADRs in older adults go unrecognized because of their nonspecific nature and their similarity to some of the subtle changes with aging and to the vague signs and symptoms of many of the chronic conditions common in later life (Kim et al, 2014).

Many such adverse reactions, however, can be serious or fatal. These serious consequences are often preventable—an estimated 27% of the ADEs in the primary care setting and 42% in the long-term care setting (American Geriatrics Society [AGS], 2012). When a response reaches the level of harm, it is referred to as an *adverse drug event* (ADE). Many of these must be reported to the U.S. Food and Drug Administration or other regulatory body. ADEs can result either from the administration of a single medication or from the interaction of multiple medications as discussed previously. Although the reporting of ADEs had previously been limited to prescribed substances, this reporting has now been expanded to include any other products (such as dietary supplements) for which health-related claims are made. Most reporting is voluntary; however, reporting ADEs and product quality problems contributes to the protection of the public from harm.

Although ADRs and ADEs continue to occur, there has been considerable progress in the development of strategies to reduce their likelihood, especially in the recognition of age-related pharmacokinetic and pharmacodynamic changes in later life. We now know that in many cases an older adult should be prescribed lower dosages of several of the medications commonly needed, especially when beginning a new medication regimen. To minimize the likelihood of an ADR, the dose can be slowly increased until it safely reaches a therapeutic level. A common adage related to medication dosing in older adults is, "Start low, go slow, but go." There has also been a recognition that the risk of ADEs is so high with some medications that the drugs are simply not recommended for use in persons with any known risk factors.

"Beers' Criteria"

The appropriate use of medications in the older adult means that such products are used only as needed, at the minimum dose necessary to achieve the desired effects, and in a manner in which the risks relative to benefits have been considered within the greater context of the person's life expectancy, health, lifestyle, and values. Beers published a list of "potentially inappropriate medications (PIMs)" for nursing home settings in 1997 (Beers, 1997). It was expanded to cover all care settings several times, and most recently in 2012 in partnership with the American Geriatrics Society (AGS, 2012; Molony and Greenberg, 2013). One of the findings noted in the recent PIM list is not only that many medications have limited effectiveness but also that they may result in poor outcomes such as delirium and gastrointestinal bleeding.

The list is divided into three broad medication groups: those to avoid in older adults regardless of disease or condition, those considered potentially inappropriate when used with certain conditions, and those that should be used with caution. The Beers' Criteria also include information about the deleterious effect of specific medications on common health problems seen in older adults.

The Beers' Criteria have been incorporated into regulatory policy for long-term care facilities via their inclusion in regulations from the Centers for Medicare and Medicaid Services. They are a part of the quality measures for the National Committee for Quality Assurance (NCQA) and the Healthcare Effectiveness Data and Information Set (HEDIS) (AGS, 2012). When one of those medications on the "do not use" portion is prescribed in the long-term care (LTC) setting without documentation of an overwhelming benefit of its use, it can be considered a form of medication misuse by the prescribing practitioner (Box 9-7). The American Geriatrics Society provides the entire list, a downloadable app, teaching slides, and a number of other tools at their website (www.americangeriatrics.org).

Psychoactive Medications

Psychoactive medications are those that affect mental function, which in turn affects behavior and how the world is experienced. The gerontological nurse, especially one working in a long-term care setting, is likely to be responsible for older adults who are receiving psychoactive medications, especially those for the treatment of depression, anxiety, and bipolar disorders (Chapter 28). Medications with psychoactive properties

> **BOX 9-7   Select Medications from the Beers' Criteria for Potentially Inappropriate Medications for Use in Older Adults (>65 Years of Age)**
>
> First-generation antihistamines
> Nitrofurantoin (Macrobid)
> Alpha$_1$-blockers
> Antiarrhythmics, especially amiodarone
> Digoxin (no dose >0.25 mg)
> Nifedipine, immediate release
> Tricyclic antidepressants
> Many of the antipsychotics
> Barbiturates
> Benzodiazepines
> Sliding scale insulin
> Sulfonylureas, long duration
> Glyburide
> Demerol
> Non–COX-selective NSAIDs*
>
> *Concurrent use of a proton pump inhibitor reduces risk, short-term use only.
> From American Geriatrics Society (AGS) Expert Panel: American Geriatrics Society updated Beers Criteria for potentially inappropriate medication use in older adults, *J Am Geriatr Soc* 60:616–631, 2012.

have a higher than usual risk for adverse events and must be prescribed and administered, especially in the older population, with an acute awareness of how age-related changes in absorption, distribution, excretion, and hepatic function affect their overall concentration in the serum. Some studies indicate that 35% to 53% of persons living in assisted living facilities were taking at least one psychoactive medication and more than half of older adults admitted from the community into a skilled nursing facility were prescribed at least one such drug within 2 weeks of admission (Lindsey, 2009).

In an effort to control the burgeoning use of psychotropic medications in nursing homes, the Centers for Medicare and Medicaid Services issued a clarification of previous instructions, which was issued to guide those who were responsible for monitoring the quality of patient care (usually state surveyors) (CMS, 2013). This classification of medications may never be used as a "quick fix" and should only be used when a thorough assessment had been completed, nonpharmacological approaches had proven ineffective, and the patient would clearly benefit from their use.

One specific class of psychoactive medications, antipsychotics, is commonly prescribed to persons with neurodegenerative disorders and behavior disturbances that place those around the person in danger, due to hallucinations and delusions. Persons taking these medications must be monitored with special care. These drugs should never be used for the convenience of the staff or to simply provide sedation; to do so is considered chemical restraint.

Antipsychotics

Antipsychotic drugs are tranquilizing medications used primarily to treat psychoses, including those associated with the dementias, and are used off-label as mood stabilizers for bipolar disorder. Their mechanism of action centers on blocking dopamine receptor pathways in the brain. Antipsychotics also affect the hypothalamic and thermoregulatory pathways. They are often ranked in relation to their side effects, especially sedation, hypotension, and extrapyramidal (and anticholinergic) side effects (EPSEs). Up to 75% of persons taking typical antipsychotic medications are affected by EPSEs (Lindsey, 2009). Other side effects of these medications include neuroleptic malignant syndrome and movement disorders.

The first such medications to be produced (in the 1950s) are now referred to as "typical antipsychotics" (e.g., Haldol, Thorazine), and the newer, second-generation medications (developed since the 1990s) are referred to as "atypicals" (e.g., Risperidone, Seroquel). The dangers associated with the use of the typical antipsychotics require that their use be significantly justified and that a careful cost/benefit analysis be done. *Typical antipsychotics can never be used for someone with the diagnosis of dementia with Lewy bodies.*

When used appropriately and cautiously, antipsychotics can provide a person with relief from what may be frightening and distressing symptoms. Inappropriate use of antipsychotic medications may mask a reversible cause for the psychosis (such as delirium, infection, dehydration, fever, or electrolyte imbalance), an adverse medication effect, or a sudden change in the environment (Medicines and Healthcare Products Regulatory Agency [MHRA], 2014). Because of the seriousness and frequency of the side effects and associated complications, these medications are prescribed at the lowest dose possible and the patient is monitored closely. When antipsychotic medications are prescribed, more caution than usual must be used.

SAFETY ALERT

Potential complications of antipsychotic medications include stroke (at three times the risk of people not taking the medications), falls, fractures, transient ischemic attacks (TIAs), and death (Hughes and Beizer, 2014).

Malignant Syndrome

Because antipsychotics affect the thermoregulatory pathway, patients taking them cannot tolerate excess environmental heat. Even mild elevations of core temperature can result in liver damage, called *neuroleptic malignant syndrome* (NMS). Acute NMS is characterized by high fever, rigidity, altered mental status, and other symptoms of autonomic instability such as tachycardia and pallor. The nurse or caregiver must therefore protect the elder affected with hyperthermia by making sure the environment is cool enough at all times. Appropriate interventions include promotion of adequate hydration, relocation to a cooler area away from direct sunlight, and use of a fan or sponge bath. Because the patient may or may not share his or her discomfort about the heat, regular assessment of body temperature is essential. Any circumstance resulting in dehydration greatly increases the risk of heat stroke, which in late life is associated with high death rates.

Movement Disorders

Neuroleptic malignant syndrome is not commonly seen in older adults taking antipsychotics. The more commonly seen significant potential side effects are movement disorders, also referred to as *extrapyramidal syndrome* (EPS). These include acute dystonia, akathisia, parkinsonian symptoms, and tardive dyskinesia. Although these side effects are much more common with the typical antipsychotics, they can occur with the atypical antipsychotics as well. The prescribing provider should be notified immediately any time such symptoms or signs are seen. Many of these are potentially life-threatening. In most cases the offending medication must be stopped immediately, with implications for the potential need for hospitalization.

Acute dystonia. An acute dystonic reaction is an abnormal involuntary movement consisting of a slow and continuous muscular contraction or spasm. Involuntary muscular contractions of the mouth, jaw, face, and neck are common. The jaw may lock (trismus), the tongue may roll back and block the throat, the neck may arch backward (opisthotonos), or the eyes may close. In an oculogyric crisis, the eyes are fixed in one position. Often this creates a feeling of needing to look up constantly without the ability to make the eyes come down. These reactions may occur hours or days after the initiation of a medication or after a dose increase and may continue as long as only a few minutes to many hours.

Akathisia. Akathisia is a compulsion to be in motion, a sense of restlessness, being unable to be still, having an unrelenting desire to move, and feeling "like crawling out of my skin." The patient is seen pacing, fidgeting, and markedly restless. Often this symptom is mistaken for worsening psychosis instead of the adverse medication reaction that it is. It may occur at any time during therapy.

Parkinsonian symptoms. The use of antipsychotics may cause a collection of symptoms that are similar to those of Parkinson's disease: a bilateral tremor (as opposed to a unilateral tremor in true Parkinson's), bradykinesia, and rigidity that may progress to the inability to move. The patient may have an inflexible facial expression and appear bored and apathetic and thus be mistakenly diagnosed as depressed. These are more common with the higher potency antipsychotics: these side effects may begin within weeks to months of initiation of antipsychotic therapy.

Tardive dyskinesia. When antipsychotics have been used continuously for at least 3 to 6 months, patients are at risk for the development of the irreversible movement disorder called tardive dyskinesia (TD). Both low- and high-potency agents have been implicated (Bullock and Saharan, 2002; Goldberg, 2002). TD symptoms usually appear first as wormlike movements of the tongue and other facial movements include grimacing, blinking, and frowning. Slow, maintained, involuntary twisting movements of the limbs, trunk, neck, face, and eyes (involuntary eye closure) have been reported. No treatment reverses the effect of TD. Therefore it is essential that the nurse be attentive for early detection so that the health care provider can make prompt changes to the psychotropic regimen. The scheduled and repeated use of a standardized monitoring instrument is recommended.

◆ PROMOTING HEALTHY AGING: IMPLICATIONS FOR GERONTOLOGICAL NURSING

The gerontological nurse is a key person in ensuring that the medication used is appropriate, effective, and as safe as possible. The knowledgeable nurse is alert for potential medication interactions and for signs or symptoms of adverse medication effects. Nurses in the long-term care setting are responsible for monitoring the overall health of the residents, including fluid and dietary intake, and for being alert to the need for laboratory tests and other measures to ensure correct medication dosage. They are responsible for prompt attention to changes in the patient's or resident's condition (such as potassium level) that either are the result of the medication regimen or are affected by the regimen. The nurse is often the person to initiate assessment of medication use, evaluate outcomes, and provide the teaching necessary for safe medication use and self-administration.

In all settings, a vital nursing function is to educate patients and to ensure that they understand the purpose and side effects of the medications and assist the patient and family in adapting the medication regimen to functional ability and lifestyle.

◆ Assessment

The initial step in ensuring that medication use is safe and effective is to conduct a comprehensive medication assessment. Although in some settings clinical pharmacists interview patients about their medication history, more often such reviews are completed through the combined efforts of the licensed nurse and the health care provider (e.g., a physician or a nurse practitioner).

The "gold standard" of assessment that is especially important to use with the older adult is the "brown bag approach," in which the person is asked to show the nurse all of the medications that he or she is taking, including OTCs, herbals, and other dietary supplements. As each product container is removed from the bag, the necessary information can be obtained and compiled. To prevent possible misunderstandings or to determine misuse, it is best to ask the person how he or she actually takes the medicine rather than to depend on how the label is written. By completing the assessment in this manner, the nurse can discover discrepancies between the prescribed dosage and the actual dosage, spot potential interactions, and identify potential or actual ADRs. The basics of the comprehensive medication assessment are the same as those for younger adults (Box 9-8). For details of the information needed in such an assessment that are particularly important for older adults, see Box 9-9.

The analysis by the nurse or the advanced practice nurse (APN) should be centered on identifying unnecessary or inappropriate medications, establishing safe usage, determining the patient's self-medication management ability, monitoring the effect of current medications and other products (e.g., herbals), and evaluating effectiveness of any education provided. Ideally, the nurse should know what resources are available for teaching about medications, such as the clinical pharmacist. The nurse is well situated to coordinate care, identify the patient's goals, determine what the patient needs to learn in order to understand his or her medications, and arrange for follow-up care to determine the outcome of medication teaching.

BOX 9-8   Analysis of Assessment Findings Related to Medication Use

1. Is the medication working to improve the patient's symptoms?
   a. What are the therapeutic effects of the medication? (What symptoms are targeted?)
   b. What is the time frame for the therapeutic effects?
   c. Have the appropriate medication and dose been prescribed?
   d. Has the appropriate time been tried for therapeutic effects?
2. Is the medication harming the patient?
   a. What physiological changes are occurring?
   b. What laboratory values are changing?
   c. What mental status changes are occurring?
   d. What functional changes are occurring?
   e. Is the patient experiencing side effects?
   f. Is the medication interacting with any other medication?
3. Does the patient understand the following?
   a. Why is the patient taking the medication?
   b. How is the medication supposed to be taken?
   c. How do you identify side effects and medication interactions?
   d. How do you reduce or manage side effects?
   e. What limitations are imposed by taking the medication (e.g., sedative effects)?

BOX 9-9   TIPS FOR BEST PRACTICE

Components of a Medication Assessment with Special Emphasis for Older Adults

- Ability to pay for prescription medications
- Ability to obtain medications and refills
- Persons involved in decision making regarding medication use
- Medications obtained from others
- Recently discontinued medications or "leftover" prescriptions
- Strategies used to remember when to take medications
- Recent medication blood levels as appropriate
- Recent measurement of liver and kidney functioning
- Ability to remove packaging, manipulate medication, and store supply

---

◆ Education

Patient education is the most common intervention used to promote safe medication use. Because of the complex needs of the older patient, education can be particularly challenging. The following tips may be helpful when the goal of the nurse is to promote healthy aging related to medication use:

Key persons: Find out who, if anyone, manages the person's medications, helps the person, or assists with decision making; and with the elder's permission, make sure that the helper is present when any teaching is done (Box 9-10).

Environment: Minimize distraction, and avoid competition with television, grandchildren, or others demanding the patient's attention; make sure the person is comfortable and is not hungry, thirsty, tired, too warm or too cold, in pain, or in need of the toilet.

Timing: Provide the teaching during the best time of the day for the person, when he or she is most engaged and energetic. Keep the education sessions short and succinct.

Communication: Ensure that you will be understood. Make sure the elders have their glasses or hearing aids on, if they are

BOX 9-10   Knowing Who You Are Talking To

M. François came to the clinic as a new patient with uncontrolled hypertension. The nurse practitioner, through an interpreter, spent a lot of time with him explaining how to take his medications, what they were for, and so on. He and his presumed caregiver sat quietly and appeared to understand. When he returned a month later his blood pressure was still out of control. There was a different person with him who asked all of the questions that were addressed at the first appointment. On further inquiry it was determined that the person who brought M. François the first time was just a neighbor helping out and not involved in his day-to-day life at all! His niece who "takes care of things" had been unavailable during the previous appointment and was now available to take him to his appointment.

BOX 9-11   TIPS FOR BEST PRACTICE

Reducing Adverse Medication Events

By paying attention to the following principles for prescribing and monitoring medications for older adults, the advanced practice nurse can reduce the risk for adverse medication events:

- Give the lowest dose possible.
- Discontinue unnecessary therapy.
- Attempt nonpharmacological interventions first.
- Give the safest medication possible.
- Assess renal function.
- Always consider the risk-to-benefit ratio when adding medications.
- Assess for new interactions with any new prescription.
- Avoid the prescribing cascade (i.e., new medications without consideration of those to be discontinued).
- Avoid inappropriate medications.

BOX 9-12   A Potentially Lethal Misunderstanding

I was making a visit to Mrs. Helena to enroll her in a research study. As we were reviewing her health and current medications she shared that she had not been feeling well and thought it was her heart, and that she had been told to "take the little white pills" until she felt better. When I looked at her pill bottle she had already taken five or more digoxin in the space of about 2 hours. I called an ambulance.

TABLE 9-3   Examples of Changes with Aging that May Interfere with Medication Self-Administration

CHANGE IN AGING	CONSEQUENCE
Sensory	
Decreased visual acuity	Greater difficulty in reading instructions
Decreased sensation	Greater difficulty in manipulating medications
Decreased salivation	Greater difficulty in swallowing
Mechanical	
Decreased fine motor coordination	Greater difficulty in manipulating medications and packaging
Stiffening of large joints	Greater difficulty in self-administering medications

used. Use simple and direct language, and avoid medical or nursing jargon (e.g., "intake"). Speak clearly, facing the person and with light on your face, at head level. Use formal language (e.g., Mr. Jones) unless you have permission to do otherwise. Do not touch the patient unless he or she indicates to you that it is acceptable to do so (e.g., patient lays his or her hand on yours, Chapter 6). If the person is blind, braille instructions may be available from the pharmacy. If the person has limited language proficiency in the country in which care is delivered, a trained medical interpreter is needed.

Reinforce teaching: Although there is a wide array of teaching tools and medication reminders available on the market today, many older adults continue to use the strategies they have developed over the years to remember to take their medications. These may be as simple as a using an egg carton as a storage box or turning a bottle upside down once it has been taken for the day, or as intense as having a family member or friend call the person at designated times. Encourage the person to use techniques that have worked in the past or to develop new strategies to ensure correct and timely medication use when needed. All education is supported by written or graphic material in the language that the person (if literate) can read or in the language of the persons who helps.

SAFE MEDICATION USE

A safe, optimal, and feasible medication plan is one to which the patient can adhere. Appropriate nursing interventions include those that minimize polypharmacy, avoid adverse medication reactions, and promote adherence to medication regimens that promote healthy aging (or comfort while dying) (Box 9-11). The responsibility of the nurse caring for frail elders is especially challenging because of the physical and social vulnerability and medical complexity common in late life; medication interactions are more likely and adverse reactions more lethal.

The promotion of safe medication use requires attention to the potential for misuse, including overuse, underuse, erratic use, and contraindicated use, all of which are referred to as nonadherence. Misuse by patients may be unintentional, such as with misunderstanding, or purposeful, such as when trying to make a prescription last longer because of cost, or believing that it is not appropriate for the believed cause of illness (Box 9-12) (Gould and Mitty, 2010). A person may have considerable difficulty adhering to a medication regimen that is inconsistent with his or her established life patterns or beliefs. For example, the individual cannot follow the instruction to take medication three times per day with meals if he or she eats only two meals each day. In late life adherence is made significantly more complicated when the complexity of a medication regimen is combined with difficulties with self-administration due to normal changes with aging (Table 9-3).

All medications have indications, side effects, interactions, and individual patient reactions. The nurse must determine whether side effects are minimal and tolerable or serious (Table 9-4). Asking subjective question and observing the patient's interactions, behavior, mood, emotional responses, and daily habits can provide essential objective data. By compiling the information obtained in this manner, patient problems can be delineated, nursing diagnoses developed, outcome criteria planned, and interventions initiated.

TABLE 9-4   Indications of Toxicity of Medications Commonly Prescribed to Older Adults

MEDICATION(S)	SIGNS AND SYMPTOMS
Benzodiazepines (e.g., Ativan)	Ataxia, restlessness, confusion, depression, anticholinergic effect
Cimetidine (Tagamet)	Confusion, depression
Digitalis (Digoxin)	Confusion, headache, anorexia, vomiting, arrhythmias, blurred vision or visual changes (halos, frost on objects, color blindness), paresthesia
Furosemide (Lasix)	Electrolyte imbalance, hepatic changes, pancreatitis, leukopenia, thrombocytopenia
Levodopa (L-Dopa)	Muscle and eye twitching, disorientation, asterixis, hallucinations, dyskinetic movements, grimacing, depression, delirium, ataxia
Nonsteroidal antiinflammatory medications (NSAIDs) such as Advil and Naprosyn	Photosensitivity, fluid retention, anemia, nephrotoxicity, visual changes, bleeding, blood pressure elevations
Ranitidine (Zantac)	Liver dysfunction, blood dyscrasias
Sulfonylureas—first generation (e.g., Diabinese)	Hypoglycemia, hepatic changes, heart failure, bone marrow depression, jaundice

From Lexicomp: *Long term-care nursing drug handbook*, ed 14, Hudson, OH, 2013, Lexi-Comp.

Lastly, it is necessary for the gerontological nurse to monitor and evaluate prescribed treatments for both side effects and efficacy (Planton and Edlund, 2010). Monitoring and evaluation involve making astute observations and documenting those observations, noting changes in physical and functional status (e.g., vital signs, performance of activities of daily living, sleeping, eating, hydrating, eliminating) and mental status (e.g., attention and level of alertness, memory, orientation, behavior, mood, emotional display and affect, content and characteristics of interactions). Monitoring also means ensuring that blood levels are measured when they are needed—for example, regular thyroid-stimulating hormone (TSH) levels for all persons taking thyroid replacement therapy, INRs for all persons taking warfarin, or periodic hemoglobin A_{1C} levels for all persons with diabetes or taking antipsychotics (see Chapter 8). Proper patient care requires nurses to promptly communicate their findings of potential problems to the patient's nurse practitioner or physician. Accurate monitoring is dependent on the nurse possessing and understanding the relevant information about the treatments and medications that are administered.

Medications occupy a central place in the lives of many older persons: cost, acceptability, interactions, untoward side effects, and the need to schedule medications appropriately all combine to create many difficulties. The nurse can promote healthy aging through knowledge of the effect of normal age-related changes on pharmacodynamics and pharmacokinetics, as well as by awareness of the key issues in medication use in older adults in all care settings.

KEY CONCEPTS

- The therapeutic goal of pharmacological intervention is to reduce the targeted symptoms and disease conditions without undesirable side effects.
- One must be alert at all times for medication-medication, medication-herb, and medication-food interactions; whereas some are known and anticipated, others are unique.
- Polypharmacy significantly increases the risk of medication interactions and adverse events. Polypharmacy increases with each prescriber seen.
- Daily or twice-daily dosing is optimal.
- Any time there is a change in the patient's status, it is reasonable to first consider the possibility of a medication effect; this is of paramount importance when caring for an older adult and those who are frail.
- Many medications have the potential to cause temporary cognitive impairment.
- Medication misuse may be triggered by prescriber practices, individual self-medication, physiological idiosyncrasies, altered biodegradability, nutritional and fluid states, and inadequate assessment before prescribing.
- Nurses must investigate medications immediately if a change in mental status is observed in an individual who is normally alert and aware.
- Patients cannot comply with a prescription or treatment when incompatibilities interfere with the practicalities of life

or are distressful to the individual's well-being or when actual misinformation or disability prevents compliance.
- The side effects of psychotropic medications vary significantly; thus these medications must be selected with care when prescribed for the older adult.
- The response of the elder to treatment with psychotropic medications should show reduced distress, clearer thinking, and more appropriate behavior.
- It is always expected that psychotropic pharmacological approaches augment rather than replace nonpharmacological approaches.
- Older adults are particularly vulnerable to developing movement disorders (extrapyramidal symptoms, parkinsonian symptoms, akathisia, dystonias) with the use of antipsychotics.
- The Health Care Financing Administration (HCFA) and the congressional Omnibus Budget Reconciliation Act (OBRA) have severely restricted the use of psychotropic medications for the elderly unless they are truly needed for specific disorders and to maintain or improve function. Careful monitoring and continued justification is required (Table 9-5).
- Any time a behavior change is noted in a person, reversible causes must be sought and treated before psychotropic medications are used.
- Antidepressant medications must be tailored to the elder, with careful observation for side effects.

TABLE 9-5   Monitoring Parameters and Evaluation of Effectiveness for Medications Commonly Prescribed to Older Adults

CLASS OF MEDICATION	MONITORING ACTIVITY
Antibiotics and antivirals	Improvement of infection: symptom reduction
Antihyperlipidemics	Lipid profile: lipids and triglycerides within normal limits for this person Liver function testing: no changes in function Blood glucose: no elevation
Cardiac medications	Measurement of heart rate and rhythm: within optimal parameters for that person
Anticoagulants	Clotting times (international normalized ratio [INR], prothrombin time): no bleeding; if using INR, kept between 2.0 and 3.0 in most cases
Antihypertensives	Measurement of blood pressure: maintained within normal limits and without the development of orthostatic hypotension Weight: no unexplained weight gain
Antihyperglycemics	Hemoglobin A_{1c}: maintained between 6.0 and 7.0 (controversy regarding a combination of goal and health status)
Antiarthritics	Relief from arthritis symptoms such as pain and inflammation
Antiparkinsonians	Improved functional status Less visible immobility; improved mobility
Analgesics	Improved symptoms of pain and inflammation

NURSING STUDY: AT RISK FOR AN ADVERSE EVENT

Rosa was a 78-year-old woman who lived alone in a large city. She had been widowed for 10 years. Her children were grown, and all were successful. She was very proud of them because she and her husband had immigrated to the United States when the children were small and had worked very hard to establish and maintain a home. She had only a few years of primary education and still clung to many of her "old country" ways. She spoke a mixture of English and her native language, and her children were somewhat embarrassed by her. They thought she was somewhat of a hypochondriac because she constantly complained to them about various aches and pains, her knees that "gave out," her "sugar" and "water" problems, and her heart palpitations. She had been diagnosed with mild diabetes and congestive heart failure. She was a devout Catholic and attended mass each morning. Her treks to church events, to the senior center at church, and to her various physicians (internist; orthopedic, cardiac, and ophthalmic specialists) constituted her social life. One day

the recreation director at the senior center noticed her pulling a paper bag of medication bottles from her purse. She sat down to talk with Rosa about them and soon realized that Rosa had only a vague idea of what most of them were for and tended to take them whenever she felt she needed them.

- What factors about Rosa's probable medication misuse would be most alarming to you?
- List two of Rosa's strengths that you have identified from the information presented in the study.
- Develop three nursing diagnoses appropriate to this nursing study. These must be stated in concrete and measurable terms.
- Plan and state one or more interventions for each diagnosed problem. Provide specific documentation of the source used to determine the appropriate intervention and how the effectiveness can be evaluated.

CRITICAL THINKING QUESTIONS AND ACTIVITIES

1. As a nurse visiting the center for a 6-week student assignment, how would you begin to help someone like Rosa?
2. Who should be responsible for teaching and monitoring medication use in persons such as Rosa? In any case?
3. Mrs. J., a patient of yours in a long-term care setting, is calling out repeatedly for a nurse; other patients are complaining, and you simply cannot be available for long periods to quiet her. Considering the setting and the OBRA guidelines, what would you do to manage the situation?
4. When you are given a prescription for medication, what do you ask about it?
5. Do you think most elders seek adequate information about their medications before taking them?

RESEARCH QUESTIONS

1. Where would you obtain sufficient medication information for persons with limited English proficiency (LEP)?
2. What symptoms do elders self-treat with OTC and herbal medicines?
3. What are nursing roles in preventing adverse medication events in elders?
4. Among the following three teaching strategies, which works the best: computer-assisted medication teaching, telephone teaching, or in-person medication teaching?
5. What aspects of Rosa's situation related to medications do you think are common among isolated elders?

REFERENCES

Ajemigbitse AA, Omole MK, Erhun WO: An assessment of the rate, types and severity of prescribing errors in a tertiary hospital in southwestern Nigeria, *Afr J Med Sci* 42(4):339–346, 2013.

American Geriatrics Society (AGS) Expert Panel: American Geriatrics Society updated Beers Criteria for potentially inappropriate medication use in older adults, *J Am Geriatr Soc* 60:616–631, 2012.

Beers M: Explicit criteria for determining potentially inappropriate medication use by the elderly. An update, *Arch Intern Med* 157:1531–1536, 1997.

Beyth RJ, Shorr RI: Medication use. In Shorr RI, Hoth AB, Rawls N, editors: *Medications for the geriatric patient*, St. Louis, MO, 2007, Saunders.

Bullock R, Saharan A: Atypical antipsychotics: experience and use in the elderly, *Int J Clin Pract* 56:515–525, 2002.

Burchum JLR: Pharmacologic management. In Meiner S, editor: *Gerontologic nursing*, ed 4, St. Louis, MO, 2011, Elsevier.

Centers for Medicare and Medicaid Services (CMS): *Dementia care in nursing homes: clarification to Appendix P State Operations Manual (SOM) and Appendix PP in the SOM for F309 – Quality of Care and F329 – Unnecessary Drugs* (Memorandum S&C: 13-35 NH), 2013. http://www.cms.gov/medicare/provider-enrollment-and-certification/survey certificationgeninfo/downloads/survey-and-cert-letter-13-35.pdf. Accessed July 2014.

Gnjidic D, Hilmer SN, Blyth FM, et al: Polypharmacy cutoff and outcomes: five or more medications were used to identify community-dwelling older men at risk of different adverse outcomes, *J Clin Epidemiol* 65(9):989–995, 2012.

Goldberg RJ: Tardive dyskinesia in elderly patients: an update, *J Am Med Dir Assoc* 3:152–161, 2002.

Gould E, Mitty E: Medication adherence is a partnership, medication compliance is not, *Geriatr Nurs* 31:290–298, 2010.

Hughes GJ, Beizer JL: Appropriate prescribing. In Ham RJ, Sloane PD, Warshaw GA, et al, editors: *Primary care geriatrics: a case-based approach*, ed 6, Philadelphia, 2014, Elsevier, pp 67–76.

Kim M, Dam A, Green J: Common GI drug interactions in the elderly, *Curr Treat Options Gastroenterol* 12(3):292–309, 2014.

Lindsey PL: Psychotropic medication use among older adults: what all nurses need to know, *J Gerontol Nurs* 35(9):28–38, 2009.

Lucado J, Paez K, Elixhauser A: *Medication-related adverse outcomes in U.S. hospitals and emergency rooms, 2008* (Statistical brief no. 109), Healthcare Cost and Utilization Project, 2011. http://www.hcup-us.ahrq.gov/reports/statbriefs/sb109.jsp. Accessed July 2014.

Medicines and Healthcare Products Regulatory Agency (MHRA): *Antipsychotic drugs*, 2014. http://www.mhra.gov.uk/Safetyinformation/Generalsafetyinformationandadvice/Product-specificinformationandadvice/Product-specificinformationandadvice-A-F/Antipsychoticdrugs/index.htm. Accessed July 2014.

Molony S, Greenberg SA: *The 2012 American Geriatrics Society updated Beers criteria for potentially inappropriate medication use in older adults*, New York, 2013, Hartford Institute for Geriatric Nursing. http://consultgerirn.org/uploads/File/trythis/try_this_16_1.pdf. Accessed October 31, 2014.

Peron EP, Gray SL, Hanlon JT: Medication use and functional status decline in older adults: a review, *Am J Geriatr Pharmacother* 9(6):378–391, 2011.

Planton J, Edlund BJ: Strategies for reducing polypharmacy in older adults, *J Gerontol Nurs* 36:8–12, 2010.

Rochon PA: *Drug prescribing for older adults*, 2014. UpToDate. http://www.uptodate.com/contents/drug-prescribing-for-older-adults. Accessed July 2014.

Saxon SV, Etten MJ, Perkins EA: *Physical change and aging*, ed 5, New York, 2010, Springer.

CHAPTER 10

The Use of Herbs and Supplements

Jo Lynne Robins and Lisa Burroughs Phipps

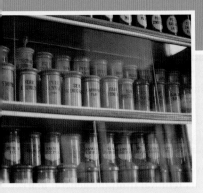

http://evolve.elsevier.com/Touhy/TwdHlthAging

A STUDENT SPEAKS

I had no idea how many different things people take. Older adults have so many remedies! All sorts of herbal teas and vitamins . . . I wonder if they work.

Kelly, age 18

AN ELDER SPEAKS

I try to take the medicines that the nurse practitioner gives me but I can't always afford them, so I ask my friend what I should do because she knows a lot about herbs and teas. I take them to supplement my medicines. Sometimes they really help.

Jean, age 65

LEARNING OBJECTIVES

On completion of this chapter, the reader will be able to:

1. Identify the legal standards that affect herb and supplement use.
2. Discuss the information that older adults should know about the use of select herbs and supplements.
3. Discuss the role of the gerontological nurse when assisting the older adult who uses herbs and supplements.
4. Describe the effects of selected commonly used herbs and supplements on the older adult.
5. Develop a nursing care plan to prevent adverse reactions related to herb or supplement use.
6. Identify the important aspects of education related to the use of herbs and supplements by older adults.
7. Describe the effects of herbal supplements on the older adult with chronic disease.

Herbs and other supplements have been used for thousands of years to promote health and treat illness, but during most of the past century, their popularity waned with the availability of prescription and over-the-counter medications. The use of herbs and supplements has resurged over the past two decades. The most recent national data available estimated that 38% of American adults spend $14.8 billion on non-vitamin herbs and supplements, and the highest use rates were for those ages 50 to 59 years (Barnes et al, 2008; Nahin et al, 2009). The most commonly used supplement among adults is fish oil/omega 3 fatty acids, followed by glucosamine, echinacea, flaxseed, ginseng, ginkgo, chondroitin, and garlic (Barnes et al, 2008). In older men and women ages 60 to 99 years, glucosamine was the most frequently used supplement followed by ginkgo, chondroitin, and garlic. Men most commonly use α-lipoic acid, ginkgo, and grape seed extract (Wold et al, 2005).Women favored black cohosh, evening primrose oil, flaxseed oil, chondroitin, ginkgo, glucosamine, grape seed extract, hawthorn, and St. John's wort.

In a survey of 445 community-dwelling older adults 28.3% reported using vitamins and 20.7% used herbal supplements (Cheung et al, 2007).

While herb and supplement use occurs across races and ethnicities, a National Health and Nutrition Examination Survey indicated the highest rate of use was in non-Hispanic white, older, normal to underweight, educated females (Radimer et al, 2004). In the United States the increasing use of herbs and dietary supplements by older adults may be related to their hopes of preventing illness, promoting and maintaining health, treating a particular health problem, or replacing some currently missing dietary component (Bruno and Ellis, 2005; Cheung et al, 2007; Yoon and Horne, 2001; Yoon et al, 2004). People perceive that such products will give them more control of their health and bodies. Herbs and supplements are typically used as a complement to, rather than a replacement for, a person's prescribed therapies (Yoon, 2006). Elders with chronic conditions are more likely to use herbs and supplements with their traditional therapies (Nieva et al, 2012;

Ryder et al, 2008). Combining herbs and supplements with prescription and over-the-counter (OTC) medications increases the likelihood of adverse reactions in older adults (Lam and Bradley, 2006; Loya et al, 2009). While historically, patients have not been likely to disclose the use of herbs and supplements to their health care providers (Bruno and Ellis, 2005; Cheung et al, 2007), persons older than 50 years of age may be more likely than younger persons to share information about their use of supplements with their providers (Durante et al, 2001; Israel and Youngkin, 2005; Ryder et al, 2008). Gerontological nurses can anticipate that older adults may use a variety of complementary and alternative therapies, including herbs and supplements, in addition to prescribed and OTC drugs. The nurse has a significant obligation to ask the right questions and obtain specific information related to use—reason, form, frequency, duration, dose, any side/adverse effects, and plans for continuing.

STANDARDS IN MANUFACTURING

Before 1962 all herbs were regarded as medications. In 1962 the U.S. Food and Drug Administration (FDA) required that all products considered "medications" be evaluated for safety, efficacy, and standardization between manufacturers of the same product. The role of the FDA also expanded to that of monitoring these products. In response, herbal manufacturers declared their products as "foods" and therefore not subject to FDA regulations (Youngkin and Israel, 1996). In 1994 some regulation was placed over herbs through the Dietary Supplement Health and Education Act (DSHEA), and they were reclassified as "dietary supplements."

By regulation, herbs and other supplements may not be labeled for prevention, treatment, or cure of a health condition of any kind unless the claim has been substantiated by research and recognized by the FDA (U.S. FDA, 2014). Of all the identified herbs, few are FDA approved as medications: aloe, psyllium, capsicum, witch hazel, cascara, senna, and slippery elm. It is required that all adverse events be reported to the FDA. The World Health Organization and regulatory agencies of individual countries are answering the call for safety and efficacy information based on scientific evaluation of herbs and supplements (Blumenthal et al, 2000; Israel and Youngkin, 2005).

Factors that make commercially marketed herbal products difficult to study systematically include the following: differences in plant products used (parts of plant, such as whole plant or extract), different combination products and proprietary blends, and differences in manufacturing processes. To help improve the quality of dietary supplements, the FDA put *Good Manufacturing Practices* (GMPs) into place in 2007. This set of guidelines for preparation and storage of dietary supplements stipulates that manufacturers are now required to guarantee the identity, purity, strength, and composition of dietary supplements. Many manufacturers today have heeded the call to standardize the production and labeling of herbs and supplements. Some manufacturers are also using standardization to ensure consistency of their products between batches. Honest marketing and the independent testing of products for purity are occurring.

Nurses can alert and educate individuals to potential risks and adverse effects, as well as drug-herb and drug-supplement interactions. Risks include the product containing the wrong parts of the herb; containing little or no active ingredient, rendering it ineffective; or being adulterated with one or more unidentified substances that may be dangerous. Mixed herbal supplements, such as some weight loss products, can also have hazardous effects on blood pressure and heart rate and rhythm and can be particularly risky because actually determining what the product contains may be difficult. For example, bitter orange (Citrus aurantium) was used to replace ephedra in many weight loss products after its removal from the general market by the FDA in 2004, but bitter orange has synephrine (epinephrine-like) effects, as did ephedra, that can lead to cardiac arrest and ventricular fibrillation and thus is still unsafe for use in some patients (Swanson, 2007).

Nurses must maintain current knowledge about herbs and other supplements so that when they conduct a complete medication review (Chapter 9), potential and actual harmful effects may be recognized. Consideration of each product's intended use, dose, possible adverse effects, and possible interactions with other substances based on the person's health or illness conditions is required. Nurses should urge their patients to be aware of these issues and to purchase products from reputable distributors and discuss dietary supplement use with their health care providers and pharmacists.

HERB FORMS

Different parts of many herbs have uses and actions that are unrelated. For example, the bulb of the garlic plant contains the active ingredient, whereas the leaf of chamomile is used (Israel and Youngkin, 2005).

Herbal products are manufactured in several forms, including teas, capsules, tablets, extracts, oils, tinctures, and salves (Khalsa, 2007). Efficacy varies and depends in part on the form of the herb that is used and how it is prepared. An *extract* is a concentrated fluid or solid form of the herb that is made by mixing the crude herb with alcohol or other solvents that are then distilled or evaporated (Khalsa, 2007). When an herb is soaked in water, alcohol, vinegar, or glycerin for a specific time and the liquid is then strained to dispose of the plant remains, a *tincture* is formed. A *salve* is a type of ointment that is used topically (Khalsa, 2007). *Essential oils* are aromatic, volatile compounds derived from various parts of the fresh plant. They are commonly used in aromatherapy or massage therapy (Tillett and Ames, 2010).

Teas

As a beverage, teas are consumed by millions around the world, second only to water. It is considered a food and regulated as such in the United States. It should be noted that the word "tea" is often used to describe preparations that do not contain a tea plant at all. True tea comes from the plant *Camellia sinensis*, which produces white, green, oolong, black, and pu-erh teas. The difference in these teas is in the processing of the *C. sinensis* plant. Maté and red teas are from different plants and are not true tea, and many herbal teas contain flowers and herbs but no *Camellia sinensis*. Some refer to these preparations as tisanes or infusions, and some still refer to them as tea. Newly reported research indicates that some teas may have very positive effects, especially related to cardiovascular disease. Women and non-smokers seemed to benefit the most from green tea. Animal studies suggest that green tea antioxidants may offer eye tissue protection (Chu et al, 2010); antioxidants in tea and raspberry juice may decrease plaque formation and help decrease the risk of atherosclerosis (Rouanet et al, 2009); and tea alone may lower serum cholesterol levels (Singh et al, 2009).

In a systematic review of the effects of tea on cardiovascular disease, potential mechanisms include antiinflammatory, antioxidant, and antiproliferative effects, but findings are confounded by lifestyle and dietary factors (Deka and Vita, 2011). In a meta-analysis of coronary heart disease, a protective effect was found for green tea (Wang et al, 2011) and both reviews highlighted the need for additional rigorous studies. Drinking green tea has also been associated with a decreased risk of some cancers, such as prostate cancer in men and breast and stomach cancers in women (Boehm et al, 2009; Inoue et al, 2009; Shrubsole et al, 2009; Tang et al, 2009). Consuming more than four cups of tea daily was associated with a reduced risk of type 2 diabetes in adults (Huxley et al, 2009), and drinking more than four cups of green tea daily was associated with a reduced risk of depression in adults 70 years of age and older (Niu et al, 2009) and in breast cancer survivors (Chen et al, 2010).

While the consumption of tea and most tisanes and infusions can be considered safe, there have been instances of high use of some that can cause problems. For instance, senna leaf may cause serious fluid and electrolyte imbalance effects if used in excess and for a prolonged period (Israel and Youngkin, 2005). Some tea and tisane preparations may have names that imply they are used for a specific purpose (e.g., detoxification, fluid retention, anxiety/stress, energy). Instructions for how much should be consumed are often found on these preparations. Consumption of more than the recommended amounts of these preparations may cause illness and possible death. For example, comfrey tea has been linked with serious liver disease (Youngkin and Israel, 1996), and drinking very hot tea too fast may be associated with an increased risk of esophageal cancer (Islami et al, 2009). For herbal teas and tisanes that state specific uses, it would be wise to check ingredients, use with care, and examine instructions carefully for any warnings or suggestions for quantity of use. As with any caffeinated beverage, consumers should be aware of caffeine content. For true *Camellia sinensis* teas, white teas have very little caffeine, green and oolong teas have some caffeine, and black tea can have almost as much or as much caffeine as a cup of coffee. These are generalities for the types of true tea, and consumers may want to check with specific vendors for the caffeine content of each product.

SELECT COMMONLY USED TEAS, HERBS, AND SUPPLEMENTS

Although potential benefits of various products have been reported, it must be noted that in many cases the scientific evidence supporting the claims is limited or inconclusive at this time (Basch and Ulbricht, 2005). It is recommended that dosing be carefully researched for the specific brand due to the inconsistencies in formulations. Doses vary widely depending on the condition being treated, so it is best to use products from a reputable source. For information about evolving research related to these products, the reader is referred to the website of the National Center for Complementary and Integrative Health (http://nccih.nih.gov/). In this section some of the most commonly used teas, herbs, and nutritional supplements are reviewed.

Chamomile

Chamomile *(Matricaria recutita* or *Chamomilla recutita)*, also known as *German chamomile* or *Hungarian chamomile,* is usually taken in tea form. It reportedly is useful as an antispasmodic (said to relax smooth muscle) and to relieve gastrointestinal upset, promote sleep, and reduce anxiety (Amsterdam et al, 2009; Israel and Youngkin, 2005; Natural Standard, 2013c). It also may have effects comparable with nonsteroidal antiinflammatory medications (NSAIDs) (Srivastava et al, 2009).

Like other herbal preparations, excessive ingestion may be dangerous. Large doses may cause gastrointestinal (GI) upset, contact dermatitis, and hypersensitivity reactions. Chamomile tea should not be used by those taking benzodiazepines and other sedative-causing drugs; it may inhibit some cytochrome P450 substrates. Taking it with warfarin may increase warfarin's effect and increase the risk of bleeding.

⚡ **SAFETY ALERT**

Chamomile may cause anaphylaxis in those allergic to ragweed, asters, or chrysanthemums.

Echinacea

Echinacea *(Echinacea angustifolia, E. purpurea, E. pallida),* also known as *Sampson root* and *purple coneflower,* is a very popular product, especially for upper respiratory infections (URIs) such as common colds (Shah et al, 2007). It is available commercially as capsules, tea, juice, extract, and tincture.

E. purpurea has been shown to be effective for the prevention of upper respiratory infections (URIs) or in decreasing the duration of URIs by 1 to 2 days if used at the onset of symptoms (Karsch-Völk et al, 2014; Natural Standard, 2013o). If the herb is used as directed, the side effects for most persons are few. However, a number of adverse reactions have been known to occur, including fever, sore throat, diarrhea, nausea and vomiting, abdominal pain, and dry eyes (Askeroglu et al, 2013; Natural Standard, 2013e). Persons allergic to daisy family plants or who have human immunodeficiency virus/acquired immunodeficiency syndrome (HIV/AIDS) or an autoimmune disease should use this herb with caution. It may interfere with the clearance of drugs eliminated by CYP3A or CYP1A2 in the liver (Gorski et al, 2004).

⚡ **SAFETY ALERT**

Combining echinacea with acetaminophen and other drugs or herbs that could cause liver damage is discouraged because it may cause liver inflammation (Natural Standard, 2013e).

Garlic

Garlic (*Allium sativum* bulb), known by names such as *clove garlic* and *camphor of the poor,* is composed of more than 200 chemicals; a sulfur compound called *allicin* is thought to be garlic's primary active health ingredient. When the garlic clove is crushed, chewed, or chopped, allicin is released. Garlic is generally well tolerated, with the main side effect being "tasting garlic."

Among the reported benefits are the ability to decrease blood clots and to reduce total serum cholesterol and low-density lipoprotein (LDL) cholesterol levels. Its effect on high-density lipoprotein (HDL) cholesterol is not clear (Natural Standard, 2013f; Ried, Toben et al, 2013). While evidence is not yet sufficient to broadly recommend its use in the treatment of hypertension (Simons et al, 2009; Stabler et al, 2012), two meta-analyses have shown that garlic helps reduce blood pressure in persons with hypertension (Reinhart et al, 2008; Ried et al, 2008; Ried, Frank et al, 2013).

Possible adverse reactions include severe allergic reactions, increased flatulence, and upper GI irritation with nausea and heartburn, the latter a special concern in persons with ulcers or acid reflux disorders (Natural Standard, 2013g; Tachjian et al, 2010).

Ginkgo biloba

Ginkgo (*Ginkgo biloba),* also known as *maidenhair tree, fossil tree,* and *wonder of the world,* is a leaf abstract from the oldest living tree species (Waddell et al, 2001). It is prepared in capsule, extract, and tablet forms and is used in tisanes and tea blends. The usual dose varies depending on its purpose and is administered in two or three oral divided doses (Natural Standard, 2013h). The flavonoids, glycosides, and terpenoids such as gingkolide B and bilobalide are considered to be the primary active ingredients (Jiang et al, 2011). It is often marketed as EGb761, a standardized extract containing 22% to 27% flavone glycosides and 5% to 7% terpenoids.

Many studies, often very small, have investigated ginkgo for conditions ranging from vertigo, tinnitus, macular degeneration, and depression to altitude sickness and acute hemorrhoids, but adequate scientific evidence to support its use for such concerns is unclear and inconsistent (Natural Standard, 2013h).

It is widely believed that ginkgo benefits cognitive function in dementia. However, there is no scientific evidence that ginkgo impacts cognitive impairment, memory, attention, language, visual-spatial ability, executive functions or reduced prevalence of dementia and Alzheimer's disease (Birks et al, 2009; Canter and Ernst, 2007; NCCIH, 2009).

One of the more serious side effects of ginkgo use is bleeding (Natural Standard, 2013h). People known to be at risk for bleeding or using medications that can increase the risk for bleeding (e.g., anticoagulants) should not start taking gingko without consulting their physicians and pharmacists because the risks likely outweigh the benefits in these cases. Many other herbs increase the risk of bleeding, such as *Panax ginseng,* ginger, and garlic (Kuhn, 2002; Natural Standard, 2013h), and should be used with caution if taken together with gingko-containing products.

> ### ⚡ SAFETY ALERT
>
> **Bleeding Risk**
> A number of herbs themselves or in combination with other herbs may cause significant changes in coagulation. Due to the high number of older adults taking anticoagulants, this is a special concern, especially for one of the newer medications such as Pradaxa for which there is no antidote for drug-related excessive bleeding. See Chapter 9 for more information.

Some of the reported side effects of ginkgo include increased blood pressure, intestinal upset, headache, palpitations, dizziness, muscle weakness, and constipation (Jalili et al, 2013). Due to the high number of serious interactions and potential side effects and the lack of demonstrated benefits, the use of *Ginkgo biloba* should be discouraged.

> ### ⚡ SAFETY ALERT
>
> *Ginkgo biloba* seeds may be toxic (Natural Standard, 2013h).

Ginseng

Two of the main categories of *ginseng* are American and Asian. *Asian ginseng* is also referred to as Chinese, Korean, and Asiatic. The Latin name is *Panax ginseng.* Another herb called *Siberian ginseng* or *eleuthero* is not true ginseng. The ginseng root is dried and used to make tablets, capsules, extracts, teas, and tinctures. The most active constituents are ginsenosides or panaxosides, but ginseng also contains other compounds that may also play a role in its efficacy (Natural Standard, 2013i). Dosages vary with the type of ginseng, the preparation, the frequency of consumption, the strength of dose, and the indication for use.

Ginseng has had numerous applications over thousands of years' use and has long been believed to improve well-being, help with stress adaptation, enhance immune function, and decrease oxidative cell damage (Chapter 25). It has also been thought to improve mental and physical performance, lower blood glucose level and blood pressure, regulate symptoms related to menopause (NCCIH, 2012a), and treat erectile dysfunction (Hong et al, 2002).

In small clinical trials it has been found that Asian ginseng may lower blood glucose levels and improve immune function (NCCIH, 2012a). There is also some evidence that the *Panax* ginsengs enhance the immune system, decrease the duration of upper respiratory tract infections, and improve mental performance (Natural Standard, 2013i). As more research is conducted ginseng may be shown to benefit persons with heart disorders by reducing LDL cholesterol, lower blood glucose levels in type 2 diabetes, and enhance the immune system (Basch and Ulbricht, 2005; Natural Standard, 2013i).

There is not enough evidence to support its use for improving memory, enhancing feelings of well-being, or affecting hyperlipidemia, arrhythmias, or stroke outcomes, as some suggest (Natural Standard, 2013i).

Short-term use for most people and at recommended doses appears to be safe; however, it is suggested that long-term use may

BOX 10-1 Potential Side Effects of Ginseng of Significance for Older Adults

- Tachycardia
- Hypertension
- Hypotension
- Hypoglycemia
- Insomnia

From Natural Standard: *Ginkgo*, 2013. http://www.naturalstandard.com Accessed May 2014; Tachjian A, Maria V, Jahangir A: Use of herbal products and potential interactions in patients with cardiovascular diseases, *J Am Coll Cardiol* 55:515–525, 2010.

result in side effects, including those that may be particularly important to older adults such as increased blood pressure and risk for bleeding (Amico et al, 2013; Jalili et al, 2013; Natural Standard, 2013; Tachjian et al, 2010) (Box 10-1). Allergic reactions are reported in people allergic to plants in the Araliaceae family.

⚡ SAFETY ALERT

Persons who have had strokes may have increased bleeding if they take ginseng and blood-thinning medications at the same time (Lee et al, 2008).

Glucosamine and Chondroitin Sulfate

Glucosamine and chondroitin sulfate are natural substances found in and around the cells of the cartilage and connective tissue. Chondroitin sulfate helps the cartilage retain water. Both are classified as nutritional supplements and therefore regulated as a food product. While they can be purchased separately, they are often combined in one formulation. They are typically used for osteoarthritis (OA) of the knees to help reduce pain and improve function (Natural Standard, 2013j). Major studies have been conducted regarding the safety and efficacy of these products both individually and together (Box 10-2).

BOX 10-2 Evidence-Based Practice

The Glucosamine/Chondroitin Arthritis Intervention Trial (GAIT) found that while well tolerated and without significant adverse effects, neither of these supplements, either alone or together, was more effective than either a placebo or celecoxib, a currently available NSAID (NCCIH, 2014; Sawitzke et al, 2010); however, they did find that one small subgroup with moderate-to-severe pain had a 20% improvement in pain (Bruyere and Reginster, 2007; Clegg et al, 2006).

From Bruyere O, Reginster JY: Glucosamine and chondroitin sulfate as the therapeutic agents for knee and hip osteoarthritis, *Drugs Aging* 24:573–580, 2007; Clegg DO, Reda DJ, Harris CL et al: Glucosamine, chondroitin sulfate, and the two in combination for painful knee osteoarthritis, *N Engl J Med* 354:795–808, 2006; Natural Medicines Comprehensive Database (NMCD): *Drug-supplement interactions*, 2014. http://naturaldatabase.therapeuticresearch.com/ce/ceCourse. aspx?s=ND&cs=CP&pc=07-34&cec=1&pm=5. Accessed October 31, 2014; Sawitzke AD, Shi H, Finco MF et al: Clinical efficacy and safety of glucosamine, chondroitin sulphate, their combination, celecoxib or placebo taken to treat osteoarthritis of the knee: 2-year results from GAIT, *Ann Rheumatol Dis* 69:1459–1464, 2010.

Because both of these supplements have demonstrated mild antiinflammatory effects, future research may further clarify their role in treating osteoarthritis and even other inflammation-related diseases such as cancer and cardiovascular disease (Kantor et al, 2012).

The nurse might advise that although glucosamine sulfate with chondroitin sulfate has generally been shown safe for use, there is currently limited evidence to support their effectiveness in decreasing OA pain or progression (Natural Standard, 2013p) and caution must be used given potential herb/supplement–drug interactions and allergic reactions. Persons with diabetes, asthma, or shellfish allergy should use glucosamine with caution. Those who eat a vegetarian or vegan diet should be informed that chondroitin is derived from cartilage of animals, in case they do not wish to consume these products.

Research is emerging investigating the use of methylsulfonylmethane (MSM) in conjunction with glucosamine and chondroitin sulfate. In a pilot study of 32 participants, this combination was found to significantly reduce pain and oxidative stress (Nakasone et al, 2011). Other clinical trials support the safety and use of MSM alone in reducing pain and functional impairment (Debbi et al, 2011; Kim et al, 2006). However, a meta-analysis of three studies indicated there was no significant benefit of MSM in osteoarthritis of the knee, indicating additional research is needed before recommending it in clinical practice (Brien et al, 2011).

A few mild side effects have been reported including gastrointestinal upset, insomnia, headache, and skin reactions. However, there are multiple drug or herb/supplement interactions, particularly those with antiglycemic or anticoagulant properties (Burks, 2005; Natural Standard, 2013q). MSM alone or in combination with glucosamine sulfate and chondroitin may be safe and useful in reducing OA pain and improving function, but additional research is needed.

Hawthorn

Hawthorn (*Crataegus monogyna, Crataegus laevigata*) is a small flowering tree or shrub in the rose family. The leaves and flowers can be put into capsules and tablets or are used to make teas or liquid extracts when combined with water and alcohol. It has been used for centuries in the treatment of heart disease and digestive and kidney problems (NCCIH, 2012b). It is reported to increase cardiac output and to have antispasmodic, antianxiety, antiinflammatory, antilipidemic, and diuretic and sedating effects (Jurikova et al, 2012).

An analysis of clinical trials indicated that benefits were significant for hawthorn use as short-term adjunctive therapy in both chronic and severe heart failure (Eggeling et al, 2011; Natural Standard, 2013k; Pittler et al, 2008).

Currently, because noted side effects have been mild and infrequent (Daniele et al, 2006), hawthorn is considered safe for short-term use (up to 16 weeks); however, given its indication and mechanisms of action, close oversight by a knowledgeable health care provider is recommended. The most common side effects are vertigo and dizziness, noteworthy problems for older adults who are already at a higher risk for falls. GI upset, allergic response with rash, palpitations, fatigue, and sweating are among the less common side effects.

Melatonin

Sleep disorders are increasingly common with aging (Chapter 17). Several medications are used to try to help the person get to sleep, stay asleep, or have a restful sleep. *Melatonin* is used as an alternative or as an adjuvant to these medications. In the natural state, melatonin is endogenously produced by the pineal gland and is an important signal in regulating the sleep-wake cycle. Melatonin levels are low during the day, increase during the evening, remain high throughout the night, and decrease again by morning. Melatonin acts at MT_1 and MT_2 receptors to promote sleep.

Numerous studies, including meta-analyses and systematic reviews, have shown supportive evidence for its use in conditions such as jet lag; insomnia in children, adults, and the elderly; and delayed sleep phase syndrome (Ferracioli-Oda et al, 2013; Krystal et al, 2013; Ramar and Olson, 2013; Wilhelmsen-Langeland et al, 2013). It is most commonly used to promote sleep.

Specifically, melatonin can decrease sleep onset latency, increase sleep duration, and improve sleep quality, although its effects are generally not as strong as those for benzodiazepines and benzodiazepine receptor agonists (Ferracioli-Oda et al, 2013). Melatonin is available in both immediate and extended release forms, and both have been found to be effective. A meta-analysis specifically looking at an extended-release melatonin preparation in patients older than 55 found that a dose of 2 mg orally 2 hours before bed was effective at decreasing sleep onset latency, improving quality of sleep, and improving morning wakefulness (Lemoine and Zisapel, 2012).

Adverse effects include dizziness, nausea, and drowsiness. Care should be taken if a patient is taking other medications that can cause drowsiness or have central nervous system depressant effects, such as antihistamines, benzodiazepines, and some pain medications. While melatonin is considered generally safe for use, as with all supplements it should only be recommended or taken when considering the patient's entire medication/supplement profile (Natural Standards, 2013n).

Red Yeast Rice

Red yeast rice is thought by many to be a dietary supplement helpful in controlling one's cholesterol level. It has been a traditional Chinese culinary and medicinal product for centuries. The medicinal effect is from monacolin K, which is chemically equivalent and as effective as the lipid-lowering drug lovastatin. The side effect profiles are similar, such as myalgias. However, if the rice includes more than a trace amount of monacolin K, it is considered an unapproved *medication* and cannot be sold legally in the United States as a dietary supplement (Natural Standard, 2013r; NCCIH, 2013). It is not known if other red yeast products that do not contain monacolin K have any effect on cholesterol levels. However, some products do contain a contaminant called citrinin, which can cause kidney failure.

> ### ⚡ SAFETY ALERT
>
> **Red Yeast Rice**
>
> Some products do contain a contaminant called citrinin, which can cause kidney failure. It is important to purchase red yeast rice from a reliable and reputable source.
>
> The composition of the rice depends on a number of factors, especially manufacturing processes. The FDA has monitored its safety and found that it contains only trace amounts, if any, of monacolin K. Red yeast rice is a food product, yet in 2009 approximately $20 million was spent on purchasing this product as a supplement.
>
> Many older adults are taking lipid-lowering products and discussions about the inclusion of red yeast rice in their diet are especially important. Patients must be advised that they should only purchase the rice from respected sources and should avoid Internet purchases because these products may be adulterated (U.S. FDA, 2007).

St. John's Wort

St. John's wort (SJW; *Hypericum perforatum*) has many names, such as *demon chaser* and *goatweed*. This yellow-flowered plant has been used for mental disorders, nerve pain, and many other problems over the years. The flowers are used to prepare teas and also can be made into tablets and capsules and concentrated into extracts and salves. The proposed active ingredients in SJW include hypericin and hyperforin. One available standardized product, known as WS® 5570, contains 0.1% to 0.3% hypericin and 3% to 6% hyperforin.

SJW is most often taken as a treatment for depression, although it is used by some without clear evidential support for a large variety of illnesses such as seasonal affective disorder, anxiety, pain relief, and premenstrual syndrome (Ernst, 2002; Lawvere and Mahoney, 2005; NCCIH, 2012c; Ravindran et al, 2009; van der Watt et al, 2008).

The only research that has been done examined the effect of SJW on depression. It has been found to be ineffective for major depression (NCCIH, 2008; Sego, 2006; Shelton, 2009). However, it may be superior to placebo and as effective as commonly used antidepressants for mild or moderate depression (Linde et al, 2008; Natural Standard, 2013t).

The concern of many experts is that its use could endanger the individual with depression by increasing the risk of suicide when other treatment is delayed. Another serious concern about the use of SJW is the interaction with other medications such as warfarin and digoxin, both medications taken by many older adults (NCCIH, 2012c).

Unless otherwise contraindicated, SJW is considered relatively well tolerated in recommended doses for 1 to 3 months (Brattström, 2009; Natural Standard, 2013t). As with standard antidepressants, side effects are fairly common but not often severe, occurring in about one out of three patients. Such side effects include dermatitis, GI upset, restlessness, anxiety, headache, dry mouth, and possible sexual dysfunction (Natural Standard, 2013t). Patients taking SJW should be aware of photosensitivity and be advised to wear sunscreen and seek shade in prolonged outdoor exposure. Hypomania with bipolar disorder has been reported, as well as suicidal and homicidal thoughts. Hypertension has been reported as well (Jalili et al, 2013).

St. John's wort is a known inducer of the cytochrome P450 3A4 enzyme and, as such, should be used cautiously with medications metabolized by this route because it may decrease the effectiveness of these medications.

> ⚡ **SAFETY ALERT**
>
> St. John's wort is a known inducer of the cytochrome P450 3A4 enzyme, more so than many other herbs; therefore it has significantly more potential herb-drug interactions.

If individuals are taking any antidepressant they will need to wait at least 2 weeks after discontinuing its use before beginning SJW or cross-taper the medication and the herb to avoid the potential for serious adverse effects. The list of possible drug-drug, drug–herb/supplement, herb-disease, and anesthesia interactions is long and the benefits small, if any; yet its use remains popular.

Saw Palmetto

Saw palmetto, a fruit-bearing palm tree known as *Serenoa repens*, grows wild in the southern United States. The ripe fruit or berries are dried and ground into tablets or capsules or made into extracts or teas. It has been used for a variety of symptoms, most notably for those related to benign prostatic hyperplasia (BPH) (Tacklind et al, 2009). It may exert some estrogenic effects and inhibit 5α-reductase and androgen receptors (Natural Standard, 2013s), and it has been noted to offer mild to modest symptom improvement for persons with benign prostatic hyperplasia (BPH) (Israel and Youngkin, 2005; Natural Standard, 2013s). However, several studies, including those funded by the NIH, have found no more effect than a placebo (Barry et al, 2011; Kim et al, 2012; MacDonald et al, 2012).

Although considered not to cause serious drug interactions or toxicity, the herb is associated with some mild side effects, such as dizziness, fatigue, rhinitis, decreased libido, headache, and GI upset, and there could be possible adverse reactions not yet seen (Agbabiaka et al, 2009; Avins et al, 2008). Saw palmetto may prolong bleeding time; therefore, its combined use with anticoagulant/antiplatelet drugs, supplements, or herbs is advised with caution and under supervision. The herb must not be taken with other drugs used for the treatment of BPH or prostate cancer or with any drug or herb/supplement that can affect male sex hormones (Natural Standard, 2013s).

USE OF HERBS AND SUPPLEMENTS FOR SELECT CONDITIONS

Hypertension

A number of herbs, minerals, and supplements may exert positive effects in lowering blood pressure but need more research to support their use in treatment. Some of these are coenzyme Q10, garlic, green tea, hawthorn, melatonin, and magnesium (Natural Standard, 2013q).

Hawthorn has been used to treat hypertension for many years (National Standard, 2013m). A British study found that

people with diabetes type 2 who were taking antidiabetic medications had a significant reduction in diastolic blood pressure when randomized to take hawthorn (Walker et al, 2006). As therapeutic levels are not established, overtreatment and undertreatment can occur when hawthorn alone is used. Caution is urged when erectile dysfunction drugs are used concomitantly with hawthorn because hypotension may result (Hong et al, 2002). Research shows that dietary calcium in enriched low-fat dairy products taken three times daily may lower blood pressure in moderate hypertension (Natural Standard, 2013q). Health care providers are urged to provide up-to-date information about the use of any such substance when counseling patients who have hypertension (Edwards et al, 2005).

> ⚡ **SAFETY ALERT**
>
> If a person adds hawthorn while already taking beta-blockers or calcium channel blockers, it may precipitate dangerous hypotension (NMCD, 2014).

Human Immunodeficiency Virus–Related Symptoms

The number of persons entering late life who are living with HIV infection is increasing. Many have been using a number of complementary and alternative therapies, including herbs, to address their symptoms. Herbal therapies were among the self-care strategies used by 92% of participants in one study for symptoms of HIV and depression (Eller et al, 2005). Of concern is the potential that some herbal products may alter the metabolic action of antiretroviral drugs used in treatment (Ladenheim et al, 2008; Walubo, 2007). For example, SJW is commonly used for depression, but research indicates it may lower the blood level of antiretroviral medications when taken together. Some studies discuss the use of herbal medicines with HIV/AIDS patients for possible antiviral benefits (Natural Standard, 2013l), and other studies in Thailand and Africa indicate significant improvement in health overall and quality of life, suggesting a need for further study (Sugimoto et al, 2005; Tshibangu et al, 2004).

Gastrointestinal Disorders

Elders with gastrointestinal problems such as irritable bowel syndrome (IBS) are likely to use alternative therapies, including herbs (Tillisch, 2006). The Chinese have used herbal therapies for thousands of years to treat IBS. A search of the literature by Liu and colleagues (2006) found 75 randomized clinical trials for IBS that indicated it was improved by some of the herbal therapies. Psyllium (*Plantago ovata* and *P. ispaghula*) is used as a bulk laxative (Natural Standard, 2013g) that is generally well tolerated and may decrease IBS symptoms, although results are conflicting (Basch and Ulbricht, 2005). Calcium is approved by the FDA and scientifically well supported for use in reducing gastric acidity; probiotic products help control harmful organisms in the gut, such as *Helicobacter pylori* (Natural Standard, 2013g). Also, as previously noted, chamomile may help in the management of GI problems. Milk thistle has been shown to improve chronic alcohol-induced and fulminant hepatitis (Basch and Ulbricht, 2005).

Cancer

In the United States, many herbs have the potential to be used in the treatment of cancer but more research is needed. Patients with cancer often use complementary and alternative therapies in self-care, including herbs and dietary supplements. Some of the herbs that need more scientific study for helping patients with cancer include milk thistle and garlic (Natural Standard, 2013b; Williams et al, 2006). Calcium, garlic, ginkgo, ginseng and psyllium may help decrease the risk for colorectal and gastric cancer (Finnegan-John et al, 2013; Natural Standard, 2013a).

Drinking green tea is thought to help prevent cancer, but evidence is conflicting and insufficient (Boehm et al, 2009). Claims are often made that a substance or an herb will "cure" or help the patient with cancer, even though no data support such claims. Clients and their families may become desperate in an effort to "do something" to help. Gerontological nurses must be sensitive to this situation and work with all concerned to provide the best evidence-based care possible.

Alzheimer's Disease

Among 82 elderly veterans with dementia and depression, nearly one fifth of the veterans and their caretakers used herbs and supplements (Kales et al, 2004). Ginkgo is often used by older persons with dementia because it increases blood supply to the brain. There is some scientific support for modest improvement in Alzheimer's and dementia symptoms, but the GEM Study (NCCIH, 2009), discussed in the earlier section on *Ginkgo biloba*, found no scientific evidence to support the use of this herb to prevent or treat Alzheimer's disease.

Further study is advised in the use of sage with dementia and Alzheimer's disease (Natural Standard, 2013a). According to William Thies, chief medical and scientific officer of the Alzheimer's Association, engaging in moderate to heavy physical activity levels, drinking tea one to four times per day, and maintaining normal serum levels of vitamin D have all been associated with decreased risk for cognitive decline (Marcus, 2010b). Currently, additional studies are needed to substantiate these associations, as well as the use of melatonin for sleep benefits and lemon balm for agitation with patients with Alzheimer's disease or dementia (Marcus, 2010b; Natural Standard, 2013a).

Diabetes

Herbal approaches to diabetes management were in place before the discovery of insulin in 1921. As many as 400 herbs and supplements have been reported as beneficial in treating diabetes (Kasuli, 2011). Much of the supportive data exist in cellular and animal models with mechanisms of actions that include increased insulin secretion and sensitivity, improved glucose uptake in adipose and muscle tissue, and decreased intestinal glucose absorption and hepatocyte glucose production and antiinflammatory actions (Li et al, 2012). However, human studies are often not well designed and have yielded negative or mixed results. Fenugreek (*Trigonella foenum-graecum),* a seed powder, when consumed as a cup of tea three times daily or taken orally in a capsule can induce a hypoglycemic response and must be used carefully (Basch and Ulbricht, 2005). It can cause diarrhea and flatulence and may increase anticoagulant activity of other drugs the person is taking. Research indicates that every additional daily cup

consumed significantly decreases the risk of diabetes, and comparable amounts of decaffeinated coffee and tea result in similar decreases (Huxley et al, 2009). The protection from coffee may be present regardless of caffeine effect (Oba et al, 2010). However, J.D. Lane, a professor at Duke Medical Center, advises that drinking that much coffee a day may amplify problems with blood sugar in individuals with diabetes (Marcus, 2010a). A number of possible adverse effects may occur with increased caffeine intake, including headache, insomnia, anxiety and nervousness, hypertension, and heart rhythm disturbance.

Cinnamon is another herb that has been linked with lowering blood glucose level, but scientific evidence is mixed and overall the results do not support its effectiveness in diabetes (Baker et al, 2008; Kirkham et al, 2009; Leach and Kumar, 2012; Natural Standard, 2013d; Pham et al, 2007). Although aloe vera has not been proven efficacious in the treatment of diabetes, in 1 study of 45 participants with prediabetes/metabolic syndrome, it was shown to significantly reduce impaired fasting glucose level and glucose tolerance (Devaraj et al, 2013). Other herbs or supplements linked with some scientific evidence of lowering blood glucose level are α-lipoic acid, American ginseng, chromium, ginseng, gymnema, melatonin, and stevia (Kasuli, 2011; Lee and Dugoua, 2011; Natural Standard, 2013d).

Numerous other substances are said to have unclear or conflicting scientific evidence for lowering blood sugar, such as astragalus, bilberry, black or green tea, red yeast rice, honey, and even the parasitic vine kudzu, but the evidence is not sufficient to support that these are effective in treating or reducing the development of diabetes type 2 (Natural Standard, 2013d). Garlic and green tea may be useful in decreasing cardiovascular risk by lowering glucose and lipid levels, but additional studies are needed (Rudkowska, 2012). To date, there are insufficient data to support the use of herbal supplements in the primary treatment of diabetes. If any herb or supplement is used by the patient for diabetes management, health care professionals need to urge careful blood glucose monitoring and direct appropriate dose adjustments for prescribed medications.

HERB AND SUPPLEMENT INTERACTIONS WITH STANDARDIZED DRUGS

A major issue in the use of herbs and other supplements is the risk for interactions. While herb-supplement and herb-drug interactions involve a relatively small subset of frequently prescribed medications such as warfarin and digoxin, among others, these interactions are of particular concern because of the number of medications already taken by elders and the potential danger of interactions (prescription, OTC, herbs, and supplements) (Tsai et al, 2012). A 22-month study of more than 3000 U.S. adults, ages 75 years or older, found that almost 2250 of the study participants combined at least 1 prescription drug with 1 dietary supplement daily, and approximately 10% to 33% combined up to 5 prescription drugs and 5 supplements daily (Nahin et al, 2009). This chapter addresses only select herb-drug interactions especially relevant to older adults because of the extensive nature of such interaction issues (Box 10-3).

The more herbs, supplements, and other drugs that the person is taking, the more likely it is that an interaction will occur

Drug-Herb Interactions

Persons taking medications that have a narrow therapeutic index such as warfarin and digoxin should be especially discouraged from using herbal remedies. Interactions may cause alterations in absorption, distribution, or metabolism. For example, aloe and rhubarb have been found to bind with digoxin and warfarin, reducing their effectiveness by limiting their absorption. In these cases, the drug should be taken at least 1 hour before the herb.

From Tsai HH, Lin HW, Pickard AS et al: Evaluation of documented drug interactions and contraindications associated with herbs and dietary supplements: a systematic literature review, *Int J Clin Pract* 66:1056–1078, 2012.

(see Chapter 9) (Kuhn, 2002). In a study of 58 women 65 years and older, nearly 75% of them were taking herbs, prescription drugs, and/or OTC drugs that could interact at a moderate- or high-risk level (Yoon and Schaffer, 2006). Of the total interactions, 63% involved NSAIDs. The authors found this worrisome because older adults are at risk for bleeding even when NSAIDs are taken properly.

Herbs that are more likely to cause a distribution-type interaction may increase the possibility of adverse effects. Metabolism-type interactions may increase or decrease the effectiveness of a medication, depending on the herb and the medication. For example, garlic and St. John's wort (SJW) have significant interactions with conventional drugs and may decrease the drug's concentration by inducing cytochrome P450s (CYPs) and P-glycoprotein, the major drug transporter and lead to adverse reactions (Izzo and Ernst, 2009; Zhou and Lai, 2008). This may be an issue in as many as 50% of drugs (NMCD, 2014). Examples of drug interactions with the herbs and supplements discussed in this section can be found Chapter 9.

The content of active herb(s) in products by different manufacturers varies considerably; therefore the therapeutic outcome and potential for herb-drug interactions vary as well.

◆ PROMOTING HEALTHY AGING: IMPLICATIONS FOR GERONTOLOGICAL NURSING

The gerontological nurse can promote healthy aging in several ways among persons who use or are considering the use of herbs and other supplements.

This begins with creating a safe and nonjudgmental relationship wherein the person feels comfortable describing his or her use and understanding of these products. Any verbal or nonverbal action from the provider that may block this openness may lead to a potentially dangerous lack of assessment data.

Once this conversation has begun, both the nurse and the elder can begin to evaluate the existing knowledge regarding safe use of the herb or supplement. This includes not only the name of the herb/supplement but also the understanding of its potential side effects and interactions. It is helpful to know what the person hopes to accomplish by using the herb/supplement. Reinforcing the positive effects and reviewing the cost of using the product may assist relaxation of the patient and open additional lines of communication. The conversation is a useful venue for teaching about the safe use of herbs and supplements.

◆ Perioperative Assessment

Including herbs and supplements in the perioperative or emergency surgery assessment is of vital importance. The reader is advised to see the article by Messina (2006) for risks associated with the use of 10 herbs by the patient who is scheduled for surgery. As discussed, hypertension, excessive and prolonged bleeding, and the increased chance for interactions between the herb and other drugs are discussed. Herbs that can affect bleeding and clotting time, such as garlic, ginger, ginkgo, and ginseng, should be especially noted and reported to the surgical team. Many older adults are electing aesthetic surgery today, and these patients must also be assessed carefully preoperatively as well (Rowe and Baker, 2009). Several select herbs and their perioperative effects are listed in Table 10-1. The American Society of Anesthesiologists suggests all herbal products be stopped 2 to 3 weeks before surgery (Kaye et al, 2004). This should be done

TABLE 10-1   Select Herbs and the Perioperative Patient

HERB	PERIOPERATIVE ISSUE	PREOPERATIVE DISCONTINUATION
Chamomile	Potential for increased sedation with anesthetics	No time advised in data; advise discussing with surgeon or anesthesiologist
Chondroitin	Potential for increased bleeding	No time advised in data; discuss with surgeon or anesthesiologist
Echinacea	Allergic reactions; decreased effectiveness of immunosuppressants	No time advised in data; discuss with surgeon or anesthesiologist
Garlic	Potential for increased bleeding; modest hypotensive effect; metabolic drug interactions	1 to 2 weeks before surgery
Ginkgo	Potential for increased bleeding	2 weeks before surgery
Ginseng	Hypoglycemia; potential for increased bleeding	1 to 2 weeks before surgery
Glucosamine	Potential for increased bleeding	No time advised in data; discuss with surgeon or anesthesiologist
Melatonin	Potential for increased sedation with anesthetics	No time advised in data; discuss with surgeon or anesthesiologist
St. John's wort	Potential for increased sedation with anesthetics	5 days before surgery*
Saw palmetto	Potential for increased bleeding	No time advised in data; discuss with surgeon or anesthesiologist

*Clients taking St. John's wort for depression must be advised to slowly taper discontinuation of the herb and to discuss with a physician when to stop taking the herb before surgery. A washout period of 3 weeks may be needed.

Data from Natural Medicines Comprehensive Database: www.naturaldatabase.com Accessed April 2014.

with provider monitoring if the herb's discontinuation may potentially cause a serious problem.

◆ Interventions

If an herb or supplement is being used in an inappropriate manner, the goal is to discontinue use or to use only the advised dosage for a specific condition. This can be done by providing needed information and asking the individual to consider the correct use of the product. The LEARN Model discussed in Chapter 4 may be particularly helpful in achieving this goal. The person may be willing to show the specific herb or supplement to the health care professional and discuss safer and better ways to use it.

If it is unclear whether the herb is beneficial or harmful, it is the health care professional's responsibility to determine this information and inform the patient. The health care professional may also observe the placebo effect with persons who are taking herbs and supplements. That is, the taking of the product, and not the action of the herb or supplement itself, may produce a positive effect on the person. In this instance, if the herb or supplement causes no harm, it may be continued. However, the safe or unsafe of a certain herb or supplement in a particular person is often difficult to determine and a placebo effect impossible to measure.

If the health care provider is not familiar with a product and its characteristics, then there are several sources of needed information. Most health care settings today have accessible computers and may have databases that can be searched. These may be in an examination room or on a tablet computer carried by the nurse at the bedside. Other times the person has already "done the search" and comes with questions. Pharmacists are an additional resource for nurses when working with patients who are taking herbs and supplements.

Important interventions of the gerontological nurse in the promotion of healthy aging include providing education; checking for side effects, adverse reactions, and interactions among herbs, supplements, medications, foods, and the illness; and negotiating a discontinuance of possibly harmful products. In instances in which an adverse reaction or harmful interaction is suspected, the person must be urged to stop taking the herb or supplement and to see his or her prescribing health care provider or seek emergency care, if indicated. Educating patients about potential side effects and interactions in realistic and understandable ways may be the most useful intervention.

◆ Education

Scientific data and information about the safe use of herbs must be provided in the context of the person's age and particular learning needs. Follow-up care is essential. The word "natural" printed on the label does not mean that it is healthy for every person, or even that the product is indeed natural. The provider must seek out the best client motivation factors for the use of herbs or supplements to provide significant help.

Several additional issues need to be addressed with persons who are taking herbs and supplements:

- Elders should be helped to understand the importance of reporting the use of all herbs and supplements to their health care provider before beginning an herb or supplement for the first time.
- Regarding product safety: (1) There is no universal standardization among manufacturers, so the amount of active ingredient per dose among brands may be inconsistent; (2) herbs and supplements should be purchased from reputable sources; (3) herbs are available in different forms, making accurate dosing difficult; (4) research on both the potential adverse and the beneficial effects of most herbs and supplements is inadequate, making recommendations about specific products difficult; and (5) persons who have allergies to certain plants may have allergies to herbs in the same plant family.
- If side effects occur within 1 or 2 hours of taking the supplement, it should be discontinued immediately. If the side effects continue or worsen, the person should report them to the health care provider or go to the nearest emergency department. Because older adults may react differently to supplements, health care providers may need to prescribe less than the recommended dose. Herbs and supplements taken with other such products may cause unpredictable effects.
- Many adults take herbs and supplements along with prescribed and OTC medications. Thus the approach with the person must be open and encouraging for effective assessment, evaluation of risks, appropriate teaching-learning applications, intervention, and monitoring. The gerontological nurse must be knowledgeable and continue to determine the latest information about herbs, supplements, OTC medications, prescribed medications, and interactions.
- Lastly, the nurse has a responsibility for maintaining a sound knowledge base, as well as having readily available sources of changing current data, regarding the treatments used by the patient, including both those prescribed and those used in self-care. At the same time, making recommendations for or against the use of herbs and supplements may be considered a form of "prescribing" in some states and settings, such as long-term and acute care. The nurse is cautioned to be aware of both state nurse practice regulations and organizational policies (Moquin et al, 2009).

▮ KEY CONCEPTS

- Many individuals continue their prescribed medications and therapies in addition to other complementary and alternative therapies including herbs and supplements.

- The renewed interest in herbal therapies is based in part on the focus on disease prevention. Herbs are often used by individuals who want to be more involved in their own health care, who are unable to afford prescription medications, or who are following long practiced traditions.

- The U.S. government has no standards in place to control the quality of herbs or herbal products or other supplements.
- Nurses and other health care providers should always ask about the use of herbs and supplements when conducting a health interview.
- Nurses and other health care providers should provide an open, nonjudgmental environment to foster disclosure of

the use of herbs, supplements, and medications, both prescribed and OTC.
- Patients should be told to discontinue herbal treatments for the prescribed period of time before scheduled surgery or certain procedures (e.g., colonoscopy); in addition, patients should receive an explanation of why it is important to discontinue these herbal preparations or treatments.

NURSE STUDY: COMMON USE OF HERBS AND SUPPLEMENTS

Anna is an 80-year-old woman of French descent who lives with her 83-year-old husband in the suburbs of a large city. They have been married for 57 years and have two grown children, six grandchildren, and five great-grandchildren. Anna is very proud of all of them. Anna taught high school English for 20 years but was raised with many of the "old country" traditions, speaking French for most of her formative years. As part of her background, she would rather use herbs and "home treatments" than prescribed "pills." She has been diagnosed with hypertension, diabetes mellitus, and arthritis. She often complains of symptoms that are related to these chronic conditions, but she refuses to consistently follow her diet or take any prescribed medications. Anna attends mass daily and, with her husband, takes part in community activities. While accompanying her husband on a visit to his health care provider, she mentions the use of herbal supplements. After some discussion, the nurse practitioner realizes that

Anna has little information about herbal supplements and has some incorrect assumptions about them.

- From these data, identify key aspects of education specific for Anna.
- Plan and state one or more interventions for each identified problem. Provide specific documentation of the source used to determine the appropriate intervention.
- Plan at least one intervention that incorporates Anna's existing strengths.
- Evaluate the success of the intervention. Interventions must correlate directly with the stated outcome criteria to measure the outcome success.
- How would you begin your discussion with Anna regarding her knowledge of herbal supplements? What information would you be especially interested in obtaining regarding herbal supplements and each of Anna's medical diagnoses? How would you prepare Anna should she need surgery?

CRITICAL THINKING QUESTIONS AND ACTIVITIES

1. Interview a member of your health care community who recommends the use of herbs and/or supplements along with traditional strategies.
2. Tour a local health food store. Read the labels of the more commonly used herbal supplements. Do the labels list the

information you expected? How would you make sure that your clients have the necessary information?
3. Visit a senior citizen center. Talk with members about their use of herbal supplements. Keep track of the more commonly used herbs and the reasons for their use.

RESEARCH QUESTIONS

1. How do elders decide which herbs or supplements to use?
2. How does one ensure standardization among products?
3. How did the older adults find out about which herb or supplement to take?
4. Are older adults aware of possible negative effects of herbs and supplements?
5. What questions do older adults ask before taking an herbal or nonherbal supplement?

6. What are the rewards (positive factors) versus the costs (negative factors) of using herbal and other supplements?
7. What strategies can health care providers use to bridge the gap between herb/supplement remedies and potential prescribed medications?

REFERENCES

Agbabiaka TB, Pittler MH, Wider B, et al: Serenoa repens (saw palmetto): a systematic review of adverse events, *Drug Saf* 32:637–647, 2009.

Amico AP, Terlizzi A, Damiani S, et al: Immunopharmacology of the main herbal supplements: a review, *Endocr Metab Immune Disord Drug Targets* 13:283–288, 2013.

Amsterdam JD, Li Y, Soeller I, et al: A randomized, double-blind, placebo-controlled trial of oral *Matricaria recutita* (chamomile) extract therapy for

generalized anxiety disorder, *J Clin Psychopharmacol* 29:378–382, 2009.

Askeroglu U, Alleyne B, Guyuron B: Pharmaceutical and herbal products that may contribute to dry eyes, *Plast Reconstr Surg* 131:159–167, 2013.

Avins AL, Bent S, Staccone S, et al: A detailed safety assessment of a saw palmetto extract, *Complement Ther Med* 16:147–154, 2008.

Baker WL, Gutierrez-Williams G, White CM, et al: Effect of cinnamon on glucose control and lipid parameters, *Diabetes Care* 31:41–43, 2008.

Barnes PM, Bloom B, Nahin R: Complementary and alternative medicine use among adults and children: United States, 2007, *Natl Health Stat Rep* 12:1–23, 2008.

Barry MJ, Meleth S, Lee JY, et al: Effect of increasing doses of saw palmetto extract on lower urinary tract symptoms, *JAMA* 306:1344–1351, 2011.

Basch E, Ulbricht C: *Natural standard herb & supplement handbook*: the clinical bottom line, St. Louis, MO, 2005, Mosby.

Birks J, Grimley Evans J: *Ginkgo biloba* for cognitive impairment and dementia, *Cochrane Database Syst Rev* 1:CD003120, 2009.

Blumenthal M, Goldberg A, Brinckmann J: *Herbal medicine*: expanded Commission E monographs, Newton, MA, 2000, Integrative Medicine Communications.

Boehm K, Borrelli F, Ernst E, et al: Green tea (*Camellia sinensis*) for the prevention of cancer, *Cochrane Database Syst Rev* 3:CD005004, 2009.

Brattström A: Long-term effects of St. John's wort (*Hypericum perforatum*) treatment: a 1-year safety study in mild to moderate depression, *Phytomedicine* 16:277–283, 2009.

Brien S, Prescott P, Lewith G: Meta-analysis of the related nutritional supplements dimethyl sulfoxide and methylsulfonylmethane in the treatment of osteoarthritis of the knee, *Evid Based Complement Alternat Med* 2011:528403, 2011.

Bruno JJ, Ellis JJ: Herbal use among U.S. elderly: 2002. National Health Interview Survey, *Ann Pharmacother* 39:643–648, 2005.

Bruyere O, Reginster JY: Glucosamine and chondroitin sulfate as the therapeutic agents for knee and hip osteoarthritis, *Drugs Aging* 24:573–580, 2007.

Burks K: Osteoarthritis in older adults: current treatments, *J Gerontol Nurs* 31:11–19, 2005.

Canter PH, Ernst E: *Ginkgo biloba* is not a smart drug: an updated systematic review of randomised clinical trials testing the nootropic effects of *G. biloba* extracts in healthy people, *Hum Psychopharmacol* 22:265–278, 2007.

Chen X, Lu W, Zheng Y, et al: Exercise, tea consumption, and depression among breast cancer survivors, *J Clin Oncol* 28:991–998, 2010.

Cheung CK, Wyman JF, Halcon LL: Use of complementary and alternative therapies in community-dwelling older adults, *J Altern Complement Med* 13:997–1006, 2007.

Chu KO, Chan KP, Wang CC, et al: Green tea catechins and their oxidative protection in the rat eye, *J Agric Food Chem* 58:1523–1534, 2010.

Clegg DO, Reda DJ, Harris CL, et al: Glucosamine, chondroitin sulfate, and the two in combination for painful knee osteoarthritis, *N Engl J Med* 354:795–808, 2006.

Daniele C, Mazzanti G, Pittler MH, et al: Adverse-event profile of *Crataegus* spp.: a systematic review, *Drug Saf* 29:523–535, 2006.

Debbi EM, Agar G, Fichman G, et al: Efficacy of methylsulfonylmethane supplementation on osteoarthritis of the knee: a randomized controlled study, *BMC Complement Altern Med* 11:50, 2011.

Deka A, Vita JA: Tea and cardiovascular disease, *Pharmacol Res* 64:136–145, 2011.

Devaraj S, Yimam M, Brownell MS, et al: Effects of aloe vera supplementation in subjects with prediabetes/metabolic syndrome, *Metab Syndr Relat Disord* 11:35–40, 2013.

Durante KM, Whitmore B, Jones CA, et al: Use of vitamins, minerals and herbs: a survey of patients attending family practice clinics, *Clin Invest Med* 24:242–249, 2001.

Edwards Q, Colquist S, Maradiegue A: What's cooking with garlic: is this complementary and alternative medicine for hypertension? *J Am Acad Nurse Pract* 17:381–385, 2005.

Eggeling T, Regitz-Zagrosek V, Zimmermann A, et al: Baseline severity but not gender modulates quantified *Crataegus* extract effects in early heart failure—a pooled analysis of clinical trials, *Phytomedicine* 18:1214–1219, 2011.

Eller LS, Corless I, Bunch EH, et al: Self-care strategies for depressive symptoms in people with HIV disease, *J Adv Nurs* 51:119–130, 2005.

Ernst E: The risk-benefit profile of commonly used herbal therapies: ginkgo, St. John's wort, ginseng, echinacea, saw palmetto, and kava, *Ann Intern Med* 136:42–53, 2002.

Ferracioli-Oda E, Qawasmi A, Bloch MH: Meta-analysis: melatonin for the treatment of primary sleep disorders, *PLoS One* 8:e63773, 2013.

Finnegan-John J, Molassiotis A, Richardson A, et al: A systematic review of complementary and alternative medicine interventions for the management of cancer-related fatigue, *Integr Cancer Ther* 12:276–290, 2013.

Gorski JC, Huang SM, Pinto A, et al: The effect of echinacea (*Echinacea purpurea* root) on cytochrome P450 activity in vivo, *Clin Pharmacol Ther* 75:89–100, 2004.

Hong B, Ji YH, Hong JH, et al: A double-blind crossover study evaluating the efficacy of Korean red ginseng in patients with erectile dysfunction: a preliminary report, *J Urol* 168:2070–2073, 2002.

Huxley R, Lee CM, Barzi F, et al: Decaffeinated coffee and tea consumption in relation to incident type 2 diabetes mellitus: a systematic review with meta-analysis, *Arch Intern Med* 169:2053–2063, 2009.

Inoue M, Sasazuki S, Wakai K, et al: Green tea consumption and gastric cancer in Japanese: a pooled analysis of six cohort studies, *Gut* 58:1323–1332, 2009.

Islami F, Pourshams A, Nasrollahzadeh D, et al: Tea drinking habits and oesophageal cancer in a high risk area in northern Iran: population based case–control study, *BMJ* 338:b929, 2009.

Israel D, Youngkin E: Herbal therapies for common health problems. In Youngkin E, Sawin KJ, Kissinger JF, et al, editors: *Pharmacotherapeutics: a primary care guide*, ed 2, Upper Saddle River, NJ, 2005, Pearson Prentice Hall.

Jalili J, Askeroglu U, Alleyne B, et al: Herbal products that may contribute to hypertension, *Plast Reconstr Surg* 131:168–173, 2013.

Jiang W, Qiu W, Wang Y, et al: Ginkgo may prevent genetic-associated ovarian cancer risk: multiple biomarkers and anticancer pathways induced by ginkgolide B in BRCA1-mutant ovarian epithelial cells, *Eur J Cancer Prev* 20:508–517, 2011.

Jurikova T, Sochor J, Rop O, et al: Polyphenolic profile and biological activity of Chinese hawthorn (*Crataegus pinnatifida* BUNGE) fruits, *Molecules* 6:14490–14509, 2012.

Kales HC, Blow FC, Welsh DE, et al: Herbal products and other supplements: use by elderly veterans with depression and dementia and their caregivers, *J Geriatr Psychiatry Neurol* 17:25–31, 2004.

Kantor ED, Lampe JW, Vaughan TL, et al: Association between use of specialty dietary supplements and C-reactive protein concentrations, *Am J Epidemiol* 176:1002–1013, 2012.

Kasuli EG: Are alternative supplements effective treatment for diabetes mellitus? *Nutr Clin Pract* 26:352–355, 2011.

Karsch-Völk M, Barrett B, Kiefer D, et al: Echinacea for preventing and treating the common cold, *Cochrane Database Syst Rev* 2:CD000530, 2014.

Kaye AD, Kucera I, Sabar R: Perioperative anesthesia clinical considerations of alternative medicines, *Anesthesiol Clin North America* 22:125–139, 2004.

Khalsa KP: Preparing botanical medicines, *J Herb Pharmacother* 7:267–277, 2007.

Kim LS, Axelrod LJ, Howard P, et al: Efficacy of methylsulfonylmethane (MSM) in osteoarthritis pain of the knee: a pilot clinical trial, *Osteoarthritis Cartilage* 14:286–294, 2006.

Kim TH, Lim HJ, Kim MS, et al: Dietary supplements for benign prostatic hyperplasia: an overview of systematic reviews, *Maturitas* 73:180–185, 2012.

Kirkham S, Akilen R, Sharma S, et al: The potential of cinnamon to reduce blood glucose levels in patients with type 2 diabetes and insulin resistance, *Diabetes Obes Metab* 11:1100–1113, 2009.

Krystal AD, Benca RM, Kilduff TS: Understanding the sleep-wake cycle: sleep, insomnia, and the orexin system, *J Clin Psychiatry* 74(Suppl 1):3–20, 2013.

Kuhn M: Herbal remedies: drug-herb interactions, *Crit Care Nurse* 22:22–28, 2002.

Ladenheim D, Horn O, Werneke U, et al: Potential health risks of complementary alternative medicines in HIV patients, *HIV Med* 9:653–659, 2008.

Lam A, Bradley G: Use of self-prescribed nonprescription medications and dietary supplements among assisted living facility residents, *J Am Pharm Assoc* 46:547–581, 2006.

Lawvere S, Mahoney MC: St. John's wort, *Am Fam Physician* 72:2249–2254, 2005.

Leach MJ, Kumar S: Cinnamon for diabetes mellitus, *Cochrane Database Syst Rev* 9:CD007170, 2012.

Lee SH, Ahn YM, Ahn SY, et al: Interaction between warfarin and *Panax ginseng* in ischemic stroke patients, *J Altern Complement Med* 14:715–721, 2008.

Lee T, Dugoua J-J: Nutritional supplements and their effect on glucose control, *Curr Diab Rep* 11:142–148, 2011.

Lemoine P, Zisapel N: Prolonged-release formulation of melatonin (Circadin) for the treatment of insomnia, *Expert Opin Pharmacother* 13:895–905, 2012.

Li GQ, Kam A, Wong KH, et al: Herbal medicines for the management of diabetes, *Adv Exp Med Biol* 771:396–413, 2012.

Linde K, Berner MM, Kriston L: St. John's wort for major depression, *Cochrane Database Syst Rev* 4:CD000448, 2008.

Liu JP, Yang M, Liu Y, Wei ML, Grimsgaard S: Herbal Medicines for treatment of irritable bowel syndrome (Review), *Cochrane Database of Systematic* 25:CD004116, 2006.

Loya AM, González-Stuart A, Rivera JO: Prevalence of polypharmacy, polyherbacy, nutritional supplement use and potential interactions among older adults living on the United States–Mexico border: a descriptive, questionnaire-based study, *Drugs Aging* 26:423–436, 2009.

MacDonald R, Tacklind JW, Rutks I, et al: *Serenoa repens* monotherapy for benign prostatic hyperplasia (BPH): an updated Cochrane systematic review, *BJU Int* 109:1756–1761, 2012.

Marcus MB: *Coffee's endless health debate is grounded in fact.* USA Today, June 14, 2010. http://www.usatoday.com/news/health/2010-06-14-coffee14_ST_N.htm. Accessed December 2010.

Marcus MB: Exercise, tea and vitamin D to ward off dementia, USA Today, July 11, 2010. http://www.usatoday.com/news/health/2010-07-12-alzheimerslifestyle12_ST_N.htm. Accessed December 2010.

Messina BA: Herbal supplements: facts and myths—talking to your patients about herbal supplements, *J Perianesth Nurs* 21:268–278, 2006.

Moquin B, Blackman MR, Mitty E, et al: Complementary and alternative medicine (CAM), *Geriatr Nurs* 30:196–203, 2009.

Nahin RL, Barnes PM, Stussman BA, et al: Costs of complementary and alternative medicine (CAM) and frequency of visits to CAM practitioners: United States, 2007, *Natl Health Stat Rep* 18:1–14, 2009.

Nakasone Y, Watabe K, Vatanabe K, et al: Effect of a glucosamine-based combination supplement containing chondroitin sulfate and antioxidant micronutrients in subjects with symptomatic knee osteoarthritis: a pilot study, *Exp Ther Med* 2:893–899, 2011.

National Center for Complementary and Integrative Health (NCCIH): *A review of St. John's wort extracts for major depression*, 2008. https://nccih.nih.gov/research/results/spotlight/120908.htm. Accessed April 2014.

NCCIH: *Ginkgo biloba does not slow cognitive decline in large cohort study of older adults*, 2009. https://nccih.nih.gov/research/results/spotlight/20091229.htm. Accessed April 2014.

NCCIH: *Asian ginseng*, 2012. https://nccih.nih.gov/health/asianginseng/ataglance.htm. Accessed April 2014.

NCCIH: *Hawthorn*, 2012. https://nccih.nih.gov/health/hawthorn. Accessed April 2014.

NCCIH: *St. John's wort*, 2015. https://nccih.nih.gov/health/stjohnswort. Accessed April 2014.

NCCIH: *Red yeast rice: an introduction*, 2013. https://nccih.nih.gov/health/redyeastrice. Accessed April 2014.

Natural Medicines Comprehensive Database (NMCD): *Drug-supplement interactions*, 2014. http://naturaldatabase.therapeuticresearch.com/ce/ceCourse.aspx?s=ND&cs=CP&pc=07-34&cec=1&pm=5. Accessed October 31, 2014.

Natural Standard: *Alzheimer's disease*, 2013. http://www.naturalstandard.com/. Accessed April 2014.

Natural Standard: *Cancer*, 2013. http://www.naturalstandard.com/. Accessed April 2014.

Natural Standard: *Chamomile (Matricaria recutita, Chamaemelum nobile)*, 2013. http://www.naturalstandard.com/. Accessed April 2014.

Natural Standard: *Diabetes*, 2013. http://www.naturalstandard.com/. Accessed April 2014.

Natural Standard: *Echinacea (Echinacea angustifolia, Echnicacea pallida, Echnicaea purpura)*, 2013. http://www.naturalstandard.com/. Accessed April 2014.

Natural Standard: *Garlic (Allium sativum)*, 2013. http://www.naturalstandard.com/. Accessed April 2014.

Natural Standard: *Gastrointestinal disorders*, 2013. http://www.naturalstandard.com/. Accessed April 2014.

Natural Standard: *Ginkgo (Ginkgo biloba)*, 2013. http://www.naturalstandard.com/. Accessed April 2014.

Natural Standard: *Ginseng (American ginseng, Asian ginseng, Chinese ginseng, Korean red ginseng, Panax ginseng: Panax spp., including P. ginseng and P. quinquefolius, excluding Eleutherococcus senticosus)*, 2013. http://www.naturalstandard.com/. Accessed April 2014.

Natural Standard: *Glucosamine*, 2013. http://www.naturalstandard.com/. Accessed April 2014.

Natural Standard: *Hawthorn (Crataegus spp.)*, 2013. http://www.naturalstandard.com/. Accessed April 2014.

Natural Standard: *HIV/AIDS*, 2013. http://www.naturalstandard.com/. Accessed April 2014.

Natural Standard: *High blood pressure*, 2013. http://www.naturalstandard.com. Accessed April 2014.

Natural Standard: *Melatonin (N-acetyl-5-methoxytryptamine)*, 2013n. http://www.naturalstandard.com. Accessed April 2014.

Natural Standard: *News: Echinacea for the common cold*, 2013. http://www.naturalstandard.com. Accessed April 2014.

Natural Standard: *News: Glucosamine may not slow osteoarthritis progression*, 2013. http://www.naturalstandard.com/. Accessed April 2014.

Natural Standard: *News: Prescription chondroitin for knee arthritis*, 2013.

http://www.naturalstandard.com/. Accessed April 2014.

Natural Standard: *Red yeast rice (Monascus purpureus)*, 2013. http://www.natural standard.com/. Accessed April 2014.

Natural Standard: *Saw palmetto (Serenoa repens, Serenoa serrulata)*, 2013. http://www.naturalstandard.com/. Accessed April 2014.

Natural Standard: *St. John's wort (Hypericum perforatum)*, 2013. http://www.natural standard.com/. Accessed April 2014.

Nieva R, Safavynia SA, Lee BK, et al: Herbal, vitamin, and supplement use in patients enrolled in a cardiac rehabilitation program, *J Cardiopulm Rehabil Prev* 32:270–277, 2012.

Niu K, Hozawa A, Kuriyama S, et al: Green tea consumption associated with depressive symptoms in the elderly, *Am J Clin Nutr* 90:1615–1622, 2009.

Oba S, Nagata C, Nakamura K, et al: Consumption of coffee, green tea, oolong tea, black tea, chocolate snacks and the caffeine content in relation to risk of diabetes in Japanese men and women, *Br J Nutr* 103:453–459, 2010.

Pham AQ, Kourlas H, Pham DQ: Cinnamon supplementation in patients with type 2 diabetes mellitus, *Pharmacotherapy* 27: 595–599, 2007.

Pittler MH, Guo R, Ernst E: Hawthorn extract for treating chronic heart failure, *Cochrane Database Syst Rev* 1:CD005312, 2008.

Radimer K, Bindewald B, Hughes J, et al: Dietary supplement use by U.S. adults: data from the National Health and Nutrition Examination Survey, 1999. 2000, *Am J Epidemiol* 160:339–349, 2004.

Ramar K, Olson EJ: Management of common sleep disorders, *Am Fam Physician* 88:231–238, 2013.

Ravindran AV, Lam RW, Filteau, MJ, et al: Canadian Network for Mood and Anxiety Treatments (CANMAT) clinical guidelines for the management of major depressive disorder in adults. V. Complementary and alternative medicine treatments, *J Affect Disord* 117(Suppl 1):S54–S64, 2009.

Reinhart KM, Coleman CI, Teevan C, et al: Effects of garlic on blood pressure in patients with and without systolic hypertension: a meta-analysis, *Ann Pharmacother* 42:1766–1771, 2008.

Ried K, Frank OR, Stocks NP, Fakler P, Sullivan T: Effect of garlic on blood pressure: a systematic review and meta-analysis, *BMC Cardiovasc Disord* 8:13, 2008.

Ried K, Frank OR, Stocks NP: Aged garlic extract reduces blood pressure in hypertensives: a dose-response trial, *Eur J Clin Nutr* 67:64–70, 2013.

Ried K, Toben C, Fakler P: Effect of garlic on serum lipids: an updated meta-analysis, *Nutr Rev* 71:282–299, 2013.

Rouanet JM, Decorde K, Del Rio D, et al: Berry juices, tea, antioxidants and the prevention of atherosclerosis in hamsters, *Food Chem* 118:266–271, 2009.

Rowe DJ, Baker AC: Perioperative risks and benefits of herbal supplements in aesthetic surgery, *Aesthet Surg J* 29:150–157, 2009.

Rudkowska I: Lipid lowering with dietary supplements: focus on diabetes, *Maturitas* 72:113–116, 2012.

Ryder PT, Wolpert B, Orwig D, et al: Complementary and alternative medicine use among older urban African Americans: individual and neighborhood associations, *J Natl Med Assoc* 100:1186–1192, 2008.

Sawitzke AD, Shi H, Finco MF, et al: Clinical efficacy and safety of glucosamine, chondroitin sulphate, their combination, celecoxib or placebo taken to treat osteoarthritis of the knee: 2-year results from GAIT, *Ann Rheumatol Dis* 69:1459–1464, 2010.

Shah, SA, Sander S, White CM, et al: Evaluation of echinacea for the prevention and treatment of the common cold: a meta-analysis, *Lancet Infect Dis* 7:473–480, 2007.

Shelton RC: St. John's wort *(Hypericum perforatum)* in major depression, *J Clin Psychiatry* 70(Suppl 5):23–27, 2009.

Shrubsole MJ, Lu W, Chen Z, et al: Drinking green tea modestly reduces breast cancer risk, *J Nutr* 139:310–316, 2009.

Simons S, Wollersheim H, Thien T: A systematic review on the influence of trial quality on the effect of garlic on blood pressure, *Neth J Med* 67:212–219, 2009.

Singh DK, Banerjee S, Porter TD: Green and black tea extracts inhibit HMG-CoA reductase and activate AMP kinase to decrease cholesterol synthesis in hepatoma cells, *J Nutr Biochem* 20: 816–822, 2009.

Srivastava JK, Pandey M, Gupta S: Chamomile, a novel and selective COX-2 inhibitor with anti-inflammatory activity, *Life Sci* 85: 663–669, 2009.

Stabler SN, Tejani AM, Huyng F, et al: Garlic for the prevention of cardiovascular morbidity and mortality in hypertensive patients, *Cochrane Database Syst Rev* 8:CD007653, 2012.

Sugimoto N, Ichikawa M, Siriliang B, et al: Herbal medicine use and quality of life among people living with HIV/AIDS in northeastern Thailand, *AIDS Care* 17: 252–262, 2005.

Swanson B: Beware bitter orange, *ADVANCE for Nurses* 43, September 4, 134–137, 2007.

Tachjian A, Maria V, Jahangir A: Use of herbal products and potential interactions in patients with cardiovascular diseases, *J Am Coll Cardiol* 55:515–525, 2010.

Tacklind J, MacDonald R, Rutks I, et al: Serenoa repens for benign prostatic hyperplasia, *Cochrane Database Syst Rev* 2:CD001423, 2009.

Tait EM, Laditka SB, Laditka JN, et al: Use of complementary and alternative medicine for physical performance, energy, immune function, and general health among older women and men in the United States, *J Women Aging* 24:23–43, 2012.

Tang N, Wu Y, Zhou B, et al: Green tea, black tea consumption and risk of lung cancer: a meta-analysis, *Lung Cancer* 65:274–283, 2009.

Tillett, J, Ames, D: The uses of aromatherapy in women's health, *J Perinat Neonatal Nurs* 24:238–245, 2010.

Tillisch K: Complementary and alternative medicine for functional gastrointestinal disorders, *Gut* 55:593–596, 2006.

Tsai HH, Lin HW, Pickard AS, et al: Evaluation of documented drug interactions and contraindications associated with herbs and dietary supplements: a systematic literature review, *Int J Clin Pract* 66:1056–1078, 2012.

Tshibangu K, Worku ZB, de Jongh MA, et al: Assessment of effectiveness of traditional herbal medicine in managing HIV/AIDS patients in South Africa, *East Afr Med J* 81:499–504, 2004.

U.S. Food and Drug Administration: *FDA warns consumers to avoid red yeast rice products promoted on Internet as treatments for high cholesterol; products found to contain unauthorized drug* (Press release), Aug 9, 2007. http://www.fda.gov/NewsEvents/Newsroom/Press Announcements/2007/ucm108962.htm. Accessed May 31, 2014.

U.S. Food and Drug Administration: *Dietary supplements*, 2014. http://www.fda.gov/Food/Dietarysupplements/default.htm. Accessed May 31, 2014.

van der Watt G, Laugharne J, Janca A: Complementary and alternative medicine in the treatment of anxiety and depression, *Curr Opin Psychiatry* 21:37–42, 2008.

Waddell DL, Hummell ME, Sumners AD: Three herbs you should get to know, *Am J Nurse* 101:48–54, 2001.

Walker AF, Marakis G, Simpson E, et al: Hypotensive effects of hawthorn for patients with diabetes taking prescription drugs: a randomized controlled trial, *Br J Gen Pract* 56:437–443, 2006.

Walubo A: The role of cytochrome P450 in antiretroviral drug interactions, *Expert Opin Drug Metab Toxicol* 3:583–598, 2007.

Wang ZM, Zhou B, Wang YS, et al: Black and green tea consumption and the risk of coronary artery disease: a meta-analysis, *Am J Clin Nutr* 93:506–515, 2011.

Wilhelmsen-Langeland A, Saxvig IW, Pallesen S, et al: A randomized controlled trial with bright light and melatonin for the treatment of delayed sleep phase disorder: effects on subjective and objective sleepiness and cognitive function, *J Biol Rhythms* 28:306–321, 2013.

Williams P, Piamjariyakul U, Ducey K, et al: Cancer treatment, symptom monitoring, and self-care in adults: pilot study, *Cancer Nurs* 29:347–355, 2006.

Wold RS, Lopez ST, Yau CL, et al: Increasing trends in elderly persons' use of nonvitamin, nonmineral dietary supplements and concurrent use of medications, *J Am Diet Assoc* 105:54–63, 2005.

Yoon SL: Racial/ethnic differences in self-reported health problems and herbal use among older women, *J Natl Med Assoc* 98:918–925, 2006.

Yoon SL, Horne CH: Herbal products and conventional medicines used by community-residing older women, *J Adv Nurs* 33:51–59, 2001.

Yoon SL, Horne CH, Adams C: Herbal product use by African American older women, *Clin Nurs Res* 13:271–288, 2004.

Yoon SL, Schaffer SD: Herbal, prescribed, and over-the-counter drug use in older women: prevalence of drug interactions, *Geriatr Nurs* 27:118–129, 2006.

Youngkin EQ, Israel DS: A review and critique of common herbal alternative therapies, *Nurse Pract* 21:39, 43–46, 49–52, 1996.

11 CHAPTER

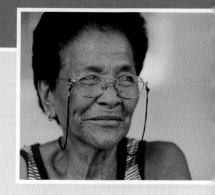

Vision

Theris A. Touhy

http://evolve.elsevier.com/Touhy/TwdHlthAging

A STUDENT SPEAKS

I kind of understand the problems vision impairment can cause as one ages. I am pretty blind without my glasses. I can't even see the alarm clock numbers. I worry about what my vision will be when I am older. I took care of a woman in the assisted living facility with macular degeneration. I asked her how the disease affects her vision. The woman put her hand in front of my face and said, "I can see your hair, the color, and some of the space around you, but I cannot see your face or the color of your skin." She seems to cope pretty well and uses low vision devices to help her manage her life. It frightened me a little but also gave me hope that even with this kind of vision loss, she is able to function and stay in pretty good spirits. I am going to get some information about how to keep my eyes healthy. I hadn't thought about the things I could do now that might help as I age.

Debbie, age 27

AN ELDER SPEAKS

One of the great frustrations is the matter of eyesight. One can get used to large print and hope for black letters on white paper, but why do modern publishers seem to prefer the shiny, slick off-white paper and pale ink in minuscule print? Thank goodness for restaurants with lighted menus and my new iPhone with a bright light. And my new prescription glasses have not restored my ability to cut my own toenails without danger of wounding myself.

Lyn, age 85

LEARNING OBJECTIVES

On completion of this chapter, the reader will be able to:

1. Identify age-related changes in the eye that affect vision and discuss recommendations to promote eye health throughout life.
2. Discuss diseases of the eye that may occur in older adults.
3. Describe the importance of screening, health education, and treatment of eye diseases to prevent unnecessary vision loss.
4. Identify effective communication strategies for older adults with vision impairments.
5. Gain awareness of assistive devices to enhance vision.

CHANGES IN VISION WITH AGE

Changes in eye structure begin early, are progressive in nature, and are both functional and structural. The structures most affected are the cornea, anterior chamber, lens, ciliary muscles, and retina. All of the age-related changes affect visual acuity and accommodation. Although presbyopia (decreased near vision as a result of aging) is first seen between 45 and 55 years of age, 80% of those older than 65 years have fair to adequate far vision past 90 years of age. Nearly 95% of adults older than 65 years wear glasses for close vision and 18% also use a magnifying glass for reading and close work.

Extraocular Changes

Like the skin elsewhere, the eyelids lose elasticity and drooping (senile ptosis) may result. In most cases, this is only a cosmetic concern. In some cases, it can interfere with vision if the lids sag far enough over the lower lid margin. Spasms of the orbicular muscle may cause the lower lid to turn inward. If it stays this way, it is called *entropion*. With the curling of the lid, the lower lashes also turn inward, causing irritation and scratching of the cornea. Surgery may be needed to prevent permanent injury. Decreases in orbicular muscle strength may result in *ectropion*, or an out-turning of the lower lid (Figure 11-1). Without the

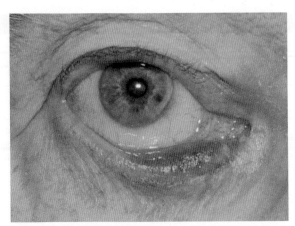

FIGURE 11-1 Ectropion. (From Swartz MH: *Textbook of physical diagnosis: history and examination,* ed 6, Philadelphia, 2009, Saunders.)

integrity of the trough of the lower lid, tears run down the cheek instead of bathing the cornea. This, and an inability to close the lid completely, lead to excessively dry eyes (xerophthalmia) and the need for artificial tears. The person also may need to tape the eyes shut during sleep. A reduction of goblet cells in the conjunctiva is another cause for drying of the eyes in the older adult. Goblet cells produce mucin, which slows the evaporation of tear film, and are essential for eye lubrication and movement.

Ocular Changes

The cornea is the avascular transparent outer surface of the eye globe that refracts (bends) light rays entering the eye through the pupil. With aging, the cornea becomes flatter, less smooth, and thicker, with the changes noticeable by its lackluster appearance or loss of sparkling transparency. The result is the increased incidence of astigmatism. The anterior chamber is the space between the cornea and the lens. The edges of the chamber include the canals that control the volume and movement of aqueous fluid within the space. With aging, the chamber decreases slightly in size and volume capacity because of thickening of the lens. Resorption of the intraocular fluid becomes less efficient and may lead to eventual breakdown in the absorption process. If the change is greater, it can lead to increased intraocular pressure and the development of glaucoma.

The iris is a ring of muscles inside the anterior chamber. The iris surrounds the opening into the eye (the pupil), gives the eye color, and regulates the amount of light that reaches the retina. With age the iris becomes paler in color as a result of pigment loss and increases in the density of collagen fibers. A normal age-related change in the iris is related to other neurological changes—that is, slowed response to sensory stimuli, in this case, to light and dark. Slowness to dilate in dark environments creates moments when elders cannot see where they are going (e.g., moving from a well-lit area to a dark area such as in a movie theater).

Because of the slow ability of the pupils to accommodate to changes in light, glare can be a major problem. Glare is caused by not only sunlight but also reflection of light on any shiny object, such as headlights or polished floors. The use of sunglasses outdoors (and indoors if considerable glare exists) can be helpful. The effect of glare from headlights of oncoming vehicles increases safety risks with driving (night blindness). Persistent pupillary constriction is known as **senile miosis**. It is often noted during the physical exam but often a normal finding if it is bilateral. At the edges of the cornea and the iris is a small ring known as the **limbus.** In some older adults, a gray-white ring or partial ring, known as **arcus senilis,** forms 1 to 2 mm inside the limbus. It does not affect vision and is composed of deposits of calcium and cholesterol salts.

The lens, a small, flexible, biconvex, crystal-like structure just behind the iris, is responsible for visual acuity as it adjusts the light entering the pupil and focuses it on the retina. Age-related changes in the lens are probably universal, but many of the changes are thought to result from exposure to ultraviolet light (Servat et al, 2011). The constant compression of lens fibers with age, the yellowing effect, and the inefficiency of the aqueous humor, which provides the lens with nutrition, all have a role in altered lens transparency. Lens cells continue to grow but at a slower rate than previously. The lens can no longer focus (refract) close objects effectively, described as decreased accommodation.

Changes to the suspensory ligaments, ciliary muscles, and parasympathetic nerves contribute to the decreased accommodation as well. Finally, light scattering increases and color perception decreases. For the person who was myopic (nearsighted) earlier in life, this change may actually improve vision. Lens opacity (cataracts) begins to develop around the fifth decade of life. The origins are not fully understood, although ultraviolet light contributes, with cross-linkage of collagen creating a more rigid and thickened lens structure.

Intraocular Changes

The vitreous humor, which gives the eye globe its shape and support, loses some of its water and fibrous skeletal support with age. Opacities other than cataracts can be seen by the person as lines, webs, spots, or clusters of dots moving rapidly across the visual field with each movement of the eye. These opacities are called "floaters" and are bits of coalesced vitreous humor that have broken off from the peripheral or central part of the retina. Most are harmless but annoying until they dissipate or one gets used to them. However, if the person sees a shower of these and a flash of light, immediate medical attention is required and is always considered an ocular emergency (retinal detachment).

The retina, which lines the inside of the eye, has less distinct margins and is duller in appearance than in younger adults. Fidelity of color is less accurate with blues, violets, and greens of the spectrum; warm colors such as reds, oranges, and yellows are more easily seen. Color clarity diminishes by 25% in the sixth decade and by 59% in the eighth decade. Some of this difficulty is linked to the yellowing of the lens and the impaired transmission of light to the retina, and the fovea may not be as bright. The average 80-year-old needs more than twice as much light as a 20-year-old to see equally well (Huether et al, 2014).

Drusen (yellow-white) spots may appear in the area of the macula. As long as these changes are not accompanied by dis-

TABLE 11-1	Changes in the Eye Caused by Aging	
STRUCTURE	**CHANGE**	**CONSEQUENCE**
Cornea	Thicker and less curved	Increase in astigmatism
	Formation of a gray ring at the edge of cornea (arcus senilis)	Not detrimental to vision
Anterior chamber	Decrease in size and volume caused by thickening of lens	Occasionally exerts pressure on Schlemm canal and may lead to increased intraocular pressure and glaucoma
Lens	Increase in opacity	Decrease in refraction with increased light scattering and decreased color vision (green and blue); decreased dark adaptation; cataracts
	Loss of elasticity	Loss of accommodation (presbyopia: loss of focus for near objects)
Ciliary muscles	Reduction in pupil diameter, atrophy of radial dilation muscles	Persistent constriction (senile miosis); decrease in critical flicker frequency*
Retina	Reduction in number of rods at periphery, loss of rods and associated nerve cells	Increase in the minimum amount of light necessary to see an object
Macula	Atrophy (age-related macular degeneration)	Loss of vision
Vitreous	Liquefaction of vitreous and decrease in gel volume	Posterior vitreous detachment causing "floaters"; risk for retinal detachment

*The rate at which consecutive visual stimuli can be presented and still be perceived as separate.
From McCance KL, Huether SE, editors: *Pathophysiology*, ed 7, St Louis, 2014, Mosby.

tortion of objects or a decrease in vision, they are not clinically significant. Finally, the number of rods and associated nerves at the periphery of the retina is reduced, resulting in peripheral vision that is not as discrete or is absent. Arteries in the back of the eye may show atherosclerosis and slight narrowing. Veins may show indentations (nicking) at the arteriovenous crossings if the person has a long history of hypertension.

Vision loss is not an inevitable part of the aging process, but age-related changes contribute to decreased vision (Table 11-1). Even older adults with good visual acuity (20/40 or better) and no significant eye disease show deficits in visual function and need accommodations to enhance vision and safety (Johnson and Record, 2014). As we age there is a higher risk of developing age-related eye diseases and other conditions (hypertension, diabetes) that can result in vision losses if left untreated.

VISUAL IMPAIRMENT

Incidence and Prevalence

Vision loss is a leading cause of age-related disability. More than two-thirds of those with visual impairment are more than 65 years of age and adults older than 80 years account for 70% of the cases of severe visual impairment Visual impairment among nursing home residents ranges from 3% to 15% higher than for adults of the same age living in the community (Johnson and Record, 2014). The World Health Organization (WHO, 2013) defines visual impairment as visual acuity worse than 20/70 but better than 20/400 (legal blindness) in the better eye, even with corrective lenses. Individuals with moderate visual impairment, combined with those with severe visual impairment, are grouped under the term "low vision." Low vision, combined with blindness, represents all visual impairment (World Health Organization, 2013).

Visual impairment worldwide has decreased since the 1990s as a result of increased availability of eye care services (particularly cataract surgery), promotion of eye care education, and improved treatment of infectious diseases. However, vision impairment is a major public health problem that is expected to increase substantially with the aging of the population. Rates of blindness and visual impairment in disadvantaged, minority populations, particularly African American and Latino subpopulations who have an increased prevalence of diabetes and hypertension, are expected to increase even further (Servat et al, 2011). Globally, uncorrected refractive errors (myopia, hyperopia, or astigmatism) and unoperated cataract and glaucoma are the leading causes of visual impairment.

In the United States, the leading causes of visual impairment are age-related macular degeneration (ARMD), cataracts, glaucoma, and diabetic retinopathy. Vision loss from eye disease is particularly a concern in the developing countries, where 90% of the world's blind individuals live. Cataracts are the leading cause of blindness in economically challenged countries, largely as a result of limited service and treatment (World Health Organization, 2013).

In 2013, the World Health Organization approved the Global Action Plan for the Prevention of Avoidable Blindness and Visual Impairment (GAP) 2014-2019. Goals of GAP are to reduce avoidable visual impairment and secure access to vision rehabilitation services by improving access to comprehensive eye care services that are integrated into health systems (World Health Organization, 2014). Estimates are that 80% of all visual impairment can be avoided or cured. Box 11-1 presents *Healthy People 2020* objectives for vision in older adults.

Consequences of Visual Impairment

Visual problems have a negative impact on quality of life, equivalent to that of life-threatening conditions such as heart disease and cancer. Loss of vision impacts a person's quality of life and ability to function in most daily activities such as driving, reading, maneuvering safely, dressing, cooking, and taking medications, as well as participating in social activities. Decreased vision has also been found to be a significant risk factor for falls and other accidents and is associated with cognitive decline and depression, as well as increased risk of

Objectives Vision—Older Adults

- Increase the proportion of adults who have had a comprehensive eye examination, including dilation, within the past 2 years.
- Reduce visual impairment due to diabetic retinopathy.
- Reduce visual impairment due to glaucoma.
- Reduce visual impairment due to cataracts.
- Reduce visual impairment due to age-related macular degeneration.
- Increase the use of vision rehabilitation services by persons with visual impairment.
- Increase the use of assistive and adaptive devices by persons with visual impairment.

Data from U.S. Department of Health and Human Services, Office of Disease Prevention and Health Promotion: *Healthy People 2020*, 2012. http://www.healthypeople.gov/2020

BOX 11-3 Promoting Healthy Eyes

- Do not smoke.
- Eat a diet rich in green, leafy vegetables and fish.
- Exercise.
- Maintain normal blood pressure and blood glucose measurements.
- Wear sunglasses and a brimmed hat anytime you are outside in bright sunshine.
- Wear safety eyewear when working around your house or playing sports.
- See an eye care professional routinely.

Source: National Eye Institute, National Eye Health Education Program: *Make vision health a priority*. http://www.nei.nih.gov/healthyeyestoolkit/pdf/VisionAndHealth_Tagged.pdf Accessed October 31, 2014.

institutionalization and death (Gopinath et al, 2013; International Federation on Ageing, 2012). "Vision loss not only severely impairs one's ability to be independent and self-sufficient, but it also has a 'snowball effect' on the health and well-being of older people, families, caregivers, and society at large. This cumulative effect is severely underestimated" (International Federation on Ageing, 2012, p. 4).

Prevention of Visual Impairment

Many age-related eye diseases have no symptoms in the early stages but can be detected early through a comprehensive dilated eye exam. However, knowledge about eye disease and treatments remains inadequate among both lay persons and medical professionals (NEI, NEHEP, 2014b,c). Only about 45% of adults with diabetes know the disease puts them at higher risk for vision problems, and only about 60% had an eye exam in the previous year (Bressler et al, 2014). Socioeconomic position and educational position are important social determinants that may influence access to and use of effective and appropriate eye care, thus influencing disease identification and treatment (MacLennan et al, 2014; Zhang et al, 2013) (Box 11-2).

BOX 11-2 RESEARCH HIGHLIGHTS

Data from the National Health Interview Survey (NHS) were used to assess the variance and trends in the use of eye care services across levels of socioeconomic position (as measured by income and educational level) for individuals older than 40 who reported age-related eye disease (ARMD, cataract, diabetic retinopathy, glaucoma). Data analysis revealed considerable differences in the use of eye care services by socioeconomic position and showed that use decreased with increasing socioeconomic disadvantage. Persons with less than a high school education were less likely than those with at least a college education to report a visit to an eye care provider or to have undergone a dilated eye examination. More research is needed to determine how income and educational inequalities affect health-seeking behavior. Appropriate public health interventions targeted at adults with low levels of education and income may reduce the disparity in eye care.

Data from Zhang X, Beckles G, Chou C-F, et al: Socioeconomic disparity among US adults with age-related eye diseases: National Health Interview Survey 2002 and 2008, *JAMA Ophthalmol* 131(9):1198–1206, 2013.

At all ages, attention to eye health and protecting your vision is important (Box 11-3). Prevention and treatment of eye disease are important priorities for nurses and other health professionals. The National Eye Health Education Program (NEHEP) of the National Eye Institute (NEI) provides a program for health professionals with evidence-based tools and resources that can be used in community settings to educate older adults about eye health and maintaining healthy vision (www.nei.nih.gov/SeeWellToolkit; see Box 11-6). The program emphasizes the importance of annual dilated eye examinations for anyone older than age 50 and stresses that eye diseases often have no warning signs or symptoms, so early detection is essential but not always possible. NEHEP provides educational materials and outreach activities targeted to populations at high risk for eye diseases, including African Americans, American Indians, Alaska natives, Hispanics/Latinos, and individuals with diabetes and a family history of glaucoma (National Eye Institute, 2014a,b).

DISEASES AND DISORDERS OF THE EYE

Glaucoma

Glaucoma affects as many as 2.3 million Americans age 40 years and older and 6% of those older than age 65. While the numbers cannot be exact, the World Health Organization reports that glaucoma affects 2% of the world's population. At least half of all persons with glaucoma are unaware they have the disease. Primary open-angle glaucoma (POAG), the most common form of glaucoma, is the second most common cause of legal blindness in the United States and the leading cause of blindness among African Americans. African Americans are at risk of developing glaucoma at an earlier age than other racial and ethnic groups, with projections of a 66% increase in the number of cases by 2030 (Johnson and Record, 2014; NEI, 2014c). Some research suggests that the anatomical microstructure of the posterior sclera in African Americans may be significantly different from that of whites, possible favoring the earlier development and severity of ocular disease (Servat et al, 2011). Other high-risk groups are Mexican Americans, people older than age 60, and persons with diabetes, hypertension, and a family history of glaucoma (NEI, 2014c). The NEI is conducting a wide range of studies to understand causes and potential areas of treatment for glaucoma.

Other types of glaucoma are congenital glaucoma, low-tension or normal-tension glaucoma, secondary glaucoma (complication of other medical conditions), and acute angle-closure glaucoma, which is an emergency. The etiology of glaucoma is variable and often unknown. However, when the natural fluids of the eye are blocked by ciliary muscle rigidity and the buildup of pressure, damage to the optic nerve occurs. Glaucoma can be bilateral, but it more commonly occurs in one eye.

POAG is characterized by progressive and asymptomatic optic neuropathy resulting in visual field loss. Intraocular pressure (IOP) increases and damages optic nerve fibers (Johnson and Record, 2014). However, if detected early, glaucoma can usually be controlled and serious vision loss prevented. Signs of glaucoma can include headaches, poor vision in dim lighting, increased sensitivity to glare, "tired eyes," impaired peripheral vision, a fixed and dilated pupil, and frequent changes in prescriptions for corrective lenses. Figure 11-2, A, shows normal vision and Figure 11-2, B, illustrates the effects of glaucoma on vision.

Angle-closure glaucoma is not as common as POAG and occurs when the angle of the iris causes obstruction of the aqueous humor through the trabecular network. It may occur as a result of infection or trauma. IOP rises rapidly accompanied by redness and pain in and around the eye, severe headaches, nausea and vomiting, and blurring of vision. It is a medical emergency and blindness can occur in 2 days. Treatment is an iridectomy to ease pressure. Many drugs with anticholinergic properties, including antihistamines, stimulants, vasodilators, and sympathomimetics, are particularly dangerous for individuals predisposed to acute-closure glaucoma.

⚡ SAFETY ALERT

Redness and pain in and around the eye, severe headaches, nausea and vomiting, and blurring of vision occur with angle-closure glaucoma. It is a medical emergency and blindness can occur in 2 days.

Screening and Treatment of Glaucoma

A dilated eye examination and tonometry are necessary to diagnose glaucoma. Adults older than age 65 should have annual eye examinations with dilation, and those with medication-controlled glaucoma should be examined at least every 6 months. Annual screening is also recommended for African Americans and other individuals with a family history of glaucoma who are older than 40 years. Although standard Medicare does not cover routine eye care, it does cover 80% of the cost for dilated eye exams for individuals at higher risk for glaucoma and those with diabetes.

Management of glaucoma involves medications (oral or topical eye drops) to decrease IOP and/or laser trabeculoplasty and filtration surgery. Medications lower eye pressure either by decreasing the amount of aqueous fluid produced within the eye or by improving the flow through the drainage angle. Beta-blockers are the first-line therapy for glaucoma followed by prostaglandin analogs. Second-line agents include topical carbonic anhydrase inhibitors and α_2-agonists

(Johnson and Record, 2014). The patient may need combinations of several types of eye drops. There is ongoing research on the development of a contact lens to deliver glaucoma medication continuously for a month (Ciolino et al, 2014).

In the hospital or long-term care setting, it is important to obtain a past medical history to determine if the person has glaucoma and to ensure that eye drops are given according to the person's treatment regimen. Without the eye drops, eye pressure can rise and cause an acute exacerbation of glaucoma. Usually medications can control glaucoma, but laser surgery (trabeculoplasty) and filtration surgery may be recommended for some types of glaucoma. Surgery is usually recommended only if necessary to prevent further damage to the optic nerve.

Cataracts

A cataract is an opacity in the lens causing the lens to lose transparency or scatter light. Cataracts are caused by oxidative damage to lens protein and fatty deposits (lipofuscin) in the ocular lens. The prevalence of cataracts increases with age, affecting as many as 70% of white individuals 80 years and older. Cataracts are categorized according to their location within the lens and are usually bilateral. Cataracts are recognized by the clouding of the ordinarily clear ocular lens; the red reflex may be absent or may appear as a black area. The cardinal sign of cataracts is the appearance of halos around objects as light is diffused. Other common symptoms include blurring, decreased perception of light and color (giving a yellow tint to most things), and sensitivity to glare. Figure 11-2, C, illustrates the effects of a cataract on vision.

The most common causes of cataracts are heredity and advancing age. They may occur more frequently and at earlier ages in individuals who have been exposed to excessive sunlight; have poor dietary habits, diabetes, hypertension, kidney disease, or eye trauma; or have a history of alcohol intake and tobacco use. Older individuals with diabetes are 60% more likely to develop cataracts than persons without diabetes. Cataracts are more likely to occur after glaucoma surgery or other types of eye surgery.

Treatment of Cataracts

The treatment of cataracts is surgical and cataract surgery is the most common surgical procedure performed in the United States. Most often, cataract surgery involves only local anesthesia, is done on an outpatient basis, and is one of the most successful surgical procedures, with 95% of patients reporting excellent vision after surgery. Surgery is performed when there is functional visual impairment. The surgery involves removal of the lens and placement of a plastic intraocular lens (IOL).

Presurgical and Postsurgical Interventions

Nursing interventions when caring for the person experiencing cataract surgery include preparing the individual for significant changes in vision and adaptation to light and ensuring that the individual has received adequate counseling regarding realistic postsurgical expectations. Following surgery, the individual needs to avoid heavy lifting, straining, and bending at the waist. Eye drops may be prescribed to aid

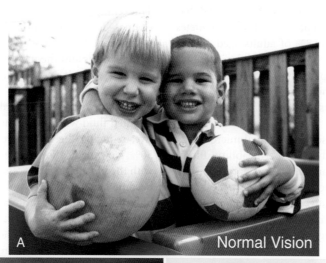

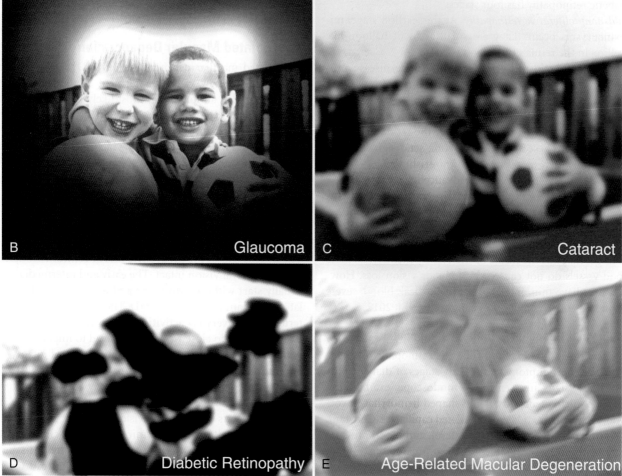

FIGURE 11-2 A, Normal vision. **B,** Simulated vision with glaucoma. **C,** Simulated vision with cataracts. **D,** Simulated vision with diabetic retinopathy. **E,** Simulated loss of vision with age-related macular degeneration (AMD). (From National Eye Institute, National Institutes of Health, 2010.)

healing and prevent infection. Teaching fall prevention techniques and ensuring home safety modifications are also important because some research suggests that the risk of falls increases after surgery, particularly between first and second cataract surgeries (Meuleners et al, 2013). The vision imbalance that can occur if the person has one "good" eye and one "bad" eye contributes to the risk of falls. If the person has bilateral cataracts, surgery is performed first on one eye with the second surgery on the other eye a month or so later to ensure healing.

Diabetic Retinopathy

Diabetes has become an epidemic in the United States, and diabetic retinopathy occurs in both type 1 and type 2 diabetes (Chapter 24). Estimates are that 40.8% of adults aged 40 and older with diabetes have diabetic retinopathy, and the incidence increases with age. Most diabetic patients will develop diabetic retinopathy within 20 years of diagnosis. Diabetic retinopathy is the leading cause of new blindness for Americans between the ages of 20 and 74.

Diabetic retinopathy is a disease of the retinal microvasculature characterized by increased vessel permeability. Blood and lipid leakage leads to macular edema and hard exudates (composed of lipids). In advanced disease, new fragile blood vessels form and hemorrhage easily. Because of the vascular and cellular changes accompanying diabetes, there is often rapid worsening of other pathologic vision conditions as well (Figure 11-2, *D*).

Diabetic retinopathy has four stages:

1. *Mild nonproliferative retinopathy.* At this earliest stage, microaneurysms occur. They are small areas of balloon-like swelling in the retina's tiny blood vessels.
2. *Moderate nonproliferative retinopathy.* As the disease progresses, some blood vessels that nourish the retina are blocked.
3. *Severe nonproliferative retinopathy.* Many more blood vessels are blocked, depriving several areas of the retina with their blood supply. These areas of the retina send signals to the body to grow new blood vessels for nourishment.
4. *Proliferative retinopathy.* At this advanced stage, the signals sent by the retina for nourishment trigger the growth of new blood vessels. This condition is called proliferative retinopathy. These new blood vessels are abnormal and fragile. They grow along the retina and along the surface of the clear, vitreous gel that fills the inside of the eye. By themselves, these blood vessels do not cause symptoms or vision loss. However, they have thin, fragile walls. If they leak blood, severe vision loss and even blindness can result (NEI, 2012).

Screening and Treatment of Diabetic Retinopathy

Early detection and treatment of diabetic retinopathy is essential. There are no symptoms in the early stages of diabetic retinopathy. Early signs are seen in the fundoscopic examination and include microaneurysms, flame-shaped hemorrhages, cotton wool spots, hard exudates, and dilated capillaries. Constant, strict control of blood glucose, cholesterol, and blood pressure measurements and laser photocoagulation treatments can halt progression of the disease. Laser treatment can reduce vision loss in 50% of patients.

Annual dilated fundoscopic examination of the eye is recommended beginning 5 years after diagnosis of diabetes type 1 and at the time of diagnosis of diabetes type 2. Nurses need to provide education to diabetic patients about the risk of diabetic retinopathy and the importance of early identification, as well as good control of diabetes. Some experts are encouraging mass screening efforts. There is good treatment that can reverse vision loss and improve vision, but individuals must have access to screenings and eye examinations.

Diabetic Macular Edema (DME)

Thickening of the center of the retina—diabetic macular edema—is the most common cause of visual loss attributable to diabetes. The disease affects 1 in 25 adults age 40 and older with diabetes and the incidence is higher in African Americans and Hispanics. It is the leading cause of legal blindness. Treatment includes medications (often cortisone-type drugs) and laser therapy to cauterize leaky blood vessels and reduce accumulated fluid within the macula. Laser treatment is very effective, reducing the risk of substantial worsening of vision by 50%. New medications under study include those that interfere with the biochemical process that allows retinal blood vessels to become leaky. Tight control of blood glucose, cholesterol, and blood pressure values; annual dilated retinal examinations; and education about eye disease and diabetes are essential. However, in a recent study, only 44.7% of adults 40 years and older with DME reported that they were told by a physician that diabetes had affected their eyes and 59.7% had received a dilated eye examination in the last year (Bressler et al, 2014).

Age-Related Macular Degeneration

Age-related macular degeneration (ARMD) is the most common cause of new visual impairment among people age 50 years and older, although it is most likely to occur after age 60 (Johnson and Record, 2014; NEI, 2013). The prevalence of ARMD increases drastically with age, with more than 15% of white women older than age 80 having the disease. Whites and Asian Americans are more likely to lose vision from ARMD than African Americans or Hispanics/Latinos. With the number of affected older adults projected to increase over the next 20 years, ARMD has been called a growing epidemic.

ARMD is a degenerative eye disease that affects the macula, the central part of the eye responsible for clear central vision. The disease causes the progressive loss of central vision, leaving only peripheral vision intact. The early and intermediate stages usually start without symptoms and only a comprehensive dilated eye exam can detect ARMD. The loss of central vision interferes with everyday activities such as the ability to see faces, read, drive, or do close work and can lead to impaired mobility, increased risk of falls, depression, and decreased quality of life (Johnson and Record, 2014; National Eye Institute, 2013). Persons in the early stage of the disease may attribute their vision problems to normal aging or cataracts. Figure 11-2, *E*, illustrates the effects of ARMD on vision.

ARMD results from systemic changes in circulation, accumulation of cellular waste products, atrophy of tissue, and growth of abnormal blood vessels in the choroid layer beneath the retina. Fibrous scarring disrupts nourishment of photoreceptor cells, causing their death and loss of central vision. Risk factors for ARMD are similar to those for coronary artery disease (hypertension, atherosclerosis). Smoking doubles the risk of ARMD. Other risk factors are thought to include genetic predisposition, inflammation, and diet. A genetic link for ARMD is suspected in 50% of new cases (Johnson and Record, 2014). Genetic studies are ongoing by the Human Genome Project and the Genome-Wide Association Studies.

There are two forms of macular degeneration—the "dry" form and the "wet" form. Dry ARMD accounts for the majority of cases (90%) and rarely causes severe visual impairment but can lead to the more aggressive wet ARMD. Dry AMRD generally affects both eyes, but vision can be lost in one eye while the other eye seems unaffected. Dry ARMD has three stages, which may occur in one or both eyes. One of the most common early signs is drusen bodies seen during an ophthalmological examination. Drusen are yellow deposits under the retina and are often found in people older than 60. The relationship between drusen and ARMD is not clear, but an increase in the size or number of drusen increases the risk of developing either advanced ARMD or wet ARMD.

Wet ARMD (also called neovascular) occurs when abnormal blood vessels behind the retina start to grow under the macula. These new blood vessels are fragile and often leak blood and fluid, which raise the macula from its normal place at the back of the eye. With wet ARMD, the severe loss of central vision can be rapid and many people will be legally blind within 2 years of diagnosis.

Screening and Treatment of ARMD

Early diagnosis is the key. An Amsler grid (Figure 11-3) is used to determine clarity of vision. A perception of wavy lines is diagnostic of beginning macular degeneration. In the advanced forms, the person may see dark or empty spaces that block the center of vision. People with ARMD are usually taught to test their eyes daily using an Amsler grid so that they will be aware of any changes. While research is ongoing related to the use of antioxidant supplements, a diet high in green leafy vegetables and fruits may protect the eyes and lower progression of macular degeneration (Chew et al, 2014).

Treatment of wet ARMD includes photodynamic therapy (PDT), laser photocoagulation (LPC), and anti-VEGF therapy. Anti-VEGF therapy is the standard treatment. Lucentis and Avastin (anti–vascular endothelial growth factor [VEGF] therapy) are biological drugs that are the most common form of treatment in advanced ARMD. Abnormally high levels of a specific growth factor occur in eyes with wet ARMD, which promote the growth of abnormal blood vessels. Anti-VEGF therapy blocks the effect of the growth factor. These drugs are injected into the eye as often as once a month and can help slow vision loss from ARMD and, in some cases, improve sight.

Detached Retina

A retinal detachment can occur at any age but is more common after the age of 40 years. Emergency medical treatment is required or permanent visual loss can result. There may be small areas of the retina that are torn (retinal tears or breaks) and will lead to retinal detachment. This condition can develop in persons with cataracts or recent cataract surgery or trauma, or it can occur spontaneously. Symptoms include a gradual increase in the number of floaters and/or light flashes in the eye. It also manifests as a curtain coming down over the person's field of vision. Small holes or tears are treated with laser surgery or a freeze treatment called *cryopexy*. Retinal detachments are treated with surgery. More than 90% of individuals with a retinal detachment can be successfully treated, although sometimes a second treatment is needed. However, the visual outcome is not always predictable and may not be known for several months following surgery. Visual results are best if the detachment is repaired before the macula detaches, so immediate treatment of symptoms is essential (National Eye Institute, 2014d).

Dry Eye

Dry eye is not a disease of the eye but is a frequent complaint among older people. Tear production normally diminishes as we age. The condition is termed *keratoconjunctivitis sicca*. It occurs most commonly in women after menopause. There may be age-related changes in the mucin-secreting cells necessary for surface wetting, in the lacrimal glands, or in the meibomian glands that secrete surface oil, and all of these may occur at the same time. The older person will describe a dry, scratchy feeling in mild cases (xerophthalmia). There may be marked discomfort and decreased mucus production in severe situations.

Medications can cause dry eye, especially anticholinergics, antihistamines, diuretics, beta-blockers, and some hypnotics. Sjögren's syndrome is a cell-mediated autoimmune disease whose manifestations include decreased lacrimal gland activity.

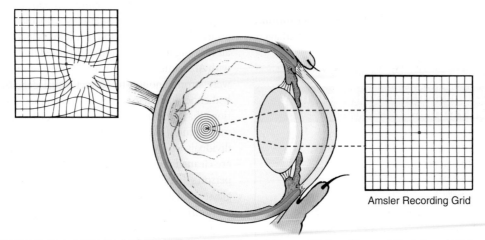

Amsler Recording Grid

FIGURE 11-3 Macular Degeneration: Distortion of Center Vision, Normal Peripheral Vision. (Illustration by Harriet R. Greenfied, Newton, Mass.)

The problem is diagnosed by an ophthalmologist using a Schirmer tear test, in which filter paper strips are placed under the lower eyelid to measure the rate of tear production. A common treatment is artificial tears or a saline gel, but dry eyes may be sensitive to them because of preservatives, which can be irritating. The ophthalmologist may close the tear duct channel either temporarily or permanently. Other management methods include keeping the house air moist with humidifiers, avoiding wind and hair dryers, and using artificial tear ointments at bedtime. Vitamin A deficiency can be a cause of dry eye, and vitamin A ointments are available for treatment.

◆ PROMOTING HEALTHY AGING: IMPLICATIONS FOR GERONTOLOGICAL NURSES

◆ Assessment

Vision impairment is common among older adults in connection with aging changes and eye diseases and can significantly affect communication, functional ability, safety, and quality of life. To promote healthy aging and quality of life, nurses who care for elders in all settings can improve outcomes for visually impaired elders by assessing for vision changes (Box 11-4), adapting the environment to enhance vision and safety, communicating appropriately, and providing appropriate health teaching and referrals for prevention, treatment, and assistive devices.

◆ Interventions

General principles in caring for persons with visual impairment include the following: use warm incandescent lighting; increase intensity of lighting; control glare by using shades and blinds; suggest yellow or amber lenses to decrease glare; suggest sunglasses that block all ultraviolet light; recommend reading materials that have large, dark, evenly spaced printing; and select colors with good contrast and intensity. Color contrasts are used to facilitate location of items. Sharply contrasting colors assist the partially sighted. For instance, a bright towel is much easier to locate than a white towel hanging on a beige wall. When choosing color, it is best to use primary colors at the top end of the spectrum rather than those at the bottom. If you think of the colors of the rainbow, it is more likely that people will see reds and oranges better than blues and greens. Figure 11-4 beautifully illustrates the use of color in a nursing home in Copenhagen,

---

BOX 11-4   Signs and Behaviors that may Indicate Vision Problems

Individual may report:
- Pain in eyes
- Difficulty seeing in darkened area
- Double vision/distorted vision
- Migraine headaches coupled with blurred vision
- Flashes of light
- Halos surrounding lights
- Difficulty driving at night
- Falls or injuries

BOX 11-5   TIPS FOR BEST PRACTICE

Communicating with Elders Who Have Visual Impairment

- Assess for vision loss.
- Make sure you have the person's attention before speaking.
- Clearly identify yourself and others with you. State when you are leaving to make sure the person is aware of your departure.
- Position yourself at the person's level when speaking.
- When others are present, address the visually impaired person by prefacing remarks with his or her name or a light touch on the arm.
- Ensure adequate lighting and eliminate glare.
- Select colors for paint, furniture, pictures with rich intensity (e.g., red, orange).
- Use large, dark, evenly spaced printing.
- Use contrast in printed material (e.g., black marker on white paper).
- Use a night light in bathroom and hallways and use illuminated switches.
- Do not change room arrangement or the arrangement of personal items without explanations.
- If in a hospital or nursing home, use some means to identify patients who are visually impaired and include visual impairment in the plan of care.
- Use the analogy of a clock face to help locate objects (e.g., describe positions of food on a plate in relation to clock positions, such as meat at 3 o'clock, dessert at 6 o'clock).
- Label eyeglasses and have a spare pair if possible; make sure glasses are worn and are clean.
- Be aware of low-vision assistive devices such as talking watches, talking books, and magnifiers, and facilitate access to these resources.
- If the person is blind, ask the person how you can help. If walking, do not try to push or pull. Let the person take your arm just above the elbow, and give directions with details (e.g., the bench is on your immediate right); when seating the person, place his or her hand on the back of the chair.
- Recommend screening for vision loss and annual dilated eye exams for older people.

Denmark. Box 11-5 presents Tips for Best Practice for elders with visual impairment.

◆ Special Considerations in Long-Term Care Settings

Nursing homes and assisted living facilities (ALFs) care for a large number of individuals who are visually impaired and many also experience hearing and cognitive impairment (Elliott et al, 2013). Cognitive impairment interferes with the person's ability to be aware of limited vision and to ask for help. One study of individuals residing in nursing homes reported that one in three residents with Alzheimer's disease was not using or did not have glasses that were strong enough to correct visual deficits. These individuals had either lost their glasses or broken them, or they had prescriptions that were no longer accurate (Koch et al, 2005). Although it may sound like common sense, it is especially important that individuals who wear glasses are wearing them and that the glasses are cleaned regularly. Also important is asking the person or the person's family/significant other if the person routinely wears glasses and if the person is able to see well enough to function.

Routine eye care is sorely lacking in nursing homes and is related to functional decline, decreased quality of life, and depression. Estimates are that approximately one third of vision impairment in this setting is reversible with currently available

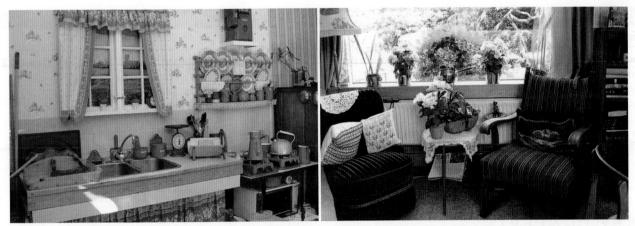

FIGURE 11-4 A, Reminiscence kitchen (Højdevang Sogns Plejejem, Copenhagen, Denmark). **B,** Sitting room (Højdevang Sogns Plejejem). (Photos courtesy Christine Williams, PhD, RN.)

treatments such as correction of refractive errors and cataract surgery (Elliott et al, 2013). Even in individuals with dementia who have clinically significant cataracts, surgery was found to improve visual acuity, slow the rate of cognitive decline, decrease neuropsychiatric symptoms, and reduce caregiver stress (Cassels, 2014).

◆ Low-Vision Optical Devices

Technology advances in the past decade have produced some low-vision devices that may be used successfully in the care of the visually impaired individual. These devices are grouped into devices for "near" activities (such as reading, sewing, writing) and devices for "distance" activities (such as attending movies, reading street signs, and identifying numbers on buses and trains). Nurses can refer individuals with low vision or blindness to vision rehabilitation services, which may include assistance with communication skills, counseling, independent living and personal management skills, independent movement and travel skills, training with low-vision devices, and vocational rehabilitation. It is important to be familiar with agencies in your community that offer these services. Persons with severe visual impairment may qualify for disability and financial and social services assistance through government and private programs including vision rehabilitation programs.

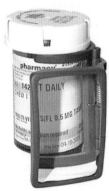

Prescription Bottle Magnifier. (Reprinted with permission from Carson Optical.)

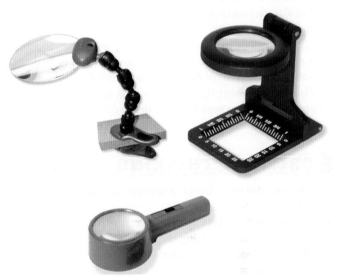

Magnifiers. (Reprinted with permission from Carson Optical.)

An array of low-vision assistive devices is now available, including insulin delivery systems, talking clocks and watches, large-print books, magnifiers, telescopes (handheld or mounted on eyeglasses), electronic magnification through closed circuit television or computer software, and software that converts text into artificial voice output. iPods have a setting for audio menus; Microsoft and Apple computer programs allow a person to change color schemes, select a high-contrast display, and magnify and enlarge print. Many websites also have an option for audio text. The e-Reader product from Kindle allows the user to increase font sizes up to 40 points in e-books and offers a Text-to-Speech feature. The iPad from Apple can enlarge text up to 56 points and includes VoiceOver, a feature that reads everything displayed on the screen for you, making it fully usable for people with low to no vision. More and more mobile phones have speech-enabled features, and the Jitterbug phone comes with a live operator whose actions can be directed. As individual needs are unique, it is recommended that before investing in vision aids, the individual consult with a low-vision center or low-vision specialist. Other vision resources are presented in Box 11-6.

BOX 11-6   RESOURCES FOR BEST PRACTICE
Vision

Centers for Disease Control and Prevention: Education, videos illustrating vision with AMD, glaucoma, diabetic retinopathy

Cacchione P: Sensory changes. In Boltz et al, editors: *Evidence-based geriatric nursing protocols for best practice*, New York, Springer, 2012, pp 48-73

Eye Care America: On-line referral center for eye care resources

Lighthouse International

Lighthouse for the Blind

National Eye Health Education Program (NEHEP) and National Eye Institute: Educational and professional resources, vision and aging program; See Well for a Lifetime Toolkit, vodcasts on common visual problems

National Federation for the Blind

USDHHS/AHRQ: Evidence-based practice guideline: care of the patient with open angle glaucoma.

Vision Aware (American Foundation for the Blind): Resources for Independent Living with Vision Loss; Getting started kit for people new to vision loss; How to walk with a guide

KEY CONCEPTS

- Vision loss is a leading cause of age-related disability.
- The leading causes of visual impairment in the United States are diseases that are common in older adults: age-related macular degeneration (ARMD), cataract, glaucoma, and diabetic retinopathy.
- Many causes of visual impairment are preventable, so attention to keeping eyes healthy throughout life and early detection and treatment of eye disease is essential.
- Visual impairment significantly affects quality of life and a person's ability to perform activities of daily living and function independently.

- Nurses who care for visually impaired elders in all settings can improve outcomes by assessing for vision changes, adapting the environment to enhance vision and safety, communicating appropriately, and providing appropriate health teaching and referrals for prevention, treatment, and assistive devices.

CRITICAL THINKING QUESTIONS AND ACTIVITIES

1. How can nurses enhance awareness and education about vision disorders?
2. Have students attempt to ambulate, read, or take simulated medications while wearing sunglasses with lenses covered in Vaseline or with one lens covered.
3. What is the role of the nurse in the acute care setting/long-term setting in screening and assessment of vision?
4. Develop a teaching plan for an individual with a new diagnosis of glaucoma.
5. What community resources are available in your area for individuals with vision impairment?

RESEARCH QUESTIONS

1. What do people think is helpful in enhancing communication with the visually impaired?
2. What content on visual impairment and nursing interventions is included in curricula of BSN nursing programs?
3. What are the factors influencing the decisions of older people to seek help for visual problems?
4. Which types of educational programs and outreach activities are most effective in educating older individuals about prevention and treatment of eye diseases?
5. Are there differences in the views about visual health in aging among diverse groups of older people?
6. What is the effect of visual rehabilitation services on performance of activities of daily living (ADLs) and instrumental activities of daily living (IADLs) and quality of life for visually impaired older individuals?

REFERENCES

Bressler N, Varma R, Doan Q, et al: Underuse of the health care system by persons with diabetes mellitus and diabetic macular edema in the United States, *JAMA Ophthalmol* 132(2):168–173, 2014.

Cassels, C: Cataract surgery may cut cognitive decline in dementia, *Medscape Medical News*, July 14, 2014. http://www.medscape.com/viewarticle/828188. Accessed July 2014.

Chew E, Clemons T, SanGiovanni J, et al: Secondary analysis of the effects of lutein/zeaxanthin on age-related macular degeneration progression: AREDS2

Report No. 3, *JAMA Ophthalmol* 132(2):142–149, 2014.

Ciolino J, Stefanescu C, Ross A, et al: In vivo performance of a drug-eluting contact lens to treat glaucoma for a month, *Biomaterials* 35(1):432–439, 2014.

Elliott A, McGwin G, Owsley C: Vision impairment among older adults residing in assisted living, *J Aging Health* 25(2):364–378, 2013.

Gopinath B, Schneider J, McMahon C, et al: Dual sensory impairment in older adults increases the risk of mortality: a population-based study, *PLOS One*, 8(1), Mar 4, 2013. doi: 10.1371/journal.pone.0055054. [Epub ahead of print]. http://www.plosone.org/article/info%3Adoi%2F10.1371%2Fjournal.pone.0055054. Accessed August 2014.

Huether S, Rodway G, DeFriez C: Pain, temperature regulation, sleep, and sensory function. In McCance K, Huether S, editors: *Pathophysiology*, ed 7, St. Louis, 2014, Elsevier, pp 516.

International Federation on Ageing: *The high cost of low vision: the evidence on ageing and the loss of sight*, 2012. http://www.ifa-fiv.org/ifa-publication/vision-ageing/the-high-cost-of-low-vision-the-evidence-on-ageing-and-the-loss-of-sight. Accessed March 1, 2014.

Johnson K, Record S: Visual impairment and eye problems. In Ham R, Sloane R, Warshaw G, et al, editors: *Primary care geriatrics*, ed 6, Philadelphia, 2014, Elsevier Saunders, pp 301–305.

Koch J, Datta G, Makhdoom S, et al: Unmet visual needs of Alzheimer's patients in long-term care facilities, *J Am Med Dir Assoc* 6:233–237, 2005.

MacLennan P, McGivin G, Heckemeyer C, et al: Eye care use among a high-risk diabetic population seen in a public hospital's clinics, *JAMA Ophthalmol* 132(2):162–167, 2014.

Meuleners L, Fraser M, Ng J, et al: The impact of first-and second-eye cataract surgery on injurious falls that require hospitalization: a whole population study, *Age Ageing*, Nov 4, 2013. doi: 10.1093/ageing/aft 177. [Epub ahead of print]. http://www.ncbi.nlm.nih.gov/pubmed/24192250. Accessed March 3, 2014.

National Eye Institute: *Facts about diabetic retinopathy*, 2012. http://www.nei.nih.gov/health/diabetic/retinopathy.asp. Accessed August 2014.

National Eye Institute: *Facts about macular degeneration*, 2013. https://www.nei.nih.gov/health/maculardegen/armd_facts.asp. Accessed March 3, 2014.

National Eye Institute, National Eye Health Education Program: *Primary care physicians and eye health*, 2014. http://www.nei.nih.gov/nehep/research/Manuscript.pdf. Accessed March 3, 2014.

National Eye Institute, National Eye Health Education Program: *Five-year agenda, 2012.2017,* 2014. https://www.nei.nih.gov/nehep/docs/NEHEP_Five-Year_Agenda_2012-2017.pdf. Accessed March 3, 2014.

National Eye Institute, National Eye Health Education Program: *Glaucoma can take your sight away*, 2014. http://www.nei.nih.gov/nehep/programs/glaucoma/materials/DropIn_GenPub_Rel_508.pdf. http://www.nei.nih.go. Accessed March 3, 2014.

National Eye Institute, National Eye Health Education Program: *Facts about retinal detachment*, 2014. http://www.nei.nih.gov/health/retinaldetach. Accessed July 2014.

Servat J, Risco M, Nakasato Y, et al: Visual impairment and the elderly: impact on functional ability and quality of life, *Clin Geriatrics* 19(7):1–12, 2011.

World Health Organization: *Visual impairment and blindness* (Fact sheet no. 282), 2013. http://www.who.int/mediacentre/factsheets/fs282/en/. Accessed March 1, 2014.

World Health Organization: *Prevention of blindness and visual impairment*. http://www.who.int/blindness/actionplan/en/. Accessed July 2014.

Zhang X, Beckles G, Chou, C-F, et al: Socioeconomic disparity among US adults with age-related eye diseases: National Health Interview Survey 2002 and 2008, *JAMA Ophthalmol* 131(9):1198–1206, 2013.

12 CHAPTER

Hearing

Theris A. Touhy

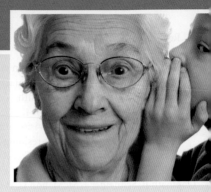

ⓔ http://evolve.elsevier.com/Touhy/TwdHlthAging

A STUDENT SPEAKS

My Dad has had a hearing problem for a couple of years and it has driven us all crazy. He won't admit he can't hear. It's always us mumbling or some other excuse. When you go in the house the TV is so loud no one can talk and visit. When I call him on his cell phone, he gets half of what I am saying. His responses are off the wall a lot of the time. I am sure there is something that would help him if he would accept it—it would sure help us!

Sophia, age 21

AN ELDER SPEAKS

A great annoyance of hearing loss is in the subtle aspects of living with a partner, who most probably has a hearing loss as well. You must often repeat what you say, and in lovemaking, whispering sweet words becomes a gesture for yourself alone.

Bob, age 80

LEARNING OBJECTIVES

On completion of this chapter, the reader will be able to:

1. Discuss changes in hearing with age and describe their impact on quality of life and function.
2. Describe the types of hearing loss and contributing factors.
3. Describe the importance of health education and screening for hearing problems.
4. Identify the components of a focused assessment to evaluate hearing and hearing loss.
5. Identify effective communication strategies for individuals with hearing impairment.
6. Increase awareness of the resources available to assist individuals with hearing loss.
7. Discuss the role of the nurse in assisting individuals to utilize hearing aids and assistive technology to improve hearing.

Although both vision and hearing impairment significantly affect all aspects of life, Oliver Sacks (1989), in his book *Seeing Voices*, presents a view that blindness may in fact be less serious than loss of hearing. Hearing loss interferes with communication with others and the interactional input that is so necessary to stimulate and validate. Helen Keller was most profound in her expression: "Never to see the face of a loved one nor to witness a summer sunset is indeed a handicap. But I can touch a face and feel the warmth of the sun. But to be deprived of hearing the song of the first spring robin and the laughter of children provides me with a long and dreadful sadness" (Keller, 1902).

HEARING IMPAIRMENT

Hearing loss is the third most prevalent chronic condition and the foremost communicative disorder of older adults in the United States. Hearing loss is an underrecognized public health issue. Among adults between the ages of 60 and 69 years of age, 31% have bilateral hearing loss of at least mild severity. In those older than 70 years of age, the prevalence is 63%, and in those older than age 85, the prevalence is 80%. In all age groups, men are more likely than women to be hearing impaired and black Americans have a lower prevalence of hearing impairment than either white or Hispanic Americans (Bainbridge and Wallhagen, 2014). Box 12-1 presents *Healthy People 2020* objectives related to hearing impairment and older adults.

Age-related hearing impairment is a complex disease caused by interactions between age-related changes (Table 12-1), genetics, lifestyle, and environmental factors. Factors associated with hearing loss include noise exposure, ear infections, smoking, and chronic disease (e.g., diabetes, chronic kidney disease, heart disease) (Bainbridge and Wallhagen, 2014). Hearing loss

BOX 12-1 HEALTHY PEOPLE 2020

Objectives Hearing—Older Adults

- Increase the proportion of persons with hearing impairment who have ever used a hearing aid or assistive listening device or who have cochlear implants.
- Increase the proportion of adults 70 years of age who have had a hearing examination in the past 5 years.
- Increase the number of persons who are referred by their primary care physician or other health care provider for hearing evaluation and treatment.
- Increase the proportion of adults bothered by tinnitus who have seen a doctor or other health care professional.
- Increase the proportion of persons with hearing loss and other sensory communication disorders who have used Internet resources for health care information, guidance, or advice in the past 12 months.

Data from U.S. Department of Health and Human Services, Office of Disease Prevention and Health Promotion: *Healthy People 2020,* 2012. http://www.healthypeople.gov/2020.

TABLE 12-1 Changes in Hearing Related to Aging

CHANGES IN STRUCTURE	CHANGES IN FUNCTION
Cochlear hair cell degeneration; Loss of auditory neurons in spiral ganglia of organ of Corti	Inability to hear high-frequency sounds (presbycusis, sensorineural loss); interferes with understanding speech; hearing may be lost in both ears at different times
Degeneration of basilar (cochlear) conductive membrane of cochlea	Inability to hear at all frequencies, but more pronounced at higher frequencies (cochlear conductive loss)
Decreased vascularity of cochlea; Loss of cortical auditory neurons	Equal loss of hearing at all frequencies (strial loss); inability to disseminate localization of sound

From McCance KL, Huether SE: *Pathophysiology,* ed 7, St Louis, MO, 2014, Mosby.

may not be an inevitable part of aging and increased attention is being given to the links between lifestyle factors (e.g., smoking, poor nutrition, hypertension) and hearing impairment (Heine et al, 2013) (Box 12-2).

Consequences of Hearing Impairment

The broad consequences of hearing loss have functional and clinical significance and should not be viewed as something a person accepts as part of aging. Hearing loss diminishes quality of life and is associated with multiple negative outcomes, including decreased function, increased likelihood of hospitalizations, miscommunication, depression, falls, loss of self-esteem, safety risks, and cognitive decline (Bainbridge and Wallhagen, 2014; Lin et al, 2013). Growing evidence supports an association between age-related hearing loss and cognitive decline and dementia (Bainbridge and Wallhagen, 2014; Lin, 2012; Lin et al, 2013).

BOX 12-2 Promoting Healthy Hearing

Avoid exposure to excessively loud noises.
Avoid cigarette smoking.
Maintain blood pressure/cholesterol levels within normal limits.
Eat a healthy diet.
Have hearing evaluated if any changes.
Avoid injury with cotton-tipped applicators and other cleaning materials.

Hearing impairment increases feelings of isolation and may cause older adults to become suspicious or distrustful or to display feelings of paranoia. Because older persons with a hearing loss may not understand or respond appropriately to conversation, they may be inappropriately diagnosed with dementia. All of these consequences of hearing impairment further increase social isolation and decrease opportunities for meaningful interaction and stimulation.

Types of Hearing Loss

The two major forms of hearing loss are conductive and sensorineural. *Sensorineural hearing loss* results from damage to any part of the inner ear or the neural pathways to the brain. *Presbycusis* (also called age-related hearing impairment or ARHI) is a form of sensorineural hearing loss that is related to aging and is the most common form of hearing loss. Presbycusis progressively worsens with age and is usually permanent. The cochlea appears to be the site of pathogenesis, but the precise cause of presbycusis is uncertain (Lewis, 2014).

Noise-induced hearing loss (NIHL) is the second most common cause of sensorineural hearing loss among older adults. Direct mechanical injury to the sensory hair cells of the cochlea causes NIHL, and continuous noise exposure contributes to damage more than intermittent exposure (Lewis, 2014). NIHL is permanent but considered largely preventable. The rate of hearing impairment is expected to rise because of the growing number of older adults and also because of the increased number of military personnel who have been exposed to blast exposure in combat situations. Noise-induced hearing loss may be reduced through the development of better ear-protection devices, education about exposure to loud noise, and emerging research into interventions that may protect or repair hair cells in the ear, which are key to the body's ability to hear (National Institute on Deafness and Other Communication Disorders [NIDCD], 2014).

Presbycusis is a slow, progressive hearing loss that affects both ears equally. Because of its slow progression, many individuals ignore their hearing loss for years, considering it "just part of aging." Only about 40% of adults aged 70 years and older who could benefit from hearing aids use them (Bainbridge and Wallhagen, 2014). It is common to hear older adults deny hearing impairment and accuse others of mumbling. Their spouse or significant other, however, often voices frustration over the hearing loss long before the individual acknowledges it.

One of the first signs of presbycusis is difficulty hearing and understanding speech in noisy environments. Presbycusis begins in the high frequencies and later affects the lower frequencies. High-frequency consonants are important to speech understanding.

Changes related to presbycusis make it difficult to distinguish among some of the sibilant consonants such as *z, s, sh, f, p, k, t,* and *g.* People often raise their voices when speaking to a hearing-impaired person. When this happens, more consonants drop out of speech, making hearing even more difficult. Without consonants, the high-frequency–pitched language becomes disjointed and misunderstood. Older people with presbycusis have difficulty filtering out background noise and often complain of difficulty understanding women's and children's speech and conversations in large groups. Sensorineural hearing loss is treated with hearing aids and, in some cases, cochlear implants.

Conductive hearing loss usually involves abnormalities of the external and middle ear that reduce the ability of sound to be transmitted to the middle ear. Otosclerosis, infection, perforated eardrum, fluid in the middle ear, tumors, or cerumen accumulations cause conductive hearing loss. Cerumen impaction is the most common and easily corrected of all interferences in the hearing of older people (Figure 12-1).

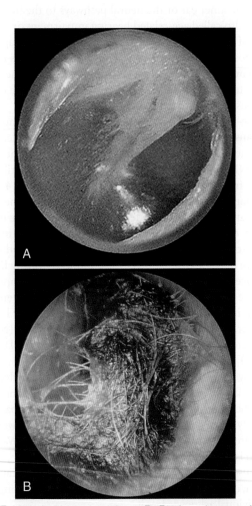

FIGURE 12-1 A, Normal eardrum. **B,** Eardrum impacted with cerumen. (**A,** from Ball JW, Dains JE, Flynn FA, et al: *Seidel's guide to physical examination,* ed 8, St Louis, 2015, Mosby. **B,** from Swartz MH: *Textbook of physical diagnosis,* ed 7, Philadelphia, 2014, Saunders.)

Cerumen interferes with the conduction of sound through air in the eardrum. The reduction in the number and activity of cerumen-producing glands results in a tendency toward cerumen impaction. Long-standing impactions become hard, dry, and dark brown. Individuals at particular risk of impaction are African Americans, individuals who wear hearing aids, and older men with large amounts of ear canal tragi (hairs in the ear) that tend to become entangled with the cerumen. Cerumen impaction has been found to occur in 33% of nursing home residents (Hersh, 2010).

When hearing loss is suspected, or a person with existing hearing loss experiences increasing difficulty, it is important first to check for cerumen impaction as a possible cause. After accurate assessment, if cerumen removal is indicated, it may be removed through irrigation, cerumenolytic products, or manual extraction (Hersh, 2010) (see Safety Alert box). Box 12-3 presents a protocol for cerumen removal.

> ### ⚡ SAFETY ALERT
>
> Do not attempt ear lavage or cerumen removal if the person has a history of ear surgery, ruptured tympanic membrane, otitis externa (swimmer's ear), or ear trauma. Use sterilized equipment to avoid infection and spreading bacteria and use caution in patients with diabetes because of an increased risk of infection.

INTERVENTIONS TO ENHANCE HEARING

Hearing Aids

A hearing aid is a personal amplifying system that includes a microphone, an amplifier, and a loudspeaker. There are numerous types of hearing aids with either analog or digital circuitry. The size, appearance, and effectiveness of hearing aids have greatly improved (decreasing stigma), and many can be programmed to meet specific needs. Digital hearing aids are smaller and have better sound quality and noise reduction, as well as less acoustic feedback; however, they are expensive. The behind-the-ear hearing aid looks like a shrimp and fits around and behind the ear; a small tube sits in the canal to direct the amplified sound. It is less commonly used now than the small, in-the-ear aid, which fits in the concha of the ear (Figure 12-2). Completely-in-the-canal (CIC) hearing aids fit entirely in the ear canal. These types of devices are among the most expensive and require good dexterity. Some models are invisible and placed deep in the ear canal and replaced every 4 months. New hearing aids can be adjusted precisely for noisy environments and telephone usage through software built into Smartphones.

Most individuals can obtain some hearing enhancement with a hearing aid. The kind of device chosen depends on the type of hearing impairment and the cost, but most users will experience hearing improvement with a basic to midlevel hearing aid. The investment in a good hearing aid is considerable, and a good fit is critical. Hearing aids can range in price from about $500 to several thousand dollars per aid, depending on the technology. The cost of hearing aids is usually not covered by health insurance or Medicare, another barrier to purchase.

BOX 12-3 Protocol for Cerumen Removal

Before Cerumen Removal

- Ask the patient if he or she has ever had a problem with his or her eardrum and is currently having ear pain or drainage. If so, refer the person to an otolaryngologist for care.
- Using an otoscope, gently insert it into the ear canal while pulling up on the auricle; while doing so, examine the canal for trauma and the presence of excess cerumen or a cerumen impaction (when the TM is not visible or only partial visible).

Cerumen Removal Procedure*

1. If the cerumen is somewhat dry and close to the canal opening, it may be easily removed with the use of a curette† specially designed for this purpose. Gently scoop the cerumen and bring it forward, being careful to avoid scratching the canal.
2. Once the cerumen is slightly extended from the canal, it can be removed easily with the use of forceps† or clamps.
3. Reexamine the canal for remaining cerumen.
4. If the cerumen is hard and cannot be removed easily, it may be necessary to soften it before further removal. Softening agents may be instilled into the ear before the removal attempt using mineral or olive oil, commercial products, or a liquid stool softener twice daily for 1 to 2 days.

5. Alternatively, hydrogen peroxide may be instilled and allowed to soften the wax several minutes before the removal is attempted. The patient will tell you when the "bubbling has stopped."
6. If it is still not possible to remove the wax safely using the curette, a water flush may be effective.
   a. Protect clothing and linens with a water-proof material.
   b. Follow the directions on a commercial ear irrigating product. This usually involves pumping a small amount of water into the canal through a small short cannula, at which time the water returns into a collection cup with dissolved cerumen (hopefully).
   c. Before the flush, test the water temperature by pumping a few drops on the external ear. The acceptable temperature for the irrigation is highly individual.
   d. Check the canal frequently for effectiveness and check with the patient for tolerability.
   e. During the irrigation, the cerumen will either be returned with the water or brought closer to the surface so that it can be removed with the curette (see procedure 1).
   f. Any time the patient expresses nausea or dizziness, stop immediately and refer to an otolaryngologist for further treatment.

*This should not be attempted without prior demonstration.
†There are now commercially available single-use curettes and ear forceps that are lighted with fiber optics, allowing clear vision of the canal during cerumen removal.
From McCarter DF, Courtney AU, Pollart SM: Cerumen impaction, *Am Fam Physician* 75(10):1523–1528, 2007.

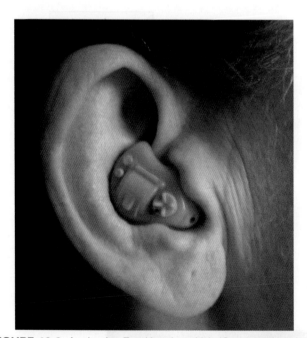

FIGURE 12-2 An In-the-Ear Hearing Aid. (Courtesy Kathleen Jett.)

Adjustment to Hearing Aids

Nearly 50% of people who purchased hearing aids either never began wearing them or stopped wearing them after a short period. Factors contributing to low hearing aid use after purchase include difficulty manipulating the device, annoying loud noises, being exposed to sensory overload, developing headaches, and perceiving stigma. Hearing aids amplify all sounds, making things sound different. People often delay acquiring hearing aids because the loss occurs gradually and they often ignore or deny the loss. Individuals wait on average 7 to 10 years between signs of hearing loss and audiological consultation (Lewis, 2014). This delay makes adjustment to the device even more challenging (Lane and Conn, 2013). More research about factors that influence the decision to seek help for hearing loss is needed (Bainbridge and Wallhagen, 2014).

Lin (2012) suggests that the impression among both the public and health care providers is that a hearing aid is all that is needed to treat hearing loss. Age-related hearing loss (ARHL) is like any other physical impairment and requires counseling, rehabilitative training, environmental accommodations, and patience. Audiology centers, often attached to hospitals, medical centers, and universities, are excellent places for aural rehabilitation programs but costs are usually not covered by Medicare. Audiological rehabilitation programs (both individual and group) may improve central processing deficits and should include auditory-cognitive training, as well as support and education regarding hearing loss and communication strategies for the individual and significant others (Anderson et al, 2013). The Internet may be a valuable tool for aural rehabilitation, as well as for improving adjustment to hearing aids and communication (Lewis, 2014).

It is important for nurses who work with individuals wearing hearing aids to be knowledgeable about the care and maintenance. They can teach the individual, family, or formal caregiver proper use and care of hearing aids (Box 12-4). Many older people experience unnecessary communication problems when in the hospital or nursing home because their hearing aids are not inserted and working properly, or they are lost.

BOX 12-4   **Hearing Aid Care and Use**

- When a hearing aid is first purchased: Initially it is advisable to wear for 15 to 20 minutes per day until one is adjusted to the new sounds.
- Gradually increase the wearing time to 10 to 12 hours.
- Be patient and realize that the process of adaptation is difficult but ultimately will be rewarding.
- Make sure your fingers are dry and clean before handling hearing aids. Use a soft dry cloth to wipe your hearing aids.
- Each day, remove any earwax that has accumulated on the hearing aids. Use the brush that is included with the aid to clean difficult-to-reach areas.
- You will be instructed how to best insert the model you purchase.
- If it is not pre-programmed, adjust the volume to a level that is comfortable for you. You may be able to adjust the volume for differing environments, depending on the model.

- Use great caution to avoid getting the aid wet; do not wear when swimming or taking a shower or bath.
- Also avoid use when around fine particles that can clog the microphone such as hair spray, make-up, or blowing sand and dirt.
- Many aids will slowly decrease in volume and may make a "peep" when it is time to change the battery. Check the battery by turning the hearing aid on, turning up the volume, cupping your hand over the ear mold, and listening. A constant whistling sound indicates that the battery is functioning. A weak sound indicates that the battery is losing power and needs replacement.
- Be sure to remove the battery and return the aid to its case when not in use. This will extend the life of the battery and protect the aid.

From Johns Hopkins Medicine: *Caring for your hearing aid,* 2007. http://www.hopkinsmedicine.org/hearing/hearing_aids/caring_for_hearing_aids.htm. Accessed March 2014.

Cochlear Implants

Cochlear implants are increasingly being used for older adults with sensorineural loss who are not able to gain effective speech recognition with hearing aids. Cochlear implants are safe and well tolerated and improve communication. The surgery is now commonly done bilaterally (Lewis, 2014). A cochlear implant is a small, complex electronic device that consists of an external portion that sits behind the ear and a second portion that is surgically placed under the skin (Figure 12-3). Unlike hearing aids that magnify sounds, the cochlear implant bypasses damaged portions of the ear and directly stimulates the auditory nerve. Hearing through a cochlear implant is different from

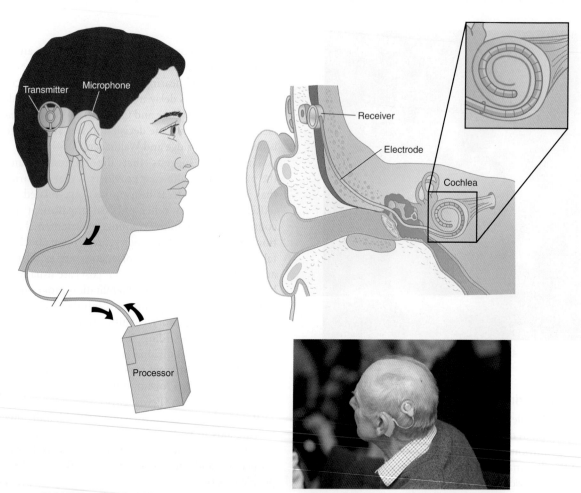

FIGURE 12-3 Cochlear implant. Photo courtesy of the patient. Available at http://ais. southampton.ac.uk/new-programme-launched-help-cochlear-implant-users-enjoy-music/.

normal hearing and takes time to learn or relearn. Most insurance plans cover the cochlear implant procedure. The transplant carries some risk because the surgery destroys any residual hearing. Therefore, cochlear implant users can never revert to using a hearing aid. Individuals with cochlear implants need to be advised to never to have an MRI because it may dislodge the implant or demagnetize its internal magnet.

Assistive Listening and Adaptive Devices

Assistive listening devices (also called personal listening systems) should be considered as an adjunct to hearing aids or used in place of hearing aids for people with hearing impairment. These devices are available commercially and can be used to enhance face-to-face communication and to better understand speech in large rooms such as theaters, to use the telephone, and to listen to television. Many movie theaters have both sound amplifiers and personal subtitle devices available. Hearing loop conduction systems are newer technology and consist of a copper wire that is installed around the periphery of a room or other venue to transmit the microphone or TV sound signal to hearing aids and cochlear implants that have "telecoil" receivers (built into most hearing aids and cochlear implants). Sound from the microphone or TV is received but not background noises. This transforms the hearing aid into loudspeakers delivering sound for one's own hearing loss. These devices are widely used in Europe and becoming more available in the United States in places such as theaters, churches, subway information booths, taxi back seats, and home TV rooms. Cost ranges from $140 to $300 for self-installed home loops (HearingLoop.org, 2014; Lewis, 2014).

Other examples of assistive listening and adaptive devices include text messaging devices for telephones and closed-caption television, now required on all televisions with screens 13 inches and larger. Alerting devices, such as vibrating alarm clocks that shake the bed or activate a flashing light, and sound lamps that respond with lights to sounds, such as doorbells and telephones, are also available. Special service dogs ("hearing dogs") are trained to alert people with a hearing impairment about sounds and intruders. Dogs are trained to respond to different sounds, such as the telephone, smoke alarms, alarm clock, doorbell/door knock, and name call, and lead the individual to the sound.

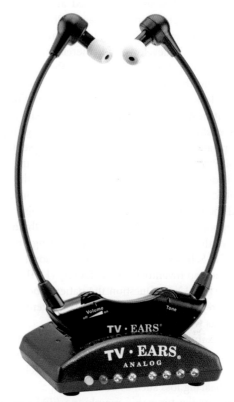

Voice-Clarifying Headset System for TV Listening. (With permission from TV Ears, Inc.)

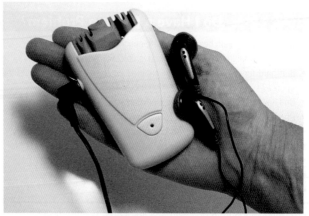

Pocket-Sized Amplifier. (With permission from Sonic Technology Products.)

Amplified Telephone. (With permission from Clarity, a division of Plantronics, Inc.)

The use of computers and email also assists individuals with hearing impairment to communicate more easily. Programs such as Skype and Face Time are also beneficial because they may allow the person to lip read and to adjust volume. Pocket-sized amplifiers (available at retail stores) are especially helpful in improving communication in health care settings, and nurses should be able to obtain appropriate devices for use with hearing-impaired individuals.

PROMOTING HEALTHY AGING: IMPLICATIONS FOR GERONTOLOGICAL NURSING

Assessment

Hearing impairment is underdiagnosed and undertreated in older people (Bainbridge and Wallhagen, 2014). Older people may be initially unaware of hearing loss because of the gradual manner in which it develops and, therefore, not report any problems. Despite gathering evidence of the consequences of hearing loss and the inadequacy of detection, the U.S. Preventive Services Task Force (USPSTF) (2012) does not recommend routine adult hearing screening due to inadequate evidence of the effectiveness. However, screening for hearing impairment and appropriate treatment are considered an essential part of primary care for older adults. Assessment of hearing includes a focused history and physical examination and also screening assessment for hearing impairment. Ask the person if he or she has any difficulty understanding speech in noisy situations, during telephone use, or in daily conversation. Obtaining information from the significant other about hearing problems can also be useful. Self-assessment instruments (Box 12-5) and the Hearing Handicap Inventory for the Elderly (HHIE-S) can also be included (Box 12-6). Question the patient about prolonged noise exposure, past ear injuries, and use of potentially ototoxic medications as well.

Physical examination includes assessing the external ear to determine any evidence of infection and using an otoscope to visualize the inner ear, looking for any possible causes of conductive hearing loss such as cerumen impaction or foreign objects. Inspect the tympanic membrane (TM) for integrity.

BOX 12-6   RESOURCES FOR BEST PRACTICE

Hearing Impairment

- **American Tinnitus Association:** Sounds of Tinnitus
- **Hartford Institute for Geriatric Nursing (Try This General Assessment Series):** Hearing Handicap for the Elderly: Screening Version (HHIT-S).
- **NIDCD (National Institute on Deafness and Other Communication Disorders):** Hearing loss and older adults; Interactive sound ruler: how loud is too loud (experience noise levels).
- **NIH Senior Health:** Hearing Loss (patient information)
- **Sight and Hearing Association:** Unfair Hearing Test/Filtered Speech (experience presbycusis).

Depending on findings, the patient may need to be referred for follow-up by a specialist. If no problems are identified, perform a few basic screening tests. These may include the Rinne and Weber tests to differentiate between conductive and sensorineural hearing loss. Other tests include the whisper and finger rub test.

Interventions

Nursing actions are based on assessment findings and may include referral to an audiologist, education on hearing loss (including prevention and consequences), hearing aids, assistive listening devices, and communication techniques. If cerumen impaction is found, cerumen removal may be indicated (see Box 12-3). There are many evidence-based resources available that can be used to educate the patient and family and assist the nurse in designing educational materials (Box 12-6). Using the information presented in this chapter, nurses can play an important role in providing older adults the information they need to improve their hearing and avoid the negative consequences of untreated hearing loss. Effective communication strategies when working with individuals who are hearing-impaired are presented in Box 12-7.

Margaret Wallhagen, director of the John A. Hartford Center for Excellence in Gerontological Nursing Education at the

BOX 12-5   Do I Have a Hearing Problem?

- Do I have a problem hearing on the telephone?
- Do I have trouble hearing when there is noise in the background?
- Is it hard for me to follow a conversation when two or more people talk at once?
- Do I have to strain to understand a conversation?
- Do many people I talk to seem to mumble (or not speak clearly)?
- Do I misunderstand what others are saying and respond inappropriately?
- Do I have trouble understanding the speech of women and children?
- Do people complain that I turn the TV volume up too high?
- Do I hear a ringing, roaring, or hissing sound a lot?
- Do some sounds seem too loud?

From National Institute on Deafness and Other Communication Disorders: *Hearing loss and older adults,* 2014. http://www.nidcd.nih.gov/health/hearing/pages/older.aspx#2. Accessed October 31, 2014.

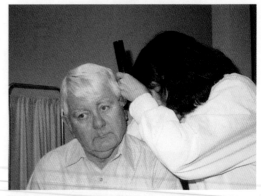

Proper Technique for an Otoscopic Examination. (From Ignatavicius DD, Workman ML: *Medical-surgical nursing: patient-centered collaborative care,* ed 6, St Louis, 2010, Saunders.)

Communication with Individuals with Hearing Impairment

- Never assume hearing loss is from age until other causes are ruled out (infection, cerumen buildup).
- Inappropriate responses, inattentiveness, and apathy may be symptoms of a hearing loss.
- Face the individual, and stand or sit on the same level; do not turn away while speaking (e.g., face a computer).
- Gain the individual's attention before beginning to speak. Look directly at the person at eye level before starting to speak.
- Determine if hearing is better in one ear than another, and position yourself appropriately.
- If hearing aid is used, make sure it is in place and batteries are functioning.
- Ask patient or family what helps the person to hear best.
- Keep hands away from your mouth and project voice by controlled diaphragmatic breathing.
- Avoid conversations in which the speaker's face is in glare or darkness; orient the light on the speaker's face.
- Lower your tone of voice, articulate clearly, and use a moderate rate of speech.
- If the person is in a hospital or nursing facility, label the chart, note on the intercom button, and inform all caregivers that the patient has a hearing impairment.
- Use nonverbal approaches: gestures, demonstrations, visual aids, and written materials.
- Pause between sentences or phrases to confirm understanding.
- Restate with different words when you are not understood.
- When changing topics, preface the change by stating the topic.
- Reduce background noise (e.g., turn off television, close door).
- Utilize assistive listening devices such as pocket talker.
- Verify that the information being given has been clearly understood. Be aware that the person may agree to everything and appear to understand what you have said even when he or she did not hear you (listener bluffing).
- Share resources for the hearing-impaired and refer as appropriate.

From Adams-Wendling L, Pimple C: Evidence-based guideline: nursing management of hearing impairment in nursing facility residents, *J Gerontol Nurs* 34(11):9–16, 2008.

University of California San Francisco School of Nursing, is one of the leading nurse researchers investigating hearing impairment in older adults. Her current research, funded by the National Institutes of Health, is a good example of the contributions nursing research makes to the care of older adults (Box 12-8).

TINNITUS

Tinnitus is defined as the perception of sound in one or both ears or in the head when no external sound is present. It is often referred to as "ringing in the ears" but may also manifest as buzzing, hissing, whistling, cricket chirping, bells, roaring, clicking, pulsating, humming, or swishing sounds. The sounds may be constant or intermittent and are more acute at night or in quiet surroundings. The most common type is high-pitched tinnitus with sensorineural loss; less common is low-pitched tinnitus with conduction loss such as is seen in Meniere's disease.

The NIH-funded study will compare the outcomes of three interventions for hearing loss for older adults who are not currently wearing hearing aids and who screen positive as at risk for hearing loss on subsequent access to and use of hearing health care services. Participants will receive one of three interventions: (1) screening only with statement that the person should obtain follow-up evaluation; (2) screening with an educational brochure on hearing loss, hearing aids, and assistive listening devices; and (3) screening with educational brochures on hearing loss, hearing aids, and assistive listening devices and brief training by a knowledgeable professional. The study will follow patients for 8 months and track and compare the costs of clinical time and the use and benefits of hearing health services by those screened. Results of studies such as this will help guide the choice of interventions to promote the best outcome.

Data from NIH Research Portfolio Online Reporting Tools: *Primary care intervention promoting hearing healthcare service* (project no. 4R33DC011510-03), 2014. http://projectreporter.nih.gov/project_info_description.cfm?aid=8607610 Accessed February 14, 2014.

Tinnitus generally increases over time. It is a condition that afflicts many older people and can interfere with hearing, as well as become extremely irritating. It is estimated to occur in nearly 11% of elders with presbycusis. Approximately 50 million people in the United States have tinnitus and about 2 million are so seriously debilitated that they cannot function on a "normal," day-to-day basis. Tinnitus is a growing problem for America's military personnel and is the leading cause of service-connected disability of veterans returning from Iraq or Afghanistan (American Tinnitus Association, 2013).

The exact physiological cause or causes of tinnitus are not known, but there are several likely factors that are known to trigger or worsen tinnitus. Exposure to loud noises is the leading cause of tinnitus, and the exposure can damage and destroy cilia in the inner ear. Once damaged, the cilia cannot be renewed or replaced. Other possible causes of tinnitus include head and neck trauma, certain types of tumors, cerumen accumulation, jaw misalignment, cardiovascular disease, and ototoxicity from medications. More than 200 prescription and nonprescription medications list tinnitus as a potential side effect, aspirin being the most common. There is some evidence that caffeine, alcohol, cigarettes, stress, and fatigue may exacerbate the problem.

Interventions

Some persons with tinnitus will never find the cause; for others the problem may arbitrarily disappear. Hearing aids can be prescribed to amplify environmental sounds to obscure tinnitus, and there is a device that combines the features of a masker and a hearing aid, which emits a competitive but pleasant sound that distracts from head noise. Therapeutic modes of treating tinnitus include transtympanal electrostimulation, iontophoresis, biofeedback, tinnitus masking with alternative sound production (white noise), cochlear implants, and hearing aids. Some have found hypnosis, cognitive behavioral therapy, acupuncture, and chiropractic, naturopathic, allergy, or drug treatment to be effective.

Nursing actions include discussions with the client regarding times when the noises are most irritating and having the person keep a diary to identify patterns. Assess medications for possibly contributing to the problem. Discuss lifestyle changes and alternative methods that some have found effective. Also, refer clients to the American Tinnitus Association for research updates, education, and support groups (see Box 12-6).

KEY CONCEPTS

- Hearing impairment is the third most prevalent chronic condition among older Americans and the foremost communicative disorder.
- Age-related hearing impairment is a complex disease caused by interactions among age-related changes, genetics, lifestyle, and environment.
- The two major forms of hearing loss are conductive and sensorineural.
- *Presbycusis* (also called age-related hearing impairment or ARHI) is a form of sensorineural hearing loss that is related to aging and is the most common form of hearing loss.

- Hearing aids and cochlear implants are used to improve hearing, and both require a period of adjustment and education.
- Hearing loss diminishes quality of life and is associated with multiple negative outcomes including decreased function, increased likelihood of hospitalizations, miscommunication, depression, falls, loss of self-esteem, safety risks, and cognitive decline.
- Screening for hearing loss is an essential component of assessment in older adults.
- Nurses need to know how to operate hearing aids and assist individuals with hearing impairment to access assistive listening devices to enhance communication.

NURSING STUDY: HEARING IMPAIRMENT

Sonya is a 66-year-old high school nurse/consultant. She retired from the Army Nurse Corps with an officer's rank after serving 20 years, much of it in the Korean conflict with heavy exposure to shelling in the early part of her career. She became aware of hearing loss at about age 45, and by age 55 years it had become severe. While in the service she had considerable assistance from noncommissioned personnel and functioned well. When she entered civilian life, it became more difficult for her to manage but she was unwilling to admit to others her major hearing deficit. During those years she simply attempted to cover it as much as possible, and some of her coworkers thought she was rather obtuse; others suspected her deafness. When she took the position with the school district, she was involved with three high schools, numerous faculty members, and students, and interpersonal communication was a major aspect of her position. When she was evaluated at the end of the first year, it was pointed out that feedback indicated she was inattentive. She did then admit her hearing problem and was advised to get a hearing aid. She said, "I've known several people over the years who have hearing aids, and none of them were really satisfied with them. I guess that is why I have not gotten them before now." She complied but, after a few weeks, rarely wore her hearing aids. The personnel officer of the school board, after hearing several more complaints of inappropriate communication, told her she must wear the hearing aids if she wished to continue in her position. Sonya knew that hearing aids were essential, not only for communication but also for safety—she had almost been hit by a car while walking because she simply did not hear it coming. Yet she did not want to go back to the audiology clinic, because they did not seem to know what they were doing, and each time she saw someone, the person gave her different information. She tried three different types of aids that seemed of little help. She lost confidence in her ear, nose, and throat specialist because he had been unable to help her resolve the ringing in her ears. Now her school district had contracted with a health maintenance organization, and she was not even sure which health care provider she should see.

On the basis of the nursing study, develop a nursing care plan using the following procedure*:

- List Sonya's comments that provide subjective data.
- List information that provides objective data.
- From these data identify and state, using accepted format, two nursing diagnoses you determine are most significant to Sonya at this time. List two of Sonya's strengths that you have identified from data.
- Determine and state outcome criteria for each diagnosis. These must reflect some alleviation of the problem identified in the nursing diagnosis and must be stated in concrete and measurable terms.
- Plan and state one or more interventions for each diagnosed problem. Provide specific documentation of the source used to determine the appropriate intervention. Plan at least one intervention that incorporates Sonya's existing strengths.
- Evaluate the success of the intervention. Interventions must correlate directly with the stated outcome criteria to measure the outcome success.

*Students are advised to refer to their nursing diagnosis text and identify possible or potential problems.

CRITICAL THINKING QUESTIONS AND ACTIVITIES

1. What are some of the possible reasons Sonya suffered severe hearing loss at so young an age?
2. Discuss the stigma of hearing loss and hearing aids.
3. Obtain a "hearing aid loaner." Instruct students to wear it for several hours and report their reactions in writing. List difficulties experienced.
4. How would you advise Sonya if you were her nurse/friend?
5. Discuss the various kinds of hearing aids and explain how they differ.
6. Discuss reasons Sonya may have discontinued wearing her hearing aids.

7. What might you suggest that would be helpful in adapting to wearing a hearing aid?
8. Which of the various sensory/perceptual changes of aging would you find most difficult to handle?
9. Discuss the meanings and the thoughts triggered by the student's and elder's viewpoints expressed at the beginning of the chapter. How do these vary from your own experience?

RESEARCH QUESTIONS

1. What do older people think is helpful in enhancing communication with individuals experiencing hearing impairment?
2. What strategies are most effective in facilitating adaptation to hearing aids?
3. What are the challenges for older people and their families/significant others in living with hearing loss?
4. What is the knowledge level of professional nurses related to hearing impairment and communication strategies to enhance communication?
5. What is the relationship between stigma and denial of hearing loss and wearing hearing aids?

REFERENCES

American Tinnitus Association: *ATA's top 10 most frequently asked questions*, 2013. http://www.ata.org/for-patients/faqs. Accessed October 31, 2014.

Anderson S, White-Schwoch T, Choi H, et al: Training changes processing of speech cues in older adults with hearing loss, *Front Syst Neurosci* 7(97):97, 2013.

Bainbridge K, Wallhagen M: Hearing loss in an aging American population: extent, impact, management, *Ann Rev Public Health* 35:139–152, 2014.

HearingLoop.org: *Getting hard of hearing people in the loop*, 2014. http://www.hearing loop.org. Accessed February 28, 2014.

Heine C, Browning C, Cowlishaw S, et al: Trajectories of older adults' hearing difficulties: examining the influence of health behaviors and social activity over 10 years, *Geriatr Gerontol Int* 13(4): 911–918, 2013.

Hersh S: Cerumen: insights and management, *Ann Longterm Care* 18:39, 2010.

Keller H: *The story of my life*, Garden City, NY, 1902, Doubleday.

Lane K, Conn V: To hear or not to hear, *Res Gerontol Nurs* 6(2):79–80, 2013.

Lewis T: Hearing impairment. In Ham R, Sloane P, Warshaw G, et al, editors: *Primary care geriatrics*, ed 6, Philadelphia, 2014, Elsevier Saunders, pp 291–300.

Lin F: Hearing loss in older adults—who's listening? *JAMA* 307(11):1147–1148, 2012.

Lin F, Yaffe K, Xia Y, et al: Hearing loss and cognitive decline in older adults, *JAMA Intern Med* 173(4):293–299, 2013.

National Institute on Deafness and Other Communication Disorders (NIDCD): *Noise-induced hearing loss* (NIH publication no. 14-4233), 2014. http://www.nidcd.nih.gov/health/hearing/pages/noise.aspx. Accessed August 2014.

Sacks O: *Seeing voices: a journey into the world of the deaf*, Berkeley, 1989, University of California Press.

U.S. Preventive Services Task Force: Screening for hearing loss in older adults, *Ann Intern Med* 157:655–661, 2012. http://www.guideline.gov/content.aspx?id=38356. Accessed October 2014.

Skin Care

Theris A. Touhy

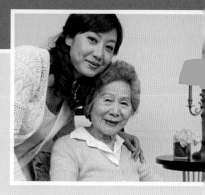

http://evolve.elsevier.com/Touhy/TwdHlthAging

A GRANDCHILD SPEAKS

An elderly woman and her little grandson, whose face was sprinkled with bright freckles,
spent the day at the zoo. Lots of children were waiting in line to get their cheeks painted by a local artist who was decorating them with tiger paws.
"You've got so many freckles, there's no place to paint!" a girl in the line said to the little fellow.
Embarrassed, the little boy dropped his head. His grandmother knelt down next to him.
"I love your freckles. When I was a little girl I always wanted freckles," she said, while
tracing her finger across the child's cheek. "Freckles are beautiful."
The boy looked up, "Really?"
"Of course," said the grandmother. "Why just name me one thing that's prettier than freckles?"
The little boy thought for a moment, peered intensely into his grandma's face, and softly
whispered, "Wrinkles."

A STUDENT SPEAKS

My mother is always on me to take care of my skin so that it will look good when I am older. Stay out of the tanning salon and the sun, wear sunscreen all the time, use moisturizer. It's hard to think that 50 years from now I might not have this beautiful skin anymore unless I take better care of it now. Mom keeps pointing to a magnet on her refrigerator: "Wrinkled was not one of the things I wanted to be when I was older."

Janine, age 19

AN ELDER SPEAKS

I have that white Irish skin and have really had a lot of problems ever since I was 40 with pre-cancerous lesions and even a basal cell skin cancer or two. Of course, we didn't know about sunscreen when I was growing up and I remember lathering myself with baby oil and iodine to get a good tan (or a bad burn). I am pretty obsessive about going to the dermatologist every 3 months and staying out of the sun. A year ago she saw an area on my back that looked suspicious, so a biopsy was done. Turned out it was a melanoma and was removed by a plastic surgeon, who told me that I was lucky it was found or I would have been dead in 6 months. The area was not unusual looking at all—no change, no irritation, no irregular borders, no elevation—looked like nothing. Best advice I can give is to make the skin checks regular. It may save your life.

Bob, age 70

A WOUND CARE NURSE SPEAKS

"Everyone wants to look at a cardiac case, but it is harder to get people interested in pressure ulcers."

Mark Collier, Tissue Viability Nurse, United Lincolnshire Hospital Trust
(Nursing Times.net, October 22, 2013).

LEARNING OBJECTIVES

On completion of this chapter, the reader will be able to:
1. Identify age-related changes in the integument.
2. Identify skin problems commonly found in later life.
3. Identify preventive, maintenance, and restorative measures for skin health.
4. Identify risk factors for pressure ulcers and design interventions for prevention and evidence-based treatment.

Gerontological nurses have an instrumental role in promoting the health of the skin of the persons who seek their care. The skin may often be overlooked when the focus is on management of disease or acute problems. However, skin problems can be challenging concerns, affecting health and compromising quality of life. Thorough assessment and intervention based on age-related evidence-based protocols is important to healthy aging and best practice gerontological nursing.

SKIN

The skin is the largest organ of the body and has at least seven physiological functions (Box 13-1). Exposure to heat, cold, water, trauma, friction, and pressure notwithstanding, the skin's function is to maintain a homeostatic environment. Healthy skin is durable, pliable, and strong enough to protect the body by absorbing, reflecting, cushioning, and restricting various substances and forces that might enter and alter its function, yet it is sensitive enough to relay subtle messages to the brain. When the integument malfunctions or is overwhelmed, discomfort, disfigurement, or death may ensue. However, the nurse can both promptly recognize and help to prevent many of the sources of danger to a person's skin in the promotion of the best possible health.

Many age-related changes in the skin are visible; similar changes in other organs of the body are not as readily observed. Although there are some changes related to the aging process, genetics and environmental factors (ultraviolet [UV] radiation, tobacco smoke, inflammatory responses, and gravity) contribute to these changes (McCann and Huether, 2014). Many skin problems are seen with aging, both in health and when compromised by illness or mobility limitations. Even though many worry about wrinkles and gray hair, the most common skin problems of aging are xerosis (dry skin), pruritus, seborrheic keratosis, herpes zoster, and cancer. Those who are immobilized or medically fragile are at risk for fungal infections and pressure ulcers, both major threats to wellness. Table 13-1 provides an overview of skin changes related to aging.

BOX 13-1 Physiological Functions of the Skin

- Protects underlying structures.
- Regulates body temperature.
- Serves as a vehicle for sensation.
- Stores fat.
- Is a component of the metabolism of salt and water.
- Is a site for two-way gas exchange.
- Is a site for the production of vitamin D when exposed to sunlight.

TABLE 13-1 Changes in the Integument Related to Aging

CHANGES	EFFECTS
Skin	
Epidermis	
Melanocytes decrease	Lightening of overall skin tone; decreased protection against UV radiation
Keratinocytes smaller; regeneration slower	Slowed wound healing
Noncancerous pigmented spots (freckles, nevi) enlarge	Mostly cosmetic
Increased lentigine ("age" or "liver" spots) and seborrheic keratosis common	Mostly cosmetic (see Figure 13-2)
Dermatosis papulosa nigra, variant of keratosis in dark skin, increases	Clinically insignificant (see Figure 13-2)
Dermis	
20% loss of thickness	Skin more transparent and fragile; skin tears/bruising occur easily
Dermal blood vessels decrease	Skin pallor and cooler skin temperature; increased susceptibility to skin cancer; diminished dermal clearance, absorption, and immunological response
Cross-linking increases; collagen synthesis decreases	Skin "gives less" under stress and tears easily
Elastin fibers thicken and fragment	Loss of stretch and elasticity; "sagging" appearance
Decreased sebum production	Skin becomes drier; risk for cracking and xerosis increases

Continued

TABLE 13-1   Changes in the Integument Related to Aging—cont'd

CHANGES	EFFECTS
Hypodermis	
Shifting of subcutaneous fat; loss of subcutaneous tissue	Skinfolds on the back of the hand diminish even with substantial weight gain; more risk for injury as cushioning decreases; wrinkling and sagging of skin
Reduced efficiency of eccrine glands	Temperature regulation compromised; risk for hyperthermia and hypothermia; moisture evaporates quickly; skin is drier
Fewer Meissner's/Pacinian corpuscles	Diminished tactile sensitivity; increased susceptibility to injury
Decreased Langerhans cells	Reduces skin's immune response
Hair	
Diminished melanocytes; loss of hair follicles	50% of population have gray or partly gray hair
Other changes	Men experience hair loss in vertex, frontal, and temporal areas; by 60 years, 80% of men are substantially bald; less pronounced in women. Race, gender, sex-linked genes, and hormonal balance influence maximum amount hair one has and the changes that occur throughout life
	Terminal hair can occur in face and chin area in women after menopause
	Amount of hair increases in ears, nose, eyebrows; axillary, extremity, and pubic hair diminishes or disappears
Nails	
Decreased circulation	Fingernails and toenails thicken and change in shape and color
	Nails become brittle, flat, or concave rather than convex; longitudinal striations; may appear yellow or grayish with poorly defined or absent lunulae; cuticle becomes thick and wide
	Onychogryphosis (thickening and distortion of nail plate) and fungal infection (onycholysis) common but not part of normal aging

COMMON SKIN PROBLEMS

Xerosis

Xerosis is extremely dry, cracked, and itchy skin. Xerosis is the most common skin problem experienced and may be linked to a dramatic age-associated decrease in the amount of epidermal filaggrin, a protein required for binding keratin filaments into macrofibrils. This leads to separation of dermal and epidermal surfaces, which compromises the nutrient transfer between the two layers of the skin. Xerosis occurs primarily in the extremities, especially the legs, but can affect the face and the trunk as well. The thinner epidermis of older skin makes it less efficient, allowing more moisture to escape. Inadequate fluid intake worsens xerosis as the body will pull moisture from the skin in an attempt to combat systemic dehydration. Box 13-2 presents Tips for Best Practice in prevention and treatment of xerosis.

Pruritus

One of the consequences of xerosis is *pruritus*, that is, itchy skin. It is a symptom, not a diagnosis or disease, and is a threat to skin integrity because of the attempts to relieve it by scratching. It is aggravated by perfumed detergents, fabric softeners, heat, sudden temperature changes, pressure, vibration, electrical stimuli, sweating, restrictive clothing, fatigue, exercise, and anxiety. Medication side effects are another common cause of pruritus. Pruritus also may accompany systemic disorders such as chronic renal failure and biliary or hepatic disease. Subacute to chronic, generalized pruritus that awakens the individual is an indication to look for secondary causes (especially lymphoma or hematological conditions) (Endo and Norman, 2014).

BOX 13-2   TIPS FOR BEST PRACTICE

Prevention and Treatment of Xerosis

Assessment
- Evaluate for dehydration, nutritional deficiencies, and systemic diseases (diabetes mellitus, hypothyroidism, renal disease), open lesions.
- Determine precipitating and alleviating factors.
- Evaluate current treatment and effectiveness.

Interventions
- Maintain environment of 60% humidity.
- Promote adequate fluid intake; skin can only be rehydrated with water.
- Creams, lubricants, emollients should be applied to towel-patted dry, damp skin immediately after a bath; water-laden emulsions without perfumes or alcohol should be used.
- Mineral oil or vaseline is effective and more economical than commercial lotions and oils.
- Use only tepid water for bathing; avoid long-duration baths; daily baths and showers may not be needed; advise sponge bathing.
- Use super-fatted soaps or skin cleansers (Cetaphil, Dove, Caress soaps; Neutrogena and Oil of Olay bath washes); avoid deodorant soaps except in places such as axilla and groin.
- In cases of extreme dryness, petroleum jelly can be applied to affected area before bed (can use cotton gloves and socks to cover hands/feet).

The gerontological nurse should always listen carefully to the patient's ideas of why the pruritus is occurring, as well as the patient's description of aggravating and relieving factors. If rehydration of the stratum corneum (outer layer of the skin) and other measures to prevent and treat xerosis are not sufficient to control itching, cool compresses or oatmeal or Epsom salt baths may be helpful. Failure to control the itching increases the risk for eczema, excoriations, cracks in the skin, inflammation, and infection arising from the usually linear excoriations resulting from scratching. The nurse should be alert to signs of infection.

Scabies

Scabies is a skin condition that causes intense itching, particularly at night. Scabies is caused by a tiny burrowing mite called *Sarcoptes scabiei.* Scabies is contagious and can be passed easily by an infested person to his or her household members, caregivers, or sexual partners. Scabies can spread easily through close physical contact in a family, childcare group, or school class. Scabies outbreaks have occurred among patients, visitors, and staff in institutions such as nursing homes and hospitals. These types of outbreaks are frequently the result of delayed diagnosis and treatment of crusted (Norwegian) scabies. Some immunocompromised, disabled, or debilitated persons are at risk for this form of scabies.

In addition, individuals with crusted scabies have thick crusts of skin that contain large numbers of scabies mites and eggs. In addition to spreading through skin-to-skin contact, crusted scabies can transmit indirectly through contamination of clothing, linen, and furniture. Because the characteristic itching and rash of scabies can be absent in crusted scabies, there may be misdiagnosis and delayed or inadequate treatment and continued transmission. To diagnose scabies, a close skin examination is conducted to look for signs of mites, including their characteristic burrows. A scraping may be taken from an area of skin for microscopic examination to determine the presence of mites or their eggs.

Scabies treatment involves eliminating the infestation with prescribed lotions and creams. Two or more applications, about a week apart, may be necessary, especially for crusted scabies. Treatment is usually provided to family members and other close contacts even if they show no signs of scabies infestation. Medication kills the mites, but itching may not stop for several weeks. Oral medications may be prescribed for individuals with altered immune systems, for those with crusted scabies, or for those who do not respond to prescription lotions and creams. All clothes and linen used at least three times before treatment should be washed in hot, soapy water and dried with high heat. Rooms used by the person with crusted scabies should be thoroughly cleaned and vacuumed (Centers for Disease Control and Prevention [CDC], 2010).

Purpura

Thinning of the dermis leads to increased fragility of the dermal capillaries and to easy rupture of blood vessels with minimal trauma. Extravasation of the blood into the surrounding tissue, commonly seen on the dorsal forearm and hands, is called *purpura.* Most cases are not related to a pathological condition. The incidence of purpura increases with age due to the normal changes in the skin. Persons who take blood thinners are especially prone to easily acquiring purpura. For those who find that they are prone to purpura, it is advisable to use protective garments—such as long-sleeved pants and shirts. Health care personnel must be advised to be gentle while providing care to persons with sensitive or easily traumatized skin.

Skin Tears

Skin tears occur commonly in persons with thin and fragile skin, and they occur to persons in all settings, from persons in long-term care to active persons in the community They are painful, acute, accidental wounds, perhaps more prevalent than pressure ulcers, and are largely preventable. Skin tears should be classified using the Payne-Martin classification system: Category 1—a skin tear without tissue loss; Category 2—a skin tear with partial tissue loss; and Category 3—a skin tear with complete tissue loss where the epidermal flap is absent (Ayello and Sibbald, 2012).

Management of skin tears includes proper assessment of skin tear category, control of bleeding, cleansing with nontoxic solutions (normal saline or nonionic surfactant cleaners) at safe pressures, use of appropriate dressings that provide moist wound healing, protection of periwound skin, management of exudate, prevention of infection, and implementation of prevention protocols and education. Skin flaps, if present, should not be removed but instead rolled back over the open, cleaned area. Steri-strips can be very useful; suturing is not recommended. Dressing recommendations can be found in the Skin Tear Tool Kit (LeBlanc and Baranoski, 2013) or online at www.skintears.org (Box 13-3). Box 13-4 presents a skin tear protocol.

BOX 13-3   RESOURCES FOR BEST PRACTICE

Pressure Ulcer Prevention and Treatment

Agency for Healthcare Research and Quality: Preventing pressure ulcers in hospitals: a toolkit for improving quality of care

Agency for Healthcare Research and Quality: Pressure ulcer prevention and treatment protocol: www.guideline.gov

Agency for Healthcare Research and Quality: On-time pressure ulcer healing project: http://www.ahrq.gov/professionals/systems/long-term-care/resources/pressure-ulcers/pressureulcerhealing/index.html

Agency for Healthcare Research and Quality: Preventing pressure ulcers in hospitals: a toolkit for improving quality of care: http://www.ahrq.gov/professionals/systems/long-term-care/resources/pressure-ulcers/pressureulcerhealing/index.htm.

Ayello E, Sibbald G: Preventing pressure ulcers and skin tears. In Boltz M, Capezuti E, Fulmer T, et al, editors: *Evidence-based geriatric nursing protocols for best practice,* New York, 2012, Springer, pp 298-323. Also available at Hartford Institute for Geriatric Nursing: *Want to know more: Nursing standard of practice protocol: pressure ulcer prevention and skin tear prevention,* consultgerirn.org

Hartford Institute for Geriatric Nursing: Braden Scale and video demonstrating use of Braden Scale; Nursing Standard of Practice Protocol: Pressure ulcer preventions and skin tear prevention

National Pressure Ulcer Advisory Panel (NPUAP): International Pressure Ulcer Prevention Guidelines (available in 17 languages); Pressure ulcer scale for healing (PUSH): PUSH Tool 3.0, Pressure Ulcer Healing Chart, Pressure Ulcer Prevention Points, Support Surface Standards Initiative, Pressure Ulcer Photos, and other educational materials on prevention and treatment also available online and via an application for iPhones, iPads, and Android devices

NICHE: Need to know for patients and families: skin care: pressure ulcers

Perry D, Borchert K, Burke S, Chick K, et al: Institute for Clinical Systems Improvement, Pressure Ulcer Prevention and Treatment Protocol. Available from Institute for Clinical Systems Improvement: www.icsi.org.

SkinTears.org: Skin Tears Tool Kit, State of the Science Consensus Statements, educational materials

BOX 13-4 TIPS FOR BEST PRACTICE

Skin Tears: Prevention and Treatment

Prevention

- Identify high-risk individuals: impaired activity, mobility, sensation, cognition. Patients who are dependent are at greatest risk. Top causes of skin tears are equipment injury, patient transfers, activities of daily living, and treatment and dressing removal.
- Have individual wear long sleeves or pants to protect extremities.
- Provide a safe environment (adequate lighting, uncluttered rooms).
- Ensure adequate hydration and nutrition; provide a nutritional consultation.
- Lubricate skin with hypoallergenic moisturizer twice daily; apply to damp skin after bathing.
- Perform careful transfers; use a lift sheet to move and turn patients.
- Pad bed rails, wheelchair arms, leg supports, and furniture edges.
- Support dangling arms and legs with pillows/blankets.
- Avoid use of adhesive products. Use nonadherent dressings and paper tape only as needed.
- Use gauze wrap, stockinettes, flexible netting, or other wraps to secure dressings.
- Use no-rinse, soapless bathing products and warm/tepid water for bathing.
- Caregivers need to keep nails short and not wear jewelry that can catch and contribute to skin tears.
- Educate patients, staff, and health care providers regarding prevention and management.

Treatment

- If skin tear occurs, assess and classify according to Payne-Martin classification system and assess size as well.
- Gently cleanse skin with normal saline.
- Air dry or pat dry carefully.
- Approximate skin tear flap if present; consider Steri-Strips; do not suture.
- Use nonadherent dressings.
- Use skin sealants to protect surrounding skin.
- Consider drawing an arrow to indicate direction of skin tear to minimize further injury during dressing removal; consider doing a wound tracing.
- Document assessment and treatment findings.

Data from Ayello E, Sibbald R: Preventing pressure ulcers and skin tears. In Boltz M, Capezuti E, Fulmer T, et al, editors: *Evidence-based geriatric nursing protocols for best practice*, ed 4, New York, 2012, Springer, pp 298–323. Also available at Hartford Institute for Geriatric Nursing: *Want to know more: Nursing standard of practice protocol: pressure ulcer prevention and skin tear prevention*, http://consultgerirn.org/topics/pressure_ulcers_and_skin_tears/want_to_know_more Accessed October 31, 2014; LeBlanc K, Baranoski S: Skin tears: state of the science: consensus statements for the prevention, prediction, assessment and treatment of skin tears, *Adv Skin Wound Care* 24(Suppl 9):2–15, 2011.

Keratoses

There are two types of keratosis: seborrheic and actinic. *Actinic keratosis* is a precancerous lesion, and *seborrheic keratosis* is a benign growth that appears mainly on the trunk, the face, the neck, and the scalp as single or multiple lesions. One or more lesions are present on nearly all adults older than 65 years and are more common in men. An individual may have dozens of these benign lesions. Seborrheic keratosis is a waxy, raised lesion, flesh colored or pigmented in various sizes. The lesions have a "stuck-on" appearance, as if they could be scraped off. Seborrheic keratoses may be removed by a dermatologist for cosmetic reasons (Figure 13-1). A variant seen in darkly

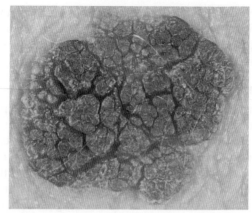

FIGURE 13-1 Seborrheic Keratosis in an Older Adult. (From Habif TP: *Clinical dermatology: a color guide to diagnosis and therapy,* ed 5, St Louis, MO, 2010, Mosby.)

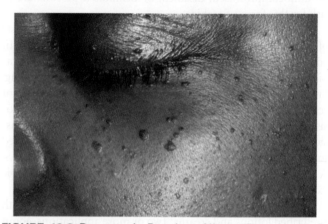

FIGURE 13-2 Dermatosis Papulosa Nigra. (From Neville B, Damm DD, Allen CM, et al: *Oral and maxillofacial pathology,* ed 3, St Louis, MO, 2009, Saunders.)

pigmented persons occurs mostly on the face and appears as numerous small, dark, possibly taglike lesions (Figure 13-2).

Actinic keratosis is a precancerous lesion that is thought to be in the middle of the spectrum between photoaging changes and squamous cell carcinoma (Endo and Norman, 2014). It is directly related to years of overexposure to UV light. Risk factors are older age and fair complexion. It is found on the face, the lips, and the hands and forearms—areas of chronic sun exposure in everyday life. Actinic keratosis is characterized by rough, scaly, sandpaper-like patches, pink to reddish-brown on an erythematous base (Figure 13-3). Lesions may be single or multiple; they may be painless or mildly tender. The person with actinic keratoses should be monitored by a dermatologist every 6 to 12 months for any change in appearance of the lesions. Early recognition, treatment, and removal of these lesions is easy and important and may be combined with topical field therapy (Endo and Norman, 2014).

Herpes Zoster

Herpes zoster (HZ), or shingles, is a viral infection frequently seen in adults older than age 50, those who have medical conditions that compromise the immune system, or people who

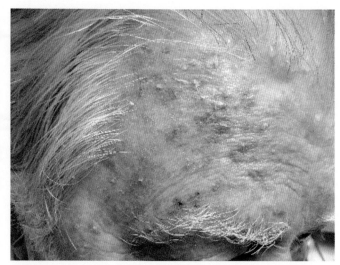

FIGURE 13-3 Actinic Keratoses. (Courtesy Dr. Robert Norman.)

receive immunosuppressive drugs. More than 90% of the world's population is infected with this virus, and by the age of 85, about 50% of the population has reactivated the virus as manifested by a rash (Langana et al, 2014). HZ is caused by reactivation of latent varicella-zoster virus (VZV) within the sensory neurons of the dorsal root ganglion decades after initial VZV infection is established.

HZ always occurs along a nerve pathway, or *dermatome.* The more dermatomes involved, the more serious the infection, especially if it involves the head. When the eye is affected it is always a medical emergency. Most HZ occurs in the thoracic region, but it can also occur in the trigeminal area and cervical, lumbar, and sacral areas. HZ vesicles never cross the midline. In most cases, the severity of the infection increases with age.

The onset may be preceded by itching, tingling, or pain in the affected dermatome several days before the outbreak of the rash. It is important to differentiate HZ from herpes simplex. Herpes simplex does not occur in a dermatome pattern and is recurrent. During the healing process, clusters of papulovesicles develop along a nerve pathway. The lesions themselves eventually rupture, crust over, and resolve. Scarring may result, especially if scratching or poor hygiene leads to a secondary bacterial infection. HZ is infectious until it becomes crusty. HZ may be very painful and pruritic. Prompt treatment with the oral antiviral agents acyclovir, valacyclovir, and famciclovir may shorten the length and severity of the illness; however, to be effective, the medications must be started as soon as possible after the rash appears. Analgesics may help relieve pain. Wet compresses, calamine lotion, and colloidal oatmeal baths may help relieve itching.

Zoster vaccine (Zostavax) is recommended for all persons aged 60 years and older who have no contraindications, including persons who report a previous episode of zoster or who have chronic medical conditions (CDC, 2014b). Older adults who are vaccinated may reduce their risk of acquiring HZ in half; and if they do get it, they are likely to have a milder case. A recent study reported that individuals with shingles face a significantly increased risk of stroke in the weeks following the onset of the painful skin rash and that the risk is increased for those who develop the rash around one or both eyes. Antiviral therapy may lead to a reduced stroke risk (Langana et al, 2014).

HZ vaccination rates are low overall: 2% of blacks and 14% of whites have been vaccinated. More public awareness and education is needed to vaccination rates (Lee et al, 2013). *Healthy People 2020* includes a goal of increasing the percentage of adults who are vaccinated against zoster (shingles) in the overall goal of reducing or eliminating cases of vaccine-preventable diseases.

A common complication of HZ that is minimized for those who are immunized is postherpetic neuralgia (PHN), a chronic, often debilitating painful condition that can last months or even years. Older adults are more likely to have PHN and to have longer lasting and more severe pain. Another complication of HZ is eye involvement, which occurs in 10% to 25% of zoster episodes and can result in prolonged or permanent pain, facial scarring, and loss of vision. The pain of PHN has been difficult to control and can significantly affect one's quality of life. Treatment should include medical, psychological, and complementary and alternative medicine options, as well as rehabilitation. The best evidence studies for medications indicate that the most effective are the tricyclic antidepressants, gabapentin and pregabalin, carbamazepine (for trigeminal neuralgia), opioids, tramadol, topical lidocaine patch, and duloxetine or venlafaxine. Relatively newer treatments for PHN include a high-concentration (8%) topical capsaicin patch, gastroretentive gabapentin, gabapentin enacarbil, and pregabalin in combination with lidocaine plaster, oxycodone, or transcutaneous electrical nerve stimulation (TENS) (Endo and Norman, 2014; Harden et al, 2013). Assessment and management of pain are discussed in Chapter 27.

Candidiasis *(Candida albicans)*

The fungus *Candida albicans* (referred to as "yeast") is present on the skin of healthy persons of any age. However, under certain circumstances and in the right environment, a fungal infection can develop. Persons who are obese or malnourished, are receiving antibiotic or steroid therapy, or have diabetes are at increased risk. *Candida* grows especially well in areas that are moist, warm, and dark, such as in skinfolds, in the axilla, in the groin area, and under pendulous breasts. It can also be found in the corners of the mouth associated with the chronic moisture of angular cheilitis. In the vagina it is also called a "yeast infection." If this is found in an older woman, it may mean that her diabetes either has not yet been diagnosed or is in poor control.

Inside the mouth a *Candida* infection is referred to as "thrush" and is associated with poor hygiene and the immunocompromised individual, such as those who have long-term steroid use (e.g., because of chronic obstructive pulmonary disease), who are receiving chemotherapy, or who test positive for or are infected with human immunodeficiency virus (HIV) or have acquired immunodeficiency syndrome (AIDS). In the mouth, candidiasis appears as irregular, white, flat to slightly raised patches on an erythematous base that cannot be removed by scraping. The infection can extend down into the throat and cause swallowing to be painful. In severely immunocompromised persons the infection can extend down the entire gastrointestinal tract.

On the skin, *Candida* is usually maculopapular, glazed, and dark pink in persons with less pigmentation and grayish in persons with more pigmentation. If it is advanced, the central area may be completely red and/or dark, and weeping with characteristic bright red and/or dark satellite lesions (distinct lesions a short distance from the center). At this point the skin may be edematous, itching, and burning.

The best approach to managing fungal infections is to prevent them, and the key to prevention is limiting the conditions that encourage fungal growth. Prevention is prioritized for persons who are obese, bedridden, incontinent, or diaphoretic (Box 13-5).

Photo Damage of the Skin

Although exposure to sunlight is necessary for the production of vitamin D, the sun is also the most common cause of skin damage and skin cancer. More than 90% of the visible changes commonly attributed to skin aging are caused by the sun (Skin Cancer Foundation, 2014). With aging one accumulates years of sun exposure and the epidermis is thinner, significantly increasing the risk for older adults. The damage (photo or solar damage) comes from prolonged exposure to ultraviolet (UV) light from the environment or in tanning booths. Although the amount of sun-induced damage varies with skin type, genetics, and geographical location, much of the associated damage is preventable. Ideally, preventive measures begin in childhood, but clinical evidence has shown that some improvement can be achieved at any time by limiting sun exposure and using sunscreens regularly regardless of skin tones.

BOX 13-5   TIPS FOR BEST PRACTICE

Candidiasis: Prevention and Treatment

- Identify high-risk individuals (e.g., obese, bedridden, incontinent, diaphoretic, immunocompromised) and limit conditions that encourage fungal growth.
- Provide adequate drying of target areas after bathing and prompt management of incontinent episodes. A hair dryer on the low setting can help dry hard-to-reach, vulnerable areas.
- A dry, folded washcloth or cotton sanitary pad can be placed under the breasts or between skinfolds to promote exposure to air and light.
- Use loose-fitting clothing and underwear; change clothing and bedding when damp.
- Avoid incontinent products that are tight or have plastic that touches the skin.
- Avoid use of cornstarch because it promotes growth of *Candida* organisms.
- Optimize nutrition and glycemic control.
- The goal of treatment is to eradicate the infection and may include the use of a prescribed antifungal medication for 7 to 14 days or until the infection is completely cleared. Antifungal preparations are available as powders, creams, and lotions. Powders are recommended because they trap moisture less than the others.

SKIN CANCERS

Facts and Figures

Currently, between 2 and 3 million nonmelanoma skin cancers and 132,000 melanoma skin cancers occur globally each year. Cancer of the skin (including melanoma and nonmelanoma skin cancer) is the most common of all cancers. Skin cancer is a major public health problem and skin cancers in the United States, unlike many other cancers, continue to rise (USDHHS, 2014). One in five Americans will develop skin cancer in the course of a lifetime (World Health Organization [WHO], 2014). Caucasian populations generally have a much higher risk of getting nonmelanoma or melanoma skin cancers than dark-skinned populations, but individuals of all skin colors should minimize sun exposure. Individuals with pale or freckled skin, fair or red hair, and blue eyes belong to the highest risk group. However, excessive exposure to intense sunlight can damage all skin types, and the risk of eye damage and heat stroke is the same for everyone (WHO, 2014).

Recent research suggests that individuals who have a nonmelanoma skin cancer before their mid-20 have a high risk of developing cancers of the bladder, brain, breast, lung, pancreas, and stomach. With age, the risk for developing cancer decreased but remained higher compared with individuals who did not have nonmelanoma skin cancer when young (Ong et al, 2014). The exact number of basal and squamous cell cancers is not known for certain because they are not reported to cancer registries, but it is estimated that there are more than 2 million basal and squamous cell skin cancers found each year. Most of these are basal cell cancers. Squamous cell cancer is less common but rates are increasing. Most of these are curable; the type with the greatest potential to cause death is melanoma.

Basal Cell Carcinoma

Basal cell carcinoma is the most common malignant skin cancer. It occurs mainly in older age groups but is occurring more and more in younger persons. It is slow growing, and metastasis is rare. A basal cell lesion can be triggered by extensive sun exposure, especially burns, chronic irritation, and chronic ulceration of the skin. It is more prevalent in light-skinned persons. It usually begins as a pearly papule with prominent telangiectasias (blood vessels) or as a scarlike area with no history of trauma (Figure 13-4). Basal cell carcinoma is also known to ulcerate. It may be indistinguishable from squamous cell carcinoma and is diagnosed by biopsy. Early detection and treatment are necessary to minimize disfigurement. Treatment is usually surgical with either simple excision or Mohs micrographic surgery (Endo and Norman, 2014).

Squamous Cell Carcinoma

Squamous cell carcinoma is the second most common skin cancer. However, it is aggressive and has a high incidence of metastasis if not identified and treated promptly. Major risk factors include sun exposure, fair skin, and immunosuppression. Individuals in their mid-60s who have been or are chronically exposed to the sun (e.g., persons who work out of

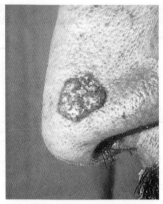

FIGURE 13-4 Basal Cell Carcinoma. (Courtesy Gary Monheit, MD, University of Alabama at Birmingham School of Medicine.)

doors or are athletes) are prime candidates for this type of cancer. Less common causes include chronic stasis ulcers, scars from injury, and exposure to chemical carcinogens, such as topical hydrocarbons, arsenic, and radiation (especially for individuals who received treatments for acne in the mid-twentieth century) (Endo and Norman, 2014).

The lesion begins as a firm, irregular, fleshy, pink-colored nodule that becomes reddened and scaly, much like actinic keratosis, but it may increase rapidly in size. It may also be hard and wartlike with a gray top and horny texture, or it may be ulcerated and indurated with raised, defined borders (Figure 13-5). Because it can appear so differently, it is often overlooked or thought to be insignificant. All persons, especially those who live in sunny climates, should be regularly screened by a dermatologist. Treatment depends on the size, histologic features, and patient preference and may include electrodesiccation and curettage, Mohs micrographic surgery, aggressive cryotherapy, or topical 5-fluorouracil (Endo and Norman, 2014). Once a person has been diagnosed with

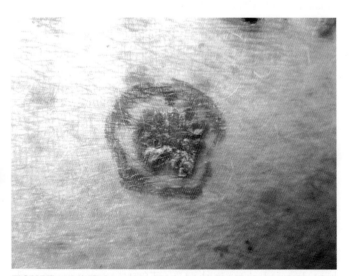

FIGURE 13-5 Squamous Cell Carcinoma. (From Ham RJ, Sloane PD, Warshaw GA, et al, *Primary care geriatrics*, ed 6, Philadelphia, 2014, Saunders. Used with permission, University of Utah Department of Dermatology.)

a squamous cell carcinoma, he or she needs to be routinely followed because the majority of recurrences are within the first few years.

Melanoma

Melanoma, a neoplasm of the melanocytes, affects the skin or, less commonly, the retina. Melanoma has a classical multicolor, raised appearance with an asymmetrical, irregular border. It may appear to be of any size, but the surface diameter is not necessarily reflective of the size beneath the surface, similar in concept to an iceberg. It is treatable if diagnosed early, before it has a chance to invade surrounding tissue. Melanoma accounts for less than 2% of skin cancer cases, but it causes most skin cancer deaths. Melanoma is highly curable if the cancer is detected in its earliest stages and treated promptly (Garrett et al, 2014).

Incidence and Prevalence

The American Cancer Society (2014) estimates that about 76,100 new cases of melanoma were diagnosed in 2014. The number of new cases of melanoma in the United States has been increasing for at least 30 years. Overall, the lifetime risk of getting melanoma is about 1 in 50 for the white population, 1 in 1000 for black individuals, and 1 in 200 for the Hispanic population. Melanoma rates among middle-aged adults, especially women, have increased in the past 4 decades (Garrett et al, 2014). Men have a higher rate of melanoma than women and a person who has already had a melanoma has a higher risk of developing another one. The risk of melanoma is more than 10 times higher for white Americans than for black Americans.

Risk Factors

Risk factors for melanoma include a personal history of melanoma; the presence of atypical, large, or numerous (more than 50) moles; sun sensitivity; history of excessive sun exposure and severe sunburns; use of tanning booths; natural blond or red hair color; diseases or treatments that suppress the immune system; and a history of skin cancer. Increasing age along with a history of sun exposure increases one's risk even further. The legs and backs of women and the backs of men are the most common sites of melanoma. Many studies have linked melanoma on the trunk, legs, and arms to frequent sunburns, especially in childhood. Blistering sunburns before the age of 18 years are thought to damage Langerhans cells, which affect the immune response of the skin and increase the risk for a later melanoma. Two-thirds of melanomas develop from preexisting moles; only one-third arise alone.

Indoor tanning. Although melanoma occurs more often in older people, it is one of the most common cancers in people younger than 30 years. Exposure to indoor tanning, common in Western countries, is thought to be contributing to the increasing rates of melanoma and other skin cancers among younger individuals. Indoor tanning increases the risk of melanoma by 75% when use started before age 35 years. Indoor tanners are 2.5 times more likely to develop squamous cell cancer and 1.5 times more likely to develop basal cell cancer. In the

United States, 35% of adults and 55% of college students have used indoor tanning devices. Worldwide, there are more skin cancer cases due to indoor tanning than there are lung cancer cases due to smoking (Wehner et al, 2013). This is considered a major public health issue with many states limiting minors' access to tanning salons. The U.S. Food and Drug Administration (FDA) has announced that it will soon require labels on tanning beds and lamps warning against use by anyone younger than 18 years of age (CDC, 2014a). *Healthy People 2020* includes objectives to reduce the proportion of adolescents and adults using indoor tanning devices.

◆ PROMOTING HEALTHY AGING: IMPLICATIONS FOR GERONTOLOGICAL NURSING

Age-related skin changes, such as thinning and diminished numbers of melanocytes, significantly increase the risk for solar damage and subsequent skin cancer. The nurse has an active role in the prevention and early recognition of skin cancers. This role may include working with community awareness and education programs, as well as screening clinics and providing direct care. By far the most important preventive nursing intervention is to provide education regarding skin cancer risk factors and adequate lifelong protective measures (Box 13-6).

Careful skin inspection is essential and the nurse is vigilant in observing skin for changes that require further evaluation. Patient education also includes teaching the individual how to examine his or her skin once a month to look for warning signs or any suspicious lesions. If the individual has a partner, partners can perform regular "checks" of each other's skin, watching for signs of change and the need to contact a primary care provider or dermatologist promptly. For the person with keratosis and multiple freckles (nevi), photographing the body parts may be a useful reference. The adage "when in doubt, get it checked" is an important one and regular screenings should be a part of the health care of all older adults. The "ABCDE" approach to assessing such potential lesions is used (Box 13-7).

BOX 13-6   Promoting Healthy Skin

Sun Protection

- Seek the shade.
- Do not burn.
- Avoid indoor tanning booths and sunlamps.
- Wear hats with a brim wide enough to shade face, ears, and neck, as well as clothing that adequately covers the arms, legs, and torso. Cover up with clothing, including a broad-brimmed hat and UV-blocking sunglasses.
- Use a broad-spectrum (UVA/UVB) sunscreen with an SPF of 30 or higher every day.
- Apply 1 ounce (2 tablespoons) of sunscreen to your entire body 30 minutes before going outdoors. Reapply every 2 hours or immediately after swimming or excessive sweating.
- Examine your skin head-to-toe every month.
- See your health care provider every year for a professional skin exam.

Modified from Skin Cancer Foundation: Prevention Guidelines, http://www.skincancer.org/prevention/sun-protection/prevention-guidelines, Accessed May 5, 2015.

BOX 13-7   Danger Signs: Remember ABCDE

Asymmetry of a mole (one that is not regularly round or oval)
Border is irregular
Color variation (areas of black, brown, tan, blue, red, white, or a combination)
Diameter greater than the size of a pencil eraser (although early stages may be smaller)
Elevation and **E**nlargement*

*Lesions that change, itch, bleed, or do not heal are also alarm signals.
From Skin Cancer Foundation: *Do you know your ABCDEs?* http://www.skincancer.org/skin-cancer-information/melanoma/melanoma-warning-signs-and-images/do-you-know-your-abcdes. Accessed March 7, 2014.

PRESSURE ULCERS

Aging carries a high risk for the development of pressure ulcers; 70% of pressure ulcers (PUs) occur in older adults (Jamshed and Schneider, 2010). Pressure ulcers are recognized as one of the geriatric syndromes (Chapter 7), and *Healthy People 2020* has addressed this issue with a goal of reducing the rate of pressure ulcer–related hospitalizations among older adults. Nurses play a key role in the prevention of pressure ulcers and selection of evidence-based treatment strategies.

Definition

The National Pressure Ulcer Advisory Panel (NPUAP) and the European Pressure Ulcer Advisory Panel (EPUAP) constitute an international collaboration convened to develop evidence-based recommendations to be used throughout the world to prevent and treat pressure-related wounds. According to this group, a pressure ulcer is a "localized injury to the skin and/or underlying tissue usually over a bony prominence, as a result of pressure, or pressure in combination with shear. A number of contributing or confounding factors are also associated with pressure ulcers; the significance of these factors is yet to be elucidated" (NPUAP and EPUAP, 2014b).

Scope of the Problem

Pressure ulcers are a major challenge worldwide and a major cause of morbidity, mortality, and health care burden globally (Wounds International, 2009). In Japan, the frequency of PUs is 23.1% for in-hospital patients; U.S. prevalence ranges from 4.7% to 32.1% in-hospital and from 8.5% to 22% in nursing homes; and in Canada, prevalence in-hospital is reported at 25.1% (Nagamachi et al, 2013). The epidemiology of PUs varies appreciably by clinical setting. Critically ill patients in the intensive care unit (ICU) are considered to be at the greatest risk for PU development as a result of high acuity and the multiple interventions and therapies they receive. In ICUs, prevalence ranges from 49% across Western Europe, 22% in North America, 50% in Australia, and 29% in Jordan (Tayyib et al, 2013). While overall prevalence rates have dropped, some in the United States in acute care, multiple studies have shown that the incidence of facility-acquired pressure ulcers remains high in ICUs (10% to 41%) (Cooper, 2013).

There is wide variation in prevalence between countries and continents. Differences in sample characteristics, definition of a PU, and study methodologies affect these statistics, but it is clear that pressure ulcers are a significant problem in all settings around the globe, particularly in ICUs. However, data from the United States and Europe suggest that pressure ulcer rates have failed to respond to prevention strategies, with many countries continuing to report double-figure percentage results (Phillips and Buttery, 2009). Concern over the global problem of PUs had led the NPUAP to establish a Pressure Ulcer Registry, the first database of its type to allow clinicians to input cases of pressure ulcers in an effort to provide statistically significant rigorous analysis of the variables associated with the development of unavoidable PUs (NPUAP, 2014a). NPUAP/EPUAP sponsors a worldwide "Stop Pressure Ulcer Day" annually with educational resources available to patients and health care professionals.

Cost and Regulatory Requirements

Treatment of pressure ulcers is costly in terms of both healthcare expenditure and patient suffering. PU treatment is estimated to cost in the range of up to $11 billion annually in the United States (Chou et al, 2013). In the United States, the Centers for Medicare and Medicaid Services (CMS) estimates that the cost per stay for hospitalized beneficiaries with a secondary diagnosis of pressure ulcer is $40,381 (Garcia and White-Chu, 2014). In Europe, PU cost accounts for up to 4% of the annual health care budget (Tayyib et al, 2013), and in one report from the Netherlands, where there are a very high percentage of older people, pressure ulcers were identified as the country's most costly condition, surpassing cancer and cardiovascular disease (Garcia and White-Chu, 2014). The actual cost of pressure ulcers is hard to determine because there is no standardization related to what is included in estimates (e.g., nursing care costs, material costs, added acute care days). However, costs are significant and have led to national and international efforts to decrease the prevalence of pressure ulcers.

In 2008, CMS included hospital-acquired pressure ulcers (HAPUs) as one of the preventable adverse events (health care–acquired conditions [HCAs]). The development of a stage/category 3 or 4 pressure ulcer is considered a "never event" (serious medical errors or adverse events that should never happen to a patient). Hospitals no longer receive additional reimbursement to care for a patient who has acquired pressure ulcers under the hospital's care, and this has the potential to greatly increase the financial strain for facilities that fail to rise to this challenge (Armstrong et al, 2008; Cooper, 2013; Gray-Siracusa and Schrier, 2011).

The Japanese government, in 2002, also introduced a scheme of financial penalties for hospitals that failed to implement a series of specified pressure ulcer prevention strategies, which has resulted in a decrease in the prevalence of PUs of all stages (Wounds International, 2009). Evaluation of the impact of governmental regulations on pressure ulcer management is one of the research priorities of the NPUAP (2013).

Characteristics

Pressure ulcers can develop anywhere on the body but are seen most frequently on the posterior aspects, especially the sacrum, the heels, and the greater trochanters. Secondary areas of breakdown include the lateral condyles of the knees and the ankles. The pinna of the ears, occiput, elbows, and scapulae are other areas subject to breakdown. Heels are particularly prone to the development of pressure ulcers because there is little soft tissue. Twenty-five to thirty percent of pressure ulcers are on the heels, and individuals with peripheral arterial disease are at high risk for heel ulcers (McGinnis et al, 2013).

> ### ⚡ SAFETY ALERT
> Approximately 25% to 35% of pressure ulcers are on heels. Those with peripheral vascular disease (PVD) are at high risk. Keep heels elevated off the bed with a pillow under calf or heel suspension boots.

Classification

The EPUAP and NPUAP recommend a four-category classification of pressure ulcers. The NPUAP also describes two additional categories for the United States that do not fall into one of the established or classifiable categories: suspected deep tissue injury and unstageable or unclassified wound (Box 13-8). The ulcer is always classified by the highest stage "achieved," and reverse staging is never used. This means that the wound is documented as the stage representing the maximal damage and depth that has occurred. As the wound heals, it fills with granulation tissue composed of endothelial cells, fibroblasts, collagen, and an extracellular matrix. Muscle, subcutaneous fat, and dermis are not replaced. A stage IV pressure ulcer that is healing does not revert to stage III and then stage II. It remains defined as a healing stage IV pressure ulcer.

Skin Changes at Life's End (SCALE)

Skin failure is defined as "an event in which the skin and underlying tissue die due to hypoperfusion that occurs concurrent with severe dysfunction or failure of other organ systems" (White-Chu and Langemo, 2012, p. 28). Skin failure is identified as a real condition that can occur in the last days or weeks of life and can occur in both acute and chronic conditions. Skin failure is a documentable condition and not the same as a pressure ulcer (Black et al, 2011).

In 2009 an interdisciplinary panel of experts in wound healing developed a consensus statement on the changes that occur to the skin at the end of life (SCALE) (European Pressure Ulcer Advisory Panel, 2014; Sibbald et al, 2010). Knowledge of this condition is limited, and further research is required. The Kennedy Terminal Ulcer, first described in 1989 and now explained as an unavoidable skin breakdown that occurs during the dying process, presents as a red, yellow, or purple lesion shaped like a pear, butterfly, or horseshoe on the coccyx or sacrum. The lesion will darken deeply and progress to a full-thickness ulcer in a few days and usually indicate that death is imminent (Sibbald et al, 2010; White-Chu and Langemo, 2012). The

BOX 13-8   Pressure Ulcer Stages/Categories

Suspected Deep Tissue Injury: Depth Unknown

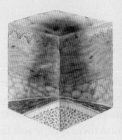 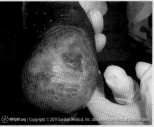

Heel, ethnic skin

Purple or maroon localized area of discolored intact skin or blood-filled blister due to damage of underlying soft tissue from pressure and/or shear. Visible damage in the area may be preceded by tissue that is painful, firm, mushy, boggy, warmer, or cooler as compared with adjacent tissue.

Further description—Deep tissue injury may be difficult to detect in individuals with dark skin tones (may appear as a bruise). Evolution may include a thin blister over a dark wound bed. The wound may further evolve and become covered by thin eschar. Evolution may be rapid, exposing additional layers of tissue even with optimal treatment.

Category/Stage I: Nonblanchable Erythema

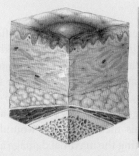 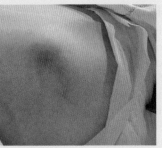

Intact skin with nonblanchable redness of a localized area, usually over a bony prominence. Darkly pigmented skin may not have visible blanching; its color may differ from the surrounding area.

Further description—The area may be painful, firm, soft, warmer, or cooler as compared with adjacent tissue. Category 1 may be difficult to detect in individuals with dark skin tones. May indicate "at risk" persons.

Category/Stage II: Partial-Thickness Skin Loss

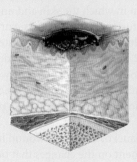 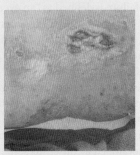

Partial-thickness loss of dermis presenting as a shallow open ulcer with a reddish pink wound bed, without slough. May also present as an intact or open/ruptured serum-filled blister.

Further description—Presents as a shiny or dry shallow ulcer without slough or bruising. Bruising indicates deep tissue injury. This stage should not be used to describe skin tears, tape burns, perineal dermatitis, maceration, or excoriation.

Category/Stage III: Full-Thickness Skin Loss

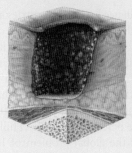 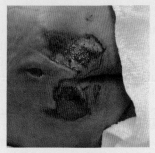

Full-thickness tissue loss. Subcutaneous fat may be visible but bone, tendon, and muscle are not exposed. Slough may be present but does not obscure the depth of tissue loss. *May* include undermining and tunneling.

Further description—The depth of a stage III pressure ulcer varies by anatomical location. The bridge of the nose, ear, occiput, and malleolus do not have subcutaneous tissue, and stage III ulcers can be shallow. In contrast, areas of significant adiposity can develop extremely deep stage III pressure ulcers. Bone or tendon is not visible or directly palpable.

Category/Stage IV: Full-Thickness Skin Loss

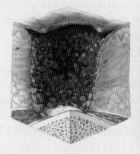 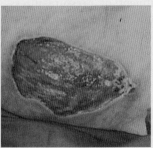

Full-thickness tissue loss with exposed bone, tendon, or muscle. Slough or eschar may be present on some parts of the wound bed. Often includes undermining and tunneling.

Further description—The depth of a stage IV pressure ulcer varies by anatomical location. The bridge of the nose, ear, occiput, and malleolus do not have subcutaneous tissue, and these ulcers can be shallow. Stage IV ulcers can extend into muscle and/or supporting structures (e.g., fascia, tendon, or joint capsule), making osteomyelitis possible. Exposed bone or tendon is visible or directly palpable.

Unstageable: Depth Unknown

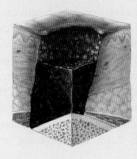 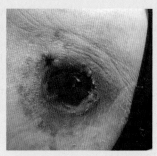

Full-thickness tissue loss in which the base of the ulcer is covered by slough (yellow, tan, gray, green, or brown) and/or eschar (tan, brown, or black) in the wound bed.

Further description—Until enough slough and/or eschar is removed to expose the base of the wound, the true depth, and therefore stage, cannot be determined. Stable (dry, adherent, intact without erythema or fluctuance) eschar on the heels serves as "the body's natural (biological) cover" and should not be removed.

From the National Pressure Ulcer Advisory Panel (NPUAP): *Updated staging system: pressure ulcer stages revised by NPUAP*. Reprinted with permission of the NPUAP, 2007. Suspected DTI photo: NPUAP. Stages I-IV photos: From Cameron MH, Monroe L, editors: *Physical rehabilitation for the physical therapist assistant,* St Louis, MO, 2011, Saunders. Unstageable photo: From Ham RJ, Sloane PD, Warshaw GA, et al, editors: *Primary care geriatrics,* ed 6, Philadelphia, 2014, Elsevier Saunders.

consensus statement concludes that these changes can be an unavoidable part of the dying process and may occur even with appropriate evidence-based interventions (Sibbald et al, 2010).

Treatment decisions are made after careful assessment of the skin and underlying physical factors such as diminished tissue perfusion, suboptimal nutrition, weakness and progressive limitation of mobility, and impaired immune function. Determination should be made if the ulcer is (1) healable within an individual's lifetime; (2) maintained; or (3) nonhealable or palliative. Determination of appropriate interventions should be made by considering the 5 P's (Box 13-9).

Risk Factors

Many factors increase the risk of pressure ulcers including changes in the skin, comorbid illnesses, nutritional status, frailty, surgical procedures (especially orthopedic/cardiac), cognitive deficits, incontinence, and reduced mobility (Box 13-10). A major risk factor is the combination of intensity and duration of pressure and tissue tolerance (Ayello and Sibbald, 2012). Individuals confined to a bed or chair, who are unable to shift weight or reposition themselves at regular intervals, are at high risk. Tissue tolerance, in addition to unrelieved pressure, contributes to the risk of a pressure ulcer. Tissue tolerance is related to the ability of the tissue to distribute and compensate for pressure exerted over bony prominences. Factors that affect tissue tolerance include moisture, friction, shear force, nutritional status, age, sensory perception, and arterial pressure.

In darker-pigmented persons, redness and blanching may not be observed as early signs of skin damage. In dark skin, early signs of skin damage can manifest as a purplish color or appear like a bruise. It is important to observe for induration, darkening, change in color from surrounding skin, or a shadowed appearance of the skin. The affected skin area, when

BOX 13-10   **Pressure Ulcer Risk Factors**

Prolonged Pressure/Immobilization
Lying in bed or sitting in a chair or wheelchair without changing position or relieving pressure over an extended period
Lying for hours on hard x-ray and operating tables
Neurological disorders (coma, spinal cord injuries, cognitive impairment, or cerebrovascular disease)
Fractures or contractures
Debilitation: elderly persons in hospitals and nursing homes
Pain
Sedation
Shearing forces (moving by dragging on coarse bed sheets)

Disease/Tissue Factors
Impaired perfusion; ischemia
Fecal or urinary incontinence; prolonged exposure to moisture
Malnutrition, dehydration
Chronic diseases accompanied by anemia, edema, renal failure, malnutrition, peripheral vascular disease, or sepsis
Previous history of pressure ulcers

Additional Risk Factors for the Critically Ill
Norepinephrine infusion
Acute Physiology and Chronic Health Evaluation (APACHE II) score
Anemia
Age older than 40 years
Multiple organ system disease or comorbid complications
Length of hospital stay

From McCance KL, Huether SE, editors: *Pathophysiology*, ed 7, St Louis, MO, 2014, Mosby.

compared with adjacent tissues, may be firm, warmer, cooler, or painful (Garcia and White-Chu, 2014). Several studies have reported a higher prevalence and incidence of pressure ulcers among black individuals in nursing homes than other race groups (Baumgarten et al, 2009; Harms et al, 2014; Howard and Taylor, 2009) (Box 13-11). These findings indicate a need for better assessment of dark skin for early signs of damage and increased attention to prevention of PUs before admission and during nursing home stays (Harms et al, 2014).

Prevention of Pressure Ulcers

The importance of prevention of pressure ulcers has been frequently emphasized and is the key to pressure ulcer treatment. A consensus paper from the International Expert Wound Care Advisory Panel (Armstrong et al, 2008) provides recommendations for prevention of pressure ulcers that include patient education, clinician training for all members of the health care team, strategies in developing communication and terminology materials, implementation of toolkits and protocols (prevention bundles), documentation checklists, outcome evaluation, quality improvement efforts, evidence-based treatment protocols, and appropriate products.

A comprehensive pressure ulcer program that includes multiple interventions (care bundle) appears to be related to better outcomes. A bundle is composed of a set of evidence-based practices that when performed collectively and reliably have

BOX 13-9   **Determining Appropriate Interventions: SCALE**

Prevention: Address excessive pressure, friction, shear, moisture, suboptimal nutrition, immobilization, tissue tolerance, comorbid conditions.
Prescription: Interventions for a treatable lesion. Even in the stress of dying, some lesions are healable after appropriate treatment. Interventions need to be aimed at treating the cause and at patient-centered concerns (pain, quality of life) before addressing the components of wound care consistent with the patient/family goals and wishes.
Preservation: If opportunity for wound healing is limited, maintenance of the wound in the present clinical state may be the outcome.
Palliation: Refers to situations in which the goal of treatment is comfort and care, not healing. In some situations, palliative wounds may benefit from interventions such as surgical debridement or support surfaces even if the goal is not to heal the wound.
Preference: Take into account the preferences of the patient and the patient's circle of care.

Data from Sibbald R, Krasner D, Lutz J, et al: SCALE: skin changes at life's end: final consensus statement, October 1, 2009, *Adv Skin Wound Care* 23(5):225–236, 2010.

BOX 13-11   RESEARCH HIGHLIGHTS

This study examined the prevalence of pressure ulcers (stages II to IV) among racial and ethnic groups of older individuals admitted to nursing homes. Results show that the number of PUs in black older adults was greater than that in Hispanic older adults, which were both higher than white older adults. The rate of PUs among admissions of black individuals was 1.7 times higher than that for white individuals. The percentages of stage III and IV PUs were higher in all groups of minority admissions compared with white admissions. The prevalence of PUs was higher among nursing homes with a lower percentage of admissions of white individuals. The sample in this study was the largest, most diverse, and nationally representative of any investigating racial/ethnic differences in PUs among nursing home admissions.

Darker skin presents challenges for detecting skin changes because redness (considered the first sign of skin damage) can manifest as a purplish color or more subtle discoloration of usual skin tone and may be missed. Clinical assessment tools for dark skin are lacking. Education must be provided about assessment of dark skin for early damage and PUs, and nursing homes with higher numbers of racially and culturally diverse individuals may need additional resources to manage PUs.

Data from Harms S, Bliss D, Garrad J, et al: Prevalence of pressure ulcers by race and ethnicity for older adults admitted to nursing homes, *J Gerontol Nurs* 40(3):20–26, 2014.

been shown to improve patient outcomes (Gray-Siracusa and Schrier, 2011). Involvement of the patient and family may enhance the effectiveness of care bundles (Gillespie et al, 2014). Core preventive strategies include risk assessment, skin assessment, nutritional assessment, repositioning, and appropriate support surfaces. The NPUAP is coordinating the development of a uniform terminology, test methods, and reporting standards for support surfaces (see Box 13-3). Interventions that addressed limited mobility, compromised skin integrity, and nutritional support have been associated with significant improvements in PU rates (Gillespie et al, 2014; Gray-Siracusa and Schrier, 2011).

Systematic prevention programs have been shown to decrease hospital-acquired pressure ulcers by 34% to 50% (Armstrong et al, 2008). Olsho et al. (2014) reported a 59% reduction in the monthly incidence of pressure ulcers in a nursing home with the use of the AHRQ On-Time Pressure Ulcer Prevention Program (see Box 13-13). However, "despite a number of national prevention initiatives and existing evidence-based protocols, pressure ulcer frequency has not declined in recent years and pressure ulcers continue to have a negative impact on patient outcomes and health care costs in a variety of care settings" (Baumgarten et al, 2009, p. 253). Several studies have reported that compliance with evidence-based protocol recommendations is a concern and less than half of at-risk patients actually receive core preventive strategies (Baumgarten et al, 2009; Gillespie et al, 2014; Spillsbury et al, 2007).

The prevention and treatment of pressure ulcers is complex and does not belong to any one specialty; a team approach that involves primary care providers, nursing staff, physical therapists, nutritionists, and other clinicians is most effective (Armstrong et al, 2008).

Consequences of Pressure Ulcers

Pressure ulcers are costly to treat and prolong recovery and extend rehabilitation. Complications include the need for grafting or amputation, sepsis, or even death and may lead to legal action by the individual or his or her representative against the caregiver. The personal impact of a pressure ulcer on health and quality of life is also significant and not well understood or researched. Findings from a study exploring patients' perceptions of the impact of a pressure ulcer and its treatment on health and quality of life suggest that pressure ulcers cause suffering, pain, discomfort, and distress that are not always recognized or adequately treated by nursing staff. Pressure ulcers had a profound impact on the patients' lives—physically, socially, emotionally, and mentally (Spillsbury et al, 2007).

◆ PROMOTING HEALTHY AGING: IMPLICATIONS FOR GERONTOLOGICAL NURSING

Nursing staff, as direct caregivers, are key team members who perform skin assessment, identify risk factors, and implement numerous preventive interventions. The nurse alerts the health care provider of the need for prescribed treatments, recommends treatments, and administers and evaluates the changing status of the wound(s) and adequacy of treatments.

◆ Assessment of Pressure Ulcer Risk

Skin assessments are performed on admission and whenever there is a change in the status of the patient (Box 13-12). In the nursing home, the MDS 3.0 provides an evidence-based assessment of skin integrity and pressure ulcers with accompanying care guidelines (Chapter 7). Assessment begins with a history, detailed head-to-toe skin examination, nutritional evaluation, and analysis of laboratory findings. Laboratory values that have been correlated with risk for the development and the poor healing of pressure ulcers include those that reflect anemia and poor nutritional status. Visual and tactile inspection of the entire skin surface with special attention to bony prominences is essential. The nurse looks for any interruption of skin integrity or other changes, including redness or **hyperemia**. Special attention must be given to the assessment of dark skin because tissue injury will appear differently. Assessment of pain related to the ulcer (dressing changes, turning) is important so that appropriate treatment can be given to relieve pain (Chapter 27).

Box 13-12   Guidelines for Skin Assessment

Acute care: On admission, reassess at least every 24 hours or sooner if patient's condition changes

Long-term Care: On admission, weekly for 4 weeks, then quarterly and whenever resident's condition changes

Home care: On admission and at every nurse visit

Data from NPUAP: *Pressure ulcer prevention points*, 2007. http://www.npuap.org/wp-content/uploads/2012/03/PU_Prev_Points.pdf. Accessed March 11, 2014.

If pressure is present, it should be relieved and the area reassessed in 1 hour. Pressure areas and surrounding tissue should be palpated for changes in temperature and tissue resilience. Blisters or pimples with or without hyperemia and scabs over weight-bearing areas in the absence of trauma should be considered suspect. Inspection is best accomplished in nonglare daylight or, if that is not possible, with focused lighting. Special attention should be directed to affected areas when an individual uses orthotic devices such as corsets, braces, prostheses, postural supports, splints, slings, or casts and to areas of skin around other devices such as endotracheal and tracheostomy tubes as well.

Early identification of risk status is critical so that timely interventions can be designed to address specific risk factors. The Braden Scale for Predicting Pressure Sore Risk, developed by nurses Barbara Braden and Nancy Bergstrom, is widely used and clinically validated. This scale assesses the risk of pressure ulcers on the basis of a numerical scoring system of six risk factors: sensory perception, moisture, activity, mobility, nutrition, and friction/shear. For a video on the use of the Braden Scale, see Box 13-3.

Because the Braden Scale does not include all of the risk factors for pressure ulcers, it is recommended that it be used as an adjunct rather than in place of clinical judgment. A thorough patient history to assess other risk factors such as age, medications, comorbidities (diabetes, peripheral vascular disease [PVD]), history of pressure ulcers, and other factors is important to fully address the risk of pressure ulcer development so that appropriate preventive interventions can be developed (Armstrong et al, 2008; Jull and Griffiths, 2010).

Most institutions have special forms or screens on their computer software for recording skin assessments. The Agency for Healthcare Research and Quality (AHRQ) provides the On-Time Pressure Ulcer Healing Project (2014) (Box 13-3). The focus of this project is on prevention and timely treatment of pressure ulcers in long-term care. Tools to document pressure ulcer healing and treatments and reports to monitor the healing process are available. The reader is referred to the NPUAP website (www.npuap.org) for more information.

Interventions

The goal of nurses is to help maintain skin integrity against the various environmental, mechanical, and chemical assaults that are potential causes of breakdown. Nursing actions include eliminating friction and irritation to the skin, such as from shearing; reducing moisture so that tissues do not macerate; managing incontinence; and displacing body weight from prominent areas to facilitate circulation to the skin. The nurse should be familiar with the types of supportive surfaces so that the most effective products are used. The nurse should assess the frequency of position change, adding pillows so that skin surfaces do not touch and establishing a repositioning and turning schedule. A comprehensive protocol for prevention and treatment of PUs is presented in Box 13-13.

⚡ SAFETY ALERT

Individuals placed on pressure redistribution mattresses continue to need turning and repositioning according to an established schedule.

Consultation with the nutritional team is important. Nutritional intake should be monitored, as well as the serum albumin, hematocrit, and hemoglobin levels (Chapters 8 and 14). Caloric, protein, vitamin, and/or mineral supplementation can be considered if there is evidence of deficiencies of these nutrients. Routine use of higher than the recommended daily allowance of vitamin C and zinc for the prevention and/or treatment of pressure ulcers is not supported by evidence (Jamshed and Schneider, 2010). The nurse promotes nutritional health by ensuring that the person receives adequate assistance with eating and that dining time is a pleasant experience for the person.

Pressure Ulcer Assessment

Ulcers are assessed with each dressing change with a detailed assessment repeated on a weekly, biweekly, and as-needed basis. The purpose is to specifically and carefully evaluate the effectiveness of treatment. If there are no signs of healing from week to week or worsening of the wound is seen, then either the treatment is insufficient or the wound has become infected; in both cases, treatment must be changed. Determining the cause of the ulcer is important so that appropriate preventive measures can be implemented. The care team, in consultation with the individual and family, reviews the assessment and care plan and determines, if possible, if the underlying cause is reversible so that appropriate treatment decisions can be made to ensure patient comfort. Consultation with a wound care specialist is advisable for wounds that are extensive or nonhealing. Specialized nurses such as enterostomal therapists or nurse practitioners, who may work with wound centers or surgeons, provide consultation in nursing homes, offices, or clinics.

The PUSH tool (Pressure Ulcer Scale for Healing) (Box 13-3) provides a detailed form that covers all aspects of assessment but contains only three items and takes a short time to complete (NPUAP, 2014c). Photographic documentation is highly recommended both at the onset of the problem and at intervals during treatment (Ahn and Salicido, 2008; Garcia and White-Chu, 2014).

Pressure Ulcer Dressings

The type of dressing selected is based on careful assessment of the condition of the ulcer; the presence of granulation, necrotic tissue, and slough; the amount of drainage; the microbial status; and the quality of the surrounding skin. If the wound has necrotic tissue, it must be debrided. Debridement methods include mechanical (whirlpool, wet-to-dry); sharp (scalpel, scissors); enzymatic (collagenase); and autolytic (hydrocolloid, hydrogel). Wound cleansing should be done with nontoxic preparations; normal saline is recommended. Other principles are presented in Box 13-14. The NPUAP and the *Prevention and Treatment of Pressure Ulcers Clinical Practice Guidelines* (AHRQ, 2009) provide guidance

BOX 13-13 TIPS FOR BEST PRACTICE

Pressure Ulcer Prevention

I. Risk Assessment

1. Consider all bed-bound and chair-bound persons, or those whose ability to reposition is impaired, to be at risk for pressure ulcers.
2. Use a valid, reliable, and age-appropriate method of risk assessment that ensures systematic evaluation of individual risk factors.
3. Assess on admission to the patient care setting, at regular intervals thereafter, and with any change in condition.
4. Inspect skin regularly for color changes such as redness in lightly pigmented persons and discoloration in darkly pigmented persons.
5. Assess surgical patients for increased risk of pressure ulcers including the following factors: length of operation, number of hypotensive episodes, and/or low-core temperatures intraoperatively, reduced mobility on first postoperative day.
6. Look at the skin under any medical devices.
7. Identify all individual risk factors (decreased mental status, exposure to moisture, incontinence, device-related pressure, friction, shear, immobility, inactivity, nutritional deficits, tissue tolerance) to guide specific preventive treatments. Modify care according to individual factors.
8. Document risk assessment subscale scores and total scores and implement a risk-based prevention plan.

II. Skin Care

1. Perform a head-to-toe skin assessment at least daily, especially checking pressure points such as sacrum, ischium, trochanters, heels, elbows, and back of the head.
2. Individualize bathing frequency. Use a mild cleansing agent. Avoid hot water and excessive rubbing. Use lotion after bathing.
3. Establish a bowel and bladder program for the patient with incontinence. When incontinence cannot be controlled, cleanse skin at time of soiling, and use a topical barrier to protect the skin. Select underpads or briefs that are absorbent and provide quick-drying action.
4. Use moisturizers for dry skin. Minimize factors leading to dry skin such as low humidity and cold air.
5. Avoid massage over bony prominences.
6. Protect high-risk areas such as elbows, heels, sacrum, and back of head from friction injury.

III. Nutrition

1. Identify and correct factors compromising protein/calorie intake consistent with overall goals of care.
2. Consider nutritional supplementation/support for nutritionally compromised persons consistent with overall goals of care.
3. If appropriate, offer a glass of water when turning to keep patient hydrated.
4. Administer multivitamin with minerals per provider order.

IV. Mechanical Loading and Support Surfaces

1. Reposition bed-bound persons at least every 2 hours and chair-bound persons every 4 hours consistent with overall goals of care. **Follow repositioning guidelines when person is on pressure-redistributing mattress.**
2. Consider postural alignment; distribution of weight, balance, and stability; and pressure redistribution when positioning persons in chairs and wheelchairs. Evaluate fit of the wheelchair.
3. Teach chair-bound persons, who are able, to shift weight every 15 minutes.
4. Use a written repositioning schedule.
5. Place at-risk person on pressure-redistributing mattress and chair cushion surfaces.
6. Avoid using donut-type devices and sheepskin for pressure redistribution.
7. Use pressure-redistributing devices in the operating room for individuals assessed to be at high risk for pressure ulcer development.
8. Use lifting devices (e.g., trapeze or bed linens) to move persons rather than drag them during transfers and position changes.
9. Use pillows or foam wedges to keep bony prominences, such as knees and ankles, from direct contact with each other. Pad skin subjected to device-related pressure and inspect regularly.
10. Use devices that eliminate pressure on the heels. For short-term use with cooperative patients, place pillows under calf to raise heel off the bed. Place heel suspension boots for long-term use.
11. Avoid positioning directly on the trochanter when using side-lying position; use the 30-degree lateral inclined position.
12. Maintain the head of the bed at or less than 30 degrees or at the lowest degree of elevation consistent with the person's medical condition.
13. Intitute a rehabilitation program to maintain or improve mobility/activity status.

V. Education

1. Implement pressure ulcer prevention educational programs that are structured, organized, comprehensive, and directed at all levels of health care providers, patients, family, and caregivers.
2. Include information on:
   a. Etiology of and risk factors for pressure ulcers
   b. Risk assessment tools and their application
   c. Skin assessment
   d. Nutritional support
   e. Program for bowel and bladder management
   f. Development and implementation of individualized programs of skin care
   g. Demonstration of positioning to decrease risk of tissue breakdown
   h. Accurate documentation of pertinent data
3. Include mechanisms to evaluate program effectiveness in preventing pressure ulcers.

Adapted with permission from NPUAP: *Pressure Ulcer Prevention Points, 2007,* http://www.npuap.org/wp-content/uploads/2012/03/PU_Prev_Points.pdf. Copyright 2007; with data from Ayello E, Sibbald R: Preventing pressure ulcers and skin tears. In Boltz M, Capezuti E, Fulmer T, et al, editors: *Evidence-based geriatric nursing protocols for best practice,* ed 4, New York, 2012, Springer, pp 298–323. Also available at Hartford Institute for Geriatric Nursing: *Want to know more: nursing standard of practice protocol: pressure ulcer prevention and skin tear prevention,* http://consultgerirn.org/topics/pressure_ulcers_and_skin_tears/want_to_know_more Accessed October 31, 2014.

BOX 13-14 Mnemonic for Pressure Ulcer Treatment: DIPAMOPI

Debride
Identify and treat infection
Pack dead space lightly
Absorb excess exudate
Maintain moist wound surface
Open or excise closed wound edges
Protect healing wound from infection/trauma
Insulate to maintain normal temperature

on selection of appropriate wound dressings based on wound characteristics. Box 13-15 presents general guidelines for PU dressings.

Provision of education to patients, families, and professional staff must also be included in any skin care program. Teach the individual and his or her family about the normal healing process and keep them informed about progress (or lack of progress) toward healing, including signs and symptoms that should be brought to the professional's attention.

BOX 13-15 Factors to Consider in Selecting Pressure Ulcer Dressing

- Shallow, dry wounds with no/minimal exudate need hydrating dressings that add or trap moisture; very shallow wounds require cover dressing only (gels/transparent adhesive dressings, thin hydrocolloid, thin polyurethane foam).
- Shallow wounds with moderate to large exudate need dressings that absorb exudate, maintain moist surface, support autolysis if necrotic tissue present, protect and insulate, and protect surrounding tissue (hydrocolloids,

semipermeable polyurethane foam, calcium alginates, gauze). Cover with an absorptive cover dressing.
- Deep wounds with moderate to large exudate require filling of dead space, absorption of exudate, maintenance of moist environment, support of autolysis if necrotic tissue present, protection, and insulation (copolymer starch, dextranomer beads, calcium alginates, foam cavity). Cover with gauze pad, ABD, transparent thin film, or polyurethane foam.

KEY CONCEPTS

- The skin is the largest and most visible organ of the body; it has multiple roles in maintaining one's health.
- Maintaining adequate oral hydration and skin lubrication will reduce the incidence of xerosis and other skin problems.
- The best way to minimize the risk of skin cancer is to avoid prolonged sun exposure.
- The primary risk factors for pressure ulcer developmen are immobility and reduced activity.
- Changes in the skin with age, comorbid illnesses, nutritional status, low body mass, shear, and friction also increase pressure ulcer risk. Individuals at greatest risk include those who are confined to a bed or chair and unable to shift weight or reposition themselves.

- Structured protocols and prevention bundles should be present in all facilities and have been shown to reduce pressure ulcer development.
- A pressure ulcer is documented by stage, which reflects the greatest degree of tissue damage, and as it heals, reverse staging is not appropriate.
- A pressure ulcer covered in dead tissue (eschar or slough) cannot be staged until it is debrided.
- Darkly pigmented skin will not display the "typical" erythema of a stage I pressure ulcer or early deep tissue injury (DTI); therefore, close vigilance is necessary.

NURSING STUDY: SKIN CHANGES

James is an 84-year-old black male admitted to the hospital for surgical repair of a fractured right hip. He lives alone and his neighbors found him lying on his bathroom floor around 8 PM. James told them he had been lying there since the afternoon but could not reach the phone to call for help and was unable to move. James has a history of hypertension and diabetes.

As the nurse is performing an assessment on the second postoperative day, he documents an area on James's right heel that is purplish in color and appears to be a bruise. The area is cooler to touch than the surrounding skin. There is no redness and there are no open areas; James denies any pain in the heel.

On the basis of the nursing study, develop a nursing care plan using the following procedure*:
- List the subjective data.
- List information that provides objective data.

- From these data, identify and state, using an accepted format, two nursing diagnoses you determine are most significant at this time.
- Determine and state outcome criteria for each diagnosis. These must reflect some alleviation of the problem identified in the nursing diagnosis and must be stated in concrete and measurable terms.
- Plan and state one or more interventions for each diagnosed problem. Provide specific documentation of the source used to determine the appropriate intervention.
- Evaluate the success of the intervention. Interventions must correlate directly with the stated outcome criteria to measure the outcome success.

*Students are advised to refer to their nursing diagnosis text and identify possible or potential problems.

CRITICAL THINKING QUESTIONS AND ACTIVITIES

1. What risk factors for pressure ulcers are present in the nursing study presented above?
2. How does skin color affect the presentation of deep tissue injury?
3. What areas of the body are susceptible to pressure ulcer development and why?
4. What education needs to be provided to the patient, staff, and family?
5. When James returns home, what interventions to enhance his safety would be appropriate?

RESEARCH QUESTIONS

1. What is the most effective strategy to inform younger people about the risk of skin cancer from sun and tanning bed exposure?
2. What is the knowledge level of older individuals about pressure ulcer risk?
3. What are the major barriers identified by nursing staff to implementation of preventive interventions for pressure ulcers?
4. How effective are current patient education materials in enhancing knowledge of pressure ulcer risk among racially and culturally diverse older individuals?

REFERENCES

Agency for Healthcare Research and Quality: *On-Time Pressure Ulcer Healing Project,* 2009. http://www.ahrq.gov/professionals/systems/long-term-care/resources/pressure-ulcers/pressureulcerhealing/index.html. Accessed March 23, 2014.

Ahn C, Salicido R: Advances in wound photography and assessment methods, *Adv Skin Wound Care* 21(2):94–95, 2008.

American Cancer Society: *Cancer facts and figures 2014,* 2014. http://www.cancer.org/research/cancerfactsstatistics/cancer-factsfigures2014. Accessed March 7, 2014.

Armstrong D, Ayello E, Capitulo K, et al: New opportunities to improve pressure ulcer prevention and treatment: implementations of the CMS inpatient hospital care present on admission (POA) indicators/hospital acquired conditions (HCA) policy, *Wounds* 20:A14, 2008.

Ayello E, Sibbald R: Preventing skin ulcers and skin tears. In Boltz M, Capezuti E, Fulmer T, et al, editors: *Evidence-based geriatric nursing protocols for best practice,* ed 4, New York, 2012, Springer, pp 298–319.

Baumgarten, N, Margolis D, Orwig D, et al: Use of pressure-redistributing support surfaces among elderly hip fracture patients across the continuum of care: adherence to pressure ulcer prevention guidelines, *Gerontologist* 50:253–262, 2009.

Black J, Edsberg L, Baharestani M, et al: Pressure ulcers: avoidable or unavoidable? Results of the National Pressure Ulcer Advisory Panel Consensus Conference, *Ostomy Wound Manage* 57(2):24–37, 2011.

Centers for Disease Control and Prevention: *Parasites-scabies,* 2010. http://www.cdc.gov/parasites/scabies/. Accessed March 6, 2014.

Centers for Disease Control and Prevention: *Indoor tanning is not safe,* 2014a. http://www.cdc.gov/cancer/skin/basic_info/indoor_tanning.htm. Accessed August 2014.

Centers for Disease Control and Prevention: *Shingles (herpes zoster),* 2014b. http://www.cdc.gov/shingles. Accessed March 6, 2014.

Chou R, Dana T, Bougatsos C, et al: Pressure ulcer risk assessment and prevention: comparative effectiveness, *Comparative Effectiveness Review* no. 87 (AHRQ publication no. 12[13]-EHC148-EF), 2013. http://www.effectivehealthcare.ahrq.gov/ehc/products/309/1489/pressure-ulcer-prevention-report-130528.pdf. Accessed March 20, 2014.

Cooper K: Evidence-based prevention of pressure ulcers in the intensive care unit, *Crit Care Nurse* 33(6):57–66, 2013.

Endo J, Norman R: Skin problems. In Ham R, Sloane P, Warshaw G, et al, editors: *Primary care geriatrics,* ed 6, Philadelphia, 2014, Elsevier Saunders, pp 573–587.

European Pressure Ulcer Advisory Panel: *SCALE—skin changes at life's end, 2009.* http://www.epuap.org/scale-skin-hanges-at-lifes-end/. Accessed March 11, 2014.

Garcia A, White-Chu E: Pressure ulcers. In Ham R, Sloane P, Warshaw G, et al, editors: *Primary care geriatrics,* ed 6, Philadelphia, 2014, Elsevier Saunders, pp 333–343.

Garrett C, Saavedra A, Reed K, et al: Increasing incidence of melanoma among middle-aged adults: an epidemiological study in Olmsted County, Minnesota, *Mayo Clin Proc* 89(1):52–59, 2014.

Gillespie B, Chaboyer W, Sykes M, et al: Development and pilot testing of a patient-participatory pressure ulcer prevention bundle, *J Nurs Care Qual* 29(1):74–82, 2014.

Gray-Siracusa K, Schrier L: Use of an intervention bundle to eliminate pressure ulcers in critical care, *J Nurs Care Qual* 26(3):216–225, 2011.

Harden R, Kaye A, Kintanar T, et al: Evidence-based guideline for the management of postherpetic neuralgia in primary care, *Postgrad Med* 125(4):191–202, 2013.

Harms S, Bliss D, Garrad J, et al: Prevalence of pressure ulcers by race and ethnicity for older adults admitted to nursing homes, *J Gerontol Nurs* 40(3):20–26, 2014.

Howard D, Taylor Y: Racial and gender differences in pressure development among nursing home residents in the southeastern United States, *J Women Aging* 21:266–278, 2009.

Jamshed N, Schneider E: Is the use of supplemental vitamin C and zinc for the prevention and treatment of pressure ulcers evidence-based? *Ann Longterm Care* 18:28–32, 2010.

Jull A, Griffiths P: Is pressure ulcer prevention a sensitive indicator of the quality of nursing care? A cautionary note, *Inter J Nurs Stud* 47:531–533, 2010.

Langana S, Minassiana C, Smeeth L, et al: Risk of stroke following herpes zoster: a self-controlled case-series study, *Clin Infect Dis,* Apr 2, 2014. doi: 10.1093/cid/ciu098. [Epub ahead of print]. http://cid.oxfordjournals.org/content/early/2014/03/25/cid.ciu098.abstract. Accessed August 2014.

LeBlanc K, Baranoski S: International skin tear advisory panel: a tool kit to aid in the prevention, assessment, and treatment of skin tears using a simplified classification system, *Adv Skin Wound Care* 26:459–476, 2013.

Lee J, Cummings H, Carpenter C, et al: Herpes zoster knowledge, prevalence, and vaccination rate by race, *J Am Board Fam Med* 26(1):45–51, 2013.

McCann S, Huether S: Structure, function, and disorders of the integument. In McCance K, Huether S, editors: *Pathophysiology,* ed 7, St. Louis, MO, 2014, Elsevier, pp 1616–1651.

McGinnis E, Greenwood D, Nelson A, et al: A prospective cohort study of prognostic factors for the healing of heel pressure ulcers, *Age Ageing* 43:267–271, 2013.

Nagamachi M, Ishihara S, Nakamura M, et al: Development of a pressure-ulcer preventing mattress based on ergonomics and Kansei engineering, *Gerotechnology* 11(4):513–520, 2013.

National Pressure Ulcer Advisory Panel: *Research priorities identified for pressure ulcer prevention,* treatment and policy (Press release), June 10, 2013. http://www.npuap.org/research-priorities-identified-for-pressure-ulcer-prevention-treatment-policy. Accessed March 10, 2014.

National Pressure Ulcer Advisory Panel: *NPUAP announces new pressure ulcer registry* (Press release), Mar 10, 2014a. http://www.npuap.org/npuap-announces-new-pressure-ulcer-registry. Accessed March 11, 2014.

National Pressure Ulcer Advisory Panel: *NPUAP Pressure ulcer stages/categories*, 2014b. http://www.npuap.org/resources/educational-and-clinical-resources/npuap-pressure-ulcer-stagescategories. Accessed March 20, 2014.

National Pressure Ulcer Advisory Panel: *PUSH tool*, 2014c. https://www.npuap.org/resources/educational-and-clinical-resources/push-tool. Accessed March 23, 2014.

Olsho L, Spector W, Williams C, et al: Evaluation of AHRQ's on-time pressure ulcer prevention program: a facilitator-assisted clinical decision support intervention for nursing homes, *Med Care* 52(3):258–266, 2014.

Ong E, Goldacre R, Hoang U, et al: Subsequent primary malignancies in patients with nonmelanoma skin cancer in England: a national record-linkage study, *Cancer Epidemiol Biomarkers Prev* 23:490–498, 2014.

Phillips L, Buttery J: Exploring pressure ulcer prevalence and preventative care, *Nurs Times* 105(16):34–36, 2009.

Skin Cancer Foundation: *Skin cancer facts*, 2014. http://www.skincancer.org/skin-cancer-information. Accessed March 7, 2014.

Sibbald R, Krasner D, Lutz J, et al: SCALE: skin changes at life's end: final consensus statement: October 1, 2009, *Adv Skin Wound Care* 23(5):225–236, 2010.

Spillsbury K, Nelson A, Cullum N, et al: Pressure ulcers and their treatment an effects on quality of life: hospital inpatient perspectives, *J Adv Nurs* 57:494–504, 2007.

Tayyib N, Coyer F, Lewis P: Pressure ulcers in the adult intensive care unit: a literature review of patient risk factors and risk assessment scales, *J Nurs Educ Pract* 3(11):28–42, 2013.

U.S. Department of Health and Human Services: *Surgeon General calls for action to prevent skin cancer*, 2014. http://www.surgeongeneral.gov/library/calls/prevent-skin-cancer. Accessed August 2014.

Wehner M, Chren C, Nameth D, et al: International prevalence of indoor tanning: a systematic review and meta-analysis, *JAMA Dermatol*, Jan 29, 2013. doi: 10:10/1001/jamadermatol.2013.6896. [Epub ahead of print].

White-Chu F, Langemo D: Skin failure: identifying and managing an underrecognized condition, *Ann Longterm Care* 20(7):28–32, 2012.

World Health Organization: *Ultraviolet radiation and the INTERSUN Programme*: Skin cancers, 2014. http://www.who.int/uv/faq/skincancer/en/index2.html. Accessed March 23, 2014.

Wounds International: *International guidelines*. Pressure ulcer prevention: prevalence and incidence in context. A consensus document, London, 2009, Medical Education Partnership (MEP) Ltd. http://www.woundsinternational.com/clinical-guidelines/international-guidelines-pressure-ulcer-prevention-prevalence-and-incidence-in-context-a-consensus-document. Accessed March 10, 2014.

14 CHAPTER

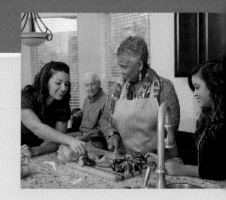

Nutrition

Theris A. Touhy

http://evolve.elsevier.com/Touhy/TwdHlthAging

A STUDENT SPEAKS

I work as a certified nursing assistant in a skilled nursing facility and I am responsible for feeding 10 residents at the dinner meal. I try to get them to eat but they are very slow and we only have a limited amount of time. Sometimes, I end up just mixing the food and getting them to take a few spoonfuls. The people with dementia need even more time and I know that they are not getting enough to eat. It makes me feel terrible and we need so much more help to do a good job.

Marcia, age 21

AN ELDER SPEAKS

If I do reach the point where I can no longer feed myself, I hope that the hands holding my fork belong to someone who has a feeling for who I am. I hope my helper will remember what she learns about me and that her awareness of me will grow from one encounter to another. Why should this make a difference? Yet I am certain that my experience of needing to be fed will be altered if it occurs in the context of my being truly known . . . I will want to know about the lives of the people I rely on, especially the one who holds my fork for me. If she would talk to me, if we could laugh together, I might even forget the chagrin of my useless hands. We would have a conversation, rather than a feeding.

From Lustbader W: Thoughts on the meaning of frailty, Generations 13:21–22, 1999.

LEARNING OBJECTIVES

On completion of this chapter, the reader will be able to:

1. Discuss nutritional requirements and factors affecting nutrition for older adults.
2. Delineate risk factors for undernutrition and identify strategies for management.
3. Describe a nutritional screening and assessment.
4. Identify evidence-based strategies to ensure adequate nutrition.
5. Describe special considerations in ensuring adequate nutrition for individuals experiencing hospitalization and institutionalization.
6. Discuss assessment and interventions for older adults with dysphagia.
7. Develop a plan of care to assist an older person in developing and maintaining good nutritional status.

The quality and quantity of diet are important factors in preventing, delaying onset, and managing chronic illnesses associated with aging. Results of studies provide growing evidence that diet can affect longevity and, when combined with lifestyle changes, reduce disease risk. "Of the top 10 leading causes of death in the United States, a lifetime of good nutrition would positively improve nine causes: heart disease, cancer, stroke, chronic respiratory disease, Alzheimer's disease, diabetes, influenza/pneumonia, nephritic syndrome/nephritis, and septicemia" (Amella and Aselage, 2012, p. 452). Additionally, about 87% of elders have diabetes, hypertension, dyslipidemia, or a combination of these diseases that have dietary implications (ADA, ASN, SNE, 2010).

Proper nutrition means that all of the essential nutrients (i.e., carbohydrates, fat, protein, vitamins, minerals, and water) are adequately supplied and used to maintain optimal health and wellness. Although some age-related changes in the gastrointestinal system do occur (Box 14-1), these changes are rarely the primary factors in inadequate nutrition. Fulfillment of nutritional needs in aging is more often affected by numerous other factors, including chronic disease, lifelong eating habits, ethnicity, socialization, income, transportation, housing, mood,

BOX 14-1   Aging-Related Changes Affecting Nutrition

Taste

Individuals have varied levels of taste sensitivity that seem predetermined by genetics and constitution, as well as age variations

The number of taste cells decreases and the remaining cells atrophy as individuals age (beginning at age 40 to 60), but they can regenerate. Lag time in regeneration may contribute to diminished taste response

Mouth produces less saliva, which can affect sense of taste

Usually salty and sweet tastes lost first, followed by bitter and sour

Dentures, smoking, and medications can affect taste

Smell

Gradual decline in number of sensor cells that detect aromas and in nerves that carry signals to the brain and in olfactory bulb that processes them; less mucus produced in nose

Increase in odor threshold and decline in odor identification

Many factors affect smell: nasal sinus disease, injury to olfactory receptors through viral infections, damage from industrial work before proper safety standards/equipment in place, smoking, medications, periodontal disease/dental problems

Changes in smell associated with Alzheimer's and Parkinson's disease

Smelling food while it is cooking and participation in preparation can stimulate appetite.

Digestive System

Changes do not significantly affect function; digestive system remains adequate throughout life

Decreased gastric motility and volume and reductions in secretion of bicarbonate and gastric mucus caused by age-related gastric atrophy, which results in hypochlorhydria (insufficient hydrochloric acid)

Decreased production of intrinsic factor can lead to pernicious anemia if stomach not able to use ingested B_{12} vitamins

Protective alkaline viscous mucus of stomach lost because of increase in stomach pH, making stomach more susceptible to *Helicobacter pylori* infection and peptic ulcer disease, particularly with use of nonsteroidal antiinflammatory drugs

Presbyesophagus (decrease in intensity of propulsive waves) may occur, forcing the lower end to dilate and may lead to digestive discomfort

Pathological processes seen with increasing frequency include gastroesophageal reflux disease (GERD) and hiatal hernia

Loss of smooth muscle in stomach delays emptying time, which may lead to anorexia or weight loss as a result of distention, meal-induced fullness, and premature satiety

Buccal Cavity

Teeth become worn, darker in color, prone to longitudinal cracks

Dentin becomes brittle and thick; pulp space decreases

Osteopenia of the facial bones and subtle changes to the connective tissues of the skin, sinuses, and oral cavity

Xerostomia (dry mouth) occurs in 30% of older individuals and can affect eating, swallowing, and speaking and lead to dental decay. More than 500 medications can affect salivary flow

Artificial saliva preparations and adequate fluid intake can help

Regulation of Appetite

Appetite depends on physical activity, functional limitations, smell, taste, mood, socialization, comfort, medications, chronic illness, oral/dental problems

Individuals may be less hungry, fuller before meals, consume smaller meals, become more satiated following meal

Gastrointestinal hormones such as cholescystokinin (CCK) regulate satiety to varying degrees. With age, CCK is increased basally and following a meal and may have a more potent satiating effect. Disease states increase cytokine levels as a result of release by diseased tissues. Increase in CCK levels also occurs in malnutrition, which further decreases appetite

Endogenous opioid feeding and drinking drive may decline and contribute to decreased appetite and dehydration

Decreased stomach fundal compliance, decreased testosterone, increased leptin and amylin also thought to contribute to decreased appetite

Ability to feed self/staff feeding techniques, and mealtime ambience also affect appetite

Body Composition

Increase in body fat, including visceral fat stores

Decrease in muscle mass

Body weight usually peaks fifth or sixth decade of life and remains stable until age 65 or 70, after which there is a slow decrease in body weight for remainder of life

---

food knowledge, functional impairments, health, and dentition. Data from the National Health and Nutrition Examination Survey (NHANES) showed that U.S. adults continue to fall short in meeting recommended dietary guidelines, and sociodemographic conditions influence food choices and overall diet quality (Ervin, 2011).

This chapter discusses the dietary needs of older adults, age-related changes affecting nutrition, risk factors contributing to inadequate nutrition, obesity, and the effect of diseases, functional and cognitive impairment, and dysphagia on nutrition. Readers are referred to a nutrition text for more comprehensive information on nutrition and aging.

GLOBAL NUTRITION CONCERNS

Adequate, affordable food supplies and improved nutrition are concerns worldwide with some differences between developed

and developing countries. In 2008, Dr. Margaret Chan, Director-General of the World Health Organization, presented a lecture on the global nutrition challenge. Her presentation beautifully summarized many of the challenges related to nutrition worldwide (Box 14-2). Although issues vary among different areas of the globe, nutrition as a major contributor to health is a universal concern. Box 14-3 presents resources on nutrition and global initiatives.

AGE-RELATED REQUIREMENTS

United States Dietary Guidelines

The *2010 Dietary Guidelines for Americans*, published by the federal government, is designed to promote health, reduce the risk of chronic diseases, an reduce the prevalence of overweight and obesity through improved nutrition and physical activity. The guidelines focus on balancing calories with physical activity

BOX 14-2   Global Nutrition

"The global nutrition situation is a picture of extremes including fasting and feasting, of wasting, stunting, and obesity. At one end, undernutrition and deficiencies in essential nutrients are the underlying cause of an estimated 3.5 million deaths each year, largely in young children and pregnant women. At the other end we have a global epidemic of obesity, increasingly starting in childhood. We have millions of people at increased risk of developing diet-related chronic diseases, like heart disease, cancer and diabetes. Long considered the companions of wealthy societies, these chronic diseases have changed place. They now impose their greatest burden in low and middle income countries. Contributing factors include longer life expectancies, urbanization, lifestyle changes, the industrialization of food production, and the globalization of food marketing and distribution."

Source: Chan M: *The global nutrition challenge: getting a healthy start* (Keynote address, Pacific Health Summit), 2008. http://www.who.int/dg/speeches/2008/20080618/en Accessed March 2014.

BOX 14-3   RESOURCES FOR BEST PRACTICE

Nutrition

American Heart Association: DASH diet; Mediterranean diet

Capezuti E, Zwicker D, Mezey M, et al, editors: *Evidence-based geriatric nursing protocols for best practice*, ed 4, New York, 2012, Springer (Nutrition, Mealtime Difficulties)

Global Alliance for Improved Nutrition (GAIN): Supports partnerships to increase access to the missing nutrients in diets necessary for people, communities, and economies

HelpGuide.com: Eating well over 50, Nutrition and Diet Tips for Healthy Eating as You Age

National Institute on Aging: What's on your plate? Smart Food Choices for Healthy Aging

Pioneer Network: New Dining Practice Standards (LTC)

The American Geriatrics Society: *Position statement: Feeding tubes in advanced dementia*

The Hartford Foundation for Geriatric Nursing: Assessing Nutrition in Older Adults (includes video of administration of MNA); Mealtime Difficulties, Preventing Aspiration in Older Adults with Dysphagia (includes video)

The Hunger Project: A global, non-profit organization committed to the sustainable end of world hunger

The Journal for Nurse Practitioners: Malnutrition Resource Center

World Health Organization: Nutrition: Educational materials, databases, global initiatives

and encourage Americans to consume more healthy foods like vegetables, fruits, whole grains, fat-free and low-fat dairy products, and seafood and to consume less sodium, saturated and *trans* fats, added sugars, and refined grains. In addition to the key recommendations, there are recommendations for specific population groups including older adults (USDA and USDHHS, 2010). *Healthy People 2020* also provides goals for nutrition (Box 14-4).

MyPlate for Older Adults

As part of the 2010 Guidelines, the new visual depiction of daily food intake, Choose MyPlate (ChooseMyPlate.gov), replaces the information formerly found on MyPyramid.gov. The USDA

BOX 14-4   HEALTHY PEOPLE 2020

Nutrition and Weight Status

- Promote health and reduce chronic disease through the consumption of healthful diets and achievement and maintenance of body weight.
- Increase the proportion of primary care physicians who regularly measure the body mass index in their adult patients.
- Increase the proportion of physician office visits made by adult patients who are obese that include counseling or education related to weight reduction, nutrition, or physical activity.
- Increase the proportion of adults who are at a healthy weight.
- Reduce household food insecurity and in so doing reduce hunger.

Data from U.S. Department of Health and Human Services, Office of Disease Prevention and Health Promotion: Healthy People 2020, 2012. http://www.healthypeople.gov/2020

Human Nutrition Research Center on Aging at Tufts University has introduced the MyPlate for Older Adults, which calls attention to the unique nutritional and physical activity needs associated with advancing years. The drawing features different forms of vegetables and fruits that are convenient, affordable, and readily available. Other unique components of the MyPlate for Older Adults include icons for regular physical activity and emphasis on adequate fluid intake, areas of particular concern for older adults (Figure 14-1).

Generally, older adults need fewer calories because they may not be as active and metabolic rates decline. However, they still require the same or higher levels of nutrients for optimal health outcomes. The recommendations may need modification for individuals who have illnesses. The Dietary Approaches to Stop Hypertension (DASH) eating plan is a recommended eating plan to assist with maintenance of optimal weight and management of hypertension. This plan consists of fruits, vegetables, whole grains, low-fat dairy products, poultry, and fish, as well as restriction of salt intake (see Box 14-3).

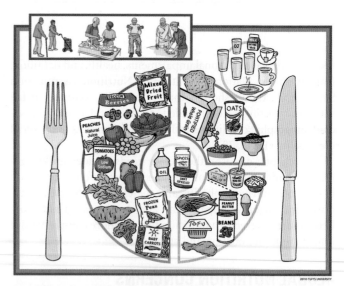

FIGURE 14-1 MyPlate for Older Adults. (From the Jean Mayer USDA Human Nutrition Research Center on Aging, Tufts University: MyPlate for older adults, 2011. http://hnrca.tufts.edu/my-plate-for-older-adults.

The Mediterranean diet has also been associated with a lower incidence of chronic illness, weight gain, impaired physical function, and improved cognition in recent studies (Martinez-Lapiscina et al, 2013; Samieri et al, 2013a,b; Slomski, 2014; Yang et al, 2014). This diet is characterized by a greater intake of fruits, vegetables, legumes, whole grains, and fish; a lower intake of red and processed meats; higher amounts of monosaturated fats, mostly provided by olive oil from Mediterranean countries; and lower amounts of saturated fats. The MIND diet, a hybrid between the Mediteranean and DASH diets, is also associated with a lower risk of Alzheimer's disease (Morris et al, 2015).

Other Dietary Recommendations
Fats

Although there has been some discussion regarding the benefits of a high intake of polyunsaturated fats and a low consumption of saturated fats (Chowdhury et al, 2014), it is recommended, similar to other age groups, that older adults should limit intake of saturated fat and trans fatty acids. High-fat diets cause obesity and increase the risk of heart disease and cancer. Recommendations are that 20% to 35% of total calories should be from fat, 45% to 65% from carbohydrates, and 10% to 35% from proteins. Monounsaturated fats, such as olive oil, are the best type of fat because they lower low-density lipoprotein (LDL) level but leave the high-density lipoprotein (HDL) level intact or even slightly raise it. A simple technique to determine how much fat a person should consume is to divide the ideal weight in half and allowing that number of grams of fat (Haber, 2010).

Protein

Presently, the Institute of Medicine's Recommended Dietary Allowance (RDA) for protein of 0.8 g/kg per day, based primarily on studies in younger men, may be inadequate for older adults. Higher protein consumption, particularly animal protein, as a fraction of total caloric intake, is associated with a decline in risk of frailty in older adults (Beasley et al, 2010; Imai et al, 2014). Protein intake of 1.5 g/kg per day, or 20% to 25% of total calorie intake, may be more appropriate for older adults at risk of becoming frail. Older people who are ill are the most likely segment of society to experience protein deficiency. Those with limitations affecting their ability to shop, cook, and consume food are also at risk for protein deficiency and malnutrition.

Fiber

Fiber is an important dietary component that some older people do not consume in sufficient quantities. A daily intake of 25 g of fiber is recommended and must be combined with adequate amounts of fluid. This amount of fiber is equivalent to eating 7 apples or 12 bananas/day, or 8 carrots/day, or 1 cup of bran or a few cups of cereal each day (Acalovschi, 2012). Insufficient amounts of fiber in the diet, as well as insufficient fluids, contribute to constipation. Fiber is the indigestible material that gives plants their structure. It is abundant in raw fruits and vegetables and in unrefined grains and cereals (Box 14-5).

Vitamins and Minerals

Older people who consume five servings of fruits and vegetables daily will obtain adequate intake of vitamins A, C, and E

BOX 14-5 TIPS FOR BEST PRACTICE
Teaching about Fiber in the Diet

Benefits of Fiber
- Facilitates absorption of water; helps control weight by delaying gastric emptying and providing feeling of fullness; improves glucose tolerance; prevents or reduces constipation, hemorrhoids, diverticulosis; reduces risk of heart disease; protects against cancer

Diet Tips to Add Fiber
- Best to get fiber from food rather than supplements because they do not contain essential nutrients found in high-fiber foods and anticancer benefits are questionable; the more refined or processed the food becomes, the lower the fiber content (e.g., apple with peel higher fiber than applesauce or juice)
- Increase consumption of fresh fruits and vegetables; eat dry beans, peas, and lentils; leave skin on fruits and vegetables; eat whole fruit rather than drink juice; eat whole-grain breads and cereals; add finely chopped veggies to pasta sauce, soups, and casseroles; add a cup of spinach or other leafy greens to a smoothie (you will not taste the spinach at all but your drink will be green); sprinkle unsweetened bran on cereals or put in soups, meat loaf, or casseroles
- Some foods naturally high in fiber: large pear with skin (7 g); 1 cup fresh raspberries (8 g); ½ medium avocado (5 g); 1 oz almonds (3.5 g); ¼ cup cooked black beans (7.5 g); 3 cups air-popped popcorn (3.6 g); 1 cup cooked pearled barley (6 g)

How Much Bran?
- Generally 1-2 tablespoons daily; begin with 1 teaspoon and increase gradually to avoid bloating, gas, diarrhea, other colon discomforts

How Much Fluid?
- 64 oz daily unless fluid restriction

and also potassium. Americans of all ages eat less than half of the recommended amounts of fruits and vegetables (Haber, 2010). After age 50, the stomach produces less gastric acid, which makes vitamin B_{12} absorption less efficient. Vitamin B_{12} deficiency is a common and underrecognized condition that is estimated to occur in 12% to 14% of community-dwelling older adults and in up to 25% of those residing in institutional settings (Ahmed and Haboubi, 2010).

Although intake of this vitamin is generally adequate, older adults should increase their intake of the crystalline form of vitamin B_{12} from fortified foods such as whole-grain breakfast cereals. Use of proton pump inhibitors for more than 1 year, as well as histamine H_2-receptor blockers, can lead to lower serum vitamin B_{12} levels by impairing absorption of the vitamin from food. Metformin, colchicine, and antibiotic and anticonvulsant agents may also increase the risk of vitamin B_{12} deficiency (Cadogan, 2010). Calcium and vitamin D are essential for bone health and may prevent osteoporosis and decrease the risk of fracture. Chapter 26 discusses recommendations for calcium and vitamin D supplementation.

OBESITY (OVERNUTRITION)

The World Health Organization (WHO, 2003) noted that an escalating global epidemic of overweight and obesity—"globesity"—is a major public health concern in both developed and developing countries. The number of obese adults worldwide is 300 million, with estimates that 115 million people in developing countries suffer from obesity-related problems. Overweight and obesity are associated with increased health care costs, functional impairments, disability, chronic disease, and nursing home admission (Felix, 2008; Newman, 2009). It is important to remember that overweight/obese individuals are also at risk for malnutrition as a result of chronic illness or diets inadequate in appropriate nutrients.

Obesity and Older Adults

In the United States, more than two-thirds of all adults are overweight (body mass index [BMI] = 25 to 29.9) or obese (BMI ≥30). There has been some slowing in the rapid increase in obesity, but prevalence has not changed in the past decade and remains very high. Since 2008, Americans aged 65 and older have seen the sharpest rise in obesity and the proportion of older adults who are obese has doubled in the past 30 years (Flicker et al, 2010). More than one-third of individuals 65 years and older are obese with a higher prevalence in those 65 to 74 years than in those 75 years and older. Rates of obesity have increased in women 60 years and older. Overweight and obesity are more prevalent among African American (82%) and Hispanic (77%) women than among white women (63%). Socioeconomic deprivation and lower levels of education have been linked to obesity (Ogden et al, 2014).

Although there is strong evidence that obesity in younger people lessens life expectancy and has a negative effect on functionality and morbidity, it remains unclear whether overweight and obesity are predictors of mortality in older adults. In what has been termed the *obesity paradox*, some research has found that for people who have survived to 70 years of age, mortality risk is lowest in those with a BMI classified as overweight (Felix, 2008; Tobias et al, 2014). Persons who increased or decreased in BMI have a greater mortality risk than those who have a stable BMI, particularly in those aged 70 to 79 (Dahl et al, 2013). For nursing home residents with severely decreased functional status, obesity may be regarded as a protective factor with regard to functionality and mortality (Kaiser et al, 2010).

Some experts have noted that BMI thresholds for overweight and obese are overly restrictive for older people (Dahl et al, 2013; Flicker et al, 2010). Recently, Tobias and colleagues (2014) questioned the obesity paradox and reported that for persons with diabetes, obesity significantly increased mortality risk. However, before any clinical recommendations can be made, further research is needed to understand how long-term intentional weight loss and associated shifts in body composition affect the onset of chronic disease.

Weight loss recommendations should be carefully considered on an individualized basis with attention to the weight history and medical conditions. The most effective weight loss program combines nutrition education, diet, and exercise with behavioral strategies (Bales and Buhr, 2008; Mathew and Jacobs, 2014). Maintaining a healthy weight throughout life can prevent many illnesses and functional limitations as a person grows older.

MALNUTRITION (UNDERNUTRITION)

Malnutrition is a recognized geriatric syndrome (DiMaria-Ghalili, 2012; Institute of Medicine, 2008). The rising incidence of malnutrition among older adults has been documented in acute care, long-term care, and the community. Malnutrition is estimated to occur in 1% to 15% of ambulatory outpatients, 25% to 60% of institutionalized patients, 35% to 65% of hospitalized patients, and 49% of patients discharged from the hospital (Buys et al, 2013; Mathew and Jacobs, 2014). These figures are expected to rise dramatically in the next 30 years (Ahmed and Haboubi, 2010). A high prevalence of hospital malnutrition has also been reported in Australia, Europe, and the UK (Jefferies et al, 2011). Malnutrition among older people is clearly a serious challenge for health professionals in all settings.

Consequences

Malnutrition is a precursor to frailty and has serious consequences, including infections, pressure ulcers, anemia, hypotension, impaired cognition, hip fractures, prolonged hospital stay, institutionalization, and increased morbidity and mortality (DiMaria-Ghalili, 2012; White et al, 2012). "Malnourished older adults take 40% longer to recover from illness, have two to three times as many complications, and have hospital stays that are 90% longer" (Haber, 2010, p. 211). Many factors contribute to the occurrence of malnutrition in older adults (Figure 14-2).

Characteristics

The understanding of malnutrition is evolving, and research is ongoing. "Malnutrition is a complex syndrome that develops following two primary trajectories. It can occur when the individual does not consume sufficient amounts of micronutrients (i.e., vitamins, minerals, phytochemicals) and macronutrients (i.e., protein, carbohydrates, fat, water) required to maintain organ function and healthy tissues. This type of malnutrition can occur from prolonged undernutrition or overnutrition. In contrast, inflammation-related malnutrition develops as a consequence of injury, surgery, or disease states that trigger inflammatory mediators that contribute to increased metabolic rate and impaired nutrient utilization" (Litchford, 2013, p. 38). Inflammation is increasingly identified as an important underlying factor that increases risk for malnutrition and a contributing factor to suboptimal responses to nutritional intervention and increased risk of mortality (DiMaria-Ghalili, 2012). Weight loss frequently occurs in both trajectories (White et al, 2012).

A consensus approach to defining adult malnutrition was developed by an international guideline committee with identification of new adult disease–related malnutrition subtypes (Jensen et al, 2010) (Box 14-6). Because there is a wide variation in approaches to the diagnosis of malnutrition, the international guideline committee also proposed criteria for identifying malnutrition (White et al, 2012) (Box 14-7).

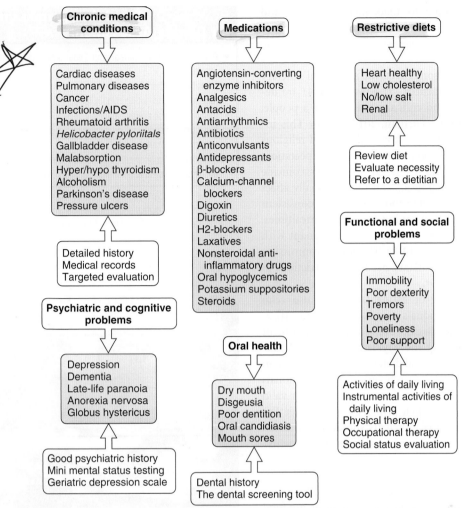

FIGURE 14-2 Risk Factors for Undernutrition and Assessment. (From Omran M, Salem P: Diagnosing undernutrition, *Clin Geriatr Med* 18:719–736, 2002.)

BOX 14-6   **Malnutrition Subtypes**

- Starvation-related malnutrition (no inflammation, pure chronic starvation, anorexia nervosa)
- Chronic disease–related malnutrition (mild to moderate inflammation, organ failure, pancreatic cancer, rheumatoid arthritis, sarcopenic obesity)
- Acute disease–related malnutrition (marked inflammatory response, major infection, burns, trauma, closed head injury)

Source: White J, Guenter P, Jensen G, et al: Consensus statement of the Academy of Nutrition and Dietetics/American Society for Parenteral and Enteral Nutrition: characteristics recommended for the identification and documentation of adult malnutrition (undernutrition), *J Acad Nutr Diet* 112:730–738, 2012.

BOX 14-7   **Criteria for Malnutrition**

Identification of two or more of the following recommended for diagnosis of malnutrition:

- Insufficient protein intake
- Weight loss
- Loss of muscle mass
- Loss of subcutaneous fat
- Localized or generalized fluid accumulation that may sometimes mask weight loss
- Diminished functional status as measured by hand-grip strength

Source: White J, Guenter P, Jensen G, et al: Consensus statement of the Academy of Nutrition and Dietetics/American Society for Parenteral and Enteral Nutrition: characteristics recommended for the identification and documentation of adult malnutrition (undernutrition), *J Acad Nutr Diet* 112:730–738, 2012.

FACTORS AFFECTING FULFILLMENT OF NUTRITIONAL NEEDS

Fulfillment of the older person's nutritional needs is affected by numerous factors including changes associated with aging, lifelong eating habits, acute and chronic illness, medication regimens, ethnicity and culture, ability to obtain and prepare food, mood, socialization, socioeconomic deprivation, transportation, housing, and food knowledge.

Age-Associated Changes

Some age-related changes in the senses of taste and smell (chemosenses) and the digestive tract (see Box 14-1) do occur as the individual ages and may affect nutrition. For most older people, these changes do not seriously interfere with eating, digestion, and the enjoyment of food. However, combined with other factors, they may contribute to inadequate nutrition and decreased eating pleasure.

Lifelong Eating Habits

The nutritional state of a person reflects the individual's dietary history and present food practices. "Foodways (2014) are defined as the eating habits and culinary practices of a people, region, or historical period" (Furman, 2014, p. 80). This includes unique eating patterns of various cultural and religious groups. Foodways influence food preferences, meal expectation, and nutritional intake. Eating habits do not always coincide with fulfillment of nutritional needs and may especially affect the ability and desire to consume food that is not consistent with individual foodways. The meaning of food and mealtimes, often established in childhood, "become more poignant with age" (Furman, 2014, p. 83) (Box 14-8). The Joint Commission (2010) specifies assessment of dietary needs and restrictions in a patient safety tool (Box 14-9).

Lifelong habits of dieting or eating fad foods also echo through the later years. Individuals may fall prey to advertisements that claim specific foods can reverse aging or rid one of chronic conditions. Following the MyPlate for Older Adults (see Figure 14-1) is best for an ideal diet, with changes based on particular problems, such as hypercholesteremia. Individuals should be counseled to base their dietary decisions on valid research and consultation with their primary care provider. For the healthy individual, essential nutrients should be obtained from food sources rather than relying on dietary supplements.

Socialization

The fundamentally social aspect of eating has to do with sharing and the feeling of belonging that it provides. All of us use food as a means of giving and receiving love, friendship, or belonging. The presence of others during meals is a significant predictor of caloric intake (Locher et al, 2008). "Food and mealtimes are

---

BOX 14-9   The Joint Commission Guidelines for Dietary Assessment

- Ask the patient "Is there anything your providers should be aware of regarding your diet?"
- Identify whether the patient's religious or spiritual beliefs or customs require or forbid eating certain foods.
- Determine if the patient routinely or periodically observes fasting practices.
- Note the dietary needs or restrictions in the medical record and communicate them to staff.
- Make sure the hospital food service accommodates the patient's preferences and cultural and religious eating customs.

From The Joint Commission: *Patient Safety Tool: Advancing effective communication, cultural competence and patient- and family-centered care: a roadmap for hospitals,* Oakbrook Terrace, IL, 2010, The Joint Commission.

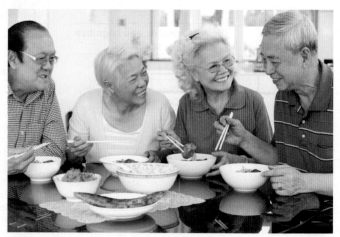

Older Adults Enjoying a Meal Together. (©iStock.com/monkeybusinessimages.)

---

associated with both personal and social identity and represent more than solids or liquids to ingest or a time and place to ingest them" (Furman, 2014, p. 83).

The meaning and enjoyment of eating can often be challenged as one ages, requires hospitalization or nursing home residence, or experiences chronic illnesses, depression, isolation, and functional limitations. Nurses need to remember this when they assess nutritional adequacy and design interventions to enhance intake.

Disinterest in food may also result from the effects of medication or disease processes. Misuse and abuse of alcohol are prevalent among older adults and are growing public health concerns. Excessive drinking interferes with nutrition. Drinking alcohol depletes the body of necessary nutrients and often replaces meals, thus making an individual susceptible to malnutrition (Chapter 28).

The elderly nutrition program, authorized under Title III of the Older Americans Act (OAA), is the largest national food and nutrition program specifically for older adults. Programs and services include congregate nutrition programs, home-delivered nutrition services (Meals-on-Wheels), and nutrition

---

🔍 BOX 14-8   RESEARCH HIGHLIGHTS

This study explored the effect of Tabinah on depression, stress and anxiety, and selected categories of mood among institutionalized older adults in Malaysia. Tabinah is a barley syrup cooked with milk and sweetened with honey that the Prophet Mohammad recommended people eat when sad events happen because it soothes hearts and relieves sadness. Among Arabs, Tabinah food has been used to relieve depression but there has been little scientific study of its effect.

Results showed that Tabinah had significant effects on reducing depression and enhancing mood. The nutritional composition of Tabinah, mainly the high carbohydrate content, differential amino acid ratio, and zinc content, may be the reason behind this positive effect. High carbohydrate content has an effect on mood and depression due to the effect of carbohydrates on serotonin synthesis. Further studies are needed, but Tabinah may be a nutritious food that could reduce depression, relieve stress, and enhance mood among institutionalized older individuals.

Source: Badrasawi M, Shahar S, Manaf Z, et al: Effect of Tabinah food consumption on depressive symptoms among elderly individuals in long term care facilities, randomized clinical trial, *Clin Interv Aging* 8: 279–285, 2013.

screening and education. The program is not means tested, and participants may make voluntary confidential contributions for meals. However, the OAA Nutrition Program reaches less than one-third of older adults in need of its program and services, and those served receive only three meals a week. With the emphasis on community-based care rather than institutional care, expansion of nutrition services should be a priority.

These nutrition programs enable older adults to avoid or delay costly institutionalization and allow them to stay in their homes and communities. An added benefit of congregate dining is the socialization provided. The American Dietetic Association (Kamp et al, 2010) estimates that the cost of 1 day in a hospital equals the cost of 1 year of OAA Nutrition Program meals, while the cost of 1 month in a nursing home equals that of providing midday meals 5 days a week in the community for about 7 years.

Chronic Diseases and Conditions

Many chronic diseases and their sequelae pose nutritional challenges for older adults. For example, heart failure and chronic obstructive pulmonary disease (COPD) are associated with fatigue, increased energy expenditure, and decreased appetite. Dietary interventions for diabetes are essential but may also affect customary eating patterns and require lifestyle changes. Conditions of the teeth and dental problems also affect nutrition (Chapter 15). More detailed information on chronic illness can be found in Chapters 21-27.

Many medications affect appetite and nutrition (Figure 14-2). There are clinically significant drug-nutrient interactions that result in nutrient loss, and evidence is accumulating that shows the use of nutritional supplements may counteract these possible drug-induced nutrient depletions. A thorough medication review is an essential component of nutritional assessment, and individuals should receive education about the effects of prescription medications, as well as herbals and supplements, on nutritional status (Chapters 9 and 10).

Gastrointestinal Disorders and Conditions

Although there are several physiological and functional changes in the gut associated with aging, the majority of the problems are the result of extrinsic factors. Polypharmacy, comorbid conditions, inactivity, and high-fat, high-volume meals are all aggravating factors. Gastroesophageal reflux disease (GERD) and diverticular disease are discussed here. Constipation is discussed in Chapter 16.

Gastroesophageal Reflux Disease

Gastroesophageal reflux disease (GERD) is a syndrome defined as mucosal damage from the movement of gastric contents backwards from the stomach into the esophagus. It is the most common gastrointestinal (GI) disorder affecting older adults. GERD is diagnosed empirically based on history and response to treatment. When the symptoms do not resolve with standard treatment, an endoscopy is indicated.

Etiology. The majority of GERD is caused by abnormalities of the lower esophageal sphincter (LES). When this muscle relaxes and allows reflux or is generally weak, GERD may occur. Risk factors include hiatal hernia, obesity, pregnancy, cigarette smoking, or inhaling second-hand smoke (Pluta et al, 2011). People of all ages can develop GERD, some for unknown reasons (National Digestive Diseases Information Clearinghouse, 2014).

Signs and symptoms. Although complaints of simple "heartburn" are often from dyspepsia, when other signs and symptoms are added it is a greater concern. The classic complaints indicative of GERD are heartburn plus regurgitation—a sensation of burning in the throat as partially digested food and stomach acid inappropriately return to the posterior oropharynx. Older adults more commonly have more atypical symptoms of persistent cough, exacerbations of asthma, laryngitis, and intermittent chest pain. Abdominal pain may occur within 1 hour of eating, and symptoms are worse when lying down with the added pressure of gravity on the LES. Consumption of alcohol before or during eating exacerbates the reflux.

Complications. Persistent symptoms may lead to esophagitis, peptic strictures, esophageal ulcers (with bleeding), and, most importantly, Barrett's esophagus, a precursor to cancer. The most serious complication is the development of pneumonia from the aspiration of stomach contents. Dental caries may be caused from chronic exposure to gastric acids.

Diverticular Disease

Diverticula are small herniations or saclike out-pouchings of mucosa that extend through the muscle layers of the colon wall, almost exclusive of the sigmoid colon. They form at weak points in the colon wall, usually where arteries penetrate and provide nutrients to the mucosal layer. Usually less than 1 cm in diameter, diverticula have thin, compressible walls if empty or firm walls if full of fecal matter. Diverticular disease is primarily a "hot" illness by those persons who subscribe to the hot/cold theory of disease causation and treatment (Giger and Davidhizar, 2003; Chapter 4). The prevalence is 5% for persons younger than age 40, and it increases to 30% for age 60 and to 50% for those older than age 80 (McQuaid, 2010). The risk factors for diverticular disease can be found in Box 14-10. Diverticulitis is an acute inflammatory complication of diverticulosis. Occasionally the fecal matter in a diverticulum will become quite desiccated, even calcified.

Etiology. Although the exact etiology of diverticular disease is unknown, it is thought to be the result of a low-fiber diet, especially one accompanied by increased intraabdominal pressure and chronic constipation. Smoking and obesity have been linked to diverticulitis and physical activity is associated with a decreased risk (Morris et al, 2014).

BOX 14-10 Risk Factors for Diverticular Disease

- Family history
- Personal history of gallbladder disease
- Low dietary intake of fiber
- Use of medications that slow fecal transit time
- Chronic constipation
- Obesity

Signs and symptoms. The majority of persons with diverticulosis are completely asymptomatic, and the condition is found only when a barium enema, colonoscopy, or computed tomography (CT) scan is performed for some other reason. Persons with uncomplicated diverticulitis complain of abdominal pain, especially in the left-lower quadrant, and may have a fever and elevated white blood cell count, although the latter symptoms may be delayed or absent in the older adult. The physical assessment may be completely negative. Rectal bleeding is typically acute in onset, is painless, and stops spontaneously.

Complications. The complications of diverticulitis are rupture, abscess, stricture, or fistula. With any perforation, peritonitis is likely. Persons with these complications may have an elevated pulse rate or are hypotensive; however, in the older adult, unexplained lethargy or confusion may be seen as well or instead. A lower-left quadrant mass may be palpated. Complicated diverticulitis is always considered an emergency and requires hospitalization for treatment and possible surgical repair.

◆ PROMOTING HEALTHY AGING: IMPLICATIONS FOR GERONTOLOGICAL NURSING

Although neither can be prevented, it may be possible to exert considerable control over exacerbation of the symptoms of GERD and diverticular disease, and to have some effect on preventing complications or, at a minimum, developing awareness of the early signs of potential complications.

The management of GERD combines lifestyle changes with pharmacological preparations, used in a stepwise fashion. Lifestyle modifications include eating smaller meals; not eating 3 to 4 hours before bed; avoiding high-fat foods, alcohol, caffeine, and nicotine; and sleeping with the head of the bed elevated. Weight reduction and smoking cessation are helpful. These strategies alone may control the majority of symptoms when complications are not present. Pharmacological preparations begin with over-the-counter antacids, such as Tums and Rolaids, and progress to H_2 blockers, such as ranitidine (Zantac), and then proton pump inhibitors, such as lansoprazole (Prevacid). In severe cases of GERD, surgical tightening of the lower esophageal sphincter may be necessary. The nurse may work with the elder to identify situations that aggravate his or her GERD (e.g., overeating, consuming alcohol at mealtime) and develop strategies to best deal with them. The nurse also teaches persons with GERD the alarm signs—the signs that should receive prompt evaluation by a physician or nurse practitioner (Box 14-11).

For persons with diverticulosis, the goal is prevention of diverticulitis. High-fiber diets (25 to 30 g/day) have been cited in American, European, and Asian studies as protective against diverticulosis. In addition, persons should strive for intake of six to eight glasses of fluid per day, preferably with little caffeine.

Acute diverticulitis can be quite painful. The nurse works with the individual to find effective and safe comfort strategies that include pain medication and creative nonpharmacological

---

BOX 14-11   Warning Signs Suggesting Possible GERD Complication

- Anemia
- Anorexia
- Dysphagia
- Hematemesis
- Odynophagia
- Weight loss

GERD, Gastroesophageal reflux disease.

---

approaches such as massage, hot or cold packs, stretching exercises, relaxation, music, or meditation techniques. Uncomplicated diverticulitis is treated with antibiotics and a clear liquid diet and is usually managed in the outpatient setting.

In the promotion of healthy aging, the nurse works with the elder to analyze diet, fluid intake, and activity level to ensure adequate motility and minimal pressure within the GI tract. If the person is overweight or obese, weight loss will decrease intraabdominal pressure and decrease the risk for the development of new diverticula and exacerbations of GERD. In all cases, the nurse is responsible for patient education regarding the appropriate use of medications, the warning signs of potential problems, and the best response to the signs or symptoms. When working with an elder in a cross-cultural setting, it is especially important for the nurse to communicate effectively and incorporate cultural expectations and habits (e.g., diet) into the plan of nursing care. The nurse works with the elder to achieve lifestyle modifications.

Socioeconomic Deprivation

There is a strong relationship between poor nutrition and socioeconomic deprivation. About 1 in 10 individuals ages 65 and older has an income below the poverty level in the United States. Rates are closer to 15% when the supplemental poverty measure is used rather than the official poverty measure (Levinson et al, 2013). Estimates are that 8.8% of households with older adults in the United States are food insecure, which means that they are not sure where or how they will get their next meal (Greenlee, 2014). Poverty rates among older African Americans and Hispanics, as well as older single women, are higher than for other groups.

Older individuals in developing countries consistently experience disproportionately high levels of poverty, with estimates that 80% have no regular income and 100 million live on less than 1 U.S. dollar a day. The economic marginalization of older people in developing countries has multiple health effects. Individuals with low incomes may need to choose among fulfilling needs such as food, heat, telephone bills, medications, and health care visits. Some older people eat only once per day in an attempt to make their income last through the month.

The Supplemental Nutrition Assistance Program (SNAP), a program of the United States Department of Agriculture (UDSA), Food and Nutrition Services, offers nutrition assistance to eligible, low-income individuals and families, but older adults are less likely than any other age group to use food assistance programs (Fuller-Thomson and Redmond, 2008). Some individuals may not see the benefit and others, especially those who lived through the Great Depression, are very reluctant to accept "welfare" (Chapter 1).

Fuller-Thomson and Redmond (2008) suggest the use of focused outreach programs and public education to destigmatize food assistance programs and encourage greater use by older individuals in need. The SNAP program works with state agencies, nutrition educators, and neighborhood and faith-based organizations to assist those eligible for nutrition assistance to make informed decisions about applying for the program and accessing benefits. Other suggestions to encourage greater use include creating mobile and satellite food assistance program offices; increasing on-line application forms; developing more user-friendly applications; providing home visits by food assistance program staff; offering more extensive multilingual services; and targeting information to those who receive Supplemental Security Income (SSI) or Medicaid, who live in public housing, and whose Social Security payments are below the poverty line (Fuller-Thomson and Redmond, 2008).

Free food programs, such as donated commodities, are also available at distribution centers (food banks) for those with limited incomes. Although this is another valuable option, use of such programs is not always feasible. One takes a chance on the types of food available on any particular day or week; quantities distributed are frequently too large for the single older person or the older couple to use or even carry from the distribution site; the site may be too far away or difficult to reach; and the time of food distribution may be inconvenient.

There are cafeterias and restaurants that provide special meal prices for older people, but costs have risen with increases in food costs. The previous advantages of eating out have diminished. Yet many single elders eat out for most meals. More elders are eating at fast food restaurants that typically do not offer low-fat/low-salt menu items. Providing education about the nutritional content of fast food and other convenient ways to enhance healthy nutritional intake is important (Box 14-3).

Transportation

Available and easily accessible transportation may be limited for older people. Many small, long-standing neighborhood food stores have been closed in the wake of the expansion of larger supermarkets, which are located in areas that serve a greater segment of the population. It may become difficult to walk to the market, to reach it by public transportation, or to carry a bag of groceries while using a cane or walker. Fear is apparent in elders' consideration of transportation. They may fear walking in the street and being mugged, not being able to cross the street in the time it takes the traffic light to change, or being knocked down or falling as they walk in crowded streets. Despite reduced senior citizen bus fares, many older people remain very fearful of attack when using public transportation. Functional impairments also make the use of public transportation difficult for others.

Transportation by taxicab may be unrealistic for an individual on a limited income, but sharing a taxicab with others who also need to shop may enable the older person to go where

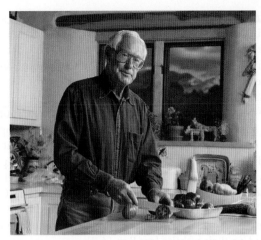

An Older Man Preparing a Meal. (Courtesy Corbis Images.)

food prices are cheaper and to take advantage of sale items. Senior citizen organizations in many parts of the United States have been helpful in providing older adults with van service to shopping areas. In housing complexes, it may be possible to schedule group trips to the supermarket. Many urban communities have multiple sources of transportation available, but the individual may be unaware of them. Resources in rural areas are more limited. It is important for nurses to be knowledgeable about transportation resources in the community.

In addition, many older adults, particularly widowed men, may have never learned to shop and prepare food. Often, individuals have to rely on others to shop for them, and this may be a cause of concern depending on the availability of support and the reluctance to be dependent on someone else, particularly family. For those who own a computer, shopping over the Internet and having groceries delivered offers advantages, although prices may be higher than those in the stores.

◆ PROMOTING HEALTHY AGING: IMPLICATIONS FOR GERONTOLOGICAL NURSING

The role of nursing in nutrition assessment and intervention should be comprehensive and include increased attention to the process of eating and the entire ritual of meals, as well as the assessment of nutritional status within the interprofessional team (Amella and Aselage, 2012).

Comprehensive nutritional screening and assessment are essential in identifying older adults at risk for nutrition problems or who are malnourished. Older people are less likely than younger people to show signs of malnutrition and nutrient malabsorption. Evaluation of nutritional health can be difficult in the absence of severe malnutrition, but a comprehensive assessment can reveal deficits. Screening and assessment of concerns identified should be conducted on admission to hospital, home health, or long-term care. Nutritional status changes as health status changes, and ongoing assessment is also important.

◆ Nutritional Screening

Nutritional screening is the first step in identifying individuals who are at risk for malnutrition, or have undetected malnutrition, and determines the need for a more comprehensive assessment and nutritional interventions. There are several screening tools specific to older individuals, and screening can be completed in any setting. The Nutrition Screening Initiative Checklist (Figure 14-3) can be self-administered or completed by a family member or any member of the health care team.

The Mini Nutritional Assessment (MNA) (Figure 14-4) is both a screening tool and a detailed assessment. Developed by Nestle of Geneva, Switzerland, the MNA is only validated for individuals older than age 65 and intended for use by professionals. If an individual scores less than 12 on the screen, then the assessment section should be completed (DiMaria-Ghalili, 2012). The MNA is recommended by the Hartford Institute for Geriatric Nursing, and a video of administration of the tool is provided on their website (see Box 14-3).

The Minimum Data Set 3.0 (MDS 3.0) (Chapter 7), used in long-term care facilities, includes assessment information that can be used to identify potential nutritional problems, risk factors, and the potential for improved function. Triggers for more thorough investigation of problems include weight loss, alterations in taste, medical therapies, prescription medications, hunger, parenteral or intravenous feedings, mechanically altered or therapeutic diets, percentage of food left uneaten, pressure ulcers, and edema.

Nutritional Assessment

When risk for malnutrition or malnutrition is detected, a comprehensive nutritional assessment is indicated and will provide the most conclusive data about a person's actual nutritional state. Interprofessional approaches are key to appropriate assessment and intervention and should involve medicine, nursing, dietary, physical, occupational, and speech therapy, and social work. The collective results provide the data needed to identify the immediate and the potential nutritional problems so that plans for supervision, assistance, and education in the attainment of adequate nutrition can be implemented. Components of a nutrition assessment include interview, history, physical examination, anthropometric data, laboratory data, food/nutrient intake, and functional assessment. A summary is presented in Box 14-12. Explanations of several components are discussed in the following sections.

Food/Nutrient Intake

Frequently a 24-hour diet recall compared with the MyPlate for Older Adults can provide an estimate of nutritional adequacy. When the individual cannot supply all of the requested information, it may be possible to obtain data from a family member or another source such as a shopping receipt. There will be times, however, when information will not be as complete as one would like, or the individual, too proud to admit that he or she is not eating, will furnish erroneous information. Even so, the nurse will be able to obtain additional data from the other three areas of the nutritional assessment.

Keeping a dietary record for 3 days is another assessment tool. What foods were eaten, when food was eaten, and the amounts eaten must be carefully recorded. Computer analysis of the dietary records provides information on energy and vitamin and mineral intake. Printouts can provide the older person and the health care provider with a visual graph of the intake. Accurate completion of 3-day dietary records in hospitals and nursing homes can be problematic, and intake may be either underestimated or overestimated. Standardized observational protocols should be developed to ensure accuracy of oral intake documentation, as well as the adequacy and quality of feeding assistance during mealtimes. Nurses should ensure that direct caregivers are educated on the proper observation and documentation of intake and should closely monitor performance in this area.

Anthropomorphic Measurements

Anthropomorphic measurements include height, weight, midarm circumference, and triceps skinfold thickness. These measurements offer information about the status of the older person's muscle mass and body fat in relation to height and

Read the statements below. Circle the number in the Yes column for those that apply to you or someone you know. For each "yes" answer, score the number listed. Total your nutritional score.

	YES
I have an illness or condition that made me change the kind or amount of food I eat.	2
I eat fewer than two meals per day.	3
I eat few fruits, vegetables or milk products.	2
I have three or more drinks of beer, liquor, or wine almost every day.	2
I have tooth or mouth problems that make it hard for me to eat.	2
I don't always have enough money to buy the food I need.	4
I eat alone most of the time.	1
I take three or more different prescriptions or over-the-counter drugs each day.	1
Without wanting to, I have lost or gained 10 pounds in the past 6 months.	2
I am not always physically able to shop, cook, and/or feed myself.	2

Total Nutritional Score

0-2 indicates good nutrition
3-5 moderate risk
6+ high nutritional risk

FIGURE 14-3 Nutrition Screening Initiative. (Courtesy The Nutrition Screening Initiative, Washington, DC.)

Mini Nutritional Assessment
MNA®

Nestlé
Nutrition Institute

Last name: _____ First name: _____

Sex: _____ Age: _____ Weight, kg: _____ Height, cm: _____ Date: _____

Complete the screen by filling in the boxes with the appropriate numbers. Total the numbers for the final screening score.

Screening

A Has food intake declined over the past 3 months due to loss of appetite, digestive problems, chewing or swallowing difficulties?

0 = severe decrease in food intake
1 = moderate decrease in food intake
2 = no decrease in food intake ☐

B Weight loss during the last 3 months

0 = weight loss greater than 3 kg (6.6 lbs)
1 = does not know
2 = weight loss between 1 and 3 kg (2.2 and 6.6 lbs)
3 = no weight loss ☐

C Mobility

0 = bed or chair bound
1 = able to get out of bed / chair but does not go out
2 = goes out ☐

D Has suffered psychological stress or acute disease in the past 3 months?

0 = yes　　　2 = no ☐

E Neuropsychological problems

0 = severe dementia or depression
1 = mild dementia
2 = no psychological problems ☐

F1 Body Mass Index (BMI) (weight in kg) / (height in m)^2

0 = BMI less than 19
1 = BMI 19 to less than 21
2 = BMI 21 to less than 23
3 = BMI 23 or greater ☐

IF BMI IS NOT AVAILABLE, REPLACE QUESTION F1 WITH QUESTION F2.
DO NOT ANSWER QUESTION F2 IF QUESTION F1 IS ALREADY COMPLETED.

F2 Calf circumference (CC) in cm

0 = CC less than 31
3 = CC 31 or greater ☐

Screening score (max. 14 points)

12 - 14 points: Normal nutritional status
8 - 11 points: At risk of malnutrition
0 - 7 points: Malnourished ☐☐

References
1. Vellas B, Villars H, Abellan G, et al. Overview of the MNA® - Its History and Challenges. *J Nutr Health Aging.* 2006;**10**:456-465.
2. Rubenstein LZ, Harker JO, Salva A, Guigoz Y, Vellas B. Screening for Undernutrition in Geriatric Practice: Developing the Short-Form Mini Nutritional Assessment (MNA-SF). *J. Geront.* 2001; **56A**: M366-377
3. Guigoz Y. The Mini-Nutritional Assessment (MNA®) Review of the Literature - What does it tell us? *J Nutr Health Aging.* 2006; **10**:466-487.
4. Kaiser MJ, Bauer JM, Ramsch C, et al. Validation of the Mini Nutritional Assessment Short-Form (MNA®-SF): A practical tool for identification of nutritional status. *J Nutr Health Aging.* 2009; **13**:782-788.
® Société des Produits Nestlé, S.A., Vevey, Switzerland, Trademark Owners © Nestlé, 1994, Revision 2009. N67200 12/99 10M
For more information: www.mna-elderly.com

FIGURE 14-4 Mini Nutritional Assessment. (®Société des Produits Nestlé S.A., Vevey, Switzerland, Trademark Owners.

BOX 14-12 Components of Nutritional Assessment

Dietary History and Current Intake
- Food preferences and habits; meaning and significance of food to the individual; do they eat alone?
- Cultural or religious food habits
- Ability to obtain and prepare food including adequate finances to obtain nutritious food
- Social activities and normal patterns; meal frequency
- Control over food selection and choices
- Fluid intake
- Alcohol intake
- Special diet
- Vitamins/minerals/supplement use
- Chewing/swallowing problems
- Functional limitations that impair independence in eating
- Cognitive changes affecting appetite/ability to feed self
- Depression screen if indicated

History/Physical
- Chief complaint, medical history, chronic conditions, presence or absence of inflammation (fever, hypothermia, signs of systemic inflammatory response), usual weight and any loss or gain, fluid retention, loss of muscle/fat, oral health and dentition, medication use

Anthropometric Measurements
- Body mass index
- Height
- Current weight and usual adult weight
- Recent weight changes
- Skinfold measurements

Biochemical Analysis
- Complete blood count
- Protein status
- Lipid profile
- Electrolytes
- BUN/creatinine ratio

Food/Nutrient Intake
- Periods of inadequate intake (NPO status)
- 24-hour or 3-day diet record

Functional Assessment
- Hand-grip strength
- Standard functional assessment (Chapter 7)

Source: Adapted from Mathew M, Jacobs M: Malnutrition and feeding problems. In Ham R, Sloane P, Warshaw G, et al, editors: *Primary care geriatrics: a case-based approach,* ed 6, Philadelphia, 2014, Elsevier Saunders, p 318.

weight. Muscle mass measurements are obtained by measuring the arm circumference of the nondominant upper arm. The arm hangs freely at the side, and a measuring tape is placed around the midpoint of the upper arm, between the acromion of the scapula and the olecranon of the ulna. The centimeter circumference is recorded and compared with standard values.

Body fat and lean muscle mass are assessed by measuring specific skinfolds with Lange or Harpenden calipers. Two areas are accessible for measurement. One area is the midpoint of the upper arm, the triceps area, which is also used to obtain arm circumference. The nondominant arm is again used. Lift the skin with the thumb and forefinger so that it parallels the humerus. The calipers are placed around the skinfold, 1 cm below where the fingers are grasping the skin. Two readings are averaged to the nearest half centimeter. If there is a neuropathological condition or hemiplegia following a stroke, the unaffected arm should be used for obtaining measurements (DiMaria-Ghalili, 2012).

◆ Weight/Height Considerations

A detailed weight history should be obtained along with current weight. Weight loss is a key indicator of malnutrition, even in overweight older adults. History should include a history of weight loss, if the weight loss was intentional or unintentional, and during what period it occurred. A history of anorexia is also important, and many older people, especially women, have limited their weight throughout life. Debate continues in the quest to determine the appropriate weight charts for an older adult. Although weight alone does not indicate the adequacy of diet, unplanned fluctuations in weight are significant and should be evaluated.

Accurate weight patterns are sometimes difficult to obtain in long-term care settings. Procedures for weighing people should be established and followed consistently to obtain an accurate representation of weight changes. Weighing procedure should be supervised by licensed personnel, and changes should be reported immediately to the provider. One might meet correct weight values for height, but weight changes may be the result of fluid retention, edema, or ascites and merit investigation. An unintentional weight loss of more than 5% of body weight in 1 month, more than 7.5% in 3 months, or more than 10% in 6 months is considered a significant indicator of poor nutrition, as well as an MDS trigger.

Height should always be measured and never estimated or given by self-report. If the person cannot stand, an alternative way of measuring standing height is knee-height using special calipers. An alternative to knee-height measurements is a demispan measurement, which is half the total arm span (DiMaria-Ghalili, 2012). BMI should be calculated to determine if weight for height is within the normal range of 22 to 27. Individuals at either extreme of BMI may be at increased risk of poor nutritional status (White et al, 2012).

◆ Biochemical Analysis/Measures of Visceral Protein

There is no single biochemical marker of malnutrition, and unintentional weight loss remains the most important indicator of a potential nutritional deficit (Ahmed and Haboubi, 2010). The relevance of laboratory tests of serum albumin and prealbumin, as indicators of malnutrition, is limited. These acute phase proteins do not consistently or predictability change with weight loss, calorie restriction, or negative nitrogen balance. They appear to better reflect severity of inflammatory response rather than poor nutritional status (White et al, 2012).

Further investigation of the significance of low protein levels is needed. Serum albumin level has been noted as a "strong prognostic marker for morbidity and mortality in the older hospitalized patient" and remains a recommendation in evaluation of nutritional status (DiMaria-Ghalili, 2012, p. 442). With continued research on biomarkers of inflammation, these may be included in future diagnostic recommendations for malnutrition.

◆ Interventions

Interventions are formulated around the identified nutritional problem or problems. Nursing interventions are centered on techniques to increase food intake and enhance and manage the environment to promote increased food intake (DiMaria-Ghalili, 2012). Jefferies et al. (2011) suggest that nurturing and nourishing describe the nurses' role in nutritional care. Nurses hold a pivotal role in ensuring adequate nutrition to promote healthy aging. Inherent in the role is (1) assessment of the individual for issues related to performance at mealtimes; (2) modification of the environment to be pleasurable for eating; (3) supervision of eating; (4) provision of guidance and support to staff on feeding techniques that enhance intake and preserve dignity and independence; and (5) evaluation of outcomes (Amella and Aselage, 2012). Collaboration with the interprofessional team (e.g., dietitian, pharmacist, social worker, occupational or speech therapist) is important in planning interventions.

For the community-dwelling elder, nutrition education and problem solving with the elder and family members or caregivers on how to best resolve the potential or actual nutritional deficit is important. Causes of poor nutrition are complex, and all of the factors emphasized in this chapter are important to assess when planning individualized interventions to ensure adequate nutrition for older people. Box 14-3 presents resources to assist older adults in planning for good nutrition.

Older adults in hospitals and long-term care are more likely to enter the settings with malnutrition, be at high risk for malnutrition (see Figure 14-2), and have disease conditions that contribute to malnutrition. Severely restricted diets, long periods of nothing-by-mouth (NPO) status, and insufficient time and staff for feeding assistance also contribute to inadequate nutrition. Older adults with dementia are particularly at risk for weight loss and inadequate nutrition (Chapter 29).

◆ Feeding Assistance

The incidence of eating disability in long-term care is high with estimates that 50% of all residents cannot eat independently (Burger et al, 2000). Inadequate staffing in long-term care facilities is associated with poor nutrition and hydration. "Certified nursing assistants (CNAs) have an impossible task trying to feed the number of people who need assistance" (Kayser-Jones, 1997, p. 19). In a study by Simmons and colleagues (2001), 50% of residents significantly increased their oral food and fluid intake during mealtime when they received one-on-one feeding assistance. The time required to implement the feeding assistance (38 minutes) greatly exceeded the time nursing staff spent assisting residents in usual mealtime conditions (9 minutes).

In response to concerns about the lack of adequate assistance during mealtime in long-term care facilities, the Centers for Medicare and Medicaid Services (CMS) implemented a rule that allows feeding assistants with 8 hours of approved training to help residents with eating. Feeding assistants must be supervised by a registered nurse (RN) or licensed practical–vocational nurse (LPN-LVN). Family members may also be willing and able to assist at mealtimes and also provide a familiar social context for the patient.

Assistance with meals in hospitals is also a concern. An innovative volunteer program to address the unique needs of older hospitalized patients was reported by Buys et al. (2013). Support for and Promotion Of Optimal Nutritional Status (SPOONS) focused on three important factors of the mealtime experience: socialization, functional assistance, and staffing challenges. Further research is needed on the effectiveness of feeding assistance programs in hospital settings.

The theory of compromised eating behavior, derived from a nursing study, suggests that the meaning of food and meals to older adults is challenged during hospitalization. As individuals age, traditional food and mealtimes become more meaningful. If food was not traditional in flavor or consistent with the older adult's acculturated foodways, the meaning of food and meal was compromised, thus influencing dietary intake. Strategies to enhance the meaning of food and mealtimes can improve the negative outcomes associated with undernutrition in the hospital setting (Box 14-13). Box 14-14 presents tips to enhance nutritional intake in hospitalized individuals.

◆ Approaches to Enhancing Intake in Long-Term Care

In addition to adequate staff, many innovative and evidence-based ideas can improve nutritional intake in institutions.

BOX 14-13   RESEARCH HIGHLIGHTS

Furman (2014) developed the Theory of Compromised Eating Behavior using grounded theory methodology. The study setting was a large, acute care hospital and participants included eight older adults and four health care providers. Interviews, mealtime observations, and document review were used to collect data. The following observations from the study can provide insights from patients that can be used to guide nurses in developing interventions to promote adequate intake in hospital settings:

"We have a meatloaf but it's turkey meatloaf and it's not really distinguished to me. It doesn't look like meatloaf to me either and these fancy dishes like shrimp Provencal. The menu describes it with these fancy descriptions. I think people are afraid to order it because they're not sure what it is."

"It depends where they leave the meal tray and how my bed goes. If my bed goes up a little maybe I can reach it or if it goes down a little, maybe I can reach it. If I can't, maybe I'll ask someone. If they come in I'll eat; if they don't I won't. I won't even look at it."

"An RN suggested that the patient try the soup. Yet, the nurse neglected to note that with his significant hand tremor, the patient would not be able to get the soup from tray to mouth without spilling. The nurse did not offer assistance nor did the patient ask for assistance. Total dietary intake for the meal consisted of a cracker, which the older adult struggled to access, in addition to sips of milk consumed during medication administration."

From Furman E: The theory of compromised eating behavior, *Res Gerontol Nurs* 7(2):78–86, 2014.

BOX 14-14   TIPS FOR BEST PRACTICE
Improving Nutritional Intake in Hospitals

- Assess nutritional and oral health status, including ability to eat and amount of assistance needed.
- Ensure proper fit and cleanliness of dentures and denture use.
- Provide oral hygiene, and allow the person to wash his or her hands before meals.
- Ensure environment is conducive to eating (remove objects such as urinals and bed pans; clear bedside tables). Ask yourself if you would want to eat the food in the environment in which it is presented.
- Position patient for safe eating (head of bed elevated or sit in a chair if possible).
- Stop non-essential clinical activity during meals (e.g., procedures, rounds, medication administration).
- Emphasize the importance of mealtimes/eating; increase presence and interaction during mealtimes; make mealtime rounds.
- Ensure that all nursing staff are aware of the patients who need assistance with eating and adequate help is provided.
- Ensure that all necessary items are on the tray; prepare all food on the tray if needed; butter bread, open containers, provide straws, provide adaptive equipment as needed.
- Consider volunteers or family members to assist with eating and train and supervise.
- Administer medication for pain or nausea on a schedule that provides comfort at mealtime.
- Determine food preferences; provide for choices in food; include foods appropriate to cultural and religious customs.
- Accurately assess dietary intake using a validated method.
- Make dietary changes/referrals readily.
- Make food available 24 hours/day—provide snacks between meals and at night.
- Limit periods of NPO status and provide food as soon as patient is able to eat.
- Consider liberalizing therapeutic diet if intake is inadequate; offer diet options/alternatives as indicated, including flavor enhancement.

Source: From Furman E: The theory of compromised eating behavior, *Res Gerontol Nurs* 7(2):78–86, 2014.

BOX 14-15   TIPS FOR BEST PRACTICE
Improving Nutritional Intake in Long-Term Care

- Assess nutritional and oral health status.
- Assess ability to eat and amount of assistance needed.
- Serve meals with the person in a chair rather than in bed when possible.
- Provide analgesics and antiemetics on a schedule that provides comfort at mealtime.
- Determine food preferences; provide for choices in food; include foods appropriate to cultural and religious customs.
- Consider buffet-style dining, use of steam tables rather than meal delivery service from trays, café or bistro type dining.
- Make food available 24 hours/day—provide snacks between meals and at night.
- Do not interrupt meals to administer medication if possible.
- Limit staff breaks to before and after mealtimes to ensure adequate staff are available to assist with meals.
- Walk around the dining area or the rooms at mealtime to determine if food is being eaten or if assistance is needed.
- Encourage family members to share the mealtimes for a heightened social situation.
- If caloric supplements are used, offer them between meals or with the medication pass.
- Recommend an exercise program that may increase appetite.
- Ensure proper fit of dentures and denture use.
- Provide oral hygiene, and allow the person to wash his or her hands before meals.
- Have the person wear his or her glasses during meals.
- Sit while feeding the person who needs assistance, use touch, and carry on a social conversation.
- Provide soft music during the meal.
- Use small, round tables seating six to eight people. Consider using tablecloths and centerpieces.
- Seat people with like interests and abilities together, and encourage socialization.
- Involve in restorative dining programs.
- Make diets as liberal as possible depending on health status, especially for frail elders who are not consuming adequate amounts of food.
- Consider a referral to occupational therapist for individuals experiencing difficulties with eating.

Many suggestions are found in the literature: homelike dining rooms; cafeteria-style service; refreshment stations with easy access to juices, water, and healthy snacks; kitchens on the nursing units; choice of mealtimes; finger foods; visually appealing pureed foods with texture and shape; music; touch. Other suggestions can be found in Box 14-15.

Attention to the environment in which meals are served is important. It is not uncommon to hear over the public address system at mealtimes: "Feeder trays are ready." This reference to the need to feed those unable to feed themselves is, in itself, degrading and erases any trace of dignity the individual is trying to maintain in a controlled environment. It is not malicious intent by nurses or other caregivers but rather a habit of convenience. Feeding older people who have difficulty eating can become mechanical and devoid of feeling. The feeding process becomes rapid, and if it bogs down and becomes too slow, the meal may be ended abruptly, depending on the time the caregiver has allotted for feeding the person. Any pleasure derived through socialization and eating and any dignity that could be maintained are often absent (see "An Elder Speaks" at the beginning of this chapter).

◆ Restrictive Diets and Caloric Supplements

The use of restrictive therapeutic diets for frail elders in long-term care (low cholesterol, low salt, no concentrated sweets) often reduces food intake without significantly helping the clinical status of the individual (Pioneer Network and Rothschild Foundation, 2011). If caloric supplements are used, they should be administered at least 1 hour before meals or they interfere with meal intake. These products are widely used and can be costly. Often, they are not dispensed or consumed as ordered. Powdered breakfast drinks added to milk are an adequate substitute (Duffy, 2010).

Dispensing a small amount of calorically dense oral nutritional supplement (2 calories/mL) during the routine medication pass may have a greater effect on weight gain than a traditional supplement (1.06 calories/mL) with or between meals. Small volumes of nutrient-dense supplement may have less of an effect on appetite and will enhance food intake during meals and snacks. This delivery method allows nurses to observe and document consumption.

Further studies and randomized clinical trials are needed to evaluate the effectiveness of nutritional supplementation (Doll-Shankaruk et al, 2008). The American Geriatrics Society (2014) recognizes that high-calorie supplements increase weight in older people but recommends avoiding the use of high-caloric supplements for treatment of anorexia or cachexia because there is no evidence that they affect other important clinical outcomes, such as quality of life, mood, functional status, or survival. See Box 14-3 for an evidence-based protocol on assessment and management of mealtime difficulties.

◆ Pharmacological Therapy

The American Geriatrics Society (2014) does not recommend drugs that stimulate appetite (orexigenic drugs) to treat anorexia or malnutrition in older people. Use of drugs, such as megestrol acetate, results in minimum improvement in appetite and weight gain, no improvement in quality of life or survival, and increased risk of thrombotic events, fluid retention, and death. Systematic reviews of cannabinoids, dietary polyunsaturated fatty acids (DHA and EPA), thalidomide and anabolic steroids, have not identified adequate evidence for the efficacy and safety of these agents for weight gain. The antidepressant drug Mirtazapine (Remeron) is likely to cause weight gain or increased appetite when used to treat depression, but there is little evidence to support its use to promote appetite and weight gain in the absence of depression. Optimizing social supports, providing feeding assistance, and clarifying patient goals and expectations are recommended interventions. Boxes 14-14 and 14-15 provide other suggestions to improve intake.

◆ Patient Education

Education should be provided on nutritional requirements for health, special diet modifications for chronic illness management, the effect of age-associated changes and medication on nutrition, and community resources to assist in maintaining adequate nutrition. Medicare covers nutrition therapy for select diseases, such as diabetes and kidney disease.

Dysphagia

Dysphagia, or difficulty swallowing, is a common problem in older adults. The prevalence of swallowing disorders is 16% to 22% in adults older than 50 years of age, and up to 60% of nursing home residents have clinical evidence of dysphagia (Tanner, 2010). Dysphagia can be the result of behavioral, sensory, or motor problems and is common in individuals with neurological disease and dementia (Box 14-16) (Chapters 23 and 29). Dysphagia is a serious problem and has negative consequences, including weight loss, malnutrition, dehydration, aspiration pneumonia, and even death.

Aspiration (the misdirection of oropharyngeal secretions or gastric contents into the larynx and lower respiratory tract) is common in older adults with dysphagia and can lead to aspiration pneumonia. Dysphagia carries a sevenfold increased risk of aspiration pneumonia and is an independent predictor of mortality (Metheny, 2012).

BOX 14-16 Risk Factors for Dysphagia

- Cerebrovascular accident
- Parkinson's disease
- Neuromuscular disorders (ALS, MS, myasthenia gravis)
- Dementia
- Head and neck cancer
- Traumatic brain injury
- Aspiration pneumonia
- Inadequate feeding technique
- Poor dentition

ALS, Amyotrophic lateral sclerosis; *MS,* multiple sclerosis.

◆ PROMOTING HEALTHY AGING: IMPLICATIONS FOR GERONTOLOGICAL NURSING

◆ Assessment

It is important to obtain a careful history of the older adult's response to dysphagia and to observe the person during mealtime. Symptoms that alert the nurse to possible swallowing problems are presented in Box 14-17. Patients referred for a dysphagia evaluation ("swallowing study") must be assumed to be dysphagic and at risk for aspiration. Nothing-by-mouth (NPO) status should be maintained until the swallowing evaluation is completed. During this period, if necessary, nutrition and hydration needs can be met by intravenous, nasogastric, or gastric tubes (Tanner, 2010). A comprehensive evaluation by a speech-language pathologist (SLP), usually including a video fluoroscopic recording of a modified barium swallow, should be considered when dysphagia is suspected.

BOX 14-17 Symptoms of Dysphagia or Possible Aspiration

- Difficult, labored swallowing
- Drooling
- Copious oral secretions
- Coughing, choking at meals
- Holding or pocketing of food/medications in the mouth
- Difficulty moving food or liquid from mouth to throat
- Difficulty chewing
- Nasal voice or hoarseness
- Wet or gurgling voice
- Excessive throat clearing
- Food or liquid leaking from the nose
- Prolonged eating time
- Pain with swallowing
- Unusual head or neck posturing while swallowing
- Sensation of something stuck in the throat during swallowing; sensation of a lump in the throat
- Heartburn
- Chest pain
- Hiccups
- Weight loss
- Frequent respiratory tract infections, pneumonia

◆ Interventions

After the swallowing evaluation, a decision must be made about the person's potential for functional improvement of the swallowing disorder and the person's safety in swallowing liquid and solid food. The goal is safe oral intake to maintain optimal nutrition and caloric needs. Nurses work closely with speech therapy and the dietitian to implement interventions to prevent aspiration. Compensatory interventions include postural changes, such as chin tucks or head turns while swallowing, and modification of bolus volume, consistency, temperature, and rate of presentation (Easterling and Robbins, 2008). Diets may be modified in texture from pudding like to nearly normal-textured solids. Liquids may range from spoon thick, to honey-like, nectar-like, and thin. Commercial thickeners and thickened products are also available (Mathew and Jacobs, 2014).

Neuromuscular electrical stimulation has received clearance by the U.S. Food and Drug Administration for treatment of dysphagia. This therapy involves the administration of small electrical impulses to the swallowing muscles in the throat and is used in combination with traditional swallowing exercises (Shune and Moon, 2012).

Aspiration is the most profound and dangerous problem for older adults experiencing dysphagia. It is important to have a suction machine available at the bedside or in the dining room in the institutional setting. Suggested interventions helpful in preventing aspiration during hand feeding are presented in Box 14-18. Research on the appropriate management of swallowing disorders in older people, particularly during acute illness and in long-term care facilities, is very limited, and additional study is essential. A protocol for preventing aspiration in older adults with dysphagia, as well as directions to access a video presentation of dysphagia, can be found in Box 14-3.

◆ Feeding Tubes

Comprehensive assessment of swallowing problems and other factors that influence intake must be conducted before initiating severely restricted diet modifications or considering the use of feeding tubes, particularly in older people with end-stage dementia or those at the end of life. However, there may be certain circumstances when providing temporary short-term tube feeding may be appropriate (e.g., individuals with stroke and resulting dysphagia and other conditions when it may be possible to resume oral nutrition at some point).

◆ Tube Feeding in End-Stage Dementia

Currently, there is no scientific study that demonstrates improved survival, reduced incidence of pneumonia or other infections, improved function, or fewer pressure ulcers with the use of feeding tubes in older people with advanced dementia who have poor nutritional intake (Teno et al, 2010; Teno et al, 2011) (Box 14-19). However, there is a continued need for

---

BOX 14-18   TIPS FOR BEST PRACTICE

Preventing Aspiration in Patients with Dysphagia: Hand Feeding

- Provide a 30-minute rest period before meal consumption; a rested person will likely have less difficulty swallowing.
- The person should sit at 90 degrees during all oral (PO) intake.
- Maintain 90-degree positioning for at least 1 hour after PO intake.
- Adjust rate of feeding and size of bites to the person's tolerance; avoid rushed or forced feeding.
- Alternate solid and liquid boluses.
- Have the person swallow twice before the next mouthful.
- Stroke under chin downward to initiate swallowing.
- Follow speech therapist's recommendation for safe swallowing techniques and modified food consistency (may need thickened liquids, pureed foods).
- If facial weakness is present, place food on the nonimpaired side of the mouth.
- Avoid sedatives and hypnotics that may impair cough reflex and swallowing ability.
- Keep suction equipment ready at all times.
- Supervise all meals.
- Monitor temperature.
- Observe color of phlegm.
- Visually check the mouth for pocketing of food in cheeks.
- Check for food under dentures.
- Provide mouth care every 4 hours and before and after meals, including denture cleaning.

BOX 14-19   Myths and Facts about Peg Tubes in Advanced Dementia and End-of-Life Care

Myths
- PEGs prevent death from inadequate intake.
- PEGs reduce aspiration pneumonia.
- PEGs improve albumin levels and nutritional status.
- PEGs assist in healing pressure ulcers.
- PEGs provide enhanced comfort for people at the end of life.
- Not feeding people is a form of euthanasia, and we cannot let people starve to death.

Facts
- PEGs do not improve quality of life.
- PEGs do not reduce risk of aspiration and increase the rate of pneumonia development. In one study, the use of feeding tubes was associated with an increased risk of pressure ulcers among nursing home residents with advanced cognitive impairment (Teno et al., 2012).
- PEGs do not prolong survival in dementia.
- Nearly 50% of patients die within 6 months following PEG tube insertion.
- PEGs cause increased discomfort from both the tube presence and the use of restraints.
- PEGs are associated with infections, gastrointestinal symptoms, and abscesses.
- PEG tube feeding deprives people of the taste of food and contact with caregivers during feeding.
- PEGs are popular because they are convenient and labor beneficial.

Data from Aparanji K, Dharmarajan T: Pause before a PEG: a feeding tube may not be necessary in every candidate, *J Am Med Dir Assoc* 11:453–456, 2010; Teno J, Gozalo P, Mitchell S, et al: Feeding tubes and the prevention or healing of pressure ulcers, *Arch Intern Med* 172(9):697–701, 2012; Vitale C, Monteleoni C, Burke L, et al: Strategies for improving care for patients with advanced dementia and eating problems: optimizing care through physician and speech pathologist collaboration, *Ann Longterm Care* 17:32–39, 2009.

randomized controlled trials to determine the benefits and risks (Glick and Jolkowitz, 2013). An estimated 5% to 30% of nursing home residents with dementia in the United States and Europe have percutaneous endoscopic gastrostomy (PEG) tubes inserted. In Japan, approximately 50% of nursing home residents receive PEG tubes, and the use of PEGs is higher in Israel than in the Western countries (Glick and Jolkowitz, 2013; Ogita et al, 2012).

The American Geriatrics Society (AGS) (2013) does not recommend feeding tubes for older adults with advanced dementia (see Box 14-3). The AGS guidelines suggest that careful hand feeding for patients with severe dementia is at least as good as tube feeding for the outcomes of death, aspiration pneumonia, functional status, and patient comfort (see Box 14-18). Further, tube feeding is associated with agitation, increased use of physical and chemical restraints, and worsening of pressure ulcers (Teno et al, 2012).

As discussed earlier in this chapter, food and eating are closely tied to socialization, comfort, pleasure, love, and the meeting of basic biological needs. Feeding is often equated with caring, and not providing adequate nutrition can seem cruel and inhumane. Decisions about feeding tube placement are challenging and require thoughtful discussion with patients and caregivers, who should be free to make decisions without duress and with careful consideration of the patient's advance directives, if available. Friedrich (2013) suggests that "many considerations factor into decisions families and providers make about enteral feeding, including the individual's wishes in an advanced directive, cultural, religious and ethical beliefs, legal and financial concerns, and emotions" (p. 31).

Decisions to place a feeding tube are often taken without completely exhausting means to maintain a normal oral intake. Research has shown that discussions surrounding the decision are often inadequate (Teno et al, 2011). Discussion about advance directives and feeding support should begin early in the course of the illness rather than waiting until a crisis develops. The best advice for individuals is to state preferences for the use of a feeding tube in a written advance directive.

Individuals have the right to use or not use a feeding tube but should be given information about the risks and benefits of enteral feeding, particularly in late-stage dementia. In difficult situations, an ethics committee may be consulted to help make decisions. It is important that everyone involved in the care of the patient be knowledgeable about the evidence related to the risks and benefits of tube feeding. The decision should never be understood as a question of tube feeding versus no feeding. No family member should be made to feel that he or she is starving his or her loved one to death if a decision is made not to institute enteral feeding. Efforts to provide nutrition should continue, and patients should be able to take any type of nutrition they desire any time they desire.

Regardless of the decision, an important nursing role is to journey with the patient's loved ones, providing support and encouraging expression of feelings. Making these decisions is very difficult and loved ones "have to make peace with their decisions" (Teno et al, 2011).

KEY CONCEPTS

- Results of studies provide growing evidence that diet can affect longevity and, when combined with lifestyle changes, reduce disease risk.
- Many factors affect adequate nutrition in later life, including lifelong eating habits, income, age-associated changes, chronic illness, dentition, mood disorders, capacity for food preparation, and functional limitations.
- An escalating global epidemic of overweight and obesity—"globesity"—is a major public health concern in both developed and developing countries. More than one-third of individuals 65 years and older are obese with a higher prevalence in those 65 to 74 years than in those 75 years and older. Rates of obesity have increased in women 60 years and older.
- The rising incidence of malnutrition among older adults has been documented in acute care, long-term care, and the community and is expected to rise dramatically in the next 30 years. It is important to remember that overweight/obese individuals are also at risk for malnutrition.
- Malnutrition is a precursor to frailty and has serious consequences, including infections, pressure ulcers, anemia, hypotension, impaired cognition, hip fractures, prolonged hospital stay, institutionalization, and increased morbidity and mortality.
- A comprehensive nutritional assessment is an essential component of the assessment of older adults.
- The role of nursing in nutrition assessment and intervention should be comprehensive and include attention to the process of eating and the entire ritual of meals, as well as the assessment of nutritional status within the interprofessional team.
- Making mealtimes pleasant and attractive for the older person who is unable to eat unassisted is a nursing challenge; mealtimes must be made enjoyable, and adequate assistance must be provided.
- Dysphagia is a serious problem and has negative consequences, including weight loss, malnutrition, dehydration, aspiration pneumonia, and even death. Nurses must carefully assess risk factors for dysphagia, observe for signs and symptoms, refer for evaluation, and collaborate with speech-language pathologists on interventions to prevent aspiration.

NURSING STUDY: NUTRITION

Helen, 77 years old, had dieted all her life—or so it seemed. She often chided herself about it. "After all, at my age who cares if I'm too fat? I do. It depresses me when I gain weight and then I gain even more when I'm depressed." At 5 feet, 4 inches tall and 148 pounds, her weight was ideal for her height and age, but Helen, like so many women of her generation, had incorporated the image of women on TV who weighed 105 pounds as her ideal. She had achieved that weight for only a few weeks three or four times in her adult life. She had tried high-protein diets, celery and cottage cheese diets, fasting, commercially prepared diet foods, and numerous fad diets. She always discontinued the diets when she perceived any negative effects. She was invested in maintaining her general good health. Her most recent attempt at losing 30 pounds on an all-liquid diet had been unsuccessful and left her feeling constipated, weak, irritable, and mildly nauseated and experiencing heart palpitations. This really frightened her. Her physician criticized her regarding the liquid diet but seemed rather amused while reinforcing that her weight was "just perfect" for her age. In the discussion, the physician pointed out how fortunate she was that she was able to drive to the market, had sufficient money for food, and was able to eat anything with no dietary restrictions. Helen left his office feeling silly. She was an independent, intelligent woman; she had been a successful manager of a large financial office. Before her retirement 7 years ago, her work had consumed most of her energies.

There had been no time for family, romance, or hobbies. Lately, she had immersed herself in reading the Harvard Classics as she had promised herself she would when she retired. Unfortunately, now that she had the time to read them, she was losing interest. She knew that she must begin to "pull herself together" and "be grateful for her blessings" just as the physician had said.

Based on the case study, develop a nursing care plan using the following procedure*:

- List Helen's comments that provide subjective data.
- List information that provides objective data.
- From these data, identify and state, using an accepted format, two nursing diagnoses you determine are most significant to Helen at this time. List two of Helen's strengths that you have identified from the data.
- Determine and state outcome criteria for each diagnosis. These must reflect some alleviation of the problem identified in the nursing diagnosis and must be stated in concrete and measurable terms.
- Plan and state one or more interventions for each diagnosed problem. Provide specific documentation of the source used to determine the appropriate intervention. Plan at least one intervention that incorporates Helen's existing strengths.
- Evaluate the success of the intervention. Interventions must correlate directly with the stated outcome criteria to measure the outcome success.

*Students are advised to refer to their nursing diagnosis text and identify possible or potential problems.

CRITICAL THINKING QUESTIONS AND ACTIVITIES

1. Discuss how you would counsel Helen regarding her weight.
2. If Helen insists on dieting, what diet would you recommend, considering her age and activity level?
3. What lifestyle changes would you suggest to Helen?
4. What are the specific health concerns that require attention in Helen's case?
5. What factors may be involved in Helen's preoccupation with her weight?
6. What are some of the reasons that fad diets are dangerous?

RESEARCH QUESTIONS

1. What are the dietary patterns of older men living alone?
2. What percentage of women and men older than age 60 are satisfied with their weight?
3. What factors influence older people to implement dietary changes suggested by nurses, dietitians, or primary care providers?
4. What nursing interventions can enhance the nutritional intake of frail older adults residing in nursing facilities?
5. What is the level of knowledge about dysphagia among acute care and long-term care nurses?

REFERENCES

Acalovschi M: What differentiates chronic constipation from constipation type irritable bowel syndrome and does it matter for dietary recommendations? In *World Gastroenterology Organisation: Digestive Health Day: a special 2012 WDHD supplement*, 2012, pp 13–14. http://www.wgofoundation.org/assets/docs/pdf/wdhd12-supplement-HI.pdf. Accessed October 31, 2014.

Ahmed T, Haboubi N: Assessment and management of nutrition in older people and its importance to health, *Clin Interv Aging* 5:207–216, 2010.

Amella E, Aselage M: Mealtime difficulties. In Boltz M, Capezuti E, Fulmer T, et al, editors: *Evidence-based geriatric nursing protocols for best practice*, ed 4, New York, 2012, Springer, pp 453–468.

American Dietetic Association, the American Society for Nutrition, and the Society for Nutrition Education: Position of the American Dietetic Association, American Society for Nutrition and Society for Nutrition Education: Food and nutrition programs for community-residing older adults, *J Am Diet Assoc* 110(3): 463, 2010.

American Geriatrics Society: *Feeding tubes in advanced dementia position statement*, May 2013.http://www.americangeriatrics.org/health_care_professionals/clinical_practice/clinical_guidelines_recommendations. Accessed April 2014.

American Geriatrics Society: *Choosing wisely: five things physicians and patients should question*, 2014.http://www.choosingwisely.org/clinician-lists/american-geriatrics-society-prescription-appetite-stimulants-to-treat-anorexia-cachexia-in-elderly/. Accessed April 2014.

Bales C, Buhr G: Is obesity bad for older persons? A systematic review of the pros and cons of weight reduction in later life, *J Am Med Dir Assoc* 9:302–312, 2008.

Beasley J, LaCroix A, Neuhouser M, et al: Protein intake and incident frailty in the Women's Health Initiative Observational Study, *J Am Geriatr Soc* 58:1063–1071, 2010.

Burger S, Kayser-Jones J, Prince J: Malnutrition and dehydration in nursing homes: key issues in prevention and treatment, 2000. http://www.commonwealthfund.org/usr_doc/burger_mal_386.pdf. Accessed January 2014.

Buys D, Flood K, Real K, et al: Mealtime assistance for hospitalized older adults: a report on the SPOONS volunteer program, *J Gerontol Nurs* 39(9):18–22, 2013.

Cadogan M: Functional consequences of vitamin B_{12} deficiency, *J Gerontol Nurs* 36:16–21, 2010.

Chowdhury R, Warmakula S, Kunutsor S, et al: Association of dietary, circulating, and supplement fatty acids with coronary risk: a systematic review and meta-analysis, *Ann Intern Med* 160(6):398–406, 2014.

Dahl A, Fauth E, Ernsth-Bravell M, et al: Body mass index, change in body mass index, and survival in old and very old persons, *J Am Geriatr Soc* 61(4):512–518, 2013.

DiMaria-Ghalili R: Nutrition. In Boltz M, Capezuti E, Fulmer T, et al, editors: *Evidence-based geriatric nursing protocols for best practice*, ed 4, New York, 2012, Springer, pp 439–452.

Doll-Shankaruk M, Yau W, Oekle C: Implementation and effects of a medication pass nutritional supplement program in a long-term care facility, *J Gerontol Nurs* 34:45–51, 2008.

Duffy E: *Malnutrition in older adults: deciphering a complex syndrome*, 2010. http://nurse-practitioners-and-physician-assistants.advanceweb.com/Article/Malnutrition-in-Older-Adults.aspx. Accessed October 2014.

Easterling C, Robbins E: Dementia and dysphagia, *Geriatr Nurs* 29:275–285, 2008.

Ervin R: Healthy eating index—2005 total component scores for adults age 20 and over: National Health and Nutrition Examination Survey, 2003–2004, *National Health Statistics Reports* no. 44, 2011. http://www.cdc.gov/nchs/data/nhsr/nhsr044.pdf. Accessed August 2014.

Felix H: Obesity, disability and nursing home admission, *Ann Longterm Care* 16:33, 2008.

Flicker L, McCaul K, Hankey G, et al: Body mass index and survival in men and women aged 70 to 75, *J Am Geriatr Soc* 58:234–241, 2010.

Friedrich L: End-of-life nutrition: is tube feeding the solution? *Ann Longterm Care* 21(10):30–33, 2013.

Fuller-Thomson E, Redmond M: Falling through the social safety net: food stamp use and nonuse among older impoverished Americans, *Gerontologist* 48:235–244, 2008.

Furman E: The theory of compromised eating behavior, *Res Gerontol Nurs* 7(2):78–86, 2014.

Gallup Healthway: *State of American Well-Being, 2014.* http://info.healthways.com/wellbeingindex. Accessed January 27, 2014.

Giger JN, Davidhizar RE: *Transcultural nursing: assessment and intervention*, ed 4, St. Louis, 2003, Mosby.

Glick S, Jolkowitz A: Feeding dementia patients via percutaneous endoscopic gastrostomy, *Ann Longterm Care* 21(1):32–34, 2013.

Greenlee K: *"Have you eaten?" ACL Blog,* 2014. http://www.acl.gov/NewsRoom/Blog/2014/2014_03_28.aspx. Accessed April 2014.

Haber D: *Health promotion and aging*, ed 5, New York, 2010, Springer.

Imai E, Tsubota-Utsugi M, Kikuya M, et al: Animal protein intake is associated with higher-level functional capacity in elderly adults: the Ohasama study, *J Am Geriatr Soc* 62:426–434, 2014.

Institute of Medicine: *Retooling for an aging America: building the health care workforce*, Washington, DC, 2008, National Academies Press.

Jefferies D, Johnson M, Ravens J: Nurturing and nourishing: the nurses' role in nutritional care, *J Clin Nurs* 20:317–330, 2011.

Jensen G, Miratallo J, Compher C, et al: Adult starvation and disease-related malnutrition: a proposal for etiology-based diagnosis in the clinical practice setting from the International Consensus Guideline Committee, *JPEN* 34:156–159, 2010.

Kaiser R, Winning K, Uter W, et al: Functionality and mortality in obese nursing home residents: an example of "risk factor paradox"? *J Am Med Dir Assoc* 11:428–435, 2010.

Kamp B, Wellman N, Russell C: Position of the American Dietetic Association, American Society for Nutrition and Society for Nutrition Education: Food and nutrition programs for community-residing older adults, *J Am Diet Assoc* 110:463–472, 2010.

Kayser-Jones J: Inadequate staffing at mealtime: implications for nursing and health policy, *J Gerontol Nurs* 23:14–21, 1997.

Levinson Z, Damico A, Cubanski J: *A state-by-state snapshot of poverty among seniors: findings from analysis of the supplemental poverty measure* (Issue brief), May 20, 2013. http://kff.org/medicare/issue-brief/a-state-by-state-snapshot-of-poverty-among-seniors. Accessed April 2014.

Litchford M: Putting the nutrition-focused physical assessment into practice in long-term care, *Ann Longterm Care* 21(11):38–41, 2013.

Locher J, Ritchie C, Robinson C, et al: A multidimensional approach to understanding under-eating in homebound older adults: the importance of social factors, *Gerontologist*, 48:223–234, 2008.

Lustbader W: Thoughts on the meaning of frailty, *Generations* 13:21, 1999.

Martinez-Lapiscina E, Clavero P, Toledo E, et al: Mediterranean diet improves cognition: the PREDIMEN-NAVARRA randomised trial, *J Neurol Neurosurg Psychiatry* 84(12):1318–1325, 2013.

Mathew M, Jacobs M: Malnutrition and feeding problems. In Ham R, Sloane P, Warshaw G, et al, editors: *Primary care geriatrics*, ed 6, Philadelphia, 2014, Elsevier Saunders, pp 315–322.

McQuaid KR: Gastrointestinal disorders. In McPhee SJ, Papadakis MA, editors: *Current medical diagnosis and treatment 2010,* New York, 2010, McGraw-Hill Lange, pp 502–597.

Metheney N: Preventing aspiration in older adults with dysphagia, *Try This: Best practices in nursing care to older adults*, 2012. http://consultgerirn.org/uploads/File/trythis/try_this_20.pdf. Accessed October 31, 2014.

Morris A, Regenbogen S, Hardman K, et al: Sigmoid diverticulitis, *JAMA* 311(3):287–297, 2014.

Morris M, Tangney C, Wang Y, et al: MIND diet associated with reduced incidence of Alzheimer's disease, Alzheimers Dement. 2015 Feb 11. pii: S1552-5260(15)00017-5. doi: 10.1016/j.jalz.2014.11.009. [Epub ahead of print

National Digestive Diseases Information Clearinghouse: *Gastroesophageal reflux (GER) and gastroesophageal reflux disease (GERD) in adults* (NIH publication no. 13-0882), 2014. http://digestive.niddk.nih.gov/ddiseases/pubs/gerd. Accessed October 2014.

Newman A: Obesity in older adults, *Online J Issues Nurs* 14(1), 2009. http://www.nursingworld.org/MainMenuCategories/ANAMarketplace/ANAPeriodicals/OJIN/TableofContents/Vol142009/No1Jan09/

Obesity-in-Older-Adults.html. Accessed April 2014.

Ogden C, Carroll M, Kit B, et al: Prevalence of childhood and adult obesity in the United States, 2011-2012, *JAMA* 311(8):806–814, 2014.

Ogita M, Utsunomiya H, Akishita M, et al: Indications and practice for tube feeding in Japanese geriatricians: implications of multidisciplinary team approach, *Geriatr Gerontol Int* 12:643–651, 2012.

Pioneer Network and Rothschild Foundation: *New dining practice standards*, 2011. http://www.pioneernetwork.net/Providers/DiningPracticeStandards. Accessed April 2014.

Pluta R, Perazza G, Golub R: Gastroesophageal reflux disease, *JAMA* 305(19):2024, 2011.

Samieri C, Grodstein F, Rosner B, et al: Mediterranean diet and cognitive function in older age, *Epidemiology* 24(4):490–499, 2013a.

Samieri C, Sun Q, Townsend M, et al: The association between dietary patterns in midlife and health in aging: an observational study, *Ann Intern Med* 159(9):584–591, 2013b.

Shune S, Moon J: Neuromuscular electrical stimulation in dysphagia management: clinician use and perceived barriers, *Contemp Issues Commun Sci Disord* 39:55–68, 2012.

Simmons S, Osterweil D, Schnelle J: Improving food intake in nursing home residents with feeding assistance: a staffing analysis, *J Gerontol A Biol Sci Med Sci* 12:M790–M794, 2001.

Slomski A: Mediterranean diet may reduce diabetes risk in older people, *JAMA* 311(8):790, 2014.

Tanner D: Lessons from nursing home dysphagia malpractice litigation, *J Gerontol Nurs* 36:41–46, 2010.

Teno J: *Families need information on feeding tubes for elderly dementia patients*, May 5, 2011. http://news.brown.edu/pressreleases/2011/05/intubation. Accessed April 2014.

Teno J, Gozalo F, Mitchell S, et al: Feeding tubes and the prevention or healing of pressure ulcers, *Arch Intern Med* 172(9):697–701, 2012.

Teno J, Mitchell S, Gozalo P, et al: Hospital characteristics associated with feeding tube placement in nursing home residents with advanced cognitive impairment, *JAMA* 303:544–550, 2010.

Teno J, Mitchell S, Kuo S, et al: Decision-making and outcomes of feeding tube insertion: a five-state study, *J Am Geriatr Soc* 59(5):881–886, 2011.

The Joint Commission: *Patient Safety Tool: Advancing effective communication, cultural competence and patient- and family-centered care: a roadmap for hospitals*, Oakbrook Terrace, IL, 2010, The Joint Commission.

Tobias D, Pan A, Jackson C, et al: Body-mass index and mortality among older adults with incident type 2 diabetes, *N Engl J Med* 370(3):233–244, 2014.

U.S. Department of Agriculture (USDA), U.S. Department of Health and Human Services (USDHHS): *2010 Dietary guidelines for Americans*, ed 7, 2010. http://www.cnpp.usda.gov/dietaryguidelines.htm. Accessed April 2014.

Vitale C, Monteleoni C, Burke L, et al: Strategies for improving care for patients with advanced dementia and eating problems: optimizing care through physician and speech pathologist collaboration, *Ann Longterm Care* 17:32, 2009.

White J, Guenter P, Jensen G, et al: Consensus statement of the Academy of Nutrition and Dietetics/American Society for Parenteral and Enteral Nutrition: characteristics recommended for the identification and documentation of adult malnutrition (undernutrition), *J Acad Nutr Diet* 112:730–738, 2012.

World Health Organization: *Nutrition: Controlling the global obesity epidemic*, 2003. http://www.who.int/nutrition/topics/obesity/en. Accessed April 2014.

Yang J, Farioli A, Korre M, et al: Modified Mediterranean diet score and cardiovascular risk in a North American working population, *PLoS ONE* 9(2):e87539, 2014. doi: 10.1371/journal.pone.0087539.

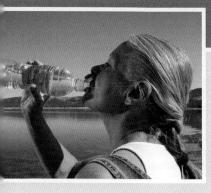

CHAPTER 15

Hydration and Oral Care

Theris A. Touhy

http://evolve.elsevier.com/Touhy/TwdHlthAging

A STUDENT SPEAKS

I never thought that part of my nursing care was brushing someone's false teeth. I didn't even know my patient had false teeth until he asked me to help him take them out. Thank goodness he was able to tell me how to do it because I had no idea. He was really worried because he said the last time he was in the hospital, no one had taken them out for several days and he got a sore under them that was very painful. Together we got them out, cleaned, and back in with no problems. Made me realize how important the little things really are.

Jeff, age 22

AN ELDER SPEAKS

I know I don't drink enough water—coffee, yes; water, no. It's hard when you are in a wheelchair and only have one arm that works. This smart little student nurse really fixed me up. She gave me a plastic water bottle and attached it to my chair on my good side. Now wherever I go, the water goes.

Jack, age 84

LEARNING OBJECTIVES

On completion of this chapter, the reader will be able to:

1. Identify factors that influence hydration management in older adults.
2. Identify the components of hydration assessment.
3. Describe interventions for prevention and treatment of dehydration.
4. Demonstrate understanding of the relationship between oral health and disease.
5. Discuss common oral problems that can occur with aging and appropriate assessment and interventions.
6. Discuss interventions that promote good oral hygiene for older people in a variety of settings.

HYDRATION MANAGEMENT

Hydration management is the promotion of an adequate fluid balance, which prevents complications resulting from abnormal or undesirable fluid levels. Water, an accessible and available commodity to almost all people, is often overlooked as an essential part of nutritional requirements. Water's function in the body includes thermoregulation, dilution of water-soluble medications, facilitation of renal and bowel function, and creation of requisite conditions for and maintenance of metabolic processes.

Daily needs for water can usually be met by functionally independent older adults through intake of fluids with meals and social drinks. However, a significant number of older adults (up to 85% of those 85 years of age and older) drink less than 1 liter of fluid per day. Older adults, with the exception of those requiring fluid restrictions, should consume at least 1500 mL of fluid per day (Mentes, 2012). Maintenance of fluid balance (fluid intake equals fluid output) is essential to health, regardless of a person's age (Mentes, 2006a).

Age-related changes (Box 15-1 and Figure 15-1), medication use, functional impairments, and comorbid medical and emotional illnesses place some older adults at risk for changes in fluid balance, especially dehydration (Mentes, 2012). Hydration habits, as described by Mentes (2006b, 2012), influence how and why individuals consume liquids and understanding these habits can be valuable in planning appropriate interventions (Box 15-2). Collaboration between the nurse and the community-dwelling elder in education about the details of fluid intake (e.g., how to measure water, how to determine personal fluid needs) and how to specifically incorporate the information into daily life is important (Palmer et al, 2014).

BOX 15-1 Age-Related Changes Affecting Hydration Status

- Thirst sensation diminishes; thirst is not proportional to metabolic needs in response to dehydrating conditions
- Creatinine clearance declines, kidneys less able to concentrate urine (particularly in individuals with illnesses affecting kidney function)
- Total body water (TBW) decreases
- Loss of muscle mass/increase in proportion of fat cells; greater in women than men because they have a higher percentage of body fat and less muscle mass; fat cells contain less water than muscle cells

Adapted from Mentes JC: Managing oral hydration. In Boltz M, Capezuti E, Fulmer T, et al, editors: *Evidence-based geriatric nursing protocols for best practice*, ed 4, New York, 2012, Springer, pp 419–438.

DEHYDRATION

Dehydration is defined clinically as "a complex condition resulting in a reduction in total body water. In older people, dehydration most often develops as a result of disease, age-related changes, and/or the effects of medication and not primarily due to lack of access to water" (Thomas et al, 2008, p. 293). Dehydration is considered a geriatric syndrome that is frequently associated with common diseases (e.g., diabetes, respiratory illness, heart failure) and frailty. It is often an unappreciated comorbid condition that exacerbates an underlying condition such as a urinary tract infection, respiratory tract infection, or worsening depression. Dehydration is a significant risk factor for delirium, thromboembolic complications, infections, kidney stones, constipation and obstipation,

BOX 15-2 RESEARCH HIGHLIGHTS

From this classic study of dehydration events in nursing home residents, a typology of hydration problems emerged that included the following four groups: (1) Can Drink; (2) Can't Drink; (3) Won't Drink; and (4) End of Life. Each group has different hydration habits that can guide assessment and interventions. Providing targeted interventions to those at greatest risk may decrease the prevalence of dehydration. The typology can be used effectively by nursing assistants, who can also be helpful in identifying residents' hydration habits. It is also valuable for nurses working in different settings to target hydration interventions.

CAN DRINK: Capable of accessing and consuming fluids but may not know what is adequate intake or may forget to drink as a result of cognitive impairment. May need education about daily fluid needs and the importance of reporting any changes; verbal encouragement and prompting; easy access to fluids

CAN'T DRINK: Physically incapable of accessing or safely consuming fluids related to physical dependence or swallowing disorders. May need dysphagia prevention interventions; physical aids to assist with drinking (e.g., sports bottle, sippy cup); swallowing evaluation and safe swallowing techniques; oral care; foods rich in fluid (smoothies); adequate assistance

WON'T DRINK: Highest risk for dehydration. Capable of consuming fluids safely but do not because of fear of being incontinent; or have lower cognitive abilities and consume limited amounts of fluid at a time (sippers). Interventions may include offering frequent small amounts of fluid at each contact (preferred beverages); providing fluid with activities; implementing toileting programs; promoting education about maintaining fluid intake

END OF LIFE: Terminally ill individuals who may have hydration patterns described in other categories. Hydration will be dependent on resident and family preference, advance directives

From Mentes JC: A typology of oral hydration, *J Gerontol Nurs* 32(1):13–19, 2006.

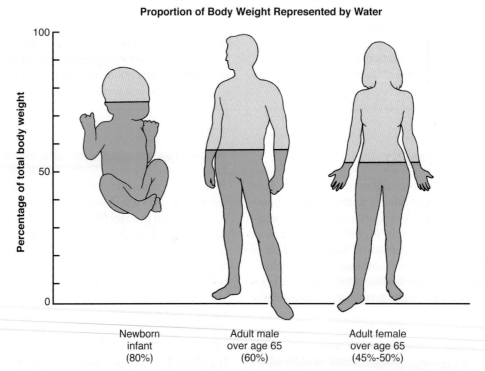

Proportion of Body Weight Represented by Water

Percentage of total body weight

Newborn infant (80%) Adult male over age 65 (60%) Adult female over age 65 (45%-50%)

FIGURE 15-1 Changes in Body Water Distribution with Age. (From Thibodeau GA, Patton KT: *Structure & function of the body*, ed 13, St Louis, MO, 2008, Mosby.)

falls, medication toxicity, renal failure, seizure, electrolyte imbalance, hyperthermia, and delayed wound healing (Faes et al, 2007; Mentes, 2012).

⚡ SAFETY ALERT

Dehydration is a problem prevalent among older adults in all settings. If not treated adequately, mortality from dehydration can be as high as 50% (Faes et al, 2007).

Thomas and colleagues (2008) comment that there are few diagnoses that generate as much concern about causes and consequences as does dehydration. Due to a lack of understanding of the pathogenesis and consequences of dehydration in older adults, the condition is often attributed to poor care by nursing home staff and/primary care providers. However, the majority of older people develop dehydration as a result of increased fluid losses combined with decreased fluid intake, related to decreased thirst. The condition is rarely due to neglect.

Risk Factors for Dehydration

The presence of physical or emotional illness, surgery, trauma, or conditions of higher physiological demands increases the risk of dehydration. When the fluid balance of older adults is at risk, the limited capacity of homeostatic mechanisms becomes significant (see Box 15-1 and Figure 15-1). Box 15-3 presents risk factors for dehydration.

BOX 15-3   Risk Factors for Dehydration

Age-related changes
Medications: diuretics, laxatives, angiotensin-converting enzyme (ACE) inhibitors, psychotropics
Use of four or more medications
Functional deficits
Communication and comprehension problems
Oral problems
Dysphagia
Delirium
Dementia
Hospitalization
Low body weight
Diagnostic procedures requiring fasting
Inadequate assistance with fluid/food intake
Diarrhea
Fever
Vomiting
Infections
Bleeding
Draining wounds
Artificial ventilation
Fluid restrictions
High environmental temperatures
Multiple comorbidities

◆ PROMOTING HEALTHY AGING: IMPLICATIONS FOR GERONTOLOGICAL NURSING

◆ Assessment

Prevention of dehydration is essential, but assessment is complex in older people. Clinical signs may not appear until dehydration is advanced. Attention to risk factors for dehydration using a screening tool (Box 15-4) is very important. In addition, the MDS 3.0 (Chapter 7) assesses for dehydration/fluid maintenance. Education should be provided to older people and their caregivers on the need for fluids and the signs and symptoms of dehydration. Acute situations such as vomiting, diarrhea, or febrile episodes should be identified quickly and treated.

◆ Signs/Symptoms of Dehydration

Typical signs of dehydration may not always be present in older people and symptoms are often atypical. Skin turgor, assessed at the sternum and commonly included in the assessment of dehydration, is an unreliable marker in older adults because of the loss of subcutaneous tissue with aging. Dry mucous membranes in the mouth and nose, longitudinal furrows on the tongue, orthostasis, speech incoherence, rapid pulse rate, decreased urine output, extremity weakness, dry axilla, and sunken eyes may indicate dehydration. However, the diagnosis of dehydration is biochemically proven (Thomas et al, 2008).

◆ Laboratory Tests

If dehydration is suspected, laboratory tests include blood urea nitrogen (BUN)/creatinine ratio, serum sodium level, serum and urine osmolarity, and specific gravity (Mentes, 2012). Although most cases of dehydration have an elevated BUN measurement, there are many other causes of an elevated BUN/creatinine ratio, so this test cannot be used alone to diagnose dehydration in older adults (Thomas et al, 2008). Attention to risk factors is important to identify possible dehydration and to intervene early. Body weight changes should also be assessed as indicators of changes in hydration (Faes et al, 2007).

◆ Urine Color

Urine color, which is measured using a urine color chart, has been suggested as helpful in assessing hydration status (not

---

BOX 15-4   Simple Screen for Dehydration

Drugs (e.g., diuretics)
End of life
High fever
Yellow urine turns dark
Dizziness (orthostasis)
Reduced oral intake
Axilla dry
Tachycardia
Incontinence (fear of)
Oral problems/sippers
Neurological impairment (confusion)
Sunken eyes

From Thomas D, Cote T, Lawhorne L, et al: Understanding clinical dehydration and its treatment, *J Am Med Dir Assoc* 9:292–301, 2008.

dehydration) in individuals in nursing homes with adequate renal function (Mentes, 2012). The urine color chart has eight standardized colors, ranging from pale straw (number 1) to greenish brown (number 8), approximating urine specific gravities of 1.003 to 1.029. Urine color should be assessed and charted over several days. Pale straw–colored urine usually indicates normal hydration status, and as urine darkens, poor hydration may be indicated (after taking into account discoloration by food or medications). For older adults, a reading of 4 or less is preferred (Mentes, 2006a). If a person's urine becomes darker than his or her usual color, fluid intake assessment is indicated, and fluids can be increased before dehydration occurs (Mentes, 2012).

◆ Interventions

Interventions are derived from a comprehensive assessment and consist of risk identification and hydration management (Mentes, 2012) (Box 15-5). Any individual who develops fever, diarrhea, vomiting, or a nonfebrile infection should be monitored closely by implementing intake and output records and providing additional fluids. NPO (nothing by mouth) requirements for diagnostic tests and surgical procedures should be as short as possible for older adults, and adequate fluids should be given once tests and procedures are completed. A 2-hour suspension of fluid intake is recommended for many procedures (Mentes, 2012).

Hydration management involves both acute and ongoing management of oral intake. Oral hydration is the first treatment approach for dehydration. Individuals with mild to moderate dehydration who can drink and do not have significant mental or physical compromise due to fluid loss may be able to replenish fluids orally. Water is considered the best fluid to offer, but other clear fluids may also be useful depending on the person's preference.

◆ Rehydration Methods

Rehydration methods depend on the severity and the type of dehydration and may include intravenous or hypodermoclysis (HDC). A general rule is to replace 50% of the loss within the first 12 hours (or 1 L/day in afebrile elders) or sufficient quantity to relieve tachycardia and hypotension. Further fluid replacement can be administered more slowly over a longer period of time. It is important to monitor for symptoms of overhydration (unexplained weight gain, pedal edema, neck vein distention, shortness of breath), especially in individuals with heart failure or renal disease. Individuals taking selective serotonin reuptake inhibitors (SSRIs) should have serum sodium levels and hydration status closely monitored due to risk for hyponatremia (Chapter 9). Increasing fluid intake may aggravate an evolving hyponatremia (Mentes, 2012).

◆ Hypodermoclysis (HDC)

HDC is an infusion of isotonic fluids into the subcutaneous space. HDC is safe, easy to administer, and a useful alternative to intravenous administration for persons with mild to moderate dehydration, particularly those patients with altered mental status. HDC cannot be used in severe dehydration or for any situation requiring more than 3 L over 24 hours. Common sites of infusion are the lateral abdominal wall; the anterior or lateral aspects of the thighs; the infraclavicular region; and the back,

---

BOX 15-5   TIPS FOR BEST PRACTICE

Ongoing Management of Oral Intake: Long-Term Care

1. Calculate a daily fluid goal.
   - All older adults should have an individualized fluid goal determined by a documented standard for daily fluid intake. At least 1500 mL of fluid/day should be provided.
2. Compare current intake to fluid goal to evaluate hydration status.
3. Provide fluids consistently throughout the day.
   - Provide 75% to 80% of fluids at mealtimes and the remainder during non-mealtimes such as medication times.
   - Offer a variety of fluids and fluids that the person prefers.
   - Standardize the amount of fluid that is offered with medication administration (e.g., at least 6 oz).
4. Plan for at-risk individuals.
   - Have fluid rounds midmorning and midafternoon.
   - Provide two 8-oz glasses of fluid in the morning and evening.
   - Offer a "happy hour" or "tea time," when residents can gather for additional fluids and socialization.
   - Provide modified fluid containers based on resident's abilities—for example, lighter cups and glasses, weighted cups and glasses, plastic water bottles with straws (attach to wheelchairs, deliver with meals).
   - Make fluids accessible at all times and be sure residents can access them—for example, filled water pitchers, fluid stations, or beverage carts in congregate areas.
   - Allow adequate time and staff for eating or feeding. Meals can provide two-thirds of daily fluids.
   - Encourage family members to participate in feeding and offering fluids.
5. Perform fluid regulation and documentation.
   - Teach individuals, if possible, to use a urine color chart to monitor hydration status.
   - Document complete intake including hydration habits.
   - Know volumes of fluid containers to accurately calculate fluid consumption.
   - Frequency of documentation of fluid intake will vary among settings and is dependent on the individual's condition. In most settings, at least one accurate intake and output recording should be documented, including amount of fluid consumed, difficulties with consumption, and urine specific gravity and color.
   - For individuals who are not continent, teach caregivers to observe incontinent pads or briefs for amount and frequency of urine, color changes, and odor, and report variations from individual's normal pattern.

Adapted from Mentes JC: Managing oral hydration. In Boltz M, Capezuti E, Fulmer T, et al, editors: *Evidence-based geriatric nursing protocols for best practice*, ed 4, New York, 2012, Springer, pp 419–438.

---

usually the interscapular or subscapular regions with a fat fold at least 1 inch thick (Mei and Auerhahn, 2009). Normal saline (0.9%), half-normal saline (0.45%), 5% glucose in water infusion (D5W), or Ringer's solution can be used (Thomas et al, 2008). Hypodermoclysis can be administered in almost any setting, so hospital admissions may be avoided. Hypodermoclysis is "an evidence-based low-cost therapy in geriatrics" (Faes et al, 2007). Other resources on hydration can be found in Box 15-6.

ORAL HEALTH

Orodental health is integral to general health. Orodental health is a basic need that is increasingly neglected with advanced age, debilitation, and limited mobility. Age-related changes in the oral cavity (see Box 14-1), medical conditions, poor dental

Hydration and Oral Care

Administration on Aging: Older adults and oral health
American Medical Directors Association: Oral Healthcare Toolkit
Mentes J: Hydration management. In Boltz M, Capezuti E, Fulmer T et al, editors: *Evidence-based geriatric nursing protocols for best practice,* ed 4, New York, 2012, Springer
O'Connor L: Oral health care. In Boltz M, Capezuti E, Fulmer T et al, editors: *Evidence-based geriatric nursing protocols for best practice,* ed 4, New York, 2012, Springer
Oral Health America: Educational materials, resources, affordable dental care
The Hartford Institute for Geriatric Nursing: Nursing Standard of Practice Protocols: Oral health care in aging, hydration management
Oral Health Assessment of Older Adults: The Kayser-Jones Brief Oral Health Status Examination (BOHSE)

BOX 15-8 HEALTHY PEOPLE 2020

Dental Health Goals for Older Adults

- Prevent and control oral and craniofacial diseases, conditions, and injuries, and improve access to preventive services and dental care.
- Reduce the proportion of adults with untreated dental decay.
- Reduce the proportion of older adults with untreated caries.
- Reduce the proportion of adults who have ever had a permanent tooth extracted because of dental caries or periodontal disease.
- Reduce the proportion of older adults 65 to 74 years of age who have lost all of their natural teeth.
- Reduce the proportion of adults 45 to 74 years of age with moderate or severe periodontitis.
- Increase the proportion of oral and pharyngeal cancers detected at the earliest stages.

Data from U.S. Department of Health and Human Services, Office of Disease Prevention and Health Promotion: Healthy People 2020, 2012. http://www.healthypeople.gov/2020

hygiene, and lack of dental care contribute to poor oral health. Poor oral health is recognized as a risk factor for dehydration and malnutrition, as well as a number of systemic diseases, including pneumonia, joint infections, cardiovascular disease, and poor glycemic control in type 1 and type 2 diabetes (Jablonski, 2010; O'Connor, 2012; Stein et al, 2014).

Poor oral health is an important public health issue and a growing burden to countries worldwide. Health disparities are evident across and within regions and result from living conditions and availability of oral health services. The World Health Organization Global Oral Health Programme encourages the development of effective and affordable strategies and programs for better oral health and increasing resources for health promotion and oral disease prevention (World Health Organization, 2014). Tips for promotion of oral health are presented in (Box 15-7). *Healthy People 2020* addresses oral health (Box 15-8).

Common Oral Problems

Xerostomia (Mouth Dryness)

Xerostomia and hyposalivation are present in approximately 30% of older adults and can affect eating, swallowing, and

BOX 15-7 TIPS FOR BEST PRACTICE

Promoting Oral Health

Encourage annual dental exams, including individuals with dentures.
Brush and floss twice daily; use a fluoride dentifrice and mouthwash.
Ensure dentures fit well and are cleaned regularly.
Maintain adequate daily fluid intake (1500 mL).
Avoid tobacco.
Limit alcohol.
Eat a well-balanced diet.
Use an ultrasonic toothbrush (more effective in removing plaque).
Use a commercial floss handle for easier flossing.
Adapt toothbrush if manual dexterity impaired. Use a child's toothbrush or enlarge the handle of an adult-sized toothbrush by adding a foam grip or wrapping it with gauze or rubber bands to increase handle size.
If medications cause a dry mouth, ask your health care provider if there are other drugs that can be substituted. If dry mouth cannot be avoided, drink plenty of water, chew sugarless gum, avoid alcohol and tobacco.

speaking and contribute to dental caries and periodontal disease. Adequate saliva is necessary for the beginning stage of digestion, helping to break down starches and fats. It also functions to clear the mouth of food debris and prevent overgrowth of oral microbes. The flow of saliva does not decrease with age, but medical conditions and medications affect salivary flow (Stein et al, 2014). More than 500 medications have a side effect of hyposalivation including antihypertensives, antidepressants, antihistamines, antipsychotics, diuretics, and antiparkinson agents.

Treatment of xerostomia. A review of all medications is important, and if medication side effects are contributing to dry mouth, medications may be changed or altered. Affected individuals should practice good oral hygiene practices and have regular dental care to screen for decay. Consumption of adequate water intake and avoidance of alcohol and caffeine are recommended. Over-the-counter saliva substitutes (Oral Balance Gel, MouthKote) and salivary stimulants such as Biotene Xylitol gum and sugarless candy can be helpful (Stein et al, 2014).

Oral Cancer

Oral cancers occur more with age. The median age at diagnosis is 61 years; men are affected twice as often as women. Oral cancer occurs more frequently in black men, and the incidence of oral cancer varies in different countries. It is much more common in Hungary and France than in the United States and much less common in Mexico and Japan (American Geriatrics Society, 2006). The 5-year survival rate is 50% and has not changed significantly in the past 50 years.

Early detection is essential, but more than 60% of oral cancers are not diagnosed until an advanced stage. Early signs and symptoms may be subtle and not recognized by the individual or health care provider (Stein et al, 2014). Oral examinations can assist in early identification and treatment. All persons, especially those older than 50 years of age, with or without dentures, should have oral examinations on a regular basis. Box 15-9 presents common signs and symptoms of oral cancer, and Box 15-10 lists risk factors. Once diagnosed, therapy options are based on diagnosis and staging and include surgery, radiation, and chemotherapy. If detected early, these cancers can almost always be treated successfully.

Oral Care

Nearly one-third of individuals older than age 65 have untreated tooth decay. About one-fourth of persons age 65 and older have no remaining teeth (edentulous), primarily as a result of periodontitis, which occurs in about 95% of those in this age group (Administration on Aging [AOA], 2014). There has been a dramatic reduction in the prevalence of tooth loss as knowledge increases and more people use fluorides, improve nutrition, engage in new oral hygiene practices, and take advantage of improved dental health care. Half of all Americans were edentulous in the 1950s, but today the rate has decreased to 18% (Stein et al, 2014). However, many individuals may not have had the advantages of new preventive treatment, and those with functional and cognitive limitations may be unable to perform oral hygiene.

Access to dental care for older people may be limited and cost prohibitive. In the existing health care system, dental care is a low priority. Medicare does not provide any coverage for oral health care services, and few Americans 75 years of age or older have private dental insurance. Medicaid coverage for dental varies from state to state, but funding has decreased and coverage can be limited. Elders have fewer dentist visits than any other age group, and dental care utilization among low-income adults has declined or remained constant in almost every state from 2000 to 2010 (Vujicic, 2013). Older Americans with the poorest oral health are those who are economically disadvantaged and lack insurance. Being disabled, homebound, or institutionalized increases the risk of poor oral health. In many undeveloped countries, there is a shortage of trained dental professionals. Dental care is nonexistent except that provided by groups such as medical and dental ministries from other countries. The World Health Organization (2014) established the Global Oral Health Programme with goals of developing global policies in oral health promotion and oral disease prevention.

◆ PROMOTING HEALTHY AGING: IMPLICATIONS FOR GERONTOLOGICAL NURSING

◆ Assessment

Good oral hygiene and timely assessment of oral health are essentials of nursing care. In addition to identifying oral health problems, examination of the mouth can serve as an early warning system for some diseases and lead to early diagnosis and treatment. Assessment of the mouth, teeth, and oral cavity is an essential part of health assessment (Chapter 7) and especially important when an individual is hospitalized or in a long-term care facility. The MDS 3.0 requires information obtained from an oral assessment. Federal regulations mandate an annual examination for residents of long-term care facilities. Although the oral examination is best performed by a dentist, nurses in health care settings can provide oral health screenings using an instrument such as The Kayser-Jones Brief Oral Health Status Examination (BOHSE) (see Box 15-6).

◆ Interventions

Nurses may be involved in promoting oral health through teaching individuals or caregivers recommended interventions, screening for oral disease, and making dental referrals, or by providing, supervising, and evaluating oral care in hospitals and long-term care facilities. Box 15-11 presents information on providing oral hygiene.

◆ Dentures

Older adults and those who may care for them should be taught proper care of dentures and oral tissue to prevent odor, stain, plaque buildup, and oral infections. All nursing staff should be knowledgeable about care of dentures (Box 15-12). Dentures are very personal and expensive possessions and the utmost care should be taken when handling, cleaning, and storing dentures, especially in hospitals and long-term care facilities. It is not uncommon to hear that dentures were lost, broken, or mixed up with those of others, or not removed and cleaned during a hospital or nursing home stay. Dentures should be marked, and many states require all newly made dentures to contain the client's identification. A commercial denture marking system called Identure, produced by the 3M Company, provides a simple, efficient, and permanent means of marking dentures.

BOX 15-11 TIPS FOR BEST PRACTICE

Provision of Oral Care

1. Explain all actions to the individual; use gestures and demonstration as needed; cue and prompt to encourage as much self-care performance as possible.

2. If the individual is in bed, elevate his or her head by raising the bed or propping it with pillows, and have the individual turn his or her head to face you. Place a clean towel across the chest and under the chin, and place a basin under the chin.

3. If the individual is sitting in a stationary chair or wheelchair, stand behind the individual and stabilize his or her head by placing one hand under the chin and resting the head against your body. Place a towel across the chest and over the shoulders.

4. The basin can be kept handy in the individual's lap or on a table placed in front of or at the side of the patient. A wheelchair may be positioned in front of the sink.

5. If the individual's lips are dry or cracked, apply a light coating of petroleum jelly or use lip balm.

6. Inspect the oral cavity to identify teeth in ill repair, pain, lesions, or inflammation.

7. Brush and floss the individual's teeth (use an electric toothbrush if possible, with sulcular brushing). It may be helpful to retract the lips and cheek with a tongue blade or fingers in order to see the area that is being cleaned. Use a mouth prop as needed if the individual cannot hold his or her mouth open. If manual flossing is too difficult, use a floss holder or interproximal brush to clean the proximal surfaces between the teeth. Use a dentifrice containing fluoride.

8. Provide the conscious individual with fluoride rinses or other rinses as indicated by the dentist or hygienist.

BOX 15-12 TIPS FOR BEST PRACTICE

Providing Denture Care

1. Remove dentures or ask individual to remove dentures. Observe ability to remove dentures.

2. Inspect oral cavity.

3. Rinse denture or dentures after each meal to remove soft debris. Do not use toothpaste on dentures because it abrades denture surfaces.

4. Once each day, preferably before retiring, remove denture and brush thoroughly.

   a. Although an ordinary soft toothbrush is adequate, a specially designed denture brush may clean more effectively. (**Caution:** Acrylic denture material is softer than natural teeth and may be damaged by being brushed with very firm bristles.)

   b. Brush denture over a sink lined with a facecloth and half-filled with water. This will prevent breakage if the denture is dropped.

   c. Hold the denture securely in one hand, but do not squeeze. Hold the brush in the other hand. It is not essential to use a denture paste, particularly if dentures are soaked before being brushed to soften debris. Never use a commercial tooth powder because it is abrasive and may damage the denture materials. Plain water, mild soap, or sodium bicarbonate may be used.

   d. When cleaning a removable partial denture, great care must be taken to remove plaque from the curved metal clasps that hook around the teeth. This can be done with a regular toothbrush or with a specially designed clasp brush.

5. After brushing, rinse denture thoroughly; then place it in a denture-cleaning solution and allow it to soak overnight or for at least a few hours. (**Note:** Acrylic denture material must be kept wet at all times to prevent cracking or warping.) In the morning, remove denture from the cleaning solution and rinse it thoroughly before inserting it into the mouth. Use denture paste if necessary to secure dentures.

6. Dentures should be worn constantly except at night (to allow relief of compression on the gums) and replaced in the mouth in the morning.

Broken or damaged dentures and dentures that no longer fit because of weight loss or changes in the oral cavity are a common problem for older adults. Many elders believe that there is no longer a need for oral care once they have dentures, but regular professional attention is important. "Only 13% of denture wearers seek annual dental care, and nearly half have not seen a dentist in 5 years" (Stein et al, 2014, p. 566). Rebasing of dentures is a technique to improve the fit of dentures. Ill-fitting dentures or dentures that are not cleaned contribute to oral problems (lesions, stomatitis), as well as to poor nutrition and reduced enjoyment of food.

◆ Oral Hygiene in Hospitals and Long-Term Care

Oral care is an often neglected part of daily nursing care and should receive the same priority as other kinds of care. When the person is unable to carry out his or her dental/oral regimen, it is the responsibility of the caregiver to provide oral care. Lack of attention to oral hygiene contributes significantly to poor nutrition and other negative outcomes such as aspiration pneumonia. There is evidence that cleaning the person's teeth with a toothbrush after meals lowers the risk of developing aspiration pneumonia (Metheny, 2012; van der Maarel-Wierink et al, 2013). In the acute care setting, good oral care is crucial to the prevention of ventilator-associated pneumonia (VAP), one of the most common hospital-acquired infections and a leading cause of morbidity and mortality in intensive care units (ICUs) (Booker et at., 2013).

Illness, acute care situations, and functional and cognitive impairments make the provision of oral care difficult. Factors contributing to less than adequate oral care include inadequate knowledge of how to provide care, lack of appropriate supplies, inadequate training and staffing, and lack of oral care protocols. Booker et al. (2013) noted that oral care practices among critical care nurses are not consistently implemented and mouth care may be perceived as a comfort measure rather than a critical component of infection control. These authors provide a comprehensive protocol for provision of oral care to ventilator-dependent patients.

Individuals residing in long-term care facilities are particularly vulnerable to problems with oral care as a result of functional and cognitive impairments. A large number are dependent on staff for the provision of oral hygiene. Individuals with cognitive impairment may be resistive to mouth care, and this is one of the reasons caregivers may neglect oral care. Placing yourself at eye level and explaining all actions in step-by-step instructions with cues and gestures may decrease mouth care–resistive behavior. Even with individuals who need help, caregivers should encourage as much self-care as possible. Caregivers can have the person hold the toothbrush but place their hand over the person's hand (hand-over-hand technique) (Jablonski, 2010).

The use of therapeutic rinses (e.g., chlorhexidine) that are broad-spectrum antimicrobial agents has been shown to help control plaque. These can be used in conjunction with brushing or in place of brushing in those unable to tolerate brushing. Xylitol products (gum, mints, toothpaste) have also been evaluated as an effective method of reducing oral pathogens (Gulkowski, 2013).

Many long-term care institutions have implemented programs, such as special training of nursing assistants for dental care teams, providing visits from mobile dentistry units on a routine basis, or using dental students to perform oral screening and cleaning of teeth. An important nursing role is to assist in the development of oral care protocols and staff education in all health care settings.

◆ Tube Feeding and Oral Hygiene

Tube feeding is associated with significant pathologic colonization of the mouth, greater than that observed in people who received oral feeding. Oral care should be provided every 4 hours for patients with gastrostomy tubes, and teeth should be brushed with a toothbrush after each feeding to decrease the risk of aspiration pneumonia (Metheny et al, 2008; O'Connor, 2012). Foam swabs are available to provide oral hygiene but do not remove plaque as well as toothbrushes. Foam swabs may be used to clean the oral mucosa of an edentulous older adult.

⚡ SAFETY ALERT

Lemon glycerin swabs should never be used for oral care. In combination with decreased salivary flow and xerostomia, they inhibit salivary production, causing dry mouth and promoting bacterial growth (Booker et al, 2013).

KEY CONCEPTS

- Age-related changes, medication use, functional impairments, and comorbid medical and emotional illnesses place some older adults at risk for changes in fluid balance, especially dehydration.
- In older people, dehydration most often develops as a result of disease, age-related changes, and/or the effects of medication; dehydration is not primarily due to lack of access to water. Dehydration is considered a geriatric syndrome that is frequently associated with common diseases (e.g., diabetes, respiratory illness, heart failure) and declining stages of the frail elderly.
- Prevention of dehydration is essential, but assessment is complex in older people. Clinical signs may not appear until dehydration is advanced and signs and symptoms may be nonspecific, making prevention and early identification important.

- Age-related changes in the oral cavity, medical conditions, poor dental hygiene, and lack of dental care contribute to poor oral health. Poor oral health is a risk factor for dehydration and malnutrition, as well as a number of systemic diseases, including pneumonia, joint infections, cardiovascular disease, and poor glycemic control in type 1 and type 2 diabetes.
- Good oral hygiene and timely assessment of oral health are essentials of nursing care.
- Nurses may be involved in promoting oral health by teaching individuals or caregivers recommended interventions, by screening for oral disease and making dental referrals, or by providing, supervising, and evaluating oral care in hospitals and long-term care facilities.

NURSING STUDY: HYDRATION STATUS

Violet Barnes is an 87-year-old woman who resides in a skilled nursing facility. Her diagnoses include dementia, hypertension, and diabetes. She is able to walk and feed herself with assistance. She knows her name and responds to conversation appropriately, although she is not oriented to time or place. Two days ago she underwent a colonoscopy on an outpatient basis in the hospital for a suspected mass in the large intestine. She was maintained NPO for 12 hours before the procedure and returned to the skilled facility following the procedure. Since she has returned, she has become very lethargic and not able to respond to familiar caregivers. She is refusing any food or fluids offered. She has had four episodes of diarrhea and her stool is being tested for *C. difficile*.

On the basis of the nursing study, develop a nursing care plan using the following procedure*:
- List information that provides objective data.
- From the data, identify and state, using an accepted format, two nursing diagnoses you determine are most significant to Violet at this time. List two of Violet's strengths that you have identified from data.

- Determine and state outcome criteria for each diagnosis. These must reflect some alleviation of the problem identified in the nursing diagnosis and must be stated in concrete and measurable terms.
- Plan and state one or more interventions for each diagnosed problem. Provide specific documentation of the source used to determine the appropriate intervention. Plan at least one intervention that incorporates Violet's existing strengths.
- Evaluate the success of the intervention. Interventions must correlate directly with the stated outcome criteria to measure the outcome success.

---

*Students are advised to refer to their nursing diagnosis text and identify possible or potential problems.

CRITICAL THINKING QUESTIONS AND ACTIVITIES

1. What risk factors for Violet's condition are present in nursing study above?
2. What preventive interventions by nursing would have been appropriate?
3. What are your suggestions for enhancing fluid intake for individuals with dementia residing in skilled nursing facilities?

RESEARCH QUESTIONS

1. What is the knowledge level of older adults about oral health practices?
2. What factors influence adequate dental care among older adults?
3. What strategies are most helpful in enhancing fluid intake of older adults in long-term care facilities?
4. What are the barriers to adequate oral care for older people in hospitals and long-term care facilities?
5. What content related to oral health is included in nursing education curricula?

REFERENCES

Administration on Aging: *Older adults and oral health*, 2014. http://aoa.acl.gov/AoARoot/AoA_Programs/HPW/Oral_Health/index.aspx. Accessed April 2014.

American Geriatrics Society: *Geriatric review syllabus*, ed 6, New York, 2006, American Geriatrics Society.

Booker S, Murff S, Kitko L, et al: Mouth care to reduce ventilator-associated pneumonia, *Am J Nurs* 113(10):24–30, 2013.

Faes MC, Spigt MG, Olde R, et al: Dehydration in geriatrics, *Geriatr Aging* 10:590–596, 2007.

Gulkowski S: Using Xylitol products and MI paste to reduce oral biofilm in long-term care residents, *Ann Longterm Care* 21(12):26–28, 2013.

Jablonski R: Examining oral health in nursing home residents and overcoming mouth-care resistive behaviors, *Ann Longterm Care* 18:21–26, 2010.

Mei A, Auerhahn C: Hypodermoclysis: maintaining hydration in the frail older adult, *Ann Longterm Care* 17:28–30, 2009.

Mentes JC: Oral hydration in older adults: greater awareness is needed in preventing, recognizing and treating dehydration, *Am J Nurs* 106:40–49, 2006a.

Mentes JC: A typology of oral hydration, *J Gerontol Nurs* 32(1):13–19, 2006b.

Mentes JC: Managing oral hydration. In Boltz M, Capezuti E, Fulmer T, et al, editors: *Evidence-based geriatric nursing protocols for best practice*, ed 4, New York, 2012, Springer, pp 419–438.

Metheny M: *Preventing aspiration in older adults with dysphagia*, New York, 2012, Hartford Institute for Geriatric Nursing. http://consultgerirn.org/uploads/File/trythis/try_this_20.pdf. Accessed April 2014.

O'Connor L: Oral health care. In Boltz M, Capezuti E, Fulmer T et al, editors: *Evidence-based geriatric nursing protocols for best practice*, ed 4, New York, 2012, Springer, pp 409–418.

Palmer M, Marquez C, Kline K, et al: Hydrate for health: listening to older adults' need for information, *J Gerontol Nurs* 40(10):24–30, 2014.

Stein P, Miller C, Fowler C: Oral disorders. In Ham R, Sloane P, Warshaw G, et al, editors: *Primary care geriatrics: a case-based approach*, ed 6, Philadelphia, 2014, Elsevier Saunders, pp 563–572.

Thomas D, Cote T, Lawhorne L, et al: Understanding clinical dehydration and its treatment, *J Am Med Dir Assoc* 9:292–301, 2008.

van der Maarel-Wierink C, Vanobbergen J, Bronkhorst E, et al: Oral health care and aspiration pneumonia in frail older people: a systematic literature review, *Gerodontology* 30(1):3–9, 2013.

Vujicic M: *Dental care utilization declined among low-income adults*, increased among low-income children in most states from 2000-2010 (Health Policy Resources Center research brief), Feb 2013. http://www.ada.org/~/media/ADA/Science%20and%20Research/HPI/Files/HPIBrief_0213_3.ashx. Accessed April 2014.

World Health Organization: *Oral health*, 2014. http://www.who.int/oral_health/en/. Accessed April 2014.

16 | CHAPTER

Elimination

Theris A. Touhy

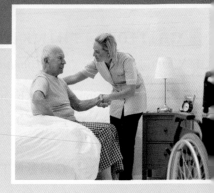

http://evolve.elsevier.com/Touhy/TwdHlthAging

A STUDENT SPEAKS

"My grandmother doesn't like to go out shopping with me anymore. She says she has to go to the bathroom all the time and can't walk fast enough to get to the bathrooms in the mall. She won't wear a protective garment or a pad because she says they smell. I hope I learn something in this class that will help her."

Molly, 20 years old

ELDERS SPEAK

"Being incontinent is like being a bad kid or a big baby."

"There's nothing that can be done. Well, I don't think there is anything else but a diaper."

"Sometimes I have to wet my bed before they get here, you know, and they are all busy and I have to wait for somebody."

"I do something that is very wrong. I try not to drink too much. How can you drink a lot, you would be soaked all the time."

Comments from participants in a study of living with urinary incontinence in long-term care (MacDonald and Butler, 2007)

A NURSE SPEAKS

"Urinary incontinence is a preventable and treatable condition and yet continence remains undervalued and UI remains underassessed. Even though UI is a basic nursing issue, nurses are not claiming it as one."

Comment from nurses in expert continence care (Mason et al, 2003, p. 3).

LEARNING OBJECTIVES

On completion of this chapter, the student will be able to:

1. Identify age-related changes and other contributing factors affecting bowel and bladder elimination.
2. Identify appropriate assessment of bowel and bladder function.
3. Explain the types of urinary incontinence and their causes.
4. Identify risk factors for accidental bowel leakage and describe appropriate nursing interventions.
5. Use evidence-based protocols in the assessment and development of interventions to promote bowel and bladder health.

The body must remove waste products of metabolism to sustain healthy function, but bladder and bowel activity are fraught with social implications. Bladder and bowel function in later life, although normally only slightly altered by the physiological changes of age (Box 16-1), can contribute to problems severe enough to interfere with the ability to continue independent living and can seriously threaten the body's capacity to function

and to survive. The effects of uncontrolled bladder and bowel action are a threat to the person's independence and well-being.

Elimination is a private matter, not publicized socially. In most cultures children are taught early to deal with their own body waste. Deviations from this may be socially unacceptable and can lead to chastisement, ostracism, and social withdrawal. Nurses are in a key position to implement evidence-based

BOX 16-1 Age-Related Changes in the Renal and Urological Systems

Kidneys

Decreased size and function begins in fourth decade; kidney is 20% to 30% smaller by end of eighth decade

Decrease in renal blood flow and GFR (less pronounced in healthy individuals)

Diverticula of renal tubules in distal portion of nephron

Glucose reabsorption decreases (more glucose in the urine)

Decline in renal activation of vitamin D decreases intestinal absorption of calcium; more vitamin D is needed to counteract diminishing renal function

Ability to concentrate urine decreases; hyperkalemia more common; sudden large changes in pH or fluid load can quickly lead to hypervolemia or hypovolemia. These changes cause a high risk for adverse events if individual exposed to changes in environment (high temperatures, renal-toxic medications) or to functional restrictions that limit ability to obtain adequate fluids

Ureters, Bladder, Urethra

Less tone and elasticity

Loss of bladder holding capacity

Total bladder capacity decreases to 300 mL from 600 mL

Urge to void occurs at lower bladder volume (160 to 300 mL)

Weakened contractions during emptying, which can lead to postvoid residual and increased risk for bladder infection

More urine produced at night; may be due to changes in circadian rhythm, output, medications, or be indicator of sleep apnea

Increased collagen content, changes in gap junctions, increased space between myocytes, and changes in sensitivity of sensory afferents, all of which may contribute to involuntary bladder contractions and overactive bladder symptoms

Sources: Gibson W, Wagg A: New horizons: urinary incontinence in older people, *Age Ageing* 43:167–163, 2014; McCance K, Huether S, editors: *Pathophysiology*, ed 7, St Louis, MO, 2014, Elsevier.

BOX 16-2 Normal Bladder Elimination

- Normal bladder function requires an intact brain and spinal cord, competent lower urinary tract function, the motivation to maintain continence, the functional ability to use a toilet, and an environment that facilitates the process (Dowling-Castronovo and Bradway, 2008).
- A full bladder increases pressure and signals the spinal cord and the brainstem center of the desire to micturate. Social training then dictates whether micturition should be addressed or should be postponed until there is an appropriate opportunity to locate toilet facilities.
- When the bladder contents reach 500 mL or more, the pressure is such that it becomes more difficult to control the urge to void. As volume increases, emptying the bladder becomes an uncontrollable act.

BOX 16-3 Promoting a Healthy Bladder

- Drink 8 to 10 glasses of water a day before 8 PM.
- Eliminate or reduce the use of coffee, tea, brown cola, and alcohol, particularly before bedtime.
- Empty bladder completely before and after meals and at bedtime.
- Urinate whenever the urge arises; never ignore it.
- Limit the use of sleeping pills, sedatives, and alcohol because they decrease sensation to urinate.
- Make sure toilet is nearby with a clear path to it and good lighting, especially at night. Consider a grab bar or a raised toilet seat if there is difficulty getting on and off the toilet.
- Maintain ideal body weight.
- Get regular physical exercise.
- Avoid smoking.
- Seek professional treatment for complaints of burning, urgency, pain, blood in urine, or difficulties maintaining continence.

assessment and interventions to enhance continence and improve function, independence, and quality of life.

AGE-RELATED CHANGES IN THE RENAL AND UROLOGICAL SYSTEMS

The renal system is responsible for excreting toxins, regulating water and salts, and maintaining the acid-base balance in the blood. The kidneys, the primary organs in the renal system, are highly vascular. They produce the hormone *erythropoietin,* which stimulates the bone marrow to produce red blood cells, and the enzyme *renin,* which helps regulate blood pressure. In aging there are both anatomical and functional changes. The age-related loss of nephrons, kidney mass, and ability to concentrate urine ordinarily leads to little change in the body's ability to regulate its body fluids and the ability to maintain adequate fluid homeostasis under usual circumstances. Renal disease or urinary tract obstruction can amplify age-related declines in function (Doig and Huether, 2014). Changes that may contribute to urinary incontinence (UI) increase in frequency, but UI should never be considered a normal part of aging. Box 16-2 describes the process of normal bladder elimination and Box 16-3 describes promotion of a healthy bladder.

URINARY INCONTINENCE = pressure sonss most common us women

Urinary incontinence (UI) is the involuntary loss of urine sufficient to be a problem (Dowling-Castronovo and Bradway, 2012). UI is a stigmatized, underreported, underdiagnosed, undertreated condition that is erroneously thought to be part of normal aging.

Two-thirds of men and women ages 30 to 70 years have never discussed bladder health with their health care providers and only one in eight who have experienced bladder control problems has been diagnosed. On average, women wait 6.5 years from the first time they experience symptoms until they obtain a diagnosis for their bladder control problems (National Association for Continence, 2014). Instead, they try to cope with the condition on their own, with variable success (Wilde et al, 2014). Older individuals are less likely to receive evidence-based care for UI complaints than younger people (Gibson and Wagg, 2014).

Individuals may not seek treatment for UI because they are embarrassed to talk about the problem or think that it is a normal part of aging. They may be unaware that successful treatments are available. Men may be unlikely to report UI to their primary care provider because they feel it is a woman's disease. Older people want more information about bladder control,

Diabetes cause may pee/urine
3 "p"

and nurses must take the lead in implementing approaches to continence promotion and public health education about UI (Palmer and Newman, 2006).

UI is an important yet neglected geriatric syndrome (Lawhorne et al, 2008). UI tends to be viewed as an inconvenience rather than a condition requiring assessment and treatment. In comparison with nurses in other health care settings, nurses in hospitals view incontinent patients more negatively (Dowling-Castronovo and Bradway, 2012). In nursing facilities, physicians, geriatric nurse practitioners, and directors of nursing evaluated and managed UI significantly less often than five other geriatric syndromes (falls, dementia, unintended weight loss, pain, and delirium). Nursing assistants were more likely to be involved in care provision for UI than any other syndrome and rated UI second only to pain with respect to its effect on quality of life (Lawhorne et al, 2008).

Without an adequate knowledge base of continence care and use of evidence-based practice guidelines, nursing care will continue to consist of just containment strategies, such as the use of pads and briefs, to manage UI. Nurses in all practice settings who care for older adults should be prepared to assess data that relate to urine control and implement nursing interventions that promote continence. There is a growing role for nurses in continence care, and advanced training and certification are available through specialty organizations such as the Society of Urologic Nurses and Associates and the Wound, Ostomy and Continence Nurses Society.

UI Facts and Figures

Inconsistencies with definitions and measurements, as well as underreporting and underassessment, make definitive statistics on prevalence and incidence of UI problematic (Dowling-Castronovo and Bradway, 2012). However, because of the high prevalence and chronic but preventable nature of UI, it is most appropriately considered a public health problem. UI affects millions of adults worldwide. As a result of the aging population, estimates are that UI will increase 22% between 2008 and 2018, affecting an estimated 546 million people. The burden of this condition is greatest in the developing countries of Asia, South America, and Africa. There is some evidence that community-dwelling women living in resource-poor settings may be more affected (Irwin et al, 2011; Seshan and Muliira, 2013). A World Continence Week occurs yearly and is sponsored by the International Continence Foundation. The purpose is to raise awareness of incontinence worldwide.

UI is more common in women with the peak incidence around the time of menopause. In men, there is a steady increase in prevalence with age (Gibson and Wagg, 2014). Twenty-five percent of young women, 44% to 57% of middle-aged and postmenopausal women, and 75% of older women in nursing homes have some involuntary urine loss (Agency for Healthcare Research and Quality, 2012). UI is more prevalent than diabetes, Alzheimer's disease, and many other chronic conditions that have prompted more attention and treatment. Incontinence is also costly; the indirect costs are estimated at

more than $16 billion annually in the United States. UI costs exceed those of coronary artery bypass surgery and renal dialysis combined (Dowling-Castronovo and Bradway, 2008).

Risk Factors for UI

Many of the risk factors associated with UI are unrelated to changes in the urinary tract (Box 16-4). "The maintenance of continence is dependent not only on a functional lower urinary tract and pelvic floor, but also on sufficient cognition to interpret the desire to void and locate a toilet, adequate mobility and dexterity to manipulate clothing and allow safe and effective walking to the toilet, and an appropriate environment in which to allow this" (Gibson and Wagg, 2014, p. 168). Older people with dementia are at high risk for UI.

Dementia does not cause urinary incontinence but affects the ability of the person to find a bathroom and recognize the urge to void. Mobility problems and dependency in transfers are better predictors of continence status than dementia, suggesting that persons with dementia may have the potential to remain continent as long as they are mobile. Drugs that increase urinary output and sedatives, tranquilizers, and hypnotics, which produce drowsiness, confusion, or limited mobility, promote incontinence by dulling the transmission of the desire to urinate.

Consequences of UI

UI affects quality of life and has physical, psychosocial, and economic consequences. UI is identified as a marker of frailty in community-dwelling older adults. UI is more common

---

BOX 16-4 Risk Factors for UI

- Age
- Immobility, functional limitations
- Diminished cognitive capacity (dementia, delirium)
- Medications (those with anticholinergic properties, diuretics)
- Smoking
- High caffeine intake
- Low fluid intake
- Obesity
- Constipation, fecal impaction
- Pregnancy, vaginal delivery, episiotomy, forceps birth, large baby
- Environmental barriers
- High-impact physical exercise
- Diabetes, stroke, Parkinson's disease, multiple sclerosis, spinal cord injury
- Hysterectomy
- Pelvic muscle weakness, pelvic organ prolapse
- Childhood nocturnal enuresis
- Prostate surgery
- Estrogen deficiency
- Arthritis and/or back problems
- Malnutrition
- Depression
- Hearing or visual impairments

Adapted from Dowling-Castronovo A, Bradway C: Urinary incontinence. In Boltz M, Capzuti E, Fulmer T, et al, editors: *Evidence-based geriatric nursing protocols for best practice,* ed 4, New York, 2012, Springer, pp 363–387.

and more severe in older people and associated with sequelae not seen in younger people, such as increased risk of falls, fractures, and hospitalization. "In a typical older person, incontinence is the end result of multiple underlying risk factors, pathophysiologies and modifiers" (Gibson and Wagg, 2014, p. 168).

UI affects self-esteem and increases the risk for depression, anxiety, loss of dignity and autonomy, social isolation, falls, skin breakdown, and avoidance of sexual activity (Xu and Kane, 2013). UI also increases the risk of admission to a nursing home in individuals older than 65 years of age. Older adults with UI experience a loss of independence and self-confidence, as well as feelings of shame and embarrassment (Dowling-Castronovo and Bradway, 2012; Wilde et al, 2014). The psychosocial impact of UI affects the individual and the family caregivers.

Types of UI

Incontinence is classified as either *transient* (acute) or *established* (chronic). *Transient* incontinence has a sudden onset, is present for 6 months or less, and is usually caused by treatable factors such as urinary tract infections (UTIs), delirium, constipation and stool impaction, and increased urine production caused by metabolic conditions such as hyperglycemia and hypercalcemia. Hospitalized older adults are at risk of developing transient UI and may also be at risk of being discharged without resolution of the condition. Use of medications such as diuretics, anticholinergic agents, antidepressants, sedatives, hypnotics, calcium channel blockers, and α-adrenergic agonists and blockers can also lead to transient UI (Dowling-Castronovo and Bradway, 2012).

Established UI may have either a sudden or a gradual onset and is categorized into the following types: (1) stress; (2) urge; (3) urge, mixed, or stress UI with high postvoid residual (PVR) (originally termed overflow UI); (4) functional UI; and (5) mixed UI (Table 16-1).

◆ PROMOTING HEALTHY AGING: IMPLICATIONS FOR GERONTOLOGICAL NURSING

◆ Assessment

Continence must be routinely addressed in the initial assessment of every older person. Health care personnel must begin to change their thinking about incontinence and acknowledge that incontinence can be cured in about 80% of individuals (Wound, Ostomy and Continence Nurses Society, 2009). If it cannot be cured, it can be treated to minimize its detrimental effects. Nurses are often the ones to identify urinary incontinence, but neither nurses nor physicians have been particularly aggressive in its management.

Nurses in all settings are expected to be able to collect and organize data about urine control, report findings to the interprofessional team, and implement evidence-based interventions to promote continence. "Nurses have long been the providers of personal hygiene information for those entrusted to their care. Therefore, it is essential that nurses play a leading role in assessing and managing UI . . . " (Dowling-Castronovo and Bradway, 2007, p. 7).

TABLE 16-1	Types and Symptoms of Urinary Incontinence
TYPE	**SYMPTOMS**
Stress	Loss of small amount of urine with activities that increase intraabdominal pressure (coughing, sneezing, exercising, lifting, bending More common in women but can occur in men after prostate surgery/treatment PVR low
Urge	Loss of moderate to large amount of urine before getting to toilet; inability to suppress need to urinate Frequency and nocturia may be present PVR low May be associated with overactive bladder (OAB) characterized by urinary frequency (>8 voids/24 hr), nocturia, urgency, with or without UI
Urge, mixed, or stress with high residuals (formerly called overflow)	Nearly constant urine loss (dribbling), hesitancy in starting urine, slow urine stream, passing small volumes of urine, feeling of incomplete bladder emptying PVR high
Functional	Lower urinary tract intact but individual unable to reach toilet due to environmental barriers, physical limitations, cognitive impairment, lack of assistance, difficulty managing belts, zippers, getting a dress up and undergarments down, or sitting on a toilet May occur with other types of UI; more common in individuals who are institutionalized
Mixed	Combination of more than one UI problem; usually stress and urge

Assessment of UI is multidimensional and targeted to identify continence patterns, alterations in continence, and contributing factors. If the individual is being admitted to a hospital, home care agency, or skilled nursing facility, it is important to document the presence or absence of UI, past continence patterns, the presence or absence of a urinary catheter, and the reasons for the catheter if present.

In the nursing home, the MDS 3.0 (Chapter 7) provides an evidence-based overview of the assessment, treatment, and evaluation of bladder continence based on the Centers for Medicare and Medicaid Services (CMS) guidelines. Residents should be assessed on admission and whenever there is a change in cognition, physical ability, or urinary tract function. An environmental assessment including the accessibility of bathrooms, the adequacy of room lighting, the availability of assistance, and the use of aids such as raised toilet seats or commodes is also important.

For individuals with UI, the nurse collaborates with the interprofessional team to (1) determine if UI is transient or established (or both); (2) determine the type of UI; and (3) identify and document possible etiologies of the UI, including a review of risk factors (Dowling-Castronovo and Bradway, 2012). Additional assessment is presented in Box 16-5,

BOX 16-5   TIPS FOR BEST PRACTICE
Continence Assessment

Screening Questions
"Have you ever leaked urine/water? If yes, how much does it bother you?"
"Do you ever leak urine/water on the way to the bathroom?"
"Do you ever use pads, tissue, or cloth in your underwear to catch urine/water?"
"Do you dribble urine/water most of the time?"
"Do you have any burning, hesitancy, or pain with urination?"

Screening Instruments
Urogenital Distress Inventory—6 (available from The Hartford Institute for Geriatric Nursing)
Incontinence Impact Questionnaire (available from The Hartford Institute for Geriatric Nursing)
Male Urinary Distress Inventory

Bladder (Voiding) Diary
Kept for 3 to 7 days by the individual or caregiver (Figure 16-1)
Voiding record for even 1 day can be helpful

Patterns of Fluid Intake
Usual fluid intake/24 hours
Types of fluids and time consumed
Decreased or increased urine output

Bowel Patterns
Frequency, consistency, straining
Use of laxatives

Exploration of Symptoms of UI
"When did UI start?"
"What have you done to manage the problem?"
"How often does it occur?"
"What things make it better or worse?"
"How severe is it?"

Focused History (Medical, Neurological, Gynecological, Genitourinary)
Review past health history: possible contributing factors to UI, pertinent diagnoses (heart failure, stroke, diabetes mellitus, multiple sclerosis, Parkinson's Disease)

Medication Review
Review all medications including OTC with focus on diuretics, anticholinergics, psychotropics, α-adrenergic blockers, α-adrenergic agonists, calcium channel blockers
Review use of alcohol

Focused Assessment
Screen for depression
Cognitive, functional

Observe Individual Using the Toilet
Ability to reach a toilet and use it, time it takes to reach the toilet, finger dexterity for clothing manipulation; character of the urine (color, odor, sediment); difficulty starting or stopping urinary stream.

Physical Examination
Abdominal, rectal, genital: Assess for suprapubic distention indicative of urinary retention
Observe for signs of perineal irritation, itching, burning, lesions, discharge, tenderness, thin and pale genital tissues (atrophic vaginitis), dyspareunia, pelvic organ prolapse
Check for fecal impaction, tenderness

Other Tests That May Be Ordered
Urinalysis; culture and sensitivity if clinically significant systemic or urinary symptoms
If indicated, PVR (bladder sonography or catheterization) 16 minutes or less post void

Adapted from Dowling-Castronovo A, Bradway C: Urinary incontinence. In Boltz M, Capzuti E, Fulmer T, et al, editors: *Evidence-based geriatric nursing protocols for best practice,* ed 4, New York, 2012, Springer, pp 363–387; Ham R, Sloane P, Warshaw G, et al, editors: *Primary care geriatrics,* ed 6, Philadelphia, 2014, Elsevier Saunders.

BOX 16-6   RESOURCES FOR BEST PRACTICE

Centers for Disease Control and Prevention: *Guideline for prevention of catheter-associated urinary tract infections,* 2009
Catheterout.org: Protocols, Educational tools, Toolkit
Di Rico N: NICHE Solution 27, 2012: A nurse-driven urinary catheter removal protocol: www.nicheprogram.org
Dowling-Castronovo A, Bradway C: Urinary incontinence. In Boltz M, Capezuti E, Fulmer T, Zwicker D: *Evidence-based geriatric nursing protocols for best practice,* ed 4, New York, 2012, Springer, pp 363-387
Hartford Institute for Geriatric Nursing (consultgerirn.org): Try This Series: Urinary incontinence assessment in older adults. Part 1: Transient Incontinence (includes link to video of assessment), Part 2: Persistent Incontinence (includes UI assessment tools - Urogenital Distress Inventory and Incontinence Impact Questionnaire)

Hartford Institute for Geriatric Nursing: Want to know more: Urinary tract infection prevention, geriatric nursing protocol: prevention of catheter-associated urinary tract infection
International Continence Society—Educational materials, product guide, research, advocacy
National Association for Continence (NAC)—Educational materials, product guide, advocacy
National Institute of Diabetes and Digestive and Kidney Disease: The NIDDK Bowel Control Awareness Campaign
Safe Care Campaign: Preventing health care and community associated infections: urinary tract infections
Simon Foundation for Continence: Educational materials, resources and products. Stool diary and Bristol Form Stool Scale

and Box 16-6 provides information on a video of a nurse conducting an assessment for transient UI. More extensive examinations are considered after the initial findings are assessed. Individuals who do not fit a simple pattern for UI should be referred promptly for urodynamic assessment (DeBeau, 2014).

◆ Interventions
◆ Behavioral Interventions

A number of behavioral interventions have a good basis in research and can be implemented by nurses without extensive and expensive evaluation. Selection of a modality and interventions will depend on a comprehensive assessment, the type of incontinence and its underlying cause, and whether the outcome is to cure or to minimize the extent and complications of the incontinence. Behavioral techniques, such as scheduled voiding, prompted voiding, bladder training, biofeedback, and pelvic floor muscle exercises (PFMEs), are recommended as first-line treatment of UI. Because UI in older adults can have multiple precipitating factors, a single intervention may not be adequate and more complex, multicomponent interventions may be required (Gibson and Wagg, 2014).

Nursing interventions focus primarily on the appropriate assessment of continence, teaching about treatments, and implementation and evaluation of supportive and therapeutic modalities to promote and restore continence and to prevent incontinence-related complications, such as skin breakdown. The nurse should share appropriate resources and explain clinical information and differences in treatment choices (Box 16-7).

Scheduled (timed) voiding. Scheduled (timed) voiding is used to treat urge and functional UI in both cognitively intact and cognitively impaired older adults. The schedule or timing of voiding is based on the person's bladder diary (Figure 16-1) or common voiding patterns (voiding on arising, before and after meals, midmorning, midafternoon, and bedtime). Many persons with UI have a very short time between voiding and leaking urine. With a program of timed voiding the goal is to slowly increase the time between voids without increasing the number, or even reducing the number, of incontinent episodes or reaching continence altogether. The person is encouraged to NOT void at an unscheduled time, thus achieving "mind over bladder."

Bladder training. Bladder training aims to increase the time interval between the urge to void and voiding. This method is appropriate for people with urge UI who are cognitively intact and independent in toileting or after removal of an indwelling catheter. Bladder training involves frequent

BOX 16-7 TIPS FOR BEST PRACTICE

Teaching about UI Interventions

- Use therapeutic communication skills and a positive and supportive attitude to help individuals overcome any embarrassment about UI.
- Teach about the range of interventions available for management of UI.
- Share helpful resources for continence management.
- Share techniques found useful by others.
- Collaborate with the individual to help him or her choose the most appropriate and acceptable intervention based on needs.
- Assist individual to develop a detailed, realistic action plan and set goals.
- Determine an evaluation plan to assess the effectiveness of interventions.
- Review progress, identify any barriers to implementation, set alternative goals, or select alternate treatments if indicated.
- Consider using various teaching formats: face-to-face counseling, small-group sessions, computer-based continence promotion systems, informative written materials.
- Make teaching collaborative and interactive.
- Reinforce effort and persistence.

Source: Wilde M, Bliss D, Booth J, et al: Self-management of urinary and fecal incontinence, *Am J Nurs* 114(2):38–45, 2014.

voluntary voiding to keep bladder volume low and suppression of the urge to void using pelvic muscle contractions, distraction, or relaxation techniques. When the individual feels the urge to urinate, the person uses the urge control techniques. After the urge subsides, the person walks at a normal pace to the toilet. The initial toileting frequency is every 2 hours and it is progressively lengthened to 4 hours, depending on tolerance, over the course of days or weeks (DeBeau, 2014; Wilde et al, 2014).

Pelvic floor muscle exercises. Pelvic floor muscle exercises (PFMEs), also called Kegel exercises, involve repeated voluntary pelvic floor muscle contraction. The targeted muscle is the pubococcygeal muscle, which forms the support for the pelvis and surrounds the vagina, the urethra, and the rectum. The goal of the repetitive contractions is to strengthen the muscle and decrease UI episodes. PFMEs are recommended for stress, urge, and mixed UI in older women and have also been shown to be helpful for men who have undergone prostatectomy. Biofeedback may improve PMFE teaching and outcomes, but further research is needed. Medicare covers biofeedback for individuals who do not improve after 4 weeks of a trial of PMFEs (DeBeau, 2014). Box 16-8 presents a protocol for PFMEs.

Although there are some nursing home residents who may benefit from PFMEs and are capable of learning and practicing, the numbers may be insufficient to justify emphasis on this approach in this setting (Johnson and Ouslander, 2006). In community-dwelling older adults, PFMEs are at least as effective as medications in treating stress and urge UI (Dowling-Castronovo and Bradway, 2012).

Vaginal weight training. Vaginal weight training was introduced in Europe as an alternative for women who have difficulty identifying the pelvic floor muscles. Graded-weight vaginal balls or cones are worn during two 16-minute periods each day or are used in addition to PFMEs. When the weighted cone is placed in the vagina, the pelvic floor muscle contractions keep it from slipping out. Although this technique involves less time and is more easily taught than PFMEs, difficulty inserting the cones and discomfort have been noted as deterrents to use.

Prompted voiding. Prompted voiding (PV) is a technique used in the nursing home that combines scheduled voiding with monitoring, prompting, and verbal reinforcement. The objective of PV is to increase self-initiated voiding and decrease the number of episodes of UI. The person is assisted to the toilet at predetermined times during waking hours if he or she requests it and receives positive feedback if he or she voids successfully (Box 16-9). PV is associated with modest short-term improvement in daytime UI and implementation of appropriate toileting programs in nursing home residents. Nighttime PV and waking program techniques have not shown to improve UI (Flanagan et al, 2012). A major advantage of PV programs is that they target residents who are likely to be successful and direct scarce staff resources to residents most likely to benefit.

Special considerations in the nursing home. Continence programs in nursing homes are required by CMS regulations. Monitoring and documentation of continence status in

Bladder Diary ("Uro-Log")

Complete one form for each day for 4 days before your appointment with a health care provider. In order to keep the most accurate diary possible, you'll want to keep it with you at all times and write down the events as they happen. Take the completed forms with you to your appointment.

Your Name: _____

Date: _____

Time	Fluids		Foods		Did you urinate?		Accidents			
							Leakage	Did you feel an urge to urinate?	What were you doing at the time?	
	What kind?	How much?	What kind?	How much?	How many times?	How much? (sm, med, lg)	How much? (sm, med, lg)		Sneezing, exercising, etc.	
Sample	Coffee	1 cup	Toast	1 slice	✓ ✓	med	sm	Yes	(No)	Running
6-7 a.m.								Yes	No	
7-8 a.m.								Yes	No	
8-9 a.m.								Yes	No	
9-10 a.m.								Yes	No	
10-11 a.m.								Yes	No	
11-12 noon								Yes	No	
12-1 p.m.								Yes	No	
1-2 p.m.								Yes	No	
2-3 p.m.								Yes	No	
3-4 p.m.								Yes	No	
4-5 p.m.								Yes	No	
5-6 p.m.								Yes	No	
6-7 p.m.								Yes	No	
7-8 p.m.								Yes	No	
8-9 p.m.								Yes	No	

FIGURE 16-1 Bladder Diary. (Provided by the National Association for Continence; 1-800-BLADDER; www.nafc.org)

relation to implemented continence care is a *quality of care indicator* for nursing homes (Shamliyan et al, 2007). Despite a growing body of evidence suggesting that toileting programs can be successful in long-term care, they are difficult to sustain. Barriers to implementation and continuation of toileting programs include inadequate staffing, lack of knowledge about UI and existing evidence-based protocols, and insufficient professional staff.

In most cases, cure of incontinence in nursing home residents may not be a realistic goal; however, every resident who is incontinent deserves appropriate medical and nursing assessment and interventions that restore continence, if possible,

or provide supportive care and prevention of complications related to incontinence (Johnson and Ouslander, 2006). Successful implementation of continence programs requires a systems-based approach with consideration of individual, group, organizational, and environmental level factors (Holroyd-Leduc and Straus, 2004).

Newly admitted nursing home residents who are incontinent (and able to use the toilet) should receive a 3- to 5-day trial of prompted voiding or other toileting programs. The trial can be helpful in demonstrating responsiveness to toileting and determining patterns of and symptoms associated with the incontinence (Figure 16-2).

BOX 16-8 Pelvic Floor Muscle Training Exercises

Purpose
Prevent the involuntary loss of urine by strengthening the muscles under the uterus, bladder, and bowel.

Who Should Perform These Exercises?
Men and women who have problems with urine leakage or bowel control

Identifying Pelvic Floor Muscles
When urinating, start to go and then stop. Feel the muscles in your vagina, bladder, or anus get tight and move up. These are the pelvic floor muscles. If you feel them tighten, you have done the exercise right.

If you are still not sure you are tightening the right muscle, keep in mind that all the muscles of the pelvic floor relax and contract at the same time. Because these muscles control the bladder, rectum, and vagina, the following tips may help:

Women: Inset a finger into your vagina. Tighten the muscles as if you are holding your urine; then let go. You should feel the muscles tighten and move up or down. These are the same muscles you would tighten if you were trying to prevent yourself from passing gas.

Men: Insert a finger into your rectum. Tighten the muscles as if you were holding your urine; then let go. You should feel the muscles tighten and move up and down. These are the same muscles you would tighten if you were trying to prevent yourself from passing gas.

Note: Nurses can teach correct muscle identification when performing a rectal or vaginal exam.

PFME Routine
1. Begin by emptying your bladder.
2. You can lie down, stand up, or sit in a chair.
3. Tighten the pelvic floor muscles and hold for a count of 10.
4. Relax the muscles completely for a count of 10.
5. Do 10 repetitions, 3 to 5 times a day.
6. Breathe deeply and relax your body when doing the exercises.
7. It is very important to keep the abdomen, buttocks, and thigh muscles relaxed when doing PFME.
8. After 4 to 6 weeks, most people see some improvement but it may take as long as 3 months. The regimen should be continued for 12 weeks.
9. After a few weeks, you can also try doing a single PFME contraction at times when you are likely to leak.

Source: U.S. National Library of Medicine, NIH National Institutes of Health: Pelvic floor muscle training exercises, *Medline Plus,* 2012. http://www.nlm.nih.gov/medlineplus/ency/article/003975.htm. Accessed March 2014.

BOX 16-9 Prompted Voiding Protocol: Long-Term Care

1. Contact resident every 2 hours from 8 AM to 9 PM (or the resident's usual bedtime).
2. Focus attention on voiding by asking if the resident is wet or dry.
3. Ask a second time if the resident does not respond.
4. Check clothes and bedding to determine if wet or dry. Give feedback on whether response was correct or incorrect.
5. Whether wet or dry, ask if the resident would like to use toilet or urinal.

If the resident says **YES:**
Offer assistance.
Record results on bladder record.
Praise for appropriate toileting.

If the resident says **NO:**
Repeat the question once or twice.

If wet and declines to use the toilet, change him or her.

Inform the resident you will be back in 2 hours and request that the resident try to delay voiding until then.

If there has been no attempt to void in the past 2 to 3 hours, repeat the request to use the toilet at least twice more before leaving.

1. Offer fluids.
2. For nighttime management, use either modified prompted voiding schedule, toilet when awake, or use padding, depending on individual's sleep pattern and preferences.
3. If the individual who has been responding well has an increase in incontinence frequency despite adequate staff implementation of the protocol, further evaluation for reversible factors is indicated.

Source: Joseph Ouslander, MD, personal communication.

Lifestyle interventions. Several lifestyle factors have been associated with either the development or the exacerbation of UI. These include increased fluid intake, weight reduction, smoking cessation, bowel management, and physical activity (Box 16-10). Some research suggests that coffee and tea consumption has limited or no effects on incontinence, but guidelines generally suggest limiting caffeine intake (Tettamanti et al, 2011) (see Box 16-4). Research has shown that women with stress UI who undergo a 5% to 10% weight loss experience a positive impact on UI symptoms. This is most likely due to the effects of reduced abdominal weight, intra-abdominal pressure, and intravesicular pressure (DeBeau, 2014; Wilde et al, 2014).

Other Interventions

Urinary catheters

Intermittent catheterization. Intermittent catheterization may be used in people with urinary retention related to a weak detrusor muscle (e.g., diabetic neuropathy), those with a blockage of the urethra (e.g., benign prostatic hypertrophy [BPH]), or those with reflux incontinence related to a spinal cord injury. The goal is to maintain 300 mL or less of urine in the bladder. Most of the research on intermittent catheterization has been conducted with children or young adults with spinal cord injuries, but it may be useful for older adults who are able to self-catheterize. It provides an important alternative to indwelling catheterization.

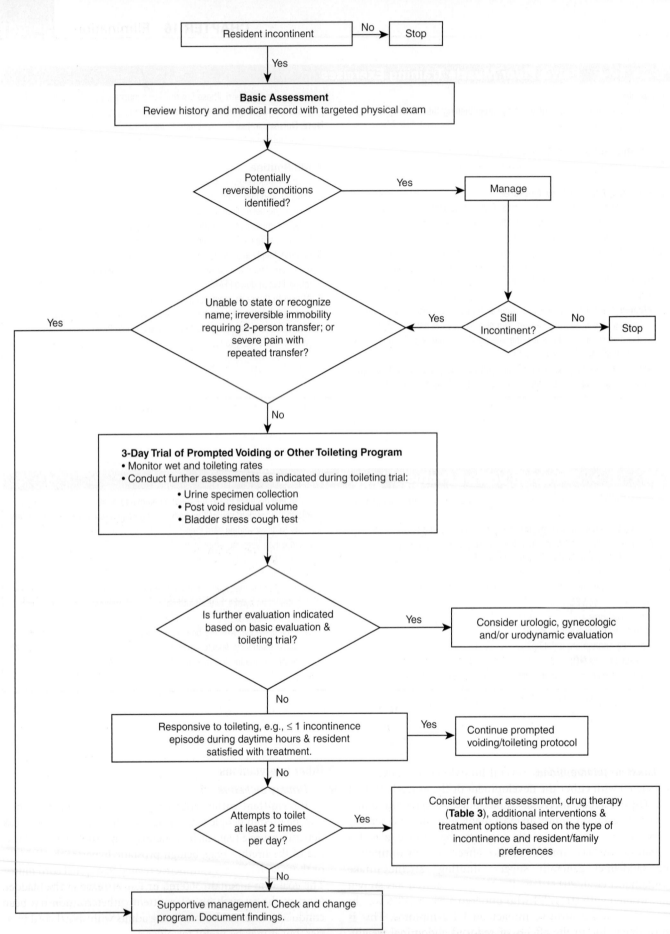

FIGURE 16-2 Diagnostic Assessment and Management of Urinary Incontinence and Overactive Bladder in the Nursing Home. (From Zarowitz B, Ouslander J: The application of evidence-based practice principles of care in older persons [issue 6]: urinary incontinence, *J Am Med Dir Assoc* 8:35–45, 2007.)

BOX 16-10 RESEARCH HIGHLIGHTS

Dancing to Treat UI

The study evaluated the feasibility of using a combination of pelvic floor muscle exercises and virtual reality rehabilitation to treat mixed UI in older women. The virtual reality program was one that involved dancing. Evaluation was done through a bladder diary, pad test, patient-reported symptoms, and quality of life and satisfaction questionnaire. Results indicated that the frequency and quantity of urine leakage decreased and the patient-reported symptoms and quality of life improved significantly. About 91% of the participants were very satisfied with the treatment. Further exploration of this type of combination therapy should be evaluated through further randomized controlled studies. The program was acceptable, efficient, and satisfying for the participants, encouraging exercise and social enjoyment while improving UI.

Source: Elliott V, de Bruin E, Dumoulin C: Virtual reality rehabilitation as a treatment approach for older women with mixed UI: a feasibility study, *Neurourol Urodyn*, Jan 10, 2014. doi: 10.1002/nau22553. [Epub ahead of print]

Indwelling catheters. Indwelling catheter use is not appropriate in any setting for long-term management (more than 30 days) except in the following clinical conditions:

- Acute urinary retention or bladder outlet obstruction
- Need for accurate measurements of urinary output in critically ill patients
- Perioperative use for selected surgical procedures: urological or other surgery on contiguous structures of the genitourinary tract; anticipated prolonged surgery duration (should be removed in postanesthesia unit); patients anticipated to receive large-volume infusions or diuretics during surgery; need for intraoperative monitoring of urinary output
- To assist in healing of open sacral or perineal wounds in incontinent patients
- Patient requires prolonged immobilization (e.g., potentially unstable thoracic or lumbar spine, multiple traumatic injuries such as pelvic fractures)
- To improve comfort for end-of-life care if needed (CDC, 2009; Johnson and Ouslander, 2006; Meddings et al, 2013)

Regulatory standards in nursing homes follow these same guidelines, and the use of indwelling catheters must be justified on the basis of medical conditions and failure of other efforts to maintain continence. In hospitals, the use of indwelling catheters is often unjustified, and they are used inappropriately or left in place too long. Between 14% and 25% of patients in the hospital setting will have an indwelling catheter, up to half of which can be inappropriate (So et al, 2014). Reasons for this include (1) convenience to manage UI; (2) lack of knowledge of risks associated with use and alternative treatments; (3) providers not tracking continued use; and (4) lack of valid continence assessment tools for older adults (DiRico, 2012).

Misuse of catheterization should be considered a medical error. Cognitive impairment and the presence of pressure ulcers almost double the risk of receiving a catheter, and severe functional decline is associated with a fourfold risk of catheter placement (Inelmen et al, 2007) (Box 16-11).

BOX 16-11 A Urinary Catheter's Perspective: The Catheter's Lament

I am a urinary catheter	That if I'm left in (a mortal sin)
Dark places I must go	You could just end up dead
My job is clear	At times, I am a useful aid
I have no fear	But my use you should not flout
I need to ease the flow	On every day
You are the one I am inside	Someone should say
It enters not your head	It's time to take me out!

Courtesy Martin Kiernan, Nurse Consultant, Infection Prevention, Southport and Ormskirk Hospital NHS Trust, Southport, UK.

⚡ SAFETY ALERT

Long-term catheter use increases the risk of recurrent urinary tract infections leading to urosepsis, urethral damage in men, urethritis, or fistula formation. Catheter-associated urinary tract infection is the most frequent health care–associated infection in the United States, and Medicare no longer reimburses hospitals for this infection. Indwelling catheters should be inserted only for appropriate conditions and must be removed as soon as possible, and alternatives should be investigated (e.g., condom catheters, intermittent catheterization, toileting programs).

External catheters. External catheters (condom catheters) are sometimes used in male patients who are incontinent and cannot be toileted. Long-term use of external catheters can lead to fungal skin infections, penile skin maceration, edema, fissures, contact burns from urea, UTIs, and septicemia. The catheter should be removed and replaced daily, and the penis cleaned, dried, and aired to prevent irritation, maceration, and the development of pressure ulcers and skin breakdown. If the catheter is not sized appropriately and applied and monitored correctly, strangulation of the penile shaft can occur.

Absorbent products. Some individuals prefer to use absorbent products in addition to toileting interventions to maintain "social continence," and a wide variety of products are available (see Box 16-6). Disposable types are available in several sizes, determined by hip and waist measurements, or as one size made to fit all. Many of these undergarments now look like regular underwear and you even see them in stylish television commercials. Nurses should avoid the use of the word diaper since it is infantilizing and demeaning to older people-the word brief is preferred. It is important that individuals are counseled to purchase proper continence products that will wick moisture away from the skin. These products are costly but they protect skin integrity. Women may tend to use menstrual pads but these do not absorb significant amounts of fluid.

◆ Pharmacological Interventions

Medications are not considered first-line treatment but can be considered in combination with behavioral strategies in some cases. Pharmacological treatment (anticholinergic, antimuscarinic agents) may be indicated for urge UI and overactive bladder (OAB). These include oxybutynin (Oxytrol, Ditropan), tolterodine (Detrol), trospium chloride (Sanctura), darifenacin (Enablex), fesoterodine (Toviaz), and solifenacin (VESIcare). All of these medications have similar efficacy in reducing urge UI frequency, and choice of medication depends on avoidance of adverse drug effects, drug-drug and drug-disease interactions, dosing frequency, titration range, and cost (DeBeau, 2014). β₃-Agonists (mirabegron) are a new class of medications for urge UI and OAB. They should not be used in patients with severe uncontrolled hypertension, hepatic insufficiency, or bladder obstruction from BPH, or in those taking antimuscarinic agents. These medications can also raise digoxin levels (DeBeau, 2014). Oxytrol for Women is the first FDA-approved over-the-counter (OTC) treatment for OAB. It is available in patch form, which is applied to the skin every 4 days.

Dosages of medications for urge UI and overactive bladder should be started low and titrated with careful attention to side effects and drug interactions. A trial of 4 to 8 weeks is adequate and recommended. If one medication is not effective, another may be tried (DeBeau, 2014). None of these medications have been evaluated in frail older people. Undesirable side effects of anticholinergic medications such as dry mouth and eyes, constipation, and cognitive impairment are problematic. People with narrow-angle glaucoma cannot use these medications, and they should not be combined with cholinesterase inhibitors. These medications can be especially problematic for those with cognitive impairment (DeBeau, 2014).

◆ **Surgical Interventions**

Surgical interventions may be indicated for stress UI and have a high cure rate. The most common procedures are colposuspension (Burch operation) and slings. Surgical suspension of the bladder neck (sling procedure) in women has proved effective in 80% to 95% of persons electing to have this surgical corrective procedure. Outcomes in older women are comparable with those in younger women. Outflow obstruction incontinence secondary to prostatic hypertrophy is generally corrected by prostatectomy. Sphincter dysfunction resulting from nerve damage following surgical trauma or radical perineal procedures is 70% to 90% repairable through sphincter implantation. Periurethral injections of collagen are also used and add bulk to the internal sphincter and close the gap that allowed leakage to occur. This is a short-term alternative and usually requires a series of injections (DeBeau, 2014).

◆ **Nonsurgical Devices**

There are a variety of intravaginal or intraurethral devices to relieve stress UI. These include intravaginal support devices, pessaries, external occlusive devices, and urethral plugs for women. For men, there are foam penile clamps. The pessary, used primarily to prevent uterine prolapse, is a device that is fitted into the vagina and exerts pressure to elevate the urethrovesical junction of the pelvic floor. The patient is taught to insert and remove the pessary, much like inserting and removing a diaphragm used for contraception. The pessary is removed weekly or monthly for cleaning with soap and water and then reinserted. Adverse effects include vaginal infection, low back pain, and vaginal mucosal erosion. Another

concern is the danger of forgetting to remove the pessary. Several of the resources in Box 16-6 provide detailed information on these devices but an evaluation of the stress UI by the health care provider should be conducted to determine if these devices woud be helpful.

URINARY TRACT INFECTIONS

Urinary tract infections (UTIs) are the most common cause of bacterial sepsis in older adults and are 10 times more common in women than in men. The clinical spectrum of UTIs ranges from asymptomatic and recurrent UTIs to sepsis associated with UTI requiring hospitalization. Assessment and appropriate treatment of UTIs in older people, particularly nursing home residents, is complex. Cognitively impaired residents may not recall or report symptoms, and older people frequently do not present with classic symptoms (fever, dysuria, flank pain) (Mody and Juthani-Mehta, 2014).

Asymptomatic bacteriuria is transient and considered benign in older women. It should not be treated with antibiotics and often resolves without treatment. Antimicrobials should not be used to treat bacteriuria in older adults unless specific urinary tract symptoms are present (American Geriatrics Society, 2014). Screening urine cultures should also not be performed in patients who are asymptomatic.

The diagnosis of symptomatic UTI is made when the patient has both clinical features and laboratory evidence of a urinary tract infection. Treatment is with antibiotics selected by identifying the pathogen, knowing local resistance rates, and considering adverse effects. Long-term suppressive antibiotics for 6 to 12 months and vaginal estrogen therapy reduce symptomatic UTI episodes and should be considered in patients with recurrent UTIs (Mody and Juthani-Mehta, 2014). An assessment and treatment algorithm for UTI in nursing homes is presented in Figure 16-3.

Catheter-Associated Urinary Tract Infections

Catheter-associated urinary tract infections (CAUTIs) refer to urinary tract infections that occur in a patient with an indwelling catheter or within 48 hours of catheter removal (Andreessen et al, 2012). CAUTIs are the most common hospital-acquired infection worldwide (So et al, 2014). CAUTIs were among the first hospital-acquired conditions (HACs) targeted for nonpayment by Medicare in 2008. They have also been further targeted as a "never event," with a national goal to reduce CAUTI by 25% and reduce urinary catheter use by 50% by 2014 (Andreessen et al, 2012; Meddings et al, 2013).

A recent study on health care–associated infections in hospitals reported a decrease with some infection types, but CAUTI rates increased by 3% between 2009 and 2012, indicating a need for better prevention efforts (CDC, 2014). One of the goals of Healthy People 2020 is to prevent, reduce, and ultimately eliminate health care associated infections. Implementation of evidence-based guidelines, catheter reminders, stop orders, nurse-initiated removal protocols, and a urinary catheter bundle can decrease CAUTIs in acute care (Andreessen et al, 2012; Shekelle et al, 2013). Box 16-12 presents Tips for Best Practice: Prevention of CAUTI.

CARE PATH *Symptoms of Urinary Tract Infection (UTI)*
(in residents without an indwelling catheter)

INTERACT
Version 4.0 Tool

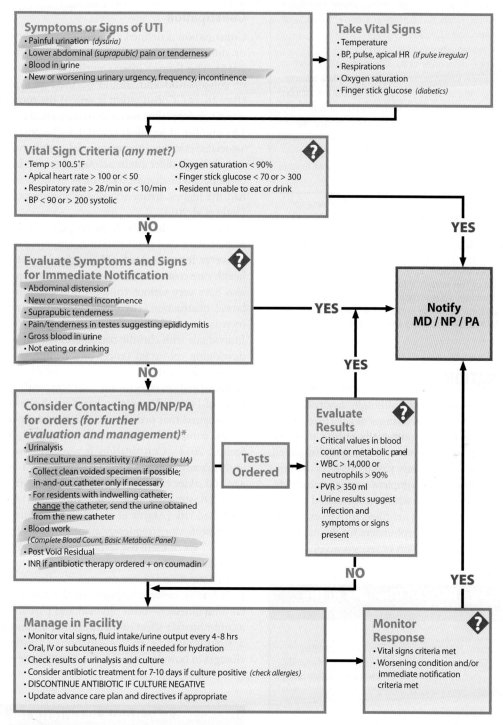

Symptoms or Signs of UTI
- Painful urination *(dysuria)*
- Lower abdominal *(suprapubic)* pain or tenderness
- Blood in urine
- New or worsening urinary urgency, frequency, incontinence

Take Vital Signs
- Temperature
- BP, pulse, apical HR *(if pulse irregular)*
- Respirations
- Oxygen saturation
- Finger stick glucose *(diabetics)*

Vital Sign Criteria *(any met?)*
- Temp > 100.5°F
- Apical heart rate > 100 or < 50
- Respiratory rate > 28/min or < 10/min
- BP < 90 or > 200 systolic
- Oxygen saturation < 90%
- Finger stick glucose < 70 or > 300
- Resident unable to eat or drink

NO / **YES**

Evaluate Symptoms and Signs for Immediate Notification
- Abdominal distension
- New or worsened incontinence
- Suprapubic tenderness
- Pain/tenderness in testes suggesting epididymitis
- Gross blood in urine
- Not eating or drinking

YES

Notify MD / NP / PA

NO

YES

Consider Contacting MD/NP/PA for orders *(for further evaluation and management)**
- Urinalysis
- Urine culture and sensitivity *(if indicated by UA)*
  - Collect clean voided specimen if possible; in-and-out catheter only if necessary
  - For residents with indwelling catheter; <u>change</u> the catheter, send the urine obtained from the new catheter
- Blood work *(Complete Blood Count, Basic Metabolic Panel)*
- Post Void Residual
- INR if antibiotic therapy ordered + on coumadin

Tests Ordered

Evaluate Results
- Critical values in blood count or metabolic panel
- WBC > 14,000 or neutrophils > 90%
- PVR > 350 ml
- Urine results suggest infection and symptoms or signs present

YES

NO

YES

Manage in Facility
- Monitor vital signs, fluid intake/urine output every 4-8 hrs
- Oral, IV or subcutaneous fluids if needed for hydration
- Check results of urinalysis and culture
- Consider antibiotic treatment for 7-10 days if culture positive *(check allergies)*
- DISCONTINUE ANTIBIOTIC IF CULTURE NEGATIVE
- Update advance care plan and directives if appropriate

Monitor Response
- Vital signs criteria met
- Worsening condition and/or immediate notification criteria met

* Please Note:
1. *Overtreatment of asymptomatic bacteriuria labeled as a "UTI" is a major problem contributing to adverse events, C. Difficile infection, and resistant organisms. Antibiotic treatment should be reserved for those who meet specific clinical criteria.*
2. *Evaluation and management of patients with indwelling catheters includes different criteria.*
See http://www.cdc.gov/nhsn/PDFs/LTC/LTCF-UTI-protocol_FINAL_8-24-2012.pdf ; or JAMDA 15 (2014) 133-139

FIGURE 16-3 Care Path: Symptoms of Urinary Tract Infection (UTI). *bid,* Twice daily; *BP,* blood pressure; *IV,* intravenous; *MD/NP/PA,* doctor/nurse practitioner/physician's assistant; *sub Q,* subcutaneous; *tid,* three times daily; *WBC,* white blood cell count. (Developed by Joe Ouslander. Copyright ©2010, Florida Atlantic University.)

BOWEL ELIMINATION

Bowel function of the older adult, although normally only slightly altered by the physiological changes of age (Box 16-13), can be a source of concern and a potentially serious problem, especially for the older person who is functionally impaired. Normal elimination should be an easy passage of feces, without undue straining or a feeling of incomplete evacuation or defecation. The urge to defecate occurs when the distended walls of the sigmoid and the rectum, which are filled with feces, stimulate pressure receptors to relax the sphincters for the expulsion of feces through the anus. Evacuation of feces is accomplished by relaxation of the sphincters and contraction of the diaphragm and abdominal muscles, which raises the intraabdominal pressure.

Constipation

Constipation is defined as a reduction in the frequency of stool or difficulty in formation or passage of stool (McKay et al, 2012). The Rome Criteria outline the operational definitions of constipation and should be used as a guide to diagnosis (Box 16-14). Constipation is one of the most common gastrointestinal complaints encountered in clinical practice in all settings. The number of inpatient hospital discharges for constipation and associated costs has increased significantly between 1997 and 2010, and although older adults accounted for the largest percentage of constipation discharges, individuals in the 1- to 17-year age group had the highest frequency of constipation per 10,000 discharges (Sethi et al, 2014).

Many individuals, both the lay public and health care professionals, may view constipation as a minor problem or nuisance. However, it is associated with impaired quality of life, significant health care costs, and a large economic burden. Constipation can also have very serious consequences including fecal impaction, bowel obstruction, cognitive dysfunction, delirium, falls, and increased morbidity and mortality (Osei-Boamah et al, 2012). Individuals with chronic constipation are also at greater risk for developing colorectal cancer and benign colorectal neoplasms (Guerin et al, 2014).

Constipation is a chronic problem worldwide with a prevalence of 14% with variation based on the definition used. Some data suggest that prevalence is higher in the Americas and Asia Pacific compared with Europe (Alayne et al, 2013; Schmidt and Santos, 2014). Constipation is associated with female gender and increasing age. Approximately 40% of people 65 years of age and older experience constipation. Women have 2-3 times more constipation than men, and black women also exhibit increased risk (Alayne et al., 2013; Markland, 2014). Constipation is seen more frequently among nursing home residents and 50% to 74% of them use laxatives on a daily basis (Foxx-Orstein and Gallegos-Orozco, 2012).

Constipation is a symptom, not a disease. It is a reflection of poor habits, delayed response to the colonic reflex, and many chronic illnesses—both physical and psychological—as well as a common side effect of medication. Diet and activity level play a significant role in constipation. Constipation and other changes in bowel habits can also signal more serious underlying problems, such as colonic dysmotility or colon cancer. Thorough assessment is important, and these complaints should not be blamed on age alone. It is important to note that alterations in cognitive status, incontinence, increased temperature, poor appetite, or unexplained falls may be the only clinical symptoms of constipation in the cognitively impaired or frail older person. Numerous precipitating factors or conditions can cause or worsen constipation (Box 16-15).

Fecal Impaction

Fecal impaction (FI) is a major complication of constipation. It is especially common in incapacitated and institutionalized older people and those who require narcotic medications (e.g., for chronic pain) and is reported to occur in more than 40% of older adults admitted to the hospital (Roach and Christie,

2008). Symptoms of fecal impaction include malaise, urinary retention, elevated temperature, incontinence of bladder or bowel, alterations in cognitive status, fissures, hemorrhoids, and intestinal obstruction. Unrecognized, unattended, or neglected constipation eventually leads to fecal impaction. Digital rectal examination for impacted stool and abdominal x-rays will confirm the presence of impacted stool. Continued obstruction by a fecal mass may eventually impair sensation, leading to the need for larger stool volume to stimulate the urge to defecate, which contributes to megacolon.

Paradoxical diarrhea, caused by leakage of fecal material around the impacted mass, may occur. Reports of diarrhea in older adults must be thoroughly assessed before the use of antidiarrheal medications, which further complicate the problem of fecal impaction. Stool analysis for *Clostridium difficile* toxin should be ordered in patients who develop new-onset diarrhea, especially for those who live in a communal setting or have been recently hospitalized.

Removal of a fecal impaction is at times worse than the misery of the condition. Management of fecal impaction requires the digital removal of the hard, compacted stool from the rectum with use of lubrication containing lidocaine jelly. In general, this is preceded by an oil-retention enema to soften the feces in preparation for manual removal. Use of suppositories is not effective because their action is blocked by the amount and size of the stool in the rectum. Suppositories do not facilitate the removal of stool in the sigmoid, which may continue to ooze once the rectum is emptied.

Several sessions or days may be necessary to totally cleanse the sigmoid colon and rectum of impacted feces. Once this is achieved, attention should be directed to planning a regimen that includes adequate fluid intake, increased dietary fiber, administration of medications if needed, and many of the suggestions presented later in the chapter for prevention of constipation. For patients who are hospitalized or residing in long-term care settings, accurate bowel records are essential; unfortunately, they are often overlooked or inaccurately completed.

Education about the importance of bowel function and the accurate reporting of size, consistency, and frequency of bowel movements should be provided to all direct care providers. This is especially important for frail or cognitively impaired elders to prevent fecal impaction, a serious and often dangerous condition for older people.

◆ PROMOTING HEALTHY AGING: IMPLICATIONS FOR GERONTOLOGICAL NURSING

◆ Assessment

Assessment and management of bowel function is an important nursing responsibility. The precipitants and causes of constipation must be included in the evaluation of the patient. A review of these factors will also determine whether the patient is at risk for altered bowel function and if any of the known risks are modifiable. Recognizing constipation can be a challenge because there may be a significant disconnect between patient definitions of constipation and those of clinicians

---

BOX 16-15 Precipitating Factors for Constipation

Physiological
Dehydration
Insufficient fiber intake
Poor dietary habits

Functional
Decreased physical activity
Inadequate toileting
Irregular defecation habits
Irritable bowel disease
Weakness

Mechanical
Abscess or ulcer
Fissures
Hemorrhoids
Megacolon
Pelvic floor dysfunction
Postsurgical obstruction
Prostate enlargement
Rectal prolapse
Rectocele
Spinal cord injury
Strictures
Tumors

Other
Lack of abdominal muscle tone
Obesity
Recent environmental changes
Poor dentition

Psychological
Avoidance of urge to defecate
Cognitive impairment

Depression
Emotional stress

Systemic
Diabetic neuropathy
Hypercalcemia
Hyperparathyroidism
Hypothyroidism
Hypokalemia
Porphyria
Uremia
Parkinson's disease
Cerebrovascular disease
Defective electrolyte transfer

Pharmacological
ACE inhibitors
Antacids: calcium carbonate, aluminum hydroxide
Antiarrhythmics
Anticholinergics
Anticonvulsants
Antidepressants
Antimuscarinics
Anti-Parkinson's medications
Calcium channel blockers
Calcium supplements
Diuretics
Iron supplements
Laxative overuse
Lipid-lowering drugs
Nonsteroidal antiinflammatories
Opiates
Phenothiazines
Sedatives
Sympathomimetics

ACE, Angiotensin-converting enzyme.
Adapted from Allison OC, Porter ME, Briggs GC: Chronic constipation: assessment and management in the elderly, *J Am Acad Nurse Pract* 6(7):311, 1994; Tabloski PA: *Gerontological nursing,* Upper Saddle River, NJ, 2006, Pearson/Prentice Hall.

(Box 16-14). Constipation has different meanings to different people. Assessment begins with clarification of what the person means by constipation. Of persons who consider themselves to be constipated, nearly half actually have a bowel movement on a daily basis but a high percentage report persistent straining and passage of hard stools on a regular basis (Foxx-Orstein and Gallegos-Orozco, 2012).

It is important to obtain a bowel history including usual patterns, frequency of bowel movements, size, consistency, any changes, and occurrence of straining and hard stools. However, recall of bowel frequency has been shown to be unreliable in establishing the presence of constipation. Having the patient keep a bowel diary and using the Bristol Stool Form Scale, which provides a visual description of stool appearance, will be more accurate (Lewis and Heaton, 1997; McKay et al, 2012). Box 16-6 provides a resource for a bowel diary and the Bristol Stool Form Scale. Assessment data are presented in Box 16-16.

◆ Interventions

The first intervention is to examine the medications the person is taking and eliminate those that are constipation producing, preferably changing to medications that do not carry that side effect. Medications are the leading cause of constipation, and almost any drug can cause it (see Box 16-15).

BOX 16-16   TIPS FOR BEST PRACTICE

Assessment of Constipation

Sample Questions
- What is your usual bowel pattern?
- How many minutes did you sit on the bedpan or toilet before you had your bowel movement?
- How much did you have to strain before you had your bowel movement?
- Do you think you are constipated? If yes, why do you think so?
- Have you had any abdominal pain, nausea, vomiting, weight loss, blood in your bowel movement, or rectal pain?
- Have you had any bowel or rectal surgery?
- What type of physical activity do you engage in and how often?

Review of Food and Fluid Intake

Medication Review (Include OTC, herbal preparations, supplements)

Psychosocial History with Attention to Depression, Anxiety, Stress Management

Review of Concurrent Medical Conditions

Other Measures
- Bowel diary
- Bristol Stool Form Survey

Focused Physical Examination
- Abdominal exam to detect masses, distention, tenderness, high-pitched or absent bowel sounds
- If these abnormalities are present, primary care provider should be contacted
- Rectal exam, following institutional policy, to identify painful anal disorders such as hemorrhoids or fissures, rectal prolapse, stool presence in the vault, strictures, masses, anal reflex

Other Tests as Indicated
- Complete blood count, fasting glucose, chemistry panel, thyroid studies
- Flexible sigmoidoscopy, colonoscopy, CT scan, abdominal x-ray

Source: McKay S, Fravel M, Scanlon C: Management of constipation, *J Gerontol Nurs* 38(7):9–16, 2014.

◆ Nonpharmacological Interventions

Nonpharmacological interventions for constipation that have been implemented and evaluated are as follows: (1) fluid and diet related, (2) physical activity, (3) environmental manipulation, (4) toileting regimen, and (5) a combination of these. Fluid intake of at least 1.5 liters per day, unless contraindicated, is the cornerstone of constipation therapy, with fluids coming mainly from water. A gradual increase in fiber intake, either as supplements or incorporated into the diet, is generally recommended. Fiber helps stools become bulkier and softer and move through the body more quickly. This will produce easier and more regular bowel movements. High fiber intake is not recommended for individuals who are immobile or do not consume at least 1.5 L of fluid per day. The importance of dietary fiber to adequate nutrition and bowel function is discussed in Chapter 14.

Physical activity. Physical activity is important as an intervention to stimulate colon motility and bowel evacuation. Daily walking for 20 to 30 minutes, if tolerated, is helpful, especially after a meal. Pelvic tilt exercises and range-of-motion (passive or active) exercises are beneficial for those who are less mobile or who are bedridden. Exercise and physical activity are discussed in Chapter 18.

Positioning. The squatting or sitting position, if the patient is able to assume it, facilitates bowel function. A similar position may be obtained by leaning forward and applying firm pressure to the lower abdomen or by placing the feet on a stool. Rocking back and forth while sitting solidly on the toilet may facilitate stool movement. Massaging the abdomen or rectum may also help stimulate the bowel.

Toileting regimen. Establishing a routine for toileting promotes or normalizes bowel function (bowel retraining). The gastrocolic reflex occurs after breakfast or supper and may be enhanced by a warm drink. Given privacy and ample time (a minimum of 10 minutes), many will have a daily bowel movement. However, any urge to defecate should be followed by a trip to the bathroom. Older people dependent on others to meet toileting needs should be assisted to maintain normal routines and provided opportunities for routine toilet use. Box 16-17 presents a bowel training program.

◆ Pharmacological Interventions

When changes in diet and lifestyle are not effective, the use of laxatives is considered. Use of these medications, both prescribed and OTC, is high. Nearly 85% of health care provider visits for constipation result in a prescription for laxatives. The annual estimated expenditure for OTC laxatives in the general population of the United States is more than $820 million annually (Markland, 2014).

The extensive use of laxatives among older adults in the United States can be considered a cultural habit. During earlier times, weekly doses of rhubarb, cascara, castor oil, and other types of laxatives were consumed and believed by many to promote health. The belief that cleaning out the colon and having a daily bowel movement is paramount to maintaining good health still persists in some groups. Providing information about normal bowel function, definition of constipation, and

Box 16-17 TIPS FOR BEST PRACTICE

Bowel Training Program

1. Obtain a bowel history and establish a schedule for the bowel training program that is normal and comfortable for the patient and conforms to his or her lifestyle.
2. Ensure adequate fiber and fluid intake (normalize stool consistency).
   a. Fiber
      i. Add high-fiber foods to diet (dried fruit, dried beans, vegetables, and wheat products).
      ii. Suggest adding one to three tablespoons of bran or Metamucil to the diet once or twice each day. (Titrate dosage on the basis of response.)
   b. Fluid
      i. Consume 2 to 3 liters daily (unless contraindicated).
      ii. Four ounces of prune, fig, or pear juice (or a warm fluid) may be given daily as a stimulus (e.g., 30 to 60 min before the established time for defecation).
3. Encourage an exercise program.
   a. Pelvic tilt, modified sit-ups for abdominal strength
   b. Walking for general muscle tone and cardiovascular system
   c. More vigorous program if appropriate
4. Establish a regular time for the bowel movement.
   a. Established time depends on patient's schedule.
   b. Best times are 20 to 40 minutes after regularly scheduled meals, when the gastrocolic reflex is active.
   c. Attempts at evacuation should be made daily within 15 minutes of the established time and whenever the patient senses rectal distention.
   d. Instruct patient about normal posture for defecation. (The patient normally sits on the toilet or bedside commode; for the patient who is unable to get out of bed, the left side–lying position is best.)
   e. Instruct the patient to contract the abdominal muscles and "bear down."
   f. Have the patient lean forward to increase the intraabdominal pressure by use of compression against the thighs.
   g. Stimulate the anorectal reflex and rectal emptying if necessary.
5. Insert a rectal suppository or mini-enema into the rectum 15 to 30 minutes before the scheduled bowel movement, placing the suppository against the bowel wall, or insert a gloved, lubricated finger into the anal canal and gently dilate the anal sphincter.

lifestyle modifications can assist in promoting healthy bowel habits without the use of laxatives.

Older persons receiving opiates need to have a constipation prevention program in place because these drugs delay gastric emptying and decrease peristalsis. Correction of constipation associated with opiate use requires senna or an osmotic laxative to overcome the strong opioid effect. Stool softeners and bulking agents alone are inadequate. Laxatives commonly used in chronic constipation are presented in Table 16-2.

◆ **Enemas.** Enemas of any type should be reserved for situations in which other methods produce no response or when it is known that there is an impaction. Enemas should not be used

TABLE 16-2 Types of Laxatives: Actions, Use, Side Effects

TYPES OF LAXATIVES	ACTIONS, USE, SIDE EFFECTS
Bulk-forming (e.g., psyllium, methylcellulose)	Usually first-line agents due to low cost and few adverse effects Do not use in presence of obstruction or compromised peristaltic activity Use with caution in frail older people, bedbound individuals, those with swallowing problems Must be taken with adequate fluid intake to avoid obstruction in esophagus, stomach, intestines Can cause abdominal distention and flatulence
Emollients and lubricants (e.g., docusate sodium)	Increase moisture content of stool Used primarily to prevent constipation in specific situations such as following surgery Use with caution in frail older people who may not have the strength to "push" when having a bowel movement since soft stool can accumulate in rectal vault The emollient laxative mineral oil should be avoided because of the risk of lipoid aspiration pneumonia
Osmotic laxatives (e.g., milk of magnesia [MOM], lactulose, sorbitol, polyethylene glycol [PEG], MiraLax)	Cause water retention in the colon Avoid MOM in individuals with renal insufficiency since use can lead to hypermagnesemia or hyperphosphatemia Lactulose and sorbitol can cause diarrhea, abdominal cramping, and flatulence. MiraLax associated with less bloating and flatulence These medications can be added if bulk laxatives are ineffective
Stimulant laxatives (e.g., senna, bisacodyl)	Stimulate colorectal motor activity May cause cramping and electrolyte or fluid losses but when used appropriately, they are a safe and effective option, especially in those with opioid-induced constipation
Chloride channel stimulating (lubiprostone [Amitiza])	Stimulate ileal secretion and increase fecal water Generally safe, well tolerated, and effective in older adults with chronic constipation Side effects include nausea, diarrhea, headaches Expense of these medications may limit use except in individuals for whom other medications have failed or who have demonstrated intolerance to other agents

Source: McKay S, Fravel M, Scanlon C: Management of constipation, *J Gerontol Nurs* 38(7):9–16, 2014; World Gastroenterology Organization: *Global guidelines constipation*, 2010. http://www.worldgastroenterology.org/constipation.html Accessed March 2014.

on a regular basis. A normal saline or tap water enema (500 to 1000 mL) at a temperature of 105° F is the best choice. Sodium citrate enemas are another safe choice. Soapsuds and phosphate enemas irritate the rectal mucosa and should not be used. Oil retention enemas are used for refractory constipation and in the treatment of fecal impaction.

⚡ **SAFETY ALERT**

Sodium phosphate enemas (e.g., Fleets) should not be used in older adults because they may lead to severe metabolic disorders associated with high mortality and morbidity (Ori et al, 2012).

◆ Alternative Treatments

Combinations of natural fiber, fruit juices, and natural laxative mixtures are often recommended in clinical practice, and some studies have found an increase in bowel frequency and a decrease in laxative use when these mixtures are used. One study (Hale et al, 2007) showed that older long-term care residents receiving the Beverley-Travis natural laxative mixture (Beverley and Travis, 1992) at a dosage of two tablespoons twice per day had a significant increase in number of bowel movements compared with residents receiving daily prescribed laxatives. The Beverley-Travis natural laxative recipe and an additional recipe for an alternative natural laxative mixture are presented in Box 16-18.

Although research is still limited, many modalities of complementary and alternative medicine, such as probiotic bacteria, traditional herbal medicines, biofeedback, and massage, are also used to treat constipation. Further study is needed but probiotic bacteria might be easiest to use and supermarkets in several countries carry brands of yogurt labeled probiotic (Cherniack, 2013).

ACCIDENTAL BOWEL LEAKAGE/FECAL INCONTINENCE

Fecal incontinence (FI) is defined by the International Continence Society as the involuntary loss of liquid or solid stool that is a social and hygienic problem (Markland, 2014). Estimates of the worldwide prevalence of FI vary widely from 5% to 24%. Prevalence varies with the study population: 2% to 17% in community-dwelling older people; 50% to 65% in older adults in nursing homes; and 33% in hospitalized older adults. Higher prevalence rates are found among patients with diabetes, irritable bowel syndrome, stroke (new onset, 30%; 16% at 3 years poststroke), multiple sclerosis, and spinal cord injury (Grover et al, 2010; Roach and Christie, 2008). A lack of consistency in the definitions used for FI and differences in populations studied and methodology affect statistics. Additionally, accurate estimates are difficult to obtain because many people are reluctant to discuss this disorder and many primary care providers do not ask about it.

Often FI is associated with urinary incontinence, and up to 50% to 70% of patients with UI also carry the diagnosis of FI. FI can be transient (episodes of diarrhea, acute illness, fecal impaction) or persistent. Fecal incontinence, like urinary incontinence, has devastating social ramifications for the individuals and families who experience it. UI and FI share similar contributing factors, including damage to the pelvic floor as a result of surgery or trauma, neurological disorders, functional impairment, immobility, and dementia. Bowel continence and defecation depend on coordination of sensory and motor innervation of the rectum and anal sphincters. Impairment of the anorectal unit, such as weakness from prolonged straining secondary to constipation, or overt anal tears seen after vaginal delivery in women (35%) are common causes of FI. Injury from obstetrical trauma is often delayed in onset, and many women do not manifest

---

BOX 16-18   Natural Laxative Recipes

Beverley-Travis Natural Laxative Mixture

Ingredients
- 1 cup raisins
- 1 cup pitted prunes
- 1 cup figs
- 1 cup dates
- 1 cup currants
- 1 cup prune concentrate

Directions
Combine contents in grinder or blender to a thickened consistency. Store in refrigerator between uses.

Dosage
Administer 2 tablespoons (tbs) twice a day (once in the morning and once in the evening). May increase or decrease according to the frequency of bowel movements.

Nutritional Composition
Each 2-tbs dose contains the following:
- 61 calories
- 137 mg of potassium
- 8 mg of sodium
- 11.9 g of sugar
- 0.5 g of protein
- 1.4 g of fiber

Power Pudding

Ingredients
- 1 cup wheat bran
- 1 cup applesauce
- 1 cup prune juice

Directions
Mix and store in refrigerator. Start with administration of 1 tbs/day. Increase slowly until desired effect is achieved and no disagreeable symptoms occur.

Beverly Travis natural laxative mixture from Hale E, Smith E, St. James J, et al: Pilot study of the feasibility and effectiveness of a natural laxative mixture, Geriatr Nurs 28(2):104–111, 2007.

symptoms until after the age of 50 years (Roach and Christie, 2008).

PROMOTING HEALTHY AGING: IMPLICATIONS FOR GERONTOLOGICAL NURSING

Assessment

An important point in assessment is the term that is chosen to describe FI. Brown et al. (2012) reported that the term accidental bowel leakage was preferred over FI. Assessment should include a complete client history as in urinary incontinence (Box 16-5) and investigation into stool consistency and frequency, use of laxatives or enemas, surgical and obstetrical history, medications, effect of FI on quality of life, focused physical examination with attention to the gastrointestinal system, and a bowel record. A digital rectal examination should be performed to identify any presence of a mass, impaction, or occult blood.

Interventions

Nursing interventions are aimed at managing and/or restoring bowel continence. Therapies similar to those used to treat urinary incontinence such as environmental manipulation (access to toilet), dietary alterations, habit training schedules, PFMEs, improving transfer and ambulation ability, sphincter training exercises, biofeedback, medications, and/or surgery to correct underlying defects are effective. Providing resources and educational information is important and will help in self-management (see Box 16-6). Other interventions are presented in Box 16-19.

Pharmacological interventions may include the use of antidiarrheal medications and fiber therapy. Dextranomer in stabilized sodium hyaluronate (Solesta) is an FDA-approved treatment that may be helpful for those who do not find relief with conservative therapies. Solesta is a sterile, injectable gel that is thought to work by thickening anal tissue. It is an outpatient procedure that is well tolerated for up to 18 months following treatment (Hoy, 2012).

Biofeedback may also be recommended and there are some surgical options. The InterStim Therapy System, also used for

UI and approved by the FDA, is a surgically implanted device that applies a small electrical stimulation to the sacral nerve that controls the anal sphincter. It is used in individuals who have failed or could not tolerate more conservative measures (U.S. Food and Drug Administration, 2013).

The effectiveness of interventions in fecal incontinence will be self-evident but will take time. As in the treatment of urinary incontinence, goals must be realistic. It cannot be stated too often or too strongly that the nurse must always provide immaculate skin care to persons with incontinence, because self-esteem and skin integrity depend on it.

BOX 16-19 TIPS FOR BEST PRACTICE
Interventions for Accidental Bowel Leakage

- Use therapeutic communication skills and a positive and supportive attitude to help individuals overcome any embarrassment.
- Use the term accidental bowel leakage rather than fecal incontinence..
- Emphasize the importance of thorough evaluation.
- Teach about the range of interventions available for management.
- Share helpful resources for continence management.
- Have individual keep a bowel diary and identify triggers. For example, if eating a meal or drinking a cup of coffee stimulates defecation, use the toilet at a given time after the trigger event. Have a regular toileting routine.
- Encourage being prepared. Schedule outings, appointments, exercise routines around anticipated bowel patterns; suggest keeping a change of underwear, clothing, and toileting supplies with them when out; use an absorbent pad and have bags to dispose of pad if soiled; deodorant sprays for odor; wear darker clothing when away from home so that if soiling occurs, it will be less noticeable; scan environment when out for toilet locations.
- Avoid greasy and flatus-producing foods, dairy products, fruits with edible seeds, acidic citrus fruits, nuts, spicy foods, and other foods that trigger leakage. Bake or broil foods instead of frying; eat meals at regular times; eat after public events to reduce likelihood of leakage.

Source: Wilde M, Bliss D, Booth J, et al: Self-management of urinary and fecal incontinence, *Am J Nurs* 114(2):38–45, 2014.

KEY CONCEPTS

- Urinary incontinence is not a part of normal aging. It is a symptom of an underlying problem and requires thorough assessment.
- Urinary incontinence can be minimized or cured, and there are many therapeutic modalities available for treatment that nurses can implement.
- Nonpharmacological treatments (PFMEs, prompted voiding, bladder training, timed voiding, lifestyle modifications) are first-line treatments for urinary incontinence.
- Asymptomatic bacteriuria is common in older women and does not need treatment.
- Indwelling catheter use is not appropriate in any setting for long-term management (more than 30 days) except in certain clinical conditions. Proper insertion, care, and timely removal of indwelling catheters can reduce the number of CAUTIs.
- Health promotion teaching, identification of risk factors, comprehensive assessment of urinary incontinence, education of formal and informal caregivers, and use of evidence-based interventions are basic continence competencies for nurses.

NURSING STUDY: CONTINENCE

Helen is an 80-year-old woman who lives in her own apartment in an assisted living residence. Helen is the mother of four adult children, whom she sees often, and enjoys family activities. She is independent in all of her activities of daily living and walks with a cane. She has osteoarthritis of her knees and although she walks slowly, she is able to get around without any difficulty. Helen is 5 feet, 2 inches tall and weighs 150 pounds. She takes an antihypertensive medication and a diuretic. She has come to see the nurse practitioner in the on-site clinic for an annual physical examination. While the nurse practitioner is obtaining Helen's health history, he asks Helen if she has any problems with control of her urine such as leaking or not getting to the bathroom before she loses urine. Helen replies: "Sometimes I do have some leaking of urine because I can't get to the bathroom quickly enough, so I wear a pad. It also sometimes happens when I cough or sneeze but I don't think at my age there is much that can be done about that."

Based on the nursing study, develop a nursing care plan using the following procedure*:

* List Helen's comments that provide subjective data.
* List information that provides objective data.
* From these data, identify and state, using an accepted format, two nursing diagnoses you determine are most significant to Helen at this time. List two of Helen's strengths that you have identified from the data.
* Determine and state outcome criteria for each diagnosis. These criteria must reflect some alleviation of the problem identified in the nursing diagnosis and must be stated in concrete and measurable terms.
* Plan and state one or more interventions for each diagnosed problem. Provide specific documentation of the source used to determine the appropriate intervention. Plan at least one intervention that incorporates Helen's existing strengths.
* Evaluate the success of the intervention. Interventions must correlate directly with the stated outcome criteria to measure the outcome success.

*Students are advised to refer to their nursing diagnosis text and identify possible or potential problems.

CRITICAL THINKING QUESTIONS AND ACTIVITIES

1. What are the risk factors for UI in this situation?
2. What should be included in a more comprehensive assessment of Helen's stated problems with urine control?
3. What type of UI do you think Helen is experiencing?
4. What type of behavioral interventions might be helpful for Helen so that she has better urine control?
5. What health teaching would you provide to Helen related to urinary problems of older women?
6. What resources would you suggest for Helen to help her be more informed about her urine control concerns and how to manage them?

NURSING STUDY: CONSTIPATION

Stella, at age 78, has never had problems with her bowel movements. They have been regular—each morning about an hour after breakfast. In fact, she hardly thought about them because they had been so regular. While hospitalized for podiatric surgery last year, she never regained her usual pattern of bowel function. She was greatly distressed by this because it had been a symbol to her of her good health. Admittedly, she did not move about as much now, or as well, and had begun to use a cane. And she had heard that pain medications sometimes make one constipated, so she tried to use them sparingly despite the pain. She tried to reestablish her pattern of having a bowel movement every morning after breakfast but with little success. She now began to worry about constipation and to use laxatives. She thought, "This constipation really upsets me. I just don't feel like myself if I don't have a bowel movement every day."

On the basis of the nursing study, develop a nursing care plan using the following procedure*:

* List Stella's comments that provide subjective data.
* List information that provides objective data.

* From these data, identify and state, using an accepted format, two nursing diagnoses you determine are most significant to Stella at this time. List two of Stella's strengths that you have identified from the data.
* Determine and state outcome criteria for each diagnosis. These criteria must reflect some alleviation of the problem identified in the nursing diagnosis and must be stated in concrete and measurable terms.
* Plan and state one or more interventions for each diagnosed problem. Provide specific documentation of the source used to determine the appropriate intervention. Plan at least one intervention that incorporates Stella's existing strengths.
* Evaluate the success of the intervention. Interventions must correlate directly with the stated outcome criteria to measure the outcome success.

*Students are advised to refer to their nursing diagnosis text and identify possible or potential problems.

CRITICAL THINKING QUESTIONS AND ACTIVITIES

1. What information will you need to obtain from Stella to help her determine the causes of her constipation?
2. What advice will you give Stella regarding the use of laxatives?
3. What dietary changes will you suggest to her, and how will you do this to encourage modifications?
4. What information regarding the relationships of medications to constipation will be useful to Stella?

RESEARCH QUESTIONS

1. Do childhood toilet training experiences and beliefs about elimination affect one's elimination functions later in life? How do these experiences vary across different cultures?
2. What is the knowledge level of graduating nursing students and practicing nurses in UI care?
3. What factors are associated with effective implementation and maintenance of PV programs in long-term care?
4. What are some of the reasons individuals do not seek professional help for incontinence concerns?
5. What types of techniques do individuals use to manage their incontinence problems and what is their level of satisfaction with the techniques?
6. How are decisions made by community-living individuals about the types of incontinence products to buy?
7. What are the specific concerns of older people related to constipation?
8. What is the knowledge level of young, middle-aged, and older individuals about normal bowel function?

REFERENCES

Agency for Healthcare Quality and Research: Experts seek better diagnosis and treatment for women's urinary incontinence and chronic pelvic pain, *AHRQ Research Activities* 383, 2012.

Alayne D, Markland D, Palsson O, et al: Association of low dietary intake of fiber and liquids with constipation, *Am J Gastroenterol* 8(5):796–803, 2013.

American Geriatrics Society Choosing Wisely Workgroup: American Geriatrics Society identifies another five things that healthcare providers and patients should question, *J Am Geriatr Soc* 62(5):950–960, 2014.

Andreessen L, Wilde M, Herrendeen P: Preventing catheter-associated urinary tract infection in acute care: the bundle approach, *J Nurs Care Qual* 27(3):209–217, 2012.

Beverley L, Travis I: Constipation: proposed natural laxative mixtures, *J Gerontol Nurs* 18(10):5–12, 1992.

Brown H, Wexner M, Segall K, et al: Accidental bowel leakage in the mature women's health study, *Int J Clin Pract* 66(11):1101–1108, 2012.

Centers for Disease Control and Prevention: *Guideline for prevention of catheter-associated urinary tract infections*, 2009. http://www.cdc.gov/hicpac/pdf/CAUTI/CAUTIguideline2009final.pdf. Accessed January 2015.

Centers for Disease Control and Prevention: *Healthcare-associated infections (HAI) progress report*, 2014. http://www.cdc.gov/hai/progress-report/index.html. Accessed March 2014.

Cherniack P: Use of complementary and alternative medicine to treat constipation in the elderly, *Geriatr Gerontol* 13(3):533–538, 2013.

DeBeau C: Urinary incontinence. In Ham R, Sloane R, Warshaw G, et al, editors: *Primary care geriatrics*, ed 6, Philadelphia, 2014, Elsevier Saunders, pp 269–280.

DiRico N: *A nurse driven urinary catheter removal protocol* (NICHE solution no. 27), 2012. https://s3.amazonaws.com/Resources2014/NICHESolutions_Dirico_27.pdf. Accessed October 31, 2014.

Doig A, Huether S: Structure and function of the renal and urologic systems. In McCance K, Huether S, editors: *Pathophysiology*, ed 7, St. Louis, MO, 2014, Elsevier, pp 1319–1339.

Dowling-Castronovo A, Bradway C: *Assessment and management of older adults with urinary incontinence*. 2007. http://hartfordign.org/uploads/File/gnec_state_of_science_papers/gnec_incontinence.pdf. Accessed March 2014.

Dowling-Castronovo A, Bradway C: Urinary incontinence (UI) in older adults admitted to acute care. In Capezuti E, Zwicker D, Mezey M, et al, editors: *Evidence-based geriatric nursing protocols for best practice*, ed 3, New York, 2008, Springer, pp 309–336.

Dowling-Castronovo A, Bradway C: Urinary incontinence. In Boltz M, Capezuti E, Fulmer T, et al, editors: *Evidence-based geriatric nursing protocols for best practice*, ed 4, New York, 2012, Springer, pp 363–387.

Flanagan L, Roe B, Jack B, et al: Systematic review of care intervention studies for the management of incontinence and promotion of continence in older people in care homes with urinary incontinence as the primary focus (1966-2010), *Geriatr Gerontol Int* 12:600–611, 2012.

Foxx-Orstein A, Gallegos-Orozco J: *Chronic constipation in the elderly*: impact, classification, mechanisms, and common contributing factors, a special 2012 WDHD supplement, 2012. http://www.wgofoundation.org/assets/docs/pdf/wdhd12-supplement-HI.pdf?utm_source=wdhd2012&utm_medium=download&utm_campaign=2012 supplement. Accessed March 2014.

Gibson W, Wagg A: New horizons: urinary incontinence in older people, *Age Ageing* 43:167–163, 2014.

Grover M, Busby-Whitehead J, Palmer M, et al: Survey of geriatricians on the effect of fecal incontinence on nursing home referral, *J Am Geriatr Soc* 58:1058–1062, 2010.

Guerin A, Mody R, Lasch K, et al: Risk of developing colorectal cancer and benign colorectal neoplasm in patients with chronic constipation, *Aliment Pharmacol Ther* 40(1):83–92, 2014.

Hale E, Smith E, St. James J, et al: Pilot study of the feasibility and effectiveness of a natural laxative mixture, *Geriatr Nurs* 28(2):104–111, 2007.

Holroyd-Leduc J, Straus S: Management of urinary incontinence in women: clinical applications, *JAMA* 291:996–999, 2004.

Hoy S: Dextranomer in stabilized sodium hyaluronate (Solesta) in adults with faecal incontinence, *Drugs* 72(12):1671–1678, 2012.

Inelmen E, Giuseppe S, Giuliano E: When are indwelling catheters appropriate in elderly patients? *Geriatrics* 62(10):18–22, 2007.

Irwin D, Kopp, Z, Agatep B, et al: Worldwide prevalence estimates of lower urinary tract symptoms, overactive bladder, urinary incontinence and bladder outlet obstruction, *BJU Int* 108:1132–1138, 2011.

Johnson T, Ouslander J: The newly revised F-Tag 316 and surveyor guidance for urinary incontinence in long-term care, *J Am Med Dir Assoc* 7:594–600, 2006.

Lawhorne L, Ouslander J, Parmelee P, et al: Urinary incontinence: a neglected geriatric syndrome in nursing facilities, *J Am Med Dir Assoc* 9:29–35, 2008.

Lewis SJ, Heaton KW: Stool form scale as a useful guide to intestinal transit time, *Scand J Gastroenterol* 32:920–924, 1997.

MacDonald DG, Butler L: Silent no more: elderly women's stories of living with urinary incontinence in long-term care, *J Gerontol Nurs* 33:14–20, 2007.

Markland A: Constipation and fecal incontinence. In Ham R, Sloane R, Warshaw G, et al, editors: *Primary care geriatrics*, ed 6, Philadelphia, 2014, Elsevier Saunders, pp 281–291.

McKay S, Fravel M, Scanlon C: Management of constipation, *J Gerontol Nurs* 38(7): 9–16, 2012.

Mason DJ, Newman DK, Palmer MH: Changing UI practice, *Am J Nurs* 103:129, 2003.

Meddings J, Krein SL, Fakih MG, et al: Reducing unnecessary urinary catheter use and other strategies to prevent catheter-associated urinary tract infections: brief update review. In *Making health care safer II: an updated critical analysis of the evidence for patient safety practices* (Evidence Reports/Technology Assessments no. 211), Rockville, MD, 2013, Agency for Healthcare Research and Quality. http://www.ncbi.nlm.nih.gov/books/NBK133354. Accessed March 2014.

Mody L, Juthani-Mehta M: Urinary tract infections in older women, *JAMA* 311(8):844–854, 2014.

National Association for Continence: *Facts and statistics*, 2014. http://www.nafc.org/media/media-kit/facts-statistics. Accessed March 2014.

Ori Y, Rozen B, Herman M, et al: Fatalities and severe metabolic distress associated with the use of sodium phosphate enema: a single center's experience, *Arch Intern Med* 172(3):263–265, 2012.

Osei-Boamah E, Chui S, Diaz C, et al: *Constipation in the hospitalized older patient*: part 2, Consultant 20(9), 2012. http://www.consultant360.com/articles/constipation-hospitalized-older-patient-part-2. Accessed August 2014.

Palmer M, Newman D: Bladder control: educational needs of older adults, *J Gerontol Nurs* 32:28–32, 2006.

Roach M, Christie J: Fecal incontinence in the elderly, *Geriatrics* 63:13, 2008.

Schmidt F, Santos V: Prevalence of constipation in the general adult population, *J Wound Ostomy Continence Nurs* 41(1):70–76, 2014.

Seshan V, Muliira J: Self-reported urinary incontinence and factors associated with symptom severity in community dwelling older women: implications for women's health promotion, *BMC Womens Health* 13:16, 2013.

Sethi S, Mikami S, Leclair J, et al: Inpatient burden of constipation in the United States: an analysis of national trends in the United States from 1997-2010, *Am J Gastroenterol* 109(2):250–256, 2014.

Shamliyan T, Wyman J, Bliss DZ, et al: *Prevention of fecal and urinary incontinence in adults*, (Evidence Report/Technology Assessment no. 161, AHRQ publication no. 08-E003), Rockville, MD, 2007, Agency for Healthcare Research and Quality.

Shekelle P, Wachter R, Pronovost P, et al: *Making healthcare safer II*: an updated critical analysis of the evidence for patient safety practices (AHRQ publication no. 13-E001-EF), Rockville, MD, 2013, Agency for Healthcare Research and Quality.

So K, Habashy D, Doyle B, Chan L: Indwelling urinary catheters: pattern of use in a public tertiary-level Australian hospital, *Urol Nurs* 34(2):69–73, 2014.

Tettamanti G, Altman D, Pedersen N, et al: Effects of coffee and tea consumption on urinary incontinence in female twins, *Urogynaecology* 118(7):806–813, 2011.

U.S. Food and Drug Administration: *Medical devices*: Medtronic Inter-Stim therapy system, 2013. http://www.fda.gov/MedicalDevices/ProductsandMedicalProcedures/DeviceApprovalsandClearances/Recently-ApprovedDevices/ucm249208.htm. Accessed March 2014.

Wilde M, Bliss D, Booth J, et al: Self-management of urinary and fecal incontinence, *Am J Nurs* 114(2):38–45, 2014.

Wound, Ostomy and Continence Nurses Society: Position statement: role of the wound, ostomy, continence nurse or continence care nurse in continence care, *J Wound Ostomy Continence Nursing* 36:529–531, 2009.

Xu D, Kane R: Effect of urinary incontinence on older nursing home residents' self-reported quality of life, *J Am Geriatr Soc* 61(9):1473–1481, 2013.

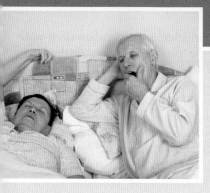

CHAPTER 17

Sleep

Theris A. Touhy

http://evolve.elsevier.com/Touhy/TwdHlthAging

A STUDENT SPEAKS

I am so stressed and tired all the time in this nursing program. The workload is so intense there is never enough time to sleep. When I have any time, I would go to bed at 7 pm and sleep until 11 in the morning if I could. When will I ever feel rested and not tired?

Marybeth, 22 years old

AN ELDER SPEAKS

The years have changed my sleep patterns. Bedtime rituals take longer. Nature wakens me two or three times a night for trips to the bathroom. Sleep returns at once unless my mind turns on and it gets launched on a needless project. The earlier remedies are called on to slow down the activities, or the next day is a disaster. My 90-year-old aunt, who slept very little and lightly and lay awake many nights, said she went to the bathroom several times just for something to do instead of just lying there.

Ricarda, 90 years old

LEARNING OBJECTIVES

On completion of this chapter, the reader will be able to:
1. Identify age-related changes that affect sleep.
2. Describe the signs, symptoms, treatment, and nursing interventions for sleep disorders: insomnia, obstructive sleep apnea, Willis-Ekbom disease (Restless Legs Syndrome—RLS), rapid eye movement sleep behavior disorder, circadian rhythm sleep disorder.
3. Use evidence-based protocols in assessment and development of nursing interventions for sleep.
4. Educate patients/families/health care staff about sleep disorders and sleep hygiene measures.

Sleep occupies one-third of our lives and is a vital function that affects cognition and performance. Research into the physiology of sleep suggests that the restorative function of sleep may be a consequence of the enhanced removal of potentially neurotoxic waste products that accumulate in the awake central nervous system (Xie et al, 2013). Sleep is a barometer of health, and sleep assessment and interventions for sleep concerns should receive as much attention as other vital signs. There is increasing awareness of the relationship between sleep problems and health outcomes, including premature mortality, osteoporosis, cardiovascular disease, diabetes, metabolic disease, impaired cognition and physical function, anxiety and depression, pain, and decreased quality of life (Chen et al, 2014; Ferrie et al, 2011; McBeth et al, 2014; Schmid et al, 2014).

Insufficient sleep is a public health epidemic and the Centers for Disease Control and Prevention (CDC, 2014) has called for continued public health surveillance of sleep quality, duration, behaviors, and disorders to monitor for sleep difficulties and their health impact. Sleep problems also constitute a global epidemic, affecting up to 45% of the world's population. Sleep problems are more common in women and older adults (Stranges et al, 2012; World Association of Sleep Medicine, 2014). Sleep problems are projected to increase in both low- and high-income countries, as the proportion of older people and the prevalence of obesity increase across the world (Ferrie et al, 2011; Stranges et al, 2012) (Box 17-1). Because of the public health burden of chronic sleep loss and sleep disorders, and the low awareness of poor sleep health, *Healthy People 2020* includes sleep health as a special topic area. Goals for adults are presented in Box 17-2.

BOX 17-1 RESEARCH HIGHLIGHTS

The study investigated the prevalence of sleep problems among older adults in low-income countries from Africa and Asia. The number of older people is escalating rapidly in the developing countries and little research has been done on the burden of sleep problems. Data were obtained from 40,000 participants in the INDEPTH WHO-SAGE study. The participating sites included Ghana, Tanzania, South Africa, India, Bangladesh, Vietnam, Indonesia, and Kenya. Sleep quality was assessed along with measures of quality of life and comorbidities. Overall, 16.6% of participants reported severe/extreme sleep problems and the prevalence was higher in women than men. Frequency of sleep problems increased with increasing age. Variations in sleep quality between countries ranged from 3.9% among male participants in Indonesia and Kenya to more than 40% among female participants in Bangladesh, one of the poorest countries in the eight-country group.

The findings indicate that the increased prevalence of sleep problems among older adults may not be due to age but may be secondary to poor health status, poorer quality of life, limited physical function or greater disability, and feelings of anxiety and depression. These findings are consistent with results of studies in high-income countries, suggesting that relationships among age, sleep complaints, and clinical characteristics of older adults may be similar regardless of differences in socioeconomic status, ethnic origin, culture, or language of participants, as well as the geography of the countries in which the older adults live.

From Stranges S, Tigbe W, Gomez-Olive, et al: Sleep problems: an emerging global epidemic? Findings from the INDEPTH WHO-SAGE study among more than 40,000 older adults from 8 countries across Africa and Asia, *Sleep* 20(2):1173–1191, 2012

BOX 17-2 HEALTHY PEOPLE 2020

Sleep Health

Goals
- Increase public knowledge of how adequate sleep and treatment of sleep disorders improve health, productivity, wellness, quality of life, and safety on roads and in the workplace.
- Increase the proportion of persons with symptoms of obstructive sleep apnea who seek medical evaluation.
- Increase the proportion of adults who get sufficient sleep.

Data from U.S. Department of Health and Human Services, Office of Disease Prevention and Health Promotion: Healthy People 2020, 2012. http://www.healthypeople.gov/2020

BIORHYTHM AND SLEEP

Our lives proceed in a series of rhythms that influence and regulate physiological function, chemical concentrations, performance, behavioral responses, moods, and the ability to adapt. It is clear that body temperature, pulse rate, blood pressure, and hormonal levels change significantly and predictably in a circadian rhythm. Circadian rhythms are linked to the 24-hour day by time cues (zeitgebers), the most important of which is the light-dark cycle. Biorhythms vary between individuals, and age-related changes in biorhythms (circadian rhythms) are relevant to health and the process of aging. With aging, there is a reduction in the amplitude of all circadian endogenous responses (e.g., body temperature, pulse rate, blood pressure, hormonal levels).

The most important biorhythm is the circadian sleep-wake rhythm. As people age, the natural circadian rhythm may become less responsive to external stimuli, such as changes in light during the course of the day. In addition, the endogenous changes in the production of melatonin are diminished, resulting in less sleep efficacy and further disruption of restorative sleep (Saccomano, 2014). Genetic research is investigating pathways linking sleep, circadian rhythm, metabolism, functioning, and disease, as well as genome-wide determinants of sleep duration (Ferrie et al, 2011).

SLEEP AND AGING

The predictable pattern of normal sleep is called **sleep architecture.** The body progresses through the five stages of the normal sleep pattern consisting of **rapid eye movement (REM)** sleep and **non–rapid eye movement (NREM)** sleep. Sleep structure is shown in Box 17-3. Most of the changes in sleep architecture in healthy adults begin between the ages of 40 and 60 years. The age-related changes include less time spent in stages 3 and 4 sleep (slow wave sleep) and more time spent awake or in stage 1 sleep. Declines in stages 3 and 4 sleep begin between 20 and 30 years of age and are nearly complete by the age of 50 to 60 years. The amount of deep sleep in stages 3 and 4 contributes to how rested and refreshed a person feels the next day.

Time spent in REM sleep also declines with age, and transitions between stages 1 and 2 are more common. REM sleep is a "critical state for sleeping elders" and is a time for the brain to replenish neurotransmitters essential for remembering,

BOX 17-3 The Stages of Sleep

Non–Rapid Eye Movement (NREM) Sleep
Stage 1
- Lightest level
- Between being awake and falling asleep

Stage 2
- Onset of sleep
- Becoming disengaged from surroundings
- Breathing and heart rates regular; body temperature drops

Stage 3 and Stage 4 (slow wave sleep)
- Deepest and most restorative sleep
- Blood pressure drops; breathing becomes slower
- Tissue growth and repair occurs
- Energy is restored

Rapid Eye Movement (REM) Sleep
- 25% of the night; first occurs about 90 minutes after falling asleep and recurs about every 90 minutes, getting longer later in the night
- Rapid eye movements are the key feature
- Breathing increases in rate and depth
- Muscle tone relaxed
- 85% of dreaming occurs in REM sleep

Adapted from National Sleep Foundation: *What happens when you sleep?* http://sleepfoundation.org/how-sleep-works/what-happens-when-you-sleep/page/0%2C1 Accessed March 17, 2014.

BOX 17-4 Age-Related Sleep Changes

- More time spent in bed awake before falling asleep
- Total sleep time and sleep efficiency are reduced
- Awakenings are frequent, increasing after age 50 years (>30 min of wakefulness after sleep onset in >50% of older subjects)
- Daytime napping
- Changes in circadian rhythm (early to bed, early to rise)
- Sleep is subjectively and objectively lighter (more stage 1, little stage 4, more disruptions)
- Rapid eye movement (REM) sleep is short, less intense, and more evenly distributed
- Frequency of abnormal breathing events is increased
- Frequency of leg movements during sleep is increased

Adapted from Teodorescu M, Husain N: Nonpharmacological approaches to insomnia in older adults, *Ann Longterm Care* 18:36–42, 2010.

learning, and problem solving. This stage of sleep also transfers short-term memories in the motor cortex to the temporal lobe, which stores long-term memories (Townsend-Roccichelli et al, 2010, p. 32). The most notable changes in sleep with aging are an increase in the number of nighttime awakenings and lower sleep efficiency (ratio of time in bed asleep to time in bed) (Teodorescu, 2014). Sleep complaints are usually linked to other health problems and sleep disorders.

Findings from a recent study suggest that the deterioration of a cluster of neurons associated with regulating sleep patterns, the ventrolateral preoptic nucleus, may be responsible for sleep decline in aging. The more neurons that are lost, the more difficult it is for the person to sleep. For individuals with Alzheimer's disease, the link between the loss of neurons is greater and causes more problems with sleep (Lim et al, 2014). The changes that occur in sleep with aging are summarized in Box 17-4.

⚡ SAFETY ALERT

Poor sleep is not an inevitable consequence of aging but rather an indicator of health status and calls for investigation (Grandner et al, 2012).

Older adults with good general health, positive moods, and engagement in more active lifestyles and meaningful activities report better sleep and fewer sleep complaints. Results of a large study (155,877 participants) that explored the prevalence of sleep-related complaints across age groups found that on average, older adults reported sleeping better than younger adults (Grandner et al, 2012).

SLEEP DISORDERS

Insomnia

Insomnia is the most common sleep disorder worldwide (Ferrie et al, 2011; Sexton-Radek, 2013). Insomnia is "a condition that interferes with sleep quality and quantity and is associated with subjective complaints of sleep disturbance that are generally characterized as a) difficulty initiating sleep, b) difficulty maintaining sleep, c) premature morning awakening, and/or d) nonrestorative sleep" (Deratnay, 2013, p. 22). The diagnosis of insomnia requires that the person has difficulty falling asleep

for at least 1 month and that impairment in daytime functioning results from difficulty sleeping.

Insomnia is classified as either primary or comorbid. Primary insomnia implies that no other cause of sleep disturbance has been identified. Comorbid insomnia is more common and is associated with psychiatric and medical disorders, medications, and primary sleep disorders, such as obstructive sleep apnea or restless legs syndrome. Comorbid insomnia does not suggest that these conditions cause insomnia but that insomnia and the other conditions co-occur and each may require attention and treatment (Bloom et al, 2009).

According to epidemiological data, the prevalence of chronic late-life insomnia ranges from 20% to nearly 50%, and is generally higher in women than in men (Haimov and Shatil, 2013). Approximately 21% of older adults report changes in cognitive functioning due to loss of sleep (Saccomano, 2014). Chronic insomnia is a significant risk factor for cognitive decline in men and a strong predictor of both mortality and long-term care placement (Teodorescu, 2014). There are many influencing factors, both physiological and behavioral (Box 17-5).

Prescription and nonprescription medications also create sleep disturbances. Drugs and alcohol are thought to account for 10% to 15% of cases of insomnia (Martin and Alessi, 2014) (Box 17-6). The times of day that medications are given can also contribute to sleep problems—for example, a diuretic given before bedtime or sedating medication given in the morning.

BOX 17-5 Risk Factors for Sleep Disturbances in Older Adults

- Age-related changes in sleep architecture
- Comorbidities (cardiovascular disease, diabetes, pulmonary disease, musculoskeletal disorders), CNS disorders (Parkinson's disease, seizure disorder, dementia), GI disorders (hiatal hernia, GERD, PUD), urinary disorders (incontinence, BPH)
- Pain
- Depression, anxiety, delirium, psychosis
- Polypharmacy
- Life stressors/response to stress
- Sleep-related beliefs
- Sleep habits (daily sleep/activity cycle, napping)
- Limited exposure to sunlight
- Environmental noises, institutional routines
- Poor sleep hygiene
- Lack of exercise
- Excessive napping
- Caregiving for a dependent elder
- Sleep apnea
- Restless legs syndrome
- Periodic leg movement
- Rapid eye movement behavior disorder
- Alcohol
- Smoking

BPH, Benign prostatic hyperplasia; *CNS,* central nervous system; *GERD,* gastroesophageal reflux disease; *GI,* gastrointestinal; *PUD,* peptic ulcer disease.
Adapted from Teodorescu M: Sleep disruptions and insomnia in older adults, *Consultant* 54(3):166–173, 2014; Subramanian S, Surani S: Sleep disorders in the elderly, *Geriatrics* 62(12):10–32, 2007.

BOX 17-6 Medications Affecting Sleep

Selective serotonin reuptake inhibitors (SSRIs)	Opiates
	Cough and cold medications
Antihypertensives (clonidine, beta-blockers, reserpine, methyldopa)	Thyroid preparations
	Phenytoin
Anticholinergics	Cortisone
Sympathomimetic amines	Levodopa
Diuretics	

Insomnia and Alzheimer's Disease

About half of individuals with dementia experience sleep dysregulation, which may be associated with agitation, wandering, comorbid illnesses, primary sleep disorders, or the medications used to treat dementia (Teodorescu, 2014). Caregivers of individuals with dementia also experience poor sleep quality, and this influences caregiver stress, as well as health problems (Rowe et al, 2010).

Results of the Nighttime Insomnia Treatment and Education for Alzheimer's Disease study (NITE-AD) (McCurry et al, 2005), a treatment program using behavioral strategies with persons with dementia and their caregivers living in the community, suggest the following behavioral techniques to enhance sleep for individuals with AD: sleep hygiene education, daily walking, and increased light exposure. A sleep education program, designed for adult family homes and derived from this research, is provided by McCurry and colleagues (2009).

◆ PROMOTING HEALTHY AGING: IMPLICATIONS FOR GERONTOLOGICAL NURSING

◆ Assessment

Sleep habits should be reviewed with older adults in all settings. Many people do not seek treatment for insomnia and may blame poor sleep on the aging process. Nurses are in an excellent position to assess sleep and suggest interventions to improve the quality of the older person's sleep. "No other group of health care providers watch more people sleep than nurses, and sleep disorders can affect all aspects of health and illness" (Chasens and Umlauf, 2012, p. 83).

Assessment for sleep disorders and awareness of contributing factors to poor sleep (pain, chronic illness, medications, alcohol use, depression, anxiety) are important. The nurse should learn how well the person sleeps at home, how many times the person is awakened at night, what time the person retires, and what rituals occur at bedtime. Rituals include bedtime snacks, watching television, listening to music, or reading—activities whose execution is crucial to the individual's ability to fall asleep. Complete sleep assessment data are presented in Box 17-7.

The sleep diary or log is also an important part of assessment (Box 17-8). This information will provide an accurate account of the person's sleep problem and help identify the sleep disturbance. A period of 2 to 4 weeks is needed to obtain a clear picture of the sleep problem. A self-rating scale, the Pittsburgh Sleep Quality Index (PSQI), can be used to measure

BOX 17-7 TIPS FOR BEST PRACTICE
Assessment of Sleep Disturbances

Basic Sleep History Questions
- Where do you sleep at night (bed, couch, recliner chair)?
- Do you have any difficulty falling asleep?
- What do you do at night before you go to bed?
- Are you having any difficulty sleeping until morning?
- Are you having difficulty sleeping throughout the night?
- How often do you awaken and how long are you awake? What prevents you from falling back to sleep?
- Have you or someone else ever noticed that you snore loudly or stop breathing in your sleep?
- Do you find yourself falling asleep during the day when you do not want to?

Follow-Up Questions
- What time do you usually go to bed? Fall asleep?
- What prevents you from falling asleep?
- Do your legs kick or jump around while you sleep?
- Are you outside in natural light most days?
- Do you have any pain, discomfort, or shortness of breath during the night?
- What type of exercise do you get during the day?
  - Individual's bed partner, family member, or caregiver can also be asked to provide information

Review intake of alcohol, nicotine, caffeine, and medications
Review risk factors (obesity, arthritis, poorly controlled illnesses)
Review of depressive symptoms; weight loss; sadness, or recent losses
Review involvement in social activities
Review functional status/ADL/IADL performance
Objective Measures
- Sleep diary (keep for 24 hours daily for 2 to 4 weeks)
- Self-rating of sleep scales—Pittsburgh Sleep Quality Index; Epworth Sleepiness Scale; Insomnia Severity Scale
- On a scale of 1 to 10 (10 the highest), how would you rate your sleep?

Adapted from Chasen E, Umlauf M: Protocol: excessive sleepiness. In Boltz M, Capezuti E, Fulmer T, et al, editors: *Evidence-based geriatric nursing protocols for best practice*, ed 4, New York, 2012, Springer, pp 74–88.

BOX 17-8 Sleep Diary

Instructions: Record the following for 2 to 4 weeks. Should be completed by the person or the caregiver if the person is unable. Record when you:
- Go to bed
- Go to sleep
- Wake up
- Get out of bed
- Take naps
- Exercise
- Consume alcohol
- Consume caffeinated beverages

From Centers for Disease Control and Prevention: *What should I do if I can't sleep?* 2013. http://www.cdc.gov/sleep/about_sleep/cant_sleep.htm Accessed March 18, 2014.

the quality and patterns of sleep in the older adult, and daytime sleepiness can be assessed with the Epworth Sleepiness Scale, both recommended by the Hartford Institute for Geriatric Nursing (Box 17-9). The Epworth Sleepiness Scale helps to distinguish between the average amount of sleep and problems with sleep deprivation that require intervention

BOX 17-9 RESOURCES FOR BEST PRACTICE

Sleep

Hartford Institute for Geriatric Nursing: Try This, General Assessment Series: Epworth Sleepiness Scale and Pittsburg Sleep Quality Index; Want to know more: Sleep: Nursing Standard Practice Protocol, Excessive Sleepiness

Chasen E, Umlauf M: Excessive sleepiness. In Boltz M, Capezuti E, Fulmer T, et al, editors: *Evidence-based geriatric nursing protocols for best practice*, New York, 2012, Springer, pp 74–88.

Qaseem A, Owens D, Dallas P, et al: *Management of obstructive sleep apnea in adults: a clinical practice guideline from the American College of Physicians*. www.hhs.gov Accessed March 17, 2014.

Willis-Ekbom Foundation: *Symptom diary*. http://www.willis-ekbom.org/about-rls-wed/publications?: Accessed March 18, 2014.

(Townsend-Roccichelli et al, 2010). The Insomnia Severity Index (ISI) is another tool to measure insomnia severity. Objective measures include polysomnography conducted in sleep laboratories, including electroencephalograms (EEGs), electromyograms (EMGs), wrist actigraphy, and direct observations.

◆ Interventions

◆ Nonpharmacological Treatment

Interventions begin after a thorough sleep history has been recorded and, if possible, a sleep log obtained. Management is directed at identifiable causes. Nonpharmacological interventions are considered first-line treatment for insomnia (Sexton-Radek, 2013). Education should be provided on changes in sleep architecture with aging and the importance of attention to sleep hygiene principles to promote good sleep habits.

Cognitive behavioral therapy for insomnia is a multidimensional approach combining psychological and behavioral therapies that include sleep hygiene, sleep restriction, stimulus control, relaxation techniques, circadian interventions, and cognitive therapy (Box 17-10). A combination of approaches is most effective and these interventions have been reported to be an effective and practical treatment for chronic insomnia in older adults (Buysse et al, 2011; Sexton-Radek, 2013; Teodorescu, 2014). Cognitive training programs (Chapter 5) may improve sleep quality and cognitive performance. New learning may be instrumental in promoting initiation and maintenance of sleep in older adults with insomnia (Haimov and Shatil, 2013). Tai chi can be considered a useful nonpharmacological approach for sleep complaints (Lo and Lee, 2014; Raman et al, 2013).

Sleep in hospitals and nursing homes. In hospital and institutional settings, promotion of a good sleep environment is important. Studies have shown that as many as 22% to 61% of hospitalized patients experience impaired sleep (Chasens and Umlauf, 2012). A multidisciplinary approach to identify sources of noise and light, such as equipment and staff interactions, could result in modification without compromising safety and quality of patient care (Box 17-11). Sleep deprivation due to

BOX 17-10 Interventions for Insomnia

Sleep Hygiene

Develop a regular physical exercise regimen for those who are able; regular exercise can deepen sleep, increase daytime arousal, and decrease depression.

Avoid exercise before bedtime.

Limit computer use before bedtime.

Limit tobacco, caffeine, and alcohol use before bedtime.

Avoid heavy meals before bedtime. If waking due to hunger, eat light carbohydrate snack.

If you have reflux, eat the evening meal 3-4 hours before bedtime.

Reduce or eliminate fluids in the evening (reduce nocturia).

Ensure bed and bed coverings are comfortable, not too restrictive.

Keep bedroom temperature comfortable, not too warm and well ventilated.

Minimize light exposure in bedroom.

Remove hearing aids/use earplugs to reduce noise.

Limit sleeping partner's disruptive nighttime activities and pets from bedroom.

Review all medications with health care provider; evaluate administration times, review side effects/interactions/effect on sleep.

Relaxation Techniques

Diaphragmatic breathing

Progressive relaxation

White noise or music

Guided imagery

Stretching

Yoga or tai chi

Sleep Restriction Measures

Limit or avoid daytime napping; napping should not exceed 2 hours.

Limit opportunities for unplanned napping or dozing, particularly in the evening.

Limit time in bed to more closely match the number of hours of actual sleep.

Stimulus Control

Create bedtime sleep rituals, such as taking a warm bath and eating a small snack.

Go to bed only when sleepy.

Avoid falling asleep in places other than own bed (e.g., couch, recliner).

If unable to fall asleep in a reasonable time (15-20 min), get out of bed and pursue relaxing activities (e.g., reading) and return to bed only when sleepy.

Use the bedroom for sleep and sex only; do not watch television from bed or work in bed.

Circadian Interventions

Reestablish connection with various environmental signals to cue the circadian rhythm (light exposure, meals, physical activity, social interactions).

Establish a regular bedtime and waking time.

Maintain stable daytime routines in regard to meals, activity, medications.

Increase duration and intensity (2500-5000 lux) of bright light or sunlight exposure during the day. In patients with dementia, evening bright light may help with advanced sleep phase disorder.

Melatonin 1-2 hours before bedtime may be helpful.

Adapted from Teodorescu M: Sleep disruptions and insomnia in older adults, *Consultant* 54(3):166–173, 2014; Saccomano S: Sleep disorders in older adults, *J Gerontol Nurs* 40(3):38–45, 2014.

BOX 17-11   TIPS FOR BEST PRACTICE

Suggestions to Promote Sleep When Hospitalized or in a Nursing Home

- Allow individual to stay out of bed and out of the room for as long as possible before bed.
- Provide 30 minutes or more of sunlight exposure in a comfortable outdoor location.
- Provide low-level physical activity three times a day.
- Keep noise level at a minimum, speak in hushed tones, do no use overhead paging, reduce light in hallways and resident rooms.
- Institute a sleep improvement protocol—"do not disturb" times, soft music, relaxation, massage, aromatherapy, sleep masks, headphones, allowing patients to shut doors. Consider having a kit that can be taken to bedside with music, aromatherapy.
- Perform necessary care (e.g., turning, changing) when the individual is awake rather than awakening the individual between the hours of 10:00 PM and 6:00 AM.
- Limit intake of caffeine and other fluids in excess before bedtime.
- Provide a light snack or warm beverage before bedtime.
- Discontinue invasive treatments when possible (Foley catheters, percutaneous gastrostomy tubes, intravenous lines).
- Encourage and assist to the bathroom before bed and as needed.
- Give pain medication before bedtime for patients with pain.
- Institute the same time for resident to arise and get out of bed every morning.
- Maintain comfortable temperature in room; provide blankets as needed.
- Provide meaningful activities (individualized and group) during the daytime.

noise can potentially exacerbate delirium. Noise from monitoring equipment alarms and infusion devices and the ringing from telephones cause an elevation of heart rate (Buxton et al, 2012). Efforts to allow sufficient time for a person to complete a full sleep cycle of 90 minutes are important and can have a positive influence on sleep effectiveness (Missildine, 2008; Missildine et al, 2010).

In institutions, there is often limited communication between night and day staff, as well as a lack of emphasis on the importance of sleep patterns. Night shift staff have the opportunity to assess sleep patterns and implement appropriate interventions to enhance sleep. Kerr and Wilkinson (2010) offer comprehensive suggestions for night staff, including the development of overnight care plans. Further research is needed on the sleep problems of older adults in the community and in acute and long-term care settings.

◆ Pharmacological Treatment

The use of over-the-counter (OTC) sleep aids, as well as the use of prescription sedative and hypnotic medications, is increasing in the United States (Preidt, 2014). Use of these medications is high for those in their 50s, as well as those in their 80 and older. Benzodiazepines represent 17% to 23% of drugs prescribed to older adults, and both opiates and benzodiazepines are the most abused drugs in the older adult population (Morgan et al, 2005; Naegle, 2008).

Women are more likely to use prescription sleep medications than men, and white people and people with higher levels of education also reported greater use (Chong et al, 2013). Adverse reactions to these medications are also increasing (Substance Abuse and Mental Health Services Administration [SAMSHA], 2013). Use of narcotic pain medications and sedatives and the use of alcohol, in combination with these medications and other prescribed medications, is a growing concern (Chapter 28). Individuals who received prescriptions for narcotic painkillers were 4.2 times more likely to also have sedative prescriptions, which place them at high risk for adverse effects, including death (Kao et al, 2014). Patients should be educated on the proper use of medications, their side effects, and their interactions with alcohol and other prescription drugs.

Pharmacological treatments for sleep disorders may be used in combination with behavioral interventions but must be managed with caution in the older population (Teodorescu, 2014; Townsend-Roccichelli et al, 2010). In long-term care settings, there are specific regulatory guidelines on the use of hypnotics, including appropriate prescribing and tapering and discontinuation of use.

⚡ SAFETY ALERT

Benzodiazepines or other sedative-hypnotics should not be used in older adults as a first choice of treatment for insomnia (American Geriatrics Society, 2014).

Over-the-counter (OTC) drugs such as diphenhydramine, found in many OTC sleep products such as Tylenol PM, are often thought to be relatively harmless but should be avoided because of antihistaminic and anticholinergic side effects. Other OTC sleep aid preparations contain ingredients such as kava kava, valerian root, melatonin, chamomile, and tryptophan. Because these ingredients are not regulated, information and outcomes of efficacy may not be known (Saccomano, 2014) (Chapter 10). Endogenous nocturnal melatonin, a major loop for circadian rhythm, may have decreased levels in older adults. Melatonin, taken 1 to 2 hours before bedtime, may replicate the natural secretion pattern of melatonin and lead to improvements in the circadian regulation of the sleep-wake cycle (Teodorescu, 2014). Melatonin is also available in a dissolving tablet, which works faster.

Routine use of OTC medications for sleep may delay appropriate assessment and treatment of contributing medical or psychological conditions, identification of sleep disorders, and appropriate counseling and treatment. The individual should report use of all OTC drugs to his or her health care provider since they may interact with other medications.

Benzodiazepine receptor agonists, such as zolpidem (Ambien), eszopiclone (Lunesta), and zaleplon (Sonata), are considered benzodiazepine-like in their action because they induce sleep easily. They can have detrimental effects, causing changes in mental status (delirium), falls and fractures, daytime drowsiness, and increased risk for motor vehicle accidents, with only minimal improvement in sleep latency and duration (American Geriatrics Society, 2014). Zolpidem is the medication most often implicated in emergency department visits for adverse drug events in adults (Hampton et al, 2014).

The U.S. Food and Drug Administration (FDA) has recommended that starting doses for zolpidem and eszopiclone be cut in half and individuals cautioned about next-day impairment and monitored closely for untoward effects (FDA, 2013). Both of these medications are on the Beers' List for Potentially Inappropriate Medication Use in Older Adults (American Geriatrics Society, 2012) (Chapter 9). The FDA has approved Belsomra (suvorexant), a new class of sedative that blocks chemicals in the brain called orexins that keep people awake. It was designed for people who have difficulty getting to sleep and staying asleep. Side effects include impaired driving and daytime drowsiness similar to the benzodiazepine receptor agonists, and the lowest possible dose should be prescribed and individuals cautioned about next-day driving or activities requiring full mental alertness.

Ramelteon, a melatonin receptor agonist that promotes sleep via action on the circadian system, is considered both a chronobiotic and a hypnotic that has been shown to promote sleep initiation and maintenance. Compared with other drugs for insomnia, ramelteon may have less next-day residual effects, withdrawal symptoms, and rebound insomnia and may cause less psychomotor and cognitive impairment in older people; however, further research is needed (Seithikurippu et al, 2011; Uchimura et al, 2011). Box 17-12 presents health teaching guidelines about sleeping medications.

Sleep Disordered Breathing and Sleep Apnea

Sleep disordered breathing (SDB) affects approximately 25% of older individuals (more men than women), and the most common form is obstructive sleep apnea (OSA) (Box 17-13). In long-term care facilities, the prevalence of OSA has been estimated to be as high as 70% to 80% (Rose and Lorenz, 2010). Untreated OSA is related to heart failure, cardiac dysrhythmias, stroke, type 2 diabetes, osteoporosis, and even death (Chen et al, 2014; Seicean et al, 2013). Older adults with OSA demonstrate significant cognitive decline compared with younger people with the same disease severity. Some research suggests that SDB may be a risk factor for Alzheimer's disease (Osorio et al, 2013). The diagnosis of OSA is often delayed in older adults and symptoms are blamed on age (Subramanian and Surani, 2007).

Age-related decline in the activity of the upper airway muscles, resulting in compromised pharyngeal patency, predisposes older adults to OSA. A high body mass index (BMI) and large neck circumference have been identified as risk factors for OSA but are not as significant in older adults (Martin and Alessi, 2014). Other risk factors are presented in Box 17-14. Symptoms of sleep apnea include loud periodic snoring, gasping and choking on awakenings, unusual nighttime activity such as

---

BOX 17-12   TIPS FOR BEST PRACTICE

Use of Sleeping Medications

Provide health education on:
1. Normal changes in sleep patterns with age
2. Importance of appropriate assessment of sleep problems before any medications are used
3. Nonpharmacological treatment of sleeping problems as first-line treatment (sleep hygiene, stimulus control, sleep restriction, relaxation techniques)
4. Avoiding OTC medications that contain diphenhydramine, which can have side effects of confusion, blurred vision, constipation, falls
5. Adverse effects of sleep medications, even OTC medications; include problems with daily function, changes in mental status, possibility of motor vehicle accidents, increase in daytime drowsiness, and increased risk of falls with only **minimal** improvement in sleep
6. Avoiding benzodiazepines (flurazepam, triazolam, temazepam) for sleep due to long-acting sedation effects
7. If sleeping medications are prescribed, the benzodiazepine receptor agonists (zolpidem, eszopiclone, zaleplon) or ramelteon is preferred; given at the lowest possible dose for short-term use only (2-3 weeks, never longer than 90 days). Medications for sleep should be taken immediately before bedtime
8. Avoiding the use of alcohol, narcotic pain relieving medications, and antianxiety medications if taking sleeping medications
9. Reviewing all medications, including OTC, with health care provider for interactions with sleeping medications
10. Using caution the day after taking sleeping medications, particularly with driving and activities that require full alertness; accidents are common

---

BOX 17-13   Abbreviations for Sleep Disorders

Sleep Disordered Breathing (SDB)
Obstructive Sleep Apnea (OSA)
Restless Legs Syndrome/Willis-Ekbom Disease (RLS/WED)
Rapid Eye Movement Sleep Behavior Disorder (RBD)
Circadian Rhythm Sleep Disorder (CRSD)
Advanced Sleep Phase Disorder (ASPD)
Irregular Sleep-Wake Disorder (ISWD)

BOX 17-14   Risk Factors For Obstructive Sleep Apnea

- Increasing age
- Increased neck circumference (not as significant in older people)
- Male gender
- Anatomical abnormalities of the upper airway
- Upper airway resistance and/or obstruction
- Family history
- Excess weight
- Use of alcohol, sedatives, or tranquilizers
- Smoking
- Hypertension

sitting upright or falling out of bed, morning headache, unexplained daytime sleepiness, poor memory and intellectual functioning, and irritability and personality change. If the person has a sleeping partner, it is often the partner who reports the nighttime symptoms. If there is a sleeping partner, he or she may move to another room to sleep because of the disturbance to his or her own rest.

PROMOTING HEALTHY AGING: IMPLICATIONS FOR GERONTOLOGICAL NURSING

Assessment

The individual with SDB may present with complaints of insomnia or daytime sleepiness and assessment should include assessment of insomnia complaints as discussed previously, including the use of screening instruments such as the Epworth Sleepiness Scale (Box 17-9). Assessment of symptoms of OSA and information from the sleeping partner, if present, are obtained. A medication review is always indicated when investigating sleep complaints. The upper airway, including the nasal and pharyngeal airways, should be examined for anatomical obstruction, tumors, or cysts. Comorbid conditions such as heart failure and diabetes should be assessed and managed appropriately.

If OSA is suspected, a referral for a sleep study should be made. A sleep study or polysomnogram is a multiple-component test that electronically transmits and records specific physical activities during sleep. The data obtained are analyzed by a qualified physician to determine whether or not the person has a sleep disorder. In most cases, sleep studies take place in a sleep lab specially set up for the test and are monitored by a technician, but they can also be conducted at home. Recognition of OSA in older adults may be more difficult because there may not be a sleeping partner to report symptoms. If presenting symptoms suggest the disorder, a tape recorder can be placed at the bedside to record snoring and breathing sounds during the night.

Interventions

Therapy will depend on the severity and type of sleep apnea, as well as the presence of comorbid illnesses. Treatment of sleep apnea may involve avoidance of alcohol and sedative-hypnotic medications, cessation of smoking, avoidance of supine sleep positions, and weight loss. The Clinical Practice Guidelines for Management of OSA recommends weight loss for obese individuals but should be combined with another treatment such as continuous positive airway pressure (CPAP) because of the low cure rate with weight loss alone (Qaseem et al, 2103). There should be risk counseling about impaired judgment from sleeplessness and the possibility of accidents when driving. Individuals need to inform health care providers of their diagnosis before any surgical procedure so that a perioperative management plan can be developed. If hospitalized, they should bring their CPAP machine with them. Further research is needed related to the preparation of individuals with OSA for surgery and the risk of perioperative complications (Memtsoudis et al, 2013).

Continuous positive airway pressure (CPAP) is recommended as initial therapy for OSA, with moderate-quality evidence (Qaseem et al, 2013). The CPAP device delivers pressurized air through tubing to a nasal mask or nasal pillows, which are fitted around the head. The pressurized air acts as an airway splint and gently opens the patient's throat and breathing passages, allowing the patient to breathe normally, but only through the nose. Teaching should be provided about the effects of untreated OSA and emphasize the need for treatment. A stepwise approach during the initiation of therapy and continued monitoring can foster better use of CPAP or prevent discontinuation of therapy. Estimates are that about half of individuals either discontinue the therapy or are nonadherent (use of <4 hours per night) (Dettenmeier et al, 2013; Schwab et al, 2013; Weaver and Sawyer, 2010).

Mandibular advancement devices are recommended as an alternative treatment for individuals who prefer this type of device or experience adverse effects with CPAP. However, this treatment has a weak recommendation with low-quality evidence (Qaseem et al, 2013). These appliances also require a stable dentition and may be problematic for individuals with dentures or extensive tooth loss (Chasens and Umlauf, 2012).

Restless Legs Syndrome/Willis-Ekbom Disease

Restless legs syndrome/Willis-Ekbom disease (RLS/WED) is a neurological movement disorder of the limbs that is often associated with a sleep complaint. Individuals with RLS/WED have an uncontrollable need to move the legs, often accompanied by discomfort in the legs. Other symptoms include paresthesias; creeping sensations; crawling sensations; tingling, cramping, and burning sensations; pain; or even indescribable sensations. RLS/WED has a circadian rhythm, with the intensity of the symptoms becoming worse at night and improving toward the morning. Symptoms may be temporarily relieved by movement.

An estimated 7% to 10% of adults in North America and Europe have the disease. The disorder is familial in about 50% of individuals, and several predisposing genes have been identified through genome-wide association studies (Silber et al, 2013). RLS/WED is less common in Asian populations. Incidence is about twice as high in women and while the disease may begin at any age (including childhood), many individuals who are severely affected are middle-aged or older. Symptoms become more frequent and last longer with age (National Institute of Neurological Disorders and Stroke [NINDS], 2010).

In most cases, RLS/WED is a primary idiopathic disorder but it also can be associated with underlying medical disorders including iron deficiency, end-stage renal disease (especially in patients requiring dialysis), diabetes, and pregnancy. Antidepressants, antihypertensives, and neuroleptic medications can aggravate RLS/WED symptoms. Increased body mass index, caffeine use, alcohol or tobacco use, sleep deprivation, and sedentary lifestyle may also be contributing factors. Other contributing factors under study include iron metabolism and neurotransmitter dysfunctions involving dopamine and glutamate (NINDS, 2010; Willis-Ekbom Disease Foundation, 2014).

Diagnosis of RLS/WED is based on symptoms and a sleep study may be indicated. Possible contributing conditions should be evaluated and all individuals with symptoms should be tested for iron deficiency with a complete iron panel (Tarsy, 2014). If iron stores are low, iron replacement is needed. Medication choice depends on the frequency of symptoms and the response to medication. Medications used include levodopa, benzodiazepines, or low-potency opioids. The chronic persistent form of the disorder may be treated with non-ergot dopamine agonists (pramipexole, ropinirole, rotigotine patch) or with gabapentin, gabapentin enacarbil, and pregabalin (Silber et al, 2013).

Nonpharmacological therapy includes stretching of the lower extremities, mild to moderate physical activity, hot baths, massage, acupressure, relaxation techniques, and avoidance of caffeine, alcohol, and tobacco. Individuals should be encouraged to keep a symptom diary for 7 to 14 days to identify triggers and aid in diagnosis. The Willis-Ekbom Disease Foundation provides a symptom diary on their website (Box 17-9).

Rapid Eye Movement Sleep Behavior Disorder

The mean age at emergence of rapid eye movement sleep behavior disorder (RBD) is 60 years and it is more common in males. Characteristics are loss of normal voluntary muscle atonia during REM sleep associated with complex behavior while dreaming. Patients report elaborate enactment of their dreams, often with violent content, during sleep. This may include violent behaviors, such as punching and kicking, with the potential for injury of both the patient and the bed partner (National Sleep Foundation, 2014).

The chronic form is usually idiopathic or associated with Parkinson's disease and dementia with Lewy bodies. The acute form of the disorder can be caused by toxic-metabolic abnormalities, drug or alcohol withdrawal, and medications (tricyclic antidepressants, monoamine oxidase inhibitors, cholinergic agents, and selective serotonin reuptake inhibitors [SSRIs]). Diagnosis is based on history, symptoms, and a sleep study to test for the key features of the disorder. Clonazepam curtails or eliminates the disorder about 90% of the time. If clonazepam is not effective, some antidepressants or melatonin may reduce the behaviors. A safe environment in the bedroom should be provided (Martin and Alessi, 2014; Murray et al, 2013; National Sleep Foundation, 2014).

Circadian Rhythm Sleep Disorders

In circadian rhythm sleep disorders (CRSDs) relatively normal sleep occurs at abnormal times. Two clinical presentations are seen: advanced sleep phase disorder (ASPD) and irregular sleep-wake disorder (ISWD). In ASPD, the individual begins and ends sleep at unusually early times (e.g., going to bed as early as 6 or 7 PM and waking up between 2 and 5 AM). Not all individuals with an advanced sleep phase have ASPD. If they are not bothered by their sleep phases and have no functional impairment, we may just consider them "morning" people. In irregular sleep-wake disorder, sleep is dispersed across the 24-hour day in bouts of irregular length. Factors contributing to these disorders are age-related changes in sleep and circadian rhythm regulation combined with decreased levels of light exposure and activity.

A combination of good sleep hygiene practices and methods to delay the timing of sleep and wake times is recommended as treatment for ASPD. Bright light therapy (2500 to 10,000 lux) for 1 to 2 hours at about 7 to 8 PM can help normalize or delay circadian rhythm patterns (Bloom et al, 2009).

In ISWD, the individual may obtain enough sleep over the 24-hour period, but time asleep is broken into at least three different periods of variable length. Erratic napping occurs during the day, and nighttime sleep is severely fragmented and shortened. Chronic insomnia and/or daytime sleepiness are present. ISWD is most commonly encountered in individuals with dementia, particularly those who are institutionalized. Sleep disturbances of individuals with dementia are often among the reasons for nursing home placement.

Increasing exposure to bright light or sunlight during the day may be helpful. For individuals with dementia, evening bright light may help with APSD. Structured activity during the day and a quiet sleeping environment may also improve the condition (Teodorescu, 2014; see Box 17-10).

KEY CONCEPTS

- Sleep is a barometer of health and can be considered one of the vital signs.
- Sleep problems constitute a global epidemic affecting up to 45% of the world's population.
- In addition to age-related changes in sleep architecture, many chronic conditions interfere with quality and quantity of sleep in older adults. Complaints of sleep difficulties should be thoroughly investigated and not attributed to age.
- Nonpharmacological interventions (sleep hygiene, sleep restriction measures, stimulus control, circadian interventions, relaxation techniques) are first-line treatment for sleep problems.
- Benzodiazepines or other sedative-hypnotics should not be used in older adults as a first choice of treatment for insomnia.
- All sleeping medications, including OTC, have adverse effects that include daytime drowsiness, changes in mental status, and increased likelihood of falls.
- If sleeping medications are prescribed, benzodiazepine receptor agonists are preferred and should be given at the lowest possible dose and used only short term (2 to 3 weeks, never more than 90 days).
- SDB affects approximately 25% of older individuals (more men than women), and the most common form is obstructive sleep apnea (OSA).
- Untreated OSA is related to heart failure, cardiac dysrhythmias, stroke, type 2 diabetes, and even death.

NURSING STUDY: REST AND SLEEP

Gerald, 80 years old, had a sleeping disorder and was tired most of the day and lonely at night. His wife of 45 years had recently moved into her sewing room, where she slept on the couch at night because she could no longer cope with his loud snoring. He sometimes even seemed to stop breathing, which kept her awake watching his abdomen rise and fall, or not. Sometimes he would awaken suddenly, gasping for air. However, Gerald had tolerated it because he thought nothing could be done for it. Because it had become a threat to his marriage, he became motivated to investigate possible solutions. Gerald said to his nurse clinician, "This isn't anything, but it upsets my wife." Although he did not admit it, he was also worried because he was beginning to feel rather weak and listless during the day. When he had consulted the clinic nurse, Gerald was diagnosed with obstructive sleep apnea. He found that some very practical means of dealing with this problem of sleep apnea were available, and if these were not effective, the nurse had reassured him that additional medical interventions could be helpful.

On the basis of the nursing study, develop a nursing care plan using the following procedure*:

- List Gerald's comments that provide subjective data.
- List information that provides objective data.
- From these data, identify and state, using an accepted format, two nursing diagnoses you determine are most significant to Gerald at this time. List two of Gerald's strengths that you have identified from the data.
- Determine and state outcome criteria for each diagnosis. These must reflect some alleviation of the problem identified in the nursing diagnosis and must be stated in concrete and measurable terms.
- Plan and state one or more interventions for each diagnosed problem. Provide specific documentation of the source used to determine the appropriate intervention. Plan at least one intervention that incorporates Gerald's existing strengths.
- Evaluate the success of the intervention. Interventions must correlate directly with the stated outcome criteria to measure the outcome success.

*Students are advised to refer to their nursing diagnosis text and identify possible or potential problems.

CRITICAL THINKING QUESTIONS AND ACTIVITIES

1. What lifestyle factors may be increasing Gerald's episodes of sleep apnea?
2. In what circumstances is sleep apnea particularly dangerous to health?
3. Compose a list of 10 questions you would ask Gerald to obtain a clear picture of factors contributing to his sleep apnea. Discuss the rationale behind each.
4. List some of the common methods for dealing with this problem that Gerald's nurse may have given to him.

RESEARCH QUESTIONS

1. Does better management of chronic disease improve sleep quality?
2. Does improving sleep quality have a favorable effect on the course of chronic illness?
3. What is the average time of the total sleep cycle as experienced by a healthy individual older than 70 years?
4. What type of exercise is effective for improved sleep?
5. Which nonpharmacological interventions are most effective for sleep and for what type of individual?
6. What are the concerns of caregivers of persons with dementia as they relate to sleep?
7. How do nurses in hospitals and nursing homes evaluate sleep quality for their patients/residents?

REFERENCES

American Geriatrics Society Choosing Wisely Group: American Geriatrics Society identifies another five things that healthcare providers and patients should question, *J Am Geriatr Soc* 62(5):950–960, 2014.

American Geriatrics Society 2012 Beers Criteria Update Expert Panel: Updated Beers Criteria for potentially inappropriate medication use in older adults, *J Am Geriatr Soc* 60(4):616–631, 2012.

Bloom H, Ahmed I, Alessi C, et al: Evidence-based recommendations for the assessment and management of sleep disorders in older persons, *J Am Geriatr Soc* 57: 761–789, 2009.

Buxton O, Ellenbogen J, Wang W, et al: Sleep disturbances due to hospital noises: a prospective evaluation, *Ann Intern Med* 157(3):170–179, 2012.

Buysse D, Germain A, Moul D, et al: Efficacy of brief behavioral treatment for chronic insomnia in older adults, *Arch Intern Med* 171(10):887–895, 2011.

Centers for Disease Control and Prevention: *Insufficient sleep is a public health epidemic*, 2014. http://www.cdc.gov/features/dssleep. Accessed March 15, 2014.

Chasens E, Umlauf M: Excessive sleepiness. In Boltz M, Capezuti E, Fulmer T, et al, editors: *Evidence-based geriatric nursing protocols for best practice*, ed 4, 2012, Springer, pp 74–88.

Chen Y, Weng S, Shen Y, et al: Obstructive sleep apnea and risk of osteoporosis: a population-based cohort study in Taiwan, *J Clin Endocrinol Metab* 99(7):2441–2447, 2014.

Chong Y, Fryar C, Gu Q: *Prescription sleep aid use among adults*: United States,

2005–2010 (NCHS data brief no. 127), August 2013. http://www.cdc.gov/nchs/data/databriefs/db127.htm. Accessed August 2014.

Deratnay P: The effect of insomnia on functional status of community-dwelling older adults, *J Gerontol Nurs* 39(10):22–30, 2013.

Dettenmeier P, Ordoz E, Espiritu J: Evaluation of a continuous positive airway pressure desensitization protocol for CPAP-intolerant patients: a pilot study, *Chest* 144:979A, 2013.

Ferrie J, Kumari M, Salo P, et al: Sleep epidemiology—a rapidly growing field, *Int J Epidemiol* 40:1431–1437, 2011.

Grandner M, Martin J, Patel N, et al: Age and sleep disturbances among American men and women: data from the U.S. behavioral risk factor surveillance system, *Sleep* 35(3):396–406, 2012. http://doi.org/10.5665/sleep.1704.

Haimov I, Shatil E: Cognitive training improves sleep quality and cognitive function among older adults with insomnia, *PLos ONE* 8(4):e61390, 2013. doi: 10.1371/journalpone.0061390.

Hampton L, Daubresse M, Chang H-Y, et al: Emergency department visits by adults for psychiatric medication adverse effects, *JAMA Psychiatry*, 79(9):1006–1014, 2014. doi: 10.1001/jamapsychiatry.2014.436.

Kao M-C, Zheng P, Mackey S: *Trends in benzodiazepine prescription and co-prescription with opioids in the United States*, 2002–2009, 2014. http://www.painmed.org/2014posters/abstract-109. Accessed March 18, 2014.

Kerr D, Wilkinson H: *Providing good care at night for older people*, London, 2010, Jessica Kingsley.

Lim A, Ellison B, Wang J, et al: Sleep is related to neuron numbers in the ventrolateral preoptic/intermediate nucleus in older adults with and without Alzheimer's disease, *Brain* 137:2847–2861, 2014. doi: 10.1093/brain/awu222, 2014.

Lo C, Lee P: Feasibility and effects of TAI CHI for the promotion of sleep quality and quality of life: a single-group study in a sample of older Chinese individuals in Hong Kong, *J Gerontol Nurs* 49(3):46–52, 2014.

Martin J, Alessi C: Sleep disorders. In Ham R, Sloane P, Warshaw G, et al, editors: *Primary care geriatrics*, ed 6, Philadelphia, 2014, Elsevier Saunders, pp 343–352.

McBeth J, Lacey R, Wilkie R: Predictors of new-onset widespread pain in older adults: results from a population-based prospective cohort study in the UK, *Arthritis Rheumatol* 66(3):757–767, 2014.

McCurry S, Gibbons L, Logsdon R, et al: Nighttime insomnia treatment and education for Alzheimer's disease: a randomized, controlled trial, *J Am Geriatr Soc* 53:793–802, 2005.

McCurry S, LaFazia D, Pike K, et al: Managing sleep disturbances in adult family homes: recruitment and implementation of a behavioral treatment program, *Geriatr Nurs* 30:36–44, 2009.

Memtsoudis S, Besculides M, Mazumdar M: A rude awakening—the perioperative sleep apnea epidemic, *N Engl J Med* 368(25):2352–2353, 2013.

Missildine K: Sleep and the sleep environment of older adults in acute care settings, *J Gerontol Nurs* 34(6):15–21, 2008.

Missildine K, Bergstrom N, Meininger J, et al: Sleep in hospitalized elders: a pilot study, *Geriatr Nurs* 31:263–271, 2010.

Morgan B, White D, Wallace A: Substance abuse in older adults. In Mellilo K, Houde S, editors: *Geropsychiatric and mental health nursing*, Sudbury, MA, 2005, Jones & Bartlett.

Murray M, Ferman T, Boeve B, et al: *REM sleep behavior disorder is associated with reduced Alzheimer's pathology*, hippocampal and parietotemporal atrophy in dementia with Lewy bodies (Abstract no. S44.006). Program and abstracts of the American Academy of Neurology 65th Annual Meeting, March 16–23, 2013, San Diego, CA.

Naegle M: Substance misuse and alcohol use disorders. In Capezuti E, Swicker D, Mezey M, et al: *Evidence-based geriatric nursing protocols for best practice*, ed 3, New York, 2008, Springer, 649–676.

National Institute of Neurological Disorders and Stroke: *Restless legs syndrome* (Fact sheet), 2010. http://www.ninds.nih.gov/disorders/restless_legs/detail_restless_legs.htm. Accessed March 17, 2014.

National Sleep Foundation: *REM behavior disorder and sleep*. http://sleepfoundation.org/sleep-disorders-problems/abnormal-sleep-behaviors/rem-behavior-disorder/page/0%2C3. Accessed March 17, 2014.

Osorio R, Ayappa I, Mantua J, et al: The interaction between sleep-disordered breathing and apolipoprotein E genotype on cerebrospinal fluid biomarkers for Alzheimer's disease in cognitively normal elderly individuals, *Neurobiol Aging*, Dec 27, 2013. doi: 10.1016/j.neurobiolaging.2013.12.030. [Epub ahead of print].

Priedt R: Study finds doctors prescribing more sedatives, *Medline Plus*,http://www.nlm.nih.gov/medlineplus/news/fullstory_144996.html. Accessed March 14, 2014.

Qaseem A, Holty J-E, Owens D, et al: Management of obstructive sleep apnea in adults: a clinical practice guidelines from the American College of Physicians, *Ann Intern Med* 159:471–483, 2013.

Raman G, Zhang Y, Minichiello V, et al: Tai Chi improves sleep quality in healthy adults and patients with chronic conditions: a systematic review and meta-analysis, *J Sleep Disord Ther* 2(6):141, 2013. http://www.omicsgroup.org/journals/tai-chi-improves-sleep-quality-in-healthy-adults-and-patients-with-chronic-conditions-a-systematic-review-and-metaanalysis-2167-0277-2-141.pdf. Accessed March 15, 2014.

Rose K, Lorenz R: Sleep disturbances in dementia: what they are and what to do, *J Gerontol Nurs* 36:9–14, 2010.

Rowe M, Kairalla J, McCrae C: Sleep in dementia caregivers and the effects of a nighttime monitoring system, *J Nurs Scholarsh* 42:338–347, 2010.

Saccomano S: Sleep disorders in older adults, *J Gerontol Nurs* 40(3):38–45, 2014.

Schmid S, Hallschmid M, Schultes B: The metabolic burden of sleep loss, *Lancet Diabetes Endocrinol*, March 25, 2014. doi: 10.1016/S2213-8587(14)70012-9. [Epub ahead of print].

Schwab R, Badr S, Epstein L, et al: An official American Thoracic Society statement: continuous positive airway pressure adherence tracking systems, *Am J Respir Crit Care Med* 184(5):613–620, 2013.

Seicean S, Strohl K, Seicean A, et al: Sleep disordered breathing as a risk of cardiac events in subjects with diabetes mellitus and normal exercise echocardiographic findings, *Am J Cardiol* 111(8):1214–1220, 2013.

Seithikurippu R, Pandi-Perumal D, Spence W, et al: Pharmacotherapy of insomnia with ramelteon: safety, efficacy and clinical applications, *J Cent Nerv Syst Dis* 3:51–65, 2011.

Sexton-Radek K: A look at worldwide sleep disturbance, *J Sleep Disorders Ther* 2:115, 2013.

Silber M, Becker P, Earley C, et al: Willis-Ekbom Disease Foundation revised consensus statement on the management of restless legs syndrome, *Mayo Clin Proc* 88(9):977–986, 2013.

Stranges S, Tigbe W, Gomez-Olive F, et al: Sleep problems: an emerging global epidemic? Findings from the INDEPTH WHO-SAGE study among more than 40,000 older adults from 8 countries across Africa and Asia, *Sleep* 35(8): 1173–1181, 2012.

Subramanian S, Surani S: Sleep disorders in the elderly, *Geriatrics* 62(12):10–32, 2007.

Substance Abuse and Mental Health Services Administration: Emergency department visits for adverse reactions involving the insomnia medication zolpidem, *The Dawn Report*, May 1, 2013. http://www.samhsa.gov/data/2k13/DAWN079/sr079-Zolpidem.htm. Accessed March 15, 2014.

Tarsy D: Clinical manifestation and diagnosis of restless legs syndrome in adults, *UpToDate*, February 11, 2014.

Teodorescu M: Sleep disruptions and insomnia in older adults, *Consultant* 54(3): 166–173, 2014.

Townsend-Roccichelli J, Sanford J, VandeWaa E: Managing sleep disorders in the elderly, *Nurse Pract* 35(5):31–37, 2010.

Uchimura N, Ogawa A, Hamamura M, et al: Efficacy and safety of remelteon in Japanese adults with chronic insomnia: a randomized, double-blind, placebo-controlled study, *Expert Rev Neurother* 11(2):215–224, 2011.

U.S. Food and Drug Administration: *FDA drug safety communication*: FDA approves new label changes and dosing for zolpidem products and a recommendation to avoid driving the day after using Ambien CR, 2013. http://www.fda.gov/drugs/drugsafety/ucm352085.htm. Accessed March 15, 2014.

Weaver T, Sawyer A: Adherence to continuous positive airway pressure treatment for obstructive sleep apnea, *Indian J Med Res* 131:245–258, 2010.

Willis-Ekbom Disease Foundation: *What is WED/RLS*.2014. http://www.willis-ekbom.org/about-wed-rls. Accessed January 18, 2014.

World Association of Sleep Medicine: *World Sleep Day*, 2014. http://worldsleepday.org. Accessed March 15, 2014.

Xie L, Kang H, Xu Q, et al: Sleep drives metabolite clearance from the adult brain, *Science* 342(6156):373–377, 2013.

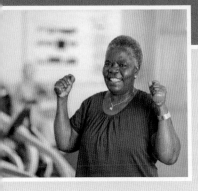

CHAPTER 18

Physical Activity and Exercise

Theris A. Touhy

ⓔ http://evolve.elsevier.com/Touhy/TwdHlthAging

A STUDENT SPEAKS

I work in a local gym on the weekends and over the last several years, I have been amazed at the number of older people who work out. We even have an older gentleman on staff who is a trainer. Some of them are really fit and look like they have been "gym rats" their whole life. Others take it a bit easier but they come a couple of times a week to lift weights or walk on the treadmill. There are also a few people recovering from knee replacements who do their exercises at the gym. I hope I can stay fit when I get old.

Jeff, age 20

AN ELDER SPEAKS

I am 82 years young. My girlfriends and I have had a walking club for 15 years. Coffee first and then our one mile walk down to the park. Now we are trying something new and are going to a yoga class at the local senior center. We've got our mats and our tights and are really enjoying ourselves. Of course, the lunch afterward is nice as well. My grandson thinks it's funny but you should see the moves we are learning!

Peggy, age 74

LEARNING OBJECTIVES

On completion of this chapter, the reader will be able to:

- Describe the relationship between physical activity and health.
- Describe the guidelines for physical activity for older adults.
- Identify components of assessment and screening to determine appropriate physical activity interventions and exercise programs.
- Identify appropriate exercise regimens for older adults and strategies to enhance adherence.
- Discuss ways to incorporate physical activity into daily life.
- Discuss adaptations for individuals with chronic illness, mobility limitations, and cognitive impairment.
- Develop a plan of care to improve the activity level of an older adult.

Few factors contribute as much to health in aging as being physically active. The adage "Use it or lose it" certainly applies to muscles and physical fitness. Regular physical activity throughout life is essential for healthy aging. Physical activity enhances health and functional status while also decreasing the number of chronic illnesses and functional limitations often assumed to be a part of growing older. Physical activity is also a protective factor for depression (Lee et al, 2014) (Box 18-1). The frail health and loss of function we associate with aging are, in large part, due to physical inactivity.

Physical activity is defined as any bodily movement produced by skeletal muscle that requires energy expenditure. This includes exercise and other activities such as playing, working, active transportation (walking, running, biking), household chores, and recreational activities. Exercise is a subcategory of physical fitness that is planned, structured, repetitive, and

BOX 18-1 Health Benefits of Physical Activity

- Reduced risk of hypertension, coronary artery disease, heart attack, stroke, diabetes, colon and breast cancers, metabolic syndrome, depression
- Reduced adverse blood lipid profile
- Prevention of weight gain
- Improved cardiorespiratory and muscular fitness
- Reduced risk of falls and hip fracture
- Improved sleep quality
- Improved bone and functional health
- Decreased risk of early death (life expectancy increased even in persons who do not begin exercising regularly until age 75)
- Improved functional independence
- Improvement in walking speed, strength, functional ability of frail nursing home residents with diagnoses ranging from arthritis to lung disease and dementia

purposeful in the sense that improvement or maintenance of one or more components of physical fitness is the objective (WHO, 2010).

PHYSICAL ACTIVITY AND AGING

Despite a large body of evidence about the benefits of physical activity to maintain and improve function, more than 60% of American adults aged 50 and older failed to achieve the recommended activity levels. With advancing age (75 years and older) participation is even lower with only 9% of men and 6% of women meeting the recommended guidelines (Taylor, 2014). Older women are sedentary for approximately two-thirds of their waking hours (Shiroma et al, 2013). For women, patterns of physical activity have been reported to decline between ages 55 and 64, and again at age 75 and older (Fan et al, 2013). These may be prime times to enhance education on the benefits of physical activity for women as they age. The levels of physical activity among older adults have not improved over the past decade in the United States.

Increasing physical activity for people of all ages is a global concern in both developed and developing countries. The World Health Organization (WHO) calls increasing physical activity a societal problem that demands a population-based, multisectoral, multidisciplinary, and culturally relevant approach (WHO, 2010). WHO identified physical inactivity as the fourth leading risk factor (high blood pressure, smoking, high blood glucose level, physical activity, obesity) for global mortality with around 3.2 million deaths each year attributable to physical inactivity (Taylor, 2014; WHO, 2010). The cardiac risk of inactive persons is comparable with that of smokers (Elsawy and Higgins, 2010).

Worldwide, it is important for governments and policy makers to initiate actions to create environments that encourage lifelong physical activity (Taylor, 2014). There are a number of global and national guidelines for physical activity, although physical activity among older adults has attracted less interest and research (Sun et al, 2013) (Box 18-2). *Healthy People 2020* goals for physical activity can be found in Box 18-3.

BOX 18-2 RESOURCES FOR BEST PRACTICE

Physical Activity

Centers for Disease Control and Prevention: *Making physical activity a part of an older adult's life* - Includes exercise program information, videos, success stories, ways to overcome barriers (Growing Stronger Program and resources for strength training including pictures/videos).

EASY: *Exercise and Screening for You:* http://easyforyou.info/ Accessed April 2014.

National Center on Health, Physical Activity and Disability: *14 Weeks to a healthier you:* http://www.ncpad.org/14weeks. Accessed April 2104.

National Institute on Aging: *Exercise & physical activity: your everyday guide from the National Institute on Aging.*

Resnick B: *Restorative care nursing for older adults: a guide for all settings,* ed 2, New York, 2011, Springer.

World Health Organization: *Global strategy on diet, physical activity and health: global recommendations on physical activity for health* Document1

♥ BOX 18-3 HEALTHY PEOPLE 2020

Physical Activity

- Reduce the proportion of adults who engage in no leisure-time physical activity.
- Increase the proportion of adults who engage in aerobic physical activity of at least moderate intensity for at least 150 minutes/week, or 75 minutes/week of vigorous intensity, or an equivalent combination.

Data from U.S. Department of Health and Human Services, Office of Disease Prevention and Health Promotion: Healthy People 2020, 2012. http://www.healthypeople.gov/2020.

Physical activity is important for all older people, not just active healthy elders. Even a small amount of time (at least 30 minutes of moderate activity several days a week) can improve health. Studies have found that increasing physical activity improves health outcomes in persons with chronic illnesses (regardless of severity) and in those with functional impairment. Among frail and mobility-limited individuals, recent reviews and meta-analyses revealed that exercise had a small to moderate positive effect on mobility and physical functioning. Strength training interventions seem most important for functional improvement, but further research is needed to determine the type of exercise necessary to maintain or improve functional ability in adults with disabilities and frail older adults (Taylor, 2014).

Walking may be a particularly beneficial activity for frail elders. In a recent study of more than 1600 inactive adults (70 to 89 years old) who were unable to walk without assistance, those who walked 20 minutes a day had an 18% lower risk of major motor disability. After 2 years, the walking group was more capable of walking without assistance for about one-fourth of a mile (Pahor et al, 2014). Regardless of age or situation, the older person can find some activity suitable for his or her condition. It is important to keep older people moving any way possible for as long as possible (Box 18-4).

BOX 18-4 Myriad of Ways to Keep Fit during Aging

- After four unsuccessful attempts, Diana Nyad, 64 years old, became the first person to swim from Cuba to Florida without the use of a shark cage.
- Nellie, 83 years old, began swimming to ease the discomfort resulting both from a short left arm, the residual effect of poliomyelitis, and from a frozen left shoulder. She became an award-winning synchronized swimmer with 20 gold medals, 12 blue ribbons, and 13 trophies to her credit. Nellie continued to exercise this way despite the need to wear cataract goggles.
- James, 72 years old, was taking 40 mg of Lipitor daily for his high cholesterol level and lisinopril 40 mg for hypertension. He was a self-proclaimed couch potato. He joined Silver Sneakers, a program through his Medicare Advantage Plan, and started going to the gym. After a year of walking on the treadmill 30 minutes 3 times a week and lifting weights, his cholesterol level and blood pressure value approached normal limits. His medications were reduced and he was 10 pounds lighter. Even his 14-year-old grandson admired his biceps.
- Em, an 86-year-old nursing home resident, jogged every morning in place for about 5 minutes and then briskly walked around outside the facility. Although she had occasional lapses of memory, she was vital, erect, and interested in life around her.

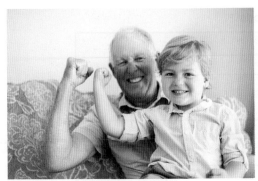

Physical Activity Is Important for All Older People. (©iStock.com/Squaredpixels)

PROMOTING HEALTHY AGING: IMPLICATIONS FOR GERONTOLOGICAL NURSING

Assessment

Assessment of function and mobility are components of a health assessment for older adults. Exercise counseling should be provided as a part of assessment. For individuals 65 years of age and older, if they are relatively fit and have no limiting health conditions, initiation of a moderate intensity exercise program is safe and does not require any type of cardiac screening (CDC, 2014). The consensus is that there is minimal cardiovascular risk to engaging in physical activity and a much greater risk in maintaining a sedentary lifestyle. Individuals with specific health conditions, such as cardiovascular disease and diabetes, may need to take extra precautions and seek medical advice before beginning an exercise program (CDC, 2014). Frail individuals will need more comprehensive assessment to adapt exercise recommendations to their abilities and ensure benefit without compromising safety.

Screening

The Exercise and Screening for You (EASY) (see Box 18-2) tool is a screening tool that can be used to determine a safe exercise program for older adults on the basis of underlying physical problems. EASY is an interactive web-based tool that can be completed by the individual or the health care provider. The tool also provides suggestions for the types of exercises that are appropriate for individuals with underlying health concerns. Resources are provided on types of exercise and programs that have all been reviewed and endorsed by national organizations such as the National Institute on Aging (Bethesda, MD) and can be printed and given to the person.

The Hendrich II Fall Risk Model (Mathias et al, 1986) (Figure 18-1) includes the Get-Up-and-Go Test, which can also be used to assess mobility, gait, and gait speed. This test is useful in fall risk assessment as well. It is a practical assessment tool that can be adapted to any setting. The client is asked to rise from a straight-backed chair, stand briefly, walk forward about 10 feet, turn, walk back to the chair, turn around, and sit down. The test can be timed as well and gait speed has been found to be a predictor of mobility. On the basis of the results of initial screening, older adults may need further evaluation.

◆ Interventions

The nurse should be knowledgeable about recommended physical activity guidelines, educate individuals about the importance of exercise and physical activity, and provide suggestions on ways to incorporate exercise into daily routines (CDC, 2014). Many older people mistakenly believe that they are too old to begin a fitness program. Older people are less likely to receive exercise counseling from their primary care providers than younger individuals. Research has noted that health care providers value the benefits of physical activity but have inadequate knowledge of specific recommendations. Giving specific advice about the type and frequency of exercise is important (CDC, 2014; Taylor, 2014). Nurses can also design and lead exercise and physical activity programs for groups of older adults in the community or in long-term care. (see Box 18-2)

◆ Physical Activity Guidelines

Guidelines for physical activity for adults 65 years of age or older who are generally fit and have no limiting health conditions are presented in Box 18-5. Recommendations for all adults include participation in 30 minutes of moderate-intensity physical activity for 5 or more days of the week. People do not have to be active for 30 minutes at a time but can accumulate 30 minutes over 24 hours. As little as 10 minutes of exercise has health benefits and three 10-minute bouts of activity have the same fitness effects as one 30-minute bout (Table 18-1). Extremely frail individuals may not be able to engage in aerobic activities and should begin with strength and balance training before participating in as little as 5 minutes of aerobic training.

◆ Incorporating Physical Activity into Lifestyle

One does not have to invest in expensive gym equipment or gym memberships to incorporate the recommended physical activity guidelines into his or her daily routine. Hand weights (or use cans of food as weights), a chair, and an exercise mat

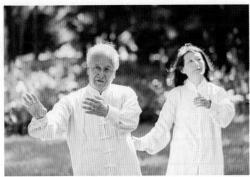

Tai Chi. Tai chi can improve flexibility and balance. (©iStock.com/Kali Nine LLC)

Hendrich II Fall Risk Model™

Confusion Disorientation Impulsivity		4	
Symptomatic Depression		2	
Altered Elimination		1	
Dizziness Vertigo		1	
Male Gender		1	
Any Administered Antiepileptics		2	
Any Administered Benzodiazepines		1	
Get Up & Go Test			
Able to rise in a single movement – No loss of balance with steps		0	
Pushes up, successful in one attempt		1	
Multiple attempts, but successful		3	
Unable to rise without assistance during test (OR if a medical order states the same and/or complete bed rest is ordered) * If unable to assess, document this on the patient chart with the date and time		4	
A Score of 5 or Greater = High Risk		**Total Score**	

FIGURE 18-1 The Hendrich II Fall Risk Model. The Hendrich II Fall Risk Model is a fall risk assessment tool recommended by the Hartford Institute for Geriatric Nursing. (©2013 AHI of Indiana Inc. All rights reserved. U.S. patent No. 7,282,031 and No. 7,682,308.

BOX 18-5   Exercise Guidelines

Older adults need at least:

- 2 hours and 30 minutes (150 minutes) of moderate-intensity aerobic activity (e.g., brisk walking, swimming, bicycling) every week *and*
- Muscle-strengthening activities on 2 or more days that work all major muscle groups (legs, hips, abdomen, chest, shoulders, and arms)

  Additionally: Stretching (flexibility) and balance exercises (particularly for older people at risk of falls) are also recommended. Yoga and tai chi exercises have been shown to be of benefit to older people in terms of improving flexibility and balance, as well as reducing pain and enhancing psychological well-being (Miller and Taylor-Piliae, 2014). Tai chi can be adapted for level of function and mobility status. Home-based balance-training exercise programs are also available.

From Centers for Disease Control and Prevention: *How much physical activity do older adults need?* 2014. http://www.cdc.gov/physicalactivity/everyone/guidelines/olderadults.html. Accessed April 2014.

can easily get the individual started (Figure 18-2). The benefits of group exercise in terms of social and emotional health have been reported, and the socialization provided may be important for individuals who live alone or do not have social networks. Adhering to a program of physical activity can be problematic for individuals. Resistance exercise programs have higher rates of adherence than aerobic exercise programs among older individuals. The high prevalence of joint diseases, such as osteoarthritis, may hamper successful performance of aerobic exercises that cause joint impact. Muscle-strengthening exercises without weight-bearing provide more joint stability (Miranda et al, 2014). Swimming is a low-risk activity that provides aerobic benefit, and water-based exercises are particularly beneficial for individuals with arthritis or other mobility limitations.

TABLE 18-1	**Guidelines for Teaching about Exercise**				
EXERCISE	**DESCRIPTION**	**BENEFITS**	**INTENSITY**	**FREQUENCY**	**EXAMPLES**
Moderate-intensity aerobic activity	Continuous movement involving large muscle groups that is sustained for a minimum of 10 min; should make your heart beat faster	Improves cardiovascular functioning, strengthens heart muscle, decreases blood glucose and triglycerides, increases HDL, improves mood	On a 10-point scale, where sitting is 0 and working as hard as you can is 10, moderate-intensity aerobic activity is a 5 or 6. You will be able to talk but not sing the words to your favorite song	30 min, 5 days/wk Perform for at least 10 min at a time	Biking, swimming and other water-based activities, dancing, brisk walking, lifestyle activities that incorporate large muscle groups (pushing a lawn mower, climbing stairs)
Muscle-strengthening activities	Activities that involve moving or lifting some type of resistance and work all major muscle groups (legs, hips, back, abdomen, chest, shoulders, arms)	Increases muscle strength, prevents sarcopenia, reduces fall risk, improves balance, modifies risk factors for cardiovascular disease and type 2 diabetes	To gain health benefits, muscle-strengthening activities need to be done to the point at which it is difficult to do another repetition without help. A repetition is one complete movement of an activity such as lifting a weight. An effort should be made to do 8-12 repetitions (1 set) per activity or continue until it would be difficult to do another repetition without help.	2 days/wk, but not consecutive days to allow muscles to recover between sessions	Lifting weights, calisthenics, working with resistance bands, Pilates, exercises that use the body's own weight for resistance (push-ups, sit-ups), heavy gardening (digging, shoveling), washing windows/floors
Stretching (flexibility)	A therapeutic maneuver designed to elongate shortened soft tissue structures and increase flexibility	Facilitates ROM around joints, prevents injury	Stretch muscle groups but not past the point of resistance or pain	At least 2 days/wk	Yoga, range-of-motion exercises
Balance exercises	Movements that improve the ability to maintain control of the body over the base of support to avoid falling	Improves lower body strength, improves balance, helps prevent falls	Safety precautions are essential (holding onto a chair, working with another person)	Can be incorporated into regularly scheduled strength exercises; more formal balance programs may be appropriate for those at high risk for falls	Tai chi, yoga Exercises such as standing on one foot, walking heel to toe or backwards or sideways, leg raises, hip extensions (can be done holding onto a chair), standing up from a sitting position without using your hands

HDL, High-density lipoprotein; *ROM,* range of motion.
Data from Centers for Disease Control and Prevention: *How much physical activity do older adults need?* 2014. http://www.cdc.gov/physicalactivity/growingstronger/exercises/index.htm. Accessed April 2014.

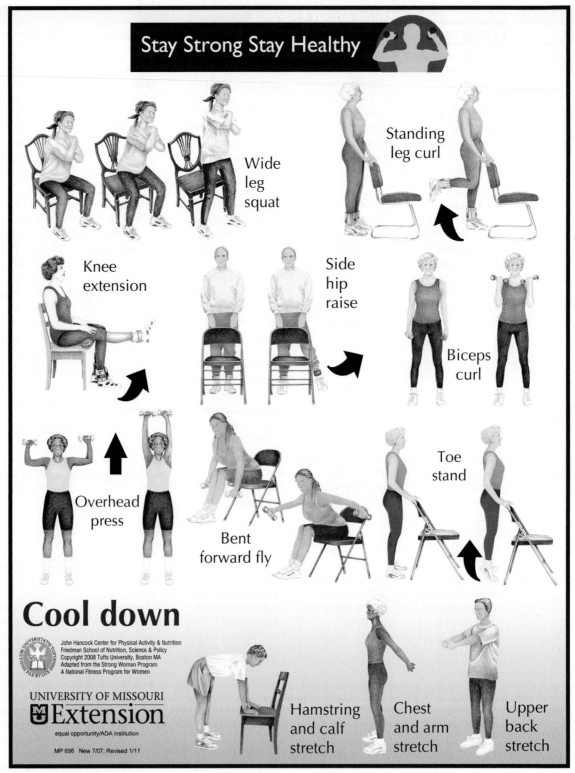

FIGURE 18-2 Stay Strong Stay Healthy. (©1993 to 2014 University of Missouri. Published by University of Missouri Extension. Used by permission of the publisher. All rights reserved.)

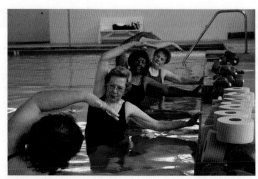

Aquatic Exercise. Aquatic programs are beneficial for elders with mobility and joint problems. They improve circulation, muscle strength, and endurance; and provide socialization and relaxation. (©iStock.com/ftwitty)

Individuals may also be able to integrate activity into daily life rather than doing a specific exercise. Examples include walking, golfing, tennis, biking, raking leaves, yard work/gardening, dancing, washing windows or floors, washing and waxing the car, and swimming and water-based exercises. One study on physical activity reported that walking is the most popular activity for women of all ages, followed by dancing, treadmill, and yoga. Dancing and treadmill offer higher-intensity structured workouts than walking and should be considered in planning programs for older women (Fan et al, 2013). If the individual is engaging in activities he or she enjoys, adherence is improved (Miranda et al, 2014).

The EASY tool offers many alternatives for those with certain conditions. Additionally, there are many excellent resources available that provide instructions, tips, pictures, videos, and stories from individuals who have embarked on fitness regimens (see Box 18-2). Box 18-6 provides helpful tips that nurses can use for encouraging individuals to adopt physical activity. Box 18-7 presents safety precautions.

Many senior living communities, as well as nursing homes, provide gym equipment for residents. The Silver Sneakers Program, the nation's leading exercise program for active community-dwelling older adults, is a membership benefit through some of the Medicare Advantage plans. Local community centers often provide exercise programs for older adults, and many gyms in the United States have reduced-cost memberships for individuals older than age 65. Some have trainers on staff with expertise in exercises appropriate for older individuals. The nurse can share resources in the community, and communities should be encouraged to provide accessible and affordable options for physical activity.

◆ Special Considerations

The benefits of physical activity extend to the more physically frail older adult, those who are nonambulatory or experience cognitive impairment, and those residing in assisted living facilities (ALFs) or skilled nursing facilities (SNFs). In fact, these individuals may benefit most from an exercise program in terms of function and quality of life (Resnick et al, 2006a). The National Center on Health, Physical Activity and Disability (see Box 18-2) provides many suggestions for adaptation of exercises for individuals with mobility limitations.

There are many creative and enjoyable ideas for enhancing physical activity such as using lower extremity cycling equipment, marching in place, tossing a ball, stretching, performing range-of-motion exercises, using resistive bands (Chen et al., 2013), and doing chair yoga. An interesting study from Finland (Back et al, 2013) presented a socially interactive robot-guided

---

BOX 18-6   TIPS FOR BEST PRACTICE

Physical Activity/Exercise Participation

- Provide appropriate screening before beginning an exercise program.
- Assess for functional abilities and discuss how exercise can enhance function.
- Provide information about the benefits of exercise, emphasizing short-term benefits such as sleeping better, improved walking ability, decreasing fall risk.
- Clarify the misconceptions associated with exercise (fatigue, injury).
- Assess barriers to exercise and provide tips on how to overcome.
- Provide an "exercise prescription" that specifies what exercises and how often the person should exercise. Include daily and long-term goals.
- Collaborate with the person to set short- and long-term goals that are specific, achievable, and match perceived needs, health, cognitive abilities, culture, gender, and interests.
- Encourage individual to keep a journal or diary to reflect experience and progress.
- Provide choices about types of exercises, and design the program so that the person can do it at home or elsewhere.
- Refer to community resources for physical fitness (e.g., YMCA, mall walking).
- Provide self-monitoring methods to assist in visualizing progress.
- Group-based programs and exercising with a buddy may be more successful.
- Try to make the program fun and entertaining (walking with favorite music, socializing with friends).
- Discuss potential exercise side effects and any symptoms that should be reported.
- Provide safety tips and situations that may require medical attention (Box 18-7).
- Share stories about the benefits of your own personal exercise program and those of older people (See Resources for Best Practice, Box 18-2)..
- Provide ongoing support and follow-up on progress; support from experts and family and peers is a significant factor in encouraging continued participation.
- Begin with low-intensity physical activity for sedentary individuals.
- Initiate low-intensity activities in short sessions (less than 10 minutes), and include warm-up and cool-down components with active stretching.
- Progression from low to moderate intensity is important to obtain maximal benefits, but activity level changes should be instituted gradually.
- Teach the importance of warming up and cooling down.
- Encourage use of proper, well-fitted footwear.
- Lifestyle activities (e.g., raking, gardening) can build endurance when performed for at least 10 minutes.

BOX 18-7   TIPS FOR BEST PRACTICE

Exercise Safety

- Always wear comfortable, loose-fitting clothing and appropriate shoes for your activity.
- Warm-up: Perform a low- to moderate-intensity warm-up for 5-10 minutes.
- Drink water before, during, and after your exercise session.
- When exercising outdoors, evaluate your surroundings for safety: traffic, pavement condition, weather, and strangers.
- Wear clothes made of fabrics that absorb sweat and remove it from your skin.
- Never wear rubber or plastic suits. These could hold the sweat on your skin and make your body overheat.
- Wear sunscreen when you exercise outdoors.

Stop Exercising Right Away if You:
- Have pain or pressure in your chest, neck, shoulder, or arm.
- Feel dizzy or sick.
- Break out in a cold sweat.
- Have muscle cramps.
- Feel acute (not just achy) pain in your joints, feet, ankles, or legs.
- Have trouble breathing. Slow down; you should be able to talk while exercising without gasping for breath.

Times Exercise Should not Be Done
- Avoid hard exercise for 2 hours after a big meal. (A leisurely walk around the block would be fine.)
- Do not exercise when you have a fever and/or viral infection accompanied by muscle aches.
- Do not exercise if your systolic blood pressure is greater than 200 mm Hg and your diastolic blood pressure is greater than 100 mm Hg.
- Do not exercise if your resting heart rate is greater than 120 beats/min.
- Do not exercise if you have a joint that you are using to exercise (such as a knee or an ankle) that is red and warm and painful.
- If you have osteoporosis, always avoid stretches that flex your spine or cause you to bend at the waist, and avoid making jerky, rapid movements.
- Stop exercising if you experience severe pain or swelling in a joint. Discomfort that persists should always be evaluated.
- Do not exercise if you have a new symptom that has not been evaluated by your health care provider, such as pain in your chest, abdomen, or a joint; swelling in an arm, leg, or joint; difficulty catching your breath at rest; or a fluttering feeling in your chest.

From Program on Healthy Aging, Texas A&M Health Science Center: *Safety tips,* 2008. http://easyforyou.info/safety.asp Accessed April 2014.

exercise program for nursing home residents. The Wii game system offers other possibilities for exercise at all levels and is increasingly being used by older people in their own homes and in senior living residences to encourage physical activity, improve balance, and provide enjoyable entertainment (Bieryla and Dold, 2013; Chao et al, 2013).

Ongoing research on alternative ways to present physical fitness programs to meet the needs of older adults and those with mobility impairments has reported many positive benefits (Box 18-8). At the Louis and Anne Green Memory and Wellness Center at Florida Atlantic University (Boca Raton, FL), 94-year-old yoga practitioner Vera Paley leads groups of cognitively impaired elders, as well as caregivers, in chair yoga sessions. Individuals with cognitive impairment are often not included in physical activity programs. While further research is needed to understand the level and intensity of exercise that is beneficial

BOX 18-8   RESEARCH HIGHLIGHTS

Nurse researcher Dr. Ruth McCaffrey and her social work colleague Dr. Juyoung Park (Florida Atlantic University) were awarded a $389,000 grant from the National Center for Complementary and Alternative Therapies to study the effects of a Sit 'N' Fit chair yoga program in community-dwelling older adults who are unable to participate in standing exercises. Effects of the 8-week program on physical function, depression, fatigue, quality of life, and life satisfaction will be measured by comparing the results of the Sit 'N' Fit chair yoga program (45 minutes twice a week) with results from an attention control group (health education program, 45 minutes twice a week for 8 weeks). The Sit 'N' Fit chair yoga program includes breathing, centering and relaxation, yoga postures to stretch and flex muscles and joints in the lower and upper body, and meditation and focusing on inner peace.

Drs. McCaffrey and Park have conducted two prior studies on chair yoga with older adults with osteoarthritis and Alzheimer's disease and reported positive changes across all physical measures. This important and creative interprofessional research will contribute to evidence about the benefits of yoga and effective interventions to improve physical function in elders who are unable to participate in regular exercise programs.

Data from Dr. Ruth McCaffrey: personal communication, April 22, 2014; National Institutes of Health: *Effect of Sit 'N' Fit chair yoga on community-dwelling elders with osteoarthritis,* 2013. https://www.collectiveip.com/grants/NIH:8573343 Accessed April 2014; McCaffrey R, Park J, Newman D, et al: The effect of chair yoga in older adults with moderate to severe Alzheimer's disease, *J Gerontol Nurs,* Feb 26, 2014. doi: 10.3928/19404921-20140218-01; Park J, McCaffrey R: Chair yoga: benefits for community-dwelling older adults with osteoarthritis, *J Gerontol Nurs* 38(5):13–20, 2012; McCaffrey R, Park J, Newman D, et al: The effect of chair yoga in older adults with moderate and severe Alzheimer's disease, *Res Gerontol Nurs* 7(4):171–177, 2014.

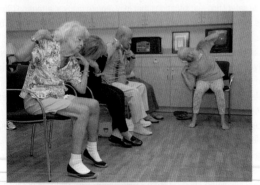

Yoga. Vera Paley leads yoga class. (Courtesy of the Louis and Anne Green Memory and Wellness Center of the Christine E. Lynn College of Nursing at Florida Atlantic University.)

for each type of dementia, exercise should be a component of the plan of care (Forbes et al, 2013).

Results of research suggest that older adults with cognitive impairment who participate in exercise programs may improve strength and endurance, cognitive function, and ability to perform activities of daily living (Forbes et al, 2013; Schwenk et al, 2014; Taylor, 2014). A growing body of research suggests that exercise programs are likely to be more successful if they are individualized, enjoyable, and involve caregivers (Yao et al, 2013). Strength-training interventions and one-component exercises seem to be more effective in increasing functional improvement in individuals with cognitive impairment (Taylor, 2014; Tseng et al, 2011). Physical activity may also have a beneficial effect on mood and behavior in cognitively impaired older people (AHRQ, 2009; Galik et al, 2009; Galik, 2010; Williams and Tappen, 2007, 2008).

◆ Maintaining Function in Acute Care Settings

Even though the focus in hospitals is on acute illness management, there is growing awareness of the need to also focus on functional status, especially in older patients. Hospitalization is associated with significantly greater loss of total, lean, and fat mass strength in older individuals. Individuals older than age 85 experience the most functional decline with hospitalization, with rates exceeding 50%. Functional decline may start preadmission and continue after discharge, depending on the individual's condition and comorbid problems.

Additional risks for functional decline include bedrest, restricted activity/low mobility, and the tendency for staff to perform ADL care rather than encouraging self-care (Boltz et al, 2012). It has been suggested that an "older adult's functional trajectory is a critical vital sign, an important prognostic marker, and an indicator to guide care delivery and transitional care (Boltz et al, 2012, p. 105).

◆ Function-Focused Care

Function-focused care (FFC), previously known as restorative care from its use in long-term care, is a comprehensive, systems-level approach that prioritizes the preservation and restoration of functional capacity. The FFC approach can be used across settings of care to maintain and improve functional abilities in older adults. FFC interactions between nurses and patients have demonstrated a decrease in overall

loss of ADL function from baseline to discharge from acute care (Boltz et al, 2012).

FFC is based on a "philosophy of care in which nurses acknowledge older adults' physical and cognitive capabilities with regard to function and integrate functional and physical activities into all care interactions" (Boltz et al, 2012, p. 111) (Box 18-9). Nurse researcher Barbara Resnick and her colleagues have conducted numerous studies evaluating the use of function-focused care in improving function and physical activity in older adults in hospitals, assisted living residences, and skilled nursing facilities. The Res-Care intervention (Resnick et al, 2006b; Resnick et al, 2009, 2011; Resnick, 2011), a self-efficacy–based approach to restore and/or maintain the residents' physical function, can be used as a model for restorative care in ALFs and SNFs.

The Res-Care intervention has been revised for use with individuals with moderate to severe cognitive impairment (Galik et al, 2009; Galik, 2010). This intervention holds promise to enhance therapeutic care of older adults with cognitive impairment and to focus interventions on quality of life rather than only on safety and behavior (Resnick et al, 2013).

BOX 18-9 TIPS FOR BEST PRACTICE

Function-Focused Care in Acute Care

- Ask or encourage the individual to move in bed and give the person time to move rather than moving the person yourself.
- Give step-by-step cues on how to move in bed (e.g., "put your right hand on the rail and pull yourself over on your left side").
- Ask or encourage the individual to transfer and wait for the individual to move rather than transferring the individual yourself or automatically using lift equipment (use of assistive equipment depends on mobility and cognitive status).
- Give step-by-step cues and use gestures/demonstration on how to transfer safely (e.g., "plant feet firmly on the floor and slide to the edge of the chair").
- Ask or encourage the individual to walk or independently propel wheelchair and give the person time to perform the activity rather than doing it yourself.
- Give step-by-step cues and use gestures/demonstration (e.g., "move your left foot forward; now move your right foot").
- Assist, ask, and/or encourage use of assistive devices; provide instruction on use and ensure that device is available and appropriate.

Adapted from Resnick B: Changing the philosophy of care—a function-focused care approach, *Aging Well* 5(2):24, 2012.

KEY CONCEPTS

- Few factors contribute as much to health in aging as being physically active.
- Physical activity enhances health and functional status while also decreasing the number of chronic illnesses and functional limitations often assumed to be a part of growing older.
- Despite a large body of evidence about the benefits of physical activity to maintain and improve function, physical activity levels of older adults remain low and have not improved over the past decade.

- Components of a health assessment for older adults include assessment of function and mobility. Exercise counseling should be provided as a part of assessment.
- The benefits of physical activity extend to the more physically frail older adult, those who are nonambulatory or experience cognitive impairment, and those residing in assisted living facilities (ALFs) or skilled nursing facilities (SNFs). In fact, these individuals may benefit most from an exercise program in terms of function and quality of life.

NURSING STUDY: EXERCISE AND ACTIVITY

Tom, 75 years old, had lost his wife Ella a year ago and had been feeling down and tired much of each day. He had retired at age 70 from his job as a housing contractor and had spent much of his time with Ella. They had been married for 50 years. He now sometimes seemed to sit in front of the television most of the day without actually remembering what it was that he had seen. Many of the couple's friends had moved away or relocated to retirement settings, and other than his daughter, who lived about 45 minutes from his house, Tom rarely saw anyone anymore. He had lived like this for nearly a year, and it had become his daily pattern of life. Tom took the initiative after a suggestion from his daughter to go to the local senior citizen center. He went and had lunch there nearly every day. At one point he was asked if he would allow a nursing student to spend time with him during her semester in a gerontology course. He agreed. In the course of her assessment, she (and he) found that his activity level was nearly completely sedentary. She gave Tom information about the ramifications of such a sedentary life. She pointed out that the center had an exercise class every day between 10 AM and 12 noon. Because he came every day (except Saturday and Sunday) for lunch, it seemed a good thing to do. Tom said to his nursing student, "This isn't anything I am really interested in doing, but I will give it a try." Though he did not admit it, he was also worried because he usually felt weak and listless during the day after his lunch. When he did attend the first class, he found that there were basic exercises and more advanced ones for elders who had participated regularly for 6 months. He found after a few weeks that he was enjoying the social aspect of the exercise, if not the exercise itself. After nearly a year of fairly regular participation, Tom began playing golf with some of the men from the center. Once he attended a dance.

On the basis of the nursing study, develop a nursing care plan for the nursing student using the following procedure*:

- List Tom's comments that provide subjective data.
- List information that provides objective data.
- From these data identify and state, using an accepted format, two nursing diagnoses you determine are most significant to Tom at this time. List two of Tom's strengths that you have identified from these data.
- Determine and state outcome criteria for each diagnosis. These must reflect some alleviation of the problem identified in the nursing diagnosis and must be stated in concrete and measurable terms.
- Plan and state one or more interventions for each diagnosed problem. Provide specific documentation of the source used to determine the appropriate intervention. Plan at least one intervention that incorporates Tom's existing strengths.
- Evaluate the success of the intervention. Interventions must correlate directly with the stated outcome criteria to measure the outcome success.

*Students are advised to refer to their nursing diagnosis text and identify possible or potential problems.

CRITICAL THINKING QUESTIONS AND ACTIVITIES

1. In the nursing study above, what lifestyle factors developed by Tom after his wife's death have become dangerous to his health?
2. Compose a list of 10 questions you would ask Tom to obtain a clear picture of factors contributing to his activity level. Discuss the rationale behind each.
3. List some of the common methods for motivating Tom that his nursing student may have used.
4. Describe the level of activity that should be Tom's starting point and discuss symptoms he might expect as he increases his activity level.

RESEARCH QUESTIONS

1. What activities and exercises are most useful in maintaining mobility in elders?
2. What factors increase adherence to an exercise program among community-dwelling older adults?
3. What are the benefits of group exercise programs?
4. What factors in the institutional environment induce immobility?
5. What are some creative ways to implement exercise in the long-term care setting?
6. How does the design of an exercise program differ for individuals with cognitive impairment?

REFERENCES

Agency for Healthcare Research and Quality: Nursing home residents with cognitive impairment are able to participate in a motivational intervention, *Research Activities*, April 2009. http://archive. ahrq.gov/news/research-activities/ apr09/0409RA14.html. Accessed April 2014.

Back I, Makela K, Kallio J: Robot-guided exercise program for rehabilitation of older nursing home residents, *Ann Longterm Care* 21(6):38–41, 2013.

Bieryla K, Dold N: Feasibility of Wii Fit training to improve clinical measures of balance in older adults, *Clin Int Aging* 8:775–781, 2013.

Boltz M, Resnick B, Galik G: Interventions to prevent functional decline in the acute care setting. In Boltz M, Capezuti E, Fulmer T, Zwicker D: *Evidence-based geriatric nursing protocols for best practice*, ed 4, New York, 2012, Springer, pp 104–121.

Centers for Disease Control and Prevention: *How much physical activity do older adults need?* 2014. http://www.cdc.gov/ physicalactivity/everyone/guidelines/old-eradults.html. Accessed April 2014.

Chao Y, Scherer Y, Wu Y, et al: The feasibility of an intervention combining self-efficacy theory and Wii Fit exergames in assisted living residents: a pilot study, *Geriatr Nurs* 34(5):377–382, 2013.

Chen K, Tseng WS, Chang YH, et al: Feasibility appraisal of an elastic band exercise program for older adults in wheelchairs, *Geriatr Nurs* 34(5):373–376, 2013.

Elsawy B, Higgins K: Physical activity guidelines for older adults, *Am Fam Physician* 1(81):55–59, 2010.

Fan J, Kowaleski-Jones L, Wen M: Walking or dancing: patterns of physical activity by cross-sectional age among U.S. women, *J Aging Health* 25:1182–1203, 2013.

Forbes D, Thiessen EJ, Blake CM, et al: Exercise programs for people with dementia, *Cochrane Database Syst Rev* 12:CD006489, 2013. doi: 10.1002/14651858.CD006489.pub3.

Galik E: Function-focused care for long-term care residents with moderate to severe cognitive impairment: a social ecological approach, *Ann Longterm Care* 18(6), 27–32, 2010.

Galik E, Resnick B, Pretzer-Aboff I: "Knowing what makes them tick": motivating cognitively impaired older adults to participate in restorative care, *Int J Nurs Pract* 15:48–55, 2009.

Lee H, Lee J, Brar J, et al: Physical activity and depressive symptoms in older adults, *Res Gerontol Nurs* 35(1):37–41, 2014.

Mathias S, Nayak US, Isaacs B: Balance in elderly patients: the "get up and go test," *Arch Phys* Med Rehabil 67(6):387–389, 1986.

Miller S, Taylor-Piliae R: Effects of Tai Chi on cognitive function in community-dwelling older adults, *Geriatr Nurs* 35: 9–19, 2014.

Miranda A, Picorelli A, Pereira D, et al: Adherence of older women with strength training and aerobic exercise, *Clin Int Aging* 9:323–331, 2014.

Pahor M, Guralnik J, Ambrosius W, et al: Effect of structured physical activity on prevention of major mobility disability in older adults: the LIFE study randomized clinical trial, *JAMA* 311(23): 2387–2396, 2014.

Resnick B, Galik E, Enders H, et al: Pilot testing of function-focused care for acute care intervention, *J Nurs Care Qual* 26(2):169–177, 2011.

Resnick B: *Restorative care nursing for older adults: a guide for all settings*, ed 2, New York, 2011, Springer.

Resnick B, Ory M, Rogers M, et al: Screening for and prescribing exercise for older adults, *Geriatrics Aging* 9:174–182, 2006a.

Resnick B, Simpson M, Bercovitz A, et al: Pilot testing of the Restorative Care Intervention: impact on residents, *J Gerontol Nurs* 32(3):39–47, 2006b.

Resnick B, Galik E, Gruber-Baldini A, et al: Implementing a restorative care philosophy of care in assisted living: pilot testing of Res-Care-AL, *J Am Acad Nurse Pract* 21:123–133, 2009.

Resnick B, Galik E, Boltz M: Function-focused care approaches: literature review of progress and future possibilities, *J Am Med Dir Assoc* 14(5):313–318, 2013.

Schwenk M, Dutzi I, Englert S, et al: An intensive exercise program improves motor performance in patients with dementia: translational model of geriatric rehabilitation, *J Alzheimers Dis* 39(3):487–498, 2014.

Shiroma E, Freedson P, Stewart G, et al: Patterns of acceleromotor-assessed sedentary behavior in older women, *JAMA* 310(23):2562–2563, 2013.

Sun F, Norman I, White A: Physical activity in older people: a systematic review, *BMC Public Health* 13:449, 2013.

Taylor D: Physical activity is medicine for older adults, *Postgrad Med J* 90:26–32, 2014.

Tseng C, Gau B, Lou M: The effectiveness of exercise on improving cognition functions in older people: a systematic review, *J Nurs Res* 19(2):119–131, 2011.

Williams C, Tappen R: Effect of exercise on mood in nursing home residents with Alzheimer's disease, *American Journal of Alzheimer's Disease and Other Dementias* 22:389–397, 2007.

Williams C, Tappen R: Exercise training for depressed older adults with Alzheimer's disease, *Aging Ment Health* 12:72–80, 2008.

World Health Organization: *Global recommendations on physical activity for health*, 2010. http://www.who.int/dietphysicalactivity/publications/9789241599979/en. http://www.who.int.or.Accessed April 2014.

Yao L, Giordani B, Algase D, et al: Fall risk-relevant functional mobility outcomes in dementia following dyadic Tai Chi exercise, *West J Nurs Res* 35(3):281–296, 2013.

19 CHAPTER

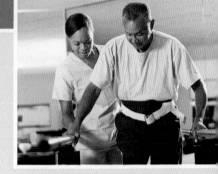

Falls and Fall Risk Reduction

Theris A. Touhy

http://evolve.elsevier.com/Touhy/TwdHlthAging

A STUDENT SPEAKS

The thought of needing someone to help me shower and dress and transfer me from a chair to bed requires more acceptance than I have ever had to muster. I'm very good at making the best out of a bad situation, but somehow adapting to something like never walking again cannot be equated with a "bad situation." It is permanent, and it is the sacrifice of my precious independence. I was born on Independence Day! Thinking about these things overwhelms me with sadness.

Holiday, age 22

AN ELDER SPEAKS

I hate to have the family see me like this. You know, I was a military man. I took pride in the way I marched . . . or just stood at attention. I never imagined a time when I wouldn't be able to walk without assistance.

Jerry, age 78

LEARNING OBJECTIVES

On completion of this chapter, the reader will be able to:
- Discuss the effects of impaired mobility on general function and quality of life.
- Identify risk factors for impaired mobility.
- Identify factors that increase vulnerability to falls.
- Describe assessment measures to determine gait and walking stability.
- List several interventions to reduce fall risks and identify those at high risk.
- Describe the effects of restraints, and identify alternative safety interventions.
- Develop a plan of care for an older adult at risk for falls.

This chapter focuses on the importance of maintaining maximal mobility; assessing gait, mobility, and fall risk factors; implementing fall risk–reduction interventions; providing restraint-free care; and implementing interventions that are useful when mobility is impaired.

MOBILITY AND AGING

Mobility is the capacity one has for movement within the personally available microcosm and macrocosm. This includes abilities such as moving oneself by turning over in bed, transferring from lying to sitting and from sitting to standing, walking, using assistive devices, or accessing transportation within the community environment. In infancy, moving about is the major mode of learning and interacting with the environment.

Throughout life, movement remains a significant means of personal contact, sensation, exploration, pleasure, and control. Retaining pride and maintaining dignity, self-care, independence, social contacts, and activity are all needs identified as important to elders, and all are facilitated by mobility. Mobility is intimately linked to health status and quality of life and healthy aging.

Mobility and comparative degrees of agility are based on muscle strength, flexibility, postural stability, vibratory sensation, cognition, and perceptions of stability. Aging produces changes in muscles and joints (Chapter 26). Individuals who maintain regular physical activity and good health habits throughout life may have fewer of these changes (Chapter 18). Prenatal and postnatal development of muscle fibers and muscle growth during puberty may have critical effects on musculoskeletal aging as well (Kuh, 2007).

Gait and mobility impairments are not an inevitable consequence of aging, but often a result of chronic diseases or past or recent trauma (Alexander, 2014). Mobility and gait impairments are caused by diseases and impairments across many organ systems. For some older people, osteoporosis, gait disorders, Parkinson's disease, strokes, and arthritic conditions markedly affect movement and functional capacities. Mobility may be limited by paresthesias; hemiplegia; neuromotor disturbances; fractures; foot, knee, and hip problems; and respiratory diseases and other illnesses that deplete one's energy. All these conditions are likely to occur more frequently and have more devastating effects as one ages. Many older adults have some of these impairments, with women significantly outnumbering men in this respect (Chapter 21).

Impairment of mobility is an early predictor of physical disability and associated with poor outcomes such as falling, loss of independence, depression, decreased quality of life, institutionalization, and death. Approximately 20% of noninstitutionalized older adults have trouble walking or require assistance from another person or equipment to ambulate. For those older than age 85, the prevalence of these limitations can exceed 54% (Alexander, 2014). Individuals residing in nursing homes have even higher rates of mobility impairment.

Maintenance of mobility and function is an essential component of best practice gerontological nursing and is effective in preventing falls, unnecessary decline, and loss of independence.

FALLS

Falls are one of the most important geriatric syndromes and the leading cause of morbidity and mortality for people older than 65 years of age. In the United States, one in three adults 65 and older falls (Centers for Disease Control and Prevention [CDC], 2014a). Among older adults, falls are the leading cause of both fatal and nonfatal injuries and the most common cause of hospital admissions for trauma (CDC, 2014a; Gray-Miceli and Quigley, 2012). Approximately 20% to 30% of people who fall suffer moderate to severe injuries (lacerations, hip fracture, traumatic brain injury [TBI]) (CDC, 2014; Gray-Miceli and Quigley, 2012). Estimates are that up to two-thirds of falls may be preventable (Lach, 2010). Box 19-1 presents further data on falls.

Falls are a significant public health problem. Worldwide, falls are the second leading cause of accidental or unintentional injury deaths. Greater than 80% of fall-related fatalities occur in low-and middle-income countries, with regions in the Western Pacific and Southeast Asia accounting for more than two-thirds of these deaths. In all regions of the world, death rates are highest among adults older than age 60 years.

The World Health Organization (WHO) recommends policies that support safer environments, promote engineering to remove the potential for falls, train health care providers on evidence-based prevention strategies, and educate individuals and communities to build risk awareness (WHO, 2014). *Healthy People 2020* includes several goals related to falls (Box 19-2).

⚡ SAFETY ALERT

The Quality and Safety Education for Nurses (QSEN) project has developed quality and safety measures for nursing and proposed targets for the knowledge, skills, and attitudes to be developed in nursing prelicensure and graduate programs. Education on falls and fall risk reduction is an important consideration in the QSEN safety competency, which addresses the need to minimize risk of harm to patients and providers through both system effectiveness and individual performance. Safe and effective transfer techniques are an important component of safety measures.

BOX 19-1 Statistics on Falls and Fall-Related Concerns

- One-third of people older than 65 years fall at least one time each year, but less than half talk to their health care provider about it.
- Of those who fall, 20% to 30% suffer moderate to serious injuries, such as hip fractures or head traumas.
- Falls account for 40% of nursing home admissions annually.
- Older adults (75 years of age and older) have the highest rates of traumatic brain injury (TBI)-related hospitalization and death. TBIs account for 46% of fatal falls among older adults.
- More than half of deaths related to falls occur within the home.
- Up to 50% of hospitalized patients are at risk for falls and almost half of those who fall suffer an injury. Between 50% and 75% of nursing home residents fall annually, twice the rate of community-dwelling older adults.
- The death rate from falls is 40% higher for men than women.
- Adults 85 years and older are 10 times more likely to experience a hip fracture than those ages 65 to 69 years.
- Rates of fall-related fractures among older adults are more than twice as high for women as for men. More than 95% of hip fractures among older adults are caused by falls. White women have significantly higher hip fracture rates than black women.
- Between 18% and 33% of older patients with hip fractures die within 1 year of their fracture.
- Up to 25% of adults who lived independently before their hip fracture have to stay in a nursing home for at least 1 year after their injury.
- In 2010, the direct medical cost of falls, adjusted for inflation, was $30 billion. By 2020, the annual and direct costs of fall injuries are expected to reach $54.9 billion (in 2007 dollars).
- Falls are considered a nursing-sensitive quality indicator.
- Falls with resultant fractures, dislocations, and crushing injuries are considered 1 of the 10 hospital-acquired conditions (HACs) that are not covered under Medicare.
- All falls in the nursing home setting are considered sentinel events and must be reported to the Centers for Medicare and Medicaid Services (CMS).
- The Joint Commission (JC) has established national patient safety goals (NPSG) for fall reduction in all JC-approved institutions across the health care continuum.

Data from Centers for Disease Control and Prevention: *Falls among older adults: an overview*, 2014. http://www.cdc.gov/homeandrecreationalsafety/falls/adultfalls.html. Accessed April 2014.

BOX 19-2 HEALTHY PEOPLE 2020

Falls, Fall Prevention, Injury

- Reduce the rate of emergency department visits due to falls among older adults.
- Reduce fatal and nonfatal injuries.
- Reduce hospitalizations for nonfatal injuries.
- Reduce fatal and nonfatal traumatic brain injuries.

Data from U.S. Department of Health and Human Services, Office of Disease Prevention and Health Promotion: Healthy People 2020, 2012. http://www.healthypeople.gov/2020.

Consequences of Falls

Hip Fractures

More than 95% of hip fractures among older adults are caused by falls. Hip fracture is the second leading cause of hospitalization for older people, occurring predominantly in older adults with underlying osteoporosis (Andersen et al, 2010). Hip fractures are associated with considerable morbidity and mortality. Only 50% to 60% of patients with hip fractures will recover their prefracture ambulation abilities in the first year postfracture. Older adults who fracture a hip have a five to eight times increased risk of mortality during the first 3 months after hip fracture. This excess mortality persists for 10 years after the fracture and is higher in men.

Contributing causes to morbidity and mortality were described in a study reporting that hip fracture patients undergo a median of four transitions across health care settings after their fracture and that their recovery is complicated by the presence of multiple comorbid conditions and potentially avoidable problems such as weight loss, delirium, pain, falls, and incontinence (Popejoy et al, 2012) (Box 19-3). Most research on hip fractures has been conducted with older women, and further studies of both men and racially and culturally diverse older adults are necessary (Andersen et al, 2010; CDC, 2010; Haentjens et al, 2010).

Traumatic Brain Injury

Older adults (75 years of age and older) have the highest rates of traumatic brain injury (TBI)-related hospitalization and death. TBI has been called the "silent epidemic" and older adults with TBIs are an even more silent population within this epidemic. Falls are the leading cause of TBI for older adults. Advancing age negatively affects the outcome after TBI, even with relatively minor head injuries. A CDC initiative, *Help Seniors Live Better Longer: Prevent Brain Injury*, provides educational resource materials on TBI for older adults, caregivers, and health care professionals in both Spanish and English (Box 19-4).

Factors that place the older adult at greater risk for TBI include the presence of comorbid conditions, use of aspirin and anticoagulants, and changes in the brain with age. Brain changes with age, although clinically insignificant, do increase the risk of TBIs and especially subdural hematomas, which are much more common in older adults. There is a decreased adherence of the dura mater to the skull, increased fragility of bridging cerebral veins, and increases in the subarachnoid space and

BOX 19-3 RESEARCH HIGHLIGHTS

The purpose of this qualitative, longitudinal, multiple case study research was to describe the number and type of transitions and problems experienced by 21 older adults in the year following surgery for repair of a hip fracture. There were three patterns of transitions identified: Pattern 1—home to hospital to inpatient rehabilitation facility; Pattern 2—home to hospital to skilled nursing facility (SNF); Pattern 3—intermediate nursing home to hospital to SNF. Participants experienced a median of 4 transitions and 4 died in the year following hip fracture; 75% of the patients in Pattern 1, 27% in Pattern 3; and 1 in Pattern 3 returned to prefracture physical functioning.

Problems common to all patterns included weight loss, delirium, depression, infections, pressure ulcers, falls, and urinary incontinence. One participant had a serious wound infection that required six additional surgical procedures; another had a second surgery to replace pins that were displaced; one had orders to ambulate to the bathroom but was supposed to be non–weight bearing; two were placed on low beds to prevent falls but were unable to maintain hip precautions as ordered; and another had a PICC line but no orders for PICC maintenance or the required intravenous antibiotic. Those admitted to SNFs experienced more infections, urinary incontinence, falls, and unrelieved pain than those in inpatient rehabilitation facilities. Participants in SNFs were more functionally impaired before the hip fracture than those in the other groups.

Families often identified problems first, so it is very important that health care staff listen and respond to family members' concerns, which often indicate impending problems. Coordination of care between settings is essential and often absent. Clinical pathways beyond the acute care setting into post discharge settings, identification of appropriate length of stay and discharge criteria, and reimbursement for case management are all needed to improve transitions of care (Chapter 2).

From Popejoy L, Marek K, Scott-Cawiezell J: Patterns and problems associated with transitions after hip fracture in older adults, *J Gerontol Nurs* 39(9):43–52, 2013.

atrophy of the brain, which create more space within the cranial vault for blood to accumulate before symptoms appear (Timmons and Menaker, 2010). Falls are the leading cause of TBI, but older people may experience TBI with seemingly more minor incidents (e.g., sharp turns or jarring movement of the head). Some patients may not even remember the incident.

In cases of moderate to severe TBI, there will be cognitive and physical sequelae obvious at the time of injury or shortly afterward that will require emergency treatment. However, older adults who experience a minor incident with seemingly lesser trauma to the head often present with more insidious and delayed symptom onset. Because of changes in the aging brain, there is an increased risk for slowly expanding subdural hematomas. TBIs are often missed or misdiagnosed among older adults (CDC, 2014).

Health professionals should have a high suspicion of TBI in an older adult who falls and strikes the head or experiences even a more minor event, such as sudden twisting of the head. For older adults who are receiving warfarin and experience minor head injury with a negative computed tomography (CT) scan, a protocol of 24-hour observation followed by a second CT scan is recommended (Mendito et al, 2012). Manifestations of TBI are often misinterpreted as signs of dementia, which can lead to inaccurate prognoses and limit implementation of

BOX 19-4 Guidelines and Protocols for Exercise, Fall Prevention, and Restraint Alternatives

- **Advancing Excellence in America's Nursing Homes:** Fast Facts: Physical Restraints
- **AHRQ:** Preventing falls in hospitals: a toolkit for improving quality of care
- **American Geriatrics Society/British Geriatrics Society:** *Clinical Practice Guideline for Prevention of Falls in Older Persons*
- **American Nurses Association:** *Safe patient handling and mobility: Interprofessional national standards across the care continuum, 2013.*
- **Bradas C, Sandhu S, Mion L:** Physical restraints and side rails in acute and critical care settings. In Boltz M, Capezuti E, Fulmer T et al, editors: *Evidence-based geriatric nursing protocols for best practice,* New York, 2012, Springer, pp 1229–1245.
- **CDC:** STEADI (Stopping Elderly Accidents, Deaths and Injuries): Educational materials for patients and providers; Check for safety: a home fall prevention checklist for older adults; Safe patient handling for schools of nursing (curricular materials)
- **Gericareonline:** Story of Your Falls

- **Gray-Micelli D, Quigley P:** Fall prevention, assessment, diagnoses, and intervention strategies. In Boltz M, Capezuti E, Fulmer T et al, editors: *Evidence-based geriatric nursing protocols for best practice,* ed 4, New York, 2012, Springer, pp 268–297.
- **HELP (Hospital Elder Life) program:** http://www.hospitalelderlifeprogram.org/public/public-main.php.
- **Hartford Institute for Geriatric Nursing** (consultgerirn.org): Fall prevention: assessment, diagnosis, intervention strategies; Avoiding restraints in hospitalized older adults with dementia; Dementia series
- **Institute for Clinical Systems Improvement:** Health care protocol: Prevention of falls (acute care)
- **NIH Senior Health:** Falls and Older Adults—Fall Proofing Your Home
- **The GROW Program:** Getting residents out of wheelchairs
- **TMF Health Quality Institute:** Restraints: Side Rail Utilization Assessment
- **VA National Center for Patient Safety:** Falls Toolkit

BOX 19-5 Signs and Symptoms of Traumatic Brain Injury in Older Adults*

Symptoms of Mild TBI
- Low-grade headache that will not dissipate
- Having more trouble than usual remembering things, paying attention or concentrating, organizing daily tasks, or making decisions and solving problems
- Slowness in thinking, speaking, acting, or reading
- Getting lost or easily confused
- Feeling tired all of the time, lack of energy or motivation
- Change in sleep pattern (sleeping much longer than usual, having trouble sleeping)
- Loss of balance, feeling light-headed or dizzy
- Increased sensitivity to sounds, lights, distractions
- Blurred vision or eyes that tire easily
- Loss of sense of taste or smell
- Ringing in the ears
- Change in sexual drive
- Mood changes (feeling sad, anxious, listless, or becoming easily irritated or angry for little or no reason)

Symptoms of Moderate to Severe TBI
- Severe headache that gets worse or does not disappear
- Repeated vomiting or nausea
- Seizures
- Inability to wake from sleep
- Dilation of one or both pupils
- Slurred speech
- Weakness or numbness in the arms or legs
- Loss of coordination
- Increased confusion, restlessness, or agitation

*NOTE: Older adults taking blood thinners should be seen immediately by a health care provider if they have a bump or blow to the head, even if they do not have any of the symptoms listed here.
From Centers for Disease Control and Prevention: *Help seniors live better, longer: prevent brain injury,* 2014. http://www.cdc.gov/traumaticbraininjury/seniors.html. Accessed April 2014.

appropriate treatment. Box 19-5 presents signs and symptoms of TBI.

Fallophobia

Even if a fall does not result in injury, falls contribute to a loss of confidence that leads to reduced physical activity, increased dependency, and social withdrawal. Fear of falling (fallophobia) may restrict an individual's life space (area in which an individual performs activities). Fear of falling is an important predictor of general functional decline and a risk factor for future falls (Hill et al, 2010; Rubenstein et al, 2003). Assessing the presence of fallophobia and referring for further assessment and management are important in all settings.

Henkel (2002) suggests that nursing staff may also contribute to fear of falling in their patients by telling them not to get up by themselves or by using restrictive devices to keep them from independently moving. More appropriate nursing responses include assessing fall risk and designing individual interventions and safety plans that will enhance mobility and independence, as well as reduce fall risk.

Fall Risk Factors

Falls are a symptom of a problem and are rarely benign in older people. The etiology of falls is multifactorial; falls may indicate neurological, sensory, cardiac, cognitive, medication, or musculoskeletal problems or impending illness. Episodes of acute illness or exacerbations of chronic illness are times of high fall risk. The presence of dementia increases risk for falls twofold, and individuals with dementia are also at increased risk of major injuries (fracture) related to falls. Deanna Gray-Miceli and colleagues (2010) developed seven types of fall classifications based on research (Box 19-6).

BOX 19-6   Fall Classifications

- Falls due to acute events such as OH, loss of balance, syncope
- Falls due to chronic events such as chronic dizziness or lower extremity weakness
- Falls due to medications
- Falls due to environmental mishaps
- Falls due to equipment malfunction
- Falls due to poor safety awareness
- Falls due to poor patient judgment

From Gray-Miceli D, Ratcliffe S, Johnson J: Use of a postfall assessment tool to prevent falls, *West J Nurs Res* 32(7):932–948, 2010.

⚡ SAFETY ALERT

A history of falls is an important risk factor and individuals who have fallen have three times the risk of falling again compared with persons who did not fall in the past year. Recurrent falls are often the result of the same underlying cause but can also be an indication of disease progression (e.g., heart failure, Parkinson's disease) or a new acute problem (e.g., infection, dehydration) (Rubenstein and Dillard, 2014).

Individual risk factors can be categorized as either intrinsic or extrinsic (Box 19-7). Intrinsic risk factors are unique to each individual and are associated with factors such as reduced vision and hearing, unsteady gait, cognitive impairment, acute and chronic illnesses, and effects of medications.

Extrinsic risk factors are external to the individual and related to the physical environment and include lack of support equipment for bathtubs and toilets, height of beds, condition of floors, poor lighting, inappropriate footwear, and improper use of assistive devices.

Falls in the young-old and the more healthy old occur more frequently because of external reasons; however, with increasing age and comorbid conditions, internal and locomotor reasons become increasingly prevalent as factors contributing to falls. The risk of falling increases as the number of risk factors increases. Most falls occur from a combination of intrinsic and extrinsic factors that combine at a certain point in time (Figure 19-1). Other factors may also influence risk for falls. A recent study reported that in a cohort of older men, stressful life events (illness, accidents, death of wife/partner or close relatives or friends, loss of pet, financial trouble, a move or change in residence, or giving up an important hobby) significantly increased risk of falls (Fink et al, 2014).

In institutional settings, extrinsic factors such as limited staffing, the lack of toileting programs, and the use of restraints and side rails also interact to increase fall risk. In hospitals, inadequate staff communication and training, incomplete patient assessments and reassessments, environmental issues, incomplete care planning or delayed care provision, and an inadequate organizational culture of safety have been reported as factors contributing to falls.

BOX 19-7   Fall Risk Factors for Elders

Conditions (Intrinsic)	Situations (Extrinsic)
Sedative and alcohol use, psychoactive medications, opioids, diuretics, anticholinergics, antidepressants, antihypertensives, anticoagulants, bowel preparations	Urinary incontinence, urgency, nocturia
Four or more medications	Environmental hazards
Unrelieved pain	Recent relocation, unfamiliarity with new environment
Previous falls and fractures	Inadequate response to transfer and toileting needs
Female, 80 years of age or older	Improper use of assistive devices
Acute and recent illness; recent hospitalization	Inadequate or missing safety rails, particularly in bathroom
Cognitive impairment (delirium, dementia)	Poorly designed or unstable furniture
Chronic pain	High chairs and beds
Dehydration	Slippery or uneven surfaces
Weakness of lower extremities	Glossy, highly waxed floors
Abnormalities of gait and balance	Wet, greasy, icy surfaces
Unsteadiness, dizziness, syncope	Inadequate visual support (glare, low wattage bulbs, lack of nightlights)
Foot problems	General clutter
Depression, anxiety	Inappropriate footwear/clothing
Decreased vision or hearing	Pets that inadvertently trip an individual
Wearing multifocal glasses while walking	Electrical cords
Fear of falling	Loose or uneven stair treads
Orthostatic hypotension	Throw rugs
Postprandial drop in blood pressure	Reaching for a high shelf
Sleep disorders	Inability to reach personal items, lack of access to call bell or inability to use it
Anemia	Side rails, restraints
Vitamin D deficiency	Lack of staff training in fall risk–reduction techniques
Osteoporosis	
Chronic conditions including arthritis, diabetes, stroke, Parkinson's disease	
Functional limitations in self-care activities	
Inability to rise from a chair without using the arms	
Slow walking speed	
Wheelchair-bound	

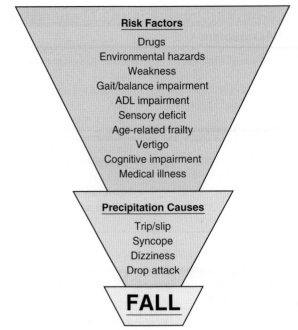

Risk Factors
Drugs
Environmental hazards
Weakness
Gait/balance impairment
ADL impairment
Sensory deficit
Age-related frailty
Vertigo
Cognitive impairment
Medical illness

Precipitation Causes
Trip/slip
Syncope
Dizziness
Drop attack

FALL

FIGURE 19-1 Multifactorial Nature of Falls. (From Ham RJ, Sloane PD, Warshaw GA, et al: *Primary care geriatrics*, ed 6, Philadelphia, 2014, Elsevier, Saunders.)

Gait Disturbances

Gait disturbances, affect between 20% and 50% of people older than 65 years, and are associated with a threefold increase in fall risk (Alexander, 2014). Marked gait disorders are not normally a consequence of aging alone but are more likely indicative of an underlying pathological condition. Arthritis of the knee may result in ligamentous weakness and instability, causing the legs to give way or collapse. Diabetes, dementia, Parkinson's disease, stroke, alcoholism, and vitamin B deficiencies may cause neurological damage and resultant gait problems. Falls were reduced 36% in those with disabling foot pain who received an enhanced podiatry program (Campbell and Robertson, 2013).

Foot Deformities

Foot deformities and ill-fitting footwear also contribute to gait problems and potential for falls. Care of the feet is an important aspect of mobility, comfort, and a stable gait and is often neglected. Little attention is given to one's feet until they interfere with walking and moving and ultimately the ability to remain independent. Foot problems are often unrecognized and untreated, leading to considerable dysfunction.

As we age, feet are subjected to a lifetime of stress and may not be able to continue to adapt, and inflammatory changes in bone and soft tissue can occur. Many individuals are limited by foot problems; approximately 90% of adults 65 and older have some form of altered foot integrity such as nail fungus, dry skin, and corns and calluses (Andersen et al, 2010). Some older persons are unable to walk comfortably, or at all, because of neglect of corns, bunions, and overgrown nails. Other causes of problems may be traced to loss of fat cushioning and resilience with aging, diabetes, ill-fitting shoes, poor arch support, excessively repetitive weight-bearing activities, obesity, or uneven distribution of weight on the feet. Table 19-1 presents common foot problems.

TABLE 19-1 Common Foot Problems

FOOT PROBLEM	PREVENTION/TREATMENT
Corns/calluses: Growths of compacted skin that occur as a result of prolonged pressure, usually from ill-fitting, tight shoes. Corns are cone-shaped and develop on the top of toe joints or between opposing surfaces of the toes from prolonged squeezing. Once formed, corns will cause pain. Unless friction and pressure are relieved, will continue to enlarge and cause increasing pain	OTC preparations may remove temporarily but may burn surrounding tissue and should not be used by diabetics or those with neurological impairment or poor circulation. For individuals with DM or PVD, foot care should be performed by a nurse with expertise in foot care, a doctor, or a podiatrist. **DO NOT** use razor blades, pocket knives, or scissors to remove corns/calluses Padding and protecting the area is the best practice (oval corn pads, gel pads, moleskin, lamb's wool, with a hole cut in the center for the corn) Daily lubrication of the feet; shoes with proper fit
Bunions: Bony deformities that develop from over the medial aspect of the joint of the great toe or at the lateral aspect of the fifth metatarsal head (little toe) Occur from long-standing squeezing of first and second toes; may be a hereditary factor	May be treated with corticosteroid injections and antiinflammatory pain medications. Surgery is also an option Use custom-made shoe(s) that provide(s) forefront space (e.g., running shoes)
Hammer toes: A permanently flexed toe with a clawlike appearance resulting from muscle imbalance and pressure from big toe slanting toward second toe; the toe contracts, leaving a bulge on top of the joint. Result of ill-fitting shoes and often seen in conjunction with bunions	Professional orthotics or specially designed protective devices; properly fitting, nonconstricting shoes and/or surgical intervention
Fungal infections: May affect skin of feet (**tinea pedis**) as well as nails. Nail fungus *(onychomycosis)* is most common nail disorder. Nail plate degenerates with color changes to yellow or brown and opaque, brittleness, and thickening of nail (Figure 19-2). Fine powdery collection of fungus forms under center of the nail, separating the layers and pushing it up, causing the sides of the nail to dig into the skin like an ingrown toenail	Wash hands after handling the feet. Culturing is the only way to diagnose; cure difficult to impossible due to limited circulation to the nails. Several oral medications available but expensive and of limited effectiveness; potentially toxic to liver and heart. Photodynamic therapy (PDT) may be helpful For *tinea pedis* keep areas between the toes clean and dry and regularly exposed to sun and air. Topical antifungal powders are usual treatment. If diabetic, glycemic control important

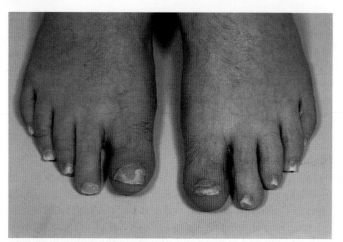

FIGURE 19-2 Onycholysis, Yellowing, Crumbling, and Thickening of the Toenails. (From Bolognia J, Jorizzo JL, Rapini RP, editors: *Dermatology*, ed 2, St Louis, MO, 2007, Mosby.)

Foot health and function may reflect systemic disease or give early clues to physical illness. Sudden or gradual changes in the condition of the nails or the skin of the feet or the appearance of recurring infections may be precursors of more serious health problems. Rheumatological disorders such as the various forms of arthritis usually affect other joints but can also affect the feet. Gout occurs most often in the joint of the great toe but is a systemic disease. Both diabetes and peripheral vascular disease (PVD) commonly cause problems in the lower extremities that can quickly become life-threatening. Estimates are that 20% of individuals with diabetes are admitted to hospitals because of foot problems and more than 60% of nontraumatic lower-limb amputations are performed in people with diabetes (Tewary et al, 2013).

◆ PROMOTING HEALTHY AGING: IMPLICATIONS FOR GERONTOLOGICAL NURSING

Care of the foot takes a team approach, including the person, the nurse, the podiatrist, and the primary health care provider. Nursing care of the person with foot problems should be directed toward providing optimal comfort and function, removing possible mechanical irritants, and decreasing the likelihood of infection. The nurse has the important function of assessing the feet for clues of functional ability and their owner's well-being (Box 19-8). Nurses can identify potential and actual problems and make referral to or seek assistance as needed from the primary care provider or podiatrist for any changes in the feet. Nurses have the opportunity to promote healthy aging by applying their knowledge of the common problems of the feet and their skills in foot care (Box 19-9).

Orthostatic and Postprandial Hypotension

Declines in depth perception, proprioception, and normotensive response to postural changes are important factors that contribute to falls, although the majority of falls occur in individuals with multiple medical problems. Clinically significant orthostatic hypotension (OH) is a common clinical finding in frail older adults. Among cognitively impaired individuals who reside in skilled

---

BOX 19-8   TIPS FOR BEST PRACTICE

Foot Assessment

Observation of Mobility
- Gait
- Use of assistive devices
- Footwear type and pattern of wear

Past Medical History
- Neuropathies
- Musculoskeletal limitations
- Peripheral vascular disease (PVD)
- Vision problems
- History of falls
- Pain affecting movement

Bilateral Assessment
- Color
- Circulation and warmth
- Pulses
- Structural deformities
- Skin lesions
- Lower-extremity edema
- Evidence of scratching
- Abrasions and other lesions
- Rash or excessive dryness
- Condition and color of toenails

BOX 19-9   TIPS FOR BEST PRACTICE

Care of the Feet

- Comprehensive annual foot examination for all persons with diabetes mellitus (DM) including identification of risk factors for ulcers and amputations, test for loss of protective sensation, assessment of pedal pulses
- Care of toenails: Trimmed after bath or shower when softened or soak 20 to 30 minutes before cutting
- Clip straight across and even with top of toe, edges filed slightly to remove sharpness but not to the point of rounding (Figure 19-3)
- Diabetic foot care done only by podiatrist or RN with expertise; persons with DM or PVD should not have pedicures from commercial establishments
- Ingrown toenails are a fragment of nail that pierces the skin at the edge of the nail; may be due to hypertrophy of the nail with onychomycosis, improper cutting, pressure on toes from tight hosiery or shoes. Should be treated by podiatrist due to risk of infection. Temporary relief can be provided by inserting a small piece of cotton under affected nail corner
- Counsel individual about proper footwear. Shoes should cover, protect, and stabilize the foot and provide maximal toe space. Feet increase in size with age and one foot is usually larger than the other. Shoes should be fitted to the largest foot and purchased in the afternoon when feet may be larger. Velcro closures are helpful for those with limited finger dexterity. Closed back shoes of low heel height and high surface contact may reduce risk of falls. Rubber-soled shoe such as sneakers may increase risk of stumbling while walking and may promote too much "sway" and affect balance if person not accustomed to shoes of this kind
- Orthotic and orthopedic shoes may be indicated for certain foot problems. Medicare Part B covers one pair of therapeutic shoes and inserts as durable medical equipment (DME) for individuals with DM

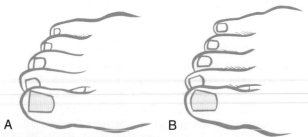

A   B

FIGURE 19-3 Cutting Toenails. A, Correct method. **B,** Incorrect method.

nursing facilities, estimates are that 50% to 60% experience OH (Momeyer, 2014). The detection of orthostatic hypotension (OH) is of clinical importance to fall prevention because OH is treatable. Evidence-based standards of care for fall prevention require OH blood pressure assessment among older adults.

OH coupled with dizziness has been found to be predictive of falls but asymptomatic OH is common. Gray-Micelli and colleagues (2012) reported that loss of balance may be predictive of OH and should trigger assessment. Orthostatic hypotension is considered a decrease of 20 mm Hg (or more) in systolic pressure or a decrease of 10 mm Hg (or more) in diastolic pressure with position change from lying or sitting to standing. However, these criteria may be too restrictive for some older adults (Gray-Micelli et al, 2012). Assessment of orthostatic hypotension in everyday nursing practice is often overlooked or assessed inaccurately (Gray-Micelli et al, 2012; Willy and Osterberg, 2014) (Box 19-10). Box 19-11 presents a protocol for care of individuals with OH in nursing homes.

BOX 19-10 Measuring Orthostatic Blood Pressure

- Orthostatic hypotension is more common in the morning, and therefore assessment should occur then.
- Have the individual lie down for 5 minutes.
- Measure the blood pressure and pulse rate in both arms. Use the arm with the higher blood pressure for measurements following position change.
- Have the individual stand (use safety precautions as needed). If unable to stand, measure blood pressure sitting with feet hanging.
- Take the blood pressure immediately after standing and ask about dizziness.
- Repeat blood pressure and pulse rate measurements after standing for 3 minutes and ask about dizziness.
- A drop in BP of ≥20 mm Hg or in diastolic BP of ≥10 mm Hg or experiencing light-headedness, dizziness, or loss of balance is considered abnormal.

From Momeyer M: Orthostatic hypotension in older adults with dementia, *J Gerontol Nurs* 40(6):22–29, 2014.

BOX 19-11 TIPS FOR BEST PRACTICE

Care of Individuals in Nursing Homes with Orthostatic Hypotension

- Keep head of bed elevated 30 degrees at all times.
- Avoid rapid changes in position, especially in the morning. When transferring out of bed, have individual sit up gradually and dangle feet on side of bed for a few minutes. After assisting to standing position, support for a few minutes before walking.
- Wear compression stockings during the daytime (thigh or knee high). Put on in the morning before getting out of bed; remove at night.
- Encourage coffee or tea with breakfast if tolerated.
- Have individual sit for 20 minutes following a meal.
- Delay physical activity from morning to afternoon or evening when blood pressure is naturally higher.
- Encourage sitting after any type of exercise.
- Avoid standing up too quickly after toileting.
- Encourage adequate fluid intake.
- Encourage dorsiflexion of feet several times before standing.
- Encourage crossing and uncrossing of legs when sitting.

From Momeyer M: Orthostatic hypotension in older adults with dementia, *J Gerontol Nurs* 40(6):22–29, 2014.

Postprandial hypotension (PPH) occurs after ingestion of a carbohydrate meal and may be related to the release of a vasodilatory peptide. PPH is more common in people with diabetes and Parkinson's disease but has been found in approximately 25% of persons who fall. Lifestyle modifications such as increasing water intake before eating or substituting six smaller meals daily for three larger meals may be effective, but further research is needed (Luciano et al, 2010). All older persons should be cautioned against sudden rising from sitting or supine positions, particularly after eating.

Cognitive Impairment

Older adults with cognitive impairment, such as dementia and delirium, are at increased risk for falls. Fall risk assessments may need to include more specific cognitive risk factors, and cognitive assessment measures may need to be more frequently scheduled for at-risk individuals. One study (Harrison et al, 2010) reported that use of the Confusion Assessment Method (CAM) to screen for delirium (Chapter 29), as well as the symptom of inattention, has the potential to improve early detection of fall risk in cognitively impaired hospitalized individuals.

Vision and Hearing

Formal vision assessment is also an important intervention to identify remediable visual problems. Although a significant relationship exists between visual problems and falls and fractures, little research has been conducted on interventions for visual problems as part of fall risk–reduction programs. Poor visual acuity, reduced contrast sensitivity, decreased visual field, cataracts, and use of nonmiotic glaucoma medications have all been associated with falls.

Hearing ability is also directly related to fall risk. For someone with only a mild hearing loss, there is a threefold increased chance of having falls (Lin and Ferrucci, 2012).

Medications

Medications implicated in increasing fall risk include those causing potentially dangerous side effects including drowsiness, mental confusion, problems with balance, loss of urinary control, and sudden drops in blood pressure with standing. These include psychotropics (benzodiazepines, sedative-hypnotics, antidepressants, neuroleptics), antiarrhythmics, digoxin, antihypertensives, and diuretics (Gray-Micelli and Quigley, 2012; Tinetti et al, 2014). All medications, including over-the-counter (OTC) and herbal medications, should be reviewed and limited to those that are absolutely essential.

In a study of the cost-effectiveness of fall prevention programs that reduce hip fracture in older adults, Frick and colleagues (2010) reported that management of psychotropics was the most effective and least expensive fall management option of those considered. The use of low-potency opioids for chronic pain, particularly codeine combinations, is increasing among older adults (Chapter 27). Higher doses of these medications result in twice the risk of injury from falls (Buckeridge et al, 2010). Further research is needed; however, if these medications are being used, patient teaching should be provided related to fall risk, appropriate dosing, and use of other medications, such as benzodiazepines, as well as alcohol use.

◆ PROMOTING HEALTHY AGING: IMPLICATIONS FOR GERONTOLOGICAL NURSING

◆ Screening and Assessment

The American Geriatrics Society/British Geriatrics Society *Clinical Practice Guideline: Prevention of Falls in Older Persons* (2010) recommends that fall risk assessment be an integral part of primary health care for the older person. All older individuals should be asked whether they have fallen in the past year and whether they experience difficulties with walking or balance. In addition, ask about falls that did not result in an injury and the circumstances of a near-fall, mishap, or misstep because this may provide important information for prevention of future falls. Older people may be reluctant to share information about falls for fear of losing independence, so the nurse must use judgment and empathy in eliciting information about falls, assuring the person that there are many modifiable factors to increase safety and help maintain independence.

The intensity of the assessment will vary with the target population:

- Low-risk community-dwelling individuals should be asked at least once a year about fall occurrence and circumstances.
- Individuals who report a single fall should be evaluated for mobility impairment and unsteadiness using a simple observational test, with those who demonstrate mobility problems or unsteadiness being referred for further assessment.
- High-risk populations (individuals who have had multiple falls in the past year, have abnormalities of gait and/or balance, have received medical attention related to a fall, or reside in a nursing home) should undergo a more comprehensive and detailed assessment (Rubenstein and Dillard, 2014).
- Comprehensive fall assessments include the following components: cognitive, nutrition, environment, medications, pathological conditions, functional assessment, feet and footwear, home safety, and a complete physical examination (including vision and hearing, as well as musculoskeletal and cardiovascular status) (Figure 19-4).

◆ Screening and Assessment in Hospital/Long-Term Care

Individuals admitted to acute or long-term care settings should have an initial fall assessment on admission, after any change in condition, and at regular intervals during their stay. Assessment is an ongoing process that includes multiple and continual types of assessment, reassessment, and evaluation following a fall or intervention to reduce the risk of a fall. "Assessment includes: (1) assessment of the older adult at risk; (2) nursing assessment of the patient following a fall; (3) assessment of the environment and other situational circumstances upon admission to a health care facility; (4) assessment of the older adult's knowledge of falls and their prevention, including willingness to change behavior, if necessary, to prevent falls" (Gray-Micelli, 2008, p. 164).

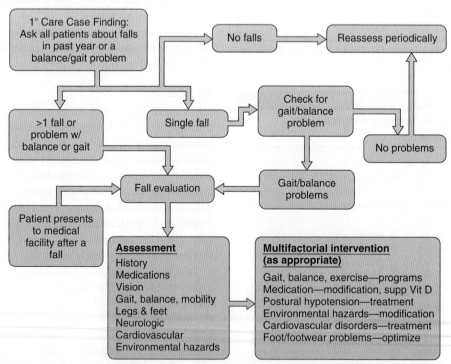

FIGURE 19-4 American Geriatrics Society Fall Assessment and Prevention Algorithm. (From Ham RJ, Sloane PD, Warshaw GA, et al: *Primary care geriatrics*, ed 6, Philadelphia, 2014, Elsevier Saunders. Adapted from Kenny RA, Rubenstein LZ, Tinetti ME, et al: AGS/BGS clinical practice guideline: prevention of falls in older persons, *J Am Geriatr Soc* 59:148–157, 2011.)

An interprofessional team (physician or nurse practitioner, nurse, risk manager, physical and occupational therapists, and other designated staff) should be involved in planning care on the basis of findings from an individualized assessment. Nurses bring expert knowledge of patient activities, abilities, and needs from a 24-hours-per-day, 7-days-per week perspective to help the team implement the most appropriate interventions and evaluate outcomes.

Fall Risk Assessment Instruments

Fall risk is formally assessed through administration of fall risk tools. However, the Institute for Clinical Systems Improvement suggests that current available literature (Degelau et al, 2012) supports using the following three questions to determine fall risk: (1) Has the patient fallen in the past year? (2) Does the patient look like he or she is going to fall (does the patient have clinically detected gait/balance abnormalities)? (3) Does the patient have additional risk factors for injurious falls (e.g., osteoporosis, anticoagulant therapy)?

Fall risk assessment instruments are still commonly included in fall prevention interventions; instruments that are utilized need to be reliable and valid and nurses need to use them judiciously (Gray-Micelli and Quigley, 2012). Often, these instruments are completed in a routine manner and risk factors are not identified or may not be known because of lack of assessment and knowledge of the individual's history. Additionally, so many patients are identified as high risk that nurses may become desensitized and have difficulty prioritizing interventions (Harrison et al, 2010; Lach, 2010). Current literature suggests that commonly used fall risk assessment tools are becoming outdated and used infrequently in assessment of community-dwelling

individuals (Hester and Wei, 2013). Additional research is needed to develop valid, reliable instruments to differentiate levels of fall risk in various settings.

The National Center for Patient Safety recommends the Morse Falls Scale, but not for use in long-term care (Box 19-4). The Performance-Oriented Mobility Assessment (Tinetti, 1986) is a well-validated tool. The Hendrich II Fall Risk Model (Hendrich et al, 2003) (see Figure 18-1), which also includes a modified Get Up and Go test, is recommended by the Hartford Foundation for Geriatric Nursing. This instrument has been validated with skilled nursing and rehabilitation populations and is also easy to use in the outpatient setting. In the skilled nursing facility, the Minimum Data Set (MDS 3.0) includes information about history of falls and hip fractures, as well as an assessment of balance during transitions and walking (moving from seated to standing, walking, turning around, moving on and off toilet, and transfers between bed and chair or wheelchair) (Chapter 7).

Fall risk assessments provide first-level assessment data as the basis for comprehensive assessment, but comprehensive postfall assessments (PFAs) (Box 19-12) must be used to identify multifactorial, complex fall and injury risk factors in those who have fallen (Gray-Micelli and Quigley, 2012). It is very important that all assessment data reported concerning an individual's risk for falls be tailored with individual assessment so that appropriate fall risk–reduction interventions can be developed and modifiable risk factors identified and managed.

Postfall Assessment

Determination of the reason(s) a fall occurred (postfall assessment [PFA]) is vital and provides information on underlying

---

BOX 19-12 Postfall Assessment Suggestions

Initiate emergency measures as indicated.

History
- Description of the fall from the individual or witness
- Individual's opinion of the cause of the fall
- Circumstances of the fall (trip or slip)
- Person's activity at the time of the fall
- Presence of comorbid conditions, such as a previous stroke, Parkinson's disease, osteoporosis, seizure disorder, sensory deficit, joint abnormalities, depression, cardiac disease
- Medication review
- Associated symptoms, such as chest pain, palpitations, light-headedness, vertigo, loss of balance, fainting, weakness, confusion, incontinence, or dyspnea
- Time of day and location of the fall
- Presence of acute illness

Physical Examination
- Vital signs: postural blood pressure changes, fever, or hypothermia
- Head and neck: visual impairment, hearing impairment, nystagmus, bruit
- Heart: arrhythmia or valvular dysfunction
- Neurological signs: altered mental status, focal deficits, peripheral neuropathy, muscle weakness, rigidity or tremor, impaired balance
- Musculoskeletal signs: arthritic changes, range of motion (ROM), podiatric deformities or problems, swelling, redness or bruises, abrasions, pain on movement, shortening and external rotation of lower extremities

Functional Assessment
- Functional gait and balance: observe resident rising from chair, walking, turning, and sitting down
- Balance test, mobility, use of assistive devices or personal assistance, extent of ambulation, restraint use, prosthetic equipment
- Activities of daily living: bathing, dressing, transferring, toileting

Environmental Assessment
- Staffing patterns, unsafe practice in transferring, delay in response to call light
- Faulty equipment
- Use of bed, chair alarm
- Call light within reach
- Wheelchair, bed locked
- Adequate supervision
- Clutter, walking paths not clear
- Dim lighting
- Glare
- Uneven flooring
- Wet, slippery floors
- Poorly fitted seating devices
- Inappropriate footwear
- Inappropriate eyewear

fall etiologies so that appropriate plans of care can be instituted. Incomplete analysis of the reasons for a fall can result in repeated incidents. "When important details are overlooked, missing information leads to an inappropriate plan of care" (Gray-Micelli, 2008, p. 33). The purpose of the PFA is to identify the clinical status of the person, verify and treat injuries, identify underlying causes of the fall when possible, and assist in implementing appropriate individualized risk-reduction interventions. For falls that happen outside the hospital or skilled nursing facility, individuals can complete the "Story of Your Falls" (see Box 19-4) to provide postfall assessment information.

Components of the PFA

PFAs include a fall-focused history; fall circumstances; medical problems; medication review; mobility assessment; vision and hearing assessment; neurological examination (including cognitive assessment); and cardiovascular assessment (orthostatic blood pressure [BP], cardiac rhythm irregularities) (Gray-Micelli and Quigley, 2012). If the older adult cannot tell you about the circumstances of the fall, information should be obtained from staff or witnesses. Because complications of falls may not occur immediately, all patients should be observed for 48 hours after a fall and vital signs and neurological status monitored for 7 days or more, as clinically indicated. Standard "incident report" forms do not provide adequate postfall assessment information. The Department of Veterans Affairs National Center for Patient Safety provides comprehensive information about fall assessment, fall risk reduction, and policies and procedures. Box 19-12 presents information for a PFA that can be used in health care institutions.

Interventions

Lach (2010) reminds us that "while there is much that the nurse can do to manage falls, it may be unrealistic to think that they can be eliminated" (p. 151). Fall risk–reduction programs are a shared responsibility of all health care providers caring for older adults. Choosing the most appropriate interventions to reduce the risk of falls depends on appropriate assessment at various intervals depending on the person's changing condition and tailoring interventions to individual cognitive function and language (American Geriatrics Society and British Geriatrics Society, 2010). A one-size-fits-all approach is not effective and further research is needed to determine the type, frequency, and timing of interventions best suited for specific populations.

Fall Risk–Reduction Programs

There is some evidence to support the effectiveness of multi-component fall risk–reduction strategies in many settings to reduce fall risks (Alexander, 2014; Cameron et al, 2010; Gillespie et al, 2012; Lee et al, 2013; Miake-Lye et al, 2013; Quigley and White, 2013; Tinetti et al, 2008). Randomized controlled trial evidence also suggests that single targeted interventions (e.g., exercise programs) might be as effective as multifactorial interventions (Campbell and Robertson, 2013). Frick and colleagues (2010) agree and suggest that multifactorial approaches aimed at all older people, or high-risk elders, are not necessarily

more cost-effective or more efficacious than focused intervention approaches and further research is needed.

The optimal bundle of interventions is not established, but common components include risk assessment, patient and staff education, bedside signs and wristband alerts, footwear assessment, scheduled and supervised toileting programs, and medication reviews (Miake-Lye et al, 2013). The components most commonly included in efficacious interventions are shown in Box 19-13

Each institution should design strategies to meet organizational needs and to match patient population needs and clinical realities of the staff (Ireland et al, 2010). Programs which utilize a system-level quality improvement approach, including educational programs for staff, realized a decrease in fall rate of 5.8% in hospitals (Box 19-14). Examples of effective programs include Acute Care of the Elderly units (ACE), Nurses Improving Care for Healthsystem Elders (NICHE), and the Geriatric Resource Nurse (GRN) model (Gray-Micelli and Quigley, 2012) (Chapter 2). The Hospital Elder Life Program (HELP) is another valuable resource in fall prevention in the hospital (see Box 19-4).

Box 19-15 presents an innovative fall risk–reduction program, designed by a nurse in an acute care facility that has been adopted around the country and included in fall risk–reduction guidelines. Other innovative programs in nursing homes include

---

BOX 19-13   Suggested Components of Fall Risk–Reduction Interventions

- Adaptation or modification of the home environment
- Withdrawal or minimization of psychoactive medications
- Withdrawal or minimization of other medications
- Management of orthostatic hypotension
- Continence programs such as prompted voiding
- Management of foot problems and footwear
- Exercise, particularly balance, strength, and gait training
- Staff and patient education

From American Geriatrics Society/British Geriatrics Society: *2010 AGS/BGS clinical practice guideline: Prevention of falls in older persons, Summary of recommendations,* 2010. http://www.americangeriatrics.org/files/documents/health_care_pros/Falls.Summary.Guide.pdf Accessed April 2014.

BOX 19-14   System-Level Interventions in Acute Care

- Nurse Champions
- Teach Backs (all patients and families receive education about their fall and injury risks)
- Comfort Care and Safety Rounds
- Safety Huddle Post Fall
- Interventions to Reduce Trauma/Protective Bundles (patients with risk factors for serious injury such as osteoporosis, anticoagulant use, history of head injury, or falls are automatically placed on high-risk fall precautions and interventions to reduce risk of serious injury; bundles may include interventions such as bedside mat on floor at side of bed, height-adjustable bed, helmet use, hip protectors, comfort and safety rounds)

From Gray-Miceli D, Quigley P: Fall prevention, assessment, diagnoses, and intervention strategies. In Boltz M, Capezuti E, Fulmer T, et al, editors: *Evidence-based geriatric nursing protocols for best practice,* ed 4, New York, 2012, Springer, pp 268–297.

the Visiting Angels and neighborhood watch teams. In the Visiting Angels program, alert residents visit and converse with cognitively impaired residents in the late afternoon and evening when fall risk starts to rise. Neighborhood watch teams involve the evening and night staff in morning reviews of any fall or incident that happened during the night (Kilgore, 2010). There are many excellent sources of information for both consumers and health care professionals on interventions to reduce fall risk (see Box 19-4).

Environmental Modifications

Environmental modifications alone have not been shown to reduce falls, but when included as part of a multifactorial program, they may be of benefit in risk reduction. However, a home safety assessment and modification interventions have been shown to be effective in reducing the rates of falls, especially for individuals at high risk of falling and those with visual impairments. It is recommended that home safety interventions be delivered by an occupational therapist (American Geriatrics Society, 2010; Gillespie et al, 2012). The CDC provides a home fall prevention checklist (see Box 19-4), and a comprehensive home safety assessment can be found in Chapter 20.

In institutional settings, the patient care environment should be assessed routinely for extrinsic factors that may contribute to falls and corrective action taken. Patients should be able to access the bathroom or be provided with a bedside commode, routine assistance to toilet, and programs such as prompted voiding (Chapter 16). The majority of falls in acute care occur in patient rooms (79.5%) followed by bathrooms (11%) and hallways (9.5%) (Tzeng and Yin, 2008). Important areas to check for safety are presented in Box 19-16.

Assistive Devices

Research on multifactorial interventions including the use of assistive devices has demonstrated benefits in fall risk reduction. Many devices are available that are designed for specific conditions and limitations. Physical therapists provide training on use of assistive devices, and nurses can supervise correct use. Improper use of these devices can lead to increased fall risk (Box 19-17). For the community-dwelling individual, Medicare may cover up to 80% of the cost of assistive devices with a written prescription. New technologies such as canes that "talk" and provide feedback to the user, sensors that detect when falls have occurred or when risk of falling is increasing, and other developing assistive technologies hold the potential to significantly improve functional ability, safety, and independence for older people (Rantz et al, 2008) (Chapter 20).

BOX 19-17 TIPS FOR BEST PRACTICE

Use of Assistive Devices

Cane Use

- Place your cane firmly on the ground before you take a step, and do not place it too far ahead of you. Put all of your weight on your unaffected leg, and then move the cane and your affected leg at a comfortable distance forward. With your weight supported on both the cane and your affected leg, step through with your unaffected leg.
- Always wear low-heeled, nonskid shoes. It is best to have the person wear the kind of shoes he or she is accustomed to wearing, and consideration should be given to properly fit orthotic shoes as appropriate.
- When using a cane on stairs, step up with the unaffected leg and down with the affected leg. Use the cane as support when lifting the affected leg. Bring the cane up to the step just reached before climbing another step. When descending, place the cane on the next step down, move the affected leg down, and then move the unaffected leg down.
- Every assistive device must be adjusted to individual height; the top of the cane should align with the crease of the wrist.
- Choose a size and shape of cane handle that fits comfortably in the palm; like a tight shoe, it will be a constant irritant if it is not properly fitted.
- Cane tips are most secure when they are flat at the bottom and have a series of rings. Replace tips frequently because they wear out, and a worn tip is insecure.

Walker Use

- When using a walker, stand upright and lift or roll the walker with both hands a step's length ahead of you. Lean slightly forward, and hold the arms of the walker for support. Step toward it with the affected leg and then bring the unaffected leg forward.
- Do not climb stairs with a walker.

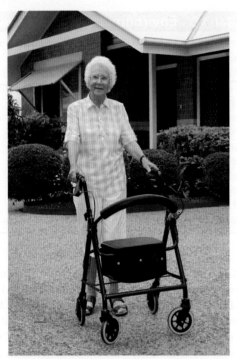

Maintaining Ambulation and Safety with Appropriate Assistive Devices. (©iStock.com/pamspix)

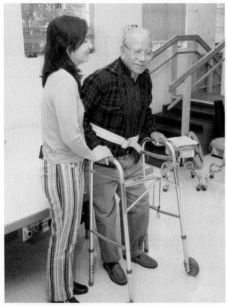

A Physical Therapist Helping a Client to Ambulate. (From Ignatavicius DD, Workman ML: *Medical-surgical nursing: patient-centered collaborative care,* ed 6, St Louis, MO, 2010, Saunders.)

Safe Patient Handling

Lifting, transferring, and repositioning patients are the most common tasks that lead to injury for health care staff and patients in hospital and nursing home environments. Handling and moving patients offers multiple challenges because of variations in size, physical abilities, cognitive function, level of cooperation, and changes in condition.

Nelson and Baptiste (2004) recommend the following evidence-based practices for safe patient handling: (1) patient handling equipment/devices; (2) patient-care ergonomic assessment protocols; (3) no lift policies; (4) training on proper use of patient handling equipment/devices; and (5) patient lift teams. Examples of helpful equipment are ceiling- and floor-based dependent lifts, sit-to-stand assists, ambulation aids, motorized hospital beds, powered shower chairs, and friction-reducing devices (American Nurses Association, 2013; Campo et al, 2013). Key aspects of patient assessment to improve safety for patients and staff are presented in Box 19-18.

Wheelchairs

Wheelchairs are a necessary adjunct at some level of immobility and for some individuals, but they are overused in nursing homes, with up to 80% of residents spending time sitting in a wheelchair every day. Often, the individual is not assessed for therapeutic treatment and restorative ambulation programs to improve mobility and function. Improperly maintained or ill-fitting wheelchairs can cause pressure ulcers, skin tears, bruises and abrasions, and nerve impingement, and they account for 16% of nursing home falls (Gavin-Dreschnack et al, 2010). It is important that a professional evaluate the wheelchair for proper fit and provide training on proper use, as well as evaluate the resident for more appropriate mobility and seating devices and ambulation programs. There are many new assistive devices that could replace wheelchairs, such as small walkers with wheels and seats.

All nursing homes need to implement programs that promote ambulation and improve function. Brief walks and repeated chair stands four times a day improved walking and endurance in frail, deconditioned, cognitively impaired nursing home residents (Gavin-Dreschnack et al, 2010). If the person is unable to ambulate without assistance, the person should be seated in a comfortable chair with frequent repositioning and

BOX 19-18	**TIPS FOR BEST PRACTICE**

Assessment of Safe Patient Handling

- Ability of the patient to provide assistance
- Ability of the patient to bear weight
- Upper extremity strength of the patient
- Ability of the patient to cooperate and follow instructions
- Patient height and weight
- Special circumstances likely to affect transfer or repositioning tasks, such as abdominal wounds, contractures, pressure ulcers, presence of tubes
- Specific physician orders or physical therapy recommendations that relate to transferring or repositioning patients (e.g., knee or hip replacement precautions)

From Nelson A, Baptiste A: Evidence-based practices for safe patient handling and movement, *Online J Issues Nurs* 9(3), 2004. http://www.seiu1991.org/files/2013/07/Audrey_Nelson_Safe_Patient_Handling.pdf. Accessed April 2014.

wheelchairs should be used for transport only. Electric scooters and wheelchairs may be appropriate for some residents as well, but instruction on safe use is necessary. At one Veterans Affairs medical center, the physical therapists held driving classes to teach safety with these devices.

The GROW initiative (Getting Residents Out of Wheelchairs) (Box 19-4) was conceived by a group of health professionals to lobby against the overuse of wheelchairs in nursing homes. The program advocates for increased ambulation whenever possible and decreasing the use of wheelchairs when regular chairs could be used for stationary seating. Their mission is to support the Advancing Excellence in America's Nursing Homes campaign, which is discussed further in Chapter 32 (Gavin-Dreschnack et al, 2010).

Osteoporosis Treatment/Vitamin D Supplementation

Other potential interventions for fall risk reduction include assessment and treatment of osteoporosis to reduce fracture rates (Chapter 26). Older people with osteoporosis are more likely to experience serious injury from a fall. The American Geriatrics Association recommends vitamin D supplementation of at least 1000 international units, as well as calcium supplementation, to community-dwelling and older adults residing in institutionalized settings to reduce the risk of fractures and falls (AGS, 2014b). In the nursing home population, more than 40% of residents have a vitamin D deficiency, defined as a level <20 ng/mL. Individuals with low levels of vitamin D have up to a 40% increased risk of hip fracture compared with those with high vitamin D levels (Li-MacDonald et al, 2014; Willy and Osterberg, 2014).

Hip Protectors

The use of hip protectors for prevention of hip fractures in high-risk individuals may be considered, and there is some evidence that they may have an overall effect on rates of hip fracture (Quigley et al, 2010), but further research is needed to determine their effectiveness. Compliance has been a concern related to the ease of application and removing them quickly enough for toileting, but newer designs that are more attractive and practical may assist with compliance issues (Willy and Osterberg, 2014).

Alarms/Motion Sensors

Alarms, either personal or chair/bed, are often used in fall prevention programs. There has been no research to support their effectiveness in prevention of a fall and "at best, it can shorten 'rescue time' " (Willy and Osterberg, 2014, p. 29). Some have suggested that the use of these alarms may increase patient agitation, especially in cognitively impaired individuals, and that their use may be more for the needs of the staff rather than the patients (Willy and Osterberg, 2014). Silent alarms, visual or auditory monitoring systems, motion detectors, and physical staff presence may be more effective. A recent study reported that use of motion sensors inside patient rooms may be a viable, cost-efficient, unobtrusive solution to prevent and detect falls (Rantz et al, 2014).

RESTRAINTS AND SIDE RAILS

Definition and History

A physical restraint is defined as any manual method, physical or mechanical device, material, or equipment that immobilizes or reduces the ability of a patient to move his or her arms, legs, body, or head freely. A chemical restraint is when a drug or medication is used as a restriction to manage the patient's behavior or restrict the patient's freedom of movement and is not a standard treatment or dosage for the patient's condition. Historically, restraints and side rails have been used for the "protection" of the patient and for the security of the patient and staff. Originally, restraints were used to control the behavior of individuals with mental illness considered to be dangerous to themselves or others (Evans and Strumpf, 1989).

Research over the past 30 years by nurses such as Lois Evans, Neville Strumpf, and Elizabeth Capezuti has shown that the practice of physical restraint is ineffective and hazardous. The use of physical restraints in long-term care settings was effectively addressed almost 25 years ago through nursing home reform legislation, resulting in a major reduction of physical restraint use in these facilities. The number of residents in nursing homes who were physically restrained dropped by more than half from 1999 to 2007 (AHRQ, 2010). The Joint Commission and the Centers for Medicare and Medicaid Services (CMS) have focused on restraint reduction strategies in acute care over the past 10 to 15 years but the use still remains common (American Geriatrics Society, 2010; Bradas et al, 2012).

Consequences of Restraints

Physical restraints, intended to prevent injury, do not protect patients from falling, wandering, or removing tubes and other medical devices. Physical restraints may actually exacerbate many of the problems for which they are used and can cause serious injury and death, as well as emotional and physical problems. "The most common mechanism of restraint-related death is by asphyxiation—that is, the person is suspended by a restraint from a bed or chair and the ability to inhale is inhibited by gravitational chest compression" (Wagner et al, 2007, p. 168).

Physical restraints are associated with higher death rates, injurious falls, nosocomial infections, incontinence, contractures, pressure ulcers, agitation, and depression. Although prevention of falls is most frequently cited as the primary reason for using restraints, restraints do not prevent serious injury and may even increase the risk of injury and death. Injuries occur as a result of the patient attempting to remove the restraint or attempting to get out of bed while restrained.

The use of restraints is a great source of physical and psychological distress to older adults and may intensify agitation and contribute to depression. Side rails may be seen as a barrier rather than a reminder of the need to request assistance with transfers. And, for some older people, especially those with a history of trauma (such as that induced by war, rape, or domestic violence), side rails may cause fear and agitation and a feeling of being jailed or caged (Sullivan-Marx, 1995; Talerico and Capezuti, 2001) (Box 19-19).

Side Rails

Side rails are no longer viewed as simply attachments to a patient's bed but are considered restraints with all the accompanying concerns just discussed. Side rails are now defined as restraints or restrictive devices when used to impede a person's ability to voluntarily get out of bed and the person cannot lower them by themselves. Restrictive side rail use is defined as two full-length or four half-length raised side rails. If the patient uses a half- or quarter-length upper side rail to assist in getting in and out of bed, it is not considered a restraint (Talerico and Capezuti, 2001).

There is no evidence to date that side rail use decreases the risk or rate of fall occurrence. There are numerous reports and studies documenting the negative effects of side rail use, including entrapment deaths and injuries that occur when the person slips through the side rail bars or between split side rails, the side rail and the mattress, or between the headboard or footboard, side rail, and mattress (Talerico and Capezuti, 2001; Wagner et al, 2007).

The Centers for Medicare and Medicaid Services (CMS) require nursing homes to conduct individualized assessments of residents, provide alternatives, or clearly document the need for restrictive side rails (Sollins, 2009). Capezuti and colleagues (1999) describe an individualized assessment tool for side rail use. A side rail utilization assessment, adapted from the work of Capezuti and colleagues (1999), is available from TMF Health Quality Institute (see Box 19-4).

Restraint-Free Care

Restraint-free care is now the standard of practice and an indicator of quality care in all health care settings, although transition to that standard is still in progress, particularly in acute care settings. Physical restraint use in acute care is now predominantly in intensive care units (ICUs), particularly for patients with medical devices and those with delirium. Older adults with delirium have higher risks of being restrained than other patients. Both the American Geriatrics Society and the American Board of Internal Medicine recommend that physical restraints should not be used to manage behavioral symptoms of hospitalized older adults with delirium (American Geriatrics Society, 2014a).

Further research is needed in ICU settings to determine the best strategies to manage delirium (Chapter 29). Daily evaluation of the necessity of medical devices (intravenous lines, nasogastric tubes, catheters, endotracheal tubes), as well as securing or camouflaging (hiding) the device, is important (American Geriatrics Society, 2010; Bradas et al, 2012) (Box 19-20). Evidence-based protocols on physical restraints and other resources on restraint alternatives can be found in Box 19-4.

Flaherty (2004) remarked that a "restraint-free environment should be held as the standard of care and anything less is substandard. The fact that it is done in some European hospitals (Bradas et al, 2012; de Vries et al, 2004) and in some U.S. hospitals, even among delirious patients, and in skilled

BOX 19-19   Being Restrained

"I felt like a dog and cried all night. It hurt me to have to be tied up. I felt like I was nobody, that I was dirt. It makes me cry to talk about it. The hospital is worse than a jail."

"I don't remember misbehaving, but I may have been deranged from all the pills they gave me. Normally, I am spirited, but I am also good and obedient. Nevertheless, the nurse tied me down, like Jesus on the cross, by bandaging both wrists and ankles . . . It felt awful, I hurt and I worried. Callers, including men friends, saw me like that and thought I lost something. I lost a little personal prestige. I was embarrassed, like a child placed in a corner for being bad. I had been important . . . and to be tied down in bed took a big toll . . . I haven't forgotten the pain and the indignity of being tied."

BOX 19-20   TIPS FOR BEST PRACTICE

Dealing with Tubes, Lines, and Other Medical Devices

- First question: "Is the device really necessary?" Remove it as soon as possible.
- Preoperative teaching about the device: Allowing the person to see the tubes may be effective in decreasing anxiety about devices.
- Use guided exploration and a mirror to help the patient understand what devices are in place and why.
- Provide comfort care to the site—oral and nasal care, anchoring of tubing, topical anesthetic on site.
- Foley catheters should be used only if the patient needs intensive output monitoring or has an obstruction.
- Weigh risks and benefits of restraint versus therapy: alternatives available—for example, replace intravenous (IV) tubing with saline lock, deliver medications intramuscularly (IM), consider intermittent IV administration or hypodermoclysis.
- Use camouflage: clothing or elastic sleeves, temporary air splint (occupational therapy can be helpful), skin sleeves to prevent IV tube dislodgement.
- Use mitts instead of wrist restraints; use roll belts instead of vest restraints.
- Use diversional activity aprons (zipping-unzipping, threading exercises, dials and knobs), busy box, therapeutic activity kit, twiddle (activity) muff.
- Hide lines by placing them in an unobtrusive place; place tubing behind the patient, out of his or her view; have patient wear long sleeves or double surgical gowns with cuffs to prevent access.
- Hang IV bags behind the patient's field of vision.
- Nasogastric (NG) tubes—replace with percutaneous endoscopic gastrostomy (PEG) tube if necessary but obtain comprehensive speech therapy swallowing evaluation. If NG tube is used, use as small a lumen as possible to minimize irritation; consider taping with occlusive dressings.
- Cover the PEG tube or abdominal incisions and other tubes with an abdominal binder and/or sweat pants.
- For men with Foley catheters—shave area just above pubis, and tape catheter to pubis. *Never* secure catheter to leg (causes discomfort and can cause a fistula). Run tubing around back and down leg to a leg bag. Patient should wear underpants and pajama pants.
- Remove restraints while working with the patient.
- Use a modified soft collar for tracheostomy protection.

nursing facilities should be evidence enough that it can be done everywhere" (p. 919). Implementing best practice nursing in fall risk reduction and restraint-free care is a complex clinical decision-making process and calls for recognition, assessment, and intervention for physical and psychosocial concerns contributing to patient safety, knowledge of restraint alternatives, interdisciplinary teamwork, and institutional commitment.

Antonelli (2008) described a comprehensive restraint management program in an acute care setting that was successful in improving care practices and reducing restraint use. Included in the program were the development of a restraint prevention cart to increase the accessibility of alternatives to restraints, rounds and consultation led by a geriatric nurse practitioner, the use of college and high school students as activity assistants, and staff education.

Removing restraints without careful attention to underlying fall risk factors and effective alternative strategies can jeopardize safety. The use of advanced practice nurse consultation in implementing alternatives to restraints has been most effective (Bourbonniere and Evans, 2002; Capezuti, 2004; Wagner et al, 2007). Important areas of focus derived from research on advanced practice nurse consultations are presented in Box 19-21.

BOX 19-21   Suggestions from Advanced Practice Nursing Consultation on Restraint-Free Fall Prevention Interventions

- Compensating for memory loss (e.g., improving behavior, anticipating needs, providing visual and physical cues)
- Improving impaired mobility; reducing injury potential
- Evaluating nocturia/incontinence; reducing sleep disturbances
- Implementing restraint-free fall prevention interventions based on conducting careful individualized assessments; what works for one individual may not necessarily be effective for another.

From Wagner L, Capezuti E, Brush B, et al: Description of an advanced practice nursing consultative model to reduce restrictive siderail use in nursing homes, *Res Nurs Health* 30:131–140, 2007.

Staff education is also important and one study reported increased knowledge, attitude change, and reduction of the use of physical restraints without any change in the incidence of falls or use of psychoactive medications after a 6-month education program (Pellfolk et al, 2010). Many of the suggestions on safety and fall risk reduction in this chapter can be used to promote a safe and restraint-free environment. Fall risk reduction and alternative strategies to restraints are presented in Box 19-22.

BOX 19-22   TIPS FOR BEST PRACTICE

Fall Risk Reduction and Restraint Alternatives

Assessment

- Work with the interdisciplinary team; nurses cannot manage these complicated challenges alone.
- Perform fall risk screening; gait, balance, and mobility assessment; and multifactorial assessment as indicated.
- Individualize the patient's plan of care based on risk factors and condition.
- Assess ambulation ability; refer to physical therapy for walking and/or strengthening programs.
- Check for postural hypotension (orthostasis).
- Use a behavior log to track when the person is trying to get up and/or when he or she seems agitated.
- Assess mental status (delirium/dementia).
- Assess vision and hearing. If the person wears glasses, hearing aid, or dentures, ensure that the assistive devices are worn.
- Assess continence status.
- Assess for pain and ensure that pain is well managed.
- Involve family and all staff in fall risk–reduction education and activities.
- Inform all staff of fall risk, and put fall risk and fall risk–reduction interventions on care plan.
- Use identification bracelet or door sign to indicate patients at risk for falling. Use red socks with treads to identify patient at risk.

Patient Room

- Lower the bed to the lowest level, or use a bed that is especially designed to be low to the floor.
- Use a concave mattress.
- Use bed boundary markers to mark the edges of the bed, such as mattress bumpers, rolled blanket, or "swimming noodles" under sheets.
- If the person is (or has been married), line the spouse's side of the bed with pillows or bolsters.

- Place a soft floor mat or a mattress by the bed to cushion any falls.
- Use a water mattress to reduce movement to the edge of the bed.
- Have the person at risk sleep on a mattress on the floor.
- Remove wheels from the bed.
- Clear the floor of debris or excessive furniture; make sure it is not wet or slippery.
- Place nonskid strips on the floor next to the bed; ensure that floors are nonskid.
- Use night lights in the bedroom and bathroom.
- Place a call bell within reach, and make sure the patient can use it—attach the call bell to the patient's garment or obtain an adapted call device.
- Provide visual reminders to encourage the patient to use the call bell.
- Have a purse (empty or without harmful items or important papers or money) in the bed with the person, if a woman.
- Ensure all personal items are within reach.
- Have ambulation devices within reach, and make sure the patient knows how to use them properly.
- Use bed, chair, or wrist alarms (the best alarm tells you only that there is an emergency; still need frequent checks, supervised areas). Apply a patient-worn sensor (lightweight alarm worn above the knee that is position-sensitive).
- Provide a trapeze or patient assist handles (transfer bars) to enhance mobility in bed.
- If the person is able, he or she should walk at every opportunity possible. If the patient walked in or could walk before hospitalization, make every effort to keep the patient walking during hospitalization.
- Do frequent bed checks, especially during the evening and at night.
- Be especially alert for falls at change-of-shift times.
- Understand that very few people spend all day in bed; activity is necessary.
- Provide diversional activities (catalogues, puzzles, therapeutic activity kit) (http://consultgerirn.org/uploads/File/trythis/try_this_d4.pdf).
- Know sleeping patterns—if the person is usually up during the night, get him or her up in a chair and keep at nursing station or involve in activities.

Continued

BOX 19-22 TIPS FOR BEST PRACTICE

Fall Risk Reduction and Restraint Alternatives—cont'd

Bathroom
- Establish toileting plan, and take the person to the bathroom frequently.
- Have the person use a bedside commode.
- Make sure the person knows the location of the bathroom—leave the door open so that he or she can see the toilet, or put a picture of a toilet on the door; clear the path to the bathroom.
- Provide grab bars in the bathroom and shower; provide a shower chair with suction bottom.
- Provide an elevated toilet seat.
- Have the person wear clothing that is easy to pull down for toileting.

On the Unit
- Assess for environmental hazards.
- Keep the person in a supervised area or room within view of the nursing station.

- Have the person sit in a reclining chair, chair with a deep seat, bean bag chair, rocker—keep close to nurses' station in the chair.
- Consider occupational therapy evaluation for seating devices.
- Provide a supervised area and meaningful activities.
- If the person is wandering or trying to exit, create a grid with masking tape on the floor in front of the doorway, use a black half-rug, and camouflage exit doors with wallpaper or window treatments. These adaptations may cause the person to stop before going out the door.
- Provide hip protectors, helmets, and arm pads for high-risk individuals.
- Investigate the Hospital Elder Life Program (HELP) and consider implementing (http://www.hospitalelderlifeprogram.org/public/public-main.ph.).
- Provide a restraint management cart with alternative restraint products arranged in order of least restrictive measures as described by Antonelli (2008).

KEY CONCEPTS

- Mobility provides opportunities for exercise, exploration, and pleasure and is the crux of maintaining independence.
- Changes in bones, muscles, and ligaments and illnesses affect balance and gait as one ages and increase instability. Gait and mobility impairments are not an inevitable consequence of aging, but often a result of chronic diseases or remote or recent trauma.
- Impairment of mobility is an early predictor of physical disability and associated with poor outcomes such as falling, loss of independence, depression, decreased quality of life, institutionalization, and death.
- Falls are one of the most important geriatric syndromes and the leading cause of morbidity and mortality for people older than 65 years of age.
- The risk of falling increases with the number of risk factors. Most falls occur from a combination of intrinsic and extrinsic factors that unite at a certain point in time.

- Fall risk assessments provide first-level assessment data as the basis for comprehensive assessment. Postfall assessments (PFAs) must be used to identify multifactorial, complex fall and injury risk factors in those who have fallen.
- Physical restraints, intended to prevent injury, do not protect patients from falling, wandering, or removing tubes and other medical devices. Physical restraints may actually exacerbate many of the problems for which they are used and can cause serious injury and death, as well as emotional and physical problems.
- Restraint-appropriate care is the standard of practice in all settings, and knowledge of restraint alternatives and safety measures is essential for nurses.

NURSING STUDY: FALL RISK REDUCTION

Jim is an 80-year-old World War II veteran who has resided in the skilled nursing facility for 2 years. His diagnoses include Alzheimer's disease, hypertension, and depression. Medications include an antihypertensive drug and an antidepressant. He is able to walk but has an unsteady gait and requires assistance. Due to his cognitive status, he often attempts to ambulate alone and today was found on the floor in the bathroom. No injuries were immediately apparent and he says he is fine. His partner of 30 years is requesting that restraints be applied to prevent him from suffering injuries from falling.

On the basis of the nursing study, develop a nursing care plan using the following procedure*:
- List information that provides objective data.
- Discuss the assessment that needs to be completed related to Jim's fall.

- From these data, identify and state, using an accepted format, two nursing diagnoses you determine are most significant to Jim at this time.
- Determine and state outcome criteria for each diagnosis. These must reflect some alleviation of the problem identified in the nursing diagnosis and must be stated in concrete and measurable terms.
- Plan and state one or more interventions for each diagnosed problem. Provide specific documentation of the source used to determine the appropriate intervention.
- Evaluate the success of the intervention. Interventions must correlate directly with the stated outcome criteria to measure the outcome success.

*Students are advised to refer to their nursing diagnosis text and identify possible or potential problems.

CRITICAL THINKING QUESTIONS AND ACTIVITIES

1. What risk factors for falls are present in the nursing study presented above?
2. What interventions are appropriate to ensure safety?
3. How would you respond to the partner's request for the use of restraints?

RESEARCH QUESTIONS

1. What types of gait disorders trigger falls and in what situations?
2. How does cognitive impairment influence risk of falls?
3. What are the psychological reactions of elders to the use of assistive devices for ambulation?
4. What factors among community-dwelling elders are most hazardous for mobility?
5. How often and in what circumstances are falls precipitated by distractions or actions of another individual?
6. What are the major reasons individuals are restrained in ICUs and what interventions are most effective in decreasing restraint use in this setting?

REFERENCES

Agency for Healthcare Research and Quality: Use of physical restraint in nursing homes cut by half in 8 years, *AHRQ New and Numbers*, July 14, 2010.http://archive.ahrq.gov/news/newsroom/news-and-numbers/071410.html. Accessed April 2014.

Alexander N: Balance, gait and mobility. In Ham R, Sloane R, Warshaw G, et al, editors: *Primary care geriatrics*, ed 6, Philadelphia, 2014, Elsevier Saunders, pp 227–234.

American Geriatrics Society: American Geriatrics Society identifies another five things that healthcare providers should question, *J Am Geriatr Soc*, Feb 27, 2014a. doi: 10.1111/jgs.12770. [Epub ahead of print].

American Geriatrics Society: Recommendations abstracted from the American Geriatrics Society Consensus Statement on vitamin D for prevention of falls and their consequences, *J Am Geriatr Soc* 62:147–152, 2014b.

American Geriatrics Society/British Geriatrics Society: *AGS/BGS clinical practice guideline*: prevention of falls in older persons, 2010.http://www.americangeriatrics.org/health_care_professionals/clinical_practice/clinical_guidelines_recommendations/prevention_of_falls_summary_of_recommendations. Accessed May 2014.

American Nurses Association: *Safe patient handling and mobility*: Interprofessional national standards across the care continuum, 2013.http://nursingworld.org/DocumentVault/Occupational Environment/SPHM-Standards-Resources/Sample-of-the-SPHM-book.pdf. Accessed January 26, 2014.

Andersen D, Osei-Boamah E, Gambert S: Impact of trauma-related hip fractures on the older adult, *Clin Geriatr* 18:18, 2010.

Antonelli M: Restraint management: moving from process to outcome, *J Nurs Care Qual* 23:227–232, 2008.

Bourbonniere M, Evans LK: Advanced practice nursing in the care of frail older adults, *J Am Geriatr Soc* 50:2062–2076, 2002.

Bradas C, Sandhu S, Mion L: Physical restraints and side rails in acute and critical care settings. In Boltz M, Capezuti E, Fulmer T, et al, editors: *Evidence-based geriatric nursing protocols for best practice*, ed 4, New York, 2012, Springer, pp 1229–1245.

Buckeridge D, Huang A, Hanley J, et al: Risk of injury associated with opioid use in older adults, *J Am Geriatr Soc* 58(9):1664–1670, 2010.

Cameron I, Murray G, Gillespie L, et al: Interventions for preventing falls in older people in nursing facilities and hospitals, *Cochrane Database Syst Rev* 1:CD005465, 2010.

Campbell A, Robertson M: Fall prevention: single or multiple interventions? Single interventions for fall prevention, *J Am Geriatr Soc* 61(2):281–284, 2013.

Campo M, Shiyko M, Margulis H, et al: Effect of patient handling program on rehabilitation outcomes, *Arch Phys Med Rehabil* 94(1):17–22, 2013.

Capezuti E: Building the science of falls-prevention research, *J Am Geriatr Soc* 52:461–462, 2004.

Capezuti E, Talerico K, Cochran I, et al: Individualized interventions to prevent bed-related falls and reduced siderail use, *J Gerontol Nurs* 25:26–34, 1999.

Centers for Disease Control and Prevention: *Hip fractures among older adults*, 2010.http://www.cdc.gov/Homeand RecreationalSafety/Falls/adulthipfx.html. Accessed October 2014.

Centers for Disease Control and Prevention: *Falls among older adults*: an overview, 2014a.http://www.cdc.gov/homeandrecreationalsafety/falls/adultfalls.html. Accessed April 2014.

Centers for Disease Control and Prevention: *Preventing traumatic brain injury in older adults*, 2014b.http://www.cdc.gov/features/braininjury. Accessed May 2014.

Degelau J, Belz M, Bungum L, et al: *Prevention of falls (acute care)*, Minneapolis, MN, 2012, Institute for Clinical Systems Improvement. https://www.icsi.org/_asset/dcn15z/Falls-Interactive0412.pdf. Accessed May 2014.

de Vries OJ, Ligthart GJ, Nikolaus T; On behalf of the participants of the European Academy of Medicine of Ageing—Course III: Differences in period prevalence of the use of physical restraints in elderly inpatients of European hospitals and nursing homes [letter], *J Gerontol A Biol Sci Med Sci* 59:M922–M923, 2004.

Evans L, Strumpf N: Tying down the elderly: a review of literature on physical restraint, *J Am Geriatr Soc* 37:65–74, 1989.

Fink H, Kuskowski M, Marshall L: Association of stressful life events with incident falls and fractures in older men: the osteoporotic fractures in men (MrOS) study, *Age Ageing* 43:103–108, 2014.

Flaherty J: Zero tolerance for physical restraints: difficult but not impossible, *J Gerontol A Biol Sci Med Sci* 59:M919–M920, 2004.

Frick K, Kung J, Parrish J, et al: Evaluating the cost-effectiveness of fall prevention programs that reduce fall-related hip fractures in older adults, *J Am Geriatr Soc* 58:136–141, 2010.

Gavin-Dreschnack D, Volicer L, Morris C: Prevention of overuse of wheelchairs in nursing homes, *Ann Longterm Care* 18:34, 2010.

Gillespie L, Robertson M, Gillespie W, et al: Interventions for preventing falls in older people living in the community, *Cochrane Database Syst Rev* 9:CD007146, Sept 12, 2012.

Gray-Micelli D: Preventing falls in acute care. In Capezuti E, Zwicker D, Mezey M, et al, editors: *Evidence-based geriatric nursing protocols for best practice*, ed 3, New York, 2008, Springer.

Gray-Micelli D, Quigley P: Fall prevention, assessment, diagnoses, and intervention strategies. In Boltz M, Capezuti E,

Fulmer T, et al, editors: *Evidence-based geriatric nursing protocols for best practice*, ed 4, New York, 2012, Springer, pp 268–297.

Gray-Micelli D, Ratcliffe S, Johnson J: Use of a postfall assessment tool to prevent falls, *West J Nurs Res* 32(7):932–948, 2010.

Gray-Miceli D, Ratcliffe S, Liu S, et al: Orthostatic hypotension in older nursing home residents who fall: are they dizzy? *Clin Nurs Res* 21:64–78, 2012.

Haentjens P, Magaziner J, Colón-Emeric C, et al: Meta-analysis: excess mortality after hip fracture among older men and women, *Ann Intern Med* 152:380–390, 2010.

Harrison B, Ferrari M, Campbell C, et al: Evaluating the relationship between inattention and impulsivity-related falls in hospitalized older adults, *Geriatr Nurs* 31:8–16, 2010.

Hendrich AL, Bender PS, Nyhuis A: Validation of the Hendrich II fall risk model: a large concurrent case/control study of hospitalized patients, *Appl Nurs Res* 16: 9–21, 2003.

Henkel G: Beyond the MDS: team approach to falls assessment, prevention and management, *Caring for the Ages* 3(4):15–20, 2002.

Hester A, Wei F: Falls in the community: state of the science, *Clin Interv Aging* 8:675–679, 2013.

Hill K, Womer M, Russell M, et al: Fear of falling in older fallers presenting at emergency departments, *J Adv Nurs* 66: 1769–1779, 2010.

Ireland S, Lazar T, Mavrak C, et al: Designing a falls prevention strategy that works, *J Nurs Care Qual* 25:198–207, 2010.

Kilgore C: Fall-prevention efforts must be multifaceted, *Caring for the Ages* 11: 26–27, 2010.

Kuh D: A life course approach to healthy aging, frailty, and capability, *J Gerontol A Biol Sci Med Sci* 62:717–721, 2007.

Kuschel B, Laflamme L, Moller J: The risk of fall injury in relation to commonly prescribed medications among older people—a Swedish case controlled study, *Eur J Public Health*, July 31, 2014. doi: 10.1093/eurpub/cku120. [Epub ahead of print]. http://eurpub.oxfordjournals.org/content/early/2014/07/31/eurpub.cku120.abstract. Accessed August 2014.

Lach H: The costs and outcomes of falls: what's a nursing administrator to do? *Nurs Admin Q* 34:147–155, 2010.

Lee H, Chang K, Tsauo J, et al: Effects of a multifactorial fall prevention program on fall incidence and physical function in community-dwelling older adults with risk of falls, *Arch Phys Med Rehabil* 94(4):606–615, 2013.

Li-MacDonald B, Pyhtila J, Brandt N: Medications and falls, *J Gerontol Nurs* 40(1): 8–14, 2014.

Lin F, Ferrucci L: Hearing loss and falls among older adults in the United States, *Arch Intern Med* 172(4): 369–371, 2012.

Luciano G, Brennan M, Rothberg M: Postprandial hypotension, *Am J Med* 123(3):281.e1–e6, 2010.

Mendito V, Lucci M, Polonara S, et al: Management of minor head injury in patients receiving oral anticoagulant therapy: a prospective study of a 24-hour observation protocol, *Ann Emerg Med* 59(6):451–455, 2012.

Miake-Lye I, Hempel S, Ganz D, et al: Inpatient fall prevention programs as a patient safety strategy, *Ann Intern Med* 158(5 Part 2):390–396, 2013.

Momeyer M: Orthostatic hypotension in older adults with dementia, *J Gerontol Nurs* 40(6):22–29, 2014.

Nelson A, Baptiste A: Evidence-based practices for safe patient handling and movement, *Online J Issues Nurs* 9(3), 2004.http://www.seiu1991.org/files/2013/07/Audrey_Nelson_Safe_Patient_Handling.pdf. Accessed April 2014.

Park M, Hsiao-Chen Tang J: Evidence-based guideline: changing the practice of physical restraint use in acute care, *J Gerontol Nurs* 33:9–16, 2007.

Pellfolk T, Gustafson Y, Bucht G, et al: Effects of a restraint minimization program on staff knowledge, attitudes, and practice: a cluster randomized trial, *J Am Geriatr Soc* 58:62–69, 2010.

Popejoy L, Marek K, Scott-Cawiezell J: Patterns and problems associated with transitions after hip fracture in older adults, *J Gerontol Nurs* 39(9):43–52, 2012.

Quigley P, Bulat T, Kurtzman E, et al: Fall prevention and injury protection for nursing home residents, *J Am Med Dir Assoc* 11:284–293, 2010.

Quigley P, White S: Hospital-based fall program measurement and improvement in high reliability organizations, *Online J Issues Nurs* 18(2), 2013.

Rantz M, Aud M, Alexander G, et al: Falls, technology, and stunt actors: new approaches to fall detection and fall risk assessment, *J Nurs Care Qual* 23:195–201, 2008.

Rantz M, Banerjee T, Cattoor E, et al: Automated fall detection with quality improvement "rewind" to reduce falls in hospital rooms, *J Gerontol Nurs* 40(1):13–17, 2014.

Rubenstein L, Dillard D: Falls. In Ham, Sloane P, Warshaw G, et al, editors: *Primary care geriatrics*, ed 6, Philadelphia, 2014, Elsevier Saunders, pp 235–242.

Rubenstein T, Alexander N, Hausdorff J: Evaluating fall risk in older adults: steps and missteps, *Clin Geriatr* 11:52–60, 2003.

Sollins H: Bed rails—be vigilant, but know the rules and guidelines, *Geriatr Nurs* 30:414–416, 2009.

Sullivan-Marx E: Psychological responses to physical restraint use in older adults, *J Psychosoc Nurs Ment Health Serv* 33: 20–25, 1995.

Talerico K, Capezuti E: Myths and facts about side rails, *Am J Nurs* 101:43–48, 2001.

Tewary S, Pandya N, Cook N: Prevention of foot problems in nursing home residents with diabetes stratified by dementia diagnosis, *Ann Longterm Care* 21(8):30–34, 2013.

Timmons T, Menaker J: Traumatic brain injury in the elderly, *Clin Geriatr* 18:20–24, 2010.

Tinetti M: Performance-oriented measurement of mobility problems in elderly patients, *J Am Geriatr Soc* 34(2):119–126, 1986.

Tinetti M, Baker D, King M, et al: Effect of dissemination of evidence in reducing injuries from falls, *N Engl J Med* 359(3):252–261, 2008.

Tinetti M, Han L, Lee D, et al: Antihypertensive medications and serious fall injuries in a nationally representative sample of older adults, *JAMA* 174(4):588–595, 2014.

Tzeng H, Yin C: The extrinsic risk factors for inpatient falls in hospital patient rooms, *J Nurs Care Qual* 23:233–241, 2008.

Wagner L, Capezuti E, Brush B, et al: Description of an advanced practice nursing consultative model to reduce restrictive siderail use in nursing homes, *Res Nurs Health* 30:131–140, 2007.

Willy B, Osterberg C: Strategies for reducing falls in long-term care, *Ann Longterm Care* 22(1):23–32, 2014.

World Health Organization: *Falls prevention in old age*, 2014.http://www.who.int/ageing/projects/falls_prevention_older_age/en. Accessed August 2014.

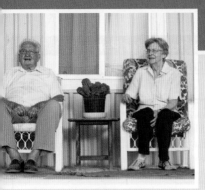

CHAPTER 20

Safety and Security

Theris A. Touhy

ⓔ http://evolve.elsevier.com/Touhy/TwdHlthAging

A STUDENT SPEAKS

During the community nursing experience my client decided to stay in her own home in spite of being barely able to shuffle around. A community program provided a homemaker for a few hours daily. She had to rely on the goodwill of neighbors when the budget for those services was discontinued. She wants so much to remain in her own home. I worry about her but don't know what I should do.

Jennifer, age 24

AN ELDER SPEAKS

I have been in my home for 50 years and widowed for 25 of those 50. The upkeep on my home is expensive and my resources are limited. I'm hoping I can manage to remain here, but I need some modifications to make it safe and I really don't know how to go about getting assistance to make the necessary changes.

Esther, age 79

LEARNING OBJECTIVES

On completion of this chapter, the reader will be able to:

1. Identify interactions of intrapersonal, interpersonal, geographical, economic, and health factors that influence environmental safety and security for older adults.
2. Discuss the effects of declining health, reduced mobility, isolation, and unpredictable life situations on the older adult's perception of security.
3. Explain the underlying vulnerability of older adults to effects of extreme temperatures, and identify actions to prevent and treat hypothermia and hyperthermia.
4. Define strategies and programs designed to prevent, detect, or alleviate crimes against older adults.
5. Consider the impact of available transportation and driving in relation to independence.
6. Discuss the use of assistive technologies to promote self-care, safety, and independence.
7. Identify the components of an elder-friendly community to enhance the ability to age in place.

ENVIRONMENTAL SAFETY

A safe environment is one in which one is capable, with reasonable caution, of carrying out activities of daily living (ADLs) and instrumental activities of daily living (IADLs), as well as the activities that enrich one's life, without fear of attack, accident, or imposed interference. Vulnerability to environmental risks increases as people become less physically or cognitively able to recognize or cope with real or potential hazards.

This chapter discusses the influence of changing health and disability on safety and security. Included are vulnerability to temperature extremes, natural disasters, crime, fire safety, driving safety, and the role of assistive technology in enhancing

independence and the ability to live safely at home. Elder-friendly communities that foster aging in place and promote safety and security are also discussed.

HOME SAFETY

Home safety assessments must be multifaceted and individualized to the areas of identified risks. They are particularly important for the older adult who is at risk for falls and are recommended in evidence-based protocols for fall risk reduction. An evidence-based home safety assessment tool is presented in Table 20-1. Box 20-1 presents resources for home safety assessments in formats easy for older adults to access and use.

TABLE 20-1   Assessment and Interventions of the Home Environment for Older Persons

PROBLEM	INTERVENTION	PROBLEM	INTERVENTION
Bathroom		**Telephone**	
Getting on and off toilet	Raised seat; side bars; grab bars	Difficult to reach	Cordless phone; cell phone; inform friends to let phone ring 10 times; answering machine and call back
Getting in and out of tub	Bath bench; transfer bench; hand-held shower nozzle; rubber mat; hydraulic lift bath seat	Difficult to hear ring	Headset; speaker phone
Hot water burns	Check water temperature before bath; set hot water thermostat to 120° F or less	Difficult to dial	Preset numbers; large button and numbers; voice-activated dialing
	Use bath thermometer		
Doorway too narrow	Remove door and use curtain; leave wheelchair at door and use walker	**Steps**	
		Cannot handle	Stair glide; lift; elevator; ramp (permanent, portable, or removable)
Bedroom		No hand rails	Install at least on one side
Rolling beds	Remove wheels; block against wall	Loose rugs	Remove or nail down to wooden steps
Bed too low	Leg extensions; blocks; second mattress; adjustable-height hospital bed	Difficult to see	Adequate lighting; mark edge of steps with bright-colored tape
Lighting	Bedside light; night-light; flashlight attached to walker or cane	Unable to use walker on stairs	Keep second walker or wheelchair at top or bottom of stairs
Sliding rugs	Remove; tack down; rubber back; two-sided tape	**Home Management**	
Slippery floor	Nonskid wax; no wax; rubber-sole footwear; indoor-outdoor carpet	Laundry	Easy to access; sit on stool to access clothes in dryer; good lighting; fold laundry sitting at table; carry laundry in bag on stairs; use cart; use laundry service
Thick rug edge/doorsill	Metal strip at edge; remove doorsill; tape down edge		
Nighttime calls	Bedside phone; cordless phone; cell phone; intercom; buzzer; lifeline	Mail	Easy-to-access mailbox; mail basket on door
Kitchen		**Safety**	
Open flames and burners	Substitute microwave; electric toaster oven	Difficulty locking doors	Remote-controlled door lock; door wedge; hook-and-chain locks
Access items	Place commonly used items in easy-to-reach areas; adjustable-height counters, cupboards, and drawers	Difficulty opening door and knowing who is there	Automatic door openers; level doorknob handles; intercom at door
Difficulty seeing	Adequate lighting; utensils with brightly colored handles	Opening and closing windows	Lever and crank handles
Living Room		Cannot hear alarms	Blinking lights; vibrating surfaces
Soft, low chair	Board under cushion; pillow or folded blanket to raise seat; blocks or platform under legs; good armrests to push up on; back and seat cushions	Lighting	Illumination 1 to 2 feet from object being viewed; change bulbs when dim; adequate lighting in stairways and hallways; night-lights
Swivel and rocking chairs	Block motion		
Obstructing furniture	Relocate or remove to clear paths		
Extension cords	Run along walls; eliminate unnecessary cords; place under sturdy furniture; use power strips with breakers		

Modified from Rehabilitation Engineering Research Center on Aging (RERC-Aging), Center for Assistive Technology, University at Buffalo, NY.

BOX 20-1   RESOURCES FOR BEST PRACTICE

Aging & Technology Research Center: On-line home safety self-assessment

American Automobile Association: Driver improvement courses, on-line defensive driving course

American Association of Retired Persons: CarFit: Helping Mature Drivers Find Their Safety Fit

Cohousing Association of the United States

National Crime Prevention Council: Safety in the Golden Years

National Fire Protection Association and the CDC: Remembering When™: A Fire and Fall Prevention Program for Older Adults

National Institute on Aging: Age Page: Hyperthermia: Too Hot for Your Health; Hypothermia: A Cold Weather Hazard

National Shared Housing Resource Center

U.S. Department of Health and Human Services, Administration on Aging: Preparing for an Emergency or Disaster, Resources for Individuals, Families, and Caregivers

Village to Village Network (Village Housing Model)

World Health Organization: Global age-friendly cities and communities: A guide; Checklist of Essential Features of Age-Friendly Cities

CRIMES AGAINST OLDER ADULTS

Risks and Vulnerability

Older individuals share many of the same fears about violent crime held by the rest of the population, but they may feel more vulnerable because of frailness or disability. Living alone; having sensory, mobility, and memory impairments; and being lonely may make elders more susceptible to crime. Property crime is the most common crime against persons age 65 years and older. Older people are more likely to be victims of consumer fraud and scams that include telemarketing fraud, email scams, and undelivered services. Older people also experience rising problems with identity theft. Resources for crime-prevention programs for older adults can be found in Box 20-1. Nurses can be instrumental in reducing fear of crime and assisting elders in exploring ways they may protect themselves and feel more secure. Box 20-2 offers crime-reduction suggestions.

BOX 20-2 Crime-Reduction Suggestions

- Do not wear flashy jewelry in public places.
- Have your key ready when approaching your front door.
- Do not dangle your purse away from your body or carry large bulky shoulder bags.
- Purse and wallet snatchers are usually not interested in injuring anyone. You are less likely to get hurt when accosted if you hand over your purse or wallet readily.
- Carry only a little money and a few personal items in your wallet or purse. Keep your car keys, larger amounts of money, and credit cards in an inside pocket of clothing.
- Do not leave your purse on the seat beside you in the car; put it on the floor where it is more difficult for someone to grab it.
- Lock bundles or bags in the trunk.
- When returning to your car, check the front seat, back seat, and floor before entering.
- Wear a small police whistle around your neck, or carry mace.
- Identify police and security personnel who are available in high-risk areas.
- Institute informal surveillance agreements with neighbors to increase security.
- Receive a home security check by police, and follow through on their security suggestions.
- Attend a crime-prevention program.
- Keep doors locked, install deadbolt locks, and choose locks that you can easily manipulate. If your key is lost or if you move, have locks replaced. Do not attach an ID tag to your key ring.
- Never open your door automatically. Use an optical viewer. Confirm authenticity of a service person's ID by calling that service agency before opening the door. Never open doors to strangers or let them know you are alone.
- Lock windows. Get fire department–approved grates installed on ground floor/fire escape windows. Keep all hidden entries locked (e.g., garage, basement, roof). Draw curtains and blinds at night.
- Protect valuables: Keep money and securities in a bank.
- Beware of phone tricks.
- Hang up on (and report) nuisance callers.
- Do not give any information to strangers over the phone.
- Consider a pet. A dog—even a small one—can provide excellent protection and good company if you are willing to care for one.
- Organize a buddy system. Neighbors can watch out for each other, go to the basement/laundry room together, and so on.
- Keep alert to stories and coverage of fraud, bogus schemes, and protective actions on the news media.
- Take advantage of self-defense courses and public awareness programs.
- Do not be afraid to report crime or suspicious activities.

Fraudulent Schemes against Elders

Fraud against elders ranges from solicitations from seemingly worthwhile charities to requests for a cash deposit to win a nonexistent prize. Increasingly common is a phone call from someone posing as a grandchild who requests money for an emergency. Trusting persons may be fooled into giving money to pen pals, Internet acquaintances, phony religious causes, or new acquaintances who "need help." Attractive prices of fraudulent door-to-door contractors, who offer services the individual cannot perform, may entice a substantial cash outlay.

According to the Internal Revenue Service (IRS), every year impersonators swindle vulnerable taxpayers out of thousands of dollars by posing as IRS agents. Older people are often targets of these frauds. Scams may involve announcements that they have won a large cash sweepstakes that requires payment of taxes before the prize is delivered. Other IRS impersonators have called on widows or widowers to pay the "back taxes" owed by their deceased spouse. These abuses often go unpunished because the individual waits too long to report the fraud or feels embarrassed over the mistake.

Medical fraud is another serious type of fraud that affects older citizens on a national scale. Medical supplies and equipment delivered to homes by various suppliers have either been grossly overpriced or charged for but never received by the client. Scams to defraud Medicare beneficiaries for the Medicare Part D benefit have also been reported. Callers ask for bank information and use the account numbers to electronically withdraw money for a Medicare card and drug plan that is not legitimate.

The Centers for Medicare and Medicaid Services (CMS) has offices to inform Medicare and Medicaid beneficiaries of ways to avoid fraud and also provides toll-free numbers to report suspected fraud. National agencies have combined forces to bring about reform. Box 20-3 presents other suggestions.

BOX 20-3 Protection against Fraud

- No one should come to your house uninvited.
- No one can ask for personal information during his or her marketing activities.
- All IRS employees carry identification and are required to show it to taxpayers when visiting a home or office.
- No check should ever be made payable to an IRS employee. Checks for federal taxes should be made payable to the Internal Revenue Service, not IRS; spelling out the full name makes it more difficult for criminals to alter the check.
- Keep personal information safe, including your Medicare number, and do not provide any information about bank accounts or credit cards to marketers.
- Legitimate Medicare drug plans will not ask for payment over the telephone or Internet and must send a bill to the beneficiary for the monthly premium.
- Most states offer the volunteer program Seniors Health Information Needs of Elders (SHINE), which offers assistance on Medicare and health insurance–related concerns, and local area agencies on aging often offer assistance to older people on completion of tax returns.

FIRE SAFETY FOR ELDERS

Fire-related death rates are three times higher in people older than 80 years than in the rest of the population. The risk of injury during a fire is greater if medication, illness, mobility, and sensory impairments slow response time or decision-making and if help is not available to contain the fire and help the person escape.

A number of factors predispose the older person to fire injuries. In home-dwelling elders, economic or climatic conditions may promote the use of ill-kept heating devices. Attempts to cook over an open flame while wearing loose-fitting clothing or inability to manage spattering grease from a frying pan can often start a fire from which the individual cannot escape. Failing vision can contribute to a person setting a cook-top burner, heating pad, or hot plate at too high a temperature, resulting in fire or thermal injury. Those living in apartment dwellings are often at the mercy of inadequate repair and safety measures and the careless behaviors of others. Many individuals living in their own homes cannot afford home repairs, placing them at risk for fire.

Most fires occur at home during the night, and deaths are attributed to smoke injury more often than burns. Smoking materials are the most common sources of residential fires. Plastic articles and other synthetics can produce noxious fumes that are deadly, particularly to persons with preexisting respiratory disorders. Even flame-retardant garments have been linked to noxious fume release when burned, and therefore they are a possible hazard. Specific fire prevention guidelines for elders appear in Box 20-4 and Box 20-5 presents information about

---

BOX 20-4   TIPS FOR BEST PRACTICE
Reducing Fire Risks in the Home

- When you smell smoke, see flames, or hear the sound of fire, evacuate everyone in the house before doing anything else.
- Use normal exits unless blocked by smoke or flames. Never use elevators unless instructed by the fire department.
- Make sure smoke alarms are installed on each level of your home and outside all sleeping areas; test smoke alarms monthly and replace batteries at least once a year.
- Know at least two exits from every room.
- Make any necessary accommodations, such as providing exit ramps and widening doorways, to facilitate an emergency exit.
- Contact your local fire department's non-emergency line and explain your special needs; they may suggest escape plan ideas and may perform a home fire safety inspection and offer suggestions about smoke alarm placement and maintenance.
- In a high-rise apartment, remain in the room with doors and hall vents closed unless smoke is in your apartment. Open or break a window to obtain fresh air.
- Rehearse what to do if clothing catches fire: do not run; lie down and then roll over and over ("stop, drop and roll"). If another person's clothing is burning, smother the flames with the handiest item such as a rug, coat, blanket, or drapes.
- If you live in a multistory home, arrange to sleep on the ground floor and near an exit.

BOX 20-5   TIPS FOR BEST PRACTICE
Preventing Fires and Burns

- Do not smoke in bed or when sleepy.
- When cooking, do not wear loose-fitting clothing (e.g., bathrobes, nightgowns, pajamas).
- Set thermostats for water heater or faucets so that the water does not become too hot.
- Install a portable hand fire extinguisher in the kitchen.
- Keep access to outside door(s) unobstructed.
- Identify emergency exits in public buildings.
- If you consider entering a boarding or foster home, check to see that it has smoke detectors, a sprinkler system, and fire extinguishers.
- Wear clothing that is nonflammable or treated with a permanent fire-retardant finish.
- Use several electrical outlets rather than overloading one outlet.

---

reducing fire risks in the home and preventing fires and burns. Box 20-1 presents fire safety resources.

VULNERABILITY TO ENVIRONMENTAL TEMPERATURES

Extreme weather events such as heat waves, cold spells, floods, storms, and droughts are increasing across the globe. These extreme events are an emerging environmental health concern and potentially affect the health status of millions of people around the globe (Green et al, 2013; Wolf and McGregor, 2013). Many individuals are exposed to temperature extremes in their own dwellings. Environmental temperature extremes impose a serious risk to older persons with declining physical health. Preventive measures require attentiveness to impending climate changes, as well as protective alternatives. Early intervention in extreme temperature exposure is crucial because excessively high or low body temperatures further impair thermoregulatory function and can be lethal.

Thermoregulation

Neurosensory changes in thermoregulation delay or diminish the individual's awareness of temperature changes and may impair behavioral and thermoregulatory response to dangerously high or low environmental temperatures (Chapter 13). These changes vary widely among individuals and are related more to general health than to age.

Additionally, many drugs affect thermoregulation by affecting the ability to vasoconstrict or vasodilate, both of which are thermoregulatory mechanisms. Other drugs inhibit neuromuscular activity (a significant source of kinetic heat production), suppress metabolic heat generation, or dull awareness (tranquilizers, pain medications). Alcohol is notorious for inhibiting thermoregulatory function by affecting vasomotor responses in either hot or cold weather.

Economic, behavioral, and environmental factors may combine to create a dangerous thermal environment in which older persons are subjected to temperature extremes from which they cannot escape or that they cannot change. Caregivers and

TABLE 20-2 Heat Syndromes

ILLNESS	SYMPTOMS	TREATMENT
Heat fatigue	Pale, sweaty skin that is still cool and moist to the touch, weakness, exhaustion Core temperature stays normal because individual can sweat	Oral hydration with electrolyte replacement Cooler, less humid environment Rest
Heat syncope	Syncope or dizziness after exercising in the heat, sweating Has lost fluids and electrolytes Pale, sweaty, weak pulse, elevated heart rate, body temperature still normal	Oral hydration with electrolyte replacement Cooler, less humid environment Rest
Heat cramps	Muscle cramps, still sweating Pulse and BP elevated May need emergency care	Cool environment Oral liquids and IV saline Rest
Heat exhaustion	Can be life-threatening Thirsty but altered mental status (dizzy, confused, weak), cool and clammy, tachycardia, nausea Core temperature slightly elevated Emergency treatment	Cool environment Oral liquids and IV saline Rest
Heat stroke	Fatal if neglected Body temperature rises quickly and out of control (often >104° F) Individual is hot and dry, confused, combative, delirious, and then comatose Tachycardia, hypotension, hyperventilation End-organ damage; acute renal failure, and hypercoagulation states occur	Need ER treatment Start by fanning patient and using tepid water sprays, aiming to cool slowly Call EMS Complex medical emergency; if untreated, can cause death Cool as rapidly as possible; consider IV infusions

Modified from Hogan T, Rios-Alba T: Emergency care. In Ham R, Sloane PD, Warshaw GA, et al, editors: *Primary care geriatrics: a case-based approach*, ed 6, Philadelphia, 2014, Elsevier, pp 177–192.

family members should be aware that persons are vulnerable to temperature extremes if they are unable to shiver, sweat, control blood supply to the skin, take in sufficient liquids, move about, add or remove clothing, adjust bedcovers, or adjust the room temperature. A temperature that may be comfortable for a young and active person may be too cold or too warm for a frail elder.

Economic conditions often play a role in determining whether an older person living in the community can afford air conditioning or adequate heating. More older people die from excessive heat than from hurricanes, lightning, tornadoes, floods, and earthquakes combined (CDC, 2006). Local governments and communities must coordinate response strategies to protect the older person. Strategies may include providing fans and opportunities to spend part of the day in air-conditioned buildings, as well as identification of high-risk individuals.

Temperature Monitoring in Older Adults

Diminished thermoregulatory responses and abnormalities in both the production and the response to endogenous pyrogens may contribute to differences in fever responses between older and younger patients in response to an infection. Up to one-third of older people with acute infections may present without a robust febrile response, leading to delays in diagnosis and appropriate treatment, as well as increased morbidity and mortality (Outzen, 2009). Careful attention to temperature monitoring in older adults is very important, and often this technical task is not given adequate consideration by professional nurses.

SAFETY ALERT

Because of thermoregulatory changes, up to one-third of older people with acute infections may present without a febrile response. Additionally, baseline temperatures in frail older people may be lower than the expected 98.6° F. If the baseline temperature is 97° F, a temperature of 98° F is a 1° degree elevation and may be significant.

Temperatures reaching or exceeding 100.94° F are very serious in older people and are more likely to be associated with serious bacterial or viral infections. Careful attention to temperature monitoring in older adults is very important and can prevent morbidity and mortality. Accurate measurement and reporting of body temperature require professional nursing supervision.

Hyperthermia

When body temperature increases above normal ranges because of environmental or metabolic heat loads, a clinical condition called heat illness, or *hyperthermia*, develops (Table 20-2). Administration of diuretics and low intake of fluids exacerbate fluid loss and can precipitate the onset of hyperthermia in hot weather. Hyperthermia is a temperature-related illness and is classified as a medical emergency. Annually, there are numerous deaths among elders from temperature extremes; therefore prevention and education are very important nursing responsibilities.

Although most of these problems occur in the home among individuals who do not have air conditioning to use during temperature extremes, older adults with multiple physical problems residing in institutions may be especially vulnerable to temperature changes. Individuals with cardiovascular disease, diabetes, or peripheral vascular disease and those taking certain medications (anticholinergics, antihistamines, diuretics,

Preventing Hyperthermia

- Drink 2 to 3 L of cool fluid daily.
- Minimize exertion, especially during the warmest times of the day.
- Stay in air-conditioned places, or use fans when possible.
- Wear hats and loose clothing of natural fibers when outside; remove most clothing when indoors.
- Take tepid baths or showers.
- Apply cold wet compresses, or immerse the hands and feet in cool water.
- Evaluate medications for risk of hyperthermia.
- Avoid alcohol.

BOX 20-7   **Factors That Increase the Risk of Hypothermia in Older Adults**

Thermoregulatory Impairment

Failure to vasoconstrict promptly or sufficiently on exposure to cold
Failure to sense cold
Failure to respond behaviorally to protect oneself against cold
Diminished or absent shivering to generate heat
Failure of metabolic rate to rise in response to cold

Conditions That Decrease Heat Production

Hypothyroidism, hypopituitarism, hypoglycemia, anemia, malnutrition, starvation
Immobility or decreased activity (e.g., stroke, paralysis, parkinsonism, dementia, arthritis, fractured hip, coma)
Thinning hair, baldness
Diabetic ketoacidosis

Conditions That Increase Heat Loss

Open wounds, generalized inflammatory skin conditions, burns

Conditions That Impair Central or Peripheral Control of Thermoregulation

Stroke, brain tumor, Wernicke's encephalopathy, subarachnoid hemorrhage
Uremia, neuropathy (e.g., diabetes, alcoholism)
Acute illnesses (e.g., pneumonia, sepsis, myocardial infarction, congestive heart failure, pulmonary embolism, pancreatitis)

Drugs That Interfere with Thermoregulation

Tranquilizers (e.g., phenothiazines); sedative-hypnotics (e.g., barbiturates, benzodiazepines); antidepressants (e.g., tricyclics); vasoactive drugs (e.g., vasodilators); alcohol (causes superficial vasodilation; may interfere with carbohydrate metabolism and judgment); others (e.g., methyldopa, lithium, morphine)

beta-blockers, antidepressants, antiparkinsonian drugs) are at risk. Interventions to prevent hyperthermia when ambient temperature exceeds 90° F (32° C) are presented in Box 20-6.

Hypothermia

Nearly 50% of all deaths from hypothermia occur in older adults (University of Maryland Medical Center, 2013). Hypothermia is produced by exposure to cold environmental temperatures and is defined as a core temperature of less than 35° C (95° F). Hypothermia is a medical emergency requiring comprehensive assessment of neurological activity, oxygenation, renal function, and fluid and electrolyte balance.

When exposed to cold temperatures, healthy persons conserve heat by vasoconstriction of superficial vessels, shunting circulation away from the skin where most heat is lost. Heat is generated by shivering and increased muscle activity, and a rise in oxygen consumption occurs to meet aerobic muscle requirements. Under normal circumstances, heat is produced in sufficient quantities by cellular metabolism of food, friction produced by contracting muscles, and the flow of blood.

Paralyzed or immobile persons lack the ability to generate significant heat by muscle activity and become cold even in normal room temperatures. Persons who are emaciated and have poor nutrition lack insulation, as well as fuel for metabolic heat-generating processes, so they may be mildly hypothermic (Hogan and Rios-Alba, 2014). Circulatory, cardiac, respiratory, or musculoskeletal impairments affect either the response to or the function of thermoregulatory mechanisms. Other risk factors include excessive alcohol use, exhaustion, poor nutrition, inadequate housing, as well as the use of sedatives, anxiolytics, phenothiazines, and tricyclic antidepressants (Box 20-7).

Older persons with some degree of thermoregulatory impairment, when exposed to cold temperatures, are at high risk for hypothermia if they undergo surgery, are injured in a fall or accident, or are lost or left unattended in a cool place. The more severe the impairment or prolonged the exposure, the less able are thermoregulatory responses to defend against heat loss.

Unfortunately, a dulling of awareness accompanies hypothermia, and persons experiencing the condition rarely recognize the problem or seek assistance. For the very old and frail, environmental temperatures less than 65° F (18° C) may cause a serious drop in core body temperature to 95° F (35° C).

All body systems are affected by hypothermia, although the most deadly consequences involve cardiac arrhythmias and suppression of respiratory function. Correctly conducted rewarming is the key to good management, and the guiding principle is to warm the core before the periphery and raise the core temperature 0.5° C to 2° C per hour. Heating blankets and specially designed heating vests are used in addition to warm humidified air by mask, warm intravenous boluses, and other measures depending on the severity of the hypothermia (Hogan and Rios-Alba, 2014).

Detecting hypothermia among community-dwelling older adults is sometimes difficult because, unlike in the clinical setting, no one is measuring body temperature. For persons exposed to low temperatures in the home or the environment, confusion and disorientation may be the first overt signs. As judgment becomes clouded, a person may remove clothing or fail to seek shelter, and hypothermia can progress to profound levels. For this reason, regular contact with home-dwelling elders during cold weather is crucial. For those with preexisting alterations in thermoregulatory ability, this surveillance should include even mildly cool weather. Because heating costs are high in the United States, the Department of Health and Human Services provides funds to help low-income families pay their heating bills. Specific interventions to prevent hypothermia are shown in Box 20-8.

BOX 20-8 TIPS FOR BEST PRACTICE

Preventing Cold Discomfort and Development of Accidental Hypothermia in Frail Elders

- Maintain a comfortably warm ambient temperature no lower than 65° F. Many frail elders will require much higher temperatures.
- Provide generous quantities of clothing and bedcovers. Layer clothing and bedcovers for best insulation. Be careful not to judge your patient's needs by how you feel working in a warm environment.
- Limit time patients sit by cold windows or air conditioners to short periods in which they are adequately dressed and covered.
- Provide a head covering whenever possible—in bed, out of bed, and particularly out-of-doors.
- Cover patients well when in bed or bathing. The standard—a light bath blanket over a naked body—is not enough protection for frail elders.
- Cover patients with heavy blankets for transfer to and from showers; dry quickly and thoroughly before leaving shower room; cover head with a dry towel or hood while wet. Shower rooms and bathrooms should have warming lights.
- Dry wet hair quickly with warm air from an electric dryer. Never allow the hair of frail elders to air-dry.
- Use absorbent pads for incontinent patients rather than allowing urine to wet large areas of clothing, sheets, and bedcovers.
- Provide as much exercise as possible to generate heat from muscle activity.
- Provide hot, high-protein meals and bedtime snacks to add heat and sustain heat production throughout the day and as far into the night as possible.

PROMOTING HEALTHY AGING: IMPLICATIONS FOR GERONTOLOGICAL NURSING

Recognition of clinical signs and severity of hypothermia and hyperthermia is an important nursing responsibility. Nurses are responsible for keeping frail elders in environments with appropriate temperatures for comfort and prevention of problems. It is important to closely monitor body temperature and pay particular attention to lower or higher than normal readings compared with the person's baseline. The potential risk of hypothermia and its associated cardiorespiratory and metabolic exertion make prevention important and early recognition vital. Nurses must advocate for resources in the community to ensure appropriate temperatures in the homes of older people and surveillance when temperature changes occur.

VULNERABILITY TO NATURAL DISASTERS

Natural disasters such as hurricanes, tornadoes, floods, and earthquakes claim the lives of many people worldwide each year. In addition, human-made or human-generated disasters include chemical, biological, radiological, and nuclear terrorism and food and water contamination. Older people are at great risk during and after disasters and have the highest casualty rate during disaster events when compared with all other age groups (Burnett et al, 2008). Older adults were 65% of the victims of the Japanese tsunami and half of the victims in Hurricane Sandy. The older and poorer the individual, the more likely he

or she is to be isolated and vulnerable (Feather, 2013). Ninety-seven percent of people killed in disasters live in developing countries (Help Age International, 2013).

Older adults at most risk include, but are not limited to, those who depend on others for daily functioning; those with limited mobility; and those who are socially isolated, cognitively impaired, or institutionalized. Older people may be less likely to seek formal or informal help during disasters and may not get as much assistance as younger individuals. A recent study found that the majority of community-living adults age 50 and older in the United States may not be prepared for a serious flood, earthquake, tornado, or other natural calamity. Individuals older than age 80 years were significantly less prepared than 65- to 79-year-old individuals (Al-Rousan et al, 2014). Nursing home residents compose a particularly vulnerable group due to their frailty and nursing homes need to be prepared for disasters.

The U.S. Department of Health and Human Services provides resources for emergency and disaster preparedness for special populations, including older adults (see Box 20-1). The World Health Organization has addressed policy implications for older people in emergencies that include mechanisms that ensure continuing development of the capacity to meet the health and safety needs of older people in emergencies and strategies to reduce vulnerability to disasters.

PROMOTING HEALTHY AGING: IMPLICATIONS FOR GERONTOLOGICAL NURSING

Gerontological nurses must be knowledgeable about disaster preparedness and assist in the development of plans to address the unique needs of older adults, as well as educate fellow professionals and community agencies about the special needs of older adults. Comprehensive planning is necessary to respond to the needs of the aging population in emergency situations around the world.

TRANSPORTATION SAFETY

Available transportation is a critical link in the ability of older adults to remain independent and functional. The lack of accessible transportation may contribute to other problems, such as social withdrawal, poor nutrition, depressive symptoms, and health decline (Dugan and Lee, 2013). Urban buses and subways can be physically hazardous and often dangerous. Rural and suburban areas may not have accessible transportation systems, making transportation by car essential. Even walking can be dangerous, and older people have more pedestrian crashes than anyone except children and are more likely to be injured or killed as pedestrians than as car drivers (Rosenbloom, 2009). Suggested pedestrian improvements include raised pavement markings, median islands, larger street signs with bigger lettering, increased time for pedestrian crossings, and lowered speed limits (Dugan and Lee, 2013).

A "crisis in mobility" exists for many older people because of the lack of an automobile, an inability to drive, limited access to public transportation, health factors, geographical location, and economic considerations. Neither public transit services nor special demand services will come anywhere near meeting the mobility needs of the country's aging population (Rosenbloom, 2009).

County, state, or federally subsidized transportation is being provided in certain areas to assist individuals in reaching social services, nutrition sites, health services, emergency care, recreational centers, day care programs, physical and vocational rehabilitation centers, grocery stores, and library services. Some senior centers also offer transportation services. Although transportation can often be found for special needs, it is virtually impossible to locate transportation for pleasure or recreation and many of these services are restricted to individuals with serious physical or mental impairments. A very small percentage of older individuals use these services.

PROMOTING HEALTHY AGING: IMPLICATIONS FOR GERONTOLOGICAL NURSING

Adequate, affordable, and convenient transportation services are essential to health and quality of life, as well as the ability to age in place. Assessment of older adults needs to include transportation needs. Referrals to local social service and aging organizations, such as Area Agencies on Aging, can be made to assist in obtaining information on transportation resources and financial assistance for services.

Suggestions to address the transportation crisis include the following: (1) adopt policies that provide substantially more funding for transit operators to develop meaningful transit services for older people without serious disabilities; (2) provide better support and financial resources for the wide variety of community transportation providers; (3) develop programs and policies to keep older people driving safely for as long as possible; (4) enhance and maintain the pedestrian network; (5) ensure that traffic regulations are enforced; and (6) focus on making neighborhoods elder friendly, including adequate transportation to needed services and recreational activities (Rosenbloom, 2009). The U.S. Department of Transportation Federal Highway Administration provides a comprehensive guideline to make roads safer for older drivers and pedestrians.

Driving

Driving is one of the instrumental activities of daily living (IADLs) for most elders because it is essential to obtaining necessary resources. Driving is the preferred means of travel for most Americans, especially older adults. Almost 90% of people 65 years of age and older continue to drive, and these numbers are expected to grow as "baby boomers" age and more people live into their 80s and 90s. For many older people, alternate transportation is not available and, consequently, they may continue driving beyond the time when it is safe. Rosenbloom (2009) suggests that the most promising mobility option would be to modify the auto-based infrastructure so that older people can drive safely longer. This would include vehicle adaptations, sensory aids, elder driving training, and driving assessment programs (Box 20-9). The CarFit program (see Box 20-1) is an educational program to improve driver-car fit.

BOX 20-9 Adaptations for Safer Driving

- Wider rear-view mirrors
- Pedal extensions
- Less complicated, larger, and legible instrument panels
- Electronic detectors in front and back that signal when the car is getting too close to other cars, drifting into another lane, or likely to hit center dividers or other highway infrastructure
- Technology that facilitates left turns by warning drivers when it is safe to make the turn
- Better protection on doors
- Booster cushions for shorter-stature drivers
- "Smart" driving assistants (under development) that automatically plan a safe driving route based on the person's driving habits
- GPS devices

Modified from Dugan E, Lee C: Biopsychosocial risk factors for driving cessation: findings from the Health and Retirement study, *J Aging Health* 25:1313–1328, 2013; Hooyman N, Kiyak H: *Social gerontology: a multidisciplinary perspective*, Boston, 2011, Allyn & Bacon.

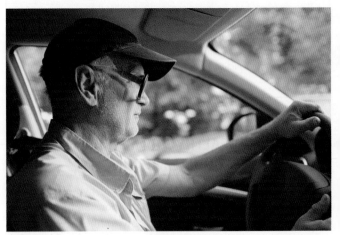

Driving is the preferred means of travel for older adults. (©iStock.com/danr13)

Driving is a highly complex activity that requires a variety of visual, motor, and cognitive skills. As individuals age, the risk for impairments that affect driving skills increases due to changes related to normal aging, as well as disease-related changes (e.g., arthritis, Parkinson's disease, stroke, dementia). Sensory impairments affect driving ability, and older drivers with dual sensory impairment are at greater accident risk than those with a visual acuity or hearing deficit alone (Dugan and Lee, 2013).

Driving Safety

Older drivers typically drive fewer miles than younger drivers and tend to drive less at night, during adverse weather conditions, or in congested areas. Generally, they choose familiar routes, and fewer older drivers speed or drive after drinking alcohol than drivers of other ages. However, when compared with younger age groups, older people have more accidents per mile driven and have a ninefold increased risk of traffic fatality (Servat et al, 2011). The leading cause of injury-related deaths among drivers 65 to 74 years of age is a motor vehicle accident; for those older than 75 years of age, motor vehicle accidents are the second leading cause of death, after falls (Hooyman and Kiyak, 2011).

The legal regulations regarding driver's license renewal in older drivers and the responsibility of medical practitioners to identify unsafe drivers vary among states and countries (Mathias and Lucas, 2009). Driver's license renewal procedures may include accelerated renewal cycles, renewal in person rather than electronically or by mail, and vision and road tests. The issues of driving in the older adult population are the subject of a great deal of public discussion. Many older drivers and their families struggle with issues related to continued safety in driving and when and how to tell older people they are no longer safe drivers.

Driving and Dementia

Driving has been identified as 1 of the top 10 tough ethical issues associated with dementia (Dobbs et al, 2009). Dementia, even in the early stages, can impair cognitive and functional skills required for safe driving. Evidence from some studies of motor vehicle crashes suggests that drivers with dementia have at least a twofold risk of crashes compared with those without cognitive impairment (Carr and Ott, 2010; Gray-Vickrey, 2010a,b). Many individuals early in the course of dementia are still able to pass a driving performance test, so a diagnosis of dementia should not be the sole justification for revocation of a driver's license (Carr and Ott, 2010). However, discussions should begin about the inevitability of driving cessation. Additionally, driving evaluations should be conducted every 6 months or as needed as the disease progresses.

Silver Alert systems. Many states have implemented the Silver Alert system. Similar to Amber Alerts for missing children, the Silver Alert is designed to create a widespread lookout for older adults who have wandered from their surroundings while driving a car. Silver Alert features a public notification system to broadcast information about missing persons, especially older adults with Alzheimer's disease or other mental disabilities, in order to aid in their return. Silver Alert uses a wide array of media outlets, such as commercial radio stations, television stations, and cable TV, to broadcast information about missing persons. Silver Alert also uses message signs on roadways to alert motorists to be on the lookout for missing elders and provides the car's make, model, and license information.

Driving Cessation

Relinquishing the mobility and independence afforded by driving one's own car has many psychological ramifications and inconveniences. Giving up driving is a major loss for an older person both in terms of independence and pleasure as well as in feelings of competence and self-worth. Driving cessation has been associated with decreased social integration, decreased out-of-home activities, increased depressive and anxiety symptoms, decreased quality of life, and increased risk of nursing home placement (Carr and Ott, 2010; Dugan and Lee, 2013).

Women are more likely than men to stop driving for less pressing reasons than health, and at a younger age (Dugan and Lee, 2013; Oxley and Charlton, 2009). Older men seem to place more value on the ability to drive, as well as owning a car, than older women. Therefore, one can expect more stress involved with the decision not to drive for older men. Other factors associated with driving cessation include IADL difficulties, poorer cognitive function, poor vision, being a member of a minority race or ethnicity, and having lower income and education (Dugan and Lee, 2013).

Planning for driving cessation should occur for all older adults before their mobility situations become urgent (Carr and Ott, 2010). Health care providers should encourage open discussion of issues related to driving with the older person and his or her family and should identify impairments that affect safe driving, correct them when possible, and offer alternatives for transportation. Matching individuals to volunteer drivers and using car-sharing programs have been successful in some communities. It is generally agreed that voluntarily giving up a driver's license, rather than having it revoked, is associated with more positive outcomes (Oxley and Charlton, 2009).

Specialized driving cessation support groups aimed at the transition from driver to nondriver may also be beneficial in decreasing the negative outcomes associated with this decision (Dobbs et al, 2009) (Box 20-10). Jett and colleagues (2005)

BOX 20-10   RESEARCH HIGHLIGHTS

Transition from Driving to Driving Cessation: The Role of Specialized Driving Cessation Support Groups for Individuals with Dementia

The loss of driving privileges due to a dementing illness is an issue that is likely to impact a sizeable number of individuals now and in the next several decades. For many individuals with dementia, the loss of driving privileges is a major occurrence in the course of their illness. Yet few, if any, interventions have been available to assist individuals in coping with the loss.

In this study, individuals with dementia (47) who had experienced a loss of driving privileges and their caregivers participated in an experimental-control design study in which they attended either in a driving cessation support group (DCSG) or in a support group offered by the Alzheimer's Society. The mean age of the participants was 77, and 57% of them were males. Of the participants, 50% had failed a formal driving assessment, and the remainder had stopped driving based on the advice of physicians, their family, or of their own accord. Before stopping driving, 25% of the participants reported having had a crash; 13% reported receiving a citation (11% received two or more) in the 6 months before driving cessation.

Participants attending the DCSGs had an improvement in depression scores, were less angry, and were happier. All participants reported that attending the DCSG had made a difference in their lives and had helped them cope with the illness and with not driving. Support groups designed specifically to deal with loss of driving privileges among individuals with dementia may be important in alleviating depressive symptoms and other negative outcomes associated with cessation of driving. DCSG interventions may represent an important step in the management of a very difficult aspect of dementia.

From Dobbs B, Harper L, Wood A: Transitioning from driving to driving cessation: the role of specialized driving cessation support groups for individuals with dementia, *Top Geriatr Rehabil* 25:73–86, 2009.

BOX 20-11 Action Strategies Used To Bring About Driving Cessation

IMPOSED TYPE	INVOLVED TYPE
Report person to division of motor vehicles for possible license suspension	All family members and individual meet, discuss the situation, and come to a mutual agreement of the problem
Use of deception or threats such as false keys, disabling the car, saying car was stolen	Dialogue is ongoing from the earliest signs of cognitive impairment about the eventuality of the need to stop driving
Attempts to order or control, such as provider writing a prescription, commands from children to stop driving	Arrangements are made for alternative transportation plans that are available when needed and acceptable to the individual

From Jett K, Tappen R, Rosselli M: Imposed versus involved: different strategies to effect driving cessation in cognitively impaired older adults, *Geriatr Nurs* 26:111–116, 2005.

provide useful strategies for driving counseling for people with dementia from a qualitative study involving guided interviews with participants (Box 20-11).

◆ PROMOTING HEALTHY AGING: IMPLICATIONS FOR GERONTOLOGICAL NURSING

Assessments of functional capacities often neglect driving ability. Assessment should include evaluation of whether an individual can drive, feels safe driving, and has a driver's license. A mnemonic, SAFE DRIVE (McGregor, 2002), addresses key components in screening older drivers (Box 20-12). Box 20-13 presents a self-assessment of driving that can be shared with individuals. The American Automobile Association also provides an interactive driving evaluation available on-line or in DVD format (see Box 20-1). These kinds of tools can be effective in raising awareness of threats to driving fitness (Dugan and Lee, 2013). Box 20-14 presents other suggestions in assessment of driving safety.

There is no gold standard for determining driving competency, but driving evaluations are offered by driver rehabilitation specialists through local hospitals and rehabilitation centers and private or university-based driving assessment programs. State Departments of Motor Vehicles (DMVs) also conduct performance-based road tests.

BOX 20-12 Safe Driving

S Safety record	**D** Drugs
A Attention skills	**R** Reaction time
F Family report	**I** Intellectual impairment
E Ethanol use	**V** Vision and visuospatial function
	E Executive functions

BOX 20-13 Driving Skills and Safety Factors

Directions

If you answer "yes" to one or more of the following questions, you may want to limit your driving or take steps to improve a problem.

If you answer "yes" to most of the questions, it may be time to consider letting someone else do your driving.

- Does driving make you feel nervous or physically exhausted?
- Do you have difficulty seeing pedestrians, signs, and vehicles?
- Do cars frequently seem to appear from nowhere?
- At night, does the glare from oncoming headlights temporarily "blind" you?
- Do you find intersections confusing?
- Are you finding it harder to judge the distance between cars?
- Do you have difficulty coordinating your hand and foot movements?
- Do you have difficulty staying in a lane?
- Are you slower than you used to be in reacting to dangerous situations?
- Do you sometimes get lost in familiar neighborhoods?
- Do other drivers often honk at you?
- Have you had any tickets?
- Have you been pulled over by the police?
- Have you had an increased number of traffic violations, accidents, or near-accidents in the past year?
- Do you have any vision problems?
- Do you have any hearing problems?
- Do you take any of the following medications: antihistamines, antipsychotics, tricyclic antidepressants, benzodiazepines, barbiturates, sleeping medications, muscle relaxants?
- Do you have any memory impairment?
- Do you have any muscle stiffness or weakness?

Adapted from Carr D, Ott B: The older adult driver with cognitive impairment: "It's a very frustrating life," *JAMA* 303:1632–1641, 2010.

BOX 20-14 TIPS FOR BEST PRACTICE

Driving Safety

- Include the person in all discussions about driving safety.
- Encourage the individual to conduct a self-assessment of driving abilities.
- Assess vision and hearing and ensure appropriate use of corrective lenses and hearing devices.
- Evaluate medical conditions that may interfere with driving ability (arthritis, Parkinson's disease, dementia, stroke) and ensure appropriate treatment, as well as adaptations that may be necessary to enhance driving safety.
- Discuss the impact of medical conditions and sensory impairments on driving safety.
- Suggest vehicle adaptations and elder driving assessment programs if indicated.
- Encourage the individual to modify driving habits, such as not driving on unfamiliar roads, during rush hour, at dusk or at night, in inclement weather, or in heavy traffic.
- Discuss strategies to decrease the need to drive including arranging for home-delivered groceries, prescriptions, and meals; having personal services provided in the home; asking a caregiver to obtain needed supplies or act as a copilot; and exploring community resources for transportation.
- If the individual has driving safety risk factors and should not be driving, ask the individual's health care provider to "prescribe" driving cessation. This may be better received than reporting the individual to the DMV.
- Ask the family to have the family lawyer discuss with the individual the financial and legal implications of a crash or injury.

From Carr D, Ott B: The older adult driver with cognitive impairment: "It's a very frustrating life," *JAMA* 303:1632–1641, 2010; Gray-Vickrey P: Enhancing driver safety in dementia, *Alzheimers Care Today* 11:147–148, 2010.

EMERGING TECHNOLOGIES TO ENHANCE SAFETY OF OLDER ADULTS

Advancements in all types of technology hold promise for improving quality of life, decreasing the need for personal care, and enhancing independence and the ability to live safely at home and age-in-place. A growing concern related to the increasing number of older people is the lack of both family and paid caregivers. The caregiver support ratio in 2010 was about 7 potential caregivers to 1 person in the high-risk years of ages 80 and older. This ratio is projected to fall to 4:1 by 2030, and to less than 3:1 by 2050, just as the youngest baby boomers enter the high-risk years for needing services (Blanchard, 2014) (Chapter 34). Emerging technologies will play a larger role in ensuring care for older people in the future.

Assistive technology is any device or system that allows a person to perform a task independently or that makes the task easier and safer to perform. Assistive technology is decreasing the number of older people who depend on others for personal care in ADLs and presents cost-effective alternatives to human services and institutionalization (Daniel et al, 2009). Gerotechnology is the term used to describe assistive technologies for older people and these technologies are expected to significantly influence how we live in the future. Health care technologies, robotics, telemedicine, mobility and activities-of-daily-living (ADL) aids, and environmental control systems (smart houses/intelligent homes) are some examples of assistive technology.

Telehealth

Telehealth (telemedicine) is defined as "the use of electronic information and telecommunication technologies to support long-distance clinical health care, patient and professional health-related education, public health, and health administration" (Grady, 2014, p. 39). Telehealth offers exciting possibilities for managing medical problems in the home or other setting, reducing health care costs, and promoting self-management of illness, particularly in rural and underserved areas. The number of telehealth programs is increasing worldwide, and these programs offer exciting possibilities for nurses, particularly advanced practice nurses (Mars, 2010; Rutledge et al, 2014; Wamala and Augustine, 2013).

Telehealth nurses may practice in any setting in which on-site access to health care providers is limited. Remote-monitoring devices allow patients to connect with telehealth nurses from their homes or from a community setting such as a senior center. Remote physical assessment (pulse oximeters, weight scales, blood glucose monitors, and intelligent toilets that collect data on weight, blood pressure, and urine glucose level) allow nurses and primary care providers to track trends in patient data. The nurse may use a digital stethoscope to auscultate lung sounds or a digital camera to assess and document wound healing. A home care telehealth nurse can "see" many more patients through virtual visits (Grady, 2014; Rutledge et al, 2014).

A number of studies have reported that telehealth technology improves patient outcomes and decreases hospital readmissions and health care costs (Grady, 2014; Rutledge et al, 2014). A recent eHealth patient survey reported that 40% of older patients want access to technology that can alert physicians and other caregivers if they are having an emergency (Morrissey, 2014). Factors driving the adoption of telehealth include rising health care costs, the desire to age in place, increasing comfort with technology, the new generation of nurses who expect to incorporate technology into their practice, and the profit motive of device manufacturers. Factors slowing widespread development include concerns about privacy, fear of diminishing human contact and caring, and limited reimbursement (Fuji et al, 2014; Grady, 2014).

Smart Homes

Smart medical homes are being studied as a way to aid in the prevention and early detection of disease through the use of sensors and monitors. These devices keep data on vital signs and other measures such as gait, behavior, and sleep and provide an interactive medical-advising system. Devices to monitor gait and detect balance problems, such as the iShoe and the "smart carpet" (a sensor system embedded in carpet that detects gait abnormalities that may predispose to falls, and also detects falls and summons assistance), are being developed (Aud et al, 2010; Rantz et al, 2008). SmartSoles, shoe insoles with an embedded GPS device, are being developed and may be an aid to locate individuals with dementia who wander from their home.

Remote-controlled houses are becoming more popular and allow the individual to control the house from anywhere (e.g., devices that turn lights on and off, automatically water plants, or feed pets; motion detectors; and leak detectors). The first of a series of smart houses to enable older people to live safely in their own homes is already on the market. An example is the QuietCare 24-hour monitoring service. This system uses an ordinary home security infrastructure to monitor the house and transfers information about the occupant's daily living activities, triggering when a normal routine is broken. Caregivers and family can perform virtual check-ins with their older relative over the Internet (Bezaitis, 2009).

The MEDCottage is a 12 × 24 foot portable and modular medical home equipped with technology and amenities for the health, safety, and comfort of older adults recovering from illness or injury. The MEDCottage provides a family communication center that allows telemetry, environmental control, and dynamic interaction to off-site caregivers through smart and robotic technology. Technology inside the home includes monitoring of the person's vital signs and safety, medication reminders, and adaptive devices. The MEDCottage can be purchased or leased and temporarily placed on the caregiver's family property.

Motion and pressure sensors may be useful in the homes of older adults with cognitive impairment. These sensors can detect movement and the absence of movement. If there has been no movement for a period of time, a monitoring system is activated and a plan of action initiated depending on the person's response or lack of response. Pressure sensors can be used under the mattress and can turn on bedside lights when the individual gets out of bed and activate an alarm if he or she does not return to bed in a specified period of time. Sensors placed in entry doors can detect if a person leaves the home and can send messages to caregivers that the individual has left the house (Daniel et al, 2009).

In hospitals and long-term care facilities, devices such as wireless pendants that track people's movements, load cells built into beds that create an alert when individuals get out of bed, as well as monitor weight and sleep patterns, and bed lifts that allow individuals to go from lying down to standing up with the push of a button are being used. Wheelchair technology that enables the user to go down stairs, move to an upright position, be reminded to change positions to alleviate pressure, or use mechanical arms to change a light bulb or get things out of the refrigerator are other developing technologies.

Robots

Robotic technology for health care is more advanced in Europe and Japan than in the United States at this time, but we can expect to see increased development and use of robotics in nursing. On the horizon are technology developments such as robots that can help lift both individuals and objects, remind patients to take their medicine or administer the medication, check a person's vital signs, provide help in the event of a fall, and assist with baths and meals. A child-size therapist robot on wheels with a humanlike torso is being developed for use in homes and long-term care facilities to assist with the high level of attention individuals with dementia require for safety and function.

A recent American film, *Robot & Frank* depicted the relationship between Frank and his robot helper that cooked, cleaned, and kept him company. Frank's son wanted him to go to an Alzheimer's facility because he was too busy to care for him but Frank resisted. Instead, the son purchased a humanoid robot for Frank. Many ethical issues have been raised about the use of robots, and nurses will play an important role in ensuring that technological competence is balanced with caring to enhance the well-being of the individual (Campling et al, 2007; Fuji et al, 2014).

As the baby boomers and future generations age, comfort with technology will be increased, and people will seek options for better, safer, and more independent ways not yet imagined. At this time, many of the assistive technologies can be cost-prohibitive for older people, but with advances in development they may be more accessible and affordable for more people. Research is needed on assistive technologies and their acceptance among older people. It is important for nurses to be aware of available technology to improve safety.

ELDER-FRIENDLY COMMUNITIES

Developing elder-friendly communities and providing increasing opportunities to age in place can lead to enhanced health and well-being. Aging in place is the ability to live in one's own home and community safely, independently, and comfortably, regardless of age, income, or ability level (CDC, 2013). Many state and local governments are assessing the community and designing interventions to enhance the ability of older people to remain in their homes and familiar environments. These interventions range from adequate transportation systems to home modifications and universal design standards for barrier-free housing.

Components of an elder-friendly community include the following: (1) addresses basic needs; (2) optimizes physical health and well-being; (3) maximizes independence for the frail and disabled; and (4) provides social and civic engagement. Figure 20-1 presents elements of an elder-friendly community.

Efforts to create physical and social urban environments that promote healthy and active aging and a good quality of life are occurring worldwide. The World Health Organization (WHO) Global Network of Age-Friendly Cities and Communities was established to foster the exchange of experience and mutual learning between cities and communities across the globe (WHO, 2007). The program helps cities and communities become more supportive of older people by addressing their needs across eight dimensions: the built environment, transport, housing, social participation, respect and social inclusion,

Addresses Basic Needs

- Provides appropriate and affordable housing
- Promotes safety at home and in the neighborhood
- Ensures no one goes hungry
- Provides useful information about available services

Promotes Social and Civic Engagement

- Fosters meaningful connections with family, neighbors, and friends
- Promotes active engagement in community life
- Provides opportunities for meaningful paid and voluntary work
- Makes aging issues a community-wide priority

Optimizes Physical and Mental Health and Well-Being

- Promotes healthy behaviors
- Supports community activities that enhance well-being
- Provides ready access to preventive health services
- Provides access to medical, social, and palliative services

Maximizes Independence for Frail and Disabled

- Mobilizes resources to facilitate "living at home"
- Provides accessible transportation
- Supports family and other caregivers

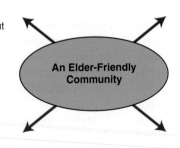

An Elder-Friendly Community

FIGURE 20-1 Essential Elements of an Elder-Friendly Community. (From AdvantAge Initiative, Center for Home Care Policy and Research, Visiting Nurse Service of New York.)

civic participation and employment, communication, and community support and health services (WHO, 2007).

Aging in Community Models

Naturally Occurring Retirement Communities (NORCs) are neighborhoods or buildings in which a large segment of the residents are older adults. They are not purpose-built senior housing or retirement communities but are places where community residents have aged in place and where they intend to spend the rest of their lives. There are approximately 50 projects across 26 states (Stone, 2013). NORCs provide a range of health and social services for the residents, as well as individual assessments of risk, coordination of nonprofessional services, and referrals and follow-up. The U.S. Administration on Aging (AoA) administers the Older Americans Act programs, including the National NORCs Initiative.

The Village model is another community program that aids in successful aging in neighborhoods. You can join an existing village in your area or create your own village with neighbors. The prototype village is Beacon Hill in Boston. Beacon Hill is an independent, self-governing, not-for-profit organization run by volunteers and paid staff who coordinate access to affordable services for older adults in their communities. Services include transportation, health and wellness programs, home repair, social and education activities and trips, and discounts on goods and services (Blanchard 2014; Stone, 2013).

Cohousing communities, a concept that originated in Denmark, are another growing option that older people may find appealing. Most of the 150 U.S. cohousing projects are intergenerational, but some also are designed specifically for individuals 50 years of age and older. According to the Cohousing Association of the United States (2014), cohousing is a type of intentional, collaborative housing in which residents actively participate in the design and operation of their neighborhoods. Communities are usually designed as attached or single-family homes along one or more pedestrian streets or clustered around a central courtyard. There is a common house where residents can gather and share a common meal or socialize. Community members work together to care for the common property. In most cases, cohousing communities are started by prospective residents, who often partner with a developer to design and finance the project. Some are started by architects and developers who then organize a group of future residents to buy into the project.

Shared housing among adult children and their older relatives has become a choice for many because of cultural preferences or need. The sharing may relieve the economic burdens of maintaining a home after widowhood or retirement on a fixed income. Chapter 34 discusses multigenerational housing. Another model of shared housing is that of opening up one's personal home to others. Older people often live in houses that were purchased in their young adult years and find that as they age, much of the space may be underused. Sharing a house can be easily implemented by locating, screening, and matching older people looking for houses to share with those who have them. The National Shared Housing Resource Center has established subgroups nationally to assist individuals interested in home sharing.

As the baby boomers age, we can expect to see more innovative housing movements that create successful opportunities for healthy aging in the community and provide a range of options for older adults beyond what is available now (Blanchard, 2014; Stone, 2013). Box 20-1 presents some resources for aging in the community.

KEY CONCEPTS

- Thermoregulatory changes, chronic illness, and medications may predispose the older adult to hypothermia and hyperthermia. Careful attention must be paid to temperature monitoring and provision of adequate heat and cooling in weather extremes.
- Transportation for older adults is critical to their physical, psychological, and social health.
- Neighborhoods change over the years, and long-term dwellers may find themselves in dangerous or crime-ridden areas as they age.
- Elders are often targets of fraud and deception.

- Reducing fire hazards is essential to feelings of security.
- Driving safety for older people is an important issue, and health care professionals must be knowledgeable about assessment, safety interventions, and transportation resources.
- Technology advances hold promise for improving quality of life, decreasing need for personal care assistance, and enhancing independence and the ability to live safely.
- Efforts to make communities more elder friendly are under way across the globe. New and innovative ideas for aging in the community will continue to change living options for older adults.

NURSING STUDY: CHANGING LIFE SITUATIONS AND ENVIRONMENTAL VULNERABILITY

Ethel had lived in one home for all her married life, but when her husband died her children worried about her safety, being alone in a big home. She could fall and lie undiscovered to die of hypothermia, the deteriorating neighborhood was no longer considered safe, and she could no longer drive and was limited in her ability to get around. They convinced her to move to a community in Phoenix near them.

They were able to find a suitable apartment that she could afford. For a while they visited her each week, but each visit became more depressing for them as she continually talked about her old home, old friends, old furniture, old priest—everything old. Their visits became less frequent. She called them faithfully each morning but detected their urge to get off the phone and on with their lives. One morning she called her daughter Gladys and said, "I'm so sick! Yesterday I walked outside and I swear I saw my friend Rose from the old neighborhood getting on the bus, but she didn't see me. I was so disappointed but managed to make it home, then couldn't find the key to my apartment so finally had to call 911 for help. They were really irritated with me when I said I had lost my key. I want to go back to Detroit. I know how things work there." After a family conclave, Ethel's family found a nice place in assisted living for Ethel and they were relieved. Ethel said, "I don't know where I am anymore. Seems I bounce around like a rubber ball." She seldom left her room except for meals, and soon she needed meals brought to her. Last week she wandered out and, when found, had suffered a serious case of heat stroke.

Based on the nursing study, develop a nursing care plan using the following procedure*:

- List Ethel's comments that provide subjective data.
- List information that provides objective data.
- From these data, identify and state, using an accepted format, two nursing diagnoses you determine are most significant to Ethel at this time. List two of Ethel's strengths that you have identified from the data.
- Determine and state outcome criteria for each diagnosis. These must reflect some alleviation of the problem identified in the nursing diagnosis and must be stated in concrete and measurable terms.
- Plan and state one or more interventions for each diagnosed problem. Provide specific documentation of the source used to determine the appropriate intervention. Plan at least one intervention that incorporates Ethel's existing strengths.
- Evaluate the success of the intervention. Interventions must correlate directly with the stated outcome criteria to measure the outcome success.

*Students are advised to refer to their nursing diagnosis text and identify possible or potential problems.

CRITICAL THINKING QUESTIONS AND ACTIVITIES

1. What alternatives could you suggest to Ethel's family as they decide on the best living situation for her?
2. How could Ethel's family have involved her in the decision making about her living situations?
3. Locate low-cost housing in your area, and assess for convenience and safety.
4. What type of support does your community provide to assist elders to safely age in place?
5. What crimes against elders are of concern in your community?
6. List several aspects of your environment that are important to you, and discuss their significance.
7. Discuss housing options that would be suitable and feasible for you if you were unable to get around without the assistance of a walker.
8. What are your city's and state's plans for disaster preparedness for disabled and older people living in the community and in institutions?
9. Compare your community to the characteristics of an elder-friendly community described in the chapter.
10. Survey the homes of elders you are serving in your clinical practice for the presence or absence of safety features.
11. Discuss how you would assist your parents in making a decision regarding a change in living situations if they become increasingly disabled and unable to care for themselves.

RESEARCH QUESTIONS

1. What criminal activities are of most concern to older people?
2. What home safety factors are most frequently causes of concern for older people?
3. What is the geographical distribution and incidence of hypothermia and hyperthermia in the United States?
4. What are the most frequent causes of fires among elders?
5. What do older people fear most in their environment?
6. What are the barriers to the use of assistive technology in institutions and personal homes?

REFERENCES

Al-Rousan T, Rubenstein L, Wallace R: Preparedness for natural disasters among US adults: a nationwide survey, *Am J Public Health* 104(3):506–511, 2014.

Aud M, Abbott C, Tyrer H, et al: Smart carpet: developing a sensor system to detect falls and summon assistance, *J Gerontol Nurs* 36:8–12, 2010.

Bezaitis A: Robot technologies: exciting new frontier, *Aging Well* 2:10, 2009.

Blanchard J: Aging in community: the communitarian alternative to aging in place, *Generations*, Feb 4, 2014. http://asaging.org/blog/aging-community-communitarian-alternative-aging-place-alone. Accessed May 2014.

Burnett J, Dyer CB, Pickins S: Rapid needs assessment for older adults in disasters, *Generations* 31:10–15, 2008.

Campling A, Tanoika T, Locsin R: Robots and nursing: concepts, relationships and practice. In Barnard A, Locsin R, editors: *Technology and nursing*, New York, 2007, Palgrave Macmillan, pp 73–99.

Carr D, Ott B: The older adult driver with cognitive impairment: "It's a very frustrating life, *JAMA* 303:1632–1641, 2010.

Centers for Disease Control and Prevention: Heat-related deaths—United States, 1999-2003, MMWR *Morb Mortal Wkly Rep* 55:796–798, 2006.

Centers for Disease Control and Prevention: *Health places terminology*, 2013. http://www.cdc.gov/healthyplaces/terminology.htm. Accessed October 2014.

Cohousing Association of the United States: *What is cohousing?* 2014. http://www.cohousing.org/what_is_cohousing. Accessed August 2014.

Daniel K, Cason CL, Ferrell S: Emerging technologies to enhance the safety of older people in their homes, *Geriatr Nurs* 30:384–389, 2009.

Dobbs B, Harper L, Wood A: Transitioning from driving to driving cessation: the role of specialized driving cessation support groups for individuals with dementia, *Top Geriatr Rehabil* 25:73–86, 2009.

Dugan E, Lee C: Biopsychosocial factors for driving cessation: findings from the Health and Retirement Study, *J Aging Health* 25:1313–1328, 2013.

Feather J: Why older adults face more danger in natural disasters, *The Blog*, Dec 18, 2013. http://www.huffingtonpost.com/john-feather-phd/why-older-adults-face-mor_b_4461648.html. Accessed May 2014.

Fuji S, Ito H, Yasuhara Y, Huang S, et al: Discussion of nursing robot's capability and ethical issues, *Information* 17(1): 349–353, 2014.

Grady J: Telehealth: a case study in disruptive innovation, *Am J Nurs* 114(4):38–45, 2014.

Gray-Vickrey P: Enhancing driver safety in dementia, *Alzheimers Care Today* 11: 147–148, 2010a.

Gray-Vickrey P: Research updates: driving and dementia, *Alzheimer's Care Today* 11:149–150, 2010b.

Green M, Prior N, Capeluto G, et al: Climate change and health in Israel: adaptation policies for extreme weather events, *Isr J Health Policy Res* 2:23, 2013.

Help Age International: *Older people in emergencies*, 2013. http://www.helpageusa.org/what-we-do/emergencies/older-people-in-emergencies. Accessed May 2014.

Hogan T, Rios-Alba T: Emergency care. In Ham R, Sloane PD, Warshaw GA, et al, editors: *Primary care geriatrics*, ed 6, 2014, Philadelphia, 2014, Elsevier, pp 177–192.

Hooyman N, Kiyak H: *Social gerontology: a multidisciplinary perspective*, Boston, 2011, Allyn & Bacon.

Jett K, Tappen R, Rosselli M: Imposed versus involved: different strategies to effect driving cessation in cognitively impaired older adults, *Geriatr Nurs* 26:111–116, 2005.

Mars M: Health capacity development through telemedicine in Africa, *Yearb Med Inform* 2010:87–93, 2010.

Mathias J, Lucas L: Cognitive predictors of unsafe driving in older drivers: a meta-analysis, *Int Psychogeriatr* 21:637–653, 2009.

McGregor D: Driving over 65: proceed with caution, *J Gerontol Nurs* 28:221–226, 2002.

Morrissey J: Remote patient monitoring: how mobile devices will curb chronic conditions, *Medical Economics*, July 8, 2014. http://medicaleconomics.modernmedicine.com/medical-economics/news/remote-patient-monitoring-how-mobile-devices-will-curb-chronic-conditions. Accessed July 2014.

Outzen M: Management of fever in older adults, *J Gerontol Nurs* 35:17–23, 2009.

Oxley J, Charlton J: Attitudes to and mobility impacts of driving cessation, *Top Geriatr Rehabil* 25:43–54, 2009.

Rantz M, Aud M, Alexander G, et al: Falls, technology, and stunt actors: new approaches to fall detection and risk fall assessment, *J Nurs Care Qual* 23:195–201, 2008.

Rosenbloom S: Meeting transportation needs in an aging-friendly community, *Generations* 33(2):33–41, 2009.

Rutledge C, Haney T, Bordelon M, et al: Telehealth: preparing advanced practice nurses to address healthcare needs in rural and underserved populations, *Int J Nurs Education Scholarship* 11(1):1–9, 2014.

Servat J, Risco M, Nakasato Y, et al: Visual impairment in the elderly: impact on functional ability and quality of life, *Clin Geriatr* 19(7), 2011.

Stone R: What are the realistic options for aging in community? *Generations* 37(4):65–70, 2013–14.

University of Maryland Medical Center: *Hypothermia*, 2013. https://umm.edu/health/medical/altmed/condition/hypothermia. Accessed April 2014.

Wamala D, Augustine K: A meta-analysis of telemedicine success in Africa, *J Pathol Inform* 4:6, 2013.

Wolf T, McGregor G: The development of a heat wave vulnerability index for London, United Kingdom, *Weather and Climate Extremes* 1:59–68, 2013.

World Health Organization: *Global age-friendly cities: a guide*, Geneva, Switzerland, 2007, WHO Press. http://www.who.int/ageing/age_friendly_cities_guide/en. Accessed May 2014.

21 CHAPTER

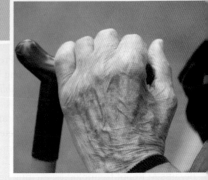

Living Well with Chronic Illness

Kathleen Jett

http://evolve.elsevier.com/Touhy/TwdHlthAging

AN ELDER SPEAKS

If I'd known I was going to live this long, I'd have taken better care of myself.

Eubie Blake, on his 100th birthday

LEARNING OBJECTIVES

On completion of this chapter, the reader will be able to:

1. Identify the most common chronic disorders of late life.
2. Describe the concept of frailty and explain how it applies to chronic disease.
3. Describe a conceptual model that may be useful for guiding the nurse in the development of strategies to promote healthy aging regardless of limitations in function.
4. Construct nursing interventions that are consistent with the Chronic Illness Trajectory.
5. Propose strategies to reduce chronic disease in the global community.

Chronic illnesses are those that are persistent regardless of treatment; they are of long duration and usually progress slowly. Their onset may be insidious and identified only during a health screening, such as when an advanced practice nurse is conducting an assessment of a person following a fall. Chronic diseases are not always obvious and may not interfere with the person's daily life until late in the disease, but they are present and require ongoing treatment, if available.

In a younger adult the initial signs of a pending chronic disease may be identified early enough to prevent later problems (e.g., the finding of an elevated cholesterol level). In older adults a chronic disease may not be diagnosed until some amount of "end organ damage" has already occurred. For example, diabetic retinopathy may be found during an annual eye exam, indicating that the diabetes has been present for some time.

If a diagnosis does not occur until late in the disease process the major goal is to "manage" it rather than "cure" it. The goals include minimizing complications, delaying the associated mortality, and optimizing health-related quality of life while attending to the person as a holistic being.

The most common chronic diseases worldwide are cardiovascular/cerebrovascular, cancer, respiratory disease, and diabetes. Together they represent 63% of all deaths, killing 36 million people a year, 80% of whom live in low- and middle-income countries. In 2014, 6 million deaths worldwide were attributed to smoking alone, a number expected to rise to 7.5 million by 2020, or 10% of all deaths due to chronic disease (WHO, 2013). In the United States the most common chronic diseases are hypertension, osteoarthritis, and heart disease (Figure 21-1). Of older adults, 92% have at least one chronic disease and 77% have at least two (NCOA, 2014).

For today's older adult with a preexisting chronic disease, its presence or absence may not be as important as its effect on function. The effect may be as little as an inconvenience or as great as an impairment of one's ability to live independently. When superimposed on the normal changes with aging, the likelihood of the person needing assistance in daily living and developing frailty increases over time.

During acute exacerbations of chronic diseases, active rehabilitation may be possible in the home or at designated rehabilitation centers, such as those found in high-income countries. Once the disease has stabilized the person may return to full function, at least until another exacerbation. If the limitations associated with a chronic condition reach a point when consistent physical, functional, or cognitive assistance is needed, informal help may be available with a move to the home of a friend or family member. Others may be able to hire the formal help of professional caregivers. Still others move to institutional settings such as assisted living facilities, nursing homes, or group homes. Unfortunately, options in the United States are highly dependent on personal financial resources; there are solutions for the very poor and the wealthy, but solutions are tenuous at

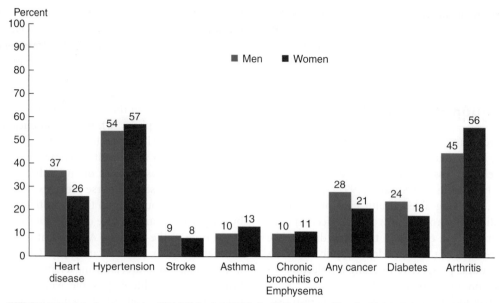

Percent

■ Men   ■ Women

NOTE: Data are based on a 2-year average from 2007–2008. See Appendix B for the definition of race and Hispanic origin in the National Health Interview Survey.
Reference population: These data refer to the civilian noninstitutionalized population.
SOURCE: Centers for Disease Control and Prevention, National Center for Health Statistics, National Health Interview Survey.

FIGURE 21-1 Chronic Health Conditions among the Population Age 65 and Older, by Sex, 2009-2010. (Redrawn from Federal Interagency Forum on Aging-Related Statistics: *Older Americans 2012: key indicators of well-being,* Washington, DC, 2012, U.S. Government Printing Office.)

best for the near poor and middle-income individuals and families

The relationship between chronic disease and aging is complex. Many diseases have been viewed as intrinsic to aging. Although chronic diseases are not normal parts of aging, the number of persons with them is growing rapidly worldwide; no country can avoid this burgeoning problem. We now know that smoking cessation as late as age 75 can reduce premature death by up to 50% (WHO, 2014). Many chronic diseases could be eliminated through preventive strategies, especially when started at a young age. For example, if the major lifestyle risk factors are eliminated (Box 21-1), all which are within control of the individual, about three-fourths of all cases of heart disease, stroke, and diabetes could be eliminated (WHO, 2013). The understanding of which preventive strategies are the most effective is becoming clearer as organizations such as the National Institutes of Health invest heavily in related research (Gupta et al, 2014).

As discussed in Chapter 1, the United States has developed multiple strategies to attempt to reduce the incidence of chronic disease and publishes their progress in the document *Healthy People 2020* (USDHHS, 2012). Strategies of particular importance

to the prevention of, and healthy living with, chronic diseases are engaging in physical activity, reducing obesity, stopping smoking, and taking medications as prescribed.

The World Health Organization has also developed a global action plan identifying multiple targets and indicators that assist countries to set national goals and policies addressing the prevention and optimal management of chronic diseases. These cover a wide range of topics and are similar to many of those found in *Healthy People 2020* (WHO, 2013) (Box 21-2).

Any consideration of chronic disease in later life leads to multiple questions. How is it that some persons develop many of the "chronic diseases of old age" and others do not? As the understanding of genomics develops, will the line between aging and chronic conditions become more blurred or more clear? We have learned that most lung disease in late life is the result of life choices earlier in life, such as smoking, yet as one ages, so does the susceptibility to pneumonia, even for the non-smoker. With the introduction of antiretroviral therapy in the

---

BOX 21-1   Major Global Lifestyle Risk Factors for the Development of Chronic Disease

Tobacco use	Physical inactivity
Unhealthy diet	Alcohol abuse

From World Health Organization (WHO): *10 facts on noncommunicable diseases,* 2013. http://www.who.int/features/factfiles/noncommunicable_diseases/en/. Accessed June 2014.

BOX 21-2   RESOURCES FOR BEST PRACTICE

World Health Organization: *10 Facts on noncommunicable diseases,* http://www.who.int/features/factfiles/noncommunicable_diseases/en.

World Health Organization: *Chronic disease and health promotion,* http://www.who.int/chp/en.

Healthy People: *Older adults,* http://www.healthypeople.gov/2020/topics-objectives/topic/older-adult.

Centers for Disease Control and Prevention: www.cdc.gov (search "frailty" and "chronic disease")

National Institute of Aging: http://www.nia.nih.go. (Research focuses on the increased risk and severity of health problems as people age).

1990s, persons are living longer than they ever had before with human immunodeficiency virus (HIV) infections. An HIV diagnosis no longer means imminent death; it has become a chronic disease instead. How will this new "collection" of diseases affect aging persons with HIV and society?

A MODEL FOR CHRONIC ILLNESS

Although there are many conceptual models from which chronic illness can be viewed, the trajectory model originally introduced by Anselm Strauss and Barney Glaser (1975), then further developed by Corbin and Strauss (1992) and Lubkin and Larsen (2012), has long aided health care providers to understand the realities of chronic illness and its effect on individuals. For each individual, even with the same disease, the trajectory is different. Using this model, chronic illness is viewed from a life course perspective or along a trajectory—a health and wellness continuum (Chapter 1).

The trajectory may include a preventive phase (pre-trajectory phase) (1) at which time preventive practices can be used by the individual before the development of a disease, such as receiving immunizations in a timely manner. The nurse advocates for health-promoting activities with individuals and in the community. Such activities are referred to as primary prevention (Chapter 1). At the beginning of the trajectory phase (2), initial signs of an illness appear and diagnoses are made. Nurses at all levels are very involved with this phase and may notice symptoms of a new chronic disease while monitoring those of another disease. In the stable phase (3), the chronic condition is present and while not curable, it is *controlled* so that the person has few, if any, symptoms and is able to maintain a high quality of life. This is the result of a combination of factors, including high-quality nursing and personal care for the person residing in a care setting such as a nursing home, and equally as high medical care provided by nurse practitioners and other health care providers including the nursing assistant. For those with more complex chronic diseases, control will require coordination among members of the health care team, often with the nurse coordinating this care. This is consistent with secondary prevention. During periods of unstable disease exacerbations (4), one or more of multiple dimensions defining the individual's strengths are stressed (Chapter 1). In the aging adult this is a particularly precarious stage because the uncontrollable chronic disease is superimposed on reduced physiological reserve, a normal change of aging. For the very frail elder, a previously controlled health condition can rapidly become acute or life-threatening because of even further age-related reduced physiological reserves that are exacerbated in the presence of a chronic disease. The nurse is instrumental in assuring that prompt care is delivered in a manner that maximizes the chance that the person can return to the highest level of wellness possible. If care is delayed for those who are frail, it may not be possible to stop the overall downward trend (see 8). In the acute phase (5), severe and unrelieved symptoms or disease complications are present. In the acute phase every effort is made to stop the escalating symptoms in the frail elder and enable the person to return to some

level of stability if at all possible. Should this phase be reached, the nurse may be the one to inform the elder and his or her family that a complete return to the trajectory phase (2) may not be possible, but symptoms can be controlled to keep the person comfortable. For those who are very ill with multiple co-morbidities, this phase may be bypassed and the person may proceed directly from the unstable phase (4) to the crisis phase (6). In the crisis phase (6), major complications of a chronic disease become critical and life-threatening. It may be triggered by an event such as an acute myocardial infarction (AMI) or even a fracture as a result of the imbalance associated with Parkinson's disease. The nurse provides or facilitates imminent emergency care but only to the point that had been expressed by the person in an advance directive or by a health care proxy at the time of the incident. Although it is unlikely that an advance directive or a health care proxy (Chapter 31) would elect not to repair a fracture, allowing a natural death to occur at the time of an AMI is highly possible. Nurses caring for frail elders need to know the content of their advance directives and understand how patients wishes you to respond in an emergency. Although less likely in frail elders, the person may be able to restore equilibrium (phase 7, the comeback phase) or a somewhat steady state for some period of time. The older one becomes and the more chronic diseases that accumulate, the less likely it is that the person will ever return to a period when symptoms are not noticeable. This is important in conversation about resuscitative efforts in frail persons or those with multiple chronic conditions. The final downward phase (9) is that which ends in death (Lubkin and Larsen, 2012). During this phase the nurse has a significant opportunity, responsibility, and privilege to provide comfort at the end of life; of reassuring those who are dying; and then of ensuring that the dying patient continues to receive the highest quality nursing and medical care possible (Table 21-1).

The shape and stability of the trajectory is influenced by the combined efforts, attitudes, and beliefs (e.g., regarding

TABLE 21-1	**The Chronic Illness Trajectory**
PHASE	**DEFINITION**
1. Pre-trajectory	Before the illness course occurs, the preventive phase, no signs or symptoms present
2. Trajectory onset	Signs and symptoms are present to some extent, includes diagnostic period
3. Stable	Controlled illness course/symptoms
4. Unstable	Illness course/symptoms not controlled by regimen but not requiring or desiring hospitalization
5. Acute	Active illness or complications that require hospitalization for management
6. Crisis	Life-threatening situation; acute threat to self-identity
7. Comeback	While this is much less likely to occur along the trajectory of those who are frail, this is a period of temporary remission from the crisis
8. Downward	Progressive decline in physical/mental status characterized by increasing disability/symptoms
9. Dying	Immediate weeks, days, hours preceding death

preventive health) held by the elder, family members, and significant others. Nurses have the opportunity to promote healthy aging at any point on the trajectory. The person's perceptions of both needs met and functional limitations are paramount to predicting movement along the illness trajectory (Corbin and Strauss, 1992).

FRAILTY

The associations between age and chronic disease and the development of frailty remain uncertain. Neither age itself nor the presence of a chronic disease is a predictor of who will become frail; however, the incidence increases with age. Old and Woolley (2014) reported on two studies: 70% of those older than 85 years of age showed some signs of frailty, and almost half still lived in the community. Many times medical and social diagnoses leading particularly to frailty are never found (primary frailty). At other times it is related to the downward progression of a specific chronic disease (secondary frailty) consistent with the downward slope of the chronic disease trajectory. For those with secondary frailty, the prognosis is poor (Old and Woolley, 2014).

The phenotype of frailty has been difficult to define. However, the phenotype that was described in 2001 is still recognized today (Fried et al, 2001; Old and Woolley, 2014). The formal diagnosis is made by the presence of at least three of the following: unintentional weight loss, self-reported exhaustion, weak grip strength, slow walking speed, and low activity (Box 21-3). In much of the geriatric literature, the signs leading to a diagnosis of frailty are referred to as "geriatric syndromes" (Nash, 2013). Together, they significantly increase the vulnerability to any challenge to the physical, cognitive, or emotional state of health (Old and Woolley, 2014). In other words, the

---

BOX 21-4 Nurses' Role in Caring for Persons with Chronic Disease

- Assessing elder and family strengths and challenges
- Teaching related to healthy lifestyle modifications, preservation of energy, and self-care strategies
- Encouraging the reduction of modifiable risk factors
- Counseling the individual in the development of reasonable expectations of self
- Providing access to resources when possible
- Referring appropriately and when needed
- Organizing and leading interdisciplinary case conferences and team meetings
- Facilitating advance care planning and palliative care when appropriate

---

normal age-related decreases in reserve capacity are exacerbated, sometimes to the point that compensation is not possible. Of note is that there is not necessarily a diagnosis in the usual sense of the word, but rather the report or observation of vague problems that cannot be explained by other means. Frailty is highly associated with falls, fractures, hospitalization, and death (Fang et al, 2012; Li et al, 2014).

Frailty, Aging, and Chronic Disease

The number of frail elders is increasing worldwide at an alarming rate. It is expected that by 2025, 1.2 billion people will be considered frail, the majority of these living in developing countries (Sourdet et al, 2012). This burgeoning population drives the need to actively address wellness in aging to prevent both chronic disease and the development of frailty in future generations.

Working with older adults who are either frail or are living with chronic illnesses means that the gerontological nurse has the opportunity to decrease both the morbidity and the mortality of older adults (Box 21-4). The next several chapters provide basic information of the most common chronic conditions the gerontological nurse will encounter in persons who are aging in today's society. Strategies will be proposed to promote healthy aging regardless of the limitations with which one lives. We do not cover all possible conditions, nor do we provide a comprehensive medical management of these disorders. However, certain disorders are encountered frequently enough in late life to merit special attention.

BOX 21-3 TIPS FOR BEST PRACTICE

Assessing Frailty

Frailty is loosely defined as evidence of three of the following: unexplained weight loss, self-reported exhaustion, weak grip strength, slow walking speed, and low activity.

It is better to ask the patient specifically about each one of these symptoms. Many people consider the signs as "just a normal part of aging."

▮ KEY CONCEPTS

- The nation's goals include increasing the span of healthy life. The challenge to this goal is to help persons find ways to promote healthy aging in the presence of chronic disease.
- The effects of chronic illness range from mild to life-limiting, with each person responding to unique circumstances in a highly individualized manner.
- Coping with chronic illness can be a physical, psychological, and spiritual challenge.
- The Chronic Illness Trajectory is a useful framework to facilitate understanding chronic illness and designing nursing interventions to promote healthy aging.

- The goals of promoting healthy aging include minimizing risk for disease and frailty, and in the presence of either, alleviating symptoms, delaying or avoiding the development of complications including end-organ damage, and maximizing function and quality of life. It also includes providing comfort to the dying.
- The gerontological nurse has the potential to serve as a leader in the promotion of health and the prevention of disease.

REFERENCES

Corbin JM, Strauss A: A nursing model for chronic illness management based upon the trajectory framework. In Woog P, editor: *The chronic illness framework: the Corbin and Strauss nursing model,* New York, 1992, Springer.

Fang X, Shi J, Song X, et al: Frailty in relation to the risk of falls, fractures and mortality rate in older Chinese adults: results from the Beijing Longitudinal Study of Aging, *J Nutr Health Aging* 16(10):903–907, 2012.

Fried LP, Tangen CM, Walston J, et al: Frailty in older adults: evidence for a phenotype, *J Gerontol A Biol Sci Med Sci* 56(3):M146–M156, 2001.

Gupta S, Sussman DA, Doubeni CA, et al: Challenges and possible solutions to colorectal cancer screening for the underserved, *J Natl Cancer Inst* 106(4): 1-12, 2014.

Li G, Ioannidis G, Pickard L, et al: Frailty index of deficit accumulation and falls: data from the Global Longitudinal Study of Osteoporosis in Women (GLOW) Hamilton cohort, *BMC Musculoskeletal Disord* 15(1):185, 2014.

Lubkin I, Larsen PD: *Chronic illness: impact and intervention,* ed 8, Burlington, MA, 2012, Jones & Bartlett.

Nash DT: Frailty: the forthcoming medical crisis, *Consultant* 53(9): 654–655, 2013.

National Council on Aging (NCOA), Center for Healthy Aging: *Chronic disease,* 2014. http://www.ncoa.org/improve-health/center-for-healthy-aging/chronic-disease. Accessed June 2014.

Old JL, Woolley D: Frailty. In Ham RJ, Sloane PD, Warshaw GA, et al, editors: *Primary care geriatrics: a case-based approach,* Philadelphia, 2014, Elsevier, pp 323–332.

Sourdet S, Rouge-Bugat ME, Vellas B, et al: Frailty and aging, *J Nutr Health Aging* 16(4):284–285, 2012.

Strauss A, Glaser B: *Chronic illness and the quality of life,* St. Louis, MO, 1975, Mosby.

U.S. Department of Health and Human Services (USDHHS): *Healthy People 2020,* 2012. http://www.healthypeople. gov. Accessed June 2014.

World Health Organization (WHO): *10 facts on noncommunicable diseases,* 2013. http://www.who.int/features/factfiles/noncommunicable_diseases/en/. Accessed June 2014.

World Health Organization (WHO): *10 facts on ageing and the life course,* 2014. http://www.who.int/features/factfiles/ageing/en/. Accessed June 2014.

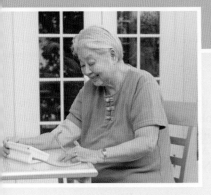

CHAPTER 22

Cardiovascular and Cerebrovascular Health and Wellness

Kathleen Jett

http://evolve.elsevier.com/Touhy/TwdHlthAging

A STUDENT SPEAKS

I thought all hearts sounded the same, but after gaining a little more experience I started hearing all sorts of differences.

Helen, a 19-year-old nursing student

AN ELDER SPEAKS

I had always been very active and healthy, and then slowly I started feeling more and more tired. I just thought it was due to growing older, but found out that my heart was no longer beating as it should.

Isabelle at 86

LEARNING OBJECTIVES

On completion of this chapter, the reader will be able to:
1. Describe the normal changes in the aging cardiovascular system.
2. Identify the most common cardiovascular disorders seen in later life.
3. Describe how the presentation of these disorders in older adults differs from that seen in younger adults.
4. Suggest interventions to promote healthy aging in the face of cardiovascular disease regardless of the stage of illness.

The cardiovascular system, composed of the heart and blood vessels, is the vehicle through which oxygenated and nutrient-rich blood is transported throughout the body and metabolic waste is carried to the excretory organs. There are several age-related changes in the system, but these have little or no effect on the lives of healthy elders. However, by the time one is in later life, the choices made earlier, such as smoking, coupled with normal changes result in a very high rate of cardiovascular disease (CVD). Both the prevalence and the incidence of CVD are so high that they are often mistaken as normal parts of aging and referred to as the "diseases of old age." In reality, while cardiovascular changes occur, cardiovascular diseases are not inevitable.

THE AGING HEART

One particular age-related change to the aging heart muscle is the progressive decline in cardiac reserve. That is, it takes longer for the heart to accelerate to meet a sudden demand for oxygen and longer to return to its resting state. This becomes quite significant when an increased cardiac response is needed in the presence of a physical or mental challenge such as acute emotional distress, infection, fluid or blood loss, or tachycardia. The associated increased pulse rate seen under these circumstances in younger adults is less likely to occur in older adults. Even a person with a presumably healthy heart may not be able to maintain heart function and failure can occur suddenly. In the presence of preexisting disease, this age-related change has the potential to increase both morbidity and mortality when it is not possible for the heart to work harder when it is taxed.

In normal aging, the heart valves separating the chambers thicken and stiffen as a result of lipid deposits and collagen cross-linking. A murmur is the sound of the backflow of blood through a valve that is no longer completely patent. *Mild systolic murmurs* (between S_1 and S_2) are expected findings in the older adult. Aortic and mitral valves are those most commonly affected. If the nurse auscultates a systolic murmur in an asymptomatic older adult, questions should be asked. Quite unlike a younger adult, most older adults will say, "Oh yes I have had that for years." If this is not the case, the person is referred to a cardiologist. If the new finding is accompanied by any signs or symptoms of distress, it is a medical emergency. *Diastolic murmurs* (heard between S_2 and S_1) are always indicative of a serious problem in cardiac hemodynamics and these persons are followed closely by a cardiologist. The nurse's ability to monitor this fragile condition is an essential skill in geriatrics and a means to work with the patient and the family to achieve the highest health-related quality of life possible.

CARDIOVASCULAR DISEASE (CVD)

In the United States 1 of every 4 deaths is related to heart disease, that is, about 600,000 deaths a year. More than half of these are the result of acute myocardial infarctions (AMIs) or heart attacks (CDC, 2014d). Although heart disease is the number 1 overall cause of death, it is second after cancer for Asian Americans, Hispanics, and Hawaiian/Pacific Islanders (Centers for Disease Control and Prevention [CDC], 2014a; Office of Minority Health [OMH], 2010) (Box 22-1). Nearly 44% of all African American men and 48% of African American women have some form of CVD (CDC, 2014c). Research has found that the risk factors for CVD are universal. They include those that the person cannot control, those in full control of the person, and those suspected to have an influence (Figure 22-1). Genetic factors influence the increased risk but do not in and of themselves cause one to develop CVD. Preventive strategies have shown to counter any genetic risk that may exist (CDC, 2014e).

Cardiovascular diseases derive from damage to the blood vessels or to the heart itself. Hypertension, coronary heart disease (CHD), heart failure (HF), atrial fibrillation (AF), and peripheral and cerebral (strokes) vascular disorders in older adults are summarized in this chapter. For more detailed examinations of these conditions, the reader is referred to geriatric medicine and nursing texts that are disease based.

Hypertension

Hypertension (HTN) is the most common chronic CVD encountered by the gerontological nurse. It occurs in 67 million people in the United States, or 1 out of every 3 persons, the majority of whom are African American and living in the Southeast (CDC, 2014e; National Heart, Lung and Blood Institute [NHLBI], 2012b).

Both the definition of and the guidelines for the treatment of HTN in the United States are provided by the Joint National Committee for the Detection, Evaluation, and Treatment of High Blood Pressure (JNC) (NHLBI, 2003). The previous guidelines did vary based on the person's age (NHLBI, 2003). The new guidelines, published in December 2013, include recommendations specifically for those ≥60 of age (Caboral-Stevens and Rosario-Sim, 2014; James et al, 2014).

Signs and Symptoms

Most persons with HTN are asymptomatic, and a diagnosis is only made during a routine health screening or after the manifestation of a disease that has developed as a result of long-standing uncontrolled hypertension (Box 22-2). Some people complain of a headache, "bad blood," light-headedness, a "swimmy head," or a "full head." These and other phrases are culture-based idioms and the nurse must first determine if the person believes that the symptoms are from an elevated or lowered blood pressure. Upon blood pressure measurement, the person may be normotensive, hypotensive, or hypertensive.

BOX 22-1	Leading Causes of Death by Racial and Ethnic Group in the United States				
AFRICAN AMERICAN	**AMERICAN INDIAN/ALASKAN NATIVE**	**ASIAN AMERICAN**	**HISPANIC OR LATINO**	**NATIVE HAWAIIAN AND OTHER PACIFIC ISLANDERS**	**WHITE**
1. Heart disease	1. Heart disease	1. Cancer	1. Cancer	1. Cancer	1. Heart disease
2. Cancer	2. Cancer	2. Heart disease	2. Heart disease	2. Heart disease	2. Cancer
3. Stroke	3. Unintentional injuries	3. Stroke	3. Unintentional injuries	3. Stroke	3. Chronic lower respiratory tract disease
4. Diabetes	4. Diabetes	4. Unintentional injuries	4. Stroke	4. Unintentional injuries	4. Stroke
5. Unintentional injuries	5. Chronic liver disease	5. Diabetes	5. Diabetes	5. Diabetes	5. Unintentional injuries
6. Kidney disease	6. Chronic lower respiratory tract disease	6. Influenza and pneumonia	6. Chronic liver disease	6. Influenza and pneumonia	6. Alzheimer's disease
7. Chronic lower respiratory tract disease	7. Stroke	7. Chronic lower respiratory tract disease	7. Chronic lower respiratory tract disease	7. Chronic lower respiratory tract disease	7. Diabetes
8. Homicide	8. Suicide	8. Kidney disease	8. Influenza and pneumonia	8. Kidney disease	8. Influenza and pneumonia
9. Septicemia	9. Influenza and pneumonia	9. Alzheimer's disease	9. Homicide	9. Alzheimer's disease	9. Kidney disease
10. Alzheimer's disease	10. Kidney disease	10. Suicide	10. Kidney disease	10. Suicide	10. Suicide

Data extracted from Centers for Disease Control and Prevention: *Black or African American populations,* 2014b. http://www.cdc.gov/minorityhealth/populations/remp/black.html Accessed June 2014; Office of Minority Health (OMH): *White population: leading causes of death,* 2010. http://www.cdc.gov/omhd/populations/White.htm Accessed June 2014.

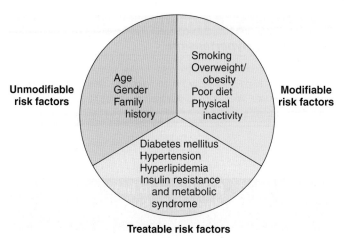

FIGURE 22-1 Risk Factors for Coronary Heart Disease. (From Grundy SM, Pasternak R, Greenland P, et al: Assessment of cardiovascular risk by use of multiple-risk-factor assessment questions, *J Am Coll Cardiol* 34(4):1348–1359, 1999.)

♥ BOX 22-2   HEALTHY PEOPLE 2020

Hypertension

Goal
Reduce the proportion of persons in the population with hypertension.

Baseline
29.9% of adults aged 18 years and older had high blood pressure/hypertension in 2005 to 2008 (age adjusted to the year 2000 standard population).

Target
26.9% of those older than 18 years of age by 2020

Data from U.S. Department of Health and Human Services, Office of Disease Prevention and Health Promotion: *Healthy People 2020,* 2012. http://www.healthypeople.gov/2020

Diagnosis

The 2014 guidelines for the diagnoses of hypertension are >140/90 mm Hg for younger adults and *now ≥150/90 mm Hg in people ≥60 of age, regardless of race.* For those with diabetes or kidney disease of any age, the upper limit is 140/90 mm Hg (James et al, 2014). Diagnosis requires two measurements, 5 minutes apart, confirmed in the contralateral arm (NHLBI, 2003). A diagnosis can never be made with a single reading. If done when sitting and standing, evidence of orthostatic hypotension will be apparent and will influence the treatment approach. Diagnosis may also be done through the analysis of self-monitoring records, especially for those who report "white coat syndrome," where readings will be artificially high in a health care situation. Many older adults in the outpatient setting monitor their blood pressure at home. If the home device is reliable and the technique is accurate (Box 22-3), then the home measurements may be the most accurate for both diagnosing and monitoring treatment effects in older adults.

Etiology   *smoking, mental health*

The exact cause of hypertension cannot be determined in the vast majority of persons (primary hypertension). We suspect that optimal mental health, stress and anger management, and a number of other protective factors can counter any genetic influence (CDC, 2014g). The normal changes in the aging vascular system (p. 293) coupled with lifelong habits, such as smoking, are the factors most likely to account for the increased incidence of HTN with aging (NHLBI, 2012a). Secondary hypertension can be caused by non–cardiac diseases, such as pheochromocytoma or Cushing's syndrome, and are relatively rare in older adults (Mayo Clinic, 2013).

Complications

While many of the complications of hypertension are preventable, there is a very low level of adequate control of blood pressure that could promote wellness (Table 22-1). In persons older than 80 years of age, only 38% of men and 23% of women in the United States have their blood pressure under adequate control with a U.S. goal of increasing that number (Box 22-4). In other countries control is even worse (Box 22-5). As a result, the ensuing complications are many, most notably increased rates of strokes, acute myocardial infarctions (AMIs), and coronary artery disease (CAD) (Table 22-2). Although there has been some discussion of the relationship between HTN and dementia, this is still under investigation (Helton, 2014).

TABLE 22-1   Examples of Complications of Uncontrolled Hypertension

COMPLICATION	CORRELATION WITH CHANGE FROM HYPERTENSION
Predictive of increased risk for stroke, heart failure, and other cardiomyopathies increased risk of stroke	Widened pulse pressure
Increased risk of stroke	Coronary artery disease
Death	Congestive heart failure
Increased incidence of microvascular complications	Diabetes
Worsening of renal insufficiency, renal failure	Chronic renal disease

Extracted from Helton M: Hypertension. In Ham RJ, Sloane PD, Warshaw GA, et al, editors: *Primary care geriatrics: a case-based approach,* ed 6, Philadelphia, 2014, Elsevier, pp 381–394.

BOX 22-4   HEALTHY PEOPLE 2020

Hypertension and Blood Pressure

Goal

Increase the proportion of adults with hypertension whose blood pressure is under control.

Baseline

43.7% of adults aged 18 years and older with high blood pressure/hypertension had it under control in 2005 to 2008 (age adjusted to the year 2000 standard population).

Target

61.2% of those with hypertension and at least 18 years of age will have their blood pressure under control by 2020.

Data from U.S. Department of Health and Human Services, Office of Disease Prevention and Health Promotion: *Healthy People 2020*, 2012. http://www.healthypeople.gov/2020

BOX 22-5   Global Issues: Uncontrolled Hypertension

In 2008, 3.5 million people in China died from CVD, especially related to HTN. Among the 1.3 billion living in rural areas, 97% had uncontrolled HTN. Through cooperative efforts of the CDC in the United States, the China-CDC, and WHO, high intake of salt was found to be a major factor.

Centers for Disease Control and Prevention: *Shaking the salt habit: sodium—hypertension control in China*, 2013. http://www.cdc.gov/globalhealth/ncd/hypertension.htm Accessed June 2014.

TABLE 22-2   Benefits of Controlling Blood Pressure

	AVERAGE PERCENT REDUCTION IN RISK FOR NEW EVENTS
Stroke decreased	30-40
Myocardial infarction decreased	20-25
Heart failure decreased	50

Treatment

Nonpharmacological interventions that promote a healthy lifestyle have been found to be highly effective in reducing blood pressure and, in doing so, minimizing or even preventing long-term complications.

There is considerable evidence regarding the influence of diet and obesity on blood pressure. Healthy eating habits have been found to irrefutably lower blood pressure (Box 22-6). Even modest reductions in sodium intake and body weight (10%) may return a person to a normotensive state, reduce the risk for other CVD or stroke, or reduce the number of medications needed (Table 22-3) (Chapter 22). If able to read, teaching people how to read food labels is an important part of preventive health education (see Chapter 14).

BOX 22-6   TIPS FOR BEST PRACTICE

Controlling Hypertension

With few exceptions the nurse promotes healthy aging by helping people maintain their blood pressure within an acceptable range. For those with late- or end-stage illness such as dementia, the range of acceptable blood pressures is broader.

TABLE 22-3   Relationship between Lifestyle Change and Reduction in Systolic Blood Pressure

LIFESTYLE CHANGE	APPROXIMATE REDUCTION IN SBP
Reduce weight	Decrease of 5-20 mm Hg per 10-lb loss
Adopt DASH diet	Decrease of 8-14 mm Hg
Lower sodium intake	Decrease of 2-8 mm Hg
Increase physical activity	Decrease of 4-9 mm Hg
Limit alcohol intake	Decrease of 2-4 mm Hg

DASH, Dietary Approaches to Stop Hypertension; *SBP*, systolic blood pressure.

Ace Inhibitors   How ACE Inhibitor works?

When hypertension is not adequately responsive to non-pharmacological approaches, pharmacological interventions are necessary. There are four types of antihypertensive medications that JNC 8 recommends for use: calcium channel blockers (CCB), thiazide diuretics, beta-blockers, angiotensin-converting enzyme inhibitors (ACEs), or angiotensin receptor blockers (ARBs). First-line treatment in the non-black population, including those with diabetes mellitus (DM), includes any of the previously mentioned interventions; however, in the black population thiazide-type diuretics and CCBs are recommended (Caboral-Stevens and Rosario-Sim, 2014). ACEs have renal protective qualities and should be prescribed to everyone with renal insufficiency; if not tolerated, an ARB can be substituted. Everything should be done to minimize the number of medications taken by older adults to reduce the risk of polypharmacy, to keep the regimen simple, and to use once-daily dosing (Chapter 9). Due to the high risk for orthostatic hypotension and related falls, the lowest dose is initially prescribed and the gerontological nurse checks the person and blood pressure frequently to assess for medication side effects and the need for a dose adjustment. By reducing or eliminating modifiable risk factors, hypertension can be controlled or prevented, leading to healthier aging.

Coronary Heart Disease *#1 Killer in US*

The heart is dependent on the coronary arteries for the oxygen and nutrients it needs to survive. Although not a normal change of aging, the incidence of coronary heart disease (CHD) rises significantly with age and is the most common form of heart disease. CHD is referred to as atherosclerosis, "hardening of the arteries," *coronary artery disease* (CAD), and ischemic heart disease.

Plaque building up. decreas Blood flow

In the United States one person dies each minute from CHD, 69% of whom are older than 75 years of age (Taffet, 2014). Those who have a complete occlusion will have an acute myocardial infarction (AMI) and more than one-third will die in the 12 months following the event (Bashore et al, 2013). While the rates of death due to CHD are declining, it remains the number 1 cause of death worldwide with variation by race, ethnicity, and gender.

Signs and Symptoms

The major symptoms of CAD are shortness of breath (dyspnea) and unexplained fatigue, identical to those symptoms that are seen in many other health problems common in late life (Box 22-7). When CAD becomes ischemic but the occlusion is incomplete, the symptoms may worsen intermittently, but over time they increase in frequency, intensity, or duration and occur with less and less provocation (unstable angina). Unstable angina is associated with arrhythmias, tachycardia, and ventricular fibrillation.

If an AMI occurs in an older adult there may be no anticipatory symptoms at all, referred to as a "silent MI." The classic symptoms such as sudden gripping chest pain with radiation to arm and chin may be present or they may be completely atypical, such as an unexplained fall or an acute change in mental status or other atypical symptoms (Table 22-4). AMIs without

---

BOX 22-7 Signs of Potential Exacerbation of Illness in an Older Adult with Coronary Heart Disease

- Light-headedness or dizziness
- Disturbances in gait and balance
- Loss of appetite or unexplained loss of weight
- Inability to concentrate or shortened attention span
- Changes in personality or mood
- Changes in grooming habits
- Unusual patterns in urination or defecation
- Vague discomfort, frequent bouts of anxiety
- Excessive fatigue, vague pain
- Withdrawal from usual sources of pleasure

TABLE 22-4 Key Differences in the Signs of Typical Cardiac-Related "Chest Pain" (Angina) in a Younger Adult Compared with Atypical Signs More Common in an Older Adult

SYMPTOM	CLASSIC	ATYPICAL
Chest pain	Present	Absent
Radiations of pain to arm or jaw	Often present	Absent
Sweating	Often present	Absent
Dyspnea	Often present	May be only symptom
Fatigue	Often present	May be only symptom

Adapted from Taffet GF: Coronary artery disease and atrial fibrillation. In Ham RJ, Sloane PD, Warshaw GA, et al, editors: *Primary care geriatrics: a case-based approach*, ed 6, Philadelphia, 2014, Elsevier, pp 395–405.

---

the classic symptoms rarely occur in younger adults. Younger adults may have no symptoms of early CAD and not know they have it until suffering an AMI, most often with the classic complaints including shortness of breath (especially for men) and the sensation of intense indigestion (especially for women).

Diagnosis

The diagnosis of CAD in the older adult may be incidental to another exam that includes a resting electrocardiogram (ECG) (e.g., annual Wellness Visit covered by Medicare) or when evaluating another problem that is found to be the result of end-organ damage, such as atrial fibrillation. If abnormalities are found on the ECG of a young adult, interventions can begin immediately (e.g., smoking cessation, weight loss) before damage occurs or to reverse the existing damage. However, there are still measures that persons can take at any age to decrease the risk of CAD (Figure 22-1).

Noninvasive diagnostic measures include a stress test; invasive tests include cardiac catheterization. If a person is suspected of having an AMI, a definitive diagnosis requires the documentation of changes in biochemical markers within 24 to 72 hours of the event (Bashore et al, 2013). Life-saving measures can be initiated if they are consistent with the patient's preexpressed wishes. Definitive testing may not always be appropriate, such as those who are very frail with limited life expectancies, when the focus of care is on optimizing quality of life and in doing so fostering healthy aging even at the end of life (Chapter 35).

Etiology

The walls of the normally pliable arteries thicken and stiffen with age; there are changes in lipid, cholesterol, and phospholipid metabolism. This may result in the formation of plaques that adhere to vessel walls and ultimately occlude the vessel or cause a spasm in the surrounding area when the heart is stressed. Once this occurs, the capacity for oxygenation of the surrounding heart tissue is reduced and will ultimately lead to tissue death (necrosis).

Complications

The most important complication of CAD is the AMI as a result of either acute or long-term cardiac anoxia. If it is witnessed, resuscitation is desired, and an automatic defibrillator is available, both the morbidity and the mortality of the person are significantly decreased.

An AMI can cause a small or extensive amount of damage to the heart muscle. The event may be triggered by a sudden increase in myocardial oxygen demand, such as from the inability of the arteries to respond adequately to an infection or bleeding, or from a sudden occlusion of an artery from a blood clot or plaque attempting to pass through a narrowed vessel. Tissue death occurs quickly.

In chronic CHD, the body attempts to compensate for the damage through a process called remodeling in which the heart enlarges and changes shape. This remodeling eventually leads to a decrease in cardiac pumping efficiency and the gradual onset of other cardiomyopathies.

Treatment

[handwritten: Cholesterol, meds, put them in blood thinner because]

Both nonpharmacological and pharmacological approaches are usually necessary to treat the person with CAD. Nonpharmacological features of treatment emphasize addressing all reversible factors. Advance practice nurses and physicians most often prescribe a combination of aspirin, clopidogrel (Plavix), and nitrates (isosorbide). Beta-blockers (e.g., metoprolol, atenolol) have been found to prolong life. Calcium channel blockers can only be used with caution (Bashore et al, 2013; Davis, 2013b). During more acute events, additional treatment is needed, usually sublingual or aerosol nitroglycerin. During intermittent chest pain (angina) or AMI, sublingual or buccal spray nitroglycerin remains the gold standard. Pharmacological interventions are geared toward minimizing symptoms and promoting health-related quality of life, including palliative care when appropriate.

(2) Atrial Fibrillation   *[handwritten: pulse feels irregular]*

Atrial fibrillation (AF or afib) is an irregular heartbeat. The irregularity may have a pattern or be completely random (paroxysmal); it may occur once, intermittently, or persistently. While it may occur in younger adults, it has a high incidence and prevalence in older adults and increases with each decade (Bashore et al, 2013). The average age of onset is 67 for men and 75 for women; it is more common in white Americans compared with those in other racial groups (Davis, 2013a).

Signs and Symptoms   *[handwritten: dizziness because poor cardiac output]*

In many cases, AF itself is completely asymptomatic and only identified by the nurse or other practitioner as part of a thorough auscultation of the heart. If symptoms occur, they are vague, such as fatigue, and since the person already has other underlying heart disease, this is difficult to attribute specifically to the AF. The fatigue may be attributed to "old age" or the onset of frailty. Occasionally people report the sensation of "palpations" and intermittent shortness of breath, or nonspecific chest pain, especially if the fibrillation is paroxysmal (Box 22-8).

Diagnosis

Diagnosis is most often based on clinical findings of an irregular heartbeat on auscultation, which may be in association with recurrent falls, episodes of syncope, "dizzy spells," and worsening

of heart failure. It may be acute (lasting <48 hours) or chronic. The frequency of the irregularity can be evaluated by a 24-hour Holter monitor. An ECG may confirm persistent AF, but may miss that which is paroxysmal.

Etiology

Atrial fibrillation is the end result of diabetes, sleep apnea, thyroid disorders, alcohol abuse, and several cardiomyopathies, including CHD and hypertension. It also may be related to the use of beta-blockers (Bowker et al, 2013). However, more than half of the incidence of AF is related to inadequate control of modifiable risk factors, identical to those associated with CAD (Figure 22-1) (Davis, 2013a; Taffett, 2014). It is associated with a heightened risk for dementia and stroke-related mortality; however, in each case the rates are highly variable (Davis, 2013a). If a younger adult has AF he or she is more likely to have it in the absence of other diseases; in an older adult it is most often a complication of another disease such as CAD.

Complications

Because the pulsations of the heart in AF are irregular to some degree, there is always a risk for pooling of blood in the atria when the time between the beats is prolonged. This pooling increases the risk for the development of emboli. The most serious complication of AF is a stroke if emboli should leave the heart and travel to the brain. In AF the risk for stroke is very high (Davis, 2013a; Taffett, 2013). If the fibrillation causes tachycardia as a compensating mechanism, then significant hypotension, myocardial ischemia, and other cardiomyopathies can develop.

Treatment

Treatment for atrial fibrillation is twofold: (1) to control heart rate and (2) to reduce stroke risk through the prevention of blood clots forming in the atria. In 2013 the American College of Cardiology Foundation/American Heart Association recommended that there was no benefit for "strict" control (i.e., <80 bpm at rest or <110 bpm during a 6-minute walk) in asymptomatic patients with stable control (Davis, 2013a). In the outpatient setting, including long-term care facilities, rate control is usually achieved through the use of beta-blockers, but bradycardia is a potential side effect. Patients can be taught to monitor their pulses. For the person at a low risk for a stroke, aspirin along with clopidogrel (Plavix) is used. For those with any higher risk, even for intermittent AF, lifelong anticoagulation therapy remains the gold standard. The anticoagulant warfarin has long been the only medication available. It must be monitored closely and regularly to ensure that the level of anticoagulation is within an appropriate range (Chapter 8). There is always a heightened risk of bleeding. Vitamin K is the antidote and can quickly inactivate the effects of warfarin. It does interact with most antibiotics and herbal products (see Chapters 9 and 10); when these medications or supplements are taken, even closer monitoring is necessary.

Several newer anticoagulants are available that do not require monitoring, making these more acceptable to some, especially

---

BOX 22-8   Sometimes I Can Feel the Palpitations

Ruth is a 75-year-old active and energetic woman with paroxysmal atrial fibrillation. Because of this condition, she takes anticoagulants—that is, she takes medication to prevent her blood from clotting and to decrease her risk of having a stroke. Most of the time Ruth's heart beats regularly and at other times it does not. When it does not, she has a sense of "chest palpitations" but they have never given her problems. One day Ruth's heart seems to be beating much more than usual. She checked it and it was at least 180 beats per minute, it was highly irregular, and she was not feeling well. She called for an ambulance and was taken immediately to the hospital where she was stabilized and then sent home.

those who spend a lot of time traveling. At the time of this writing no antidotes were available should bleeding occur (Ogbonna and Clifford, 2011). A person who is taking one of these anticoagulants should be directed to promptly seek emergency support with any obvious bleeding or the potential of bleeding (e.g., following trauma to the head following a fall).

Nurses have important roles in helping patients understand the dangers and benefits of anticoagulation therapy, the impact of medication/food/herb/nutritional supplement interactions (see Chapters 9 and 10), the need for strict adherence, and the effect of high and low vitamin K diets on warfarin. Nurses often perform point-of-care warfarin monitoring, and advanced practice nurses adjust doses as needed. Nurses are often involved in the conversations regarding the risk/benefit ratio of continuing anticoagulation therapy for the person at risk for falling or with a history of falling.

Heart Failure

Heart failure (HF) is a general term used to describe the end result of other disorders, particularly CHD, hypertension, and diabetes. It is not a normal part of aging, but like other heart diseases, it is so common that it is often considered normal. It is the most common cause for hospitalization, rehospitalization, and disability among persons older than age 65 (Ding et al, 2013) (Box 22-9).

As more persons live longer with heart disease, more failure is seen in both men and women; more than 8 million are expected to have HF by 2030. Of the new cases each year, 75% to 80% occur in persons older than 65 and approximately 50% of these die within 5 years (Bashore et al, 2013; CDC, 2013; Ding et al, 2013). African Americans are at the highest risk for HF, both to develop it at a younger age and to die from it (NHLBI, 2014).

Clinical heart failure is categorized as systolic failure, diastolic failure, or both. End-stage HF and acute HF are known as congestive heart failure (CHF). The extent of illness is in proportion to the person's ejection fraction, or the amount of blood leaving the ventricle. A normal ejection fraction is between approximately 55% and 70% (Taffett, 2014).

Acute HF (previously referred to as CHF) can appear quickly in persons with underlying CAD, especially those who have already had at least one AMI, and more slowly in persons with long-standing hypertension. Accurately attributing the signs and symptoms reported by the patient to HF is complicated in the older adult because any one of these symptoms can also be caused by other chronic diseases, geriatric syndromes, or commonly prescribed medications. The signs and symptoms are often atypical in the older adult (Box 22-10). Heart failure symptoms are ranked by their effect on function and activity (Box 22-11).

Left-Sided Failure

Left-sided failure is that in which left ventricular (LV) *systolic* function remains within normal limits in the presence of LV *diastolic dysfunction*. The heart is unable to relax enough to allow adequate diastolic function, yet the ejection fraction remains ≥50% and persons may be only minimally symptomatic

BOX 22-9 HEALTHY PEOPLE 2020

Hospitalizations for Heart Failure

Goal
Reduce hospitalizations of older adults with heart failure as the principal diagnosis.

Ages 65-74
Baseline
9.8 hospitalizations for heart failure per 1000 people aged 65 to 74 years occurred in 2007.

Target
No more than 8.8 hospitalizations per 1000 people aged 65 to 74 years will occur by 2020.

Ages 75-84
Baseline
22.4 hospitalizations for heart failure per 1000 people aged 75 to 84 years occurred in 2007.

Target
No more than 20.2 hospitalizations per 1000 people aged 75 to 84 years will occur by 2020.

Ages 85+
Baseline
42.9 hospitalizations for heart failure per 1000 people aged 85 years and older occurred in 2007.

Target
No more than 38.6 hospitalizations per 1000 people aged 85 and older will occur by 2020.

Data from U.S. Department of Health and Human Services, Office of Disease Prevention and Health Promotion: Healthy People 2020, 2012. http://www.healthypeople.gov/2020.

BOX 22-10 Classic and Atypical Signs of Heart Failure in Older Adults

CLASSIC (NONCEREBRAL)	ATYPICAL	ATYPICAL (CEREBRAL)
Dyspnea	Chronic cough	No history
Orthopnea	Insomnia	Falls
Paroxysmal nocturnal	Weight loss	Anorexia, dyspnea
Peripheral edema	Nausea	Behavioral disturbances
Unexplained weight gain	Nocturia	Decreased functional status
Weakness	Syncope	
Poor exercise tolerance		
Abdominal pain		
Fatigue		

From Ham RJ, Sloane PD, Warshaw GA, et al, editors: *Primary care geriatrics*, ed 6, Philadelphia, 2014, Elsevier.

in day-to-day life. Symptoms may only occur when the heart is stressed, i.e. when there is a need to increase stroke volume.

Right-Sided Failure

In contrast to left-sided failure, *right-sided heart failure* is associated with LV systolic *dysfunction;* the ejection fraction is

BOX 22-11   Classification of Heart Failure by the American College of Cardiologists Combined with that of the New York Heart Association*

Stage A
High risk but no symptoms or structural disorder (e.g., CAD, HTN)

Class 1 Mild
No evidence of symptoms at rest or during activity

Stage B
No symptoms but with structural disorder (e.g., LVH, hx MI)

Class 2 Mild
Ordinary activities result in fatigue, palpitation, or dyspnea

Stage C
Current or past symptoms and structural disorder
Especially dyspnea from LVSD

Class 3 Moderate
Less than ordinary activities cause symptoms

Stage D
End-stage disease
Symptomatic at rest despite optimal treatment

Class 4 Severe
Symptoms at rest, any activity increases discomfort

*Text in italics is from the New York Heart Association.
CAD, Coronary artery disease; *HTN*, hypertension; *hx*, history; *LVH*, left ventricular hypertrophy; *LVSD*, left ventricular systolic dysfunction; *MI*, myocardial infarction.
From Horsley L: Practice guidelines: ACC and AHA update on chronic heart failure guidelines, *Am Fam Physician* 81(5):654–665, 2010. American Heart Association: Classes of heart failure, 2011. http://www.heart.org/HEARTORG/Conditions/HeartFailure/AboutHeartFailure/Classes-of-Heart-Failure_UCM_306328_Article.jsp Accessed July 2014.

≤40%, and the person is always symptomatic, may be very ill, and has a poor prognosis. The typical chronic illness trajectory is one of steady decline. Long-standing left-sided failure will eventually cause right-sided failure as well.

Signs and Symptoms

Early in left-sided failure, the only symptom may be shortness of breath, especially on exertion (dyspnea on exertion [DOE]). However, it will eventually progress to orthopnea, paroxysmal nocturnal dyspnea, and dyspnea at rest (Bowker et al, 2013). It is common for the person to find ways to compensate for declining cardiac function without realizing it. For example, a person slowly reduces their activity level saying they are "not so fit anymore," "just not feeling right," or have a case of "the dwindles," all of which the person may attribute to advancing age. It is much more likely to be a pathological condition that would benefit from treatment. The typical chronic illness trajectory of a person with left-sided failure is periods of minimal symptoms interspersed with exacerbations, often leading to

hospitalizations for stabilization until this is no longer possible or desired.

The predominant signs and symptoms of right-sided failure are breathlessness, fatigue and malaise, dependent edema, sleep problems, and hepatic congestion (Ding et al, 2013). Changes in edema can be notable and the nurse works with the person to weigh himself or herself at the same time every day and look for a gain of 5 pounds as an indicator of pending changes in symptoms and the need to contact the health care provider.

Etiology

Heart failure is the end-organ damage from preexisting conditions, especially hypertension that developed into CAD. To compensate for the damage, the heart, especially the ventricles, enlarges and dilates. The enlargement decreases heart muscle function as the walls are remodeled and weakened. Eventually, the heart cannot compensate for the lost stroke volume, and evidence of failure appears.

Secondary causes of heart failure include drug and alcohol abuse, uncontrolled hyperthyroidism, and valvular heart disease. Persons with CHD who have already had extensive damage have a very high risk of developing heart failure. Its onset can be acute—often within the first few hours or days after a myocardial infarction, but even a moderate amount of muscle damage will lead to eventual heart failure.

Diagnosis

The diagnosis of early heart failure in older adults can be very difficult. All other diseases with similar signs and symptoms must be ruled out, such as thyroid disturbances and uncontrolled atrial fibrillation. While the working diagnosis is often made empirically, there are many false-positives, and a definitive diagnosis through an echocardiogram (to determine the ejection fraction) can be the best guide to devise a treatment plan and establish the prognosis (Ding et al, 2013). Measurement of serum levels of brain natriuretic peptide (BNP) or NT-proBNP is potentially useful in differentiating shortness of breath due to heart failure with that caused by other conditions (see Chapter 8) (Bashore et al, 2013).

Complications

As the severity increases and heart failure advances into intermittent or chronic heart failure, the pulse pressure narrows and signs of impaired tissue perfusion develop, such as cool skin and central or peripheral cyanosis. Diminished cognition, perhaps to the point of delirium, is common. Recurrent hospitalization is usually required until the point is reached when only palliative care is possible or desired. An episode of syncope, ventricular tachycardia, or uncontrolled fibrillation should be regarded as a harbinger of sudden death. Increased jugular venous pressure is the most reliable way to determine the prognosis (Ding et al, 2013).

Treatment

Because heart failure is indicative of end-organ damage, the goals of treatment are to prevent more damage, control symptoms, and increase health-related quality of life to the extent possible. The nurse works with the person to find ways to minimize fatigue and teaches the person how to recognize signs and symptoms indicating the early or pending onset of acute heart failure. Nurses work with persons and their significant others to determine their wishes related to medical crises and their desire for aggressive measures, such as hospitalization, intubation, and resuscitation. For those with HF in the last stages, treatment is one of palliative care (Chapter 35). Pharmacological interventions and goals are based on the level of symptoms as recommended by the American Heart Association; levels range from A (asymptomatic) to D (Refractory).

THE AGING PERIPHERAL VASCULAR SYSTEM

The younger heart propels oxygen-rich blood through highly elastic and flexible arteries that expand and contract depending on the body's need for oxygen. Deoxygenated blood returns to the heart by way of the veins, propelled by contractions of the surrounding muscles. The blood is prevented from moving backward (by the pull of gravity) by a series of valves. Several of the same age-related changes seen in the skin and muscles affect the blood vessels.

The most significant age-related changes in the arteries are reduced elasticity and narrowing. Elastin fibers fray, split, straighten, and fragment. For those without CVD or diabetes, there is little change in blood flow to the coronary arteries or brain. However, perfusion of other tissues and organs is reduced and can be significant in relationship to medication metabolism and excretion, as well as fluid and electrolyte balance (Chapters 8). The veins become stretched and the valves less efficient. Pooling of the blood leads to increased venous pressure and edema develops more quickly.

PERIPHERAL VASCULAR DISEASE

Peripheral vascular disease (PVD) is that in which there is partial or complete occlusion of the veins or arteries. The two major types of PVD are chronic venous insufficiency (CVI) and peripheral arterial disease (PAD). The reported incidence and prevalence of each disorder vary widely, but overall they increase with age (Rapp et al, 2013; Robertson et al, 2008, 2013).

Signs and Symptoms

The major signs and symptoms of CVI and PAD are pain, changes to the skin, and wounds that do not heal. Early complaints of CVI may include numbness or tingling in the affected extremity or mild edema with standing. There is a pooling of blood with venous stasis, and the affected limb is bluish or purple in lighter-pigmented persons and has a dull gray appearance in more darkly pigmented persons. The reverse blood flow through the incompetent valves results in increased hydrostatic pressure and pain during ambulation.

Over time, long-standing stasis of blood leads to the deposition of hemosiderin, giving the skin a speckled brown appearance, especially in the lower calf. Varicosities of the superficial veins are obvious. Dependent edema, dermatitis, and firm induration are

common signs of CVI. Pain is present when the extremity is dependent and during ambulation.

Because arterial disease reduces the blood flow into a limb, the early symptom of insufficiency is pain when the limb is elevated. It is classically described as an ache, numbness, or squeezing sensation, especially in the arch of the foot and toes but also in the calf, thigh, or buttocks. The pain may be instantly relieved when the limb is moved to a dependent position, when gravity helps pull the blood back into the ischemic limb. While temporarily relieved, pain returns with exertion as the tissue demands more oxygen and is relieved again by rest. This is referred to as intermittent claudication. When elevated, the extremity may be pale and cool, consistent with ischemia, and usually red or purple with dependency (Kohlman-Trigoboff, 2013). See Table 22-5 to assist with the differentiation of these two very different disorders.

TABLE 22-5 Comparison of Arterial and Venous Insufficiency of the Lower Extremities

CHARACTERISTICS	ARTERIAL	VENOUS
Pain	Pain with elevation of LE Pain initially relieved when legs become dependent Pain returns when walking short distances (claudication) but is relieved by rest (legs still dependent)	Deep ache, relieved by elevation Deep muscle pain with acute deep vein thrombosis
Pulses	Absent or weak	Normal
Skin	Thin, shiny, dry skin Thickened toenails Absence of hair growth Cool Pallor with elevation Rubor with dependency	Firm ("brawny") edema Reddish brown discoloration (hyperpigmentation) Evidence of healed ulcers Presence of varicose veins Progressive edema Dark erythema with acute deep vein thrombosis
Ulcer location	Between toes or at tips of toes Metatarsal or phalangeal heads Heels, sides, or soles of feet Lateral malleolus Pretibial area	Medial malleolus
Ulcer characteristics	Well-defined edges Necrotic tissue Deep, pale base Nonbleeding	Uneven edges Ruddy granulation tissue Superficial Bleeding

Etiology

The majority of the changes to both the arteries and the veins are attributable to CVD, especially hypertension and the development of plaques, superimposed on normal age-related changes and exacerbated by smoking. CVI may begin as a result of the development of varicose veins or the consequence of a deep vein thrombosis, both of which cause permanent damage to the vessel walls and the valves (Zhang and Melander, 2014). The development of varicose veins has a familial influence (Robertson et al, 2008). PAD is an atherosclerotic disease like that found in other parts of the body that impair circulation to the tissue distal to the plaque.

Diagnosis

PVD may be completely asymptomatic early in the disease, making prompt diagnosis difficult and delaying interventions that have the potential to prevent complications. The gerontological nurse may be the first one to notice the symptoms or hear the concerns from the elder leading to a diagnosis, especially in the inpatient or other institutional setting. Diagnosis of all of the vascular disorders discussed here begins with a good history, physical, and review of "symptoms" (Chapter 7). While the type of problem appears evident, confirmatory testing includes an ankle-brachial index (ABI) to differentiate between PAD and CVI and to determine the most appropriate treatment.

Complications

The most serious complications of peripheral vascular diseases are the development of a deep vein thrombosis (DVT) or a pulmonary embolism or an amputation from a wound that does not heal.

A DVT is the formation of a thrombus on the vein wall, most often near a valve (Johanning, 2014). It may be asymptomatic, but if it progresses to the point where it completely occludes the vein, the person will have acute pain. If a DVT is suspected, there is a difference in the circumference between the legs (Rapp et al, 2013). A venous Doppler confirms a DVT. Once the acute clot is resolved the person will have postembolic syndrome due to irreversible damage to the vessel wall, increasing the risk for another DVT. The person may require preventive extended or lifetime anticoagulation.

Any time a clot from an injured vessel or DVT is detached, a life-threatening pulmonary embolism (PE) can result. A PE should be suspected anytime the person has recently had a DVT or is at risk for one, and complains of sudden shortness of breath and has a low oxygen saturation rate. A PE will be confirmed with a chest x-ray or magnetic resonance imaging (MRI), but even the suspicion of one should be treated as a potential medical emergency. Both DVTs and PEs require hospitalization to resolve the clots.

Wounds that result from PVD may never heal. When ischemia is present long enough, especially from PAD, the surrounding tissue deteriorates, with or without trauma, and skin ulcers develop. If an ulcer is not found or treated early enough, infection may develop to the point of gangrene, necessitating amputation to save the remaining part of the limb above the lesion.

Treatment

CVI and PAD are end-organ diseases. Consequently, prevention is tied to addressing the modifiable risk factors of the original disorders. However, there are specific strategies that can be used to reduce the risk of PVD and the nurse has a major role in working with persons to adopt day-to-day preventive care strategies. For example, the nurse can encourage weight reduction to decrease the pressure on the veins from obesity or smoking cessation to reduce arterial constriction (Zhang and Melander, 2014).

For persons with *arterial* insufficiency, exercise rehabilitation and protection of the skin are paramount. Daily skin inspection and protection against the effects of pressure, friction, shear, and maceration are essential for the early detection and prevention of wounds. The nurse is usually the leader in planning and implementing patient education related to skin care.

Nothing should be done to limit circulation to the affected limb. Wearing restrictive clothing and using compression stockings are contraindicated. Exercise rehabilitation includes establishing a walking program to slowly and steadily increase the pain-free walking distance. The person is asked to walk until maximal tolerable pain occurs, rest, and then continue.

Although the person with chronic *vascular* insufficiency will need intermittent courses of diuretics for severe edema, the mainstay of management is the use of customized compression stockings. Compression facilitates wound healing, reduces venous dermatitis, improves sclerotic changes, and counteracts venous pressure. In addition to compression stockings, other devices that have been found useful to improve venous return include Unna boots (or equivalent), pneumatic compression pumps, and orthotic devices. Elevation of the legs above the heart for 30 minutes three to four times a day can reduce edema and improve skin microcirculation.

Although the principles of the management of PVD-related ulcers are similar to those of pressure ulcers, special care must be taken to ensure that venous stasis ulcers and arterial ulcers are differentiated and treated appropriately. Because of the potentially limb-threatening nature of these ulcers, it is recommended that the nurse consult with colleagues who are wound care specialists to develop the most appropriate treatment plans.

CEREBROVASCULAR DISORDERS

The major cerebrovascular disorders include the transient ischemic attack (TIA), the ischemic stroke, and both the subarachnoid and subdural hemorrhagic strokes. All are characterized by acute-onset neurological changes from anoxic damage to the brain. Both morbidity and mortality are dependent on the type of event and the time between onset and treatment (Box 22-12). Because the immediate neurological deficits appear the same but the treatment and prognoses are dramatically different, an urgent and accurate diagnosis is essential. Only when the cause is known can appropriate therapy be implemented. All strokes are medical emergencies.

BOX 22-12 Quick Assessment of the Person Who May Be Having a Stroke

If you think someone may be having a stroke, act F.A.S.T. and do the following simple test:

F—Face: Ask the person to smile. Does one side of the face droop?

A—Arms: Ask the person to raise both arms. Does one arm drift downward?

S—Speech: Ask the person to repeat a simple phrase. Is the person's speech slurred or strange?

T—Time: If you observe any of these signs, call 9-1-1 immediately.

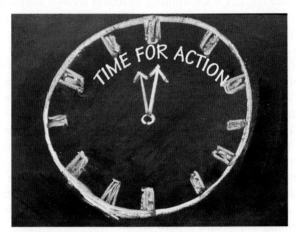

Time to Treatment Is the Most Important Factor in Surviving an Acute Myocardial Infarction. (©iStock.com/flytosky11)

BOX 22-13 HEALTHY PEOPLE 2020

Stroke Deaths

Goal

Reduce stroke deaths.

Baseline

43.5 stroke deaths per 100,000 population occurred in 2007 (age adjusted to the year 2000 standard population).

Target

No more than 34.8 deaths per 100,000 population.

Data from U.S. Department of Health and Human Services, Office of Disease Prevention and Health Promotion: Healthy People 2020, 2012. http://www.healthypeople.gov/2020

BOX 22-14 Factors for Increased Risk for Stroke (in addition to those for CVD)

Older than age 75

Previous TIA

Heart disease, especially coronary heart disease and atrial fibrillation

Prior embolic event

From Centers for Disease Control and Prevention: *Conditions that increase risk for stroke*, 2014c. http://www.cdc.gov/stroke/conditions.htm Accessed July 2014; Bashore TM, Granger CB, Hranitzky P, et al: Heart disease. In Papadakis MA, McPhee SJ, editors: *Current medical diagnosis and treatment 2013*, New York, 2013, McGraw-Hill Lange, pp 324–432.

Worldwide, 3 million women and 2.5 million men die of strokes each year, most commonly in China, India, and the Russian Federation and least commonly in the Southern Caribbean, Guyana, and Surinam. In the United States, someone dies every 1 to 4 minutes from a stroke; this computes to about 130,000 people a year, with most older than 65 years of age. One of the goals of *Healthy People 2020* is to reduce this number (Box 22-13) (CDC, 2013b, 2014h; WHO, 2014). *Age is the most important risk factor for stroke* (CDC, 2014b). There are also racial, ethnic, and geographical differences. The U.S. death rates are highest in the 11 "stroke belt" states of the Southeast and lowest in the Northeast and Southwest. African Americans, Hispanics, American Indians, and Alaskan Natives have a greater chance of having a stroke than do non-Hispanic whites or Asians Americans. The risk of having a first stroke and to die from the stroke is nearly twice as high for African American than for non-Hispanic whites (Mozaffarian et al, 2012). The most common (85%) type of stroke is ischemic (CDC, 2014b). The risk factors are those of any of the other cardiovascular diseases, especially hypertension and atrial fibrillation. See Box 22-14 for other factors that increase the risk for stroke.

Signs and Symptoms

The signs and symptoms of cerebrovascular events are a large part of both the ultimate diagnosis and the prognosis. The most common symptom of an ischemic stroke is a severe headache followed by sudden weakness, tingling, and other neurological deficits consistent with the area of the brain affected, most often on one side of the body. The whole side may be affected or just a part (e.g., a side of the face or unilateral arm). The signs and symptoms last at least 24 hours (Bowker et al, 2013).

The signs of TIAs are those of ischemic strokes but transient, as little as 1 to 5 minutes or several hours, and in most cases appear to resolve completely on their own (Bowker et al, 2013; Bowling and Weinhart, 2014). The signs often resolve before the person is even seen by a health care provider. Instead, the person reports, "I think I had a small stroke last week."

The headache of some hemorrhagic strokes is both sudden and explosive. There are more focal neurological changes, a more depressed level of consciousness, and a potential for seizures. Like the ischemic stroke, the types of neurological deficits indicate the parts of the brain affected but are usually much broader. They include alterations in motor, sensory, and visual function; coordination; cognition; and language. Nausea and vomiting suggest increased cerebral edema. Loss of consciousness indicates a very poor prognosis.

Etiology

Cerebrovascular events are the result of an occlusion in blood vessels, and therefore oxygenation, to the brain. As a result of the anoxia, brain tissues die quickly. "*One minute of brain ischemia can kill 2 million nerve cells and 14 billion synapses!"* (Luchi and Taffett, 2014, p. 427). As an embolic disorder, there are several types of contents that form the occlusions, including blood clots, plaques, or particles such as calcium or bacteria (Bowling and Weinhart, 2014).

The main causes of ischemic strokes (including TIAs) are arterial disease, cardioembolism, hematological disorders, and hypoperfusion. Arterial disease in the form of arteriosclerosis is probably most common (Figure 22-2). Cardioembolism is caused by an arrhythmia such as atrial fibrillation, frequently seen in coronary heart disease. Hematological causes include coagulation disorders and hyperviscosity syndromes. Hypoperfusion can occur from dehydration, hypotension (including overtreatment of HTN), cardiac arrest, or syncope. The blockage is complete in the ischemic stroke and will persist until it is removed or dissolved. Even though the TIA is also an ischemic event, the blockage is only partial; it lasts only a few minutes to several hours and resolves on its own (Bowling and Weinhart, 2014).

In a subdural (intracerebral) hemorrhagic stroke, a vessel ruptures within the brain and quickly fills a space between the dura and the subarachnoid matter with blood. The rupture is usually at the site of an embolus. If the person is also receiving anticoagulant medications, the bleeding will be more rapid (Bowling and Weinhart, 2014). The most important contributing factors for the incidence of hemorrhagic stroke in older adults are hypertension, the use of anticoagulants (iatrogenic strokes), acute inflammatory illness, contusions (e.g., from falls), and central cerebral thrombi.

The subarachnoid hemorrhagic stroke is triggered by an embolism as well. A blood vessel in the subarachnoid space of the brain ruptures and rapidly fills the space with blood. Either could be a small leak, especially the subdural rupture, and eventually reabsorb on its own; on the other hand, it could be a leak that advances rapidly and quickly becomes life-threatening (CDC, 2014f).

Diagnosis and Treatment

It is not possible to easily determine the treatment from the diagnosis, or even the signs and symptoms of the differing cerebrovascular disorders; many of the early signs and symptoms are similar to those of other acute health problems, such as metabolic disturbances. The need for a simultaneous evaluation for the possibility of a stroke is done at the same time. Diagnosis begins with the analysis of the presenting signs as a clue to the cause and moves quickly to a CT scan (computed tomography) whenever possible to differentiate the hemorrhagic from the ischemic stroke. If MRI is available it will provide information about the level of damage. It is also imperative that the cause of the stroke be determined to prevent a succession of these events whenever possible (Bowling and Weinhart, 2014).

Since the TIA is self-limiting, treatment revolves around the prevention of a subsequent stroke through the adoption of any of the preventive measures discussed in this chapter or in Chapter 1 (e.g., smoking cessation or never smoking).

The initial treatment of a confirmed ischemic stroke is the administration of recombinant tissue plasminogen activator (rtPA) within 3 hours of the event to dissolve the clot (Gumbinger et al, 2014).

A very small subarachnoid hemorrhagic stroke may resolve on its own. However, as there is no treatment, a subarachnoid hemorrhage has a very poor prognosis, with death likely. In this case the goal is palliative care for the patient and support for the family. The escalating potential of any stroke as one ages increases the responsibility of the nurse to ensure that the person's wishes regarding resuscitation in such circumstances are known.

Complications

In an ischemic stroke, the occlusion is complete; but in some cases, the occlusion is reversible with prompt treatment, even if the resultant damage may be permanent. The greater the occlusion and the longer time before treatment, the greater amount of damage to the brain (i.e., the greater the effect). Rehabilitation (third level prevention) will be necessary for any chance of restoring full function or functioning to the degree possible. While these services are available in high-income countries, they are not always available to all in lower-income countries. Although not all persons with TIAs have strokes, more than one-third have a major stroke within 1 year and 10% to 15% within 3 months without treatment (CDC, 2013b). Anticoagulation therapy is often the treatment of choice but is not without its own risk, such as potentially life-threatening bleeding with any trauma.

For those few who have survived a hemorrhagic stroke, brain edema is a problem and could result in obstructive hydrocephalus (Aminoff, 2010). The long-term effects of a stroke include depression, paralysis and hemiparesis, dysarthrias, dysphagias, and aphasias, depending on type, extent, and area affected (Hackett et al, 2014). Whenever paralysis results, the development of spasticity in the affected limb(s) is a risk. Spasticity can lead to contractures if it is not managed. Iatrogenic-type complications include DVT in a flaccid lower limb or contractures, aspiration pneumonia, and urinary tract infections (Bowker et al, 2013). The person with a period of nonresponsiveness is unlikely to survive (Boss and Brashers, 2014). Strokes are the

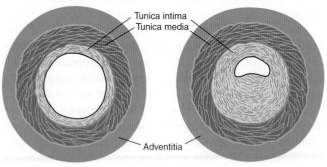

Tunica intima
Tunica media
Adventitia

Normal artery   Diseased (occluded) artery

FIGURE 22-2 Arteriosclerosis. (From Huether SE, McCance KL: *Understanding pathophysiology,* ed 5, St Louis, MO, 2012, Mosby.)

number 1 cause of disability in the United States (Bowling and Weinhart, 2014).

PROMOTING HEALTHY AGING: IMPLICATIONS FOR GERONTOLOGICAL NURSING: CARDIOVASCULAR DISEASE

Due to the prevalence and incidence of cardiovascular diseases, the role of the nurse is broad and complex. First and foremost is prevention—in individual encounters with persons in every setting; as family members, colleagues, or neighbors; and in the community at large (Chapter 1). The nurse conducts expert assessments for the early detection of both CVDs and their exacerbations.

Assessment

The gerontological nurse participates in the accurate assessment of the person in wellness and with cardiovascular disease. In advanced practice, the nurse may have the additional responsibility of assessment for the purpose of evidence-based pharmacological interventions.

Review of "Symptoms"

The cardiovascular assessment begins with the subjective review of "symptoms." This should include the onset, location (for pain), duration, characteristics, alleviating and aggravating factors, and all measures taken to relieve them (e.g., prescribed medications, fasting, herbal and over-the-counter products, prayer). Symptoms of particular importance in the cardiovascular assessment include dyspnea, strength, fall history, dizziness, changes to usual functioning, and other signs and symptoms discussed throughout this chapter.

Observation

The nurse is able to make informed observations: ease of movement, skin color and evidence of hemosiderin deposition, presence or absence of varicosities, presence or absence of wounds and their location, and presence of edema. If the person's heart is markedly enlarged, pulsations may be visible. While the finding of an absence of lower extremity (LE) hair is important in a younger adult, this is not a significant finding in later life due to the increasing loss of body hair in the normal course of aging. If a DVT is suspected, the assessment of a comparative measurement of calf circumference is necessary (Rapp et al, 2013).

Palpation

The nurse examines the skin for temperature and degree of edema if present. Edema is assessed as firm or pitting and the degree of pitting. A small amount of pitting is a normal change of aging when the legs have been dependent for an extended period of time but is not expected to be present after the legs have been elevated. It is important to attempt to palpate the pulses. Testing of capillary refill time (should be <3 seconds) becomes even more important when pulses are not palpable. Unless the skin is broken, the nurse must make a judgment whether or not to wear gloves, especially for the assessment of temperature.

Auscultation

Auscultation is the most detailed aspect of assessment of the cardiovascular system. It begins with laying the stethoscope lightly on the carotid arteries for a sign of bruits or a "swishing" sound. Peripheral pulses are palpated for presence or absence and their quality. They include the femoral, popliteal, posterior tibial, and dorsalis pedis. There are several reasons that a pulse may not be easily palpable, especially in the presence of edema; other measures of circulatory health must be used in this case. Unless the limb has acute ischemia, it is not that there is "no pulse" but that the pulse is "not palpable."

While assessment for jugular venous pressure is standard in the complete assessment of a younger adult, this is not always possible or appropriate in the older adult due to difficulty in assuming the needed recumbent position and to changes of the neck tissue that lead to inaccurate readings.

Auscultation of the heart. It is important to auscultate the heart for at least 60 seconds to determine if any irregularities are heard. It is ideal to be able to auscultate all four areas (aortic, pulmonic, tricuspid, and mitral) of the heart, with the length of time in each area dependent on what is heard. For example, if a murmur or irregular rhythm is detected in the aortic area, then 60 seconds would be a reasonable time to auscultate; if the nurse auscultates for less time, the irregularity may be missed. In the older woman the first three areas are often easier to auscultate than in a younger woman because of the age-related increased laxity of the breast tissue. Due to changes in the rib cage and spine, auscultation of the mitral area may not be possible. In someone with cardiac enlargement, the point of maximal impulse (PMI) will be found more lateral than where it is in the younger adult. The quality, rate, and rhythm of the pulsations of the carefully auscultated heart are evaluated. As noted earlier, the auscultation of a mild systolic murmur is a "normal" finding in approximately 50% of older adults (Jarvis, 2014). They are heard most often in the aortic and less so in pulmonic areas. An occasional ectopic beat may be heard and is usually completely insignificant. The rhythm may be irregularly irregular (IRIRR) or regularly irregularly (RIRR) in those with atrial fibrillation.

If the person is being seen in the outpatient setting with minimal or no symptoms of active heart disease or has significant positioning problems, such as from orthopedic deformities, assessment may need to take place in the sitting position. While it is ideal to auscultate on exposed skin, this may not be possible for a number of reasons. In that case, listening through one thin layer of a smoothed cotton fabric may be adequate for the nurse with experience and advanced skills. In a symptomatic person or a person who has any positive findings, skin to stethoscope contact is required.

The assessment includes the practice of both preventive measures and those that are in the presence of disease or disease progression, such as smoking status, level of ongoing emotional distress, current intensity of exercise (and changes in this ability), and diet. Unless the person is nearing the end of life, the importance of diabetes control is often an essential point of patient education (Chapter 24).

Despite the normal age-related changes, the healthy older heart and blood vessels are able to sustain adequate function for everyday life. At the same time, the gerontological nurse must recognize that the increased heart rate expected in a younger person who is physiologically, psychologically, or emotionally distressed is not usually found in the older adult. Additionally, due to the high rate of heart disease in today's population older than 60 or 65 years of age, the gerontological nurse must be alert to signs of rapid decompensation of both the well and the fragile elder.

◆ Intervention: The Nurse as Advocate

In addition to the nursing interventions discussed throughout this chapter, the role of an advocate will advance healthy aging for persons with CVD and cerebrovascular disease and for those at risk for these diseases by promoting preventive activities and ensuring that early signs and symptoms of both disease states and exacerbations are addressed promptly. Primary prevention includes promoting smoking cessation (or never smoking), healthy eating, exercise, and maintaining an appropriate body weight (Chapter 1). Secondary prevention includes doing everything possible to control the conditions already present (e.g., hypertension). These activities cannot be overstated and can improve health-related quality of life and in many cases slow the progression of the chronic diseases (Box 22-15 and Table 22-6). The nurse advocate is involved in introducing evidence-based programs to communities and organizations such as regional stroke centers and other programs (Box 22-16). The nurse can volunteer in mobile clinics and work with the many people with cardiovascular health problems, including older adults with more advanced disease. The nurse identifies those at high risk or stroke-prone elders. The nurse advocate serves as a healthy role model.

TABLE 22-6 Promoting Healthy Aging for the Person with PVD

Give Legs a Rest	Take Care of the Skin
Elevate the feet above heart level while sleeping, while sitting, and several times a day.	Examine feet daily, including the soles, sides, and between the toes.
Change Positions Frequently	Wash lower legs and feet regularly with mild soap and
Avoid activities that require standing or sitting with feet dangling for long periods.	water.
Give Legs Support (as directed only)	Use moisturizing cream and emollients after washing.
As directed, wear professionally made compression stockings that apply even pressure from ankles to knees or ankles to hip.	Do **not** use lanolin or petroleum-based creams when wearing support hose made with latex.
Replace hose as needed to maintain usefulness.	Avoid activities that can injure the legs or feet.
Put hose on early in the morning; wear all day; remove at bedtime.	Monitor legs for skin changes: Persistent edema
If a compression pump has been prescribed, follow the instructions.	Discoloration
	Dryness and/or itching
	Any bruises or wounds that do not go away in 1 week

BOX 22-16 RESOURCES FOR BEST PRACTICE

Promoting Healthy Hearts

USDHHS: *Million hearts: the initiative*, 2012. Available at http://millionhearts.hhs.gov/index.html
CDC: *WISEWOMAN*, 2013a. Available at http://www.cdc.gov/wisewoman.
DASH Diet: www.nhlbi.nih.gov

BOX 22-15 Nursing Interventions to Promote Healthy Aging for Persons with Heart Disease

1. Activities: pacing and tolerance
2. Exercise: strategizing adherence to prescribed program
3. Medications: timing, side effects, evaluation of effectiveness, obstacles to adherence
4. Disease self-management: signs and symptoms of exacerbation; intake, output; weight management; when to call for help and who to call with questions or questions; interpreting laboratory values; diet
5. Diet: low cholesterol, fat, and sodium
6. Fluid restriction if necessary
7. Help person develop strategies to maintain:
   a. Blood pressure ≤150/90 mm Hg
8. Help the person maintain individually tailored cholesterol and triglycerides control
9. Optimal control of diabetes as appropriate

In the long-term care setting, the nurse is the key health care provider to promote healthy aging and to advocate and secure appropriate interventions for the elder who is dependent on others. The nurse alerts the resident's nurse practitioner or physician about observed changes including atypical signs and symptoms and indicators of iatrogenesis. The provider is then responsible for the prescriptive interventions that are consistent both with the latest evidence-based practice and with the patient and family wishes and advance directives.

The nurse advocate listens carefully to the stories that are being told and is often the first to identify the progression of cardiovascular disease, such as both slow and sudden decompensation of the older adult, and the prevention of these. The nurse counters the expectation that problems that have been evaluated are not attributed to "just getting older."

KEY CONCEPTS

- Cardiovascular diseases are the leading cause of death and a frequent cause of disability in the older adult.
- The presentation of many cardiovascular diseases or nuances of these in older adults differ from those in younger adults (e.g., the "silent MI").
- The goals of promoting healthy aging include minimizing risk for disease and, in the presence of disease, alleviating symptoms, delaying or avoiding the development of complications including end-organ damage, and maximizing function and quality of life.

- The gerontological nurse is involved with the assessment of persons with CVD in daily practice.
- The gerontological nurse has the potential to serve as a leader in the promotion of health and the prevention of CVD and in the improvement of the lives of those with CVD.
- Embolic and hemorrhagic strokes must be differentiated before treatment can be initiated.

NURSING STUDY: ADHERING TO MRS. LEWIS'S WISHES

Mrs. Lewis is an 85-year-old widowed woman with three sons and a daughter. Although her husband was not of the Jewish faith, she raised her children in the practices and traditions in which she had been raised. None of her children live nearby, but she does have a very close friend from her synagogue who has been at her side during a long and difficult battle with congestive heart failure. She has been admitted to the subacute unit in the skilled nursing home where you are employed. Her prognosis is very poor and death is imminent. She has a living will in place designating her friend as her decision-maker and also has a DNR order. Between breaths she tells you that most of the time in the last 2 months she has been in the hospital and has been told there was nothing left to do but to allow a natural death. She is adamant that under no circumstances should she be returned to the hospital.

- What is the priority of care for Mrs. Lewis if you are the RN assigned to provide care to her?

- What are your priorities if you are an APN providing "medical" care to her?
- After you have thought about Mrs. Lewis's situation, discuss with a classmate how you would feel about caring for her. Could you care for her and respect her wishes?
- What symptoms do you expect she will develop in the hours or days between her admission and her death? What are your responsibilities related to them?
- Is Mrs. Lewis' decision consistent with her faith?

CRITICAL THINKING QUESTIONS AND ACTIVITIES

1. A patient's family member disagrees with that of the patient. What is the role of the nurse?
2. In a discussion with other students, describe your personal feelings about caring for someone who declines treatment.
3. In this same discussion, consider how you might reconcile personal feelings and professional responsibilities if they differ.

RESEARCH QUESTIONS

1. Are there any rituals or customs that are expected at the time nearing death or at the time of death in the Jewish faith?
2. Is a person with heart disease ever considered eligible for hospice services, and if so, under what circumstance?

REFERENCES

Aminoff MJ: Nervous system disorders. In McPhee SJ, Papadakis MA, editors: *2010 Current medical diagnosis and treatment,* New York, 2010, McGraw-Hill Lange, pp 872–936.

Bashore TM, Granger CB, Hranitzky P, et al: Heart disease. In Papadakis MA, McPhee SJ, editors: *Current medical diagnosis and treatment 2013,* New York, 2013, McGraw-Hill Lange, pp 324–432.

Boss BJ, Brashers SE: Disorders of the central and peripheral nervous systems

and the neuromuscular junction. In: McCance KL, Huether SE, editors: *Pathophysiology: the biologic basis for disease in adults and children,* ed 7, St. Louis, MO, 2014, Elsevier, pp. 581–640.

Bowker LK, Price JD, Smith SC: *Oxford handbook of geriatric medicine,* ed 2, Oxford, 2013, Oxford University Press.

Bowling SM, Weinhart J: Transient ischemic attacks and strokes. In Ham RJ, Sloane PD, Warshaw GA, et al, editors: *Primary care geriatrics: a case-based approach,*

ed 6, Philadelphia, 2014, Elsevier, pp 422–430.

Caboral-Stevens MF, Rosario-Sim M: Review of the Joint National Committee's recommendation in the management of hypertension, *J Nurse Pract* 10(5): 325–330, 2014.

Centers for Disease Control and Prevention (CDC): *Black or African American populations,* 2014a. http://www.cdc.gov/minorityhealth/populations/remp/black.html. Accessed June 2014.

CDC: *Conditions that increase the risk for stroke*, 2014b. http://www.cdc.gov/stroke/conditions.htm. Accessed July 2014.

CDC: *Genomics and health*, 2014c. http://www.cdc.gov/genomics/resources/diseases/heart.htm. Accessed June 2014.

CDC: *Heart disease facts*, 2014d. http://www.cdc.gov/heartdisease/facts.htm. Accessed June 2014.

CDC: *Heart failure fact sheet*, 2013, Division for heart disease and stroke prevention. http://www.cdc.gov/dhdsp/data_statistics/fact_sheets/fs_heart_failure.htm. Accessed June 2014.

CDC: *High blood pressure*. 2014e. http://www.cdc.gov/bloodpressure. Accessed June 2014.

CDC: *Stroke signs and symptoms*, 2014f. http://www.cdc.gov/stroke/signs_symptoms.htm. Accessed June 20014.

CDC: *Stroke statistics and maps*, 2014g. http://www.cdc.gov/stroke/statistics_maps.htm. Accessed July 2014.

CDC: *Strokes*, 2014h. http://www.cdc.gov/stroke. Accessed July 2014.

CDC: *Types of strokes*, 2013i. http://www.cdc.gov/stroke/types_of_stroke.htm. Accessed June 2014.

Davis LL: Contemporary management of arterial fibrillation, *J Nurse Pract* 9(110):643–652, 2013a.

Davis LL: Using the latest evidence to manage hypertension, *J Nurse Pract* 9(10):621–628, 2013b.

Ding Q, Yehle KS, Edwards NE, et al: Geriatric heart failure: awareness, evaluation, and treatment in primary care, *J Nurse Pract* 10(1):49–54, 2013.

Go AS, Mozaffarian D, Roger VL, et al: Heart disease and stroke statistics—2013 update: a report from the American Heart Association, *Circulation* 2012:e2–241, 2014.

Gumbinger C, Reuter B, Stock C, et al: Time to treatment with recombinant tissue plasminogen activator and outcome of stroke in clinical practice: retrospective analysis of hospital quality assurance data with comparison results from randomized clinical trials, *BMJ* 30(348):g3429, 2014.

Hackett ML, Köhler S, O'Brien, et al: Neuropsychiatric outcomes of stroke, *Lancet Neurol* 13(5):525–534, 2014.

Helton M: Hypertension. In Ham RJ, Sloane PD, Warshaw GA, et al, editors: *Primary care geriatrics: a case-based approach,* ed 6, Philadelphia, 2014, Elsevier, pp 381–394.

James PA, Oparil S, Carter BL, et al: 2014 Evidence-based guideline for the management of high blood pressure in adults: report from the panel members appointed to the Eighth Joint National Committee (JNC 8), *JAMA* 311(5): 507–520, 2014.

Jarvis C: *Physical examination and health assessment.* ed 6, St. Louis, MO, 2014, Elsevier.

Johanning JM: Peripheral vascular disease. In Ham RJ, Sloane PD, Warshaw GA, et al, editors: *Primary care geriatrics: a case-based approach,* ed 6, Philadelphia, 2014, Elsevier, pp 413–421.

Kohlman-Trigoboff D: Management of lower extremity peripheral arterial disease: interpreting the latest guidelines for nurse practitioners, *J Nurse Pract* 9(10):653–660, 2013.

Mayo Clinic: *Secondary hypertension,* 2013. http://www.mayoclinic.org/diseases-conditions/secondary-hypertension/basics/causes/con-20033994. Accessed June 2014.

National Heart, Lung, and Blood Institute (NHLBI): *The seventh report of the Joint National Committee on prevention,* detection, evaluation and treatment of high blood pressure—complete report, 2003. http://www.nhlbi.nih.gov/guidelines/hypertension/jnc7full.htm. Accessed June 2014.

NHLBI: *How can high blood pressure? be prevented.* 2012a. http://www.nhlbi.nih.gov/health/health-topics/topics/hbp/prevention.html. Accessed June 2014.

NHLBI: *Who is at risk for high blood pressure?* 2012b. http://www.nhlbi.nih.gov/health/health-topics/topics/hbp/atrisk.html. Accessed June 2014.

NHLBI: *Who is at risk for heart failure?* 2014. http://www.nhlbi.nih.gov/health/health-topics/topics/hf/atrisk.html. Accessed June 2014.

Office of Minority Health (OMH): *White population: leading causes of death, 2010.* http://www.cdc.gov/omhd/populations/White.htm. Accessed June 2014.

Ogbonna KC, Clifford KM: Moving beyond warfarin—are we ready? *J Gerontol Nurs* 39(7):8–13, 2011.

Rapp JH, Owens CD, Johnson MD: Blood vessels and lymphatic disorders. In Padadakis MA, McPhee SJ, editors: *Current medical diagnosis and treatment 2013,* New York, 2013, McGraw-Hill Lange, pp 464–489.

Robertson L, Evans C, Fowkes FG: Epidemiology of chronic venous disease, *Phlebology* 23(3):103–111, 2008.

Robertson L, Lee AJ, Evans CJ, et al: Incidence of chronic venous disease in the Edinburg Vein Study, *J Vasc Surg Venous and Lymphat Disord* 1:59–67, 2013.

Taffet GE: Coronary artery disease and atrial fibrillation. In Ham RJ, Sloane PD, Warshaw GA, et al, editors: *Primary care geriatrics: a case-based approach,* ed 6, Philadelphia, 2014, Elsevier, pp 395–405.

World Health Organization (WHO): *The atlas of heart disease and stroke,* 2014. http://www.who.int/cardiovascular_diseases/resources/atlas/en. Accessed October 31, 2014.

Zhang S, Melander S: Varicose veins: diagnosis, management and treatment, *J Nurse Pract* 10(6):417–424, 2014.

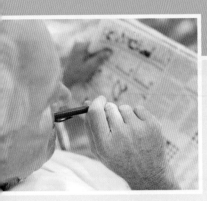

CHAPTER 23

Neurodegenerative Disorders

Kathleen Jett

🅔 http://evolve.elsevier.com/Touhy/TwdHlthAging

A STUDENT SPEAKS

It is so frustrating taking care of someone who has Parkinson's disease. Some of them just never seem to smile and seem so depressed. I try to be extra cheerful but it just doesn't seem to make any difference!

Helen, age 20

AN ELDER SPEAKS

I always kept active and healthy. I had lots of friends and we had lots of fun together. Now it seems like I am just fading away!

Ruth, age 82

LEARNING OBJECTIVES

On completion of this chapter, the reader will be able to:

1. Differentiate Parkinson's disease from the neurocognitive disorders due to Alzheimer's disease and the presence of Lewy bodies.
2. Describe the signs and symptoms that suggest the need for neurocognitive testing.
3. Identify the key aspects of the evaluation of the person with signs of cognitive limitations.
4. Identify the key characteristics of Parkinson's disease.
5. Describe the definitive test for the presence of Parkinson's disease.
6. Describe the recent genomic advances in an understanding of the mechanisms of neurodegenerative disorders.
7. Differentiate the key pharmacological interventions and their efficacy in Parkinson's disease and the neurocognitive disorders due to Alzheimer's disease and the presence of Lewy bodies.
8. Describe the nurse's role in the promotion of healthy aging in persons with neurodegenerative disorders.

Neurodegenerative disorders are seen in older adults more than any other age group. All are terminal conditions and characterized by a progressive decline in function. The declines may be barely noticeable in the beginning, with slight exacerbations and remissions, but the ultimate trajectory is always a downward slope. The impairments become so severe that the person cannot meet even his or her most basic self-care needs. However, there are interventions available to promote the healthiest aging possible for both the elder and significant others while the diseases progress. The three neurodegenerative disorders addressed in this chapter are the movement disorder Parkinson's disease, Alzheimer's disease, and dementia with Lewy bodies. There are several neurocognitive disorders of importance that are not necessarily terminal conditions, but they are beyond what is possible in this text (Box 23-1).

The recently published fifth edition of the *Diagnostic and Statistical Manual of Mental Health Disorders* (American Psychiatric Association [APA], 2013) redefined dementia in a number of ways. The word "dementia" has been replaced with the phrase "neurocognitive disorder (NCD)" and further subdivided into mild versus major. NCDs occur worldwide with the majority in low- and middle-income countries (Figure 23-1).

Although they rarely occur to persons younger than the age of 60, NCDs are not normal parts of aging (Box 23-2). The most common forms are NCD due to Alzheimer's disease (50% to 70%) and NCD due to Lewy bodies (LB) (10% to 22%) (National Institute on Aging [NIA], 2013). Both are characterized by impairments in memory, thinking, language, judgment, and behavior. A distinct difference in the two is that persons with LB will eventually develop motor symptoms as well, and the use of traditional (typical) antipsychotics (e.g., Haldol) is always contraindicated.

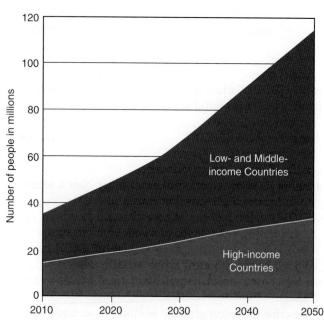

FIGURE 23-1 Number of People with Dementia. (From Alzheimer's Disease International: *World Alzheimer report 2010: the global economic impact of dementia,* 2010. http://www.alz.co.uk/research/files/WorldAlzheimerReport2010.pdf. Accessed October 31, 2014.)

DIAGNOSIS

The evaluation leading to a diagnosis of a presumed neurodegenerative disorder is initiated by the person, significant other, or a health care provider, when changes are noted in comparison to a prior state of cognition, especially memory or physical stability, such as balance or tremors. All signs are insidious in onset, often delaying diagnosis (Box 23-3). People with an undiagnosed NCD may remark that they are having a "senior moment," when it may be something far more serious than the very slight memory loss of normal aging. The symptoms that

initiate the diagnostic process in Parkinson's disease (PD) are often asymmetrical resting tremor, especially in the arm or hand or unexplained falls.

The diagnostic process begins with the assessment of all potentially reversible causes for the changes such as delirium, infection, vitamin deficiencies, or endocrine disturbances (Box 23-4). If a reversible cause is not found, or the signs remain after treatment, a more expanded, comprehensive exam is necessary to make a diagnosis and establish a baseline. This will include all of the components described in Chapter 7, tests of gait and balance (Chapter 19), and a detailed neurological and psychological examination, using highly reliable and sensitive screening instruments (see http://www.alz.or. for recommended instruments). When available, a magnetic resonance imaging (MRI) or a functional positron emission tomography (PET) scan may be done. Although diagnoses of neurodegenerative disorders cannot be confirmed until autopsy, the abilities of clinicians to do so empirically are improving.

The evaluation of people with signs or symptoms of neurodegenerative disorders increases in complexity when the person has other confounding chronic diseases, is very frail, or has sensory limitations. Expert care, including treatment of reversible conditions, may not be possible for persons with symptoms of Parkinson's disease or an NCD of any kind living in low- or middle-income countries.

PARKINSON'S DISEASE

Parkinson's disease (PD) was first described by James Parkinson in 1817. It is the fourteenth cause of death, affecting 6.3 million people worldwide (National Parkinson Foundation [NPF], 2014). In the United States, about half a million people have PD, with about 60,000 newly diagnosed each year (European Parkinson's Disease Association [EPDA], 2014; National Institute on Aging [NIA], 2012b). It is more common in men than women. Rarely occurring in those younger than age 60, the incidence increases with each decade. Persons of all races and ethnicities throughout the world are affected; however, a number of studies have found a higher prevalence in high-income countries (Khandelwal and Kaufer, 2014).

PD is the second most common *neurodegenerative* disease after Alzheimer's disease. In very late stages many develop a neurocognitive disorder as well, referred to as Parkinson disease dementia (PDD). PDD can be confused with other disorders that have parkinsonian-like symptoms, such as NCD due to Lewy bodies (Walter et al, 2014). PDD affects only 9% of those with an onset of PD before age 70 but almost 40% of those when onset is after the age of 70 (Walter et al, 2014).

Diagnosis

As a movement disorder, the diagnosis of PD can eventually be done with a reasonable level of certainty by considering the presence or absence of classic signs and symptoms. A diagnosis is confirmed by a "challenge test"—when symptoms improve dramatically after the administration of the medication levodopa (Khandelwal and Kaufer, 2014). Early falls, poor response to levodopa, symmetry of motor symptoms, lack of tremor, and early autonomic dysfunction are characteristic of other movement disorders (Box 23-5). In particular, when cognitive impairments occur before any movement symptoms appear, NCD due to Lewy bodies must be strongly considered.

Etiology

PD is the result of a deficiency of the neurotransmitter dopamine, a reduction of dopamine receptors, and the accumulation of Lewy bodies, especially in the basal ganglia. The severity of the illness is associated with the degree of neuron loss. However, by the time a person becomes overtly symptomatic, 70% to

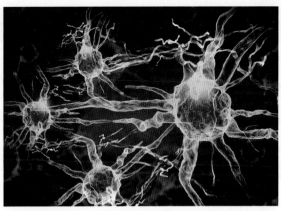

Neurons. (©iStock.com/Sergey Nivens)

90% of the dopamine-producing cells are lost (Boss and Huether, 2014; Nolden et al, 2014).

The epigenetic factors influencing the development of PD are speculated to include such things as head trauma (e.g., boxers), stroke, encephalitis, tumors, and exposure to toxins such as pesticides (National Institute of Environmental Health Services [NIEHS], 2014). Although several genes associated with PD have been identified, it is not yet known what causes them to be "activated" or "turned on," initiating the onset of the disease. However, this activation may be inherited in some way; an estimated 15% to 25% of those who develop PD have a relative with PD (NIA, 2012b) (Box 23-6).

Signs and Symptoms

The four core signs of PD are *resting tremor* (hands, arms, legs, jaw, face), *muscular rigidity, bradykinesia,* and *asymmetrical* onset (Box 23-7) (NIA, 2012b; Stallworth-Kolinas, 2014). Resting tremor is the first sign in 70% of those with PD. When present, tremors are asymmetrical and rhythmic, are of low amplitude, and disappear briefly during voluntary movement. The arm and hand are most commonly affected—the leg, foot, and head less often. They are not present during sleep but increase with stress and anxiety.

Rigidity can be assessed with passive range of motion. Instead of smooth movement, it is "cogwheel" in nature. That is, movement alternates with resistance. Severe muscle cramps may occur in the toes or hands due to lack of free and regular

---

BOX 23-5   Movement Disorders Other Than Parkinson's Disease

Essential tremor
Drug-induced parkinsonism
Progressive supranuclear palsy
Multiple system atrophy
Dementia of the Lewy body type
Normal pressure hydrocephalus

From Stallworth-Kolinas M: Parkinson's disease. In Ham RJ, Sloane D, Warshaw GA, et al, editors: *Primary care geriatrics: a case-based approach,* ed 6, Philadelphia, 2014, Elsevier, pp 554–562.

BOX 23-6   An Eye into the Brain: Genetics and Parkinson's Disease

While the exact cause is not yet known for the body's destruction of the neurons in the brain that lead to PD, scientists have identified several genes that are linked to PD. One gene *(LRRK2)* is the most common cause of the disease, about 10% inherited and 4% without genetic influence. However, a mutation of this gene *(G2019S)* is thought to cause 30% to 40% of PD cases in persons of North African Arabic descent.

From National Institutes of Health: *Insights into mutations that cause Parkinson's disease,* 2014. http://www.nih.gov/researchmatters/april2014/04282014parkinson.htm Accessed July 2014.

movement. Bradykinesia affects the person's ability to perform fine motor tasks. This early sign may have the most effect on the person's ability to independently perform day-to-day self-care functions.

As muscle rigidity and bradykinesia worsen, all of the striated muscles in the extremities, trunk, and ocular areas will ultimately be affected, including the muscles of mastication (chewing), deglutition (swallowing), and articulation (speaking). In the later stages, the person blinks infrequently and the face shows little animation, including that of emotion *(masked facies)*.

Other motor symptoms of special importance to independent functioning and safety and the need for assistance with ADLs (activities of daily living) are related to movement and positioning. Downward gaze becomes more difficult and there is an involuntary flexion of the head and neck, a stooped posture, and postural instability. The characteristic gait consists of very short steps and minimal arm movements (festination). Initiating and restarting movement is difficult (freezing) later in the disease, but once it starts the person moves forward with small steps and a forward lean, further increasing the person's risk for falling (Chapter 19). Turning is difficult and may require many steps. If off balance, correction is very slow. There are many other symptoms that are of particular importance to persons with PD, all of which decrease their quality of life (Box 23-8).

Symptoms and their intensity vary from person to person; some become severely disabled early in the disease and others experience only minor motor disturbances until much later. However, the number of symptoms and the degree to which they will affect a person's life and function will always increase over time.

Treatment

Currently there is no cure for PD, but when the symptoms are such that they interfere with the person's functioning, pharmacological interventions are initiated, sometimes providing dramatic relief. Drug therapy focuses on replacing or mimicking dopamine or slowing its breakdown.

The first-line medication is levodopa; it is especially effective in reducing bradykinesia and rigidity. It is converted to dopamine in the basal ganglia and therefore increases the amount of dopamine in the brain and inhibits hyperactive cholinergic activity. Carbidopa is usually added to the levodopa to limit peripheral breakdown of the levodopa. To maximize effectiveness, levodopa/carbidopa must be taken on an empty stomach (30 to 60 minutes before or 45 to 60 minutes after a meal). Although it can be highly and rapidly effective, its efficacy decreases with long-term use and higher doses are needed more often, increasing the side effects, such as the risk for hallucinations. Dopamine agonists such as pramipexole and ropinirole are sometimes used early in the disease or concurrently with levodopa/carbidopa. These are usually prescribed and monitored by neurologists.

When medications do not provide relief from disabling symptoms, some persons elect surgical interventions. These include deep brain stimulation (DBS) or ablation (pallidotomy). The latter is rarely done and then only in the severest of cases. DBS is only indicated for those who had some relief from medications for their motor symptoms, but they are no longer effective. It specifically addresses motor symptoms. It is highly unlikely that these would be appropriate for persons with other serious chronic conditions as is the case with many older adults. Caring for persons with Parkinson's disease requires a combination of pharmacological and nonpharmacological approaches (Nolden et al, 2014). Early nonpharmacological approaches include gait training and muscle strengthening.

ALZHEIMER'S DISEASE

Alzheimer's disease (AD) was first described by Dr. Alois Alzheimer in 1906. The incidence increases dramatically with age—from 5% of those between 65 and 75 to 50% of those 85 and older. About 5 million people in the United States have an NCD at this time, the majority of which are due to AD (Walter et al, 2014). By 2050 this number is expected to grow to 16 million (Centers for Disease Control and Prevention [CDC], 2011). It is expected that the actual number of persons diagnosed will escalate as they take advantage of the free annual wellness visit now available through the Affordable Care Act, where cognitive screening is part of the overall assessment (Chapter 30).

Researchers found distinct ethnic and racial differences among persons with AD. They may have identified a gene placing African Americans at about twice the risk for developing AD compared with their white American counterparts (Alzheimer's Association [AA], 2013). It is possible that additional risk factors are a part of this, specifically, a higher rate of cardiovascular disease (Khandelwal and Kaufer, 2014). While persons who self-identify as Hispanic are 1½ times more likely to develop AD, no known genetic factors have yet been found to explain this. Information about other groups or subgroups of people is not yet known. In the United States, AD is the sixth leading cause of death for whites, tenth for blacks, and ninth for Asian Americans and Native Hawaiian/Pacific Islanders (CDC, 2014; Office of Minority Health [OMH], 2010). The research findings regarding the effect of gender and education are mixed (NIA, 2012a).

Research has become increasingly intense in the last 30 years, fueled by the anticipation of the influx of the aging "baby boomers" (Chapter 1). Of particular interest has been the identification of a means to prevent and more adequately treat this now terminal condition. See Chapter 5 for a discussion of promoting brain health while aging.

Etiology

Through advances in genomic science, we now know the influence of the specific genes in the development of a neurocognitive disorder due to AD. Less than 5% of all persons have what is referred to as "early onset" or familial Alzheimer's disease (FAD) that is diagnosed between 30 and 60 years of age. FAD is caused by a single gene mutation on one of three chromosomes: 21, 14, or 1. The mutations result in the development of abnormal amyloid precursor proteins, presenilin 1 or presenilin 2. A child whose mother or father carries a genetic factor for FAD has a 50/50 chance of developing FAD (NIA, 2011).

Most AD is diagnosed in persons older than age 60, likely due to a number of factors including genetic risk. Everyone inherits one form of the *APOE* gene found on chromosome 19. There are three forms: ε2, ε3, and ε4. *APOE* ε3 is the most common and believed to be a neutral factor, neither increasing nor decreasing one's risk. The inheritance of either *APOE* ε2 or ε4 is much less common. *APOE* ε2 appears to have a protective influence, decreasing one's risk, while ε4 increases the risk, especially that of early onset. The ε4 form of *APOE* is present in about 25% to 30% of the general population but found in 40% of those with late-onset AD (NIA, 2014a). Genetic testing is now available to identify any one person's risk of developing AD by determining which *APOE* allele a person has. While testing is not recommended for general use, it may be especially helpful for those with one or both parents with AD to determine the presence of the ε4 form of *APOE*. It is important to note that not all persons with *APOE* ε4 develop AD.

Persons with neurocognitive dementia due to AD also have an increased number of beta-amyloid proteins (plaques) outside the neurons and an accumulation of abnormal tau proteins inside the neurons (neurofibrillary tangles), which damage the cortical areas of the brain. As a result, the number of synapses that normally connect the neurons decreases, and the neurons are deprived of nutrients, malfunction, and eventually die. As the number of beta-amyloid and tau proteins increases, more and more brain cells die. The initial memory loss seen in all persons with AD is the result of damage to the part of the brain where memories are stored.

While there is increasingly convincing evidence of the association between epigenetics and neurocognitive dementias, the exact influence is not yet clearly understood. Emotional stress, diet, and exposure to toxins are those factors that appear to "turn on" or "activate" the genes, which may explain why one member in a family develops AD and another does not (AA, 2014; NIA, 2014a).

Symptoms

The initial symptom of NCD due to AD is memory loss, specifically the ability to remember new information. As time goes on, additional signs and symptoms develop. Functional decline correlates with cognitive decline. Geriatrician Barry Reisberg has developed an excellent tool to "stage" persons with NCDs to provide anticipatory guidance to both the individual and the future caregivers (see also Chapter 7, Table 7-2).

Diagnosis

A diagnosis of an NCD due to AD requires the following: (1) there has been a decline from a previous level of functioning; (2) the onset was insidious; and (3) there has been gradual regression in cognitive abilities. Of important note is that the changes are "greater than expected for the person's age and educational background" and these changes can be documented with standardized neuropsychological testing.

Neurocognitive disorders are now categorized as possible or probable, and major or minor. Persons with a "possible" diagnosis have no genetic mutations indicative of AD or family history. Those with probable mild AD have either genetic evidence or positive family history and have only modest impairment in one or more of the cognitive domains (Walter et al, 2014). In an amnestic form, memory loss is isolated, but the person is at a higher risk (6% to 22%) of advancing to a severe dementia, compared with those with the nonamnestic variation where the impairments are in areas other than memory (Stallworth-Kolinas, 2014). A person with any type of major NCD has a substantial impairment and is still ranked in functioning as mild (difficulty with IADLs), moderate (difficulty with ADLs), or severe (completely dependent) (Walter et al, 2014) (referred to as major cognitive impairment [MCI]).

Pharmacological Treatment

Because cure is not possible, pharmacological therapy for those with AD is aimed at slowing cognitive decline. In doing so, it has the potential to help persons continue to function to the best of their ability longer and therefore maximize their quality of life and that of their loved ones. The effectiveness of the medications varies from person to person.

First-line treatment for AD continues to be cholinesterase inhibitors (CIs). They may not only help slow the speed of cognitive decline but also help control any behavioral difficulties the person may be having as a consequence of the brain damage (NIA, 2014b) (Chapter 29). CIs are begun as soon as the person is diagnosed, even for those with mild, possible disease (Walter et al, 2014).

The CIs work by blocking the breakdown of acetylcholine, a chemical believed to be important for memory and thinking. The most common side effects of the CIs are nausea and diarrhea.

Donepezil (Aricept) can be used at all stages; galantamine (Razadyne) and rivastigmine (Exelon) are indicated for mild to moderate neurocognitive decline. Exelon is now available in a patch that may be more convenient to use, has fewer side effects, and provides consistent 24-hour effectiveness.

Memantine HCl (Namenda) is approved for use in moderate to severe AD; it may be given alone or with one of the CIs. Namenda works by regulating the activity of glutamate, a brain chemical that regulates learning and memory. The major side effects are headache, constipation, confusion, and dizziness. Nonetheless, Namenda may temporarily delay worsening of symptoms (AA, 2014). Dosages are slowly titrated to decrease side effects (NIA, 2014b). Namenda has been available in both the XR (extended release) and the twice-daily formulations. However, as of the summer of 2014, only the XR was being manufactured (Forest Laboratories, 2014). As with any medications, a trial to determine both effectiveness and ability of the person to tolerate side effects should be done at repeated intervals. Depression and other mental health issues are common in persons with AD. They may go unrecognized and untreated, but the person should be monitored for these and treated appropriately and promptly should they be found (Chapters 7, 9 and 28).

NEUROCOGNITIVE DEMENTIA WITH LEWY BODIES

What has long been referred to as dementia with Lewy bodies (DLB) was named after Dr. Friederich Lewy, who discovered a new type of abnormal proteins in the brain neurons of persons with Parkinson's disease, both those who had developed a neurocognitive decline and those who had not. What we now call NCD due to LB, affects 1.3 million people in the United States and 20% of persons with cognitive disorders worldwide (Stallworth-Kolinas, 2014). It is second in prevalence to that of AD. It is often confused with PD but distinctly different in chronology of symptomatology. In PD, movement disorders always precede cognitive changes (if they occur), and in LB the cognitive changes always precede movement disorders, which *will* occur (Khandelwal and Kaufer, 2014). Men are affected slightly more than women and there is an increasing incidence with age. The life expectancy ranges broadly from 2 to 20 years, with an average of 5 to 7 years after diagnosis.

Signs and Symptoms

Although some memory may stay intact, the person with an NCD due to LB will develop severe loss of the ability to think, especially problem solving and the use of language and numerical concepts. A common symptom is fluctuating attention and alertness—that is, periods of time when the flow of ideas is illogical interspersed with periods of clarity. Unlike AD, about 80% of persons with LB have hallucinations (NIA, 2013). These may lead to delusions and paranoia. Factors contributing to psychiatric disturbances include misidentifying objects and visuospatial problems, such as in judging distance or depth.

Disordered sleep is a problem specific for persons with NCD due to LB and may appear long before other signs become obvious to anyone other than the sleep partner. The majority of the time "asleep" is spent in the REM stage (Chapter 17) in which the person actively dreams and may talk in his or her sleep, thrash about, and even fall out of bed (Mayo Clinic Staff, 2014). Restless legs syndrome (also known as Willis-Ekbom disease) may occur during nighttime sleep and there may be a significantly increased need for daytime sleep (Chapter 17). Problems in mood occur, similar to those with PD: depression, apathy, anxiety, and agitation. Some of the conditions we refer to as "geriatric syndromes" occur as the disease advances. They are the result of damage to the part of the brain controlling the autonomic nervous system (Box 23-9). It is important to recognize the difference because their treatment varies. However, clear differentiation between cognitive declines due to PD and those due to LB is necessary to avoid inadvertent but life-threatening treatment.

Etiology

In normal healthy brains alpha-synuclein proteins (which are estimated to comprise 1% of the cytosolic protein in the nervous system) help neurons communicate with each other at their synapse (Stefanis, 2012). However, Lewy bodies are abnormal spherical protein aggregates found within neurons in persons with both dementia and PD. Alpha-synuclein is highly expressed within these bodies, which can displace other cellular structures, and may contribute to cell death (Aminoff and Kerchner, 2013). In DLB these proteins are found in the brainstem, midbrain, olfactory bulb, and neocortex. The progression of this disease leads to significant deficits in neurotransmitter production along the cholinergic and dopaminergic pathways. The acetylcholine deficit leads primarily to cognitive dysfunction, and the deficit in dopamine production is responsible for the motor dysfunction that appears as the disease advances (Walter et al, 2014). Although mutations have been identified that are associated with the risk for developing Parkinson's disease, neither familial nor lifestyle factors have been found to influence the development of the neurocognitive dementia due to LB; based on our knowledge at this time, the etiology of this disease is unknown (Vigneswara et al, 2013).

Diagnosis

According to the new *DSM-5* diagnostic criteria, the person identified as one with NCDLB (neurocognitive disorder due to Lewy bodies) must first meet all of the initial mild or moderate criteria for the other NCDs and then is classified as "possible" or "probable" based on the presentation of the core features (see Box 23-3).

Pharmacological Treatment

Persons with NCDLB have a wide range of symptoms over time; changes in these symptoms result in a change in priority of treatment. Those taking a cholinesterase inhibitor (CI), especially rivastigmine (Exelon), may show more dramatic improvements in cognitive status than those with AD (Latoo and Jan, 2008). The CIs have also been found to be helpful with

---

BOX 23-9   Autonomic Signs and Symptoms of NCD Due to DLB

Frequent falls	Unexplained loss of consciousness
Syncope	Incontinence
Orthostatic hypotension	Eating disorder/risk for aspiration

other symptoms more unique to DLB (e.g., fluctuations in cognition and mood, incidence of hallucinations). It may be tempting to use a dopamine medication such as Sinemet for the motor symptoms, but since these drugs on their own can cause hallucinations, their use may precipitate these and other psychotic symptoms common in NCDLB. Antipsychotics may be helpful but have been found to increase the risk for death.

> ### ⚡ SAFETY ALERT
>
> Typical antipsychotics (e.g., Haldol) can never be used in persons with NCD due to Lewy bodies because of the very high rate of irreversible side effects and possible death.

Benzodiazepines may also be useful but increase the risk for falling and increased confusion. The use of clonazepam (Klonopin) at very low doses may be the most beneficial and replace the need for the antipsychotics (Walter et al, 2014).

COMPLICATIONS

For patients in the late stages of neurodegenerative diseases, complications are consistent with any person in later life who is medically fragile (Box 23-10). Complications include pressure ulcers, pneumonia, dysphagia, aspiration, and other problems associated with geriatric frailty. Undernutrition and weight loss occur even with adequate caloric consumption. Weight loss is an indication that the terminal stage is approaching. Behavioral disturbances can be frightening and at times dangerous to the person affected, as well as those in the immediate environment. These are brought about by the extent of and location of brain damage, as well as side effects of medications.

◆ PROMOTING HEALTHY AGING: IMPLICATIONS FOR GERONTOLOGICAL NURSING

Everyone, especially those with strong family histories of neuro-degenerative disorders, would like to find ways to prevent them. Unfortunately, at this time this is not possible. For those with neurocognitive disorders due to AD and LB, factors have been proposed that may somewhat decrease the risk (Box 23-11). It is of special note that research related to the effect of preventive strategies is still inconclusive. Unfortunately factors to decrease the risk of PD have not yet been proposed.

Most of the potentially preventive strategies and nonpharma-cological interventions to promote healthy aging in persons with neurodegenerative disorders involve the nurse working with the individual and those who are either already providing care or will be doing so. Early comprehensive health, fall risk, and gait assessments are important to help the caregivers and nursing staff provide the highest quality and most empowering care possible. The assessment is repeated periodically to monitor changes and make modifications to the plan of care as needed. In the skilled nursing setting periodic reassessments are done through the RAI process (see Chapter 7); however, it is just as important in the outpatient setting. This information guides the discussions around end-of-life care, including legal preparation when the point of cognitive incapacity is reached (Chapter 31).

To prepare those with Parkinson's disease for anticipated changes in muscular flexibility, early training in relaxation such as modified yoga or Zen techniques and exercises may be helpful. Tai chi has been found to increase balance skills (Gao et al, 2014; Li et al, 2014; Pickut et al, 2013).

Persons with neurodegenerative disorders eventually experience changes in roles and may avoid social situations due to the accompanying signs and symptoms. For those with PD, tremors may produce embarrassing movements such as spilling food when eating in public. Drooling, a common problem with those with PD, is a socially unacceptable "behavior" in most societies. The expressionless face, slowed movement, and soft, monotone speech or aphasias may give the impression of apathy, depression, and disinterest and therefore others are discouraged to continue long-time relationships. A sensitive nurse is aware that the visible symptoms produce an undesired façade that may hide an alert and responsive individual who wishes to interact but is trapped in a body or brain that no longer cooperates.

Nowhere in the care of elders is a skilled and caring multidisciplinary team more essential than in the care of persons with neurodegenerative disorders. It includes a nurse; a neurologist; a physiatrist; speech, occupational, and physical therapists; an ophthalmologist; a rehabilitation specialist; a psychologist; a movement disorders' specialist; and the hospice team. Ideally it includes a physician and a nurse practitioner working as a primary care team. It also may include a spiritual advisor or indigenous healer. It always includes the person's significant other(s), who will be involved in day-to-day life at some point in time.

Occupational therapists can assist with teaching the person how to use adaptive equipment, such as weighted utensils,

---

BOX 23-10   Potential Complications of Those with Neurodegenerative Disorders

Pneumonia
Pressure ulcers
Abuse or neglect from excess burden to caregiver
Untreated pain
Unable to report symptoms of another health problem
Unable to follow any prescribed treatment plan
Injuries from falls
Untreated depression
Malnutrition or dehydration

BOX 23-11   TIPS FOR BEST PRACTICE
Decreasing Risk for Neurocognitive Disorders

- Maintain blood pressure within normal limits
- LDL cholesterol ≤100 mg/dL
- Hemoglobin A_{1c} ≤7%
- Aspirin (81 mg enteric coated) for persons with risk for heart disease and without contraindications
- Maintain optimal control of heart failure
- Stop smoking or never start

From Khandelwal C, Kaufer DI: Alzheimer's disease and other dementias. In Ham RJ, Sloane D, Warshaw GA, et al, editors: *Primary care geriatrics: a case-based approach,* ed 6, Philadelphia, 2014, Elsevier, pp 201–213.

nonslip dinnerware, and other self-care aids. Speech therapy is beneficial for dysarthria and dysphagia; patients can be taught facial exercises and swallowing techniques to lower the risk for aspiration-related pneumonia and weight loss.

The nurse has an active role in prevention of complications (Clarke, 2007). The nurse works to actively prevent skin breakdown and falls and identifies exacerbation of confusion or function, which may indicate the development of a treatable condition such as an infection. The nurse is alert for problems with sleep and depression as the disease progresses.

Treatment focuses on relieving symptoms with medication, increasing functional ability, preventing excess disability, and decreasing the risk of injury. In caring for persons with neurodegenerative disorders, regular pain assessments and appropriate management are essential (see Chapter 27). In PD, rigidity, contractures, and dystonia may cause a considerable amount of pain. There is also a recognized but not well-understood central-pain syndrome associated with the disease itself. Persons with any of the NCDs may not be able to verbally express their pain but

nonetheless experience it as anyone else would under the same circumstances. The nurse is aware of this and uses alternative means to observe for potential pain (Chapter 27).

Persons with neurodegenerative disorders watch their own decline over time, challenging self-esteem. The nurse can direct the person and care partners to formal programs in stress management or group support and urge them to attempt to maintain former relationships (Chapters 29 and 34) (NIA, 2003).

The key factors in the care of those with neurodegenerative disorders are (1) appropriate use of available nonpharmacological and pharmacological interventions, (2) prompt treatment of all reversible conditions (e.g., infections) at any time, and (3) coordination between all care providers, including family members or partners.

In light of the current inability to enact a cure for any of the neurodegenerative disorders, the goals of care are to maximize quality of life, promote self-esteem, and maintain independent function for as long as possible. The goal of treatment is to preserve self-esteem, retain self-care abilities, and prevent complications.

KEY CONCEPTS

- Neurodegenerative conditions are those that have a downward trajectory and for which there is no cure. The conditions discussed in this chapter are limited to Alzheimer's disease, dementia with Lewy bodies, and Parkinson's disease (PD).
- The American Psychiatric Association has renamed several conditions: Alzheimer's disease is now referred to as Neurocognitive Disorder (NCD) due to Alzheimer's disease; dementia with Lewy bodies is called NCD due to Lewy Bodies.
- A significant number of persons with PD develop late-stage cognitive disorders.
- The diagnostic process for any of these conditions is extensive and complex.
- A key difference in an NCD due to LB and PD is timing of symptoms. An NCDLB begins with cognitive declines and movement disorders develop later. PD is a movement disorder that may or may not lead to an NCD.

- Although neurocognitive changes can be measured using currently available tools, diagnoses can only be confirmed on autopsy.
- At least some of the genes associated with each of these disorders have been identified.
- The NCD may be mild or major; all have memory loss as a signal characteristic.
- The signal characteristics of PD include a resting tremor and bradykinesia.
- Treatment of each condition must be individually tailored and will likely change over time.
- The nurse has a key role in monitoring changes that indicate increased risk for poor outcomes and in developing interventions to maximize quality of life and healthy aging at all points along the wellness continuum.

NURSING STUDY: "IT IS SO HARD TO WATCH . . . HE WAS LOST TO ME SO LONG AGO!"

Helen's husband Sam had been slowly dying over a period of about 5 years from Alzheimer's disease. As it progressed, he began to have what are called "behavioral disturbances." He lashed out at those around him one moment and was affectionate the next. This was especially painful for his wife. During brief moments of lucidity he would kiss her and tell her how much he loved her, but moments later would physically hurt her in some way. Most of the time he was completely disoriented, and the nurses caring for him charted Sam as "disoriented × 4" (person, place, time, and situation). After a long and steady decline in cognitive and functional ability, one day he simply stopped eating and drinking

and he began to fail rapidly. We all knew that death was imminent. His wife carefully shared that while she was glad for him that he would no longer suffer, she whispered, "and it will bring an end to my suffering as well, is that terrible to think that??? He was lost to me so long ago . . . "

- What are the subjective and objective data found in the case study?
- If you were one of the nurses caring for Sam, how would your plan of care change over time?
- If you were Helen, what would be the hardest part of your husband's illness?
- What strengths might Helen bring to such a situation?

CRITICAL THINKING QUESTIONS AND ACTIVITIES

1. Have a classroom discussion about resources in the community that would be particularly helpful for persons with neurodegenerative disorders and the persons who care for them.

2. Discuss or write a paper about the skills the nurse must have to be able to provide expert care to persons with neurocognitive disorders of any kind.

RESEARCH QUESTIONS

1. What is the average life expectancy of someone with Alzheimer's disease?
2. Are there parts of the country that have unusually high or low rates of neurodegenerative conditions? What are the areas of the country and what might be the cause of this variation?
3. Has any genomic progress been made in understanding any of the other neurodegenerative disorders that are not addressed in this chapter?

REFERENCES

Alzheimer's Association (AA): *Alzheimer's and public health spotlight: race, ethnicity and Alzheimer's disease,* 2013. http://www.alz.org/documents_custom/public-health/spotlight-race-ethnicity.pdf. Accessed July 2014.

Alzheimer's Association (AA): 2014 Alzheimer's disease facts and figures, *Alzheimers Dement* 10(2):1–80, 2014. http://www.alz.org/downloads/facts_figures_2014.pdf. Accessed July 2014.

American Psychiatric Association (APA): *Diagnostic and statistical manual of mental disorders,* ed 5, Arlington, VA, 2013, American Psychiatric Publishing.

Aminoff MJ, Kerchner GA: Nervous system disorders. In Papadakis MA, McPhee SJ, editors: *Current medical diagnosis and treatment 2013,* New York, 2013, McGraw Hill, pp 962–1037.

Boss BJ, Huether SE: Alterations in cognitive systems, cerebellar hemodynamics, and motor function. In McCance KL, Huether SE, editors: *Pathophysiology: the biological basis for disease in adults and children,* ed 7, St. Louis, 2014, Elsevier, pp 527–580.

Centers for Disease Control (CDC): *Alzheimer's disease,* 2011. http://www.cdc.gov/aging/aginginfo/alzheimers.htm. Accessed July 2014.

Centers for Disease Control (CDC): *Minority health: black or African American populations,* 2014. http://www.cdc.gov/minorityhealth/populations/remp/black.html. Accessed June 2014.

Clarke CE: Parkinson's disease, *BMJ* 335(7617):441–445, 2007.

European Parkinson's Disease Association (EPDA): *The number of people with Parkinson's disease in the most populous nations, 2005 through 2030,* 2014. http://www.epda.eu.com/en/resources/life-with-parkinsons/part-3/the-number-of-people-with-parkinsons-in-the-most-populous-nations-2005-through-2030. Accessed July 2014.

Forest Laboratories: *Namenda: letter to healthcare providers,* 2013. http://www.namenda.com/. Accessed July 2014.

Gao Q, Leung A, Yanung A, et al: Effects of Tai Chi on balance and fall prevention in Parkinson's disease: a randomized controlled trial, *Clin Rehabil,* Feb 11, 2014: 1-6. [Epub ahead of print].

Khandelwal C, Kaufer DI: Alzheimer's disease and other dementias. In Ham RJ, Sloane D, Warshaw GA, et al, editors: *Primary care geriatrics: a case-based approach,* ed 6, Philadelphia, 2014, Elsevier, pp 201–213.

Latoo J, Jan F: Dementia with Lewy bodies: clinical review, *BJMP* 1(1):10–14, 2008.

Li F, Harmer P, Liu Y, et al: A randomized controlled trial of patient-reported outcomes with tai chi exercise in Parkinson's disease, *Mov Disord* 29(4):539–545, 2014.

Mayo Clinic Staff: *Diseases and conditions: dementia,* 2014. http://www.mayoclinic.org/diseases-conditions/dementia/basics/causes/con-20034399. Accessed July 2014.

National Institute of Environmental Health Services (NIEHS): *Parkinson's disease.* 2014. http://www.niehs.nih.gov/health/topics/conditions/parkinson. Accessed July 2014.

National Institute on Aging (NIA): *Alzheimer's disease and end-of-life issues,* 2003. http://www.nia.nih.gov/alzheimers/features/alzheimers-disease-and-end-life-issues. Accessed July 2014.

NIA: *Alzheimer's disease: unraveling the mystery,* 2011. http://www.nia.nih.gov/alzheimers/publication/alzheimers-disease-unraveling-mystery/preface. Accessed July 2014.

NIA: *2011-2012 Alzheimer's disease progress report: intensifying the research effort,* 2012a. http://www.nia.nih.gov/alzheimers/publication/2011-2012-alzheimers-disease-progress-report. Accessed July 2014.

NIA: *What is Parkinson's disease.* 2012b. http://nihseniorhealth.gov/parkinsonsdisease/whatisparkinsonsdisease/01.html. Accessed July 2014.

NIA: *Lewy body dementia: information for patients, families, and professionals* (Publication no. 13-7907), 2013. http://www.nia.nih.gov/alzheimers/publication/lewy-body-dementia/types-lewy-body-dementia. Accessed July 2014.

NIA: *Alzheimer's disease genetics fact sheet,* 2014a. http://www.nia.nih.gov/alzheimers/publication/alzheimers-disease-genetics-fact-sheet#genetics. Accessed July 2014.

NIA: *Alzheimer's disease medication fact sheet,* 2014b. http://www.nia.nih.gov/alzheimers/publication/alzheimers-disease-medications-fact-sheet. Accessed July 2014.

National Parkinson Foundation (NPF): *Parkinson's disease overview.* 2014. http://www.parkinson.org/parkinson-s-disease.aspx. Accessed July 2014.

Nolden LF, Tartavoulle T, Porche DJ: Parkinson's disease: assessment, diagnosis, and management, *J Nurse Pract* 10(7): 500–506, 2014.

Office of Minority Health (OMH): *White population: leading causes of death,* 2010. http://www.cdc.gov/omhd/populations/White.htm. Accessed June 2014.

Pickut BA, Van Hecke W, Kerchofs E, et al: Mindfulness based intervention in Parkinson's disease leads to structural brain changes on MRI: a randomized controlled longitudinal trial, *Clin Neurol Neursurg* 115(12):2419–2425, 2013.

Stallworth-Kolinas M: Parkinson's disease. In Ham RJ, Sloane D, Warshaw GA, et al, editors: *Primary care geriatrics: a case-based approach,* ed 6, Philadelphia, 2014, Elsevier, pp 554–562.

Stefanis L: α-Synuclein in Parkinson's disease, *Cold Spring Harb Perspect Med* 2(2):a009399, 2012.

Vigneswara V, Cass S, Wayne D, et al: Molecular aging of alpha- and beta-synucleins: protein damage and repair mechanisms, *PLoS One,* 8(4):e61442, 2013.

Walter C, Edwards NE, Griggs R, et al: Differentiating Alzheimer's disease, Lewy body, and Parkinson's disease using DSM-5, *J Nurse Pract* 10(4):262–270, 2014.

24 | CHAPTER

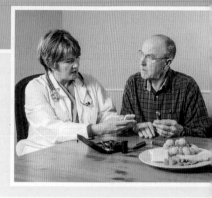

Endocrine and Immune Disorders

Kathleen Jett

AN ELDER SPEAKS

I had been wondering why I was so tired. I just could not get enough sleep. I went to my primary care provider, who did a bunch of tests and discovered I had a problem with my thyroid gland. Now that it is being treated, I cannot believe how much better I feel. Just like my old self again.

Ruth, age 72

A STUDENT SPEAKS

The immune system is so complex and affects so many other systems it is difficult to grasp. However, I see now how important my understanding is in order to provide the highest quality of care I can.

Tamara, age 30, a nurse practitioner student

LEARNING OBJECTIVES

On completion of this chapter, the reader will be able to:

1. Discuss the effects of the aging immune system on the body's ability to respond to potential infectious agents.
2. Discuss common conditions that may be related to changes in the aging immune system.
3. Describe at least two methods of diagnosing diabetes.
4. Determine how diabetes is different in older adults compared with those who are younger.
5. Identify the nurse's response to the older adult with fluctuations in glycemic levels.
6. Identify the most common pharmacological agents used to treat diabetes and explain how their use may differ in older adults.
7. Differentiate between the two major types of thyroid disorders.
8. Describe how the signs and symptoms of thyroid disorders differ in younger adults compared with older adults.
9. Describe the nurse's role in advancing healthy aging in persons with immune and endocrine disorders.

THE IMMUNE SYSTEM

The immune system functions to protect the host (the human body) from invasion by foreign substances and organisms through the activity of lymphocytes, particularly, T and B cells. T cells scan the body for invading substances such as infections and contribute to the body's immunity in a number of ways. While the total number of circulating T cells does not change with aging, the relative proportion of the types of cells does (Rote and McCance, 2014). The thymus, where T cells mature, may be only 15% of the size in late life that it was in mid-life (Rote, 2014).

B cells secrete antibodies in response to the presence of antigens such as infectious agents and other foreign substances. In aging, this function decreases, resulting in a reduced ability to produce antibodies. For example, there is a decreased ability to develop adequate immunity after an infection or after an immunization such as that for influenza (Box 24-1).

At the same time, there is an increase in the number of circulating autoantibodies in which the B cells are less sensitive to self-antigens; that is, they are less able to differentiate self cells from non-self cells. Although their effect is not well understood, there is an increase in the number of immunoglobulins leading to a decrease in innate immunity and more common autoimmune responses; autoimmune disorders are much more likely to occur in aging. These changes are referred to as *immunosenescence*. Although they can occur at any age, being alert for signs and symptoms of autoimmune disorders is probably as important as prevention and protection from infection for the older adult (Box 24-2).

BOX 24-1 TIPS FOR BEST PRACTICE

Reduced Immune Response

Early studies found that oral temperature norms in healthy older adults were significantly lower in women younger than age 80 compared with younger women. Older men consistently had an even lower temperature than women of comparable age. The old-old may have a temperature of 96.8° F with an average range of 95° to 97° F. By tympanic membrane thermometer, the temperature may be 96° F. These findings emphasize the need to carefully evaluate the basal temperature of older adults and recognize that even low-grade fevers (98.6° F) in the elderly may signify serious illness. Due to age-related delayed immune response, a lack of fever (temperature greater than 98.6° F) cannot be used to rule out an infection.

From Stengel GB: Oral temperatures in the elderly, *Gerontologist* 23:306, 1983 (special issue).

BOX 24-2 The Aging Immune System and Immune Disorders: Possible Connections

Diabetes
Insulin resistance
Hypothyroidism (chronic autoimmune thyroiditis)
Pernicious anemia
Renal insufficiency
Environmental allergies

THE ENDOCRINE SYSTEM

The endocrine system works with multiple body organs through the release of hormones to regulate and integrate body activities. Hormones are responsible for, and control, reproduction, growth and development, maintenance of homeostasis, response to stress, nutrient balance, cell metabolism, and energy balance. The primary glands of the endocrine system are the pituitary, thyroid, parathyroid, adrenal, pineal, and thymus. The pancreas, ovaries, and testes are not glands, but they contain endocrine tissue. With the exception of the ovaries, age-related changes in the endocrine system are thought to be very mild and most likely due to the autoimmunity described earlier in this chapter.

Endocrine disorders can occur at any age. However, the complex interrelationships between these, the changes attributed to normal aging, and the number of concurrent chronic conditions (including frailty) make it almost impossible to specifically attribute any endocrine disease to the aging process itself. As with most other systems, the signs and symptoms of a problem are often subtle and nonspecific. Its presence may only become known during a routine screening, laboratory exam, or the evaluation for another problem such as confusion or an unexplained fall resulting in an injury. In this chapter diabetes and thyroid disturbances as seen in the older adult are addressed.

Diabetes Mellitus

There are two main types of diabetes mellitus (DM) (type 1 and type 2) and also those related to steroid use and pregnancy. Type 1 is the result of absolute insulin deficiency due to the autoimmune destruction of beta-cells in the pancreas. Type 2 is a more complex disease and has been attributed to a combination of relative insulin deficiency and insulin resistance. It is the most common type of DM seen in older adults (Razzaque et al, 2014). Genetics, epigenetics, lifestyle, and aging are all significant contributing factors. Studies have shown that variants of the *TCF7L2* gene increase one's likelihood to develop DM type 2. If one inherits the gene from both parents, the risk of developing it is 80% higher than in those who do not carry the gene variant (National Diabetes Information Clearinghouse [NDIC], 2014).

Diabetes mellitus (DM) is now viewed on a continuum from asymptomatic prediabetic insulin resistance, to mild postprandial hyperglycemia and/or mild fasting hyperglycemia, to diagnosable diabetes (Box 24-3). The incidence of new diabetes in older adults is exacerbated by an increased resistance to insulin-mediated glucose disposal and decreased non–insulin-mediated glucose uptake (Razzaque et al, 2014). Due to the high prevalence and incidence of DM in older adults, when suspicions are suggested by clinical signs and symptoms, diagnostic testing should be done. The U.S. Preventive Services Task Force (USPSTF) recommends that screening for DM always be done for those whose blood pressure (BP) is consistently >135/80 mm Hg and with any risk factors for cardiovascular (CV) disease (USPSTF, 2008) (Chapter 22).

In the United States, the *total number* of persons with DM *decreases* with age; however, the *percentage increases* among those older than 65 years of age (Table 24-1) (CDC, 2014).

BOX 24-3 Criteria for the Diagnosis of Diabetes: Confirmed by Repeat Testing

One fasting hemoglobin A$_{1C}$ value of ≥6.5% tested by a certified laboratory*

or

One random plasma glucose ≥200 mg/dL

or

Fasting plasma glucose (FPG) ≥126 mg/dL (**NOTE:** This does not include blood glucose levels that are obtained with a fingerstick.)

or

Oral glucose tolerance test (OGTT) ≥200 mg/dL 2 hours after glucose administration

or

When classic symptoms of hyperglycemic or hypoglycemic crisis are present

*Controversy remains regarding the exact cutoff that should be used. From American Diabetes Association: Standards of medical care in diabetes—2013, *Diabetes Care* 36:S11–S66, 2013.

TABLE 24-1 Number of People with Diabetes in the United States, 2012

	NUMBER (MILLIONS)	PERCENTAGE (UNADJUSTED)
Total number >20	28.9	12.3
20-44	4.3	4.1
45-64	13.4	16.2
65+	11.2	65.9

Source: 2009-2012 National Health and Nutrition Examination Survey estimates applied to 2012 U.S. Census data.

There is a wide variation of the prevalence of diabetes among ethnic/racial groups and subgroups (Table 24-2). In the United States, American Indians alone have the highest rate of diabetes of all other groups (24.1%). This is influenced by the high prevalence of DM in the Pima Indians of the Southwest (National Institute of Diabetes and Digestive and Kidney Diseases [NIDDK], 2002). Another group at high risk is veterans who were exposed to Agent Orange and other herbicides (Box 24-4). Although many of these individuals are younger at this time, they will expand the number of those with DM as they age.

Worldwide 347 million people have diabetes; 90% of those with diabetes around the world have type 2, attributed to obesity and physical inactivity (WHO, 2013). Eighty percent of those with DM live in low- and middle-income countries. The number of persons who die from the consequences of hyperglycemia is expected to double between 2005 and 2030. The World Health Organization (WHO) predicts that diabetes will become the seventh leading cause of death by 2030 (WHO, 2014).

Signs and Symptoms

The classic signs of both DM type 1 and DM type 2 are polyuria, polyphagia, and polydipsia (the three "Ps") in younger adults. However, they are rarely presenting symptoms in later life (Razzaque et al, 2014). Polyuria does not occur due to

normal age-related increases in the renal threshold for glucose. Instead the person may develop urinary incontinence or find that it has worsened. Polydipsia is not present due to a normal age-related reduced thirst reflex. Any indication of polyphagia is reduced by age-related decreased appetite. Weight loss may occur instead of weight gain. Women may present with recurrent candidiasis as the first sign. Due to the absence or delayed signs and symptoms, the person may be found obtunded in a hyperglycemic-hyperosmolar nonketotic coma before an initial diagnosis is made. The older adult with DM should be screened regularly for the development of signs and complications that are more likely to occur in this population (Box 24-5).

Complications

The development of complications in older adults with DM is compounded by the presence of multiple comorbid diseases and disorders (Box 24-6). Although the same types of macro- and microvascular complications occur in both older and younger adults, the risk of heart disease is two to four times higher and the life expectancy is up to 15 years shorter in later life (CDC, 2014). Prolonged periods of hyperglycemia lead to glycosylation of proteins and the production of by-products, which, in turn, cause tissue damage. Functional declines are more likely unless proactive measures are taken to promote wellness (Box 24-7). Diabetes is associated with a high rate of depression, and those who are depressed have a higher mortality rate.

Too often a diagnosis is not made until evidence of end-organ damage becomes visible (Box 24-8). Worldwide, 50% of the persons with DM die of a stroke or heart disease (WHO, 2014). It is the leading cause of blindness, amputation, and kidney failure. The combined macrovascular and microvascular

TABLE 24-2	Diabetes by Race/Ethnicity
RACE/ETHNICITY	**PERCENTAGE OF DIAGNOSED DIABETES**
Non-Hispanic whites	7.6
Asian Americans	9.0
Chinese	4.4
Filipinos	11.3
Asian Indians	13.0
Other Asian Americans	8.8
Hispanics	12.8
Central and South Americans	8.5
Cubans	9.3
Mexican Americans	13.9
Puerto Ricans	14.8
Non-Hispanic blacks	13.2
American Indians/Alaskan Natives	15.9

From American Diabetes Association: *Statistics about diabetes,* June 2014. http://www.diabetes.org/diabetes-basics/statistics. Accessed October 20, 2014.

BOX 24-5   Complications of DM More Common in Older Adults

Dry eyes	Anorexia
Dry mouth	Dehydration
Confusion	Delirium
Incontinence	Nausea
Weight loss	Delayed wound healing

From Razzaque I, Morley JE, Nau KC, et al: Diabetes mellitus. In Ham RJ, Sloane PD, Warshaw GA, et al, editors: *Primary care geriatrics: a case-based approach,* ed 6, Philadelphia, 2014, Elsevier, pp 431–439.

BOX 24-4   Diabetes from Exposure to Toxins?

Veterans who were exposed to Agent Orange or other herbicides during their military service and who have developed diabetes are eligible to receive health care and disability compensation. Surviving spouses, children, and *parents* may be eligible for survivor benefits. For more information, see the following website below.

From U.S. Department of Veterans Affairs: *Public health,* 2013. Available at http://www.publichealth.va.gov/exposures/agentorange/conditions/diabetes.asp

BOX 24-6   Metabolic Syndrome (Insulin Resistance Syndrome)

A group of conditions common in persons with insulin resistance:
- Higher than normal glucose levels
- Increased waist size due to excess abdominal fat
- High blood pressure
- Abnormal levels of cholesterol and triglycerides in the blood

From National Diabetes Information Clearinghouse (NDIC): *Causes of diabetes,* 2014. http://diabetes.niddk.nih.gov/dm/pubs/causes/index.aspx Accessed August 2014.

BOX 24-7 Functional Disability Associated with Diabetes

Mobility impairment	Muscle weakness
Falls	Fatigue
Incontinence	Weight loss
Cognitive impairments	

From Razzaque I, Morley JE, Nau KC, et al: Diabetes mellitus. In Ham RJ, Sloane PD, Warshaw GA, et al, editors: *Primary care geriatrics: a case-based approach,* ed 6, Philadelphia, 2014, Elsevier, pp 431–439.

BOX 24-8 Signs of End-Organ Damage in DM

Decreased visual acuity	Heart disease
Paresthesia	Stroke
Neuropathy	Periodontal disease

From Razzaque I, Morley JE, Nau KC, et al: Diabetes mellitus. In Ham RJ, Sloane PD, Warshaw GA, et al, editors: *Primary care geriatrics: a case-based approach,* ed 6, Philadelphia, 2014, Elsevier, pp 431–439.

complications cause nerve damage ranging from peripheral neuropathy to gastroparesis and sexual dysfunction (American Diabetes Association [ADA], 2014). Impotence in men results from reduced vascular flow, peripheral neuropathy, and uncontrolled circulating blood glucose levels. Sexual dysfunction is two to five times greater in this group than in the general population.

Persons with DM commonly have problems with their lower extremities, which can have a considerable impact on functional status. Warning signs of foot problems include cold feet and intermittent claudication, neuropathic burning, tingling, hypersensitivity, and numbness of the extremities (Chapters 23). Infections are common and difficult to treat. Both the infections and the needed antibiotics often result in unstable glucose control.

Hypoglycemia (blood glucose level <60 mg/dL) can occur from many causes, such as unusually intense exercise, alcohol intake, or medication mismanagement (Rote and McCance, 2014). Signs in the older adult include tachycardia, palpitations, diaphoresis, tremors, pallor, and anxiety. Later symptoms may include headache, dizziness, fatigue, irritability, confusion, hunger, visual changes, seizures, and coma. Immediate care involves giving the patient glucose either orally or intravenously.

Hyperglycemia in older adults is harder to detect than that in a younger adult. With aging there is a higher tolerance for elevated levels of circulating glucose. It is not unusual to find persons with fasting glucose levels of 200 to 600 mg/dL or higher. This level of unrecognized hyperglycemia increases the risk for hyperosmolar hyperglycemic nonketotic coma. This is especially important in persons who are otherwise medically frail and should be considered in any older adult with diabetes who is difficult to arouse (ADA, 2013). This is always a medical emergency.

◆ PROMOTING HEALTHY AGING: IMPLICATIONS FOR GERONTOLOGICAL NURSING

The gerontological nurse has a major role in promoting healthy aging in people with diabetes. Ideally the nurse helps the person move toward all of the goals of *Healthy People 2020* (Box 24-9) and ensures that the standards of diabetic care are obtained (Box 24-10). The focus is on prevention, early identification, and delay of complications for as long as possible. Prevention includes identifying those persons at greatest risk (e.g., obese or with a positive family history), encouraging regular exercise, and maintaining excellent control of other chronic conditions.

Although glycemic control is important, more emphasis is now on the prevention and treatment of cardiovascular diseases (Box 24-11). Research has indicated that it may take 8 years of glycemic control before benefits are seen, while the benefits of better control of blood pressure and lipid levels are seen as early as 2 to 3 years. Promoting cardiovascular (CV) health has the potential to be the most efficacious in the minimization of complications in persons with DM (Razzaque et al, 2014). At all times, interventions must be considered in the context of the life expectancy and cost/benefit ratio for the individual.

Screening for DM by fasting plasma and random blood glucose testing is important for early identification of prediabetes or actual disease. Nurses participate in screenings at community health fairs and in clinical settings. Nurses also participate in community education about the need for early diagnosis, glycemic control, and prompt treatment of complications. Some nurses choose to develop particular expertise in working with those who have diabetes and become certified diabetes educators and clinicians.

Promoting healthy aging in the person with diabetes requires an array of interventions and an interdisciplinary team working together. This includes ancillary nursing staff and

♥ BOX 24-9 HEALTHY PEOPLE 2020

Goals

Reduce annual number of new cases.
Reduce death rate.
Reduce number of lower extremity amputations.
Improve glycemic control.
Improve lipid control.
Increase the proportion of persons with controlled hypertension.
Increase the number of persons with at least annual dental, foot, and dilated eye exams.
Increase the proportion of persons with at least biannual glycosylated hemoglobin measurement.
Increase the proportion of persons who obtain an annual micro-albumin measurement.
Perform self-monitoring blood glucose measurement at least twice a day.
Receive formal diabetes education.
Increase the number of persons who have been diagnosed.
Increase preventive measures in persons at high risk.

Data from U.S. Department of Health and Human Services, Office of Disease Prevention and Health Promotion: Healthy People 2020, 2012. http://www.healthypeople.gov/2020.

BOX 24-10 Evidence-Based Care: Minimum Standards of Care for the Person with Diabetes

At each visit:
- Monitor weight and BP.
- Inspect feet.
- Review self-monitoring glucose record.
- Review/adjust medications as needed.
- Review self-management skills/goals.
- Assess mood.
- Counsel on tobacco and alcohol use.

Quarterly visits:
- Obtain hemoglobin A_{1c} measurement for those whose medications have changed or who are unstable.

Annual visits:
- Obtain fasting lipid profile and serum creatinine level measurement.
- Obtain serum creatinine level to estimate glomerular filtration rate and stage level of kidney disease (Chapter 8).
- Refer for dilated eye exam (every 2 to 3 years).
- Perform comprehensive foot exam.
- Refer to dentist for annual comprehensive exam and cleaning.
- Administer influenza vaccination.

Once in lifetime:
- Administer pneumococcal vaccinations (consider (Pneumovax and Prevnar) repeat Pneumovax if longer than 5 to 10 years).

From National Diabetes Education Program: *Diabetes numbers at a glance,* 2012. http://ndep.nih.gov/publications/PublicationDetail. aspx?PubId=114 Pocket guide available. Accessed August 2014.

BOX 24-11 Minimizing Cardiovascular Risk in Persons with Diabetes

Eat a healthy diet (lower carbohydrate, lower sodium).
Get regular exercise.
Keep the BP <130/80 mm Hg for most people.
Stop smoking.
Maintain Hb A_{1c} <7% for most people.
Attain and maintain acceptable lipid levels:
- Cholesterol <200 mg/dL
- LDL <100 mg/dL
- HDL >40 mg/dL (men), >50 mg/dL (women)
- Triglycerides <150 mg/dL

From National Diabetes Education Program: *Diabetes numbers at a glance,* 2012. Available at http://ndep.nih.gov/publications/ PublicationDetail.aspx?PubId=114 Pocket guide available. Accessed August 2014.

licensed nurses, nutritionists, pharmacists, podiatrists, ophthalmologists, physicians, nurse practitioners, certified diabetes educators, and counselors working in collaboration with the patient and his or her family/significant others in culturally appropriate ways (Chapter 4). The nurse serves as team leader, educator, care provider, supporter, and guide. If the person's disease is hard to control, endocrinologists are involved, and as complications develop, more specialists are utilized, such as nephrologists, cardiologists, and wound care specialists. Nurses

are expected to advocate for older adults and encourage them to expect and receive quality care to prevent the devastating end results of poor management.

◆ Assessment

Health promotion for older adults with DM begins with a comprehensive geriatric assessment (Chapter 7). Assessment of painless neuropathy requires a careful neurological examination with an emphasis on sensation and history of functioning. Clinical guidelines suggest that the best means of testing neurological and sensory intactness is the use of the Semmes-Weinstein type monofilament (Feng et al, 2009) (Figure 24-1). The measurements of height, weight, and waist circumference may be used to calculate the body mass index (BMI) (Chapter 18); however, for the very old, BMI measurement is less useful because of the replacement of muscle mass with adipose tissue. Physical assessment includes a careful inspection of the feet, skin, and mouth for signs of injury or the presence of lesions.

Use of herbal products (Chapters 9 and 10) and nutritional supplements, over-the-counter and prescription drugs, and alcohol and tobacco are all components of the assessment of someone with diabetes (Box 24-12). All have a direct or indirect effect on renal, circulatory, neurological, and nutritional health.

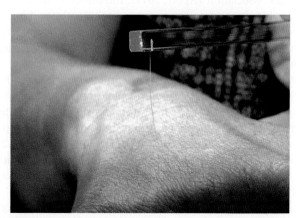

FIGURE 24-1 Semmes-Weinstein–type monofilament. (Courtesy AliMed, Dedham, Mass.)

BOX 24-12 Evidence-Based Practice: Herbs and Diabetes

One of the common herbs that is thought to help control diabetes is cinnamon. There is high-quality evidence that cinnamon has no health benefits related to diabetes or heart disease. In fact, use may worsen liver disease. Cinnamon decreases clotting time and must be used with utmost caution in persons taking blood thinners such as warfarin. Other herbal supplements that have been studied include aloe vera, bitter melon, Chinese herbal medicines, fenugreek, garlic, milk thistle, nettle, prickly pear cactus, and sweet potato. None have proven to be effective.

Available from National Complementary and Alternative Medicine at www.nih.nccam.gov search "diabetes." Accessed August 2014.

Due to the high association of depression, the assessment includes a screen for this at the time of diagnosis, at intervals thereafter, or at any time depression is suspected or reported by the patient (Chapter 7 & 28). There are depression assessment tools specific to later life available for use in persons with and without cognitive impairment (see Chapter 7).

The nurse uses the results of the assessment to work with the older adult and significant others to develop the plan of care related to both pharmacological and nonpharmacological approaches to everyday life. The regular assessment of mood and coping ensures that timely and effective interventions can be initiated.

◆ Management

The goals of health promotion for older adults with DM are often different than those of younger adults. Multiple factors confound decision-making about almost every aspect, including comorbid conditions, life expectancy, and ability to comply with the treatment plan. If the person is frail, management is difficult; and if there is not a consistent caregiver or one who has obtained the necessary diabetes education on behalf of, or with, the older adult, diabetes control will be impossible. The periodic measurement of a glycated hemoglobin test (Hb A_{1C}) is the best measure of ongoing glycemic control. While the Hb A_{1C} goal in younger persons is less than 6%, a consensus panel has recently recommended that the goal is dependent on the patient characteristics (Table 24-3) (Sinclair et al, 2012).

◆ Pharmacological Management

Care of the older adult with DM requires that the bedside or community nurse develop a knowledge base of the commonly used pharmacological interventions. These include the antiglycemics and preventive adjuvant therapy, such as angiotensin-converting enzyme (ACE) inhibitors and aspirin. All have been demonstrated to improve outcomes. The advanced practice nurse is expected to have expertise in the spectrum of pharmacological approaches to assist persons in the appropriate management of their disease and its complications.

Metformin (Glucophage) is commonly prescribed as first-line therapy; it does not cause hypoglycemia or weight gain. However, it is contraindicated in persons with renal insufficiency (serum creatinine $\geq$1.5 mg/dL in men and $\geq$1.4 mg/dL in women). It is necessary to ensure that the person's creatinine level is checked annually and if the person is more than 80 years of age with reduced muscle mass, the cystatin C level (Chapter 8) should be measured instead (Razzaque et al, 2014).

Sulfonylureas have been used for many years as first-line agents for all persons with DM type 2. They increase secretion of insulin from the pancreas and increase sensitivity in the periphery. However, they are associated with hypoglycemia and can only be used in persons who can either be aware of the signs themselves or have a caregiver capable of doing so. GLP-1 agonists (e.g., Byetta) are not appropriate due to the side effects of gastrointestinal upset and weight loss (Razzaque et al, 2014).

> ### ⚡ SAFETY ALERT
> **Do Not Use**
>
> The sulfonylureas Chlorpropamide (Diabinese) and glyburide are contraindicated due to their long half-lives and can cause prolonged hypoglycemia (American Geriatrics Society [AGS], 2012).

Insulin is used when all other strategies have failed to maintain the glycemic goals for that person. There are long-acting preparations (e.g., Lantus) now available, but they cannot be used until the required daily total dose is determined. This is done using shorter acting preparations until this is known. After that time the traditional "Sliding-scale" adjustments are not recommended (AGS, 2012). The use of insulin requires manual dexterity in the person or caregiver to ensure that glucose levels are monitored and doses are administered at the correct times. Preset syringes can be obtained and therefore could be used by someone with visual limitations; however, the cost of these is often prohibitive.

TABLE 24-3	Diabetes Treatment Goals in Consideration of Health Status					
PATIENT HEALTH	**POTENTIAL A$_{1C}$ (%) IN CONSIDERATION OF BURDEN AND RISK**	**FASTING GLUCOSE (MG/DL)**	**BEDTIME GLUCOSE (MG/DL)**	**BLOOD PRESSURE (MM HG)**	**USE OF STATIN**	**RATIONALE**
Healthy, few coexisting conditions	<7.5	90-130	90-130	<140/80	Unless contraindicated	Longer life expectancy
Complex/intermediate coexisting illnesses with ADL impairments or mild to moderate cognitive impairments	<8.0	90-150	90-150	<140/80	Unless contraindicated	Intermediate life expectancy with high treatment burden
Very complex, poor health, long-term care or end-stage, ADL impairments, moderate to severe cognitive impairment	<8.5	100-180	100-180	<150/90	Consider benefit	Limited life expectancy, uncertain benefit

From Kirkman MS, Briscoe VJ, Clark N, et al: Diabetes in older adults: a consensus report, *J Am Geriatr Soc* 60:2342–2356, 2012.

◆ Nonpharmacological Management

The cornerstones of nonpharmacological management of DM are nutrition, exercise, and self-management.

◆ *Nutrition.* Adequate and appropriate nutrition is a key factor in healthy living and aging with DM. An initial nutrition assessment with a 24-hour recall will provide some clues to the patient's dietary habits, intake, and style of eating (see Chapter 14). It is part of the nurse's responsibility to learn if access to appropriate food is possible, including necessary funds and a means of food preparation. The nurse works with the individual to identify culturally specific foods that can be translated into a "diabetic diet."

Helping people who have developed eating patterns over a lifetime is always challenging. If the older adult is from an ethnic group different from that of the nurse, the nurse will need to learn more about the usual ingredients and methods of food preparation to be able to give reasonable instructions related to adjustments for diets optimal for persons with DM. Meal planning with a diabetes specialist is a "covered service" under Medicare (Table 24-4) (Chapter 30) (Medicare, 2014). Healthy eating rather than weight loss is recommended since the latter has been shown to increase mortality among older persons with diabetes (Razzaque et al, 2014)

◆ *Exercise.* Exercise improves tissue sensitivity to insulin and promotes cardiac health. Walking is an inexpensive and beneficial way to exercise; however, it needs to be done in a safe location, which cannot be assumed to be in the person's neighborhood (Chapter 18). A more intensive exercise program, such as aerobics, should not be started until the health care provider has been consulted. Those who have limited mobility can still do chair exercises or, if possible, use exercise machines that enable sitting and holding onto something for support. In some cases exercise in conjunction with an appropriate diet may be sufficient to maintain blood glucose levels within normal range. If the person is using insulin, exercise needs to be done on a regular rather than an erratic basis, and blood glucose level must be checked before and after exercise to avoid, or respond promptly to, hypoglycemia.

◆ *Self-Care.* Due to the complexity of DM in late life, maximum wellness is difficult to achieve without considerable self-care skills. The nurse is often the professional who is responsible for working with the older adult in developing such skills (Box 24-13).

Self-management essentials for diabetes include knowing the signs of hypoglycemia and hyperglycemia, as well as actions to take if these complications arise. An identification bracelet is recommended because confusion or delirium may be a manifestation of low blood glucose level and misinterpreted as dementia, which delays treatment. Self-care also includes preventive care practices for the heart, eyes, kidneys, and feet. Nurses support patients in obtaining the needed services. Annual diabetes self-management training and a number of other diabetes-specific services are available through Medicare (Table 24-4). A large number of resources are available about diabetes through the National Diabetes

TABLE 24-4 Medicare Coverage for Supplies and Services for Those with Diabetes

SUPPLY/SERVICE	FREQUENCY	COST
Screening	Twice a year for those at risk	No cost
Self-management training	One-time teaching of decreasing risks or managing diabetes	20% of approved amount after deductible met
Equipment needed for home glucose monitoring	Some restrictions to amount of quarterly supplies	20% of Medicare-approved amount after annual deductible
Flu/pneumococcal immunizations	Annually: usually once in a lifetime	No cost
Foot exams and treatment	For those with peripheral neuropathy	20% of Medicare-approved amount after annual deductible
Glaucoma testing	Annually	20% of Medicare-approved amount after annual deductible
Insulin	As needed	Per prescription plan
Medical nutrition services	Initial assessment and follow-up as needed	No cost
Therapeutic shoes or inserts	For those with severe diabetic foot disease	20% of Medicare-approved amount after annual deductible

For more information and details, see Centers for Medicare and Medicaid Services (CMS): *Medicare's coverage of diabetes supplies and services,* 2013. http://www.medicare.gov/Pubs/pdf/11022.pdf

BOX 24-13 Self-Care Skills Needed for the Person with Diabetes

Glucose Self-Monitoring
Obtaining a blood sample correctly
Using the glucose monitoring equipment correctly
Troubleshooting when results indicate an error
Recording the values from the machine
Understanding the timing and frequency of self-monitoring
Understanding what to do with the results

Medication Self-Administration
Where Appropriate, Insulin Use
Selecting appropriate injection site
Using correct technique for injections
Disposing of used needles and syringes correctly
Storing and transporting insulin correctly

Oral Medication Use
Knowing drug, dose, timing, and side effects
Knowing drug-drug and drug-food interactions
Recognizing side effects and knowing when to report

Foot Care and Examination
Selecting and using appropriate and safe footwear

Handling Sick Days
Recognizing the signs and symptoms of both hyperglycemia and hypoglycemia

Information Clearing House (http://diabetes.niddk.nih.gov/dm/a-z.aspx?control=Pubs). This site provides links to a multitude of other sites, including those specific to ethnic and racial groups and in a variety of languages.

◆ Implications for the Frail Elder and Those Living in Residential Care Settings

Many of those who are frail also have DM. Due to their own limitations they are often dependent on others for various self-care activities. This may include meal preparation, assistance with exercise, or even help with physical movement of any kind. In a residential care setting such as a nursing home or assisted living facility, the nurse assesses the person for signs of hypoglycemia and hyperglycemia and evidence of complications. The nurse ensures that the standards of care for the person with DM are met. The nurse monitors the effect and side effects of diet, exercise, and medication use. The nurse administers or supervises the safe administration of medications.

In the home care setting the nurse works with the individual if he or she is capable, and if not, the nurse identifies the caregiver(s) who are providing the support and care for the person. In this case, the caregiver is the de facto nurse with the support of professionals in providers' offices or home health staff.

Thyroid Disease

There are slight changes in thyroid function with aging, but the evidence of their effect is contradictory. The incidence of disturbances, especially hypothyroidism, is seen with increasing frequency, especially in later life. While a number of the symptoms mirror those of other nonthyroid conditions, screening for thyroid disease is a component of the primary health care assessment of older adults, especially for persons with depression, anxiety, or evidence of cognitive or cardiovascular diseases. A thyroid screen is also often done when signs of atrial fibrillation are found, but their association is equivocal (Kim et al, 2014; Tänase et al, 2013). A fully functioning thyroid gland (or its replacement) is necessary to maintain life.

Thyroid diseases are diagnosed by the clinical presentation combined with laboratory findings and considerations of the subtleties of both the total and free T_3 (triiodothyronine) levels, the free T_4 (thyroxine) levels, and the concentration of TSH (thyroid-stimulating hormone). However, the accuracy of the laboratory findings is easily affected by laboratory errors, acute illness and frailty, concurrent environmental conditions, and drug intake, making an accurate diagnosis somewhat difficult (Table 24-5).

While the prevalence of hyperthyroidism in those older than 65 is about 2.7%, that of hypothyroidism is up to 20%, especially among older women. Many of those who are very ill and hospitalized may also have a transient elevation in TSH level. This may be in part due to the amount of iodine they are exposed to in the form of contrast products and the high use of amiodarone (Sehgal et al, 2014). If the illness resolves, many will return to a euthyroid state (Campbell, 2014).

Thyroid dysfunction, especially hypothyroidism, can have a significantly detrimental effect on the person's quality of life. If any signs or symptoms are noted, a thyroid panel should be done, which can guide the diagnosis and treatment plan in the context of other clinical findings. Diagnosis may be delayed or never made because many of the signs and symptoms are incorrectly attributed to normal aging, another disorder, a geriatric syndrome, or to side effects of medications.

Hypothyroidism

Hypothyroidism, insidious in onset, is thought to be most commonly caused by chronic autoimmune thyroiditis (previously called Hashimoto's disease). The TSH level is elevated (>10 units/mL) in definitive hypothyroidism as the pituitary gland tries to stimulate the underfunctioning thyroid (Campbell, 2014). It may be iatrogenic, resulting from radioiodine treatment, subtotal thyroidectomy, or a number of medications, especially amiodarone. It is important to always note that while there are a number of signs and symptoms of hypothyroidism, they are more subtle or vague in older adults and may be very different than those seen in younger adults (Box 24-14). The signs are often evaluated for other causes with consideration of possible hypothyroidism as a "rule out."

TABLE 24-5	Examples of Factors Affecting Laboratory Testing of Thyroid Functioning	
TEST	**INCREASED RESULT**	**DEPRESSED RESULT**
TSH	Potassium iodide and lithium, laboratory error, autoimmune disease, strenuous exercise, acute sleep deprivation	Severe illness, aspirin, dopamine, heparin, and steroids
T_3	Estrogen and methadone	Anabolic steroids, androgens, phenytoin, naproxen, propranolol, reserpine, and salicylates
T_4	Estrogen, methadone, and clofibrate	Anabolic steroids, androgens, lithium, phenytoin, and propranolol (see T_3)

TSH, Thyroid-stimulating hormone; T_3, triiodothyronine; T_4, thyroxine. From Chernecky CC, Berger BJ: *Laboratory tests and diagnostic procedures*, ed 6, St Louis, MO, 2013, Elsevier; Fitzgerald PA: Endocrine disorders. In Papadakis MA, McPhee SJ, editors: *Current medical diagnosis and treatment 2013*, New York, 2013, McGraw-Hill, pp 1093–1191.

BOX 24-14 Symptoms of Hypothyroidism

Probably Less Common in Older Adults
- Fatigue
- Weakness
- Depression
- Dry skin

Significantly Less Common
- Weight gain
- Cold intolerance
- Muscle cramps

From Campbell JW: Thyroid disorders. In Ham RJ, Sloane PD, Warshaw GA, et al, editors: *Primary care geriatrics: a case-based approach*, ed 6, Philadelphia, 2014, Elsevier, p 442.

Subclinical hypothyroidism. Subclinical hypothyroidism is defined as a normal serum T_4 level and a somewhat elevated TSH level (5 to 10 units/mL). At this time there is controversy regarding the treatment of subclinical hypothyroidism in older adults. Only a small percentage of persons have been found to convert to true hypothyroidism. Treatment is not innocuous, including a decrease in bone mass from prolonged thyroid replacement therapy (use of levothyroxine), particularly problematic for women who already have a high incidence of osteoporosis (Chapter 26). There is also some evidence that not treating subclinical hypothyroidism will actually decrease associated mortality (Campbell, 2014).

Hyperthyroidism

The prevalence of hyperthyroidism in older adults is low (0.5% to 4%) (Campbell, 2014). It is most often caused by the autoimmune disorder Graves' disease with multinodular or uninodular goiter. It can also result from ingestion of iodine or iodine-containing substances, such as seafood, exposure to contrast agents, and the use of certain medications, especially amiodarone. The onset of hyperthyroidism may be quite abrupt.

The manifestations of hyperthyroidism are often atypical, and it may not be diagnosed until the person has unexplained atrial fibrillation, heart failure, or even dementia. The presence of any of the geriatric syndromes such as constipation, anorexia, or muscle weakness and other vague complaints may also be noted. However, on further examination the causative factor in any of these complaints may be hyperthyroidism. On examination, the person is likely to have tachycardia, tremors, and weight loss. However, in later life, a condition known as apathetic thyrotoxicosis, rarely seen in younger persons, may occur in which usual hyperkinetic activity is replaced with slowed movement and depressed affect.

Complications

Complications occur both as the result of treatment and as a result of delayed diagnosis; therefore, failure to treat thyroid disorders in a timely manner can be detrimental to the person's health. Myxedema coma is a serious complication of untreated hypothyroidism in the older patient. Rapid replacement of the missing thyroxine is not possible due to risk of drug toxicity. Even with the best treatment, death may ensue. Because thyroid replacement is necessary to maintain life, the person has to learn to minimize the side effects, especially increased bone loss

(Chapter 26). Over-replacement with thyroxine increases myocardial oxygen consumption. It may result in exacerbation of angina in persons with preexisting coronary artery disease or precipitate congestive heart failure.

◆ PROMOTING HEALTHY AGING: IMPLICATIONS FOR GERONTOLOGICAL NURSING

As advocates, nurses can ensure that a thyroid screening test be done anytime there is a possibility of concern. The nurse caring for frail older adults can be attentive to the possibility that the person who is diagnosed with anxiety, dementia, or depression may instead have a thyroid disturbance. All persons suspected as having a depressive disorder must be checked for hypothyroidism (Demartini et al, 2013).

Although the nurse may understand that little can be done to prevent thyroid disturbances in late life, organizations such as the Monterey Bay Aquarium have launched campaigns to inform consumers of the iodine and mercury levels found in seafood (www.seafoodwatch.org) because of their association with thyroid disease.

The nurse may be instrumental in working with the person and family to understand both the seriousness of the problem and the need for very careful adherence to the prescribed regimen. If the elder is hospitalized for acute management, the life-threatening nature of both the disorder and the treatment can be made clear so that advanced planning can be done that will account for all possible outcomes.

The management of hypothyroidism is one of careful pharmacological replacement and, in the case of hyperthyroidism, one of surgical or chemical ablation followed by replacement—both with the medication thyroxine. The nurse works with the person and significant others in the correct self-administration of medications and in the appropriate timing of monitoring blood levels and signs or symptoms indicating an exacerbation (Box 24-15).

BOX 24-15   TIPS FOR BEST PRACTICE

Specific Instructions for Administration

Levothyroxine should always be taken early in the morning, on an empty stomach, and at least 30 minutes before a meal. It should be taken with a full glass of water to ensure it does not begin to dissolve in the esophagus. It cannot be taken within 4 hours of anything containing a mineral, such as calcium (including fortified orange juice), antacids or iron supplements. It is always dosed in micrograms, and care must be taken that it is not confused with milligrams; 12.5 to 25 mcg/day (or 0.125 to 0.25 mg/day) is the most common dose used in those older than age 50.

From Lexi-Comp: *PharMerica specialized long-term care nursing drug handbook*, Hudson, OH, 2013, Lexicomp.

KEY CONCEPTS

- Although there are relatively few age-related changes in the immune system, the decreased ability to mount a defense against antigens increases the risk for infections.
- With aging, there is an increase in autoimmunity leading to an increase in autoimmune disorders.
- The majority of diabetes cases seen worldwide among older adults is type 2.
- The prevalence of diabetes increases with age.
- While the incidence of hyperthyroidism in late life is rare, but hypothyroidism is seen with increasing frequency, especially among older women.

- There is a high association between thyroid disease and heart disease. A person with either should be screened on a regular basis.
- Undiagnosed or inadequately treated and monitored thyroid disorders have a significant effect on the person's quality of life.
- The nurse can play active roles in the early detection of autoimmune disorders and infections.
- The nurse facilitates the person's receipt of the standards of care based on evidence-based practice and the utilization of benefits available to the person to help control and treat the disease.

NURSING STUDY: "THERE IS NOTHING WRONG WITH ME, I AM JUST A LITTLE TIRED!"

Ms. P., an 82-year-old single woman, lives in a life-care community in her own apartment but has the reassurance of knowing her medical and functional needs will be taken care of, regardless of the extent of these needs. This is the primary reason she chose to sell her home and move. She is at present independent. She has been gaining weight steadily since she moved into the community and attributes that to the fact that she eats much better now that she joins others in the congregate dining room for meals. She has diabetes, which she manages with diet, exercise, and oral medications; heart failure; and mild arthritis. Although she says she feels fine, lately she has noticed some increased fatigue and that her toes are cold and somewhat numb. The great toe on her left foot seems to be discolored. Because of the lack of feeling, she often walks around her apartment barefoot because it seems to increase the sensation in her feet. She has not needed to use the health care center and goes to the clinic only to pick up her medication. Her niece stopped by last week to see her and called the clinic and spoke with the nurse. The niece reported that her aunt seemed a little confused and lethargic. The niece accompanied Ms. P. to the clinic, where the nurses checked her blood pressure and blood sugar and found them to be 170/80 mm Hg and 280 mg/dL, respectively. Ms. P. said, "Oh, I don't think it is anything to worry about! I am just a little tired."

- Of all of the symptoms that Ms. P. reports, which one should the nurse be most concerned about related to Ms. P.'s long-term health?
- Of all of the symptoms that Ms. P. reports, which one should the nurse be most concerned about related to Ms. P.'s ability to live alone?

CRITICAL THINKING QUESTIONS AND ACTIVITIES

1. What commonly held beliefs about aging would lead a person to believe that the changes in her health did not warrant seeking health care?
2. You are assigned to teach a patient the basics of diabetes care. You have one day to do this before the person is discharged home. When you walk in the room and begin talking with the person you find out that she is from a culture completely different from yours. How will you begin?
3. Expanding on the question above, discuss with a classmate how you would approach the same situation when you find out that your patient is responsible for cooking for the whole family

RESEARCH QUESTIONS

1. Is there any information that explains the differences in the incidence and prevalence of diabetes in various ethnic groups?
2. What types of nutritional food supplements are used by persons with diabetes?
3. Consult the latest research to determine any more current information and the implications of such, related to the increased number of circulating autoantibodies over time (page 310).

REFERENCES

American Diabetes Association (ADA): *Hyperosmolar hyperglycemic nonketotic syndrome (HHNS)*. 2013. http://www.diabetes.org/living-with-diabetes/complications/hyperosmolar-hyperglycemic.html. Accessed July 2014.

American Diabetes Association (ADA): *Complications.* 2014. http://www.diabetes.org/living-with-diabetes/complications. Accessed July 2014.

American Geriatrics Society (AGS) Expert Panel: American Geriatrics Society updated Beers Criteria for potentially inappropriate medication use in older adults, *J Am Geriatr Soc* 60:616–631, 2012.

Campbell JW: Thyroid disorders. In Ham RJ, Sloane PD, Warshaw GA, et al, editors: *Primary care geriatrics: a case-based approach*, ed 6, Philadelphia, Elsevier, 2014, pp 440–444.

Centers for Disease Control (CDC): *Diabetes home: resources center*. 2014. http://www.cdc.gov/diabetes/library/index.html. Accessed September 2014.

Demartini B, Ranieri R, Masu A, et al: Depressive symptoms and major depressive disorder in patients affected by subclinical hypothyroidism: a cross-sectional study, *J Nerv Ment Dis* 202(8):603–607, 2013.

Feng Y, Schlösser FJ, Sumpio BE: The Semmes Weinstein monofilament examination as a screening tool for diabetic peripheral neuropathy, *J Vasc Surg* 50:675–682, 2009.

Kim EJ, Lyass A, Wang N, et al: Relation of hypothyroidism and incident atrial fibrillation (from the Framingham Study), *Am Heart J* 167(1):123–126, 2014.

Medicare: *Your Medicare coverage: diabetes screenings.* http://www.medicare.gov/coverage/diabetes-screenings.html. Accessed October 31, 2014.

National Diabetes Information Clearinghouse (NDIC): *Causes of diabetes* (NIH publication no. 14-5164). 2014. http://diabetes.niddk.nih.gov/dm/pubs/causes/index.aspx. Accessed July 2014.

National Institute of Diabetes and Digestive and Kidney Diseases (NIDDK): *The Pima Indians: pathfinders for health.* 2002. http://diabetes.niddk.nih.gov/dm/pubs/pima/index.htm. Accessed July 2014.

Razzaque I, Morley JE, Nau, KC, et al: Diabetes mellitus. In Ham RJ, Sloane PD, Warshaw GA, et al, editors: *Primary care geriatrics: a case-based approach*, ed 6, Philadelphia, 2014, Elsevier, pp 431–439.

Rote NS: Adaptive immunity. In McCance KL, Huether SE, editors: *Pathophysiology: the biological basis for disease in adults and children*, ed 7, St. Louis, MO, 2014, Elsevier, pp 224–261.

Rote NS, McCance KL: Alterations in immunity and inflammation. In McCance KL, Huether SE, editors: *Pathophysiology: the biological basis for disease in adults and children*, ed 7, St. Louis, MO, 2014, Elsevier, pp 262–297.

Sehgal V, Sukhminder JSB, Sehgal R, et al: Clinical conundrums in management of hypothyroidism in critically ill geriatric patients, *Int J Endocrinol Metab* 12(1):13759, Jan 2014.

Sinclair A, Morley JE: Rodriguez-Mañas L, et al: Diabetes mellitus in older people: position statement on behalf of the International Associations of Gerontology and Geriatrics (IAGG), the European Diabetes Working Party for older people (EDWPOP), and the International Task Force on Experts in Diabetes, *J Am Med Dir Assoc* 13:497–502, 2012.

Tänase DM, Ionescu SD, Ouatu A, et al: Risk assessment in the development of atrial fibrillation at patients with associate thyroid dysfunctions, *Rev Med Chir Soc Med Nat Iasi* 117(3):623–629, 2013.

U.S. Department of Health and Human Services, Office of Disease Prevention and Health Promotion: *Diabetes, HealthyPeople 2020.* 2012. http://www.healthypeople.gov/2020/topicsobjectives2020/overview.aspx?topicid=8. Accessed July 2014

U.S. Preventive Services Task Force (USSPTF): *Screening for type 2 diabetes in adults.* 2008. http://www.uspreventiveservicestaskforce.org/uspstf08/type2/type2rs.htm.

World Health Organization (WHO): *Diabetes programme.* 2014. http://www.who.int/diabetes/en. Accessed July 2014.

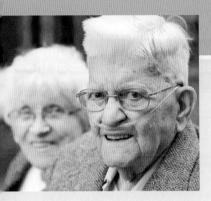

CHAPTER 25

Respiratory Health and Illness

Kathleen Jett

http://evolve.elsevier.com/Touhy/TwdHlthAging

AN ELDER SPEAKS

I have smoked since I was 12 or 13. I started coughing a little now and then when I was in my 40's. Now that I am in my 50's, I am having more and more trouble breathing when I walk too fast. They say it is something called COPD. I don't quite understand that and what it has to do with my cigarettes. I certainly could not give them up after all of these years!

Helen, age 56

A STUDENT SPEAKS

Sometimes I have to take care of someone who smokes. When they return from the smoking area the smell is so strong I can hardly stand getting close to them. But I am a nurse and that comes first, but it is so hard!

La'Shawn, age 18

LEARNING OBJECTIVES

On the completion of this chapter the reader will be able to:

1. Describe the normal changes with aging that affect the respiratory system and discuss how these affect the goal of achieving healthy aging.
2. Identify the most important factors influencing respiratory health.
3. Develop strategies to promote respiratory health.

The respiratory system is the vehicle for gas exchange, especially the transfer of oxygen into and the release of carbon dioxide out of the blood (Box 25-1). Respiration depends on cardiac health, musculoskeletal structures, and the nervous system for full function. Although there are a number of age-related changes, they are insignificant when one is free of respiratory disorders, cardiovascular illnesses, or musculoskeletal deformities of the chest. If skeletal defects such as kyphoscoliosis or arthritic costovertebral joints occur in the presence of normal age-related changes, the chest cavity can be significantly reduced. Specific age-related changes include loss of elastic recoil, stiffening of the chest wall, and increased resistance to airflow. Total lung capacity is not altered, but instead redistributed. Residual capacity increases with the diminished inspiratory and expiratory muscle strength of the thorax (Figure 25-1). The auscultation of slight bibasilar atelectasis is common due to incomplete lung expansion. Age-related changes lead to more effort required for movement of the diaphragm. Like all other systems, there is a reduced capacity to respond to sudden changes, and when confronted with a sudden demand for increased oxygen or exposed to noxious or infectious agents, a respiratory deficit may become evident and can quickly become life-threatening (Table 25-1).

NORMAL AGE-RELATED CHANGES

Among the most significant age-related changes is lowered efficiency of gas exchange and reduced ability to handle secretions. The cilia, which normally act as brushes to repel foreign substances or propel mucus out of the trachea, become less responsive and less effective. Compounded by age-related diminished cough reflex and immune response, there is a high risk for infections such as bronchitis and pneumonia. When impairments such as dysarthria, dysphagia, or decreased esophageal motility are superimposed, the risk for infection such as aspiration pneumonia increases even further. Overall, the changes are especially dangerous for those who have limited mobility, who have muscular changes to the oropharyngeal muscles due to injury such as stroke or chronic disease such as Parkinson's disease, or those who already have chronic respiratory disorders.

Gas Exchange and Aging

The effectiveness of gas exchange is measured by blood gas analysis and reported as pH, P_{CO_2}, and P_{O_2}. Whereas the pH and P_{CO_2} do not change with aging, P_{O_2} declines. The maximal P_{O_2} possible at sea level can be estimated by multiplying the person's age by 0.3 and subtracting the product from 100. For example, the maximal P_{O_2} of a 60-year-old is 82 as calculated $(100 - [60 \times 0.3])$, compared with 73 in a 90-year-old $(100 - [90 \times 0.3])$.

Data from Brashers VL: Alterations of pulmonary function. In McCance KL, Huether SE, editors: *Pathophysiology: the biological basis for disease in adults and children*, ed 7, St Louis, 2014, Mosby, pp 1225–1247.

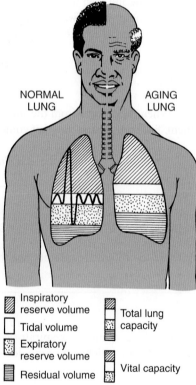

Inspiratory reserve volume

Tidal volume

Expiratory reserve volume

Residual volume

Total lung capacity

Vital capacity

FIGURE 25-1 Changes in Lung Volume with Aging. (From McCance KL, Huether SE: *Pathophysiology: the biologic basis for disease in adults and children*, ed 7, St Louis, MO, 2014, Mosby.)

RESPIRATORY DISORDERS

Normal age-related changes increase the risk for respiratory problems, and when they occur, the mortality rate is higher in older adults than in younger adults. Diseases of the respiratory system can be classified as acute or chronic, obstructive or restrictive. Obstructive disease prevents airflow out of the lungs as a result of obstruction or narrowing of the respiratory structures. In restrictive disease there is a decrease in total lung capacity as a result of limited expansion of the chest wall or the bronchial tubes, which prevents air from leaving the lungs without effort.

TABLE 25-1 Normal Changes with Aging and Potentially Serious Consequences at the Time of Illness

CHANGE	POTENTIAL CONSEQUENCE
Ossification of the costal cartilage, less compliant rib cage	Potential for less expansion such as when exercising or when increased respirations are needed
Loss of elastin attachment in the alveolar walls	Collapse of the small airways and uneven alveolar ventilation, trapping air and increasing dead space, decreasing vital capacity, and decreasing expiratory flow
Chemoreceptor function is altered or blunted at the peripheral and central chemoreceptor sites	Compensatory responses to hypercapnia and hypoxia are decreased while perception of dyspnea is intact or even enhanced. This response is independent of mechanical lung changes and is attributed to alterations in the neuromuscular drive to breathe. Compensatory responses may be significantly hindered in situations of stress

Data from U.S. Department of Health and Human Services, Office of Disease Prevention and Health Promotion: Healthy People 2020, 2012. http://www.healthypeople.gov/2020.

Chronic Obstructive Pulmonary Disease

Chronic obstructive pulmonary disease (COPD) is characterized by persistent and irreversible obstruction of airflow either into or out of the lungs. COPD includes emphysema and chronic bronchitis. Emphysema is an advanced state of COPD in which there is damage to the terminal bronchiole and is associated with destruction of the alveolar wall (Brashers and Huether, 2014).

Each year 3.1 million people worldwide die from COPD, the third most common cause of death behind ischemic heart disease and stroke (WHO, 2014). In 2011 approximately 15 million adults were estimated to have COPD in the United States, with significant age and geographic variability (Kravchenko et al, 2014). Approximately 50% of those with low pulmonary function are not aware they have COPD (CDC, 2013). Although chronic bronchitis affects persons at any age, it is most common in those older than 65 years of age. Continuing to smoke and physical inactivity are the primary factors attributed to activity limitations for persons with COPD (Garcia-Aymerich et al, 2009).

COPD is the one noninfectious chronic disease that is increasing in prevalence despite the efforts to combat it. The increase is attributed to the rise in the number of women who are affected. Since 2000, the number of women diagnosed with COPD increased fourfold, to more than 7 million. They are more often hospitalized and *die* from the disease (American Lung Association [ALA], 2014).

Spirometry is the gold standard for diagnosis. As a standardized and reproducible test, the results can objectively confirm the presence of airflow obstruction (Chesnutt et al, 2013). Measurement of the diffusing capacity for carbon monoxide may help differentiate emphysema from chronic bronchitis. Chronic or recurrent bronchitis is diagnosed clinically by a productive cough for 3 months in 2 consecutive years or 6 months in 1 year (Amin and Smith, 2014).

Etiology

The airway obstruction of COPD is caused from inhalation of toxins and pollutants earlier in life, such as dust, chemicals, and especially tobacco smoke, either directly or indirectly from secondhand smoke (Box 25-2). Tobacco use or exposure accounts for 80% to 90% of all cases of COPD (Amin and Smith, 2014). This exposure causes airway and lung destruction. Additional factors influence the likelihood that someone with such exposure will develop COPD (Box 25-3). In rare cases it appears that the development of COPD is related to a deficiency of α_1-antitrypsin, but this is still under investigation. One of the complexities of this science is the frequent comorbid condition of lung cancer (Tang et al, 2014).

Chronic or recurrent bronchitis is caused by irritation of the lungs and characterized by ongoing or intermittent symptoms. The airflow obstruction in chronic bronchitis is caused by a combination of thickening and inflammation of bronchial walls, hypertrophy of mucous glands, constriction of smooth muscle, and production of excess mucus, all of which cause lumen compromise stimulated by exposure to toxins, including both viruses and bacteria (Figure 25-2) (Amin and Smith, 2014; Chesnutt et al, 2013).

Signs and Symptoms

COPD has a long asymptomatic stage; symptoms may not appear until 50% of lung function has been irretrievably lost (Stoller, 2002). The most common symptoms of COPD are wheezing, cough, dyspnea on exertion, and increased phlegm production (Amin and Smith, 2014). Later signs include prolonged expiration with pursed-lip breathing, barrel chest, air

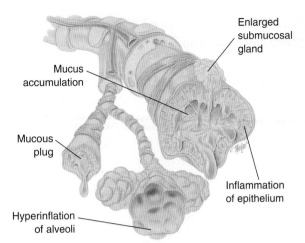

FIGURE 25-2 Chronic Bronchitis. Inflammation and thickening of mucous membrane with accumulation of mucus and pus leading to obstruction characterized by productive cough. (From McCance KL, Huether SE: *Pathophysiology: the biologic basis for disease in adults and children,* ed 7, St Louis, MO, 2014, Mosby. Modified from Des Jardins T, Burton GG: *Clinical manifestations and assessment of respiratory disease,* ed 3, St Louis, MO, 1995, Mosby.)

trapping, hyper-resonant on percussion, pale lips or nail beds, fingernail clubbing, and use of accessory muscles for breathing.

Cough is the primary symptom, affecting the majority of smokers. Unfortunately, the cough is often dismissed as insignificant because early in the disease there is no measurable airflow obstruction. In advanced disease, cyanosis, evidence of right-sided heart failure, and peripheral edema are present. In older adults, a high level of fatigue is found, and this in turn significantly decreases functional status (Stridsman et al, 2013).

Complications

COPD is a progressively debilitating condition characterized by exacerbations and remissions in symptoms. Exacerbations are worsening of the baseline signs, symptoms, and function; they may be insidious or acute and are characterized by significant worsening of dyspnea and increasing volume and changes in sputum color (Amin and Smith, 2014). Spirometry results of less than 150 mL, worsening orthopnea, paroxysmal nocturnal dyspnea, and respirations greater than 30 per minute signal an emergent exacerbation. These have numerous inciting factors, including viral or bacterial infections, air pollution or other environmental exposures, and changes in the weather. Exacerbations must be differentiated from congestive heart failure, arrhythmias, a pulmonary embolism, cor pulmonale pneumonia, or a pneumothorax so that the appropriate response can be initiated.

Exacerbations frequently precipitate the need for changes in medications, hospitalization, or respiratory support (Box 25-4). Pneumonia is a frequent and serious complication. Invasive endotracheal intubation may be needed for patients with respiratory acidosis that progresses despite therapy or for those with impaired consciousness. In the older adult, sudden altered mental status may indicate acute hypoxemia or hypercapnia.

BOX 25-2 Chronic Respiratory Problems and the Environment

Chronic respiratory problems are common but are almost always attributed to exposure to environmental toxins earlier in life (especially cigarette smoke) rather than the aging process itself.

BOX 25-3 Those Most Likely to Have COPD

Persons 65 to 75 years of age
Non-Hispanic whites
Women
Those who are unemployed, retired, or do not work
Less than a high school education
Lower incomes
Current or former smokers
History of asthma

Adapted from CDC: *What is COPD?* 2013. http://www.cdc.gov/copd/

BOX 25-4   HEALTHY PEOPLE 2020
COPD Hospitalizations

Goal
Reduce hospitalizations for chronic obstructive pulmonary disease (COPD)

Baseline
56.0 hospitalizations for COPD per 10,000 adults aged 45 years and older occurred in 2007 (age adjusted to the year 2000 standard population)

Target
50.1 hospitalizations per 10,000 by 2020

Data from U.S. Department of Health and Human Services, Office of Disease Prevention and Health Promotion: *Healthy People 2020,* 2012. http://www.healthypeople.gov/2020

 BOX 25-5   HEALTHY PEOPLE 2020
COPD Deaths

Goal
Reduce deaths from chronic obstructive pulmonary disease (COPD) among adults

Baseline
113.9 COPD deaths per 100,000 adults aged 45 years and older occurred in 2007 (age adjusted to the year 2000 standard population)

Target
102.6 deaths per 100,000 by 2020

Data from U.S. Department of Health and Human Services, Office of Disease Prevention and Health Promotion: *Healthy People 2020,* 2012. http://www.healthypeople.gov/2020

Although the acute phase (Chapter 21) of an exacerbation is usually resolved in 10 days to 2 weeks, lung function may take 4 to 6 weeks to return to baseline, if ever. In the advanced stages the prognosis is very poor (Box 25-5).

Asthma

Asthma is an inflammatory airway disease that is closely linked to allergic mechanisms and viral or bacterial infections. It may be chronic or intermittent following exposure to triggers. Asthma is characterized by variable and reoccurring airway hyper-responsiveness, bronchoconstriction, and inflammation (Rance and O'Laughlen, 2014). Asthma affects millions of people in the United States. While adults older than 65 make up a small percentage of those with asthma, they have the highest associated death rate than any other group. Although older men have asthma significantly more often than women, women die from the disease more often than men (Hanania et al, 2011).

Asthma is both underdiagnosed and undertreated in older adults. Instead, the symptoms are attributed to normal changes with aging or cardiovascular disease, or are simply labeled "COPD." The person with asthma may have developed a tolerance to the bronchorestriction and minimizes the reports of symptoms, despite the potentially significant respiratory compromise actually present.

There is still a significant gap in knowledge in this area, complicated by the number of comorbid conditions and socioeconomic factors involved in its presentation and treatment (Box 25-6). It is recognized that there are at least two asthma phenotypes in later life: long-standing and late onset. Those who have had asthma for many years have more severe airflow obstruction with less reversibility than those with late-onset asthma.

Asthma and its treatment are staged from mild to severe based on the frequency of symptoms—from dyspnea only with activity to dyspnea at rest. Clinically significant asthma is present when the FEV-1 increases by 12% or 200 mL in the first second after the administration of a bronchodilator such as albuterol (Amin and Smith, 2014; Rance and O'Laughlen, 2014). Reducing the number of older adults with asthma and decreasing the number of related hospitalizations and deaths are part of the U.S. plan to improve health by 2020 (Boxes 25-7 and 25-8) (U.S. Department of Health and Human Services [USDHHS], 2014).

Etiology

The development of asthma is influenced by genetics, environment, and lifestyle. A positive family history and atopy are positive predictors, that is, a genetic predisposition to develop symptoms of allergies.

After a susceptible person is exposed to an antigen, a cascade of reactions occurs with immediate, late, and recurrent effects.

BOX 25-6   **Those at Increased Risk for Asthma**

Children
Those older than age 65
Women (among adults) and boys (among children)
Multiracial and African Americans
Puerto Ricans
People living in the Northeast United States
People living below the U.S. federal poverty level
Employees with certain exposures in the workplace

Adapted from USDHHS: Respiratory diseases. *HealthyPeople 2020,* 2014. http://www.healthypeople.gov/2020/topicsobjectives2020/overview.aspx?topicid=36

 BOX 25-7   HEALTHY PEOPLE 2020
Asthma Hospitalizations

Goal
Reduce hospitalizations for asthma among adults aged 65 years and older

Baseline
25.3 hospitalizations for asthma per 10,000 adults aged 65 years and older occurred in 2007 (age adjusted to the year 2000 standard population)

Target
20.3 hospitalizations per 10,000 by 2020

Data from U.S. Department of Health and Human Services, Office of Disease Prevention and Health Promotion: *Healthy People 2020,* 2012. http://www.healthypeople.gov/2020

Asthma Deaths

Goal
Reduce asthma deaths among adults aged 65 years and older

Baseline
43.4 asthma deaths per million adults aged 65 years and older occurred in 2007

Target
21.5 deaths per million by 2020

Data from U.S. Department of Health and Human Services, Office of Disease Prevention and Health Promotion: *Healthy People 2020*, 2012. http://www.healthypeople.gov/2020

These reactions not only have effects on airway smooth muscle and mucous secretion but also recruit the participation of monocytes, lymphocytes, neutrophils, and eosinophils into the cells lining the airways. Repeated exposure potentiates the person's inflammatory response or desensitizes the person to the antigens to which he or she has become susceptible (Box 25-9) (Rance and O'Laughlen, 2014).

Signs and Symptoms

Although the signs and symptoms may be less obvious in older adults, they are the same as they are in younger adults. The classic presentation is one of recurrent episodes of wheezing, dyspnea on exertion, shortness of breath, nonproductive cough, and chest tightness. The wheezing is characteristically limited to expiratory respirations and may increase in intensity during the night, interrupting sleep or causing paroxysmal nocturnal dyspnea. The cough may sound identical to that caused by nonsteroidal antiinflammatories, angiotensin-converting enzyme (ACE) inhibitors, or beta-blockers (Rance and McLaughlen, 2014).

Asthmatic symptoms are usually worse at night or in the early morning hours but may begin any time following exposure. The frequency of symptoms provides a reliable measure of a person's need for, and response to, therapy. Day-to-day variations of respiratory function in persons with asthma are often measured by home peak (expiratory) flow meters (PFMs) as long as the person can manipulate the devices; the tolerance of symptoms varies greatly from one person to another. For those with mild to moderate disease, there are often periods of asymptomatic remission.

Complications

Asthma can interfere with the quality of one's life, and acute or severe exacerbations may require repeated hospitalizations. Those older than 65 have the highest asthma-related death rate of all age groups. When asthma is long-standing, untreated, or undertreated, structural changes to the airway occur (remodeling), such as thickening of the airway wall and peribronchial fibrosis. Those with obstructive sleep apnea (OSA) are more at risk for asthma and, in turn, those with asthma are more at risk for OSA (Rance and McLaughlen, 2014). When a person has asthma, he or she is at significantly higher risk for lower respiratory tract infections, including pneumonia, and prolonged associated debility than those without asthma.

◆ PROMOTING HEALTHY AGING: IMPLICATIONS FOR GERONTOLOGICAL NURSING

As with most chronic conditions, a team approach is needed to maximize the quality of life and functional capacity for persons with respiratory disorders. The core team may include the nurse, a pulmonologist, a respiratory therapist, and a pharmacist. It may also include an occupational therapist to help the person adapt to declines in functional capacity as appropriate or to learn how to slowly increase exercise capacity if the person has become unnecessarily debilitated. Management of respiratory disorders in older adults is often complicated by the presence of other chronic disorders and side effects from the medications themselves. Caring for persons with respiratory disorders requires complex nursing skills (Box 25-10). For chronically ill patients who exhibit frequent exacerbations or significantly deteriorated health, carefully planned advance care directives are recommended. This planning should include discussion of how long rehospitalizations should be continued and the conditions under which intubation is desired, especially for the patient with end-stage COPD.

The goals of health promotion for the person with COPD include optimizing pulmonary function, controlling cough, maximizing functional status, preventing exacerbations (especially through exposure to viruses), promptly recognizing exacerbations, and knowing when to seek care. Each of these goals may be more difficult to attain for older adults in light of other concurrent conditions, especially cardiovascular disorders, which frequent accompany COPD. For those who are very frail or cognitively impaired, the promotion of respiratory health is the responsibility of the nurse and other caregivers.

In chronic bronchitis the routine use of antibiotics is controversial because the causal role of bacterial infection is often difficult to document. Antibiotics are generally indicated in frail elders when *the possibility* of pneumonia or an acute exacerbation of bronchitis is suspected. The classic symptoms of new

BOX 25-9 Triggers for Onset of Asthmatic Episode

Tobacco smoke
Dust mites
Outdoor air pollution
Cockroach allergen
Pets
Mold
Smoke from burning grass or wood
Upper respiratory tract infections
Strong odors
Cold air

Adapted from Centers for Disease Control and Prevention: *Basic information: what is asthma?* 2009. http://www.cdc.gov/asthma/faqs.htm

BOX 25-10   TIPS FOR BEST PRACTICE

Caring for the Person with COPD

Emotional Support
Accept/encourage expression of emotions.
Be an active listener.
Be cognizant of conversational dyspnea; do not interrupt or cut off conversations.

Education
Teach breathing techniques:
- Pursed-lip breathing
- Diaphragmatic breathing
- Cascade coughing (series)

Teach postural drainage.
Teach about medications: what, why, frequency, amount, side effects, and what to do if side effects occur.
Teach use and care of inhalers and spacers and equipment.
Teach signs and symptoms of respiratory tract infection.
Teach about sexual activity:
- Sexual function improves with rest.
- Schedule sex around best breathing time of day.
- Use prescribed bronchodilators 20 to 30 minutes before sex.
- Use positions that do not require pressure on the chest or support of the arms.

COPD, Chronic obstructive pulmonary disease.

pulmonary infiltrates on chest x-ray and fever may not be initially detected. However, purulent sputum, a sudden increase in the volume of the expectorant, or dyspnea can suddenly become a life-threatening condition in an older adult. At the same time the normal age-related decreased immune response may delay the presentation of classic symptoms, especially a fever. Although the use of pharmacological interventions in the day-to-day life of the person with COPD may increase comfort and functional status, they do not affect mortality (Chesnutt, 2013). However, the use of long-term oxygen therapy in hypoxemic patients has been shown to improve survival, and smoking cessation at any age slows the rate of decline in lung capacity.

In 2007, through collaboration among the National Heart, Lung and Blood Institute; the National Asthma Education and Prevention Program; the Global Initiative for Asthma; and the World Health Organization, the 2003 asthma guidelines were updated (NHLBI, 2007). These offer evidence-based practice guides for the diagnosis and management of asthma. Both are based on the manifestations of the illness and, in particular, the frequency of symptoms and response to treatment. They are very useful for the advanced practice nurse (APN), who may be providing pharmacological treatment, and for the nurse who is working with the person to describe the level of symptoms experienced and the efficacy of self-managed care. The new guidelines can be downloaded at http://www.nhlbi.nih.gov/health-pro/guidelines/current/asthma-guidelines/summary-report-2007.ht.

Medications the APN may prescribe include "rescue inhalers" (i.e., short-acting bronchodilators such as albuterol) and those offering longer control (e.g., for persons with nocturnal

symptoms). Inhaled medications may be taken a number of ways, including metered-dose inhalers (MDIs), electric nebulizers, and dry-powder inhalers. There are also long-acting oral medications, such as Singulair, that may be an effective alternative for some. Because asthma is an inflammatory disorder, inhaled steroids are often used, requiring more attention to side effects and drug interactions.

Several devices are available to facilitate effective drug administration, such as spacers for helping persons with hand limitations to manage medication cylinders. All of these require manual dexterity to some extent and the cognitive ability to follow directions. The nurse helps determine which of these devices has the greatest chance to be used successfully and works with the caregivers to help the person who would benefit from their use.

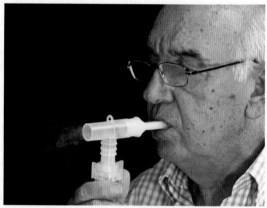

Older Adult Using an Inhaler Device. (©iStock.com/Juanmonino)

Nurses actively promote healthy respiratory aging through prevention. This means primary prevention by promoting or conducting smoking cessation programs and community intervention, including organizational efforts to promote and administer preventive vaccinations such as those for influenza and pneumonia (Box 25-11). Primary prevention includes political activism with industry leaders and environmental agencies to push for clean air and water. In occupational settings, the nurse can contribute to the health of the workers by promoting healthy work environments and, in some cases, monitoring patients, residents, and employees for exposure to, and adequate treatment of, any of the respiratory disorders, especially infections. In doing so, the nurse

BOX 25-11   Promoting Healthy Lungs

Primary Prevention

- Obtain pneumonia immunizations.
- Obtain annual influenza immunization.
- Avoid exposure to smoke and pollutants.
- Do not smoke.
- Avoid persons with respiratory illnesses.
- Seek prompt treatment of respiratory tract infections.
- Wash hands frequently.

can decrease the prevalence of respiratory diseases and their associated morbidity and mortality in older adults. At all times, the nurse is instrumental in facilitating palliative care when it is appropriate.

The nurse advances self-care when teaching the person how to be alert to exacerbations, use at-home peak flow meters to monitor disease, and know when to use "rescue inhalers" for quick, short-term use. The person should be taught that rescue medications should never be used regularly and that long-acting medications can never be used in acute situations. If rescue medications are needed on a regular basis, a reevaluation of the plan of care is needed to improve control of chronic symptoms. Nurses can work with individuals to identify what triggers their COPD exacerbations and to learn how to respond to these and, in doing so, promote healthy aging.

KEY CONCEPTS

- Two important normal changes with aging in the respiratory system are the decreased effectiveness of gas exchange and the reduced ability to handle secretions.
- COPD is almost exclusively the result of long-term exposure to tobacco smoke.
- Chronic bronchitis is characterized by repeated infections.
- Although asthma affects persons of all ages, those with the highest mortality rate are older women.
- The nurse can have a large impact on the quality of life for the elder with respiratory problems and his or her family members.
- The nurse helps the person learn to monitor symptoms and their effect on function and educates the person about the appropriate use of medications, oxygen, exercise, and the avoidance of triggers.
- The nurse encourages the person with respiratory disorders to remain as active as possible for as long as possible and to function as fully as possible within the limitations of his or her disease.

NURSING STUDY: HAS MRS. CHU BEEN UNDIAGNOSED?

One of your assigned patients in the acute care hospital where you are working is being prepared for an elective hip replacement due to long-standing arthritis. In your assessment, you find that Mrs. Chu seems to become slightly short of breath when she is speaking. This had been attributed to her advanced age and heart disease, even though her heart disease is well controlled at the time. As you gently proceed in your assessment she admits that she has a cough that seems to "come and go a lot" and that she is no longer doing many of the things she used to do because she is easily fatigued. When you inquire, she tells you that she was a heavy smoker but that was "many years ago."

- What is your nursing priority in caring for Mrs. Chu at this time?
- Discuss with another student two nursing diagnoses that can be drawn from this case.
- Develop a nursing intervention for the diagnoses and then compare them with another student's interventions.

CRITICAL THINKING QUESTIONS AND ACTIVITIES

1. Are end-of-life topics appropriate when caring for someone with COPD?
2. Think about the last place you either worked as a nurse or were assigned to as part of your nursing studies. Discuss any strategies that were used in the facility to minimize the development of respiratory illnesses among patients.
3. What additional strategies would you recommend?

RESEARCH QUESTIONS

1. What are three key reasons that chronic diseases are undiagnosed in older adults?
2. Which chronic diseases are some of those that are the most undertreated?
3. Are there any changes with aging that have a direct effect on the development of respiratory disorders?
4. Explore reliable sources to determine if older adults are subject to the development of iatrogenic respiratory tract infections while in an acute care setting. (HINT: The AHRQ and CDC websites might be good places to start.) If so, to what extent are older adults affected?

REFERENCES

American Lung Association (ALA): *COPD*, 2014. http://www.lung.org/lung-disease/copd/. Accessed October 2014.

Amin P, Smith AM: Pulmonary diseases. In Ham RJ, Sloane PD, Warshaw GA, et al, editors: *Primary care geriatrics: a case-based approach*, ed 6, Philadelphia, 2014, Elsevier, pp 497–511.

Brashers VL, Huether SE: Alterations of pulmonary function. In McCance KL, Huether SE, editors: *Pathophysiology: the biological basis for disease in children and adults*, ed 7, St. Louis, MO, 2014, Mosby, pp 1248–1289.

Centers for Disease Control (CDC): *What is COPD?* 2013. http://www.cdc.gov/copd/index.htm. Accessed August 2014.

Chesnutt MS, Prendergast TJ, Tavan ET: Pulmonary disorders. In Papadakis MA, McPhee SJ, editors: *Current medical diagnosis and treatment 2013*, New York, 2013, McGraw-Hill Lance, pp 242–323.

Garcia-Aymerich J, Serra I, Gomez FP, et al: Physical activity and clinical functional status in COPD, *Chest J* 136(1):62–70, 2009.

Hanania NA, King MJ, Braman SS, et al: Asthma in the elderly: current understanding and future needs, *J Allergy Clin Immunol* 128(Suppl 3):S4–S24, 2011.

Kravchenko J, Akushevich I, Abernethy AP, et al: Long-term dynamics of death rates of emphysema, asthma, and pneumonia and improved air quality, *Int J Chron Obstruct Pulmon Dis* 9:613–627, 2014.

National Heart Lung and Blood Institute (NHLBI): *Expert panel report 3: guidelines for the diagnosis and treatment of asthma, 2007.* http://www.nhlbi.nih.gov/health-pro/guidelines/current/asthma-guidelines/summary-report-2007.htm. Accessed August 2013.

Rance K, O'Laughlen M: Managing asthma in older adults, *J Nurse Pract* 10(1):1–9, 2014.

Stoller JK: Clinical practice: acute exacerbations of chronic obstructive pulmonary disease, *N Engl J Med* 346:988–994, 2002.

Stridsman C, Müllerova H, Skär L, et al: Fatigue in COPD and the impact of respiratory symptoms and heart disease—a population-based study, *COPD* 10(2):125–132, 2013.

Tang W, Kowgier M, Loth DW, et al: Large-scale genome-wide association studies and meta-analysis of longitudinal change in adult lung function, *PLoS One* 9(7):e100776, 2014.

U.S. Department of Health and Human Services (USDHHS): *Respiratory diseases, HealthyPeople 2020*, 2014. http://www.healthypeople.gov. Accessed August 2014.

World Health Organization (WHO): *The top 10 causes of death* (Fact sheet no. 310), 2014. http://www.who.int/mediacentre/factsheets/fs310/en. Accessed August 2014.

CHAPTER 26

Common Musculoskeletal Concerns

Kathleen Jett

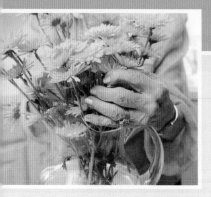

http://evolve.elsevier.com/Touhy/TwdHlthAging

AN ELDER SPEAKS

These old bones just aren't what they used to be. I sound like a rocker just a creakin' away.

Jesse, age 92

A STUDENT SPEAKS

I thought that if you were 75 you would be all crippled up and could not do anything anymore, but some of the elders I have gotten to know are still playing tennis. They say their hands hurt them afterward, but that is not going to keep them down!

Rebecca, 20-year-old nurse

LEARNING OBJECTIVES

On completion of this chapter the reader will be able to:

1. Identify the normal changes in the aging musculoskeletal system that have the potential for the greatest effect on functional status.
2. Describe a "frailty fracture" and explain its relationship to osteoporosis.
3. Differentiate the signs and symptoms of osteoarthritis, rheumatoid arthritis, and gout as manifested in older adults.
4. Describe the key aspects of promoting musculoskeletal health while aging.
5. Describe the key areas of patient education related to both nonpharmacological and pharmacological approaches for the treatment of common musculoskeletal disorders.

THE AGING MUSCULOSKELETAL SYSTEM

A functioning musculoskeletal system is necessary for the body's movement in space, responses to environmental forces, and the maintenance of posture and activity level. A fully functioning musculoskeletal system is needed to independently meet the activities of daily living (Chapter 7). Although none of the age-related changes are life-threatening, any of them could affect one's ability to remain independent, to be comfortable, and to maintain an acceptable quality of life. As the changes become visible to self and others, they have the potential to affect the individual's self-esteem.

Structure and Posture

Changes in stature and posture are two of the obvious outward signs of aging. They occur very gradually and are caused by multiple developmental factors involving skeletal, muscular, and subcutaneous and fat tissue. Vertebral disks become thinner as a result of gravity and dehydration, and spontaneous and unknown spinal fractures may occur as a result of osteoporosis causing a shortening of the trunk. When combined with a slight curving of the cervical vertebrae, height is lost; loss of up to 3 inches is indicative of significant osteoporosis (Hannafon and Cadogan, 2014). A stooped, slightly forward-bent posture is common and may be accompanied by slightly flexed hips and knees and somewhat flexed arms, bent at the elbows. To maintain eye contact, it may be necessary to slightly extend the head, which makes it appear that the person is jutting forward. Posture and structural changes occur primarily because of age-related bone calcium loss and atrophic cartilage and muscle (Figure 26-1).

Bones

Bones are composed of both organic tissue and inorganic products, especially minerals. Bone is a constantly changing tissue. There is ongoing and cyclic resorption (into the bloodstream) and renewal (into the bone) of minerals, especially calcium. Bone mass peaks at about the age of 20; the ability to achieve peak bone mass is influenced by nutrition, hormonal and genetic factors,

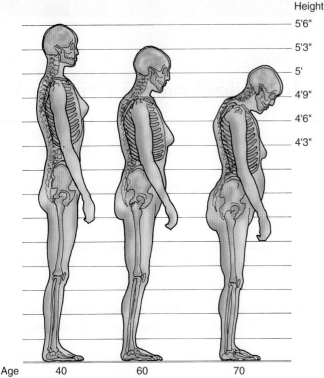

FIGURE 26-1 Age-Related Changes in the Spine as a Result of Bone Loss. Normal spine at age 40 years and osteoporotic changes at ages 60 and 70 years. These changes can cause a potential loss of as much as 6 to 9 inches in height. Note the exaggerated thoracic and lumbar curves at age 70 years. (From Ignatavicius DD, Workman ML: *Medical-surgical nursing: patient-centered collaborative care,* ed 6, Philadelphia, 2010, Saunders. Data from Sattin RW, Easley KA, Wolf SL, et al: Reduction in fear of falling through intense tai chi exercise training in older, transitionally frail adults, *J Am Geriatr Soc* 53:1168–1178, 2005.)

BOX 26-1   Factors Affecting Degree of Bone Loss While Aging

Genetics
Hormonal factors (estrogen and estradiol levels)
Decreased bone development
Nutritional deficiencies (especially calcium, magnesium, and vitamin D)
Underlying conditions (e.g., immune disorders, thyroid diseases)
Lifestyle choices (e.g., physical inactivity, smoking, alcohol intake)

From Crowther-Radulewicz CL: Structure and function of the musculo-skeletal system. In McCance KL, Huether SE, editors: *Pathophysiology: the biological basis for disease in adults and children,* ed 7, St Louis, 2014, Elsevier, p 1536.

and possibly calcium pyrophosphates. Cellular cross-linkage affects the cartilage, ligaments, and tendons. As joints dry, movement is less fluid. Pain may result if these changes progress to the extent where bone rubs on bone, as in the case of arthritis.

Muscles

The three types of muscles are smooth, skeletal, and cardiac. Smooth muscles are responsible for the contractibility of hollow organs such as the blood vessels. Skeletal muscles are essential for movement, posture, and heat production; much of it is under voluntary control. For each year after age 50, approximately 1% of the bulk and strength of skeletal muscle declines (Crowther-Radulewicz, 2014). These changes are referred to as *sarcopenia* and are seen almost exclusively in the skeletal muscle. Accelerated loss occurs with disuse and deconditioning.

MUSCULOSKELETAL DISORDERS

The most common musculoskeletal disorders are osteoporosis (OP), osteoarthritis (OA), rheumatoid arthritis (RA), and gout. Pseudogout and polymyalgia rheumatica are significant but occur much less often. Pain or problems with function associated with these and other musculoskeletal problems are among the most common reasons older adults seek medical care. In this chapter we address osteoporosis, osteoarthritis, rheumatoid arthritis, and gout.

Osteoporosis

Osteoporosis means "porous bone." In 2007 the World Health Organization (WHO) reported that osteoporosis affected 75 million people in the United States, Europe, and Japan combined (WHO, 2007). Osteoporosis is present in about 15% of those between the ages of 50 and 55 but increases to 70% by the age of 80 (WHO, 2014). In the United States about 34 million people, including 12 million men, have reduced bone mass. An estimated 5.3 million people older than 50 (0.8 million men) have osteoporosis, and the rest have osteopenia (*Healthy People,* 2014). While bone loss occurs slowly after reaching peak mass in the early 20s, it declines rapidly in women after menopause and in anyone who takes steroids for an extended period of time.

and weight-bearing exercises. Without exercise, premature bone loss will occur (Smeltzer and Qi, 2014).

When aging bone renewal cannot keep pace with resorption, reduced bone mineral density (BMD) results and the bones become brittle and fracture more easily. Reduced BMD is four times more common in older women than in men. Women may lose up to 50% of their cortical bone mass by the time they are 70 years old, the extent of which is dependent on a number of factors (Box 26-1) (Crowther-Radulewicz, 2014). In men, reduced BMD is primarily due to prolonged steroid use. Excessive loss of BMD leads to *osteopenia* or *osteoporosis.*

Joints, Tendons, and Ligaments

The joints make movement possible. Tendons and ligaments are bands of connective tissue that bind the bones to each other and allow the joints to articulate. Cartilage is a fibrous tissue that lines the joints and supports specific body parts, such as the ears and nose.

Age-related deterioration in articular cartilage results from biochemical changes: increases in the levels of transglutaminase

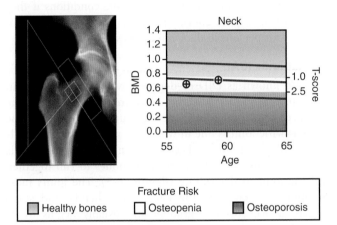

FIGURE 26-2 DEXA Scan: Determining the Presence of Reduced Bone Mineral Density. T-score = −1.4 = osteopenia. (Radiograph from Colledge NR, Walker BR, Ralston SH: *Davidson's principles and practice of medicine,* ed 21, London, 2010, Elsevier.)

Low bone density is diagnosed either following a fragility fracture (Box 26-2) or through the results of a dual-energy x-ray absorptiometry (DXA/DEXA) scan of the femoral neck and spine (Figure 26-2). The DXA/DEXA scan, where available, is still considered the "gold standard" in the diagnosis of osteoporosis and osteopenia. The results of the DEXA scan indicate the individual's BMD in comparison to a healthy reference group. *Osteopenia,* or a moderate amount of decreased BMD, is diagnosed if a "T-score" is between −1 and −2.5 standard deviations from the norm, and *osteoporosis,* or a significant amount of loss of bone density, is diagnosed if the T-score is greater than −2.5 standard deviations from the norm (WHO, 2007). The greatest implications for reduced BMD are the associations with fractures and subsequent morbidity and mortality (Chapter 19).

The National Osteoporosis Foundation (NOP) and the U.S. Preventive Services Task Force (USPSTF) recommend that all women be screened for OP at the age of 65. The NOF further recommends that all men at risk >70 years of age be screened as well (NOP, 2013; USPSTF, 2011). Medicare covers the cost of an initial scan and repeat scans at 24-month intervals if the person is diagnosed with osteoporosis or osteopenia and receiving treatment (Box 26-3) (Centers for Medicare and Medicaid Services [CMS], 2015). Although there are a number of risk factors, the prevalence of osteoporosis is highest among Caucasians (Box 26-4).

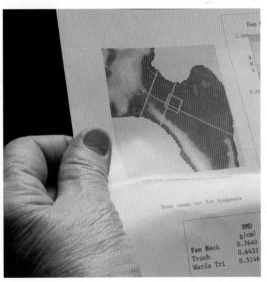

A DEXA scan provides useful information about bone health and fracture risk. (©iStock.com/kgerakis)

Etiology

OP is the result of a gradual loss of cortical (outer shell) and trabecular bone (inner spongy meshwork) and micro-architectural deterioration. Primary osteoporosis is likely a normal change of aging, particularly in postmenopausal women who do not take hormone replacement therapy. Secondary osteoporosis, which occurs much less often, can be caused by a number of factors including dietary deficiencies of calcium and vitamin D, medications such as corticosteroids and thyroid replacement, depression, and autoimmune disorders (Nelson, 2014; National Institute of Arthritis and Musculoskeletal Diseases [NIAMS], 2014).

Signs and Symptoms

Osteoporosis (OP) is a silent condition and a person may never have symptoms of any kind and not be diagnosed until a fracture occurs. Some of the more subtle signs suggestive of reduced BMD are a nontraumatic injury (fragile fracture) and loss of height of more than 3 cm from kyphosis (the development of a C shape to the cervical vertebrae) (see Figure 26-1). The nurse may be the one to identify the changes to the spine or realize that the person had a fracture or unexplained back pain but has not received a medical diagnosis. Without a diagnosis the person does not have access to the full treatments that are available.

Complications

The most serious health consequence of OP is the morbidity and mortality resulting from an osteoporosis-related fall. The most common sites for such fractures are hips, vertebra, wrist, and pelvis. Hip fractures lead to a high degree of morbidity and premature mortality (Chapter 19). Many people suffer another fracture, require long-term care, or never walk unassisted again. Wrist fractures can, and often do, result in severe limitations in self-care. The FRAX Tool™ is a computerized calculator for the determination of the 10-year probability of a fracture using a combination of risk factors and T-score. It is available in many formats including applications for tablets and iPhones (see http://www.shef.ac.uk/FRAX/).

Vertebral fractures are often not recognized by clinicians. The person may not attribute back pain to a potentially pathological process and instead accept it as a "normal change of aging." Usual therapy is bed rest, with variable success and the possible complications of deep venous thrombosis (DVT), pneumonia, and further bone loss. Effective pain management will allow early mobilization and prevent complications. Nonsteroidal antiinflammatory drugs (NSAIDs) may provide the analgesia needed, but due to the intensity of pain, the short-term use of narcotics is usually necessary. However, NSAIDs themselves have high risks for complications, especially in those who are already frail or have comorbid conditions.

Arthritis

Arthritis is common worldwide, with a dramatic increase in prevalence anticipated due to the aging population (Chapter 1). Based on 2013 data, arthritis affects 67 million (25%) of all adults at least 18 years old in the United States. It is estimated that 25 million people will report an arthritis-associated disability by 2030 (Centers for Disease Control and Prevention [CDC], 2013). The prevalence of arthritis and the type and activity limitations vary by race/ethnicity (Tables 26-1 and 26-2).

The number of persons with arthritis increases with age, especially after the age of 45. It occurs more commonly in women (CDC, 2010; CDC, 2013). Data drawn from surveys between 2010 and 2012 indicate that 49.7% of those older than age 65 have reported that they have been diagnosed with arthritis. Many of those with arthritis also have other chronic conditions (comorbidities) (Figure 26-3). Still others are at higher risk for the development of other chronic conditions if they have arthritis (Figure 26-4). Arthritis is the leading cause of disability for persons in the United States (CDC, 2015).

Osteoarthritis (OA)

OA, also known as DJD or degenerative joint disease, is an inflammatory process affecting an entire joint; it involves the cartilage, joint lining, ligaments, and underlying bones. The osteoarthritic joint is one in which the normal soft and resilient cartilaginous lining becomes thin and damaged. This causes the joint space to narrow, the bones to rub together, and the joint to deteriorate (Figure 26-5). The joints most commonly affected are the knees, hips, hands, and spine (Figure 26-6). Onset is gradual and usually begins to be noticed after the age of 40. Worldwide it is estimated that 9.6% of men and 18% of women have symptomatic OA. In the United States, OA affects 33.6% (12.4 million) persons older than age 65 (2005 data) (CDC, 2011a).

TABLE 26-1   Prevalence of Arthritis by Race/Ethnicity

RACE/ETHNICITY	PREVALENCE
Non-Hispanic white	23.8%
Non-Hispanic black	19.4%
Hispanic	11.1%
American Indian/Alaskan native	25.2%
Asian/Pacific Islander	8.4%
Multiracial/other	20.7%

From Centers for Disease Control and Prevention: *Racial/ethnic differences* (Data from National Health Interview Survey 2002, 2003, 2006), 2011. http://www.cdc.gov/arthritis/data_statistics/race.htm

TABLE 26-2   Prevalence of Activity Limitation among Adults by Race/Ethnicity

RACE/ETHNICITY	PREVALENCE
Non-Hispanic white	36.2%
Non-Hispanic black	44.6%
Hispanic	43.2%
American Indian/Alaskan native	39.1%
Asian/Pacific Islander	38.2%
Multiracial/other	49.5%

From Centers for Disease Control and Prevention: *Racial/ethnic differences* (Data from National Health Interview Survey 2002, 2003, 2006), 2011. http://www.cdc.gov/arthritis/data_statistics/race.htm

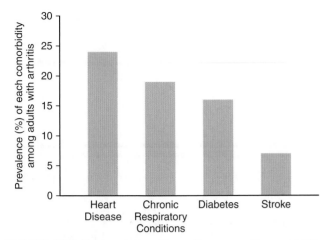

FIGURE 26-3 Four of the Most Common Comorbidities among Adults with Arthritis. (Data from Murphy L, Bolen J, Helmick CG, et al: *Comorbidities are very common among people with arthritis* [Poster 43], 20th National Conference on Chronic Disease Prevention and Control, Feb 2009.)

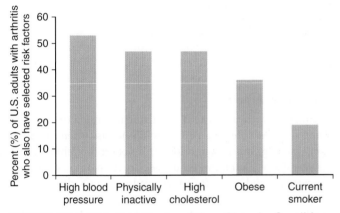

FIGURE 26-4 Risk Factors for Other Chronic Conditions among U.S. Adults with Arthritis. (Data from Murphy L, Bolen J, Helmick CG, et al: *Comorbidities are very common among people with arthritis* [Poster 43], 20th National Conference on Chronic Disease Prevention and Control, Feb 2009.)

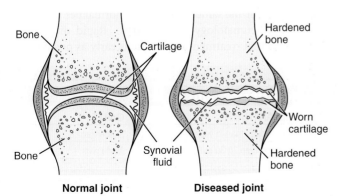

FIGURE 26-5 Normal Joint and Arthritic Joint.

What Areas Does Osteoarthritis Affect?

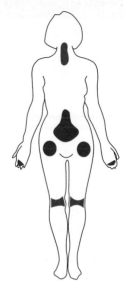

FIGURE 26-6 Common Locations for Osteoarthritis. (Source: National Institutes of Health: *Handout on health: osteoarthritis,* 2013. www.niams.nih.gov/hi/topics/arthritis/oahandout.htm Accessed July 29, 2004.)

OA is the most common cause for arthritis-related hospitalizations (69.9%), many of which are for joint replacements. Those who are non-Hispanic blacks and those with low incomes have lower rates of hip replacements but higher rates of complications and mortality. OA of the knee is 1 out of 5 of the leading causes of disability among noninstitutionalized adults in the United States and is ranked 1 of the 10 most disabling conditions in developed countries, especially for farmers (WHO, 2014). Eighty percent of those with OA will have limitations in movement at some time and 25% will not be able to meet their daily needs independently (CDC, 2014; Hootman et al, 2012; WHO, 2014).

Etiology. The specific causes of OA are unknown; however, it is now believed to be a combination of mechanical forces (e.g., trauma, obesity) and molecular events in the affected joint (Box 26-5). It is classified as idiopathic or secondary

BOX 26-5   **Risk Factors for Osteoarthritis**

Modifiable
- Obesity (especially for OA of the knee)
- Joint injury
- Knee pain
- Occupation requiring excessive or repeated mechanical stress
- Muscle weakness

Nonmodifiable
- Sex (female)
- Age (increases until about 75)
- Race (Asians with lowest risk)
- Genetic predisposition
- Poor proprioception

From Centers for Disease Control and Prevention (CDC): *Osteoarthritis,* 2014. http://www.cdc.gov/arthritis/basics/osteoarthritis.htm

(CDC, 2014). Osteoarthritis is most frequently determined by an empirical diagnosis (Box 26-6).

Signs and symptoms. In classic OA, there is stiffness with inactivity and pain with activity that is relieved by rest. The stiffness is greatest in the morning after the immobility of the joint during sleep but usually resolves within 20 to 30 minutes after movement begins (Crowther-Radulewicz and McCance, 2014). As the breakdown advances, so does the pain and stiffness. The stiffness is characterized as difficulty initiating joint movement, immobility, and loss of range of motion, all quite significant to the older adult and the maintenance of independence. On exam, subluxation and joint instability may be found and crepitus is common (both indicators of the deterioration of the synovial covering of the joints). Two-thirds of those older than 65 show joint space narrowing evident on x-rays (Nakasato and Christensen, 2014).

As the disease advances, spinal stenosis develops in the lumbar region and osteophytes develop in the joints of the fingers. Those in the distal joints are Heberden's nodes and those in the proximal joints are Bouchard's nodes. If present, they appear as deformities in the flexion of these joints. Heberden's nodes are thought to have a hereditary component (Figure 26-7).

Complications. Because OA is a disease of the joints, the complications are limited to the effect of the degenerative changes on function and the side effects of treatment of related pain. Fortunately, for advanced disease of the knees (the most common site) and hips, replacements are available and in many cases very successful. Persons with advanced OA of the spine often require the support of pain centers (see Chapter 27). A serious potential complication with the diagnosis of OA, or presumed diagnosis, is determining if the signs and symptoms are not atypical manifestations of other common conditions, for example, the attribution of shoulder pain to OA rather than to an acute myocardial infarction.

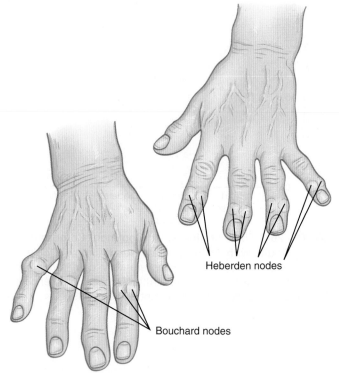

FIGURE 26-7 Nodes and Arthritis. (From McCance KL, Huether SE, editors: *Pathophysiology: the biologic basis for disease in adults and children,* ed 7, St Louis, 2014, Elsevier.)

Rheumatoid Arthritis

Rheumatoid arthritis (RA) is a systemic inflammatory autoimmune disorder affecting primarily the joints, where it causes pain, swelling, stiffness, and loss of function. Inflammation of the synovium (joint lining) causes destruction of the surrounding cartilage and bone. It can also cause anemia, dry eyes and mouth, vasculitis, and pleurisy (NIAMS, 2013).

Although the onset of OA is always insidious, the onset of RA may be acute, especially in older adults compared with younger persons (Table 26-3). A diagnosis is made through consideration of the number and types of joints involved (must include one small joint), select serological studies, and the presence of symptoms for at least 6 weeks (Boxes 26-7 and 26-8). However, laboratory findings are less specific in persons with multiple chronic diseases (e.g., most older adults) because there may be multiple other reasons for the same serological abnormalities (American College of Rheumatology [ACR], 2010). Rapid diagnosis is necessary so that treatment can begin as early as possible and

TABLE 26-3   Comparison of Osteoarthritis, Rheumatoid Arthritis, and Gout

	OSTEOARTHRITIS	RHEUMATOID ARTHRITIS	GOUT
Onset	Insidious	More acute in older adults than in younger adults	Sudden/acute
Classic symptoms	Stiffness of joint resolved in <20 minutes after rest	Stiffening lasting more than 20-30 minutes after rest	Acute pain
Classic signs	Affects distal interphalangeal joints, knees, hips, and vertebrae	Affects proximal joints, may be systemic	Inflammation, especially at the base of the great toe
Key management	Initial treatment may be nonpharmacological such as heat and exercise; later acetaminophen and NSAIDs	Use of DMARDs as soon as diagnosis is made	NSAIDs

therefore provide the greatest chance the joints can be preserved as long as possible.

Although it can occur at any age, the incidence of RA peaks in the sixth decade (Woodworth et al, 2013). It is estimated that it affects approximately 1.5 million people in the United States or 0.6% of the population and women two to three times more often than men (NIAMS, 2013).

Worldwide the prevalence is 0.3% to 1% and more often begins in those ages 20 to 40. Within 10 years of onset, up to 50% of those affected may be unable to work full time (WHO, 2014).

Etiology. A number of risk factors have been associated with the development of RA in older adults. These include smoking, periodontitis, and viral infections. (Woodworth et al, 2013). The etiology is unknown but now believed to be the result of interaction between environmental exposures, genetic factors, and age-related increased autoimmunity. The understanding of autoimmunity (Chapter 25) is advancing as scientific developments have allowed us to look into the gene itself. Of the more than 30 genes studies, the strongest genetic factors appear to be the gene variation "single nucleotide polymorphism" (SNP) (found within the enzyme PTPN22), which has been found to have an important role in the body's autoimmune system. When a person inherits one or two copies of this enzyme, T cells and other immune cells respond vigorously and may cause joint inflammation and damage. The presence of the enzyme PTPN22 has been associated with several other autoimmune diseases such as diabetes (CDC, 2012). These and additional studies are under way.

Signs and symptoms. Three variations of RA may occur: monocyclic, polycyclic, or progressive. In the monocyclic variation, the person has one episode lasting 3 to 5 years with no further episodes. In the polycyclic variation, the levels (intensity of symptoms) vary over time. In the progressive variety, RA continues to increase in severity and is present at all times (CDC, 2012).

Because RA affects joints and the system as a whole, pain, fatigue, malaise, weakness, and fever may be present (CDC, 2012). It can be initially confused with OA or concurrent geriatric syndromes. However, RA is characterized by symmetrical polyarticular limitations affecting five or more joints. The joints are erythematous, painful, and swollen; morning stiffness lasts longer than 30 minutes, compared with the few minutes seen in OA.

RA usually affects the small joints of the wrist, ankle, and hand, although it can also affect the large joints such as the knee. As the disease progresses, pain increases and joint deformities occur, with more than 10% of persons developing hand deformities within 2 years. Older adults who have had RA for many years may present with multiple deformities (Figure 26-8), especially of the hands and feet, and may have to undergo palliative joint replacement or repair surgeries.

Complications. As with OA, the complications of RA are largely a consequence of orthopedic deformities, pain, and, in RA especially, the side effect of medications. The most common deformity in RA is the boutonnière deformity or hyperextension of the distal interphalangeal (DIP) joint with flexion of the proximal interphalangeal (PIP) joint, followed by a "swan neck" deformity or flexion of the DIP and extension of the PIP, and a

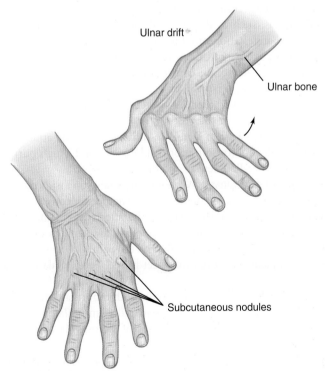

FIGURE 26-8 Rheumatoid Arthritis Deformities. (From McCance KL, Huether SE, editors: *Pathophysiology: the biologic basis for disease in adults and children,* ed 7, St Louis, 2014, Elsevier.)

vagus deformity of the knee and volar subluxation of the metatarsophalangeal (MTP) joints. Persons with RA are most likely to die from heart disease and at a higher rate than the general population, but the association is unexplained (Hellmann and Imboden, 2013).The most common comorbidities are cardiovascular disease, infections such as tuberculosis (up to one-fourth of the deaths of persons with RA), depression and anxiety, and lymphoproliferative malignancies (CDC, 2012).

Gout

Gout is an inflammatory (rheumatic) arthritis characterized by the deposition of uric acid crystals in the tissues and fluids in the body. It may either be a one-time acute illness or become chronic, with intermittent (and unpredictable) acute attacks. The joint of the great toe is the most typical site; however, it also may occur in the ankle, knee, wrist, or elbow. Gout affects approximately 6.1 million people in the United States (Nakasato and Christensen, 2014). Men between the ages of 40 and 50 are most commonly affected, but the prevalence increases significantly with age. Black men in the United States have gout about two times more often than white men (CDC, 2011b). Gout may be exacerbated by concurrent conditions and medications commonly used in later life, particularly thiazide diuretics and salicylates (even in small doses) (Stamp and Jordan, 2011). Among women, increasing age, obesity, alcohol consumption, hypertension, and diuretic use were found to be associated with a higher risk for gout (Bhole et al, 2010).

Etiology. Gout is a cytokine-mediated inflammatory response to the accumulations of uric acid in the blood and other body fluids, such as the synovial fluid of joints. Gout is the clinical manifestation of either overproduction of uric acid or inadequate excretion. Underexcretion is thought to account for about 80% to 90% of the cases of hyperuricemia (CDC, 2011b). Up to 70% of all persons with gout have a genetic component (Köttgen et al, 2012). At least 11 genes have been identified as being involved with the risk for, or the manifestation of, the disorder. Other known factors to influence an acute attack are excessive alcohol consumption, lead toxicity, and a high purine diet (Crowther-Radulewicz and McCance, 2014).

Signs and symptoms. While gout may develop insidiously, it typically starts with an acute attack. The person complains of what they call "exquisite" pain in the affected joint or joints, often starting in the middle of the night, awakening one from sleep. The joint is bright red, hot, and too painful to touch. They may complain that "even the sheet hurts." Fever, malaise, and chills may also be present. A laboratory test finding of elevated uric acid is likely, but it also may be within normal limits. The pain of gout may be very responsive to oral antiinflammatories such as NSAIDs and short courses of steroids or colchicine (Tausche et al, 2009).

Complications. With prolonged elevations of uric acid, it crystallizes, forming insoluble precipitates that gather in subcutaneous tissue. They are seen as small, white tophi that may be quite painful. If they collect in the kidneys, they can form urate renal stones and cause renal failure.

◆ PROMOTING HEALTHY AGING: IMPLICATIONS FOR GERONTOLOGICAL NURSING

Gerontological nurses have a direct impact on promoting musculoskeletal health in a number of ways. They are active at all levels of health promotion and disease prevention (Box 26-9).

◆ Osteoporosis

Nurses have an impact on osteoporosis in its prevention, worsening of existing disease, and the prevention of related complications, specifically bone fractures and pain. Preventive strategies include the promotion of healthy diets and appropriate supplementation, encouragement of physical activity, and protection from injury. The nurse's role includes education about these preventive strategies and the correct use of the medications that are available for the prevention and treatment of OP.

◆ Nutrition

While an overall nutritious diet promotes healthy aging, an adequate intake of calcium and vitamin D is especially important in the prevention and treatment of osteoporosis.

◆ *Calcium.* A lifetime of adequate intake of calcium is necessary to achieve and maintain bone health (Box 26-10). While one's diet should include calcium-enriched food, supplementation is always recommended. Calcium carbonate is the least expensive form of calcium and should be taken with meals to enhance absorption. If the person is also taking H_2 blockers, then calcium citrate should be taken instead. Teaching includes discussion of the factors that inhibit calcium absorption (e.g., excess alcohol, protein, or salt); enhance excretion (e.g., caffeine, excess fiber, phosphorus in meats, sodas, and preserved

---

♥ BOX 26-9　HEALTHY PEOPLE 2020
Goals for Musculoskeletal Wellness

- Reduce the mean level of joint pain among adults with doctor-diagnosed arthritis.
- Reduce the number of adults with diagnosed arthritis who find it "very difficult" to perform joint-related activities.
- Reduce the number of adults with diagnosed arthritis who have difficulty in performing two or more personal care activities, thereby preserving independence.
- Increase the proportion of adults with diagnosed arthritis who receive health care provider counseling.
- Reduce hip fractures among older adults.

Data from U.S. Department of Health and Human Services, Office of Disease Prevention and Health Promotion: Healthy People 2020, 2012. http://www.healthypeople.gov/2020.

BOX 26-10　Amount of Daily Calcium Needed

51-70 years of age: 1000 mg (male); 1200 mg (female)
71+ years of age: 1200 mg for both males and females

From National Institutes of Health, Office of Daily Supplements: *Calcium: daily supplement fact sheet,* 2013. http://ods.od.nih.gov/factsheets/Calcium-HealthProfessional/#h2

foods); and influence the body's response to stress (decreased calcium absorption, increased excretion of calcium in the urine). A careful consideration of the timing of when the calcium supplement is taken in relation to other medications and foods is very important. Many find calcium supplements very constipating and may need to take routine stool softeners. Calcium supplements are necessary even if someone is being treated for osteoporosis in some other way.

Vitamin D. In order to optimize the body's ability to minimize bone loss associated with the development of osteoporosis, intake of an adequate amount of vitamin D is necessary. It is essential for calcium uptake into the bones. Sunlight (ultraviolet rays) on the skin stimulates the production of vitamin D. In order to get an adequate amount of vitamin D, it is necessary to have the face, back, or arms exposed for 10 to 15 minutes three times a week. Sunscreen of SPF 8 or higher prevents the production of vitamin D but also helps prevent skin cancer. Depending on a number of factors, such as skin tone, geographic location, weather patterns, ability to leave parts of the skin uncovered for some period of time each day, and the ability to obtain sun exposure (e.g., not bedbound), supplementation may or may not be necessary. However, supplements are recommended for all persons except those who have regular sun exposure, such as those who work outside for long periods of time. The recommended supplements (800 to 1000 units a day for those older than 65) are based on the presumption that adequate naturally produced vitamin D is not possible (National Osteoporosis Foundation [NOF], 2014). Vitamin D and calcium supplements should be used at the same time for optimal bone health.

Exercise

Regular exercise is recommended at any age, but especially for those at risk for, or with, osteoporosis. Weight-bearing and muscle-strengthening exercises reduce the rates of falls and fractures (Chapter 19). Weight-bearing activity is that in which bones and muscles work against gravity. This may include walking, jogging, tai chi, stair climbing, dancing, and tennis. There are yoga and Pilates programs that have been designed especially for those who are frailer (NOF, 2014).

Education

Promoting bone health also includes education about fall prevention (see Chapter 19). Risk reduction measures should also be included in all patient or caregiver teaching. Hip protectors can be considered for frail older adults with OP.

Pharmacological Approaches

For those at risk for OP or those with existing OP, pharmacological interventions are often used. While ensuring adequate intake of vitamin D and calcium, the currently available medications include bisphosphonates (e.g., alendronate or Fosamax®), selective estrogen reception modifiers (SERMs) (e.g., raloxifene and bazedoxifene, estrogen, parathyroid hormones PTH[1-34], and teriparatide), and the RANKL inhibitor denosumab. If no other medications can be tolerated or used, the prescribing provider may consider the use of calcitonin-salmon. It has recently been reviewed by the Food and Drug Administration for possible complications (FDA, 2014). The medications for OP range from oral to nasal spray to intravenous formulations, and dosing from daily to yearly. Each has very specific administration instructions that must be followed precisely. The nurse needs to be aware of the correct techniques when educating patients or administering the medication at the bedside or clinic. Many of the medications are contraindicated in persons who cannot comply with the procedures needed for safe use. It is no longer the standard of practice to take these indefinitely, and the nurse can work with the patient and provider to determine the appropriate duration of treatment.

> **⚡ SAFETY ALERT**
>
> Due to the risk for esophageal erosions, ulceration, or possible rupture, oral bisphosphonates must be taken on an empty stomach (when first awake) with a full glass of water, and the person must remain in an upright position for at least 30 minutes and not eat or drink for at least 30 minutes.

Osteoarthritis and Rheumatoid Arthritis

In caring for those with any form of arthritis, the goals are to minimize disability by preventing further damage and ensuring adequate pain relief (Chapter 27) (Box 26-11). To minimize disability, all affected joints must be used and strengthened, but protected. In the case of RA, protection includes the prompt initiation of appropriate joint-saving medications such as the DMARDs (disease-modifying antirheumatic drugs). Adequate pain relief will allow the person to function at as high a level as possible for as long as possible.

Nonpharmacological Approaches

Nonpharmacological approaches are very important for persons with arthritis. This includes the use of heat and cold, joint support and protection, exercise, and diet. The use of heat and cold is well-known for management of arthritic pain. Heat will provide temporary relief in osteoarthritis, but ice will reduce inflammation. Devices and techniques are available that relieve some of the pressure to the joints and in doing so may decrease pain and improve balance. For example, canes and walkers relieve hip stress. A shoe lift can improve lumbar pain. A knee brace is useful for knees, especially if there is lateral instability (the knee "gives out"). If the person is no longer able to ambulate, he or she may qualify for mobility assistive devices, including electric wheelchairs and other power mobility devices

> **BOX 26-11   Goals of Nursing Care for the Person with Arthritis**
>
> Minimize or prevent pain
> Balance rest and activity of joint
> Maintain self-esteem
> Minimize swelling and inflammation
> Maintain function of affected joints

(PMDs) (CMS, 2014). Paraffin baths for the hands have been found to be very soothing. These can be purchased or may be part of the physical therapist's plan of care. The person can also avoid carrying packages by the fingers, using a cart instead, and use adaptive devices on utensils and household equipment to make a larger grip surface. A variety of adaptive equipment is available to make daily activities less problematic to the person and traumatic to the joints.

Exercise is essential for the maintenance of joint function and therefore independence. A skilled physical therapist or rehabilitation nurse specialist can provide an individualized exercise plan to maximize strengths. When performed regularly they will improve flexibility and increase muscle strength, which in turn better support the affected joints, reduce pain, improve function, and reduce falls (Egan and Mentes, 2010). Water exercise is recommended as a gentle way to exercise joints and muscles.

If pain is not adequately controlled (Chapter 27), the person will decrease activity, become deconditioned rapidly, and may gain weight. The weight puts more stress on the joints, leading to more pain, less activity, and more debility. A dietitian and nurse can work with the person to identify weight and caloric goals and develop meal plans that are culturally acceptable but still balanced and healthy.

The simplest approaches may make a big difference in helping the person remain independent. This may include easy-to-use zipper pulls, extension devices to pick up things from a distance (e.g., the floor), or devices to slide on shoes from a sitting position. Velcro closures on clothing are useful for those whose hands are no longer fully functional. Book holders, chairs to sit on while preparing foods, larger light switch changes, and secure stair railings, or even moving heavier objects or those used frequently to lower cabinet shelves, may all be very effective measures.

◆ Surgery

Surgical replacement of the joint (arthroplasty) may be highly successful in reducing intractable pain and restoring all or at least some function to the joint. Surgical replacements are recommended for even the very old with a reasonable life expectancy and when comorbid conditions are well controlled.

◆ Pharmacological Approaches

In many cases the first-line treatment for arthritis-related pain is use of a nonsteroidal antiinflammatory drug (NSAID). However, although they may be effective, they may present considerable risk and are contradicted in some cases such as those with hypertension or taking anticoagulants. COX-2 inhibitors are sometimes recommended, but they have been found to be no more effective than the NSAIDs and have their own risks (Nakasato and Christensen, 2014). For intractable pain in the knees, joint injections with either steroids or intraarticular hyaluronans may be necessary for pain management (Brzusek and Petron, 2008).

A third group of medications that are specific for the treatment of RA are the disease-modifying antirheumatic drugs (DMARDs). The DMARDs take several weeks to months to provide relief, but they are used specifically to stop the progression of the disease and resultant cartilage damage and bone loss. The DMARD methotrexate is considered first-line treatment, although a number of others are now available. All DMARDs are potentially toxic, and the nurse must work closely with the patient and family to be aware of early danger signs (Box 26-12).

For many years, it was thought that people with RA should rest their joints to protect them from damage; however, both rest and exercise are necessary. Therapeutic exercise programs are designed to help maintain or improve the ability to perform activities of daily living (ADLs). Even a warm, inflamed joint can be given ROM exercises to maintain movement in the joint. A physical or occupational therapist should be consulted for developing a program of rest and exercise. Splints and assistive devices, such as those discussed earlier, will enhance self-care ability and consequently self-esteem.

◆ Gout

The first goal of treatment during an acute attack of gout is to stop it as promptly as possible and thereby achieve pain relief. This may include NSAIDs, colchicine, and sometimes an injection of long-acting steroids into the joint. The nurse ensures that the person drinks an adequate amount of fluids (about 2 L/day) to help flush the uric acid through the kidneys if not contraindicated. During drug therapy, the person should not take salicylates, such as aspirin, which may inhibit the effectiveness of other medications being taken.

After the acute attack, the goal is to prevent another attack, systemic spread of the disease, and the development of chronic gout. This may be done by avoiding drugs or foods that are high in purine (Box 26-13) and alcohol, both of which increase uric acid levels, and by taking medications to either decrease uric acid production, such as xanthine oxidase inhibitors (e.g., allopurinol or febuxostat), or increase its excretion (e.g., probenecid) (Crowther-Radulewicz and McCance, 2014). The nurse's role includes teaching the person how to decrease the likelihood of another attack by employing preventive measures.

BOX 26-12　Potential Side Effects of Methotrexate Therapy

Hepatic cirrhosis	Mild alopecia and hair thinning
Interstitial pneumonitis	Headache
Severe myelosuppression (rare)	Fatigue
Stomatitis and oral ulcers	Nauseas or diarrhea

From Bingham C, Ruffing V: *Rheumatoid arthritis treatment,* 2013. http://www.hopkinsarthritis.org/arthritis-info/rheumatoid-arthritis/ra-treatment.

BOX 26-13　Foods High in Purine

Meat, poultry, and fish (limit to 4-6 oz a day)
Organ meats such as herring, anchovies, mackerel, brains, testicles (severely limit)
Alcohol (limit or avoid)
Foods sweetened with high-fructose corn syrup (limit or avoid)

KEY CONCEPTS

- Although several changes occur in the musculoskeletal system, they are not life-threatening but do affect overall mobility, independence and may affect self-esteem.
- Osteoporosis is diagnosed through the result of a DEXA scan or the person suffering a fragility fracture.
- The most important reason to be concerned about osteoporosis and osteopenia is their association with the risk for fractures and subsequent increased mortality and morbidity.
- The majority of persons with osteoarthritis will have significant limitations at some point, including the inability to care for themselves.
- A major nursing concern in caring for someone with arthritis is helping the person manage pain and thereby preserve function as long as possible.

- One of the differences between osteoarthritis and rheumatoid arthritis is the relationship of time to the development of joint stiffening. In osteoarthritis, stiffening occurs after a period of disuse and resolves 20 to 30 minutes after activity resumes. In rheumatoid arthritis, the stiffness lasts at least 30 minutes.
- The differentiation between osteoarthritis and another common and potentially serious condition is often difficult.
- Rheumatoid arthritis affects the joints but can also affect the body in other ways.
- Gout is the result of the deposition of uric acid crystals in a joint or joints. The onset is most often acute.

NURSING STUDY: DOES MRS. SVÖLD NEED A CALCIUM SUPPLEMENT?

Mrs. Svöld is an 80-year-old woman of Scandinavian descent. She is a very petite woman who moved to a nursing home several years ago. She is dependent on others for her mobility. She is only able to get outside at the rare times her sister visits. As you review her medication list you notice that she is not taking any supplements, including calcium and vitamin D. She does, however, take Fosamax.

- Is your patient at risk for osteoporosis?
- Since she already takes Fosamax, does she need to take supplements?
- What can you do, if anything, to foster bone growth in Mrs. Svöld, and is it necessary since she lives in a nursing home and is immobile?
- Is Mrs. Svöld at any more risk for osteoporosis than some of your other patients? Why or why not?

CRITICAL THINKING QUESTIONS AND ACTIVITIES

1. Analyze your own diet and activities and determine your relative risk for osteoporosis.

RESEARCH QUESTIONS

1. When should women begin to have DEXA scans done?
2. Under what circumstances are DEXA scans appropriate for men?
3. Review the website for Medicare (www.cms.gov) and determine if there is insurance (Medicare) coverage for activities related to bone health.

REFERENCES

American College of Rheumatology (ACR): *2010 Rheumatoid arthritis classification*, 2010. http://www.rheumatology.org/practice/clinical/classification/ra/ra_2010.asp. Accessed August 2014.

Bhole V, de Vera M, Rahman MM, et al: Epidemiology of gout in women: fifty-two-year follow-up of a prospective cohort, *Arthritis Rheum* 62(4):1069–1076, 2010.

Brzusek D, Petron D: Treating knee osteoarthritis with intra-articular hyaluronans, *Curr Med Res Opin* 24:3307–3322, 2008.

Centers for Disease Control and Prevention (CDC): Chronic disease and health promotion: arthritis, 2015. http://www.cdc.gov/chronicdisease/resources/publications/aag/arthritis.htm Accessed May 2015.

CDC: *Arthritis-related statistics*, 2011a. http://www.cdc.gov/arthritis/data_statistics/arthritis_related_stats.htm. Accessed August 2014.

CDC: *Gout*, 2011b. http://www.cdc.gov/arthritis/basics/gout.htm. Accessed August 2014.

CDC: *Rheumatoid arthritis*, 2012. http://www.cdc.gov/arthritis/basics/rheumatoid.htm. Accessed August 2014.

CDC: Prevalence of doctor-diagnosed arthritis and arthritis-attributable activity limitation—United States, *MMWR Morb Mortal Wkly Rep* 2010-2012, 62(44): 869–873, 2013.

CDC: *Osteoarthritis*, 2014. http://www.cdc.gov/arthritis/basics/osteoarthritis.htm. Accessed August 2014.

Centers for Medicare and Medicaid Services (CMS): Preventive services: bone mass measurements, 2015. http://www.cms.gov/

Medicare/Prevention/PrevntionGenInfo/Downloads/MPS_QuickReference Chart_1.pdf Accessed May 2015

CMS: *PMD documentation requirements (nationwide)*, 2014. http://www.cms.gov/Research-Statistics-Data-and-Systems/Monitoring-Programs/Medicare-FFS-Compliance-Programs/Medical-Review/PMDDocumentationRequirements Nationwide.html. Accessed February 2015.

Crowther-Radulewicz CL: Structure and function of the musculoskeletal system. In McCance KL, Huether SE, editors: *Pathophysiology: the biological basis for disease in adults and children*, ed 7, St. Louis, 2014, Elsevier, pp 1510–1539.

Crowther-Radulewicz CL, McCance KL: Alterations of musculoskeletal function. In McCance KL, Huether SE, editors:

Pathophysiology: the biological basis for disease in adults and children, ed 7, St. Louis, 2014, Elsevier, pp 1540–1590.

Egan BA, Mentes JC: Benefits of physical activity for knee osteoarthritis, *J Gerontol Nurs* 36(9):9–14, 2010.

Food and Drug Administration (FDA): *Questions and answers: changes to the indicated population for Miacalcin (calcitonin-salmon)*, 2014. http://www.fda.gov/Drugs/DrugSafety/PostmarketDrugSafetyInformationforPatientsandProviders/ucm388641.htm. Accessed August 2014.

Hannafon F, Cadogan MP: Recognition and treatment of postmenopausal osteoporosis, *J Gerontol Nurs* 40(3):10–14, 2014.

Healthy People: *Arthritis, osteoporosis, and chronic back conditions*, 2014. https://www.healthypeople.gov/2020/topics-objectives/topic/Arthritis-Osteoporosis-and-Chronic-Back-Conditions. Accessed August 2014.

Hellman DR, Imboden JB: Musculoskeletal and immunological disorders. In Papadakis MA, McPhee SJ, editors: *Current medical diagnosis and treatment 2013*, New York, 2013, McGraw-Hill Lange, pp 809–869.

Hootman JM, Helmick CG, Brady TJ: A public health approach to addressing arthritis in older adults: the most common cause of disability, *Am J Public Health* 102(3):426–433, 2012.

Köttgen A, Albrecht E, Teumer A, et al: Genome-wide association analyses identify 18 new loci associated with serum urate concentration, *Nat Genet* 45:145–154, 2012.

Nakasato Y, Christensen M: Arthritis and related disorders. In Ham RJ, Sloane PD, Warshaw GA, et al, editors: *Primary care geriatrics: a case-based approach*, ed 6, Philadelphia, 2014, Elsevier, pp 456–465.

National Institute of Arthritis and Musculoskeletal Diseases (NIAMS): *What is rheumatoid arthritis*, 2013. http://www.niams.nih.gov/Health_Info/Rheumatic_Disease/default.asp#ra_13. Accessed August 2014.

NIAMS: *Osteoporosis*, 2014. http://www.niams.nih.gov/Health_Info/Bone/Osteoporosis/. Accessed October 31, 2014.

National Osteoporosis Foundation (NOF): *Clinician's guide to prevention and treatment of osteoporosis*, Washington, DC, 2014, National Osteoporosis Foundation.

Nelson HD: Osteoporosis. In Ham RJ, Sloane PD, Warshaw GA, et al, editors: *Primary care geriatrics: a case-based approach*, ed 6, Philadelphia, 2014, Elsevier, pp 445–455.

Smeltzer SC, Qi BB: Practical implications for nurses caring for patients being treated for osteoporosis, *Nursing (Auckl)* 4:19–33, 2014.

Stamp LK, Jordan S: The challenges of gout management in the elderly, *Drugs Aging* 28(8):591–603, 2011.

Tausche AK, Jensen TL, Schröder HE, et al: Gout—current diagnosis and treatment, *Dtsch Arztebl Int* 106(34–35):549–555, 2009.

U.S Prevention Services Task Force (USPSTF): *Screening for osteoporosis*, 2011. http://www.uspreventiveservicestaskforce.org/uspstf10/osteoporosis/osteors.htm. Accessed August 2014.

Woodworth T, Ranganath V, Furst DE: Rheumatoid arthritis in the elderly: recent advances in understanding the pathogenesis, risk factors, comorbidities and risk-benefit of treatments, *Aging Health* 9(2):167–178, 2013.

World Health Organization (WHO): *WHO scientific group on the assessment of osteoporosis at primary health care level*: summary meeting report, Geneva Switzerland, 2007, WHO Press.

WHO: *Chronic rheumatic conditions*, 2014. http://www.who.int/chp/topics/rheumatic/en. Accessed August 2014.

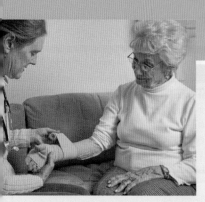

CHAPTER 27

Pain and Comfort

Kathleen Jett

http://evolve.elsevier.com/Touhy/TwdHlthAging

A STUDENT SPEAKS

I know she has pain all of the time, but if I give her too many pills she will get addicted and that would be a bad thing, right?

Ana, age 23, regarding Molly, age 89

AN ELDER SPEAKS

It seems to have crept up on me—first one joint, now the other. I wouldn't call it pain really, just an ache that never goes away and keeps me from dancing like I used to.

Gloria, age 78

LEARNING OBJECTIVES

On completion of this chapter the reader will be able to:
1. Define the concept of physical pain.
2. Identify factors that affect the elder's pain experience.
3. Identify barriers that interfere with pain assessment and treatment.
4. Describe data to include in a pain assessment.
5. Discuss pharmacological and nonpharmacological pain management therapies.
6. Develop a nursing plan of care for an elder with pain.

The International Association for the Study of Pain (IASP) defines pain as "an unpleasant sensory and emotional experience associated with actual or potential tissue damage, or described as such" (IASP, 2014). The Society has updated its 1994 taxonomy and now includes at least 28 different named types, such as hyperesthesia (increased sensitivity to stimulation), neuralgia (related to distribution of the nerves or a nerve), peripheral neuropathic pain (caused by a lesion or disease of the peripheral somatosensory nervous system), and nociceptive pain (arising from actual or threatened damage to non-neural tissue) (IASP, 2014). All pain is multidimensional with sensory, physical, psychosocial, emotional, and spiritual components. How we respond to it is part of who we are. Even the words used to describe it are many: an *ache*, a *burn*, a *pester*, or a sense of *despair*—with the language and the willingness to express it a manifestation of the person's cultural heritage and relationship with whom he or she is conversing (Box 27-1) (Campbell et al, 2009; Narayan, 2010). Pain can be a fleeting discomfort or something so pervasive that it wears heavily on one's spirit.

Pain is often categorized as either acute or persistent. Acute pain is most often the result of an acute event. The cause is clear (e.g., a fracture or infection), expected, temporary, and usually controllable with adequate analgesic treatment based on the intensity of the pain. It resolves when the underlying cause is resolved. For example, the acute pain of a myocardial infarction is temporarily relieved with nitroglycerin and permanently resolved when oxygen is restored to the myocardium. Everyone experiences acute physical pain at some point in their lives. Those at midlife and beyond continue to experience the pain of an acute event, but providing comfort becomes more complex due to concurrent conditions including those that are psychological in nature such as depression (Molton and Terrill, 2014). As one ages, acute pain is most often superimposed on the persistent pain of pre-exisiting chronic conditions.

The most common type of pain in late life is pain that has become persistent. As one ages, there are distinct pathological processes causing changes to the nervous system that worsen over time (Epplin et al, 2014). While the intensity of this type of pain may vary from day to day or hour to hour, it is always present to some extent. It is often felt in more than one area of the body, such as a knee in the case of osteoarthritis (Chapter 26). The perception of pain is altered by many factors, including the person's prior experience and expressions of pain of all types and the person's cultural, emotional, cognitive, and functional status (Horgas and Ahn, 2013; Narayan 2010). Persons with persistent pain are more likely than others to be depressed and to have sleep disorders, but not all who are depressed have physical pain (Molton and Terrill, 2014). Inadequately treated persistent pain will almost always lead to impaired functional status and in some cases cognitive impairments (Jansen, 2008) (Box 27-2).

BOX 27-1   Possible Effect of Culture on Expressions of Pain

Stoic and non-emotive
   "Grin and bear it" approach—withdrawn, prefers to be alone
   When asked about pain, it is minimized or denied
   Generalized to Northern European and Asian heritage
Emotive
   Wants others around to validate feelings
   Readily cries out in pain
   Generalized to Hispanic, Middle Eastern, Mediterranean

Data from Carteret M: *Cultural aspects of pain management,* http://www.dimensionsofculture.com/2010/11/cultural-aspects-of-pain-management. Accessed October 29, 2014.

BOX 27-2   Consequences of Untreated Pain

Falls and other accidents
Functional impairment
Slowed rehabilitation
Mood changes
Increased health care costs
Caregiver strain
Sleep disturbance
Changes in nutritional status
Impaired cognition
Increased dependency and helplessness
Depression, anxiety, fear
Decline in social and recreational activities
Increased health care utilization and costs

Data from American Geriatrics Society: Pharmacological management of persistent pain in older persons, *J Am Geriatr Soc* 57:1331–1346, 2009.

BOX 27-3   Barriers to Pain Management in Older Adults

Health Care Professional Barriers
Lack of education regarding pain assessment and management
Concern regarding regulatory scrutiny
Fears of opioid-related side effects/addiction
Belief that pain is a normal part of aging
Belief that cognitively impaired elders have less pain; lack of ability to assess pain in cognitively impaired
Personal beliefs and experiences with pain
Inability to accept self-report without "objective" signs

Patient and Family Barriers
Fear of medication side effects
Concerns related to addiction
Belief that pain is a normal part of the aging process
Belief that nothing can be done for pain in "old people"
Fear of being a "bad patient" if complaining/fear of what pain may signal

Health Care System Barriers
Cost
Time
Cultural and political bias regarding opioid use

Modified from Hanks-Bell M, Halvey K, Paice JA: Pain assessment and management in aging, *Online J Issues Nurs* 9:8, 2004. http://www.nursingworld.org/MainMenuCategories/ANAMarketplace/ANAPeriodicals/OJIN/TableofContents/Volume92004/No3Sept04/ArticlePreviousTopic/PainAssessmentandManagementinAging.html Barber JB, Gibson SJ: Treatment of chronic non-malignant pain in the elderly: safety considerations, *Drug Saf* 32:457–474, 2009.

BOX 27-4   TIPS FOR BEST PRACTICE
Potential Impact of Persistent Pain in the Older Adult

Depression
Sleep disturbances
Loss or worsening of physical function and fitness
Loneliness due to loss of social support/withdrawal from social activities
Loss of ability to perform usual role activities
Loss of ability to perform prior leisure activities
Potential for drug/alcohol abuse or misuse

Adapted from Epplin JJ, Higuchi M, Gajendra N, et al: Persistent pain. In Ham RJ, Sloane PD, Warshaw GA, et al, editors: *Primary care geriatrics: a case-based approach,* ed 6, Philadelphia, 2014, Elsevier, pp 306–314.

PAIN IN THE OLDER ADULT

Anywhere between 25% and 50% of older adults living in the community are thought to have persistent pain, and 65% of those in nursing homes have undertreated pain (Epplin et al, 2014). The barriers to adequate pain management in older adults are many (Box 27-3), and the impact is significant (Box 27-4).

The most common types of non–cancer pain in late life are nociceptive and neuropathic (Box 27-5). Both occur frequently. Nociceptive pain can often be at least temporarily relieved by the common nonpharmacological and pharmacological approaches available today. Neuropathic pain may be very difficult to adequately treat.

There is much debate over the question of elders "feeling less pain" than younger adults, especially those who are cognitively impaired. There is now evidence that there is indeed a difference in both pain perception and pain tolerance. With aging there is a decrease in the density of both myelinated and unmyelinated nerve fibers that very slightly delays the sensation of pain from the periphery. At the same time, there is slower resolution once pain is triggered. Although physical pain may not be felt as quickly, it also is less tolerated to some extent (Epplin et al, 2014).

In later life, acute pain is often superimposed on persistent pain, and in an effort to treat either we add an iatrogenic source of new pain. An example follows:

97-year-old Helen Thomas lives alone, considers herself well, and is almost always bright and cheerful. She has had osteoarthritis for the last 30 years. Her hips ache most of the time and keep her from doing everything she wants to do, but she "does pretty good for an old lady." She takes over-the-counter NSAIDs every day to take away the "sharp" pain in her hip. When walking her dog in the snow, she falls and breaks a hip. She has considerable postoperative hip pain, but she does not want to "bother the nurses." She becomes

BOX 27-5 Common Conditions that Produce Neuropathic Pain

Stroke
Diabetes
Peripheral vascular disease
Herpes zoster
Degenerative disk disease

BOX 27-6 Pain Cues in the Person with Communication Difficulties

Changes in Behavior
Restlessness and/or agitation or reduction in movement
Repetitive movements
Physical tension such as clenching teeth or hands
Unusually cautious movements, guarding

Activities of Daily Living
Sudden resistance to help from others
Decreased appetite
Decreased sleep

Vocalizations
Person groans, moans, or cries for unknown reasons
Person increases or decreases usual vocalizations

Physical Changes
Pleading expression
Grimacing
Pallor or flushing
Diaphoresis (sweating)
Increased pulse, respirations, or blood pressure

less talkative, irritable, and declares that she "just wishes they would give me that pill I take at home." When the nurse conducts a thorough assessment, she finds that Ms. Thomas is slightly confused, is getting very little sleep, and now has a pressure ulcer on her coccyx. She complains that her repaired hip hurts most of the time, as does her "good side" and now her "tail bone." Ms. Thomas has been prescribed Tylenol with codeine as needed but she takes very little of it. She is resistive to rehabilitation.

Ms. Thomas had been living with persistent pain when a traumatic event occurred that would ordinarily (in anyone) result in acute pain. While she was cheerful, there was no reasonable expectation that the persistent pain in the other hip had disappeared. When assessed, she reports ongoing pain but was not being given medications on a regular basis, and therefore her pain was undertreated. It is reasonable to believe that the lack of pain management led to her staying in one position for long periods of time, which is now a cause for iatrogenic pain—an immobility-related pressure ulcer. It is most likely that her cognitive status is being compromised by her sleeplessness, undertreated pain, and immobility. Unless there is an interruption in this cycle, Ms. Thomas will likely continue to deteriorate and quickly lose her independence.

Pain in Elders with Cognitive Impairments

Persons with cognitive impairments are consistently untreated or undertreated for pain (Corbett et al, 2014). Studies have shown that older adults who are cognitively impaired receive less pain medication, even when they experience the same acutely painful events, such as fractures, that would cause pain in others. Many cognitively impaired adults also have both nociceptive and neuropathic persistent painful conditions such as arthritis or post-herpetic neuralgia to add to their neurocognitive condition. However, according to Herr and Decker (2004, pp. 47-48):

There is no convincing evidence that peripheral nociceptor responses of pain transmission are impaired in people with dementia, although controversy does exist about central nervous system changes that influence or diminish interpretation of pain transmission. Those with dementia may have altered affective responses to pain, probably due to their inability to cognitively process the painful sensation in the context of prior pain experience, attitudes, knowledge, and beliefs.

As a result, responses to painful experiences may be different from the "typical" response of a person who is cognitively intact (Ahn and Horgas, 2013). It is best to practice under the

"assumption that any condition that is painful to a cognitively intact person would also be painful to those with advanced dementia who cannot express themselves" (Herr et al, 2010). Self-report scales have been found to be useful to some individuals, even those with mild to moderate cognitive impairment. Suspected pain should always be treated.

Research has suggested that communication of pain by persons who are nonverbal, either from dementia or from dysarthria following a stroke, is usually through changes in behavior, such as agitation, aggression, increased confusion, or passivity (Corbett et al, 2014). Although self-report scales may be possible, those with severe impairment or complete loss of language skills may be unable to communicate the presence of pain in a manner that is easily understood. Instead, the careful observations by those most familiar with the person can provide the assessment information that is needed (Herr and Decker, 2004; Herr et al, 2006; Kovach et al, 2006; Ware et al, 2006). Both formal and informal caregivers can be educated to be particularly alert for passive behaviors because they are less disruptive and may not be recognized as changes that may signal pain (Corbett et al, 2014). Providing comfort to those who cannot express themselves requires careful observation of behavior and attention to caregiver reports and knowing when subtle changes have occurred (Box 27-6). In nursing homes and other care settings, certified nursing assistants play an important role in making these observations.

◆ PROMOTING HEALTHY AGING: IMPLICATIONS FOR GERONTOLOGICAL NURSING

Pain management is that in which both pharmacological and nonpharmacological interventions work in harmony. The basic approach to pain management and control is one suggesting that whatever has worked in the past and been effective without causing harm should be encouraged. This is particularly applicable for older adults with a lifetime of experience at managing pain with both the approaches used in Western medicine and those learned through their cultural heritage.

◆ Assessment

The nurse is often the first one to hear the person's call for comfort of any kind, regardless of the setting, the type of nursing practice, or the means of expression. The assessment provides the information needed to guide the nurse, the older adult, and the caregiver(s) to find a means to address the pain in a culturally acceptable manner. Depending on culture, the elder may not relate pain complaints unless directly asked specific questions such as, "Do you hurt anywhere?" "Do you have pain now?" "Where is your pain?" "Do you have pain every day?" "Does pain keep you from sleeping at night or doing your daily activities?" It is of utmost importance that the language used by the nurse is consistent with that of the patient.

The use of standardized, evidence-based instruments and the unbiased communication of the results forms the basis to the provision of the highest quality care for the person experiencing pain. The assessment should be used whenever it is reasonable to presume pain (e.g., after an acute event such as a fracture or at the time of high risk of neuropathic pain such as from an outbreak of shingles). In skilled nursing facilities an assessment is a required part of the "MDS" (Chapter 7) (Centers for Medicare and Medicaid Services [CMS], 2014). It should be repeated at intervals to consistently measure the pain trajectory.

A high-quality comprehensive instrument (Figure 27-1) incorporates the most important aspects of the assessment in the order most often acceptable to the person. It includes the person's self-reported assessment of both qualitative and quantitative measures of comfort. For the cognitively intact elder, the first part of the assessment may begin with identifying the location of the pain (or other word used by the person). The identification of the intensity of the pain can be determined verbally when the person is asked to describe the intensity of pain from the worst pain the person can imagine to the least pain on a verbal scale of 1 to 10, with 10 being the highest level of pain (referred to as a Numerical Rating Scale [NRS]) and include qualifiers (e.g., sharp, dull, aching). There are a number of other very useful and tested pain intensity rating scales that can be used. Traditional aspects of the nursing assessment are used to determine the onset, duration, relieving and aggravating factors, and effect on quality of life. A comprehensive pain assessment includes the identification of the factors influencing the pain experience, especially depression since it is frequently a comorbid condition. If the cause is something for which there is little control, such as one of the pain syndromes, a "pain" or "comfort" goal is set (Box 27-7). With this information the nurse can help the patient work to achieve a level of pain that is no more than they find tolerable.

Since it is likely that an older adult has had previous experiences with pain, it is important to discuss these to increase the

opportunity to provide comfort. The discussion includes what has hurt in the past and what has helped and how the pain affected function and role (Box 27-8). Awareness of the individual's health and wellness paradigm is especially important in pain assessment (see Chapter 4). What does the pain mean? Is the pain believed to be the result of imbalance, a form of punishment, or an infection? A good pain assessment includes a determination of the cause for this pain, what has already been attempted to relieve the pain, and what additional strategies may be used to provide comfort. Detailed pain assessment protocols and videos are available through the Hartford Geriatric Nursing Institute at http://consultgerirn.org/topics/pain/want_to_know_more.

Travis and colleagues (2003) use the term iatrogenic disturbance pain (IDP) to describe a type of pain that can be caused by the care provider, such as turning the bedbound patient or even providing personal care. The authors suggest that, in some circumstances, tasks such as application of a blood pressure cuff, transfers out of bed, bathing, and moving and repositioning patients in the bed may cause an unacceptable level of discomfort. Patients with severe physical limitations (e.g., contractures) and significant cognitive impairment and persons at the end of life may be particularly likely to experience IDP. They suggest the use of a 5-day IDP tracking sheet for assessment and monitoring of IDP. It is helpful to have at least one of those days during the weekend. If realistic, a 7-day tracking record may provide more information. Other suggestions provided include gentle handling, adequate staffing, appropriate lifting devices and techniques, analgesic administration before care or treatments that may cause discomfort, education of staff on proper lifting and moving techniques, and assessment of discomfort during the provision of routine care.

Rating the Intensity of Pain

A key element in the assessment of pain is the *intensity of pain as perceived by the person; it is always what the person says it is.* Judgment by the nurse, such as "oh that should not hurt that much" is now a completely unacceptable and unethical practice. The use of rating scales has become the standard of care. If the person is reticent in verbal self-reporting of intensity of pain, visional scales may prove more acceptable. Scales have been found to be useful for persons who are cognitively intact and in those with mild to moderate cognitive impairment. Scales that are currently available and tested may not be reliable for persons with delirium or more severe impairments (Herr et al, 2010). The same scale must be used each time the pain is reassessed (Box 27-9).

Most often used is either a Numerical Rating Scale (NRS), as recently described, or an easy-to-use, drawn format as shown in Figure 27-2, which uses a physical object such as a lined or unlined ruler. The use of an NRS requires that the person has numerical fluency and this can never be assumed. The Verbal Descriptor Scale (VDS) and the Pain Thermometer, an adaptation of the VDS, are also good choices and have been shown to be effective in the older adult population (Herr, 2002). They are also appropriate for those without numerical skills. The VDS includes adjectives describing pain, such as mild, moderate,

INITIAL PAIN ASSESSMENT TOOL

Date_____

Patient's name_____ Age _____ Room _____

Diagnosis_____ Physician _____

Nurse _____

I. LOCATION: Patient or nurse mark drawing.

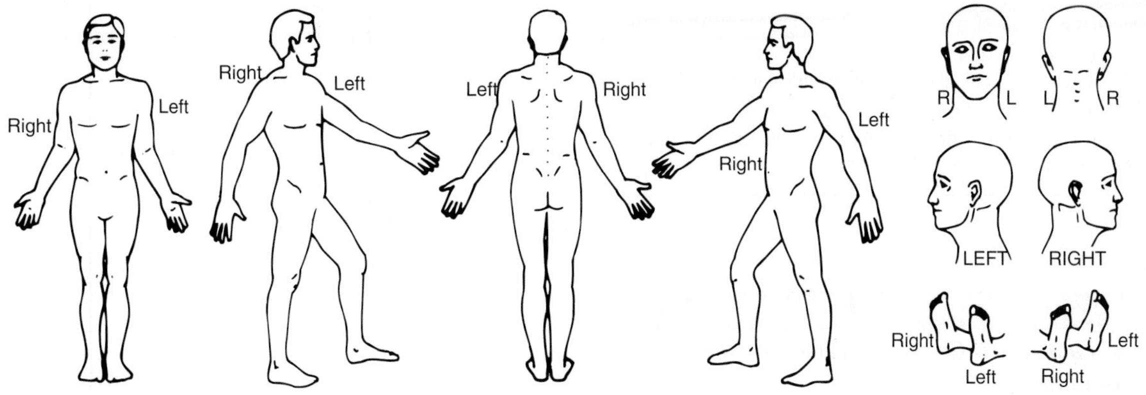

II. INTENSITY: Patient rates the pain. Scale used _____

　　Present:_____
　　Worst pain gets:_____
　　Best pain gets:_____
　　Acceptable level of pain: _____

III. QUALITY: (Use patient's own words, e.g., *prick, ache, burn, throb, pull, sharp.*) _____

IV. ONSET, DURATION VARIATIONS, RHYTHMS: _____

V. MANNER OF EXPRESSING PAIN: _____

VI. WHAT RELIEVES THE PAIN? _____

VII. WHAT CAUSES OR INCREASES THE PAIN? _____

VIII. EFFECTS OF PAIN: (Note decreased function, decreased quality of life.) _____
　　Accompanying symptoms (e.g., nausea) _____
　　Sleep_____
　　Appetite _____
　　Physical activity_____
　　Relationship with others (e.g., irritability)_____
　　Emotions (e.g., anger, suicidal, crying)_____
　　Concentration _____
　　Other _____

IX. OTHER COMMENTS: _____

X. PLAN: _____

FIGURE 27-1 Initial Pain Assessment Tool. (From McCaffery M, Bebee A: *Pain: clinical manual of nursing practice,* St Louis, MO, 1989, Mosby.)

severe, and worst pain imaginable. The Pain Thermometer is a diagram of a thermometer with word descriptions that show increasing pain intensities that can be read aloud. The Faces Pain Scale Revised (FPS-R) shows a series of faces, with each depicting a different facial expression, and may also be a useful alternative (Figure 27-3) (Hicks et al, 2001). Although it was developed for use with children, it has been found useful for adults as well. However, it can also be perceived by the person as an affective scale (e.g., emotional distress as in depression or anxiety) and must be used with caution. A scale of any kind is of no use when working with someone whose culture prohibits both the acknowledgement and expression of pain.

Setting Pain Goals

Mrs. Smith is a 92-year-old widow who lives alone. Her 74-year-old son lives next door and makes sure she has everything she needs. She has had stomach cancer for the past year. As her tumor enlarged, her pain increased, and eventually around-the-clock morphine was needed in order for her to continue her usual activities, including baking cakes for the hospice staff! The associated constipation was controlled with a stool softener, but she also had dose-related visual hallucinations. Despite efforts to lower the dose to rid her of these side effects, it was not possible to do so and maintain her pain relief. She finally declared, "I guess I will just have to learn to live with these puppies running around at my feet, better that than hurting. As least I know they are not real!"

Additional Factors to Consider When Assessing Pain in the Elderly

Function: How is the pain affecting the elder's ability to participate in usual activities, perform activities of daily living, and perform instrumental activities of daily living?

Alternative expression of pain: Have there been recent changes in cognitive ability or behavior, such as increased pacing, grimacing, or irritability? Is there an increase in the number of complaints? Are they vague and difficult to respond to? Has there been a change in sleep-wake patterns? Is the person resisting certain activities, movements, or positions?

Social support: What are the resources available to the elder in pain? What is the role of the elder in the social system, and how is pain affecting this role? How is pain affecting the elder's relationship with others?

Pain history: How has the elder managed previous experiences with pain? What is the perceived meaning of the past and present pain? What are the cultural factors that affect the elder's ability to express pain and receive relief?

For a comprehensive review of pain in older adults including copies of the tools and instructions for their use, see http://www.geriatricpain.org/Content/Assessment/Intact/Pages/default.asp.

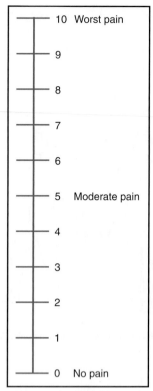

FIGURE 27-2 Numerical Rating Scale (NRS). (From Pasero C, McCaffery M: *Pain assessment and pharmacologic management,* St Louis, MO, 2011, Mosby.)

Assessment of Pain in Cognitively Impaired, Nonverbal Older Adults

The comprehensive pain assessment described previously is only possible when caring for an elder who is cognitively intact or minimally to moderately impaired. For all others, an alternate approach is needed (Box 27-10). Instead, the nurse and caregiver rely on the sometimes subtle and always confusing cues regarding the person's needs and experiences, including pain. This has been a system fraught with potential errors as the assessment varies from nurse to nurse and from shift to shift.

A consensus statement on the assessment of pain in older adults was published in 2007 by a group of international experts in the understanding of pain (Hadjistavropolous, 2007). It is recommended that attempts are made to use standard

FIGURE 27-3 Faces Pain Scale—Revised (FPS-R). Instructions: "The faces show how much pain or discomfort someone is feeling. The face on the left shows no pain. Each face shows more and more pain, and the last face shows the worst pain possible. Point to the face that shows how bad your pain is right NOW." Scoring: Score the chosen face as 0, 2, 4, 6, 8, or 10, counting left to right so 0 = "no pain" and 10 = "worst pain possible." Swartz MH: *Textbook of physical diagnosis,* ed 7, St. Louis, 2014, Saunders.

BOX 27-10 TIPS FOR BEST PRACTICE

Assessment of Pain in Persons with Impaired Communication Skills and Noncommunicative Patients

- Attempt to obtain a self-report of pain from the patient; a yes/no response is acceptable.
- If unable to obtain a self-report, document why it cannot be used and report that further observation and investigation are indicated.
- Look for possible causes of pain or discomfort, such as common conditions and procedures that cause pain (e.g., arthritis, surgery, wound care, history of persistent pain, constipation, lifting/moving).
- Medicate before performing any procedure that can cause discomfort.
- Observe and document patient behaviors that may indicate pain or distress or that are unusual from the person's normal patterns and responses. Behavioral observation scales may be used but should be used consistently and with proper training.
- Surrogate reports (family members, caregivers) of pain and behavior changes, as well as patient's usual patterns and responses to pain and discomfort. This must be from a person who knows the patient well and should be combined with the other assessment techniques.
- If comfort measures and attention to basic needs (e.g., warmth, hunger, toileting) are not effective, attempt an analgesic trial based on the intensity of the pain and analgesic history. For mild to moderate pain, administer acetaminophen every 6 hours for 24 hours. If behaviors improve, continue and add appropriate nonpharmacological interventions. If inappropriate behaviors continue, consider a single low-dose, short-acting opioid and observe effect. May titrate dose upward 25% to 50% if no change in behavior from initial dose. Continue to explore possible causes of behavior; observe for side effects and response.

From Herr K et al: Pain assessment in the nonverbal patient: position statement with clinical practice recommendations. *Pain Manag Nurs* 7:44-52, 2006.

assessment instruments first even when the person has advanced dementia. However, it is recognized that this will not likely be adequate. Alternative aspects of the assessment will be necessary and should be completed by someone who is not only familiar with the tool but also very familiar with the person.

The Pain Assessment in Advanced Dementia Scale (PAINAD Scale) was developed to be used with those who either cannot express or cannot reliably express their pain. It can be used by the nurse, the certified nursing assistant (CNA), informal caregivers, or other health care providers. It is a simple, short, focused tool that can be used on a frequent basis; it has been found to demonstrate sensitivity to change with intervention (Table 27-1). The Pain Assessment Checklist for Seniors with Limited Ability to Communicate (PACS-LAC) or the revised PACSLAC-2 is also recommended (Chan et al, 2013). They are complementary to the detailed assessment that is already required for use in skilled nursing facilities (Chapter 7). Due to the complexity of assessing pain in a nonverbal adult, the group recommended that both tools be used to determine the presence or absence of pain (i.e., at assessment and during monitoring of symptoms). Although the presence of pain may be inferred, the evaluation of the intensity of the pain for these persons is not always possible.

The PACSLAC-2 is a comprehensive behavioral assessment tool that may be very useful as an initial pain screen, as well as an interval measure. There are six domains of observation: facial expression, verbalizations and vocalizations, body movement, changes in interpersonal interactions, changes in activity patterns or routines, and mental status changes (Chan et al,

TABLE 27-1 Pain Assessment IN Advanced Dementia—PAINAD

ITEMS	0	1	2	SCORE
Breathing independent of vocalization	Normal	Occasional labored breathing Short period of hyperventilation	Noisy labored breathing Long period of hyperventilation Cheyne-Stokes respirations	
Negative vocalization	None	Occasional moan or groan Low level of speech with a negative or disapproving quality	Repeated trouble calling out Loud moaning or groaning Crying	
Facial expression	Smiling or inexpressive	Sad Frightened Frowning	Facial grimacing	
Body language	Relaxed	Tense Distressed pacing Fidgeting	Rigid Fists clenched Knees pulled up Pulling or pushing away Striking out	
Consolability	No need to console	Distracted or reassured by voice or touch	Unable to console, distract, or reassure	
			TOTAL*	

*Total scores range from 0 to 10 (based on a scale of 0 to 2 for five items), with a higher score indicating more severe pain (0 = no pain to 10 = severe pain).

From Warden V, Hurley AC, Volicer V: Development and psychometric evaluation of the Pain Assessment IN Advanced Dementia (PAINAD) Scale, *J Am Med Dir Assoc* 4:9–15, 2003.

2013). The PACSLAC-2 can serve as a guide for care regardless of who is providing it.

Detailed instructions and downloads of the PACSLAC-2 are available at www.geriatricpain.org/Content/Assessment/Impaired/Pages/default.aspx

Interventions: Providing Comfort

Working with older adults in pain and helping them achieve optimal comfort are especially challenging. Clinical manifestations are complex with multiple potential sources and sites for the pain and confounding variables such as chronic diseases, frailty, and depression. Both acute and persistent pain always interferes with health-related quality of life.

Relief of both acute and persistent pain takes commitment and determination for achievement, both on the part of the elders and on the part of formal care providers, informal care providers (as appropriate), and close family or friends. The frequency of polypharmacy and the chance of interactions cause some to hesitate, increasing the potential for undertreated or untreated pain. Persons with persistent pain are often afraid of becoming "addicted," when in reality they may need pharmacological intervention for the rest of their lives in order to maintain some level of comfort, function, and independence. Finally, there is often a societal expectation that pain is a natural part of aging or that full relief is not possible, even when quality of life is compromised.

Nonpharmacological Measures

Although pharmacological interventions have been the mainstay of the Western model of pain management, it is now well recognized that nonpharmacological measures alone, or combined with pharmacological approaches, are the most effective and appropriate way to control pain, especially the persistent pain common in later life. Most approaches have been used for dozens or even thousands of years, but more frequently the nonpharmacological measures are gaining acceptance by both patients and insurers such as Medicare. Several are described here, acknowledging that whole chapters could be devoted to any one approach. The data to support the efficacy of any one approach vary (see www.nih.nccam.gov).

Energy/touch therapies. Some say the use of touch therapies is a legacy in nursing. Over the years, different kinds of touch have been formalized to include those referred to as the contact therapy of massage (Box 27-11) (Townsend et al, 2014) and noncontact therapies such as healing touch (HT), therapeutic touch (TT), and Reiki. A review of all of the literature

---

BOX 27-11   RESEARCH NOTES

In a review of the effectiveness of massage as a form of therapeutic touch, many positive effects have been found. These include reduced pain of rheumatoid arthritis, increased immune response, and reduced depression and anxiety. Resultant changes have been evidenced in the parts of the brain controlling stress and emotional regulation.

From Field T: Massage therapy research review, *Complement Ther Clin Pract*, Aug 1, 2014. doi: 10.1016/j.ctcp.2014.07.002. [Epub ahead of print]

---

indicated modest pain relief, but the sample sizes were small (Hammerschlag et al, 2014). The acceptability of touch by individual and culture varies considerably. Some physical contact may never be acceptable, such as cross-gender touch in strict Muslim or Orthodox Jewish traditions. The culturally sensitive nurse makes no assumptions and always requests permission before touching a patient.

Transcutaneous electrical nerve stimulation. Transcutaneous electrical nerve stimulation (TENS) and transcutaneous vagal nerve stimulation have been studied for a number of years. Although there have been promising results in the treatment of acute pain, especially as an adjuvant to pharmacological approaches, there remains limited conclusive evidence related to its use (Cherian et al, 2014). Patients often anecdotally report that at least they were doing "something" for their chronic pain. TENS units are now available commercially (i.e., without prescriptions).

Acupuncture and acupressure. It is theorized that acute pain messages are sent to the brain through impulses along the nerve endings and by the production of stimulating hormones and other chemicals as they pass through a theoretical "pain gate." The "Pain Gate Theory" is one of the explanations for how acupuncture and acupressure work. It is thought that acupuncture and acupressure stimulate nerve clusters that cause the "gate to close" and block the pain from getting to the brain and then trigger the release of the body's own opiate substances, enkephalins (endorphins).

Acupuncture uses tiny needles inserted along specific meridians or pathways in the body. Acupressure is pressure applied with the thumbs or tips of the index finger at the same locations as those used in acupuncture. Acupuncture and acupressure have been used for thousands of years. Scientific evidence of their effectiveness in the treatment of persistent pain is growing and may be particularly helpful for the management of chronic pain (Hao and Mittelman, 2014; Vickers et al, 2012; Witt et al, 2006).

Relaxation, meditation, and guided imagery. Pain is often accompanied by a strong affective component. Pain is not experienced alone, but with the emotions of anger or frustration or despair (anxiety and depression). We now know that all of these emotional stressors stimulate the sympathetic nervous system, releasing norepinephrine: the strength of the mind-body connection. The norepinephrine in turn increases the sensation of pain. Hence, reducing emotional stressors lessens muscle tension and other physiological manifestations of pain. Distraction, relaxation, and meditation all enable the quieting of the mind and muscles, providing the release of tension and anxiety. Relaxation should be adjunctive to all pharmacological interventions. Meditation, mindfulness meditation, and guided imagery are methods of promoting relaxation. Imagery uses the person's imagination to focus on settings full of happiness and relaxation rather than on stressful situations. Several studies using guided imagery indicate some effect on reducing some types of pain (Meeus et al, 2014).

Music. In a review of studies of the effect of music on pain, the results were very slight but differed greatly in part due to the heterogeneity of the studies. All showed a decrease in the intensity of pain and/or opioid requirements for those with pain who listened to music (Parlac et al, 2014). McCaffrey and Freeman (2003) found music as a form of distraction to be helpful when dealing with pain from osteoarthritis, and Park (2010) found some relief for persons with dementia who listened to their preferred music.

Activity. Activity can be helpful in several ways. It is thought that the less active an individual is, the less tolerable activity becomes. Anyone who becomes inactive may feel more general discomfort than the active person. However, some activities can stimulate pain. Use of analgesics in conjunction with activity may be necessary. The administration of an analgesic medication 20 to 30 minutes before a specific activity may lessen or eliminate discomfort and fear of discomfort during and after the activity and greatly enhance the individual's capacity for that activity. The nurse should learn the patient's body tolerance for activity and work within those parameters.

Cognitive-behavioral therapy. Through cognitive-behavioral therapy (CBT), the elder learns that self-efficacy and self-care skills are both powerful mediators of pain (Linden et al, 2014; Tan et al, 2009). CBT is central to all other approaches to pain management—this means finding ways of best coping with one's circumstances. Through the setting of self-identified goals and treatment contracts with the nurse, the helplessness, hopelessness, and anxiety that often accompany persistent pain can be replaced with determination to expertly manage one's pain and increase the individually controlled interventions for comfort and prevention (Davis and White, 2008).

Pharmacological Interventions to Promote Comfort

All pharmacological interventions block pain signals from the site of pain to the brain or change its interpretation (Byrd, 2013). While treatment regimens vary, all are guided by the same underlying principles (Box 27-12). Analgesics (nonopioid and opioid agents) and many adjuvant medications (antidepressants, anticonvulsants, herbal preparations) have been found to have a role in promoting comfort in older adults in pain. In 1986 the World Health Organization introduced a

progressive three-step "ladder" as a framework for the treatment of pain as it increases in intensity or as modalities are found to be ineffective (WHO, 2014) (Figure 27-4). Although it was designed to address cancer pain, it is now applied to all pain, regardless of the type. Use of the ladder is accompanied by five recommendations: use oral formulations whenever possible; analgesics should be given at regular intervals; a pain scale of intensity should be used; dosing is based on individual needs; and formulations should be prescribed with a "constant concern for detail" (Vargas-Schaffer, 2010). The WHO three-step ladder has long been considered the standard of treatment, but there are now discussions of the appropriateness of adding a fourth step, indicating qualitative measures of the opioids (e.g., mild, moderate, strong) and taking into account the approaches that were not available when the ladder was developed, such as neurosurgical stimulators, nerve blocks, and other invasive procedures (Vargas-Schaffer, 2010).

To achieve the highest level of pain control, it is helpful to ease the "memory of pain," especially for those whose persistent pain is intense (e.g., some neuropathic pain or cancer-related pain). This means that it is necessary to prevent the pain, not simply relieve it. The most effective way to do this is to provide around-the-clock (ATC) dosing, at the appropriate dosage; it provides a more stable therapeutic plasma level of the analgesics and eliminates the extremes of overmedication and undermedication (WHO, 2014). Additional analgesics are prescribed on an as-needed basis (PRN) and should be used freely for pain that "breaks through" the ATC management (Portenoy et al, 2006). The medications that are used and the dosing will need to be determined, but with long-acting and sustained-release formulations currently available, some level of ATC relief should be possible.

Nonopioid analgesics. Acetaminophen is considered the initial treatment for persistent mild to moderate pain (American Geriatrics Society [AGS], 2009; Epplin et al, 2014; Sandvik et al, 2014). It has been found to be effective for the most

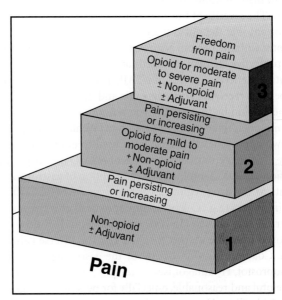

FIGURE 27-4 WHO Step Ladder. World Health Organization (WHO) three-step analgesic ladder. (Redrawn from World Health Organization: *Cancer pain relief,* ed 2, Geneva, 1996, WHO.)

common causes of pain such as osteoarthritis and back pain. With few side effects or drug interactions, it can be used for ATC dosing if this provides relief. While a maximum of 4 grams (g) in a 24-hour period is appropriate for younger adults, a maximum of only 3 g a day should be considered for older adults, especially in those with renal or hepatic compromise. A current problem is that the marketed dosing is 500-mg "extra strength" (interpreted as extra relief) tablets, caplets, gel caps, or topical preparations. Extended-release 650-mg tablets are also available. When older adults are accustomed to taking two tablets of the 325-mg tablets, the maximum dose may be quickly and inadvertently reached. The maximum of 3 g (or 4 g) includes all sources. For those with moderate pain who are also taking medications containing acetaminophen, such as hydrocodone, this must be taken into account.

Nonsteroidal antiinflammatory drugs (NSAIDs) block the pain message from the site to the sensation point in the brain and reduce inflammation. They have been highly useful when persistent pain is of an inflammatory nature (e.g., rheumatoid arthritis) or during a short inflammatory flair such as following a muscle strain. Unlike acetaminophen, NSAIDs have a higher side effect profile and drug and disease interactions, all of which are particularly dangerous to older adults. They may affect blood pressure, renal function, and heart failure and therefore may be contraindicated. The severity of gastrointestinal (GI) toxicity increases with age (Epplin et al, 2014). NSAIDs bind with proteins and may induce toxic responses in elders if serum albumin levels are low (e.g., those who are frail or with protracted chronic diseases). Other drugs that elders routinely take compete for the same protein receptor sites and may be displaced by the NSAID, creating unstable therapeutic effects. In some persons, nonacetylated NSAIDs (e.g., trisalicylate) may be alternatives but are associated with more GI toxicity.

The two formulations most commonly used are ibuprofen and naproxen (Naprosyn). Many people have ibuprofen available to them at home or it is easily accessible to them (Wehling, 2014). The severity of the GI toxicity increases with age and it is important that the nurse shares this information with each encounter with the person. Naprosyn is a COX-1/COX-2 inhibitor (GI protective element included) and therefore has fewer detrimental GI effects. The use of NSAIDS is contraindicated in use by persons receiving anticoagulants and must be used with extreme caution by those with hypertension. When used with acetaminophen there is a high death rate (Wehling, 2014).

Two approaches that have been used to address the potentially life-threatening consequences of NSAID use are the introduction of COX-2 inhibitors or the addition of gastroprotective agents to the drug regimen. Cyclooxygenase-2 (COX-2) selective inhibitors (e.g., Celebrex) appear to be as effective and have fewer GI side effects. However, two others in this group were removed from the market for their risk for adverse cardiac effects. Coadminstriion of any of the gastric agents available (misoprostol, H_2 antagonists, or proton pump inhibitors) may be helpful and reasonable, especially for persons at a higher risk for GI bleeding. However, serious concerns remain, including an alert by the U.S. Food and Drug Administration and the American Geriatrics Society.

SAFETY ALERT

NSAID Use

In 2006, the Food and Drug Administration in the United States issued a warning regarding the concomitant use of aspirin (81 mg) and ibuprofen. When taken together, the aspirin is less cardioprotective (i.e., there is less antiplatelet effect), and the person's risk for a cardiac event increases.

For persons who take immediate-release aspirin, even a single dose of ibuprofen (400 mg), the ibuprofen should be taken at least 30 minutes after or 8 hours before the aspirin.

FDA: *Information for healthcare professionals: concomitant use of ibuprofen and aspirin,* 2006. No updated information available is from the FDA at this time. Available at http://www.fda.gov/drugs/drugsafety/postmarketdrugsafetyinformationforpatientsandproviders/ucm110510.ht.

Opioid analgesics. If long-term management of moderate to severe pain is needed, opioids are recommended (e.g., tramadol, oxycodone, hydromorphone). They have lower or more predictable adverse reactions, especially in comparison with the NSAIDs. The use of opioids is always accompanied by a multipronged approach and is often the first line of approach for neuropathic pain (Vargas-Schaffer, 2010). Due to a number of age-related changes, opioids may produce a greater analgesic effect, a higher peak, and a longer duration of action (Chapter 9). When moderate to severe acute pain or persistent pain is assessed, a short trial with clear goals is recommended along with careful clinical observation of effect. Sedation, altered mental status, and impaired cognition are common side effects when opioid analgesics are started or doses increased. Although these side effects may cause great concern to patients, families, and nurses, most are transient and may be necessary to achieve the goal of pain relief. Safety measures, such as fall precautions, are needed until the person is stabilized.

SAFETY ALERT

Meperidine (Demerol), which is used in younger adults in acute pain, is always contraindicated in the older adult.

Opioid treatment should begin with "as-needed" doses of short-acting medications and should be titrated based on the amount needed, response obtained, and side effects over at least a 24-hour period then changed to an around-the-clock (ATC) formulation (e.g. MS Contin). Current recommendations are to start with the lowest anticipated effective dose, monitor the response frequently, and increase the dose slowly to desired effect: "Start low, go slow, but go!"

If a change is needed from one drug to another, and the dose of active ingredient is known, then conversion resources are available so that the patient can remain pain free. A conversion table is available at http://clincalc.com/Opioids/

Additional nonopioids and adjuvant medications or short-acting opioids can be used for breakthrough PRN treatment. However, if PRN medications are needed regularly, the long-acting opioid dosage should be adjusted accordingly. Unfortunately, too often the titration is not done (i.e., dosages are not adjusted after the original prescription) and pain relief is inadequate, especially in the long-term care setting (Hutt et al, 2006).

Side effects of opioids are significant to older adults; they include gait disturbance, dizziness, sedation, falls, nausea, pruritus, and constipation (Shorr et al, 2007). Several of these will resolve on their own as the body develops tolerance to the drug. Some side effects may be prevented when the prescribing provider works closely with the patient and the nurse to slowly increase the dose of the drug to a point where the best relief can be obtained with the fewest side effects. Because constipation is almost universal when opioids are used, the nurse should ensure that an appropriate bowel regimen is begun at the same time as the opioids. A daily dose of a combination stool softener and mild laxative may be very helpful, and adequate fluid intake is essential. Prophylactic use of an antiemetic may be helpful for associated nausea until tolerance develops.

Adjuvant drugs. There are a number of drugs developed for other purposes that have been found to be useful in pain management, sometimes alone, but more often in combination with an analgesic; these are referred to as *adjuvant drugs*. They include steroids, anxiolytics, hypnotics, antidepressants, and anticonvulsants. The antidepressants in the selective serotonin reuptake inhibitor (SSRI) class have not been effective in the management of nociceptive pain (AGS, 2009). Cannabinoids are being used more and more often as adjuvant drugs, especially for those with cancer pain, acquired immunodeficiency syndrome (AIDS), and other types of persistent pain. They have also been effective with neuropathic pain (Vargas-Schaffer, 2010).

The very old tricyclic antidepressants in low doses (to avoid the considerable side effects) have been found to provide relief to some with neuropathic pain. However, today the anti-epileptic–like drugs such as gabapentin are used more often. While the mechanism is unknown, the mixed serotonin and norepinephrine reuptake inhibitors (SNRIs) such as duloxetine (Cymbalta) and venlafaxine (Effexor) seem to be effective as well.

Pain Clinics

Pain clinics provide a specialized, often comprehensive and multidisciplinary approach to the management of pain that has not responded to the usual, more standard approaches as described herein. Their use should be encouraged when appropriate. The number and types of pain clinics and programs have increased in response to continued poor pain management in general health care practice. Pain center programs may be inpatient, outpatient, or both. They are generally one of three types: syndrome-oriented, modality-oriented, or comprehensive. Syndrome-oriented centers focus on a specific chronic pain problem, such as headache or arthritis pain. Modality-oriented centers focus on a specific treatment technique, such as relaxation or acupuncture/acupressure. The comprehensive centers tend to be larger and associated with medical centers. These centers include many services and provide a thorough initial assessment (physical, mental, psychosocial) of the person in pain. A comprehensive treatment plan is developed utilizing multiple modalities and a multidisciplinary team of interventionists. The nurse should be familiar with the types of pain management clinics available in their communities to provide the patient and family with necessary information to make a knowledgeable decision in selecting a reputable center.

Evaluation of Effectiveness

While the effectiveness of any intervention designed to relieve pain is quantitatively measured with the repeated use of the intensity scale, qualitative observations by the nurse supplement this. Qualitative indicators of better management or relief include physical changes such as relaxation of muscles that were tense and rigid or a relaxed position rather than one that was constricted. There is an increase in activity and expressions of self-worth. The person is better able to concentrate and focus and has an increased attention span, regardless of cognitive status. The individual is better able to rest, relax, and sleep, initially for what might seem like excessively long periods, but this is in response to the exhaustion that pain imposes on the body.

The nurse works to advocate for the person so that adjustments of treatment regimens and interventions are based on reassessment findings. Treatment must always begin with low doses but they should be increased until relief is obtained. In no other circumstances is it more important than to adequately relieve pain and discomfort than it is in older adults especially those who cannot communicate their needs.

KEY CONCEPTS

- The gerontological nurse can advocate for and work with the elder and significant others to prevent needless suffering and achieve a high level of pain relief and health-related quality of life.
- Multiple modalities are available today to promote comfort, and when used together, pain can be relieved in most cases.
- The experience of pain is multifactorial with physical, psychological, and spiritual components.
- Pain is a subjective experience that is unique to each individual.
- It is the responsibility of the health care professional to address the needs of the person in pain.

- The pain most common in later life is that which is persistent.
- The undertreatment of pain in older adults, especially those in long-term care facilities, is well documented.
- A careful assessment of the presence or absence of pain is possible regardless of the cognitive status of the person who may be in pain.
- If it is reasonable to expect a person in a particular circumstance to experience pain, it is reasonable to expect that pain is being felt by the person regardless of his or her ability to express this.
- It is never acceptable to fail to treat pain (or the expectation of pain) to the extent possible.

- In many cases, acetaminophen is recommended as the first-line approach for the pharmacological management of mild to moderate pain.
- Around-the-clock dosing of the appropriate dose of the appropriate medication will most likely optimize pain relief.
- The use of NSAIDs for pain relief in the older adult must be done with caution, with knowledge of the contraindications

and the awareness of the increased risk for associated cardiac events.
- The use of opioids has been found to be very effective and has the potential to significantly restore function to persons with persistent pain.
- Optimal pain management incorporates both pharmacological and nonpharmacological approaches.

NURSING STUDY: PAIN IN ELDERS

Ms. P. was a 66-year-old woman with diabetes and, after a stroke, had to relocate to a nursing facility. In a short time her diabetes began to have uncontrollable fluctuations. Her blood glucose level ranged from 20 to 800 mEq/mL. Some of this was caused by erratic eating habits, almost no exercise, frequent urinary tract infections, and considerable stress related to her condition and her future. She bumped her toe while being assisted into her wheelchair after occupational therapy. In a few days, the bruise had sloughed skin, and an open sore was evident. In spite of appropriate treatment, the sore became necrotic and was debrided. Ms. P., who rarely complained, began to moan while she was sleeping and cry a lot during the day. She complained of a continuous burning sensation and said that it felt as if her toe was "on fire." One day she threw her coffee cup

across the room complaining that it was not hot enough. Various pain medications were given by mouth on an inconsistent basis, but the relief she experienced was minimal. She began to beg to die. The nurses thought perhaps she was right—after all, her general condition was poor, and life held little satisfaction for her.

- What is the objective and subjective information in the above nursing study?
- Discuss Ms. P.'s situation and her probable prognosis.
- What could be done, on the information you have, to improve Ms. P.'s condition?
- Do you think nurses are concerned about addiction in cases like that of Ms. P.?

CRITICAL THINKING QUESTIONS AND ACTIVITIES

1. Discuss the reasons for sporadic pain medication and inattention to the patient's signals and requests.
2. In what situations do you believe addiction to pain medications is a priority concern?

3. Discuss issues of power and control related to pain management.

RESEARCH QUESTIONS

1. Do pain perceptions generally diminish as one ages?
2. What type of persistent pain do elders find most intolerable?
3. How do elders describe the pain of arthritis?
4. What nonpharmacological means of pain control do elders use most frequently?
5. What nonpharmacological means of pain control are effective, and in what circumstances do they provide pain relief?

6. How effective is patient-controlled analgesia (PCA) use by elders?
7. For whom and under what circumstances should the various modalities of pain management be used?
8. How does culture influence pain expression and treatment?
9. What culturally based remedies for pain are used and what is their efficacy?

REFERENCES

Ahn H, Horgas A: Does pain mediate or moderate the effect of cognitive impairment on aggression in nursing home residents with dementia? *Asian Nurs Resc (Korean Nurs Sci)* 8(2):105–109, 2014.

American Geriatrics Society (AGS): Pharmacological management of persistent pain in older persons: American Geriatrics Society Panel on the Pharmacological Management of Persistent Pain in Older Persons, *J Am Geriatr Soc* 57:1331–1346, 2009. Accessed August 2014.

Byrd L: Managing chronic pain in older adults: a long-term care approach,

online *Ann Longterm Care* 21(12), 2013. http://www.annalsoflongtermcare.com/article/managing-chronic-pain-older-adult-long-term-care. Accessed August 2014.

Campbell LC, Andrews N, Scipio C, et al: Pain and coping in Latino populations, *J Pain* 10(10):1012–1019, 2009.

Centers for Medicare and Medicaid (CMS): *Quality measures: what's new,* 2014. http://www.cms.gov/Medicare/Quality-Initiatives-Patient-Assessment-Instruments/NursingHomeQualityInits/NHQIQualityMeasures.html.

Chan S, Hadjistavropoulos T, Williams J, et al: Evidence-based development and initial validation of the Pain Assessment Checklist for Seniors with Limited Ability to Communicate-II (PACSLAC-II), *Clin J Pain,* November 2013. [Epub ahead of print].

Cherian JJ, Kapadia BH, Bhave A, et al: Use of transcutaneous nerve stimulation in early arthritis of the knee, *J Knee Surg* August 27, 2014. [Epub ahead of print].

Corbett A, Husebo BS, Achterberg WP, et al: The importance of pain management in older people with dementia, *Br Med Bull* 111(1):139–148, 2014.

Davis GC, White TL: A goal attainment pain management program for older adults with arthritis, *Pain Manag Nurs* 9:171–179, 2008.

Epplin JJ, Higuchi M, Gajendra N, et al: Persistent pain. In Ham RJ, Sloane PD, Warshaw GA, et al, editors: *Primary care geriatrics: a case-based approach*, ed 6, Philadelphia, Elsevier, 2014, pp 306–314.

Hadjistavropoulos T, Herr K, Turk DC, et al: An interdisciplinary expert consensus statement on assessment of pain in older persons, *Clin J Pain* 23 (Suppl 1):S1–43, 2007.

Hammerschlag R, Marx BL, Aickin M: Nontouch biofield therapy: a systematic review of human randomized controlled trials reporting use of only nonphysical contact treatment, *J Complement Med*, September 2, 2014. [Epub ahead of print].

Hao JJ, Mittleman M: Acupuncture: past present and future, *Glob Adv Health Med* 3(4):6–8, 2014.

Herr K: Chronic pain: challenges and assessment strategies, *J Gerontol Nurs* 28:20–27, 2002.

Herr K, Bursch H, Ersek M, et al: Use of pain-behavioral assessment tools in the nursing home: expert consensus recommendations for practice, *Gerontol Nurs* 36:18–29, 2010.

Herr K, Coyne PJ, Key T, et al: Pain assessment in the nonverbal patient: position statement with clinical practice recommendations, *Pain Manag Nurs* 7:44–52, 2006.

Herr K, Decker S: Assessment of pain in older adults with severe cognitive impairment, *Ann Longterm Care* 12:46–52, 2004.

Hicks CL, von Baeyer CL, Spafford PA, et al: The Faces Pain Scale—revised: toward a common metric in pediatric pain measurement, *Pain* 93:173–183, 2001.

Horgas A, Ahn H: The relationship between pain and disruptive behavior in nursing home residents with dementia, *BMC Geriatr* 13:14, 2013.

Hutt E, Pepper GA, Vojir C, et al: Assessing the appropriateness of pain medication prescribing practices in nursing homes, *J Am Geriatr Soc* 54:231–239, 2006.

International Association for the Study of Pain (IASP): *IASP taxonomy*, 2014.

http://www.iasp-pain.org/Education/Content.aspx?ItemNumber=1698#Nociceptivepain. Accessed August 2014.

Jansen MP: Pain in older adults. In Jansen MP, editor: *Managing pain in the older adult*, New York, 2008, Springer.

Kovach C, Logan BR, Noonan PE, et al: Effects of the Serial Trial Intervention on discomfort and behavior of nursing home residents with dementia, *Am J Alzheimers Dis Other Dement* 21:147–155, 2006.

Linden M, Scherbe S, Cicholas B: Randomized controlled trial on the effectiveness of cognitive behavior group therapy in chronic back pain patients, *J Back Musculoskelet Rehabil*, Aug 5, 2014. [Epub ahead of print].

McCaffrey R, Freeman E: Effect of music on chronic osteoarthritis pain in older people, *J Adv Nurs* 44:517–524, 2003.

Meeus M, Nijs J, Vanderheiden T, et al: The effect of relaxation therapy on autonomic functioning, symptoms and daily functioning in patients with chronic fatigue syndrome or fibromyalgia: a systematic review, *Clin Rehabil*, September 8, 2014. [Epub ahead of print].

Molton IR, Terrill AL: Overview of persistent pain in older adults, *Am Psychol* 69(2):197–207, 2014.

Narayan MC: Culture's effect on pain assessment and management, *Am J Nurs* 110 (4):38–47, 2010.

Parlac KS, Karadag G, Oyucu S, et al: Effect of music on pain, anxiety, and patient satisfaction in patients who present to the emergency department in Turkey, *Jpn J Nurs Sci*, March 26, 2014. [Epub ahead of print].

Park H: Effect of music on pain for home-dwelling persons with dementia, *Pain Manag Nurs* 11:141–147, 2010.

Portenoy RK, Bennett DS, Rauck R, et al: Prevalence and characteristics of breakthrough pain in opioid-treated patients with chronic cancer pain, *J Pain* 7:583–591, 2006.

Sandvik RK, Selbaek G, Seifert R, et al: Impact of a stepwise protocol for treating pain on pain intensity in nursing home patients with dementia: a cluster randomized trial, *Eur J Pain*, May 13, 2014. [Epub ahead of print].

Shorr RI, Hoth AB, Rawls N: *Drugs for the geriatric patient*, St. Louis, MO, 2007, Saunders.

Tan EP, Tan ES, Ng BY: Efficacy of cognitive behavioral therapy for patients with chronic pain in Singapore, *Ann Acad Med Singapore* 38:952–959, 2009.

Townsend CS, Bonham E, Chase L, et al: A comparison of still point induction to massage therapy in reducing pain and increasing comfort in chronic pain, *Holistic Nurs Pract* 28(2):78–84, 2014.

Travis SS, Menscer D, Dixon SO, et al: Assessing and managing iatrogenic disturbance pain for frail, dependent adults in long-term care situations, *Ann Longterm Care* 11:33, 2003.

Vargas-Schaffer G: Is the WHO analgesic ladder still valid? *Can Fam Physician* 56(6):514–517, 2010.

Vickers AJ, Chronin AM, Maschino AC, et al: Acupuncture for chronic pain: individual patient data meta-analysis, *Arch Intern Med*, September 10, 2012. [Epub ahead of print].

Warden V, Hurley AC, Volicer L: Development and psychometric evaluation of the pain assessment in advanced dementia (PAINAD) scale, *J Am Med Dir Assoc* 4:9–15, 2003.

Ware LJ, Epps CD, Herr K, et al: Evaluation of the Revised Faces Pain Scale, Verbal Descriptor Scale, Numeric Rating Scale, and Iowa Pain Thermometer in older minority adults, *Pain Manag Nurs* 7:117–125, 2006.

Wehling M: Non-steroidal anti-inflammatory drugs use in chronic pain conditions with special emphasis on the elderly and patients with relevant comorbidities: management and mitigation of risks and adverse effects, *Eur J Clin Pharmacol* 70(10):1159–1172, 2014.

Witt CM, Jena S, Brinkhaus B, et al: Acupuncture in patients with osteoarthritis of the knee or hip: a randomized, controlled trial with an additional nonrandomized arm, *Arthritis Rheum* 54:3485–3493, 2006.

World Health Organization (WHO): *WHO's cancer pain ladder for adults*, 2014. http://www.who.int/cancer/palliative/painladder/en/. Accessed August 2014.

28 CHAPTER

Mental Health

Theris A. Touhy

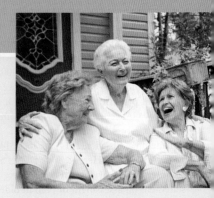

🅔 http://evolve.elsevier.com/Touhy/TwdHlthAging

A STUDENT SPEAKS

I find it a bit depressing to think about getting old. This is such a fun time in my life. But, when you think about it, older people don't have to worry about school or a job. Some of the elders I met at the retirement community are busier than I am and don't seem depressed. But, then there are those who are in nursing homes and I am sure they are depressed and lonely. I think it's important to enjoy each day now because you just don't know what life will bring when you're old.

Roseanna, age 23

AN ELDER SPEAKS

An older man wrote his philosophy succinctly:

I have no idea about what would constitute happiness for anyone else, considering the differences in taste and preferences, and no spate of ideas about improving the lot of the aged. But I am sure that among other things, a calm acceptance of the facts of life is a great help. I consider serenity and peace of mind two of the greatest gifts I have, although I cannot tell you where they came from or how to get them.

(Burnside, 1975)

LEARNING OBJECTIVES

On completion of this chapter, the reader will be able to:

1. Discuss factors contributing to mental health and wellness in late life.
2. Discuss the effect of chronic mental health problems on individuals as they age.
3. List symptoms of anxiety and depression in older adults, and discuss assessment, treatment, and nursing interventions.
4. Recognize elders who are at risk for suicide, and utilize appropriate techniques for suicide assessment and interventions.
5. Specify several indications of substance abuse in elders, and discuss appropriate nursing responses.
6. Evaluate interventions aimed at promoting mental health and wellness in older adults.
7. Develop an individualized nursing plan of care for an older person with depression and bipolar disorder.

Mental health is not different in later life, but the level of challenge may be greater. Developmental transitions, life events, physical illness, cognitive impairment, and situations calling for psychic energy may interfere with mental health in older adults. These factors, though not unique to older adults, often influence adaptation. However, anyone who has survived 80 or so years has been exposed to many stressors and crises and has developed tremendous resistance. Most older people face life's challenges with equanimity, good humor, and courage. It is our task to discover the strengths and adaptive mechanisms that will assist them to cope with the challenges.

Well-being in late life can be predicted by cognitive and affective functioning earlier in life. Thus, it is very important to know the older person's past patterns and life history (Chapter 6). Qualls (2002) offered the following comprehensive definition of mental health in aging: A mentally healthy person is "one who accepts the aging self as an active being, engaging available strengths to compensate for weaknesses in order to create personal meaning, maintain maximum autonomy by mastering the environment, and sustain positive relationships with others" (p. 12).

Mental, neurological, and substance abuse disorders (MNS) are prevalent in all regions of the world and are major contributors to morbidity and premature mortality. In both the developed and developing world, mental health care for older adults lags behind that for other age groups and mental disorders have not received adequate attention in global health (Baxter et al, 2014; Pachana, 2013). Low-and lower-middle income countries have most of the global burden of MNS disorders and also the most limited human and financial resources (World Health Organization [WHO], 2013). In response to these needs, the World Health Organization created the Mental Health Gap Action Programme (mhGAP) to increase activities and programs for mental, neurological, and substance abuse disorders, particularly in low-and lower-middle income countries (World Health Organization, 2014).

In the United States, including older adults with dementia, nearly 20% of people older than age 55 experience mental health disorders that are not part of normal aging. Global data on mental health are lacking when compared with data on other important health problems, but data on older people appear to mirror the data in the United States (WHO, 2014). For most of the world's population, mental disorders are invisible and remain a low priority (Baxter et al, 2013). The prevalence of mental health disorders may be even higher than reported statistics because these disorders are both not always reported and not well researched, especially among non-white populations. Predictions are that the number of older people with mental illness will soon overwhelm the mental health system.

Many individuals in the baby boomer generation have experienced mental health consequences from military conflict, and the 20th century drug culture will also add to the burden of psychiatric illnesses in the future. The baby boomer generation is also more aware of mental health concerns and more comfortable seeking treatment, which will add to the challenges facing the mental health care system. The most prevalent mental health problems in late life are anxiety, severe cognitive impairment, and mood disorders. Alcohol abuse and dependence are also growing concerns among older adults. Mental health disorders are associated with increased use of health care resources and overall costs of care. *Healthy People 2020* (U.S. Department of Health and Human Services [USDHHS], 2012) includes mental health and mental health disorders as a topic area (Box 28-1).

The focus of this chapter is on the differing presentation of mental health disturbances that may occur in older adults and the nursing interventions important in maintaining the mental health and self-esteem of older adults at the optimum of their capacity. Readers should refer to a comprehensive psychiatric–mental health text for more in-depth discussion of mental health disorders. A discussion of cognitive impairment and the behavioral symptoms that may accompany this disorder is found in Chapter 29.

STRESS AND COPING IN LATE LIFE

Stress and Stressors

To understand mental health and mental health disorders in aging, it is important to be aware of stressors and their effect on the functioning of older people. The experience of stress is an internal state accompanying threats to self. Healthy stress levels motivate one toward growth, whereas stress overload diminishes

BOX 28-1   HEALTHY PEOPLE 2020

Mental Health and Mental Disorder (Older Adults)

- Reduce the suicide rate.
- Reduce the proportion of persons who experience major depressive episodes.
- Increase the proportion of primary care facilities that provide mental health treatment on-site or by paid referral.
- Increase the proportion of adults with mental disorders who receive treatment.
- Increase the proportion of persons with co-occurring substance abuse and mental disorders who receive treatment for both disorders.
- Increase depression screening by primary care providers.
- Increase the proportion of homeless adults with mental health problems who receive mental health services.

From U.S. Department of Health and Human Services, Office of Disease Prevention and Health Promotion: *Healthy People 2020,* 2012. http://www.healthypeople.gov/2020

one's ability to cope effectively. As a person ages, many situations and conditions occur that may create disruptions in daily life and drain one's inner resources or create the need for new and unfamiliar coping strategies. The narrowing range of biopsychosocial homeostatic resilience and the changing environmental needs that occur with aging may produce a stress overload (Evans, 2008).

Effects of Stress

There is ongoing research about the connection between emotions and health and illness, but it is known that the mind and body are integrated and cannot be approached as separate entities. Stress may reduce one's coping ability and negatively impact neuroendocrine responses that ultimately impair immune function, and older adults show greater immunological impairments associated with distress or depression. Research on psychoneuroimmunology has explored the relationship between psychological stress and various health conditions such as cardiovascular disease, type 2 diabetes, certain cancers, Alzheimer's disease, frailty, and functional decline. The production of proinflammatory cytokines influencing these and other conditions can be directly stimulated by negative emotions and stressful experiences.

Older people often experience multiple, simultaneous stressors (Box 28-2). Some older people are in a chronic state of grief because new losses occur before prior ones are fully resolved; stress then becomes a constant state of being. The ability to tolerate stress varies between individuals and is influenced by current and ongoing stressors, by health, and also by coping ability. For example, if an elder has lost a significant person in the previous year, the grief may be manageable. If he or she has lost a significant person and developed painful, chronic health problems, the consequences may be quite different and can cause stress overload. In the older adult, stress may appear as a cognitive impairment or behavior change that will be alleviated as the stress is reduced to the parameters of the individual's adaptability. Regardless of whether stress is physical or emotional, older people will

BOX 28-2   Potential Stressors in Late Life

Abrupt internal and external body changes and illnesses
Other-oriented concerns: children, grandchildren, spouse, or partner
Loss of significant people
Functional impairment
Sensory impairments
Memory impairment (or fear of)
Loss of ability to drive (particularly men)
Acute discomfort and pain
Breach in significant relationships
Retirement (lost social roles, income)
Ageist attitudes
Fires, thefts
Injuries, falls
Major unexpected drain on economic resources (house repair, illness)
Abrupt changes in living arrangements to a new location (home, apartment, room, or institution)
Identity theft and fear of scams

BOX 28-3   Factors Influencing Ability to Manage Stress

- Health and fitness
- A sense of control over events
- Awareness of self and others
- Patience and tolerance
- Resilience
- Hardiness
- Resourcefulness
- Social support
- A strong sense of self

require more time to recover or return to prestress levels than younger people.

Any stressors that occur in the lives of older people may actually be experienced as a crisis if the event occurs abruptly, is unanticipated, or requires skills or resources the individual does not possess. Through a lifetime of coping with stress, some individuals have developed a tremendous stress tolerance, whereas others will be thrown into crisis by changes in their lives with which they feel unable to cope. Important to remember is that there is great individual variability in the definition of a stressor. For some, the loss of a pet canary is a major stressor; others accept the loss of a good friend with grief but without personal disorganization.

Factors Affecting Stress

Researchers concerned with the effects of stress in the lives of older people have examined many moderating variables and have concluded that cognitive style, coping strategies, social resources (social support, economic resources), personal efficacy, and personality characteristics are all significant to stress management. Social relationships and social support are particularly salient to stress management and coping. Social relationships may reduce stress and boost the immune system by providing resources (information, emotional, or tangible) that promote adaptive behavioral or neuroendocrine responses to acute or chronic stressors (Holt-Lunstad et al, 2010). In fact, individuals with adequate social relationships have a 50% greater likelihood of survival compared with those with poor or insufficient social relationships, an effect comparable with quitting smoking and exceeding many known risk factors for mortality (e.g., obesity, physical inactivity) (Holt-Lunstad et al, 2010; Umberson and Montez, 2010).

Some factors that influence one's ability to manage stress are presented in Box 28-3. Resilience and resourcefulness have been associated with coping with stress and crisis and may explain the ability of some individuals to withstand stress. We know the qualities associated with resilience and resourcefulness, but it is

not clear if they are personality traits or processes by which the individual responds to the environment. Further research is needed to more fully understand these concepts and their relationship to positive outcomes.

Resilience

Resilience is a concept closely related to hardiness that is associated with coping with stress and crisis. Resilience is defined as "flourishing despite adversity" (Hildon et al, 2009, p. 36). The process of resilience is characterized by successfully adapting to difficult and challenging life experiences, especially those that are highly stressful or traumatic. Resilient people "bend rather than break" during stressful conditions and are able to return to adequate (and sometimes better) functioning after stress ("bouncing back"). Characteristics associated with resilience include positive interpersonal relationships; a willingness to extend oneself to others; optimistic or positive affect; keeping things in perspective; setting goals and taking steps to achieve these goals; high self-esteem and self-efficacy; determination; a sense of purpose in life; creativity; humor; and a sense of curiosity. These are considered personality traits, as well as ways of responding to difficult events that have been learned and developed over time (Resnick and Inguito, 2011).

Individuals who have the ability to use personal resources and see the world beyond their own concerns are most likely to be resilient. Older people may demonstrate greater resilience and ability to maintain a positive emotional state under stress than younger individuals. Social support from the community, family, and professionals; access to care; and availability of resources can facilitate resilience (van Kessel, 2012).

Resourcefulness

Resourcefulness has also been linked to positive coping with life stressors. Resourcefulness is characterized as a "cognitive behavioral repertoire of self-control skills accompanied by a belief in one's ability to cope effectively with adversity" (Zauszniewski et al, 2007, p. 576). Nursing studies examining resourcefulness training (RT) for older adults suggest that RT may enhance positive affect and cognition, promote independence, and improve function in older adults (Zauszniewski et al, 2007, 2012). RT teaches and reinforces the cognitive and behavioral skills that strengthen personal and social resourcefulness. Personal resourcefulness skills include coping strategies, problem solving, positive self-talk, priority setting, and decision-making. Social resourcefulness skills involve assisting older people to make decisions about when and how to seek help from formal and informal sources, as well as strategies to strengthen internal (self-help) and external (help-seeking) resources for maintenance of healthy functioning.

Coping

Coping is a complex developmental and multifaceted process that develops over the life span. Some experts suggest that coping may be less effective in older individuals because of increased vulnerability to health problems and other stressors. Others postulate that older adults may use more constructive coping strategies in response to stress than younger adults (Clapp and Beck, 2012). Coping may also contribute more to the health of older than younger individuals because older adults utilize it to optimize their resources. Further research with older adults is needed, but coping may be a significant component of optimal aging.

Coping Strategies

Coping strategies are the stabilizing factors that help individuals maintain psychosocial balance during stressful periods. Coping strategies involve the identification, coordination, and appropriate use of personal and environmental resources to deal with stressors. Coping is a process that begins with appraisal of the stressor's potential impact and the tools available for dealing with it. The appraisal of the stressor as benign, threat, harm/loss, or challenge guides the choice of coping strategies (Lazarus and Folkman, 1984; Yancura and Aldwin, 2008). Individuals use a mixture of coping strategies depending on the situation and their skills and experience. Individuals with more personal (cognition) and environmental resources (social network) use more varied coping strategies, and this may be related to longer life expectancy (Demers et al, 2009) (Boxes 28-4 and 28-5).

BOX 28-4 Coping Strategies of Older Adults

- Use more active strategies to avoid negative situations in the first place. When uncontrollable stress occurs, older adults do not add to this by getting involved in other stressful situations.
- Use good cognitive strategies to manage negative emotions. Keep things in perspective and avoid overreacting.
- Stay focused on positive things that can be done or positive events happening at the same time.
- Actively compare current stressors to things you have experienced and coped with in the past.
- Maximize good emotional experiences by selecting activities with familiar positive impact—turn to the really meaningful people and activities in your life during hard times.

©2007 by the American Psychological Association. Adapted with permission from the American Psychological Association: *Fostering resilience in response to terrorism: for psychologists working with older adults* (Fact sheet), 2007. http://www.apa.org/pi/aging/resources/older-adults.pdf.

BOX 28-5 Coping Strategies and Actions

1. **Problem-focused:** Behaviors and cognitions targeted toward solving or managing a problem. Involves formulating and implementing a plan.
   Types of actions: Considering alternatives, drawing on past experience, stepping back from the situation and being more objective, finding out more about the situation, learning new skills, making a plan of action.
2. **Emotion-focused:** Efforts to manage one's emotional reaction to the problem.
   Types of actions: Expressing emotions, distraction, meditation, relaxation, exercise, taking one day at a time.
3. **Social support:** Efforts to seek help and guidance from friends, family, professionals.
   Types of actions: Asking for advice, help, or assistance; seeking help from persons or groups with similar experiences; providing support to others.
4. **Religious coping:** Seeking help from a higher power.
   Types of actions: Praying for strength and guidance, attending services.
5. **Cognitive reframing:** Trying to make meaning of the situation.
   Types of actions: Focusing on the positive aspects, trying to make sense of the problem, reminding self that things could be worse, expressing gratitude for what one does have.

Adapted from Yancura L, Aldwin C: Coping and health in older adults, *Curr Psychiatry Rep* 10:10–15, 2008.

◆ PROMOTING HEALTHY AGING: IMPLICATIONS FOR GERONTOLOGICAL NURSING

◆ Assessment

General issues in the psychosocial assessment of older adults involve distinguishing among normal, idiosyncratic, and diverse characteristics of aging and pathological conditions. Baseline data are often lacking from an individual's earlier years. Using standardized tools and functional assessment is valuable, but the data will be meaningless unless placed in the context of the patient's early life and hopes and expectations for the future. An understanding of past and present history, the person's coping ability, the degree of social support, and the effect of life events are all part of a holistic assessment. Careful listening to the person's life story, an appreciation of the person's strengths, and coming to know each person in his or her own uniqueness are the cornerstones of assessment (Chapter 6).

Assessment of mental health includes examination for cognitive function and conditions of anxiety and adjustment reactions, depression, paranoia, substance abuse, and suicidal risk. Assessment of mental health must also focus on social intactness and affective responses appropriate to the situation. Attention span, concentration, intelligence, judgment, learning ability, memory, orientation, perception, problem solving, psychomotor ability, and reaction time are assessed in relation to cognitive intactness and must be considered when making a psychological assessment. Assessment includes specific processes that are intact, as well as those that are diminished or compromised. Assessment for specific mental health concerns is discussed throughout this chapter and in Chapter 7. Assessment of cognitive function is discussed in Chapters 7, 23, and 29.

Obtaining assessment data from elders is best done during short sessions after some rapport has been established. Performing repeated assessments at various times of the day and in different situations will give a more complete psychological profile. It is important to be sensitive to a patient's anxiety, special needs, and disabilities and vigilant in protecting the person's privacy. The interview should be focused so that attention is given to strengths and skills, as well as deficits.

◆ Interventions

Nurses can design individualized interventions to enhance coping ability such as reinforcing the characteristics of resilience and resourcefulness. Enhancing functional status and independence, promoting a sense of control, fostering social supports and relationships, and connecting to resources are all important nursing interventions. Practices such as meditation, yoga, exercise, and spirituality and religiosity can enhance coping ability. Mind-body therapies that integrate cognitive, sensory, expressive, and physical aspects are most helpful. Reminiscence is useful in understanding the coping style of an elder, helping the elder to remember how he or she coped successfully, suggesting how these strategies might be applied to the current situation, and enhancing self-esteem and feelings of self-worth (Chapter 6).

FACTORS INFLUENCING MENTAL HEALTH CARE

Attitudes and Beliefs

Older individuals with evidence of mental health disorders, regardless of race or ethnicity, are less likely than younger people to receive needed mental health care (Institute of Medicine, 2012; Jiminez et al, 2012). Nearly half of people older than age 65 with a recognized mental or substance use disorder have unmet needs for services (Mental Health America, 2014b). Some of the reasons for this include reluctance on the part of older people to seek help because of pride of independence, stoic acceptance of difficulty, unawareness of resources, lack of geriatric mental health professionals and services, and lack of adequate insurance coverage for mental health problems. Stigma about having a mental health disorder ("being crazy"), particularly for older people, discourages many from seeking treatment. Ageism also affects identification and treatment of mental health disorders in older people.

Symptoms of mental health problems may be looked at as a normal consequence of aging or blamed on dementia by both older people and health care professionals. In older people, the presence of comorbid medical conditions complicates the recognition and diagnosis of mental health disorders. Also, the myth that older people do not respond well to treatment is still prevalent.

Other factors—including the lack of knowledge on the part of health care professionals about mental health in late life; inadequate numbers of geropsychiatrists, geropsychologists, and geropsychiatric nurses; and limited availability of geropsychiatric services—present barriers to appropriate diagnosis and treatment (Institute of Medicine, 2012). Increased attention to the preparation of mental health professionals specializing in geriatric care is important to improve mental health care delivery to older adults.

Geropsychiatric Nursing

Geropsychiatric nursing is the master's level subspecialty within the adult-psychiatric mental health nursing field. The *Geropsychiatric Nursing Collaborative*, a project of the American Academy of Nursing funded by the John A. Hartford Foundation, has developed geropsychiatric nursing competency enhancements for entry and advanced practice level education and will be developing a range of training materials and learning tools to improve the current knowledge and skills of nurses in mental health care for older adults.

Culture and Mental Health

Mental illness is found in all societies, but the frequencies of different types of mental illness vary as do the social connotations. The standards that define "normal" behavior for any culture are determined by that culture itself. What may be defined as mental illness in one culture may be viewed as normal behavior in another. Different cultures and communities also exhibit and explain symptoms of mental distress in various ways (Box 28-6). Cultural beliefs also influence who makes health care decisions, help-seeking behavior, preferences for type of treatment, and provider characteristics (Jimenez et al, 2012, 2013).

In the United States, disparities in mental health service use by racial and ethnic minority groups are well documented. Regardless of age, African American, Latino, and Asian American individuals have lower mental health treatment initiation, receive a lower quality of care, and experience a greater burden of

---

BOX 28-6 Cultural Variations in Expressing Mental Distress

- **Ataque de nervios (attack of nerves):** A syndrome among individuals of Latin descent, characterized by symptoms of intense emotional upset, including acute anxiety, anger, grief; screaming and shouting uncontrollably; attacks of crying, trembling, heat in the chest rising into the head; verbal and physical aggression. May include seizure-like or fainting episodes, suicidal gestures. Attacks frequently occur as a result of a stressful event relating to the family (such as death of a relative, conflict with spouse/children, witnessing an accident involving a family member). Symptoms are similar to acute anxiety, panic disorder. Related conditions are "blacking out" in southern United States and "falling out" in West Indies.
- **Susto (fright):** A cultural expression for distress and misfortune prevalent among some Latinos in the United States and among people in Mexico, Central America, and South America. Illness is attributed to a frightening event that causes the soul to leave the body and results in unhappiness, sickness, and difficulty functioning in social roles. Symptoms include appetite and sleep disturbances, feelings of sadness, low self-worth, lack of motivation. Symptoms are similar to PTSD, depression, and anxiety.
- **Khyâl cap (wind attacks):** A syndrome found among Cambodians in the United States and Cambodia. Symptoms include dizziness, palpitations, shortness of breath, and cold extremities. Concern that khyâl (a wind-like substance) may rise in the body, along with blood, and cause serious effects such as entering the lungs to cause shortness of breath/asphyxia or entering the brain to cause dizziness, tinnitus, and a fatal syncope. Attacks frequently brought about by worrisome thoughts. Symptoms include those of panic attacks, generalized anxiety disorder, and PTSD.

unmet mental health needs than do non-Latino whites. African Americans and Latinos utilize mental health services at half the rate of non-Latino whites (Kim et al, 2012). These differences persist even when controlling for individual factors (language) and other considerations such as economic deprivation and education. This suggests that there are other psychological barriers to receiving adequate mental health care (Jimenez et al, 2012, 2013). Disparities may result from cultural variation in beliefs about the causes of mental illness and the effects of treatment, past discrimination, and the lack of mental health treatments that are congruent with preferences, values, and beliefs (Jimenez et al, 2012, 2013) (Box 28-7).

Disparities are found in many groups. While not well researched, sexual minority individuals, particularly older gay men, demonstrate higher rates of mental disorders, substance abuse, suicidal ideation, and deliberate self-harm than heterosexual populations. Sexual minority stress (gay-related stigma, discrimination or prejudice, concealment of sexual preferences, excessive human immunodeficiency virus [HIV] bereavements) and aging-related stress are thought to contribute to the unique mental health challenges of these individuals. The effect of minority stress on health disparities in sexual minority individuals, as well as individuals of different races, ethnicities, and cultures, is an important area of research (Wright et al, 2012). Research is also needed on the effect of other stressors such as war, terrorism, displacement, and immigration on mental health.

The newest version of the *Diagnostic and Statistical Manual of Mental Disorders (DSM-5)* (American Psychiatric Association, 2013) has an increased emphasis on culture and mental health, including the range of psychopathology across the globe, not just illnesses common in the United States, Western Europe, and Canada. In other words, it is less ethnocentric (Foundation for Psychocultural Research, 2014; Warren, 2013). Another significant change in the *DSM-5* is the developmental approach and examination of disorders across the life span. This is particularly relevant for older individuals because symptoms of mental distress present differently from the presentation in younger individuals (Katz et al, 2013).

Some of the cultural components in the *DSM-5* are presented in Box 28-8. A Cultural Formulation Interview (CFI), including Kleinman's (1980) explanatory model, guides health care providers in culturally relevant assessment (Box 28-9). An increased understanding of the importance of cultural perspectives for individuals across the life span will facilitate more accurate assessment of mental health, wellness, and illness and lead to less misdiagnosis. Enhancing the cultural proficiency of health care professionals will assist in structuring more culturally appropriate services, thus improving treatment outcomes and decreasing disparities (Warren, 2013). Box 28-10 presents best practice tips for culture assessment. Research on all aspects of culture and mental health is critical. Chapter 4 discusses culture in more depth.

Availability of Mental Health Care

Dedicated financing for older adult mental health is limited even though about 20% of all Medicare beneficiaries experience some mental disorder each year. Medicare spends five times more on beneficiaries with severe mental illness and substance abuse disorders than on similar beneficiaries without these diagnoses. More than half of dual-eligible persons (those with both Medicare and Medicaid) have mental or cognitive impairments. The 2008 mental health parity legislations ended Medicare's discriminatory practice of imposing a 50% coinsurance requirement for outpatient mental health services. In 2014, coinsurance was reduced to 20%, bringing payments for mental health care in line with those required for all other Medicare Part B services (Center for Medicare Advocacy, 2014).

BOX 28-7 RESEARCH HIGHLIGHTS

The purpose of the study was to identify cultural beliefs about the causes of mental illness and treatment preferences for mental health service use among a large sample of older adults. A total of 1257 non-Latino whites, 536 African Americans, 112 Asian Americans, and 303 Latinos completed a questionnaire regarding cultural attitudes toward health care and mental illness as part of a larger study (Primary Care Research in Substance Abuse and Mental Health for the Elderly). African Americans viewed mental illness as caused by loss of family and friends, stress over money, and general stress more than non-Latino whites. A greater proportion of Asian Americans believed that family issues, medical illness, and cultural differences caused mental illness. In comparison to non-Latino whites, Latinos stated that mental illness was caused by the loss of family and friends, family issues, and moving to a different place. Compared to non-Latino whites, African Americans said they would seek spiritual advice to help them with mental health problems and were less likely than non-Latino whites to talk to psychiatrists or psychologists. Latinos were more likely to endorse a preference for medications. Knowledge of cultural beliefs about mental illness and treatment will assist in developing interventions that are more culturally appropriate.

Data from Jimenez D, Bartels S, Cardenas V, et al: Cultural beliefs and mental health treatment preferences of ethnically diverse older adult consumers in primary care, *Am J Geriatr Psychiatry* 20(6):533–542, 2012.

BOX 28-8 Cultural Components of the *DSM-5*

- Cross-cultural variations in presentations
- Cultural concepts of distress
- Cultural formulation interview (CFI)
- Questions that can be used during a cultural assessment of particular groups such as older adults and immigrants

---

BOX 28-9 Components of the Cultural Formulation Interview in *DSM-5*

- **16-question interview:** Cultural Definition of the Problem; Perceptions of Cause, Context, and Support; Cultural Factors Affecting Self-Coping and Past Help-Seeking; and Cultural Factors Affecting Current Help-Seeking
- **12 supplementary modules:** Explanatory Model; Level of Functioning; Psychosocial Stressors; Social Network; Cultural Identity; Spirituality, Religion, and Moral Traditions; Coping and Help Seeking; Patient-Clinician Relationship; Immigrants and Refugees; School-Age Children and Adolescents; Older Adults and Caregivers

Cultural Interview Questions

- "Sometimes people have different ways of describing their problem to their family, friends, or others in the community. How would you describe your problem to them?"
- "What troubles you most about your problem?"
- "Why do you think this is happening to you?" "What do you think are the causes of your problem?"
- "What do others in your family, friends, or others in your community think are the causes of your problem?"
- "Are there aspects of your background or identity that are causing other concerns or difficulties for you?"
- "Sometimes people have various ways of dealing with problems like your problem. What have you done to cope with your problems?"
- "Often people look for help from many different sources, including different kinds of doctors, helpers, or healers. In the past what kinds of treatment, help, advice, or healing have you sought for your problem? What have others advised?"
- "What do you think would be helpful?"
- "Do you have any concerns about the therapist-patient relationship?"

Adapted from Lim R: What's new in *DSM-5* for cultural psychiatry? *Psychiatric News* 48(20), 2013. doi: 10.1176/appi.pn.2013.10b12. http://psychnews.psychiatryonline.org/newsarticle.aspx?articleid=1757008 Accessed June 2014.

The Affordable Care Act will improve access to important psychiatric medication by closing the "donut hole" coverage gap in Medicare Part D (in 2020) and will also offer incentives to enhance integration of physical and behavioral health services. Medicare also covers a yearly depression screening at no cost to beneficiaries. Concerns remain about the 190-day lifetime limit for care in inpatient psychiatric facilities and the high out-of-pocket costs of prescription drugs. More comprehensive and integrated mental health care is needed, especially in light of the aging of the "baby boomer" generation (Center for Medicare Advocacy, 2014). Nurses will need to assist older people to access appropriate mental health services and understand reimbursement issues.

Psychiatric services may be provided by a psychiatrist, psychologist, licensed clinical social worker, nurse practitioner, or geropsychiatric clinical nurse specialist. Primary care providers must routinely screen for mental health problems in older adults and develop working relationships with mental health practitioners in their area to improve access and communication (Knight, 2011). New models of providing mental health care in primary care settings, many utilizing advanced practice nurses with geropsychiatric preparation, show promise for improving access and outcomes (Reuben et al, 2013).

Settings of Care

Older people receive psychiatric services across a wide range of settings, including acute and long-term inpatient psychiatric units, primary care, and community and institutional settings. More than 55% of older persons treated for mental health services receive care from primary care providers. Less than 3% receive treatment from mental health professionals. It is critical to integrate mental health and substance abuse

with other health services including primary care, specialty care, home health care, and residential-community–based care. Successful models include mental health professionals in primary care offices; care managers; community-based, multidisciplinary geriatric mental health treatment teams; and use of advanced practice nurses (Mental Health America, 2014b; Reuben et al, 2013).

In acute care settings, nurses will encounter older adults with mental health disorders in emergency departments or in general medical-surgical units. Admissions for medical problems are often exacerbated by depression, anxiety, cognitive impairment, substance abuse, or chronic mental illness. Medical patients present with psychiatric disorders in 25% to 33% of cases, although they are often unrecognized by primary care providers. Nurses who can identify mental health problems early and seek consultation and treatment will enhance timely recovery. Advanced practice psychiatric nursing consultation is an important and effective service in acute care settings.

Nursing Homes and Assisted Living Facilities

Nursing homes and, increasingly, residential care/assisted living facilities (RC/ALFs), although not licensed as psychiatric facilities, are providing the majority of care given to older adults with psychiatric conditions. Estimates of the proportion of nursing home residents with a significant mental health disorder range from 65% to 91%, and only about 20% receive treatment from a mental health clinician (Grabowski et al, 2010). Nursing homes are also caring for younger individuals with mental illness, and the number of individuals admitted with mental illness other than dementia has surpassed the dementia admissions (Splete, 2009). Medicaid beneficiaries' ages 40 to 64 years with schizophrenia are four times more likely to be admitted to a nursing home compared with Medicaid beneficiaries in the same group without a mental illness (Grabowski et al, 2010). It is often difficult to find placement for an older adult with a mental health problem in these types of facilities, and few are structured to provide best practice care to individuals with mental illness.

Along a range of different measures of quality, the treatment of mental illness in nursing homes and residential care facilities is substandard (Grabowski et al, 2010). The following are some of the obstacles to mental health care in nursing homes and RC/ALFs: (1) shortage of trained personnel; (2) limited availability and access for psychiatric services; (3) lack of staff training related to mental health and mental illness; and (4) inadequate Medicaid and Medicare reimbursement for mental health services. An insufficient number of trained personnel affects the quality of mental health care in nursing homes and often causes great stress for staff.

New models of mental health care and services are needed for nursing homes and RC/ALFs to address the growing needs of older adults in these settings. Psychiatric services in nursing homes, when they are available, are commonly provided by psychiatric consultants who are not full-time staff members and are inadequate to meet the needs of residents and staff. Training and education of frontline staff who provide basic care to residents is essential. There is an urgent need for well-designed controlled studies to examine mental health concerns in both nursing homes and RC/ALFs and the effectiveness of mental health services in improving clinical outcomes.

MENTAL HEALTH DISORDERS

Anxiety Disorders

A general definition of anxiety is unpleasant and unwarranted feelings of apprehension, which may be accompanied by physical symptoms. Anxiety itself is a normal human reaction and part of a fear response; it is rational, within reason. Anxiety becomes problematic when it is prolonged, is exaggerated, and interferes with function.

Prevalence and Characteristics

Approximately 10% of adults aged 65 and older experience a diagnosable anxiety disorder. Epidemiological studies indicate that anxiety disorders are common in older adults; however, anxiety is not well studied in older adults and is often under-recognized and undertreated by health care professionals (Bryant et al, 2013). Anxiety symptoms that may not meet the *Diagnostic and Statistical Manual of Mental Disorders (DSM-5)* (American Psychiatric Association, 2013) criteria for anxiety disorders (subthreshold symptoms) are even more prevalent, with estimated rates from 15% to 20% in community samples, with even higher rates in medically ill populations (Byers et al, 2010; Friedman et al, 2013).

The prevalence of anxiety disorders is higher among individuals with physical illnesses, particularly those in need of home health care or who live in residential settings such as nursing homes and assisted living facilities (Friedman et al, 2013). Anxiety symptoms are common in visually impaired older adults; approximately one-third of visually impaired older adults experience mild but clinically significant anxiety or depressive symptoms (van der Aa et al, 2013). Women have higher prevalence rates of symptoms of anxiety and coexisting depression-anxiety than men. Hispanic older adults are slightly more likely to report a lifetime diagnosis of an anxiety disorder compared with white non-Hispanics and African Americans.

Anxiety disorders are not considered part of the normal aging process, but the changes and challenges that older adults often face may contribute to the development of anxiety symptoms and disorders or reactivate prior anxiety disorders. Increasing frailty, medical illness, losses, pain, lack of social support, traumatic events, medications, poor self-rated health, the presence of another psychiatric illness, and an early-onset anxiety disorder are all risk factors for late-life anxiety disorders.

Late-life anxiety is often comorbid with major depressive disorder (MDD), cognitive decline and dementia, and substance abuse (Friedman et al, 2013). Almost half of older adults diagnosed with major depression also meet the criteria for anxiety. Current evidence suggests that anxiety is even more common than depression in community-dwelling older adults and may precede depressive disorders. Comorbid anxiety and depression have a poorer outcome than either condition alone (Bryant et al, 2013). There is some evidence to suggest anxiety may be predictive of cognitive decline, but anxiety also develops in response to cognitive decline (Bryant et al, 2013). Symptoms of anxiety may occur in 75% of individuals diagnosed with dementia (Clifford et al, 2015). Further investigation is needed on all aspects of anxiety in older adults.

Consequences of Anxiety

Geriatric anxiety is associated with more visits to primary care providers and increased average length of visit. Anxiety symptoms and disorders are associated with many negative consequences including increased hospitalizations, decreased physical activity and functional status, sleep disturbances, increased health service use, substance abuse, decreased life satisfaction, and increased mortality (Brenes et al, 2014; Bryant et al, 2013).

◆ PROMOTING HEALTHY AGING: IMPLICATIONS FOR GERONTOLOGICAL NURSING

◆ Assessment

Data suggest that approximately 70% of all primary care visits are driven by psychological factors (e.g., panic, generalized anxiety, stress, somatization) (American Psychological Association, 2014). This means that nurses often encounter anxious older people and can identify anxiety-related symptoms and initiate assessments that will lead to appropriate treatment and management. Whether symptoms represent a diagnosable anxiety disorder is perhaps less important than the fact that the individual will suffer needlessly if assessment and treatment are not addressed. Assessment of anxiety in older people focuses on physical, social, and environmental factors, as well as past life history, long-standing personality, coping skills, and recent events.

The general and pervasive nature of anxiety may make diagnosis difficult in older adults. In addition, older adults tend to deny the psychological symptoms, attribute anxiety-related symptoms to physical illness, and have co-existent medical conditions that mimic symptoms of anxiety. Because older people are more sensitive to the stigma associated with disclosing psychiatric symptoms, they are less likely than younger adults to report symptoms of anxiety unless prompted to do so by a well-informed clinician (Bryant et al, 2013). Avoiding previously enjoyed activities and increasing social isolation are major signs of both anxiety and depression. Often, health care providers may attribute these symptoms to "getting older" as a result of age-related stereotypes.

Some of the medical disorders that cause anxiety include cardiac arrhythmias, delirium, dementia, chronic obstructive pulmonary disease (COPD), heart failure, hyperthyroidism, hypoglycemia, postural hypotension, pulmonary edema, and pulmonary embolism. The presence of cognitive impairment also makes diagnosis complicated (Friedman et al, 2013). Anxiety is also a common side effect of many drugs (Box 28-11). A review of medications, including over-the-counter (OTC) and herbal or home remedies, is essential with elimination of those that cause anxiety if possible.

It is important to investigate all possible causes of anxiety, such as medical conditions and depression. Diagnostic and laboratory tests may be ordered as indicated to rule out medical problems. Cognitive assessment, brain imaging, and neuropsychological evaluation are included if cognitive impairment is

BOX 28-11   Medications that may Cause Anxiety Symptoms

- Anticholinergics
- Digitalis
- Theophylline
- Antihypertensives
- Beta-blockers
- Beta-adrenergic stimulators
- Corticosteroids
- Over-the-counter (OTC) medications such as appetite suppressants and cough and cold preparations
- Caffeine
- Nicotine
- Withdrawal from alcohol, sedatives, and hypnotics

suspected. When comorbid conditions are present, they must be treated.

Few assessment instruments are designed and evaluated for older adults, and if such instruments are used, they should be weighed carefully with other data—complaints, physical exam, history, and collateral interview data. When assessing anxiety reactions in individuals residing in nursing homes, look for daily disturbances, such as with staff or caregiver changes, room changes, or events over which the individual feels a lack of control or influence. By themselves, these circumstances seldom provoke an anxiety reaction, but they may be "the straw that breaks the camel's back," particularly in frail elders. Nurses must be alert to the signs of anxiety in frail older people or those with dementia because they may be unable to tell us how they are feeling. Carefully observing behavior and searching for possible reasons for changes in behavior or patterns are important (Chapter 29).

◆ Interventions

Although further research is needed to provide evidence to guide treatment, existing studies suggest that anxiety disorders in older people can be treated effectively. Treatment choices depend on the symptoms, the specific anxiety diagnosis, comorbid medical conditions, and any current medication regimen. Nonpharmacological interventions are preferred, but treatment may include a combination of psychotherapy, pharmacotherapy, and complementary and alternative therapies (Eells, 2014). If the individual has more than one anxiety disorder or suffers from comorbid depression, substance abuse, or medical problems, treatment may be complicated.

◆ Pharmacological Interventions

Pharmacotherapy is an important treatment option for many patients with anxiety disorders, either in combination with cognitive-behavioral therapy (CBT) or as stand-alone treatment. Pharmacotherapy should never be prescribed without additional educational materials (Katz et al, 2013). However, research on the effectiveness of medication in treating anxiety in older people is limited. Age-related changes in pharmacodynamics and issues of polypharmacy make prescribing and monitoring in older people a complex undertaking. Antidepressants in the form of selective serotonin reuptake inhibitors (SSRIs) are

usually the first-line treatment. Within this class of drugs, those with sedating rather than stimulating properties are preferred. Careful monitoring of response and side effects is important. A recent study found that older adults with generalized anxiety disorder who were taking escitalopram in combination with cognitive-behavioral therapy were anxiety-free for a longer time than those who received either medication or counseling alone (Wetherell et al, 2013).

Second-line treatment may include short-acting benzodiazepines (alprazolam, lorazepam, mirtazapine). Treatment with benzodiazepines should be used for short-term therapy only (less than 6 months) and relief of immediate symptoms, but it must be used carefully in older adults. Current guidelines recommend the use of benzodiazepine agents as a bridge to manage anxiety symptoms acutely until the long-term first-line medications (e.g., escitalopram) and treatments (e.g., CBT) reach therapeutic efficacy (Cliifford et al, 2015). Chronic use of benzodiazepines in older individuals can cause cognitive impairment, falls, and other serious side effects. Use of older drugs, such as diazepam or chlordiazepoxide, should be avoided because of their long half-lives and the increased risk of accumulation and toxicity in older people. Non-benzodiazepine anxiolytic agents (buspirone) may also be used. Buspirone has fewer side effects but requires a longer period of administration (up to 4 weeks) for effectiveness (Chapter 9). Antianxiety medications must be monitored closely, and this class of drugs accounts for a significant portion of adverse drug effect emergency department visits among adults (Hampton et al, 2014).

◆ Nonpharmacological Interventions

Psychotherapeutic approaches include CBT, exposure therapy mindfulness-based stress reduction (MBSR), and interpersonal therapy. Increasing evidence supports the effectiveness of psychotherapy in treating anxiety in older adults, often in combination with pharmacotherapy. CBT is designed to modify thought patterns, improve skills, and alter the environmental states that contribute to anxiety. CBT may involve relaxation training and cognitive restructuring (replacing anxiety-producing thoughts with more realistic, less catastrophic ones) and education about signs and symptoms of anxiety (Katz et al, 2013). MBSR is a new technique that introduces the concept of mindfulness through the practice of techniques such as yoga, mindful breathing, and other forms of meditation (Clifford et al, 2015). Exposure therapy, also used in treatment of PTSD that is discussed later in this chapter, involves controlled exposure to events/situations that cause anxiety until anxiety lessens and the body and mind are trained to view the situation with less distress than it is perceived to be.

Continued research is needed related to the effectiveness of psychotherapeutic approaches for older adults, particularly in community settings and for older adults from minority backgrounds living in underserved areas. Jameson et al. (2012) report on an innovative project (Calmer Life Project) in the African American community that offers individuals the option to explicitly incorporate their religious/spiritual beliefs into psychotherapy. The intervention is offered in neighborhood community centers, faith-based organizations, and churches. Sessions are also offered in the home or via phone.

Telephone-delivered and Internet-based CBT are increasingly available, and preliminary evaluation has shown good results and patient satisfaction comparable to face-to-face psychotherapy (Jameson et al, 2012; Katz et al, 2013).

Complementary and alternative therapies include biofeedback, progressive relaxation, acupuncture, yoga, massage therapy, art therapy, music therapy, dance therapy, meditation, prayer, and spiritual counseling. Music and singing have been found effective in reducing anxiety levels in older adults in a variety of setting and can be a valuable therapeutic nursing intervention (Eells, 2013). Suggested interventions for anxiety in older adults are presented in Box 28-12.

The therapeutic relationship between the patient and the health care provider is the foundation for any intervention. Support from family, referral to community resources and support groups, and provision of educational materials are other important interventions.

Posttraumatic Stress Disorder (PTSD)

Athough originally considered an anxiety disorder, the *DSM-5* removed PTSD from the classification of anxiety disorders and included it in a new chapter, Trauma- and Stressor-Related Disorders. In addition to PTSD, this *DSM-5* chapter covers acute stress disorder, adjustment disorders, and reactive attachment disorder. PTSD was once considered a psychological condition of combat veterans who were "shocked" by and unable to face their

BOX 28-12 TIPS FOR BEST PRACTICE
Interventions for Anxiety in Older Adults

- Establish a therapeutic relationship and come to know the person.
- Listen attentively to what is said and unsaid; pay attention to nonverbal behavior; use a nonjudgmental approach.
- Support the person's strengths and have faith in his/her ability to cope, drawing on past successes.
- Encourage expression of needs, concerns, questions.
- Screen for depression.
- Evaluate medications for anxiety side effects; adjust as needed.
- Manage physical conditions.
- Accept the person's defenses; do not confront, argue, or debate.
- Help the person identify precipitants of anxiety and their reactions.
- Teach the person about anxiety, symptoms, and their effects on the body.
- If irrational thoughts are present, offer accurate information while encouraging the expression of the meaning of events contributing to anxiety; reassure of safety and your presence in supporting them.
- Intervene when possible to remove the source of anxiety.
- Encourage positive self-talk, such as "I can do this one step at a time" and "Right now I need to breathe deeply."
- Teach distraction or diversion tactics; progressive relaxation exercises; deep breathing.
- Encourage participation in physical activity, adapted to the person's capabilities.
- Encourage the use of community resources such as friends, family, churches, socialization groups, self-help and support groups, and mental health counseling.

From Flood M, Buckwalter K: Recommendations for the mental health care of older adults: Part 1—an overview of depression and anxiety, *J Gerontol Nurs* 35:26–34, 2009.

experience on the battlefield. Individuals with PTSD were labeled as weak, faced rejection from their military peers and society in general, and were removed from combat zones or discharged from the military. Today we know that PTSD is a psychobiological mental disorder associated with changes in brain function and structure and can affect survivors of combat experience but also terrorist attacks, natural disasters, serious accidents, assault or abuse, and even sudden and major emotional losses (National Institute of Mental Health, 2014). The *DSM-5* criterion for PTSD has been expanded to include both direct and indirect exposure to potentially traumatic experiences (Uher et al, 2014).

Prevalence

Most of the research on PTSD has been conducted with male veterans of military combat. In the cohort of Vietnam veterans (now in the "baby boomer" cohort), 3 out of 10 experience PTSD. Among Afghanistan and Iraq veterans, 11% to 20% experience PTSD (United States Department of Veterans Affairs, 2014). Only recently realized is the fact that many World War II veterans have lived most of their lives under the shadow of PTSD without its being recognized. PTSD occurs increasingly in women, although research is scarce. Rape, child abuse, and domestic violence are the most likely traumas that will result in PTSD in women. With more women serving in the military, combat-induced PTSD among women is expected to increase (Kaiser et al, 2014a).

Prevalence rates of PTSD among older adults have not been adequately studied, but estimates are that between 3% and 5% of individuals older than age 60 experience PTSD. Many older individuals may not meet the full criteria for a PTSD diagnosis but may still exhibit symptoms (partial or subdromal PTSD) (Chopra et al, 2014). The percentage of older individuals with subclinical levels of PTSD symptoms ranges from 7% to 15% (Kaiser et al, 2014a).

In addition to military combat, seniors in our care now have also experienced the Great Depression, the Holocaust, and racism—events that also may precipitate PTSD. Although they may have managed to keep symptoms under control, a person who becomes cognitively impaired may no longer be able to control thoughts, flashbacks, or images. This can be the cause of great distress that may be exhibited by aggressive or hostile behavior. Older individuals who are Holocaust survivors may experience PTSD symptoms when they are placed in group settings in institutions. Bludau (2002) described this as the concept of second institutionalization. Older women with a history of rape or abuse as a child may also experience symptoms of PTSD when institutionalized, particularly during the provision of intimate bodily care activities, such as bathing. Box 28-13 provides some clinical examples of PTSD.

Symptoms

The *DSM-5* includes four major symptom clusters for diagnosis of PTSD: (1) reexperiencing; (2) avoidance; (3) persistent negative alterations in cognition and mood; and (4) alterations in arousal and receptivity (including irritable or aggressive behavior and reckless or self-destructive behavior) (American Psychiatric Association, 2013). Individuals often reexperience and relive the traumatic event in episodes of fear and experience symptoms

BOX 28-13 Clinical Examples of PTSD in Older Adults

Ernie's Story

Ernie may have had PTSD, although it was only speculative after his suicide. On his 18th birthday, Ernie joined the U.S. Army Air Corps (precedent to our present U.S. Air Force) in 1941. He was quickly trained and sent to Burma, China, and India. During his 3-year stint, Ernie survived two airplane crashes, saw several of his companions mutilated in crashes, watched the torture of captured Japanese soldiers, and witnessed the capture of some of his friends. When Ernie returned to the United States, his hair had turned from deep auburn to pure white. He retired from the service after 20 years but was never really able to work after his retirement.

Ernie's life was filled with episodes of alcoholic binges, outbursts of anger, and episodes of abusing others, all seemingly quite out of his control. One friend remained from his service days and visited him periodically until his death in 1996. Other relationships seemed to have been superficial and to have had little meaning for Ernie. On his 78th birthday, which he spent alone, Ernie shot himself. One must wonder how many of the elderly veterans of World War II (WWII), the most highly suicidal group in the United States, are suffering from PTSD.

Jack's Story

An 80-year-old WWII veteran resident with dementia was admitted to a large Veterans Administration (VA) nursing home. Jack's wife told the staff that he had been a high school principal who was very successful in his position. He had recurring frightening dreams throughout his life related to his war experiences and he would always turn off the radio or TV when there were programs about WWII. Now, due to his dementia, he was unable to control his thoughts and feelings. While in the nursing home, he would became very agitated and attempt to hit other residents around him when placed in the large day room. The staff recognized this as a PTSD reaction from his years as a prisoner of war. They always placed him in a smaller day room near the nursing station away from other residents, where he remained calm and pleasant. The aggression stopped without the need for medication.

PTSD, Posttraumatic stress disorder.

such as helplessness, flashbacks, intrusive thoughts, dreams, images, avoidance of thoughts or situations that remind them of the traumatic event, poor concentration, irritability, increased startle reactions, and numbing of emotional responsiveness (detachment, flattened or absent affect) (Clapp and Beck, 2012; Khouzam, 2013).

Consequences

PTSD often co-occurs with physical illness, substance use disorders, depression, and chronic pain. Depression is present in half of individuals with PTSD, making it very important to routinely assess for depression. Co-occurring PTSD and depression is associated with greater symptoms, reduced quality of life, and increased health care utilization than PTSD alone (Rytwinski et al, 2014). A recent study reported that a diagnosis of PTSD among Vietnam War veterans more than doubled the likelihood that they would develop heart disease (Vaccarino et al, 2013). There may be some association between PTSD and a greater incidence and prevalence of dementia. Data from a large Veterans Administration (VA) cohort study indicated that individuals diagnosed with PTSD were almost twice as likely to

develop dementia, when compared with those not diagnosed with PTSD (Kaiser et al, 2014a; Qureshi et al, 2010).

◆ PROMOTING HEALTHY AGING: IMPLICATIONS FOR GERONTOLOGICAL NURSING

Assessment

PTSD prevention and treatment are only now getting the research attention that other illnesses have received over the years. The care of the individual with PTSD involves awareness that certain events may trigger inappropriate reactions, and the pattern of these reactions should be identified when possible. Knowing the person's history and life experiences is essential in understanding behavior and implementing appropriate interventions. The Hartford Institute for Geriatric Nursing recommends the Impact of Event Scale–Revised (IES-R) (Christianson and Marren, 2013) (Box 28-14).

Assessment of trauma and related symptoms should be routine in older patients because they may not report traumatic experiences or may minimize their importance. Similar to other mental health concerns, elders may be more likely to report physical concerns, pain, sleep difficulties, or cognitive problems than emotional problems. Asking about issues or concerns may prompt a description of emotional reactions. Reports of physical issues should be followed with questions about changes in mood and activities. Cognitive screening for delirium/dementia is important, as well as assessment for depression and suicide (Kaiser et al, 2014b).

◆ Interventions

Effective coping with traumatic events seems to be associated with secure and supportive relationships; the ability to freely express or fully suppress the experience; favorable circumstances immediately following the trauma; productive and active lifestyles; strong faith, religion, and hope; a sense of humor; biological integrity, and resilience. Research on resiliency may lead to ways to predict who is most likely to develop PTSD following highly stressful events (National Institute of Mental Health Senior Health, 2014).

BOX 28-14 RESOURCES FOR BEST PRACTICE

- **American Academy of Nursing**: Geropsychiatric Nursing Collaborative
- **Hartford Institute for Geriatric Nursing**: Geriatric nursing protocol: Depression in Older Adults; Impact of Event Scale-Revised (IES-R); Nursing standard of practice protocol: Substance misuse and alcohol use disorders
- **National Alliance on Mental Illness**
- **National Center for PTSD**
- **National Institute of Mental Health**: Older Adults and Mental Health
- **NIH Senior Health**: Anxiety, Depression, PTSD, Alcohol Abuse (including educational videos for older adults: Problem drinking in older adults; Getting help for alcohol addiction; How can I cut back my drinking?)
- **Substance Abuse and Mental Health Services Administration**: Promoting Mental Health and Preventing Suicide: A Toolkit for Senior Living Communities (SPARK Kit)
- **University of Iowa Hartford Center for Geriatric Nursing Excellence**: Detection of depression in cognitively intact older adults

The understanding of how to treat PTSD among older adults is still developing (Clapp and Beck, 2012). There are no randomized controlled trials on the effectiveness of PTSD treatment in older adults, but recommendations are that older patients can benefit from CBT and prolonged exposure (PE) therapy (Kaiser et al, 2014b). Other therapies shown to improve PTSD symptoms include cognitive processing therapy, eye movement desensitization and reprocessing, and narrative exposure therapy (Agency for Healthcare Research and Quality [AHRQ], 2013).

Cognitive therapy aims to isolate dysfunctional thoughts and assumptions about the trauma that seem to cause distress. Individuals are encouraged to challenge the truth of the beliefs and to substitute them with more balanced thoughts. Exposure therapy involves recalling distressing memories of the trauma/event via controlled exposure to reminders of the event. Exposure can be done by imagining the trauma, reading descriptions of the event, or visiting the site of the trauma until distress associated with the memory lessens and your body and mind are retrained to view the situation less dangerous than it was perceived to be.

Evidence-based psychospiritual interventions may also be effective in the treatment of veterans with PTSD and may be more acceptable among those who have a fear of mental illness–related stigma (Bormann et al, 2008; Khouzam, 2013). Individuals able to find meaning and purpose in their traumatic experiences are less likely to develop chronic PTSD. Providers should inquire about the spiritual component of PTSD and help the individual to find meaning in his or her life (Chapter 36). Pharmacological therapy is also used, and sertraline and paroxetine have received approval by the U.S. Food and Drug Administration (FDA) to treat PTSD. Careful monitoring of these medications is necessary in older patients (Chapter 9).

Therapies should be individualized to meet the specific concerns and needs of each unique patient and may include individual, group, and family therapy (Khouzam, 2013). Internet-based therapy, self-help therapy, and telephone-assisted therapy are other creative formats to make interventions more widely available, particularly for improving response to mass trauma events (NIH, 2014). Further research is necessary to understand the various presentations of PTSD in late life and validate and improve the effectiveness of available treatment approaches (Bottche et al, 2012; Thorp et al, 2009).

SCHIZOPHRENIA

Prevalence

Older adults are the fastest growing segment of the total schizophrenia population, and the numbers are expected to grow in the coming decades with the increased longevity of the population (Meesters, 2014). Although the onset of schizophrenia usually occurs between adolescence and the mid-30s, it can extend into and first appear in late life. The prevalence of schizophrenia in older people is estimated to be approximately 0.6%—about half of the prevalence in younger adults.

There is limited research on schizophrenia in older adults and until the middle of the 20th century, it was assumed that mental illness was a part of the aging process. In fact, schizophrenia was originally conceptualized as a dementing illness in younger people and labeled dementia praecox (Collier and Sorrell, 2011).

Types

Distinction is made between early-onset schizophrenia (EOS), occurring before age 40; midlife onset (MOS), between ages 40 and 60; and late onset (LOS), after age 60. There is some suggestion that there may be neurobiological differences between LOS and EOS and LOS may be a subtype of schizophrenia (Wetherell and Jeste, 2011). LOS appears to have a better prognosis and requires lower daily doses of antipsychotics than EOS (Jeste and Maglione, 2013).

Patients with LOS are more likely to be women, and paranoia is the dominant feature of the illness. They tend to have a greater prevalence of visual hallucinations, less prevalence of a formal thought disorder, fewer negative symptoms, less cognitive impairment, and less family history of schizophrenia (Wetherell and Jeste, 2011). Individuals with EOS who have grown older may experience fewer hallucinations, delusions, and bizarre behavior, as well as inappropriate affect. Positive symptoms may wane, substance abuse becomes less common, and mental health functioning often improves (Osterweil, 2012).

Consequences

Individuals with severe persistent mental illnesses such as schizophrenia form a disenfranchised group whose access to medical care has been limited, leading to greater functional declines, morbidity, and mortality, as demonstrated by statistics that individuals with schizophrenia have a life expectancy 20 to 23 years shorter than that of an unaffected person. People with schizophrenia in their 40s and 50s may be comparable medically to those in the 60s and 70s in the general population (Jeste and Maglione, 2013). A concerning finding is that the incidence of dementia is twice as high in individuals with schizophrenia (Meesters, 2014). There have been few studies of the health status of older adults with schizophrenia and the effect of aging-related illnesses on their mental health–related disabilities (Hendrie et al, 2014). Research in the field has been limited mainly to North American study sites and more global studies are necessary (Meesters, 2014).

Schizophrenia is a costly disease both in terms of personal suffering and with regard to medical care costs. An estimated 41% of older people with schizophrenia now reside in nursing homes (Leutwyler and Wallhagen, 2010). Interventions to improve independent functioning, irrespective of age, and in conjunction with community services, would decrease the expenses associated with institutionalization. The management of older adult patients with schizophrenia is expected to become a serious burden for our health care system, requiring the development of integrated models of care across the continuum.

◆ PROMOTING HEALTHY AGING: IMPLICATIONS FOR GERONTOLOGICAL NURSING

◆ Interventions

Treatment for schizophrenia includes both medications and environmental interventions. Conventional neuroleptic medications (e.g., haloperidol) have been effective in managing the positive symptoms but are problematic in older people and carry a high risk of disabling and persistent side effects, such as tardive dyskinesia (TD). The abnormal involuntary movement scale (AIMS) is useful for evaluating early symptoms of TD (Chapter 23). The newer atypical antipsychotic medications (e.g., risperidone, olanzapine, quetiapine), given in low doses, are associated with a lower risk of extrapyramidal symptoms (EPS) and TD. As a result of the tendency for improvement in schizophrenia symptoms with age, reductions in dose or gradual tapering or discontinuation of antipsychotics may be possible in older patients (Jeste and Maglione, 2013). Federal guidelines for the use of antipsychotic medications in nursing homes provide the indications for use of these medications in schizophrenia.

Other important interventions include a combination of support, education, physical activity, and CBT. A positive approach on the part of health care professionals, patients, and their families, combined with interventions to enhance positive psychological traits such as resilience, optimism, social engagement, and wisdom, is important (Meesters, 2014; Osterweil, 2012).

Families of older people with schizophrenia experience the burden of caring for a family member with a chronic disability, as well as dealing with their own personal aging. Community-based support services that include assistance with housing, medical care, recreation services, and services that help the family plan for the future of their relative are necessary. There are relatively few services in the community for older persons with schizophrenia. The National Alliance on Mental Illness (NAMI) (see Box 28-14) is an important resource for clients and their families.

PSYCHOTIC SYMPTOMS IN OLDER ADULTS

The onset of true psychiatric disorders is low among older adults, but psychotic manifestations may occur as a secondary syndrome in a variety of disorders, the most common being Alzheimer's disease and other dementias, as well as Parkinson's disease. Psychosis of Alzheimer's disease is common and as many as half of patients develop psychotic symptoms (Wetherell and Jeste, 2011) (Chapter 29).

Paranoid Symptoms

New-onset paranoid symptoms are common among older adults and can present in a number of conditions in late life. Paranoid symptoms can signify an acute change in mental status as a result of a medical illness or delirium, or they can be caused by an underlying affective or primary psychotic mental disorder. Paranoia is also an early symptom of Alzheimer's disease, appearing approximately 20 months before diagnosis. Medications, vision and hearing loss, social isolation, alcoholism, depression, the presence of negative life events, financial strain, and PTSD can also be precipitating factors of paranoid symptoms.

Delusions

Delusions are beliefs that guide one's interpretation of events and help make sense out of disorder, even though they are inconsistent with reality. The delusions may be comforting or threatening, but they always form a structure for understanding situations that otherwise might seem unmanageable. A delusional disorder is one in which conceivable ideas, without foundation in fact, persist for more than 1 month.

Common delusions of older adults are of being poisoned, of children taking their assets, of being held prisoner, or of being deceived by a spouse, partner, or lover. In older adults, delusions often incorporate significant persons rather than the global grandiose or persecutory delusions of younger persons. Fear and a lack of trust originating from a basis in reality may become magnified, especially when one is isolated from others and does not receive reality feedback. It is always important to determine if what "appears" to be delusional ideation is, in fact, based in reality. Box 28-15 presents some clinical examples.

Hallucinations

Hallucinations are best described as sensory perceptions of a nonexistent object and may be spurred by the internal stimulation of any of the five senses. Although not attributable to environmental stimuli, hallucinations may occur as a combined result of environmental factors. Hallucinations arising from psychotic disorders are less common among older adults, and those that are generated are thought to begin in situations in which one is feeling alone, abandoned, isolated, or alienated.

BOX 28-15   Clinical Examples of Delusions

Maggie's Story

Maggie persistently held onto the delusion that her son was a very important attorney and was coming to force the administration to discharge her from the nursing home. Her son, a factory worker, had been dead for 10 years. The events of her day, her hopes, and her status were all organized around this belief. It is clear that without her delusion she would have felt forlorn, lost, and abandoned.

Herman's Story

Herman was an 88-year-old man in a nursing home who insisted that he must go and visit his mother. His thoughts seemed clear in other respects (often the case with people who are delusional), and one of the authors (P. Ebersole) suspected that he had some unresolved conflicts about his dead mother or felt the need for comforting and caring. P.E. did not argue with him about his dead mother because arguing is never a useful approach to persons with delusions. Rather, she used the best techniques she could think of to assure him that she was interested in him as a person and recognized that he must feel very lonely sometimes. He continued to say that he must go and visit his mother. When P.E. could delay his leaving no longer, she walked with him to the nurses' station and found that his 104-year-old mother did indeed live in another wing of the institution and that he visited her every day.

To compensate for insecurity, a hallucinatory experience is stimulated, often an imaginary companion. Imagined companions may fill the immense void and provide some security, but they may also become accusatory and disturbing.

The character and stages of hallucinatory experiences in late life have not been adequately defined. Many hallucinations are in response to physical disorders, such as dementia, Parkinson's disease, sensory disorders, and medications. Older people with hearing and vision deficits may also hear voices or see people and objects that are not actually present (illusions). Some have explained this as the brain's attempt to create stimulation in the absence of adequate sensory input. If illusions or hallucinations are not disturbing to the person, they do not necessitate treatment.

One older woman in a nursing home who had Alzheimer's disease and was experiencing agnosia would look in the mirror and talk to "the nice lady I see in there." "Do you want to eat or go out for a walk with me?" she would ask. It was comforting to her, and therefore she did not need medication for her "hallucination," as some would have labeled her behavior. As is the case with many disease symptoms, frail elders do not typically manifest the cardinal signs we have been taught to associate with certain physical and mental disorders. Diagnostic criteria, and often evidence-based practice guidelines, have been developed out of observation and research with younger people and may not always fit the older person. Until knowledge and research on the unique aspects of aging increase, nurses and other health care professionals are urged to individualize their assessment and treatment of older people using available guidelines specific to older people.

◆ PROMOTING HEALTHY AGING: IMPLICATIONS FOR GERONTOLOGICAL NURSING

◆ Assessment

The assessment dilemma is often one of determining if paranoia, delusions, and hallucinations are the result of medical illnesses, medications, dementia, psychoses, sensory deprivation or overload because the treatment will vary accordingly. Treatment must be based on a comprehensive assessment and on a determination of the nature of the psychotic behavior (primary or secondary psychosis) and the time of onset of first symptoms (early or late). Treating the underlying cause of a secondary psychosis caused by medical illnesses, dementia, substance abuse, or delirium is a priority.

Assessment of vision and hearing is also important because these impairments may predispose the older person to paranoia or suspiciousness. Psychotic symptoms and/or paranoid ideation also present with depression, so depression screening should also be conducted. Assessment of suicide potential is also indicated because individuals experiencing paranoid symptoms are at significant risk for harm to self. It is never safe to conclude that someone is delusional or paranoid or experiencing hallucinations unless you have thoroughly investigated his or her claims, evaluated physical and cognitive status, and assessed the environment for contributing factors to the behaviors.

◆ Interventions

Frightening hallucinations or delusions, such as feeling that one is being poisoned, usually arise in response to anxiety-provoking situations and are best managed by reducing situational stress; being available to the person; providing a safe, nonjudgmental environment; and attending to the fears more than the content of the delusion or hallucination. Direct confrontation is likely to increase anxiety and agitation and the sense of vulnerability; it also may disrupt the relationship. A more useful approach is to establish a trusting relationship that is nondemanding and not too intense.

It is important to identify the client's strengths and build on them. Demonstrating respect and a willingness to listen to complaints and fears is important. It is important that the nurse be trustworthy, give clear information, and present clear choices. Do not pretend to agree with paranoid beliefs or delusions, but rather ask what is troubling to the person and provide reassurance of safety. It is important to try to understand the person's level of distress, as well as how he or she is experiencing what is troubling. Other suggestions are to avoid television, which can be confusing, especially if the person awakens and finds it on or has a hearing or vision impairment. In addition, reduce clutter in the person's room and eliminate shadows that can appear threatening. Provide glasses and hearing aids to maximize sensory input and decrease misinterpretations.

If symptoms are interfering with function and interpersonal and environmental strategies are not effective, antipsychotic drugs may be used. The newer atypical antipsychotics (risperidone, olanzapine) are preferred but must be used judiciously, with careful attention to side effects and monitoring of response. In cognitively impaired individuals with paranoid ideation, there is some evidence suggesting that treatment with cognitive enhancer medications (cholinesterase inhibitors) may be of benefit. If symptoms interfere with function and safety and nonpharmacological interventions are not effective, antipsychotic medications may be used. However, none of the antipsychotic medications are approved for use in treatment of behavioral responses in dementia. The benefits are uncertain,

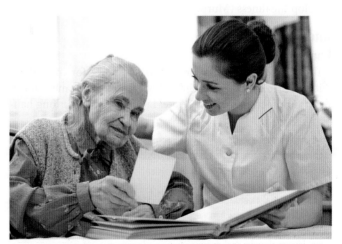

Demonstrating respect and a willingness to listen is the foundation for a caring nurse-patient relationship. (©iStock.com/AlexRaths)

and adverse effects offset any advantages. See Chapter 29 for further discussion of behavior and psychological symptoms in dementia and nonpharmacological interventions.

BIPOLAR DISORDER (BD)

The *DSM-5* defines bipolar disorder as a recurrent mood disorder that includes periods of mania or mixed episodes of mania and depression. The length of the phases of depression and mania varies, lasting from days to weeks (Carson and Yambor, 2012; Dols et al, 2014; Murphy, 2013). BD is a lifelong disease that usually begins in adolescence, but 20% of older patients with BD experience their first episode after 50 years of age. With the aging of the population, predictions are that there will be a drastic increase of older individuals with BD in the coming decades. Bipolar disorders often stabilize in late life, and individuals tend to have longer periods of depression. Mania is a more frequent cause of hospitalization than depression, but depression may account for more disability. Similar to other psychiatric disorders in older adults, comorbidities often mask the presence of the disorder and it is frequently misdiagnosed, underdiagnosed, and undertreated.

◆ PROMOTING HEALTHY AGING: IMPLICATIONS FOR GERONTOLOGICAL NURSING

◆ Assessment

Assessment includes a thorough physical examination and laboratory and radiological testing to exclude physical causes of the symptoms and identify comorbidities. A medication review should be conducted because symptoms can be a side effect of medications. Obtaining an accurate history from the individual, as well as the family, is important and should include assessment of symptoms associated with depression, mania, hypomania, and a family history of bipolar disorder. Episodes of mania combined with depressed features and a family history of bipolar disorder are highly indicative of the diagnosis. There is a strong hereditary component to BD, and a person with a parent or sibling with BD is four to six times more likely to develop the illness (Murphy, 2013) (Box 28-16).

◆ Interventions
◆ Pharmacotherapy

Lithium, the most commonly used substance for individuals with bipolar disorders, has neurological effects that make it difficult for older people to tolerate. Lithium also has a long half-

life (more than 36 hours), and dosing needs to be adjusted based on renal function. Medications that can affect urine production (diuretics) can alter lithium levels. Lithium levels, blood urea nitrogen (BUN) levels, and creatinine plasma levels need to be monitored closely (Murphy, 2013). Anticonvulsant medications such as valproic acid, divalproex sodium, and lamotrigine are more commonly used in BD treatment. Medication levels must be monitored, as well as liver function. Many of the anticonvulsant medications have an FDA warning that their use may increase suicide risk, so careful monitoring for changes in mood and behavior and signs of suicidal ideation is important.

Antidepressants such as fluoxetine, paroxetine, and venlafaxine can be used to treat depression in BD disorder in combination with other medications. Because these medications can trigger mania, careful assessment is important. Atypical antipsychotic drugs are also sometimes used, but with the same safety warnings discussed earlier, and are not to be used if dementia is suspected. Olanzapine, aripiprazole, and seroquel are all approved for the treatment of bipolar disorder and may relieve symptoms of severe mania and psychosis. Electroconvulsive therapy (ECT) may also be used when medication and/or psychotherapy is not effective (Murphy, 2013).

◆ Psychosocial Approaches

Patient and family education and support are essential, and the family must understand that the individual is not able to control mania and irritating behaviors because of a chemical imbalance in the brain. Treatment with medication and intensive psychotherapy; CBT; interpersonal and rhythm therapy (improving relationships with others and managing regular daily routines); and family-focused therapy have been reported to be effective in improving recovery rates (Crowe et al, 2010; Dols et al, 2014).

Psychoeducation is an important component of all psychosocial interventions, and nurses can assist patients in learning about BD and its treatment. Psychoeducation should include developing an acceptance of the disorder, becoming aware of factors influencing symptoms and signs of relapse, learning how to communicate with others, and establishing regular sleep and activity habits. Teaching patients to keep a log to monitor mood changes, activity levels, stressors, and amount of sleep is important. Medication regimens can be complicated, and many individuals struggle to remain adherent. An important nursing intervention is educating patients and families about the benefits and risks of prescribed medications, the importance of monitoring therapeutic effects and side effects, and the value of medication management systems (Carson and Yambor, 2012).

DEPRESSION

Depression is not a normal part of aging, and studies show that most older people are satisfied with their lives, despite physical problems (National Institute of Mental Health [NIMH], 2014). To understand depression, the nurse must understand the influence of late-life stressors and changes and the beliefs older

---

BOX 28-16   Focus on Genetics

Research on the genetic basis for mental health disorders such as depression, schizophrenia, and bipolar disorder is being conducted by the National Institute of Mental Health Center for Collaborative Genetic Studies on Mental Disorders (https://www.nimhgenetics.org/). The latest genome-wide study identified shared genetic risk factors between schizophrenia and bipolar disorder, bipolar disorder and depression, and schizophrenia and depression, the first evidence of overlap between these disorders. Continuous research on gene discovery for mental health disorders is ongoing.

people, society, and health professionals may have about depression and its treatment.

Prevalence

Depression remains underdiagnosed and undertreated in the older population and is considered a significant public health issue (Abbasi and Burke, 2014; Woodward et al, 2013). Depression is the fourth leading cause of disease burden globally and is projected to increase to the second leading cause by 2030 (World Health Organization, 2014). The prevalence of depression is increasing in the baby boomer generation, which will increase the rates of depression in the coming years (Harvath and McKenzie, 2012). Approximately 1% to 2% of adults 65 years and older are diagnosed with major depressive disorder. An additional 25% have significant depressive symptoms that do not meet the criteria for major depressive disorder (Avari et al, 2014).

Symptoms that do not meet the criteria for major depressive disorder have been referred to as minor depression, subsyndromal depression, dysthymic depression, and mild depression. The *DSM-5* replaced the term *dysthymia* with the term *persistent* depressive disorder to describe symptoms that are long standing (lasting 2 years or longer) but do not meet the criteria for major depressive disorder. Recognition and treatment are important because persistent depressive disorder has a negative impact on physical and social functioning and quality of life for many older people and is associated with an increased risk of a subsequent major depression (Harvath and McKenzie, 2012; Uher et al, 2014).

Rates of depression are higher in older adults who experience physical illness, who have cognitive impairment, or who reside in institutional settings. Fourteen percent of patients receiving home care meet the criteria for depression, and nearly half of all nursing home residents receive antidepressants for depression (Abbasi and Burke, 2014; Mitsch, 2013; Smith et al, 2015). Depression is a major reason why older people are admitted to nursing homes.

Prevalence rates of depression in older adults likely underestimate the extent of the problem. The stigma associated with depression may be more prevalent in older people, and they may not acknowledge depressive symptoms or seek treatment. Perceived stigma may be less of a concern for the future older population who are more aware of mental health concerns and more likely to seek treatment. However, in a 2012 survey, almost 1 in 3 individuals believed that depression was a natural part of the aging process (John A. Hartford Foundation, 2012). Many elders, particularly those who have survived the Great Depression, both world wars, the Holocaust, and other tragedies, may see depression as shameful, evidence of flawed character, self-centered, a spiritual weakness, and sin or retribution.

Health professionals often expect older people to be depressed and may not take appropriate action to assess for and treat depression. The differing presentation of depression in older people, as well as the increased prevalence of medical problems that may cause depressive symptoms, also contributes to inadequate recognition and treatment. Primary care providers accurately recognize depression in less than half of individuals with depression (Mental Health America, 2014a). Even if depression is identified, only about 25% of patients receive treatment consistent with current guidelines (Unutzer et al, 2013). It is important that all health care professionals receive adequate education about depression in older adults.

Racial, Ethnic, and Cultural Considerations

Racial, ethnic, and gender differences in mental illness, as well as differences within racial groups, have not received adequate attention in the United States. Hispanic adults aged 50 and older are reported to experience more depression than white, non-Hispanic adults; black, non-Hispanic adults; or other, non-Hispanic adults. Gender differences are also present in depression prevalence, and older women suffer depression at twice the rate of older men (Hall and Reynolds, 2014).

Studies have consistently found that older racial and ethnic minorities are less likely to be diagnosed with depression than their white counterparts but are also less likely to get treated (Akincigil et al, 2012; Woodward et al, 2013). A study investigating differences in depression among black Americans, as well as between blacks and whites, reported that older whites and Caribbean blacks have a significantly higher lifetime prevalence of depression than African Americans. Caribbean black men may be particularly vulnerable to mental health problems, including schizophrenia, anxiety disorders, and suicide attempts. Reasons proposed for these differences include having negative immigration experiences, being separated from family and friends, and adapting to a new culture (Woodward et al, 2013). Higher rates of depression have also been reported for older Asian immigrants and linked to gender, recentness of immigration, English proficiency, acculturation, service barriers, and social support (Harvath and McKenzie, 2012).

Differences in the prevalence of major depressive disorder and other mental disorders may be due to differences in the presentation of self-reported symptoms or other aspects of cultural context (see Box 28-6). The new criteria in the *DSM-5* addressing culturally based explanatory models will assist in better understanding differences in presentation, help-seeking behavior, and provision of more culturally appropriate treatment for all individuals (see Boxes 28-8 and 28-9).

Consequences

Depression is a common and serious medical condition second only to heart disease in causing disability and harm to an individual's health and quality of life. Depression and depressive symptomatology are associated with negative consequences, such as delayed recovery from illness and surgery, excess use of health services, cognitive impairment, exacerbation of coexisting medical illnesses, malnutrition, decreased quality of life, and increased suicide and non–suicide-related deaths (Abbasi and Burke, 2014; Alexopoulos, 2014). It is highly likely that nurses will encounter a large number of older people with depressive symptoms in all settings. Recognizing depression and enhancing access to appropriate mental health care are important nursing roles to improve outcomes for older people.

Etiology

The causes of depression in older adults are complex and must be examined in a biopsychosocial framework. Factors of health, gender, developmental needs, socioeconomics, environment, personality, losses, and functional decline are all significant to the development of depression in later life. Depression can occur for the first time in late life or can be part of a long-standing mood disorder with onset in earlier years (Harvath and McKenzie, 2012). Compared with patients with early-life depression, older patients with late-onset major depression have less frequent family history of mood disorders. Biologic causes, such as neurotransmitter imbalances, have a strong association with many depressive disorders in late life. This may be a factor in the high incidence of depression in individuals with neurological conditions such as stroke, Parkinson's, and Alzheimer's disease (Alexopoulos, 2014; Abbati and Burke, 2014).

Serious symptoms of depression occur in up to 50% of older adults with Alzheimer's disease, and major depression occurs in about 25% of cases. Depression in individuals with Alzheimer's disease may be due to an awareness of progressive decline, but research suggests that there may be a biological connection between depression and Alzheimer's disease as well (Harvath and McKenzie, 2012). Among patients who have suffered a cerebral vascular accident, the incidence of major depressive disorder is approximately 25%, with rates being close to 40% in patients with Parkinson's disease.

Medical disorders and medications can also result in depressive symptoms (Boxes 28-17 and 28-18). Other important factors influencing the development of depression are alcohol abuse, loss of a spouse or partner, loss of social supports, lower income level, caregiver stress (particularly caring for a person with dementia), and gender. Some common risk factors for depression are presented in Box 28-19.

BOX 28-17   Medical Conditions and Depression

Cancers
Cardiovascular disorders
Endocrine disorders, such as thyroid problems and diabetes
Neurological disorders, such as Alzheimer's disease, stroke, and Parkinson's disease
Metabolic and nutritional disorders, such as vitamin B_{12} deficiency, malnutrition, diabetes
Viral infections, such as herpes zoster and hepatitis
Vision and hearing impairment

BOX 28-18   Medications and Depression

Antihypertensives	Anticholesteremics
Angiotensin-converting enzyme (ACE) inhibitors	Antibiotics
	Analgesics
Methyldopa	Corticosteroids
Reserpine	Digoxin
Guanethidine	L-Dopa
Antiarrhythmics	

BOX 28-19   Risk Factors for Depression in Older Adults

- Chronic medical illnesses, disability, functional decline
- Alzheimer's disease and other dementias
- Bereavement
- Caregiving
- Female (2:1 risk)
- Socioeconomic deprivation
- Family history of depression
- Previous episode of depression
- Admission to long-term care or other change in environment
- Medications
- Alcohol or substance abuse
- Living alone
- Widowhood

◆ PROMOTING HEALTHY AGING: IMPLICATIONS FOR GERONTOLOGICAL NURSING

◆ Assessment

Making the diagnosis of depression in older people can be challenging, and symptoms of depression present differently in older people. Older people who are depressed report more somatic complaints such as insomnia, loss of appetite, weight loss, memory loss, and chronic pain. It is often difficult to distinguish somatic complaints from the physical symptoms associated with chronic illness. In medically ill individuals, assessment should focus on nonsomatic complaints such as sadness, helplessness, hopelessness, difficulty making decisions, and irritability (Avari et al, 2014). Hypochondriasis is also common, as are constant complaining and criticism, which may actually be expressions of depression. Older depressed individuals also have a higher rate of psychotic and severe depression with more weight loss and decreased appetite (Abbasi and Burke, 2014).

Decreased energy and motivation, lack of ability to experience pleasure, increased dependency, poor grooming and difficulty completing activities of daily living (ADLs), withdrawal from people or activities enjoyed in the past, decreased sexual interest, and a preoccupation with death or "giving up" are also signs of depression in older people. Feelings of guilt and worthlessness, seen in younger depressed individuals, are less frequently seen in older people.

Individuals often present with complaints of memory problems and a cognitive impairment of recent onset that mimics dementia but subsides upon remission of depression (previously called pseudodementia). It is important to note that a large percentage of these patients progress into irreversible dementia within 2 to 3 years, so recognition and treatment of depression are important. High rates of depression are seen in individuals with dementia, and depression is also a risk factor for dementia, particularly early-onset, recurrent, severe depression (Morimoto et al, 2014). It is essential to differentiate between dementia and depression, and older people with memory impairment should be evaluated for depression. Symptoms such as agitated behavior

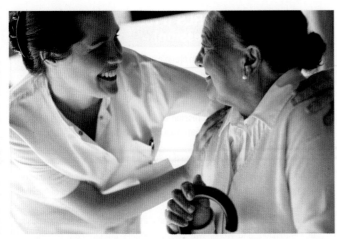

Creating hopeful environments in which meaningful activities and supportive relationships can be enjoyed is an important nursing role in the treatment of depression. (©iStock.com/Yuri)

and repetitive verbalizations in persons with dementia may be an indicator of depression (Chapter 29).

Comprehensive assessment involves a systematic and thorough evaluation using a depression screening instrument, interview, psychiatric and medical history, physical (with focused neurological exam), functional assessment, cognitive assessment, laboratory tests, medication review, determination of iatrogenic or medical causes, and family interview as indicated (Avari et al, 2014). Assessment for depressogenic medications, for alcohol and substance abuse, and for related comorbid physical conditions that may contribute to or complicate treatment of depression must also be included (Box 28-20).

Screening of all older adults for depression should be incorporated into routine health assessments across the continuum of care—in hospitals, primary care, long-term care, home care, and community-based settings. The Geriatric Depression Scale (GDS) was developed specifically for screening older adults and has been tested extensively in a number of settings. The Cornell Scale for Depression in Dementia (CSDD) is recommended for the assessment of depression in older adults with dementia (Chapter 7).

Interventions

The goals of depression treatment in older adults are to decrease symptoms, reduce relapse and recurrence, improve function and quality of life, and reduce mortality and health care costs (Harvath and McKenzie, 2012). When compared with younger individuals, older people demonstrate comparable treatment response rates, although they may have higher rates of relapse following treatment. As a result, treatment may need to be longer to prevent recurrences (Abbasi et al, 2014). If depression is diagnosed, treatment should begin as soon as possible and appropriate follow-up should be provided. Depressed people are usually unable to follow through on their own and without appropriate treatment and monitoring may be candidates for deeper depression or suicide. Interventions are individualized and are based on history, severity of symptoms, concomitant illnesses, and level of disability.

Nonpharmacological Approaches

The most effective treatment is a combination of pharmacological therapy and psychotherapy or counseling with psychotherapy alone recommended as a first-line treatment in mild major depression (Alexopoulos, 2014). Athough antidepressant medications are believed to be the best established treatment for major depressive disorder, when compared with placebos in patients with mild or moderate symptoms, their effects may be minimal or non-existent. However, for patients with severe depression, the benefits of medication over placebo are substantial (Fournier et al, 2010). The healing effects of interpersonal relationships and nonpharmacological interventions should not be underestimated for individuals with mild or moderate symptoms.

Types of nonpharmacological treatment that have been found to be helpful in depression include family and social support, education, grief management, exercise, humor, spirituality, CBT, brief psychodynamic therapy, interpersonal therapy, reminiscence, life review therapy (Chapter 6), problem-solving therapy, and complementary therapy (e.g., tai chi) (Abbasi and Burke, 2014; Chan et al, 2014; DeKeyser and Jacobs, 2014).

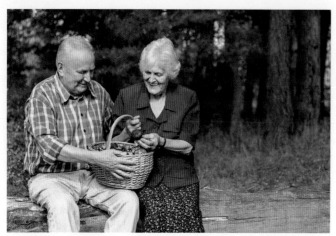
Elders enjoying an activity together. (©iStock.com/FredFroese)

BOX 28-21   PEARLS (Problem-Solving to Overcome Depression)

- Targets homebound elders with chronic conditions to provide "house-calls" for depression, particularly in underserved communities.
- Incorporates program into existing community-based programs that deliver care and resources to clients.
- Designed to treat minor depression and persistent depressive disorder by teaching behavioral and problem-solving techniques and pleasant activities scheduling.
- Utilizes the Chronic Care and Collaborative Care Models.
- Uses a psychiatrist-led team with trained counselors to work one-on-one with participants in eight in-home sessions followed by a series of maintenance telephone session contacts.
- A supervising psychiatrist reviews cases regularly, addresses other causes of depression, and works with the individual's primary care provider to assess treatment effectiveness and need for more formal depression treatment including medications.
- Results show reduction in depression symptoms, lower rates of hospitalization, and improved function, emotional well-being, and quality of life.
- Program included in SAMSHA's National Registry of Evidence-Based Programs and Practices and Agency for Healthcare Research and Quality Innovation Exchange.

Source: PEARLS: www.pearlsprogram.org

For individuals with depression and cognitive impairment, problem-adaptive therapy (PATH), a home-delivered intervention that also involves caregivers, has been found to reduce depressive symptoms. Another intervention, behavior therapy-positive events (BT-PE), teaches caregivers to increase the patient's engagement in pleasant activities and positive interactions (McGovern et al, 2014).

Despite evidence-based guidelines calling for combined pharmacological and psychotherapeutic treatment, and the fact that older adults often prefer psychotherapy to psychiatric medications, psychological interventions are often not offered as an alternative (American Psychological Association, 2014). Reasons for this include time, reimbursement constraints, and a limited well-trained geriatric mental health workforce (McGovern et al, 2014). The development of effective, simplified, and accessible psychotherapeutic approaches geared toward older adults is important (Alexopoulos, 2014) (Box 28-21). Also important is the development of telephone or Internet-based programs.

Collaborative care. Few older adults with mental health disorders receive care from mental health specialists and prefer treatment in primary care settings. More than 70 randomized controlled trials have shown collaborative care, an evidence-based approach for integrating physical and behavioral health services in primary care, is more effective and cost-efficient than usual care across diverse practice settings and patient populations (Hall and Reynolds, 2014; Unutzer et al, 2013). Some research suggests that collaborative care may improve ethnic and economic disparities in the diagnosis and treatment of depression (Hall and Reynolds, 2014).

Collaborative care models include a primary care provider (PCP, an MD or NP), care management staff (often nurses), and a psychiatric consultant working in an interprofessional team. Care managers are trained to provide evidence-based care coordination, brief behavioral interventions/psychotherapy, and treatment support initiated by the PCP, such as medications. The psychiatric consultant, either through face-to-face or by telemedicine consult, advises the team and provides guidance on patients who present diagnostic challenges or who are not yet showing improvement (Hall and Reynolds, 2014; Unutzer et al, 2013).

◆ Pharmacological Approaches

Choice of medication depends on comorbidities, drug side effects, and the type of effect desired. People with agitated depression and sleep disturbances may benefit from medications with a more sedating effect, whereas those who are not eating may do better taking medications that have an appetite-stimulating effect. There are more than 20 antidepressants approved by the FDA for the treatment of depression in older adults.

The most commonly prescribed antidepressants are the selective serotonin reuptake inhibitors (SSRIs). These agents work selectively on neurotransmitters in the brain to alleviate depression. The SSRIs are generally well tolerated in older people. Many are now available in both tablet and oral concentrate forms for easier use. Side effects are manageable and usually resolve over time; most cause initial problems with nausea, vomiting, dizziness, dry mouth, or sedation. Hyponatremia can also occur. If sexual dysfunction occurs, it will resolve only with discontinuation; therefore if the person is or plans to become sexually active, a different drug may be necessary (Chapter 9).

For those who do not respond to an adequate trial of SSRIs, there is another group of antidepressants that combines the inhibition of both serotonin and norepinephrine reuptake inhibitors (SNRIs) (e.g., venlafaxine [Effexor]). These also may be preferred by those who are engaged in or who anticipate sexual activity because they are less likely to have sexual side effects. One of the atypical antidepressants, such as bupropion [Wellbutrin] or trazodone, may be used. In the context of reducing polypharmacy, Wellbutrin also reduces nicotine dependency, and trazodone is sedating—for the person who has difficulty getting to or staying asleep.

Since the development of the SSRIs and SNRIs, the older monoamine oxidase (MAO) inhibitors and tricyclic antidepressants are no longer indicated due to their high side effect profile including risk for falls. If depression is immobilizing, psychostimulants may be used but cardiac function must be monitored closely because there are limited data on safe use in the older adult (Abbasi and Burke, 2014).

All antidepressant medications must be closely monitored for side effects and therapeutic response. Side effects can be especially problematic for older people with comorbid conditions and complex drug regimens. There are a wide range of antidepressant medications, and several may have to be evaluated. Only about one-third of depressed older adults achieve remission with any single agent (McGovern et al, 2014). Similar to other medications for older people, doses should be lower at first (50% of the target does) and titrated as indicated while adequate treatment effect is ensured.

A patient who has responded to antidepressant treatment should continue treatment for approximately 1 year for a first depressive episode because recurrence rates are high after earlier discontinuation. After a second or third episode, treatment should be extended after remission and some may require lifelong treatment. Often, older people may be resistant to take medication for depression, and it is helpful to stress that although there may be circumstances precipitating the depression, the final effect is a biochemical one that medications can correct (Abbasi and Burke, 2014).

◆ Other Treatments

Electroconvulsive therapy (ECT) is considered an excellent, safe therapy for older people with depression that is resistant to other treatments and for patients at risk for serious harm because of psychotic depression, suicidal ideation, or severe malnutrition. ECT results in a more immediate response in symptoms and is also a useful alternative for frail older people with multiple comorbid conditions who are unable to tolerate antidepressant treatment. ECT is much improved, but older people will need a careful explanation of the treatment because they may have many misconceptions.

Rapid transcranial magnetic stimulation (rTMS) is a treatment approved in 2008 by the FDA to treat major depressive disorder in adults for whom medication was not effective or tolerated. The treatment consists of administering brief magnetic pulses to the brain by passing high currents through an electromagnetic coil adjacent to the patient's scalp. The targeted magnetic pulses stimulate the circuits in the brain that are underactive in patients with depression with the goal of restoring normal function and mood. For most patients, treatment is administered in 30- to 40-minute sessions over a period of 4 to 6 weeks. The effectiveness of the treatment is still being evaluated in older adults (Abbasi and Burke, 2014). Box 28-22 presents suggestions for families and professionals caring for older adults with depression.

SUICIDE

Even though the suicide rates in older people have been decreasing over the past 8 years, the rate of suicide among older adults in

BOX 28-22   TIPS FOR BEST PRACTICE
Family and Professional Support for Depression

- Provide relief from discomfort of physical illness.
- Enhance physical function (i.e., regular exercise and/or activity; physical, occupational, recreational therapies).
- Develop a daily activity schedule that includes pleasant activities.
- Increase opportunities for socialization and enhance social support.
- Provide opportunities for decision-making and the exercise of control.
- Focus on spiritual renewal and rediscovery of meanings.
- Reactivate latent interests, or develop new ones.
- Validate depressed feelings as aiding recovery; do not try to bolster the person's mood or deny his or her despair.
- Help the person become aware of the presence of depression, the nature of the symptoms, and the time limitation of depression.
- Emphasize depression as a medical, not mental, illness that must be treated like any other disorder.
- Provide easy-to-use educational materials to older adults and family members, such as those available through NIMH.
- Involve family in patient teaching, particularly younger family members who may have different life experiences related to depression and its treatment.
- Provide an accepting atmosphere and an empathic response.
- Demonstrate faith in the person's strengths.
- Praise any and all efforts at recovery, no matter how small.
- Assist in expressing and dealing with anger.
- Do not stifle the grief process; grief cannot be hurried.
- Create a hopeful environment in which self-esteem is fostered and life is meaningful.

most countries is higher than that for any other age group—and the suicide rate for white males 85 years and older is the highest of all—four times the national age-adjusted rate (Abbasi and Burke, 2014). Older widowers are thought to be the most vulnerable because they have often depended on their wives to maintain the comforts of home and the social network of family and friends. Women in all countries have much lower suicide rates, possibly because of greater flexibility in coping skills based on multiple roles that women fill throughout their lives. However, Chinese American women aged 65 years and older have the highest suicide rate of all women older than the age of 65 years in the United States (National Alliance on Mental Illness, 2011). Despite these alarming statistics, there is little research on suicide ideation and behavior among older adults.

Recent data from the Centers for Disease Control and Prevention (CDC) (2013b) show a significant increase in suicides for adults ages 50 to 64. The suicide rate for men in this age group rose 48% between 1999 and 2010, and in women the rise was 60%. Among racial/ethnic populations, American Indian/Alaska Natives showed the greatest increases. Possible contributing factors include the economic downturn, intentional overdoses associated with the increase in use of prescription opioids, other substance abuse, and a cohort effect based on the high suicide rates of this age group in their adolescent years. These statistics contribute to the concern about the increasing mental health problems in future generations of older people and call for increased prevention efforts in this age group.

In most cases, depression and other mental health problems, including anxiety, contribute significantly to suicide risk. Common precipitants of suicide include physical or mental illness, death of a spouse or partner, substance abuse, and chronic pain (Abbasi and Burke, 2014; Draper, 2014). One of the major differences in suicidal behavior in the old and the young is the lethality of method. Eight out of 10 suicides for men older than 65 were with firearms. Older people rarely threaten to commit suicide; they just do it.

Many older adults who die by suicide reached out for help before they took their own life. Seventy percent visited a physician within 1 month before death; 40% visited within 1 week of the suicide, and 20% visited the physician on the day of the suicide (American Psychological Association, 2014). Depression is frequently missed, and older people with suicide ideation or with other mental health concerns often present with somatic complaints. The statistics suggest that opportunities for assessment of suicidal risk are present, but the need for intervention is not seen as urgent or even recognized. Consequently, it is very important for providers in all settings to inquire about recent life events, implement depression screening for all older people, evaluate for anxiety disorders, assess for suicidal thoughts and ideas based on depression assessment, and recognize warning signs and risk factors for suicide. Behavioral clues and risk and recovery factors are presented in Box 28-23.

BOX 28-23   **Warning Signs and Suicide Risk and Recovery Factors**

Risk Factors and Signs

Male gender
Physical illness
Functional impairment
Depression
Alcohol and substance misuse and abuse
Major loss, such as the death of a spouse or partner
History of major losses
Recent suicide attempt
History of suicide attempts
Major crises or transitions, such as retirement or relocation to an assisted living or nursing facility
Major crises in the lives of family members
Social isolation
Preoccupation with death
Poorly controlled pain
Expression of the belief that one is in the way, a burden
Giving away favorite possessions, money

Recovery Factors

A capacity for the following:
  Understanding
  Relating
  Benefiting from experience
  Benefiting from knowledge
  Accepting help
  Being loving
  Expressing wisdom
  Displaying a sense of humor
  Having a social interest
  Accepting a caring and available family
  Accepting a caring and available social network
  Accepting a caring, available, and knowledgeable professional and health network

---

◆ PROMOTING HEALTHY AGING: IMPLICATIONS FOR GERONTOLOGICAL NURSING

◆ Assessment

Older people with suicidal intent are encountered in many settings. It is our professional obligation to prevent, whenever possible, an impulsive destruction of life that may be a response to a crisis or a disintegrative reaction. The lethality potential of an elder must always be assessed when elements of depression, disease, and spousal loss are evident. Any direct, indirect, or enigmatic references to the ending of life must be taken seriously and discussed. In the nursing home setting, the MDS (Chapter 7) includes screening for suicide risk and mandates that long-term care facilities have effective protocols for managing suicide risk (O'Riley et al, 2013).

The most important consideration for the nurse is to establish a trusting and respectful relationship with the person. Because many older people have grown up in an era when suicide bore stigma and even criminal implications, they may not discuss their feelings in this area. It is also important to remember that in older people, typical behavioral clues such as putting personal affairs in order, giving away possessions, and making wills and funeral plans are indications of maturity and good judgment in late life and cannot be construed as indicative of suicidal intent. Even statements such as "I won't be around long" or "I'm ready to die" may be only a realistic appraisal of the situation in old age.

If there is suspicion that the elder is suicidal, use direct and straightforward questions such as the following:

- Have you ever thought about killing yourself?
- How often have you had these thoughts?
- How would you kill yourself if you decided to do it?

⚡ SAFETY ALERT

Always ask direct questions of the patient and family about suicide risks and suicide ideation.

◆ Interventions

It is important to have a suicide protocol in place that clearly defines how the nurse will intervene if a positive response is obtained from any of the questions. The person should never be left alone for any period of time until help arrives to assist and care for him or her. Patients at high risk should be hospitalized, especially if they have current psychological stressors and/or access to lethal means. Patients at moderate risk may be treated as outpatients provided they have adequate social support and no access to lethal means. Patients at low risk should have a full psychiatric evaluation and be followed up carefully.

Suicide is a taboo topic for most of us, and there is a lingering fear that the introduction of the topic will be suggestive to the patient and may incite suicidal action. Precisely the opposite is true. By introducing the topic, we demonstrate interest in the individual and open the door to honest human interaction and connection on the deep levels of psychological need. It is the nature of our concern and our ability to connect with the alienation and desperation of the individual that will make a difference. Working with isolated, depressed, and suicidal elders challenges the depths of nurses' ingenuity, patience, and self-knowledge.

SUBSTANCE USE DISORDERS

Substance use disorders among older adults are a growing public health concern. There are few international studies and little data on these disorders among older adults in developing countries, but the prevalence of substance use disorders is increasing in North America and Europe (Wang and Andrade, 2013; World Health Organization, 2014). With the aging of the baby boomer generation, the number of adults older than age 50 with substance abuse problems is projected to double by 2020 (CDC, 2013a). The baby boomer generation has had more exposure to alcohol and illegal drugs in their youth and has a more lenient attitude about substance abuse. Additionally, psychoactive drugs became more readily available for dealing with anxiety, pain, and stress. The use of illicit drugs, such as cocaine, heroin, and marijuana, is becoming more prevalent, and baby boomer marijuana users will triple in the next decades (Wang and Andrade, 2013). Marijuana is more common than nonmedical use of prescription-type drugs among adults aged 50 to 59 years while nonmedical use of prescription-type drugs is as common as use of marijuana among adults aged 60 and older (Substance Abuse and Mental Health Services Administration, 2011). Box 28-24 presents *Healthy People 2020* objectives for substance abuse in adults.

Alcohol Use Disorder
Prevalence and Characteristics
In the United States, alcohol use disorders are reported in 11% of adults aged 54 to 64 years and about 6.7% of those older than 65 years. Alcoholism is the third most prevalent psychiatric disorder (after dementia and anxiety) among older men. The prevalence of

alcohol abuse among older adults who are hospitalized for general medical and surgical procedures and institutionalized elders is approximately 18%. Most severe alcohol abuse is seen in people ages 60 to 80 years, not in those older than 80 years. Two-thirds of elderly alcoholics are early-onset drinkers (alcohol use began at age 30 or 40), and one-third are late-onset drinkers (use began after age 60). Late-onset drinking may be related to situational events such as illness, retirement, or death of a spouse and includes a higher number of women (Campbell et al, 2014). Alcohol-related problems in the elderly often go unrecognized, although the residual effects of alcohol abuse complicate the presentation and treatment of many chronic disorders of older people.

Gender Issues
While men (particularly older widowers) are four times more likely to abuse alcohol than women, the prevalence in women may be underestimated. The number and impact of older female drinkers are expected to increase over the next 20 years as the disparity between men's and women's drinking decreases. Women of all ages are significantly more vulnerable to the effects of alcohol misuse including faster progression to dependence and earlier onset of adverse consequences. Even low-risk drinking levels (no more than one standard drink per day) can be hazardous for older women. Older women also experience unique barriers to detection of and treatment for alcohol problems. Health care providers often assume that older women do not drink problematically, so they do not screen for this. Often, alcohol abuse in women is undetected until the consequences are severe (Wang and Andrade, 2013).

Physiology
Older people, especially females, develop higher blood alcohol levels because of age-related changes (increased body fat, decreased lean body mass, and total body water content) that alter absorption and distribution of alcohol. Decreases in hepatic metabolism and kidney function also slow alcohol metabolism and elimination. A decrease in the gastric enzyme alcohol dehydrogenase results in slower metabolism of alcohol and higher blood levels for a longer time. Risks of gastrointestinal ulceration and bleeding related to alcohol use may be higher in older people because of the decrease in gastric acidity that occurs in aging (Nogueira et al, 2013).

Consequences
The health consequences of long-term alcohol use disorder include cirrhosis of the liver, cancer, immune system disorders, cardiomyopathy, cerebral atrophy, and dementia and delirium. Effects of alcohol on cognitive function are receiving greater attention, and a recent study reported that middle-aged men who drink more than 2½ standard drinks a day are more likely to experience faster decline in all cognitive areas, especially memory (Sabia et al, 2014). It is estimated that 10% of dementia is alcohol related (Campbell et al, 2014).

Other effects of alcohol in older people include urinary incontinence, which results from rapid bladder filling and diminished neuromuscular control of the bladder; gait disturbances from alcohol-induced cerebellar degeneration and peripheral neuropathy; depression; functional decline, increased risk for injury; and sleep disturbances and insomnia. Alcohol misuse has also been

---

♥ **BOX 28-24   HEALTHY PEOPLE 2020**

Substance Abuse Objectives for Adults

- Increase the proportion of persons who need alcohol and/or illicit drug treatment and received specialty treatment for abuse or dependence in the past year.
- Increase the proportion of persons who are referred for follow-up care for alcohol problems, drug problems after diagnosis, or treatment for one of these conditions in a hospital emergency department.
- Increase the number of Level 1 and Level II trauma centers and primary care settings that implement evidence-based alcohol Screening and Brief Intervention (SBI).
- Reduce the proportion of adults who drank excessively in the previous 30 days.
- Reduce average alcohol consumption.
- Reduce the past-year nonmedical use of prescription drugs (pain relievers, tranquilizers, stimulants, sedatives, any psychotherapeutic drug).
- Decrease the number of deaths attributable to alcohol.

From U.S. Department of Health and Human Services, Office of Disease Prevention and Health Promotion: *Healthy People 2020,* 2012. http://www.healthypeople.gov/2020

implicated as a major factor in morbidity and mortality as a result of trauma, including falls, drownings, fires, motor vehicle crashes, homicide, and suicide (U.S. Preventive Services Task Force, 2013).

Alcohol use also exacerbates conditions such as osteoporosis, diabetes, hypertension, and ulcers. The rate of hospitalization of older adults for alcohol-related conditions is similar to those admitted for myocardial infarction (Flores, 2014). Many drugs that elders use for chronic illnesses cause adverse effects when combined with alcohol (Box 28-25). All older people should be given precise instructions regarding the interaction of alcohol with their medications.

Alcohol Guidelines for Older Adults

The possible health benefits of alcohol in moderation have been reported in the literature (reduced risk of coronary artery disease, ischemic stroke, Alzheimer's disease, and vascular dementia). As a result, older people may not perceive alcohol use as potentially harmful, but clinically significant adverse effects can occur in some individuals consuming as little as two to three drinks per day over an extended period. A drink is defined as 5 ounces of wine, 12 ounces of beer, or 1.5 ounces of 80-proof distilled spirits or liquor.

> ### BOX 28-25   Medications Interacting with Alcohol
>
> Analgesics
> Antibiotics
> Antidepressants
> Antipsychotics
> Benzodiazepines
> H_2-receptor antagonists
> Nonsteroidal antiinflammatory drugs (NSAIDs)
> Herbal medications (echinacea, valerian)
> Acetaminophen taken on a regular basis, when combined with alcohol, may lead to liver failure
> Alcohol diminishes the effects of oral hypoglycemics, anticoagulants, and anticonvulsants

Because of the increased risk of adverse effects from alcohol use, the National Institute of Alcohol Abuse and Alcoholism defines "at-risk drinking" for men and women aged 65 years and older as more than one drink per day. The American Geriatrics Society guidelines indicate that two or more drinks on a usual drinking day within the past 30 days is considered "at-risk drinking" and five or more drinks on the same occasion as "binge drinking" (Wang and Andrade, 2013). Health professionals must share information with older people about safe drinking limits and the deleterious effects of alcohol intake.

◆ PROMOTING HEALTHY AGING: IMPLICATIONS FOR GERONTOLOGICAL NURSING

◆ Assessment

Reasons for the low rate of alcohol detection among older adults by health care professionals include poor symptom recognition, inadequate knowledge about screening instruments, lack of age-appropriate diagnostic criteria for abuse in older people, and ageism. The diagnosis may be missed in three out of four older hospitalized patients with alcohol dependence (Campbell et al, 2014). Alcohol-related problems may be overlooked in older people because they do not disrupt their lives or are not clearly linked to physical disorders. Health care providers may also be pessimistic about the ability of older people to change long-standing problems.

The U.S. Preventive Services Task Force (2013) recommends that clinicians screen adults 18 years and older in primary care for alcohol misuse. Screening should be a part of health visits for people older than the age of 60 years in primary, acute, and long-term care settings. Although alcohol is the drug most often used among older adults, assessment should include all substances used (recreational drugs, prescription, nicotine, and OTC medications) (Snyder and Platt, 2013). The Hartford Institute of Geriatric Nursing recommends that the Short Michigan Alcoholism Screening Test–Geriatric Version be used with older adults because it is more age appropriate than other instruments (Campbell et al, 2014) (Table 28-1). A single

TABLE 28-1   Short Michigan Alcoholism Screening Test—Geriatric Version (S-MAST-G)

	YES (1)	NO (0)
1. When talking with others, do you ever underestimate how much you drink?		
2. After a few drinks, have you sometimes not eaten, or been able to skip a meal, because you didn't feel hungry?		
3. Does having a few drinks help decrease your shakiness or tremors?		
4. Does alcohol sometimes make it hard for you to remember parts of the day or night?		
5. Do you usually take a drink to relax or calm your nerves?		
6. Do you drink to take your mind off your problems?		
7. Have you ever increased your drinking after experiencing a loss in your life?		
8. Has a doctor or nurse ever said they were worried or concerned about your drinking?		
9. Have you ever made rules to manage your drinking?		
10. When you feel lonely, does having a drink help?		
TOTAL S-MAST-G SCORE (1-10)		

*Scoring: 2 or more "Yes" responses indicate an alcohol problem.
From the Regents of the University of Michigan: Ann Arbor, 1991, University of Michigan Alcohol Research Center.

question can also be used for alcohol screening: "How many times in the past year have you had 5 or more drinks in a day (if a man), or 4 or more drinks (if you are a woman older than 65 years of age)? If the individual acknowledges drinking that much, follow-up assessment is indicated.

Assessment of depression is also important because depression is often comorbid with alcohol abuse. Alcohol and depression screenings should be offered routinely at health fairs and other sites where older people may seek health information. A medication review should be conducted, and screening should be done both before prescribing any new medications that may interact with alcohol and as needed after life-changing events. Alcohol abuse should be suspected in an older person who presents with a history of falling, unexplained bruises, or medical problems associated with alcohol abuse problems.

Alcoholism is a disease of denial and not easy to diagnose, particularly in older people with psychosocial and functional decline from other conditions that may mask decline caused by alcohol. Early signs such as weight loss, irritability, insomnia, and falls may not be recognized as indicators of possible alcohol problems and may be attributed to "just getting older." Box 28-26 presents signs and symptoms that may indicate the presence of alcohol problems in older adults.

Alcohol users often reject or deny the diagnosis, or they may take offense at the suggestion of it. Feelings of shame or disgrace may make elders reluctant to disclose a drinking problem. Families of older people with substance abuse disorders, particularly their adult children, may be ashamed of the problem and choose not to address it. Health care providers may feel helpless over alcoholism or uncomfortable with direct questioning or may approach the person in a judgmental manner. A caring and supportive approach that provides a safe and open atmosphere is the foundation for the therapeutic relationship. It is always important to search for the pain beneath the behavior.

Interventions

Alcohol problems affect physical, mental, spiritual, and emotional health. Interventions must address quality of life in all of these spheres and be adapted to meet the unique needs of the older adult. Abstinence from alcohol is seen as the desired goal, but a focus on education, alcohol reduction, and reducing harm is also appropriate. Increasing the awareness of older adults about the risks and benefits of alcohol consumption in the context of their own situation is an important goal. Treatment and intervention strategies include cognitive-behavioral approaches, individual and group counseling, medical and psychiatric approaches, referral to Alcoholics Anonymous, family therapy, case management and community and home care services, and formalized substance abuse treatment. Treatment outcomes for older people have been shown to be equal to or better than those for younger people (Campbell et al, 2014). Providing education about alcohol use to older people and their families and referring to community resources are important nursing roles and essential to best practices.

Unless the person is in immediate danger, a stepped-care intervention approach beginning with brief interventions followed by more intensive therapies, if necessary, should be used. The U.S. Preventive Services Task Force (2013) recommends brief counseling interventions to reduce alcohol use for adults. Brief intervention is a time-limited, patient-centered strategy focused on changing behavior and assessing patient readiness to change. Sessions can range from one meeting of 10 to 30 minutes to four or five short sessions. The goals of brief intervention are to (1) reduce or stop alcohol consumption and (2) facilitate entry into formalized treatment if needed. Research results indicate that this type of intervention, with counseling by nurses in primary care settings, is effective for reducing alcohol consumption, and older people may be more likely to accept treatment given by their primary care provider.

Long-term self-help treatment programs for elders show high rates of success, especially when social outlets are emphasized and cohort supports are available. A significant concern is the lack of programs designed specifically for older people, particularly older women, whose concerns are very different from those of a younger population who abuse drugs or alcohol. Health status, availability of transportation, and mobility impairments may further limit access to treatment. Development of treatment sites in senior centers and assisted living facilities and telemedicine programs would increase accessibility. Pharmacological treatment has not played a major role in the long-term treatment of alcohol-dependent older adults, but two medications, naltrexone (Revia) and acamprosate (Campral), are approved for treatment and have been used effectively with older adults. Disulfiram (Antabuse) is seldom used in older patients due to concerns about cardiovascular adverse effects (Campbell et al, 2014). Additional resources are presented in Box 28-14.

Acute Alcohol Withdrawal

When there is significant physical dependence, withdrawal from alcohol can become a life-threatening emergency. Detoxification should be done in an inpatient setting because of the potential medical complications and because withdrawal symptoms in older adults can be prolonged. Older people who drink are at

---

BOX 28-26 Signs and Symptoms of Potential Alcohol Problems in Older Adults

Anxiety	Family conflict, abuse
Irritability (feeling worried or "crabby")	Headaches
	Incontinence
Blackouts	Memory loss
Dizziness	Poor hygiene
Indigestion	Poor nutrition
Heartburn	Insomnia
Sadness or depression	Sleep apnea
Chronic pain	Social isolation
Excessive mood swings	Out of touch with family or friends
New problems making decisions	Unusual response to medications
Lack of interest in usual activities	Frequent physical complaints and physician visits
Falls	
Bruises, burns, or other injuries	Financial problems

risk of experiencing acute alcohol withdrawal if admitted to the hospital for treatment of acute illnesses or emergencies. All patients admitted to acute care settings should be screened for alcohol use and assessed for signs and symptoms of alcohol-related problems. Older people with a long history of consuming excess alcohol, previous episodes of acute withdrawal, and/or a history of prior detoxification are at increased risk of acute alcohol withdrawal.

Symptoms of acute alcohol withdrawal vary but may be more severe and last longer in older people. Minor withdrawal (withdrawal tremulousness) begins 6 to 12 hours after a patient has consumed the last drink. Symptoms include tremor, anxiety, nausea, insomnia, tachycardia, and increased blood pressure and frequently may be mistaken for common problems in older adults. Major withdrawal is seen 10 to 72 hours after cessation of alcohol intake, and symptoms include vomiting, diaphoresis, hallucinations, tremors, and seizures (Letizia and Reinboltz, 2005).

Delirium tremens (DTs) is the term used to describe alcohol withdrawal delirium; it usually occurs 24 to 72 hours after the last drink but may occur up to 10 days later. DTs occur in 5% of patients with acute alcohol withdrawal and are considered a medical emergency, with a mortality rate from respiratory failure and cardiac arrhythmia as high as 15%. Other signs and symptoms include confusion, disorientation, hallucinations, hyperthermia, and hypertension. The Clinical Institute Withdrawal Assessment (CIWA) scale is recommended as a valid and reliable screening instrument (www.pubs.niaa.nih.gov) (Letizia and Reinboltz, 2005).

Recommended treatment is the use of short-acting benzodiazepines at one-half to one-third the normal dose around-the-clock or as needed during withdrawal. The use of oral or intravenous alcohol to prevent or treat withdrawal is not established.

The CIWA aids in medication adjustments. Other interventions include assessing mental status, monitoring vital signs, and maintaining fluid balance without overhydrating. Calm and quiet surroundings, no unnecessary stimuli, consistent caregivers, frequent reorientation, prevention of injury, and support and caring are additional suggested interventions. Nutritional assessment is indicated, as well as addition of a multivitamin containing folic acid, pyridoxine, niacin, vitamin A, and thiamine (Campbell et al, 2014; Letizia and Reinboltz, 2005).

Other Substance Abuse Concerns

A more common concern seen among older people is the misuse and abuse of prescription psychoactive medications. Dependence on sedative, hypnotic, or anxiolytic drugs, often prescribed for anxiety or insomnia, and taken for many years with resulting dependence, is especially problematic for older women, who are more likely than men to receive prescriptions for these drugs (Institute of Medicine, 2012). Opioids are ranked second only to benzodiazepines among abused prescription drugs in the older adult population (Naegle, 2012).

Some of the reasons for the abuse of psychoactive prescription medications may be inappropriate prescribing and ineffective monitoring of response and follow-up. In many instances, older people are given prescriptions for benzodiazepines or sedatives because of complaints of insomnia or nervousness, without adequate assessment for depression, anxiety, or other conditions that may be causing the symptoms. Older people may not be informed of the side effects of these medications, including interactions with alcohol, dependence, and withdrawal symptoms. More importantly, conditions such as anxiety and depression may not be recognized and treated appropriately (Wang and Andrade, 2013).

KEY CONCEPTS

- Mental health is a fluctuating situation for most individuals, with peaks and valleys of happiness and pain.
- The prevalence of mental health disorders is expected to increase significantly with the aging of the baby boomers.
- Mental health disorders are underreported and underdiagnosed among older adults. Somatic complaints are often the presenting symptoms of mental health disorders, making diagnosis difficult.
- The incidence of psychotic disorders with late-life onset is low among older people, but psychotic manifestations can occur as secondary symptoms in a variety of disorders, the most common being Alzheimer's disease. Psychotic symptoms in Alzheimer's disease necessitate different assessment and treatment than do long-standing psychotic disorders.
- Anxiety disorders are common in late life, and reestablishing feelings of adequacy and control is the heart of crisis resolution and stress management.
- Depression remains underdiagnosed and undertreated in the older population and is considered a significant public

health issue. Depression in older adults can be effectively treated. Unfortunately, it is often neglected or assumed to be a condition of aging that one must "learn to live with." An important nursing intervention is assessment of depression.
- Suicide is a significant problem among older men, particularly widowers. Many come to be seen by the health care professional with physical complaints shortly before they commit suicide, and assessment of depression and suicidal intent is important.
- Substance abuse, particularly alcohol, and misuse of psychoactive prescription drugs are often underrecognized and undertreated problems of older adults, particularly older women. Screening and appropriate assessment and intervention are important in all settings.
- Treatment outcomes for substance abuse for older people are equal to or better than those for younger people.
- Further research is needed to fully understand the racial, cultural, and ethnic differences in mental health concerns, as well as appropriate assessment and treatment.

NURSING STUDY: BIPOLAR DISORDER

Myra is a 71-year-old white woman who was admitted to the geropsychiatry inpatient unit for alcohol abuse and noncompliance with her lithium, which had been prescribed for a diagnosed bipolar disorder. Myra's primary mode of coping with her depression and mood swings has been to drink alcohol, meet abusive men, and play bingo. However, when she stops taking her dose of lithium, she begins to have flights of ideas, argues with her daughters, and tries to pick up men in her apartment complex. After seeing her at home, you discover that she has a long history of being physically abused by her husband, now deceased for 8 years, and has been living with one daughter who also has emotionally and physically abused her, causing Myra to be hospitalized. Myra's ability to test reality is compromised because of years of denial and low self-esteem. She says, "I used to have lots of times when I felt really good in between the depressions. Now I feel depressed most of the time." She tells you that her daughters harass her and interfere in her life. Your goals as a community-based nurse are to facilitate her independence (being able to live in her own apartment), to assist her with medication compliance, and to intervene with Myra to improve relationships with her daughters. Home visits are approved through Medicare for 1 month after hospital discharge.

Based on the case study, develop a nursing care plan using the following procedure*:
- List Myra's comments that provide subjective data.
- List information that provides objective data.
- From these data, identify and state, using an accepted format, two nursing diagnoses you determine are most significant to Myra at this time. List two of Myra's strengths that you have identified from the data.
- Determine and state outcome criteria for each diagnosis. These criteria must reflect some alleviation of the problem identified in the nursing diagnosis and must be stated in concrete and measurable terms.
- Plan and state one or more interventions for each diagnosed problem. Provide specific documentation of the sources used to determine the appropriate intervention. Plan at least one intervention that incorporates Myra's existing strengths.
- Evaluate the success of the intervention. Interventions must correlate directly with the stated outcome criteria to measure the outcome success.

*Students are advised to refer to their nursing diagnosis text and identify possible or potential problems.

CRITICAL THINKING QUESTIONS AND ACTIVITIES

1. How will you evaluate Myra's ability to live independently?
2. What particular strategies are necessary to meet the goals of the nursing care plan?
3. Given that Myra's primary coping strategy is drinking alcohol, how will you facilitate her sobriety and help her deal with stress?
4. How much involvement with Myra's daughters do you believe is necessary to assist with her transition back into her own apartment?
5. Given the limited number of visits covered by Medicare, what information does Myra need to provide self-care? In other words, the nurse must be teaching Myra how to live independently after discharge from home health care. What does Myra need to know?
6. Discuss the meanings and thoughts triggered by the student's and the elder's viewpoints expressed at the beginning of the chapter. How do these vary from your own experience?

NURSING STUDY: DEPRESSIVE DISORDER WITH SUICIDAL THOUGHTS

Depressive Disorder with Suicidal Thoughts

Jake had cared for his wife Emma during a long and painful illness until she died 4 years ago. He found that alcohol provided a way to cope with the stress. Within a year after her death, Jake met a lady to whom he was very attracted, and a few months later she moved in with him. Jake managed to move his things around until some space was made for her personal items, but neither of them was very comfortable with this. He really did not like to move his things from their usual place and, because her allotted space was so small, she felt like an intruder. He collected guns, and she shuddered when she saw them. He was an avid fan of John Wayne movies, and she preferred going to the symphony. He liked meat and potatoes, and she was a vegetarian. She also disapproved of his increasing reliance on alcohol. The blending of two such different lifestyles proved difficult. In a few months she moved out, and Jake blamed himself. He said over and over, "I should have done more for her. I'm not good for anything anymore." His friends began to pull away from him, just when he needed them most, because he seemed to talk of nothing but his various aches, pains, and pills and his general discouragement with life. Jake's consumption of alcohol increased markedly.

He had some health problems: a mild heart failure, a lack of exercise, dairy products gave him diarrhea, he was somewhat obese, and his knees were painful most of the time. He routinely visited his allergist, his internist, his orthopedist, and his cardiologist. However, it seemed the more he went to these specialists, the worse he felt. He was taking several medications, and each time he saw one of his clinicians, he came away with another prescription. No one asked about his drinking, and he never

mentioned it. He awoke one morning feeling very dizzy, so he went to his internist later in the day. He began to share the litany of his discomforts, and the physician reminded him that at 76 years of age he could not expect to always feel in top shape.

When he returned from seeing the physician, Jake called his daughter and surprised her by saying he had just decided he would take a week off and go to Hawaii to see if the sun and sand would revive him. Jake was not usually impulsive. His daughter, fortunately, was a psychiatric nurse and was concerned about the change in his behavior.

Based on the case study, develop a nursing care plan using the following procedure*:
- List Jake's comments that provide subjective data.
- List information that provides objective data.
- From these data, identify and state, using an accepted format, two nursing diagnoses you determine are most significant to Jake at this time. List two of Jake's strengths that you have identified from the data.
- Determine and state outcome criteria for each diagnosis. These criteria must reflect some alleviation of the problem identified in the nursing diagnosis and must be stated in concrete and measurable terms.
- Plan and state one or more interventions for each diagnosed problem. Provide specific documentation of the source used to determine the appropriate intervention. Plan at least one intervention that incorporates Jake's existing strengths.
- Evaluate the success of the intervention. Interventions must correlate directly with the stated outcome criteria to measure the outcome success.

*Students are advised to refer to their nursing diagnosis text and identify possible or potential problems.

CRITICAL THINKING QUESTIONS AND ACTIVITIES

1. Discuss the variations in symptoms of depression in the old and the young.
2. Describe some of the reasons that may make elders vulnerable to depression.
3. Describe a time when you were depressed and the feelings you had. What did you do about it?
4. Given the situation in this case, discuss what your thoughts would be if you were Jake's daughter.
5. Given his daughter's background, what are her responsibilities in this case?
6. What is the responsibility of a student nurse in the case of suspected suicidal thoughts?
7. Would you address the possibility of suicidal thoughts if you were the nurse in a primary care setting? When and how would you take on this task?
8. What action should be taken for Jake's protection?
9. Would you expect that Jake is still grieving over the death of his wife? What are your thoughts about this situation?
10. What are the clues or indications that an elder is thinking of committing suicide?
11. What are some of signs of suicidal intent in young adults? How are these signs different from those of elders?
12. Under what conditions do you think a person has a right to take his or her life?
13. What are your thoughts about Jake's use of alcohol?
14. Do you think suicide is a sign of weakness or strength?
15. Do you agree or disagree with the following statements on the basis of the evidence about depression and suicide in older adults?
    - Normally older people feel depressed much of the time.
    - Older people are more likely than young people to admit to depression.
    - Most older people talk about suicide but rarely try to kill themselves.
    - Depression of the elderly is helped by medications.
    - Depression may be the cause of forgetfulness.
    - Depression in the elderly is often linked with illness and alcoholism.

RESEARCH QUESTIONS

1. What is the prevalence of mental health disorders in community-dwelling older adults? What mental health care is nursing able to provide in the home?
2. How common is alcohol abuse a strategy of self-care used by the older adult with emotional concerns?
3. What types of interventions are most appropriate for older adults with alcohol or drug abuse problems?
4. Is psychiatric home care a more cost-effective alternative than institutional care?
5. What are the cardinal symptoms of depression in the oldest-old?
6. How many PCPs consider or evaluate for the presence of depression in elders who see them for physical complaints?
7. What are the most reliable tools for identifying depression in cognitively intact and cognitively impaired elders?
8. What is the meaning of depression in older people of different races, cultures, and ethnicities?
9. What modifications need to be made in assessment and treatment of mental health disorders to enhance cultural appropriateness?

REFERENCES

Abbasi O, Burke W: Depression. In Ham R, Sloane P, Warshaw G, et al, editors: *Primary care geriatrics*, ed 6, Philadelphia, 2014, Elsevier, pp 214–226.

Agency for Healthcare Research and Quality: *Certain therapies and medications improve outcomes of adults with post-traumatic stress disorder. Research Activities*, July 2013. http://www.ahrq.gov/news/newsletters/research-activities/13jul/0713RA3.html. Accessed July 2014.

Akincigil A, Olfson M, Siegel M, et al: Racial and ethnic disparities in depression care in community-dwelling elderly in the United States, *Am J Pub Health* 102(2):319–328, 2012.

Alexopoulos G: Clinical and neurobiological findings, treatment developments in late-life depression, *Psychiatr Ann* 44(3):126–129, 2014.

American Psychiatric Association: *Diagnostic and statistical manual of mental disorders*, ed 5, Arlington, VA, 2013, American Psychiatric Publishing.

American Psychological Association: *Mental and behavioral health and older Americans*, 2014. http://www.apa.org/about/gr/issues/aging/mental-health.aspx. Accessed July 2014.

Avari J, Yuen G, AbdelMalak B, et al: Assessment and management of late-life depression, *Psychiatr Ann* 44(3):131–137, 2014.

Baxter A, Patton G, Scott K, et al: Global epidemiology of mental disorders: what are we missing? *PLoS One*, June 24, 2013, DOI: 10.1371/journal.pone.0065514.

Baxter A, Scott K, Ferrari A, et al: Challenging the myth of an "epidemic" of common mental disorders: trends in the global prevalence of anxiety and depression between 1990 and 2010, *Depress Anxiety* 31:506–516, 2014.

Bludau J: Second institutionalization: impact of personal history on patients with dementia, *Caring Ages* 3(5):3–4, 2002.

Bormann J, Thorp S, Wetherell J, et al: A spirituality based group intervention for combat veterans with posttraumatic stress disorder: feasibility study, *J Holist Nurs* 26:109–116, 2008.

Bottche M, Kuwert P, Knaevelsrud C: Post-traumatic stress disorder in older adults: an overview of characteristics and treatment approaches, *Int J Geriatr Psychiatry* 27(3):230–239, 2012.

Brenes G, Danhauer S, Lyles M, et al: Telephone-delivered psychotherapy for rural-dwelling older adults with generalized anxiety disorder: study protocol of a randomized controlled trial, *BMC Psychiatry* 14:34, 2014.

Bryant C, Mohlman J, Gum A, et al: Anxiety disorders in older adults: looking to DSM5 and beyond, *Am J Ger Psychiatry* 21(9):872–876, 2013.

Burnside I: Listen to the aged, *Am J Nurs* 75(10):1800–1803,1822, 1975.

Byers A, Yaffe K, Covinsky K, et al: High occurrence of mood and anxiety disorders among older adults, *Arch Gen Psychiatry* 67:489–496, 2010.

Campbell J, Resnick B, Warshaw G: Alcoholism. In Ham R, Sloane P, Warshaw G, et al, editors: *Primary care geriatrics*, ed 6, Philadelphia, 2014, Elsevier, pp 365–371.

Carson V, Yambor S: Managing patients with bipolar disorder at home, *Home Healthc Nurse* 30(5):280–291, 2012.

Center for Medicare Advocacy: *Medicare and mental health*, 2014. http://www.medicareadvocacy.org/medicare-and-mental-health. Accessed June 2014.

Centers for Disease Control and Prevention: *The state of aging and health in America 2013*, Atlanta GA, 2013a, U.S. Department of Health and Human Services.

Centers for Disease Control and Prevention: Suicide among adults aged 35-64 years—United States, 1999-2010, *MMWR Morb Mortal Wkly Rep* 62(17):321–325, 2013b.

Chan M, Leong K, Heng B, et al: Reducing depression among community-dwelling older adults using life-story review: a pilot study, *Geriatr Nurs* 35:105–110, 2014.

Chopra M, Zhang H, Kaiser A, et al: PTSD is a chronic, fluctuating disorder affecting the mental quality of life in older adults, *Am J Ger Psychiatry* 22(1):86–96. 2014.

Christianson S, Marren J: *Impact of Event Scale-Revised (IES-R)*, New York, 2013, Hartford Institute for Geriatric Nursing.

Clapp J, Beck J: Treatment of PTSD in older adults: do cognitive-behavioral interventions remain viable? *Cogn Behav Pract* 19(1):126–135, 2012.

Clifford K, Duncan N, Heinrich K, Shaw J: Update on managing generalized anxiety disorder in older adults, *Jour Gerontol Nurs* 41(4):10-20, 2015.

Collier E, Sorrell J: Schizophrenia in older adults, *J Psychosoc Nurs Ment Health Serv* 49(11):17–20, 2011.

Crowe M, Whitehead L, Wilson L, et al: Disorder-specific psychosocial interventions for bipolar disorder—a systematic review of the evidence for mental health nursing practice, *Int J Nurs Studies* 47:896–908, 2010.

DeKeyser F, Jacobs J: The effect of humor on elder mental and physical health, *Geriatr Nurs* 35(3):205–211, 2014.

Demers L, Robichaud L, Gelinas I, et al: Coping strategies and social participation in older adults, *Gerontology* 55:233–239, 2009.

Dols A, Rhebergen D, Beckman A, et al: Psychiatric and medical comorbidities: results from a bipolar elderly cohort study, *Am J Geriatr Psychiatry* 22:1066–1074, 2014.

Draper B: Suicidal behaviour and suicide prevention in later life, *Maturitas* 79: 179–183, 2014.

Eells K: The use of music and singing to help manage anxiety in older adults, *Ment Health Pract* 17(5):10–17, 2014.

Evans L: *Mental health issues in aging*, 2008. http://hartfordign.org/uploads/File/gnec_state_of_science_papers/gnec_mental_health.pdf. Accessed October 31, 2014.

Flores D: *Geriatric gems and palliative pearls: alcohol use among older adults*, University of Texan Health Science Center at Houston. http://www.uth.tmc.edu/HGEC/GemsAndPearls/index.html. Accessed July 2014.

Foundation for Psychocultural Research: *DSM-5 on culture: a significant advance*, 2013. http://thefprorg.wordpress.com/2013/06/27/dsm-5-on-culture-a-significant-advance. Accessed June 2014.

Fournier J, DeRubeis R, Hollon S, et al: Antidepressant drug effects and depression severity: a patient-level meta-analysis, *JAMA* 303(1):47–53, 2010.

Friedman M, Furst L, Gellis Z, et al: Anxiety disorders in older adults, *Social Work Today* 13(4):10, 2013.

Grabowski D, Aschbrenner K, Rome V, et al: Quality of mental health care for nursing home residents: a literature review, *Med Care Res Rev* 67(6):627–656, 2010.

Hall C, Reynolds C: Late-life depression in the primary care setting: challenges, collaborative care, and prevention, *Maturitas*, June 7, 2014. http://www.maturitas.org/article/S0378-5122(14)00195-9/fulltext. Accessed July 2014.

Hampton L, Daubresse M, Chang H-Y, et al: Emergency department visits by adults for psychiatric medication adverse effects, *JAMA Psychiatry*, Jul 9, 2014. doi: 10.1001/jamapsychiatry.2014.436. [Epub ahead of print].

Harvath T, McKenzie G: Depression in older adults. In Boltz M, Capezuti E, Fulmer T, et al, editors: *Evidence-based geriatric nursing protocols for best practice*, ed 4, New York, 2012, Springer, pp 135–162.

Hendrie H, Tu W, Tabbey R, et al: Health outcomes and cost of care among older adults with schizophrenia: a 10-year study using medical records across the continuum of care, *Am J Geriatr Psychiatry* 22(5):427–435, 2014.

Hildon Z, Montgomery S, Blane D, et al: Examining resilience of quality of life in the face of health-related and psychosocial adversity at older ages: what is "right" about the way we age? *Gerontologist* 50:36–47, 2009.

Holt-Lunstad J, Smith T, Layton J: Social relationships and mortality risk: a meta-analytic review, *PLoS Med* 7:e1000316, 2010.

Institute of Medicine (IOM): *The mental health and substance use workforce for older adults: in whose hands?* 2012. http://www.iom.edu/Reports/2012/The-Mental-Health-and-Substance-Use-Workforce-for-Older-Adults.aspx. Accessed June 2014.

Jameson J, Shrestha S, Escamilla M, et al: Establishing community partnerships to support late-life anxiety research: lessons learned from the calmer life project, *Aging Ment Health* 16(7):874–883, 2012.

Jeste D, Maglione J: Treating older adults with schizophrenia: challenges and opportunities, *Schizophr Bull* 39(5):966–968, 2013.

Jimenez D, Bartels S, Cardenas V, et al: Cultural beliefs and mental health treatment preferences of ethnically diverse older adult consumers in primary care, *Am J Geriatr Psych* 20(6):533–542, 2012.

Jimenez D, Cook B, Bartels S, et al: Disparities in mental health service use of racial and ethnic minority elderly adults, *J Am Geriatr Soc* 61:18–25, 2013.

John A. Hartford Foundation: *Public poll: "Silver and blue – the unfinished business of mental heatlh care for older adults,"* Dec 10, 2012. http://www.jhartfound.org/learning-center/john-a-hartford-foundation-national-public-poll-silver-and-blue-the-unfinished-business-of-mental-health-care-for-older-adults. Accessed July 2014.

Kaiser A, Wachen J, Potter C, et al: *Posttraumatic stress symptoms among older adults: a review*, 2014a. http://www.ptsd.va.gov/professional/PTSD-overview/index.asp. Accessed July 2014.

Kaiser A, Wachen J, Potter C, et al: *PTSD assessment and treatment in older adults*, 2014b. http://www.ptsd.va.gov/professional/treatment/older. Accessed July 2014.

Katz C, Stein M, Sareen J: Anxiety disorders in the DSM-5: new rules on diagnosis and treatment, *Mood Anxiety Disord Rounds* 2(3), 2013. http://www.moodandanxietyrounds.ca/crus/144-010%20English.pdf. Accessed July 2014.

Khouzam H: Posttraumatic stress disorder: psychological and spiritual interventions, *Consultant* 53(10):720–725, 2013.

Kim G, Parton J, DeCoster J, et al: Regional variations of racial disparities in mental health service use among older adults, *Gerontologist* 53(4):618–626, 2012.

Kleinman A: *Patient and healers in the context of culture: an exploration of the borderland between anthropology, medicine, and psychiatry*, Berkeley, 1980, University of California Press.

Knight M: Access to mental health care among older adults, *Jour Gerontol Nurs* 37(3):16–21, 2011.

Lazarus R, Folkman S: *Stress appraisal and coping*, New York, 1984, Springer.

Letizia M, Reinboltz M: Identifying and managing acute alcohol withdrawal in the elderly, *Geriatr Nurs* 26(3):176–183, 2005.

Leutwyler H, Wallhagen M: Understanding physical health of older adults with schizophrenia: building and eroding trust, *J Gerontol Nurs* 36 (5):38–45, 2010.

McGovern A, Kiosses D, Raue P, et al: Psychotherapies for late-life depression, *Psychiatr Ann* 44(3):147–152, 2014.

Meesters P: Late-life schizophrenia: remission, recovery, resilience, *Am J Geriatr Psychiatry* 22(5):423–426, 2014.

Mental Health America: *Depression in older adults*, 2014a. http://www.mentalhealthamerica.net/conditions/depression-older-adults. Accessed July 2014.

Mental Health America: *Position statement 34: Aging well*, 2014b. http://www.mentalhealthamerica.net/positions/aging-well. Accessed June 2014.

Mitsch A: Antidepressant adverse drug reactions in older adults: implications for RNs and APNs, *Geriatr Nurs* 34:53–61, 2013.

Morimoto S, Kanellopoulos T, Alexopoulos G: Cognitive impairment in depressed older adults: implications for prognosis and treatment, *Psychiatr Ann* 44(3):138–142, 2014.

Murphy K: The ups and downs of bipolar disorder, *Am J Nurs* 11(4):44–50, 2013.

Naegle M: Substance misuse and alcohol use disorders. In Boltz M, Capezuti E, Fulmer T, et al, editors: *Evidence-based geriatric nursing protocols for best practice*, ed 4, New York, 2012, Springer, pp 516–537.

National Alliance on Mental Illness: *Chinese American mental health facts*, 2011. https://www.nami.org/Template.cfm?Section=Fact_Sheets1&Template=/ContentManagement/ContentDisplay.cfm&ContentID=129323. Accessed July 2014.

National Institute of Mental Health: *Posttraumatic stress disorder (PTSD)*, 2014. http://www.nimh.nih.gov/health/topics/post-traumatic-stress-disorder-ptsd/index.shtml#part1. Accessed July 2014.

National Institute of Mental Health Senior Health: *Depression*, 2014. http://nihseniorhealth.gov/depression/aboutdepression/01.html. Accessed July 2014.

Nogueira E, Neto A, Cauduro M, et al: Prevalence and patterns of alcohol misuse in a community-dwelling elderly sample in Brazil, *J Aging Health* 25:1340–1357, 2013.

O'Riley A, Nadorff M, Conwell Y, et al: Challenges associated with managing suicide risk in long-term care facilities, *Ann Longterm Care* 21(6):28–34, 2013.

Osterweil N: Older adults with schizophrenia can achieve remission, *Clin Psychiatry News*, Nov 12, 2012. http://www.clinicalpsychiatrynews.com/single-view/older-adults-with-schizophrenia-can-achieve-remission/ded3b0fff74af27314348d657b26309c.html. Accessed May 12, 2015.

Pachana N: A global snapshot of mental health issues, services, and policy, *Generations* 37(1):27–32, 2013.

Qualls S: Defining mental health in later life, *Generations* 26(7):9–13, 2002.

Qureshi S, Kimbrell T, Pyne J, et al: Greater prevalence and incidence of dementia in older veterans with posttraumatic stress disorder, *J Am Geriatr Soc* 58:1627–1633, 2010.

Resnick B, Inguito P: The resilience scale: psychometric properties and clinical applicability in older adults, *Arch Psychiatr Nurs* 25(1):11–20, 2011.

Reuben D, Ganz D, Roth C, et al: Effect of nurse practitioner comanagement on the care of geriatric conditions, *J Am Geriatr Soc* 61(6):857–867, 2013.

Rytwinski N, Scur M, Feeny N, et al: The co-occurrence of major depressive disorder among individuals with posttraumatic stress disorder: a meta-analysis, *J Trauma Stress* 26:299–309, 2014.

Sabia S, Elbaz A, Britton A, et al: Alcohol consumption and cognitive decline in early old age, *Neurology* 82(4):332–339, 2014.

Smith M, Haedtke C, Shibley D: Evidence-based practice guideline: Late-life depression detection, *Jour Gerontol Nurs* 41(2):18-25, 2015.

Snyder M, Platt L: Substance use and brain reward mechanisms in older adults, *J Psychosoc Nurs* 51(7):15–20, 2013.

Splete H: Mentally ill eclipse residents with dementia, *Caring Ages* 10(12):11, 2009.

Substance Abuse and Mental Health Services Administration, Center for Behavioral Health Statistics and Quality: *The NSDUH report: illicit drug use among older adults*, Rockville, MD, Sept 1, 2011, SAMHSA.

Thorp S, Ayers C, Nuevo R, et al: Meta-analysis comparing different behavioral treatments for late-life anxiety, *Am J Geriatr Psychiatry* 17:105–115, 2009.

Uher R, Payne J, Pavlova B, et al: Major depressive disorder in DSM-5: implications for clinical practice and research of changes from DSM-IV, *Depress Anxiety* 31:459–471, 2014.

Umberson D, Montez J: Social relationships and health: a flashpoint for health policy, *J Health Soc Behav* 51(Suppl):S54–S66, 2010.

Unutzer J, Harbin H, Schoenbaum M, et al: *The collaborative care model: an approach for integrating physical and mental health care in Medicaid health homes* (Health Home Resource Center brief), May 2013. http://www.medicaid.gov/State-Resource-Center/Medicaid-State-Technical-Assistance/Health-Homes-Technical-Assistance/Downloads/HH-IRC-Collaborative-5-13.pdf. Accessed July 2014.

U.S. Department of Health and Human Services (USDHHS), Office of Disease Prevention and Health Promotion: *Healthy People 2020*, 2012. http://www.healthypeople.gov/2020 Accessed May 12, 2015.

U.S. Department of Veterans Affairs, Office Research and Development: *Heart-mind mystery*, VA Research Currents, Feb 28, 2014. http://www.research.va.gov/currents/spring2014/spring2014-1.cfm. Accessed July 2014.

U.S. Preventive Services Task Force: *Alcohol misuse: screening and behavioral counseling interventions in primary care*, 2013. http://www.uspreventiveservicestaskforce.org/uspstf12/alcmisuse/alcmisusefinalrs.htm. Accessed July 2014.

Vaccarino V, Goldberg J, Rooks C, et al: Posttraumatic stress disorder and incidence of coronary heart disease: a twin study, *J Am Coll Cardiol* 62(11):970–979, 2013.

van der Aa H, van Rens G, Comijs H, et al: Stepped-care to prevent depression and anxiety in visually impaired older adults—design of a randomized controlled trial, *BMC Psychiatry* 13:209, 2013.

van Kessel G: The ability of older people to overcome adversity: a review of the resilience concept, *Geriatr Nurs* 34(2):122–127, 2012.

Wang Y, Andrade L: Epidemiology of alcohol and drug use in the elderly, *Curr Opin Psychiatry* 26(4):343–348, 2013.

Warren B: How culture is assessed in the DSM-5, *J Psychosoc Nurs* 51(4):40–45, 2013.

Wetherell J, Jeste D: Older adults with schizophrenia, *Elder Care* 3(2):8–11, 2011.

Wetherell J, Perkus A, White K, et al: Antidepressant medication augmented with cognitive-behavioral therapy for generalized anxiety disorder in older adults, *Am J Psychiatry* 170:782–789, 2013.

Woodward A, Taylor R, Abelson J, et al: Major depressive disorder among older African-Americans, Caribbean Blacks, and non-Hispanic Whites: secondary analysis of the national survey of American life, *Depress Anxiety* 30:589–597, 2013.

World Health Organization: *Mental health and older adults* (Fact sheet no. 381), Sept 2013. http://www.who.int/mediacentre/factsheets/fs381/en. Accessed July 2014.

World Health Organization: *Mental Health Gap Action Programme: Scaling up care for mental, neurological, and substance abuse disorders*, 2014. http://www.who.int/mental_health/mhgap/en. Accessed May 2014.

Wright R, LeBlanc A, deVries B, et al: Stress and mental health among midlife and older gay-identified men, *Am J Public Health* 102(3):503–509, 2012.

Yancura L, Aldwin C: Coping and health in older adults, *Curr Psychiatry Rep* 10:10–15, 2008.

Zauszniewski J, Au T, Musil C: Resourcefulness training for grandmothers raising grandchildren, *Issues Ment Health Nurs* 33(10):680–686, 2012.

Zauszniewski J, Bekhet A, Lai C, et al: Effects of teaching resourcefulness and acceptance of affect, behavior, and cognition of chronically ill elders, *Issues Ment Health Nurs* 28:575–592, 2007.

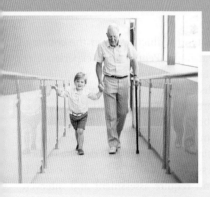

CHAPTER 29

Care of Individuals with Neurocognitive Disorders

Debra Hain, María Ordóñez, and Theris A. Touhy

http://evolve.elsevier.com/Touhy/TwdHlthAging

A STUDENT SPEAKS

I imagine I am in my late 80s and my husband and I live with our daughter. I am experiencing an unpleasant physical change; I am losing my memory. I can sharply remember all details about events that happened a long time ago but often fail to recall what happened 2 hours ago. Although this situation scares me and I wonder what will happen if my family gets tired of my forgetfulness, I remind myself that I live with the people who love and care for me very much and will not desert me when I need them the most.

Tatyana, age 30

AN ELDER SPEAKS

LIVING WITH ALZHEIMER'S DISEASE: A REQUEST

Do not ask me to remember; don't try to make me understand.

Let me rest and know you're with me, kiss my cheek and hold my hand.

I'm confused beyond your concept; I'm sad and sick and lost. All I know is that I need you to be with me at all cost.

Do not lose patience with me, do not scold or curse or cry. I can't help the way I'm acting; I can't be different though I try.

Just remember that I need you, that the best of me is gone.

Please don't fail to stand beside me, love me, till my life is gone.

Author Anonymous

LEARNING OBJECTIVES

On completion of this chapter, the reader will be able to:

1. Identify the characteristics of delirium and differentiate between delirium and mild and major neurocognitive disorders (dementia) and depression.
2. Discuss prevention, treatment, and nursing interventions for individuals with delirium.
3. Describe nursing models of care for persons with mild and major neurocognitive disorders.
4. Discuss common concerns in care of persons with mild and major neurocognitive disorders (communication, behavior, personal care, safety, nutrition) and nursing interventions.
5. Discuss strategies to enhance well-being and quality of life for both individuals with mild and major neurocognitive disorders and their caregivers.

CARING FOR INDIVIDUALS WITH NEUROCOGNITIVE DISORDERS

This chapter focuses on care of older adults living with mild and major neurocognitive disorders (dementia) and delirium with an emphasis on nursing interventions. The term dementia has been replaced with mild and major neurocognitive disorders in the *DSM-5* (American Psychiatric Association, 2013), but the terms *dementia* and *cognitive impairment* will also be

used in this chapter. Chapter 23 presents information about neurocognitive disorders including classification, etiology, disease-specific information, and pharmacological treatment.

The concept of person-centered care for people with mild and major cognitive disorders will guide health promotion strategies in this population. Person-centered care is one of the six major aims in the redesign of the U.S. health care system. Person-centered care considers what "matters most" to individuals by being respectful and responsive to an individual's preference, needs, and values and ensuring that these are considered in shared decision-making between the nurse and the person (Institute of Medicine, 2001).

All older adults with neurocognitive disorders (NCDs) are deserving of active nursing intervention to maintain the highest practicable level of physical and cognitive function and quality of life. To improve health outcomes of older adults with NCDs, it is essential that gerontological nurses embrace evidence-based practice to support person-centered interventions. Evidence-based practice takes the best available research, clinician expertise, and person/family preferences for clinical decision-making.

NEUROCOGNITIVE DISORDER: DELIRIUM

Although delirium is common in older adults, it often goes unrecognized, which increases the risk of functional decline, mortality, and health care costs (Inouye et al, 2014). Nurses play a key role in early identification and implementation of interventions aimed at reducing delirium and associated risks. Depression, delirium, and the mild and major neurocognitive disorders (dementia) are called the *three D's* of cognitive impairment because they occur frequently in older adults. These important geriatric syndromes are not a normal consequence of aging, although incidence increases with age. Because cognitive and behavioral changes characterize all *three D's*, it can be difficult to diagnose delirium, delirium superimposed on mild or major neurocognitive disorder (dementia) (DSD), or depression (Chapter 28).

Differences among Delirium, Dementia (Mild and Major Neurocognitive Disorder), and Depression

Delirium is characterized by an acute or subacute onset, with symptoms developing over a short period of time (usually hours to days). Symptoms tend to fluctuate over the course of the day, often worsening at night. People often experience reduced ability to focus, sustain, or shift attention, which leads to cognitive or perceptual disturbances (O'Mahony et al, 2011). Perceptual disturbances are often accompanied by delusional (paranoid) thoughts and behavior and hallucinations.

In contrast, major and mild neurocognitive disorder typically has a gradual onset and a slow, steady pattern of decline without alterations in consciousness. These disorders represent serious pathological alterations and require assessment and interventions. However, a change in cognitive function in older adults is often seen as "normal" and not investigated. Any change in mental status in an older person requires appropriate assessment (Chapters 5, 7, and 23). Knowledge about cognitive function in aging and appropriate assessment and evaluation are keys to differentiating these three syndromes. Table 29-1 presents the clinical features and the differences in cognitive and behavioral characteristics in delirium, mild and major neurocognitive disorders, and depression. The accepted criteria for a diagnosis of delirium are presented in the *Diagnostic and Statistical Manual of Mental Disorders* (American Psychiatric Association, 2013).

Etiology

The development of delirium is a result of complex interactions among multiple causes. Delirium results from the interaction of predisposing factors (e.g., vulnerability on the part of the individual due to predisposing conditions, such as underlying cognitive impairment, functional impairment, depression, acute illness, sensory impairment) and precipitating factors/insults (e.g., medications, procedures, restraints, iatrogenic events, sleep deprivation, bladder catheterization, pain, and

TABLE 29-1 Differentiating Delirium, Depression, and Dementia (Mild and Moderate Neurocognitive Disorders)

CHARACTERISTIC	DELIRIUM	DEPRESSION	DEMENTIA
Onset	Sudden, abrupt	Recent, may relate to life change	Insidious, slow, over years and often unrecognized until deficits obvious
Course over 24 hours	Fluctuating, often worse at night	Fairly stable, may be worse in the morning	Fairly stable, may see changes with stress
Consciousness	Reduced	Clear	Clear
Alertness	Increased, decreased, or variable	Normal	Generally normal
Psychomotor activity	Increased, decreased, or mixed Sometimes increased, other times decreased	Variable, agitation or retardation	Normal, may have apraxia or agnosia
Duration	Hours to weeks	Variable and may be chronic	Years
Attention	Disordered, fluctuates	Little impairment	Generally normal but may have trouble focusing
Orientation	Usually impaired, fluctuates	Usually normal; may answer "I don't know" to questions or may not try to answer	Often impaired; may make up answers or answer close to the right thing or may confabulate but try to answer
Speech	Often incoherent, slow, or rapid; may call out repeatedly or repeat the same phrase	May be slow	Difficulty finding word, perseveration
Affect	Variable but may look disturbed, frightened	Flat	Slowed response, may be labile

Modified from Sendelbach S, Guthrie PF, Schoenfelder DP: Acute confusion/delirium, *J Gerontol Nurs* 35(11):11–18, 2009.

environmental factors). Although a single factor, such as an infection, can trigger an episode of delirium, several co-existing factors are also likely to be present. A highly vulnerable older individual requires a lesser amount of precipitating factors to develop delirium (Inouye et al, 2014; Voyer et al, 2010).

The exact pathophysiological mechanisms involved in the development and progression of delirium remain uncertain. One single cause or mechanism is not likely, but rather emerging evidence supports the theory of complex interaction of biological factors leading to the disruption of neuronal networks (Inouye et al, 2014). Delirium is thought to be related to disturbances in the neurotransmitters in the brain that modulate the control of cognitive function, behavior, and mood. Existing evidence indicates that cholinergic dysfunction and neuroinflammation are associated with delirium pathophysiology (Cerejeira et al, 2012). The causes of delirium are potentially reversible; therefore accurate assessment and diagnosis are critical. Delirium is given many labels: acute confusional state, acute brain syndrome, confusion, reversible dementia, metabolic encephalopathy, and toxic psychosis.

Incidence and Prevalence

Delirium is a prevalent and serious disorder that occurs in older adults across the continuum of care. Among medical inpatients, delirium is present on admission to the hospital in 10% to 31% of older patients. During hospitalization, 11% to 42% of older adults develop delirium. The highest incidence rates have been in intensive care units and in postoperative and palliative care areas (Inouye et al, 2014; Tullmann et al, 2012). Up to 80% of patients in the intensive care unit (ICU) develop delirium (Bledowski and Trutia, 2013). In subacute settings, a 16% delirium rate in patients newly admitted to subacute care has been reported. More than 50% of these patients are still delirious 1 month after admission (Marcantonio et al, 2010). The prevalence of delirium in the community is low (about 1% to 2%), but the development of delirium often leads to an emergency department visit, where the prevalence is about 8% to 17% of all older adults and 40% of nursing home residents (Inouye et al, 2014).

Delirium Superimposed on Mild and Major Neurocognitive Disorders (Dementia)

Older patients with mild and major neurocognitive disorders are three to five times more likely to develop delirium, and it is less likely to be recognized and treated than delirium without mild and major NCD. DSD can accelerate the trajectory of cognitive decline in individuals and is associated with high mortality among hospitalized older people. Changes in the mental status of older adults with dementia are often attributed to underlying dementia, or "sundowning," and not investigated. Despite its prevalence, DSD has not been well investigated and there are only a few relevant studies in either the hospital or community setting (Inouye et al, 2014).

Recognition of Delirium

Delirium is a medical emergency and one of the most significant geriatric syndromes. However, it is often not recognized by health care practitioners. A comprehensive review of the literature suggested that "nurses are missing key symptoms of delirium and appear to be doing superficial mental status assessments" (Steis and Fick, 2008, p. 47). Factors contributing to the lack of recognition of delirium among health care professionals include inadequate education about delirium, limited use of formal assessment methods, a view that delirium is not as essential to the patient's well-being in light of more serious medical problems, and ageist attitudes (Kuehn, 2010a,b; Waszynski and Petrovic, 2008). Failure to recognize delirium, identify the underlying causes, and implement timely interventions contributes to the negative sequelae associated with the condition (Kuehn, 2010a,b; Tullmann et al, 2012).

Dahlke and Phinney (2008) investigated interventions nurses use to assess, prevent, and treat delirium, as well as the challenges and barriers nurses face in caring for patients with delirium in the acute care setting. The authors concluded that cognitive changes in older people are often labeled confusion by health care practitioners, are frequently accepted as part of normal aging, and are rarely questioned. If the nurse believed that confusion was normal in older adults, he or she would be less likely to recognize symptoms of delirium as a medical emergency necessitating attention and intervention. Confusion in a child or younger adult would be recognized as a medical emergency, but confusion in older adults may be accepted as a natural occurrence, "part of the older person's personality" (p. 46).

In the Dahlke and Phinney study, nurses reported that caring for patients with delirium was seen as "annoying, frustrating and not interesting" (2008, p. 45). Nurses expressed that the care of older patients with delirium interfered with what was perceived as the "real work" of caring for a medical or surgical patient. Insufficient knowledge and inadequate time and resources also influenced appropriate care. The authors conclude that nurses are faced with the predicament of fitting care for older adults into a system that does not recognize the unique needs of this population. Clearly, education and attitudes about older people must be addressed if we want to improve care outcomes for the growing number of older adults who will need care.

Risk Factors for Delirium

There are many predisposing and precipitating factors for delirium (Box 29-1). The risk of delirium increases with the number of risk factors present. The more vulnerable the individual is, the greater the risk. Identification of high-risk patients, risk factors, early and appropriate assessment, and continued surveillance are the cornerstones of delirium prevention. Among the most predictive risk factors are immobility, functional deficits, use of restraints or indwelling catheters, medications, acute illness, infections, alcohol or drug abuse, sensory impairments, malnutrition, dehydration, respiratory insufficiency, surgery, and cognitive impairment. Unrelieved or inadequately treated pain significantly increases the risk of delirium. Invasive equipment, such as nasogastric tubes, intravenous (IV) lines, catheters, and restraints, also contributes to delirium by interfering with normal feedback mechanisms of the body. Medications can contribute to delirium, and all medications, particularly

---

BOX 29-1   Precipitating Factors for Delirium

- Total number of medications >6
- Pharmacological agents, especially narcotics, anticonvulsants, psychotropics, anticholinergics, hypnotics, anxiolytics. Be suspect of any new medications or increased dosages. Consider OTC drugs and alcohol
- Hypoxemia and metabolic disturbances
- Infection, especially respiratory and urinary tracts
- Injury (often a covert fall)
- Dehydration, with and without electrolyte disturbances
- Electrolyte imbalances
- Volume overload
- Intravenous catheter complications
- Prolonged bleeding
- Transfusion reaction
- New pressure ulcer
- Emergency admission or admission from a long-term care facility
- Prolonged emergency department stay (>12 hours)
- Withdrawal syndromes (alcohol and sedative-hypnotic agents)
- Major medical and surgical treatments (especially hip fracture)
- Nutritional deficiencies

- Dementia
- Circulatory disturbances (congestive heart failure [CHF], myocardial infarction [MI], cerebrovascular accident [CVA])
- Anemia
- Pain (either unrelieved or inadequately treated)
- Sensory deficits
- Social isolation, lack of family contact
- Retention of urine and feces
- Use of invasive equipment
- Use of restraint or immobilizing device
- Prolonged immobility
- Functional deficits
- Depression
- Sensory overstimulation or understimulation
- Abrupt loss of a significant person
- Multiple losses in a short span of time
- ICU stay
- Move to a radically different environment (hospitalization, nursing home)
- Multiple moves in a short period of time

BOX 29-2   Drugs that can Cause or Contribute to Delirium in Older Adults

High Risk
Anticholinergics/antihistamines
Benzodiazepines
Dopamine agonists
Meperidine

Moderate to Low Risk
Antibiotics (e.g., quinolones, antimalarials, isoniazid, linezolid, macrolides)
Anticonvulsants
Medication for dizziness
Antiemetics
Antihypertensives (e.g., beta-blockers, clonidine)
Antivirals (e.g., acyclovir, interferon)
Antimicrobials
Antiparkinsonism drugs

Alcohol
Cardiovascular drugs
  Antiarrhythmics
  Digoxin
Corticosteroids
H_2-receptor antagonists
Metoclopramide
Narcotics other than meperidine
Nonsteroidal antiinflammatory drugs
Psychotropic drugs
  Antianxiety drugs
  Antidepressants
  Sedatives/hypnotics
Skeletal muscle relaxants

Adapted from Kalish VB, Gillham JE, Unwin BK: Delirium in older persons: evaluation and management, *Am Fam Physician* 90:150–158, 2014.

---

those with anticholinergic effects and any new medications, should be considered suspect (Box 29-2). The Beers Criteria for potentially inappropriate medication use in older adults (Chapter 9) is a resource for potential problem medications (American Geriatrics Society, 2012).

Clinical Subtypes of Delirium

Delirium is categorized according to the level of alertness and psychomotor activity. The clinical subtypes are hyperactive, hypoactive, and mixed. Box 29-3 presents the characteristics of each of these clinical subtypes. Because of the increased severity of illness and the use of psychoactive medications, hypoactive delirium may be more prevalent in the intensive care unit (ICU). Although the negative consequences of hyperactive delirium are serious, the hypoactive subtype may be more often missed and is associated with a worse prognosis because of the development of complications such as aspiration, pulmonary

embolism, pressure ulcers, and pneumonia. Box 29-4 presents additional delirium symptom assessment.

Consequences of Delirium

Delirium has serious consequences and is a "high priority nursing challenge for all nurses who care for older adults" (Tullmann et al, 2008, p. 113). Delirium is a terrifying experience for the individual and his or her family, and significant others and people often think they are "going crazy." Delirium is associated with increased length of hospital stay and hospital readmissions, increased services after discharge, and increased morbidity, mortality, and institutionalization, independent of age, co-existing illnesses, or illness severity (Balas et al, 2012).

Posttraumatic stress disorder (PTSD) symptoms (Chapter 28), although often not recognized, may occur in adults with delirium. In one study exploring PTSD in people with acute lung injury, the researchers showed that the effects of delirium were

BOX 29-3   Clinical Subtypes of Delirium

Hypoactive Delirium
- "Quiet or pleasantly confused"
- Reduced activity
- Lack of facial expression
- Passive demeanor
- Lethargy
- Inactivity
- Withdrawn and sluggish state
- Limited, slow, and wavering vocalizations

Hyperactive Delirium
- Excessive alertness
- Easy distractibility
- Increased psychomotor activity
- Hallucinations, delusions
- Agitation and aggressive actions
- Fast or loud speech
- Wandering, nonpurposeful repetitive movement
- Verbal behaviors (yelling, calling out)
- Removing tubes
- Attempting to get out of bed
- Unpredictable fluctuations between hypoactivity and hyperactivity

BOX 29-4   TIPS FOR BEST PRACTICE

Recognizing Delirium

Alteration in level of consciousness: Does the patient fall asleep during assessment or general patient care? Is there lethargy or hypoactivity?

Disorientation: Check orientation to time, place, and person. Does the individual respond to reorientation efforts? With delirium, the individual is often unable to be **reoriented and cannot retain information.**

Short-term memory impairment: Memory loss will be sudden rather than long-standing. Know the individual's usual mental status (question family or caregivers). Question the patient about his or her care earlier in the day. Those who forget family visits, bathing, or eating may have memory impairments.

Agitation: Pulling out medical devices, refusing care, screaming, attempting to get out of bed, frightened affect.

Attention impairment: The patient may be unable to maintain attention or complete a task or follow directions.

Perceptual disturbances: Visual and auditory hallucinations may be present and very distressing to the individual.

Delusions: A persistent false thought can be present and difficult to dispel in the individual with delirium. He or she may ask for a loved one who has died many years ago and accuse the nursing staff of preventing him or her from coming to the hospital or the patient may refuse medication for fear of being poisoned.

Sleep-wake cycle disturbance: Sleeping more in the daytime and awake at night. Lack of access to daytime light (window) or lights on all the time in the nursing unit can make this worse.

Modified from Waszynski D: *Confusion assessment method,* New York, 2012, Hartford Institute for Geriatric Nursing.

long-lasting and associated with psychiatric treatment the first 2 years following the event. PTSD symptoms may also be present in patients experiencing delirium in the ICU with other medical conditions. Risk factors include depression before lung injury, duration of stay, sepsis in the ICU, ventilator use, and administration of high-dose opiates (Bienvenu et al, 2013).

Patients suffered from nightmares, flashbacks, and memories and dreams that they were not able to comprehend (Box 29-5). Box 29-6 presents resources including video descriptions of delirium by patients. Family members of the patient with delirium may also be at risk of developing PTSD (Jones et al, 2012).

Although the majority of hospital inpatients recover fully from delirium, a substantial minority will never recover or recover only partially. Each episode of delirium increases vulnerability of the brain, which further enhances the risk of dementia (Inouye et al, 2014). Initial and ongoing assessments should include evaluation of medications and cognitive function. It is

BOX 29-5   Patient Descriptions of Delirium Experiences

Being handcuffed to a railing among criminals in the city jail, fighting to get free and guards standing by to shoot him if he escaped

Children running around without heads; kids with animal heads

Seeing helicopters evacuating patients from an impending tornado, leaving her behind

Blood seeping through holes and cracks in my skin, forming a puddle of red around me

A horror show of people trying to kill her, ants crawling on faces, finding herself on a raft, in a space pod, in the Arctic, in the desert—each with its own terrible narrative

Sources: Amoss M: Treating the trauma of intensive care, *Johns Hopkins Magazine,* 2013, http://hub.jhu.edu/magazine/2013/summer/ptsd-intensive-care Accessed October 2014; Edmunds L: Delirium, *Johns Hopkins Medicine,* 2014, http://www.hopkinsmedicine.org/news/publications/hopkins_medicine_magazine/features/delirium Accessed October 2014; Hoffman J: Nightmares after the ICU, *The New York Times,* July 22, 2013, http://well.blogs.nytimes.com/2013/07/22/nightmares-after-the-i-c-u Accessed October 2014.

BOX 29-6   RESOURCES FOR BEST PRACTICE

Delirium and Dementia

Centers for Medicare and Medicaid Services: Hand in Hand: A Training Series for Nursing: Educational program for staff on how to employ non-pharmacological alternatives in caring for individuals with BPSD: http://www.cms-handinhandtoolkit.info/

European Delirium Association: Patient Experiences of Delirium: Teaching Video

Hartford Institute for Geriatric Nursing: Delirium: Nursing Standard of Practice Protocol: Prevention, early recognition, and treatment; Assessment and management of delirium in older adults with dementia; CAM, CAM ICU

Hartford Institute for Geriatric Nursing: Dementia Series

Hospital Elder Life Program (HELP): Program materials, Family-HELP program, The Family Confusion Assessment Method (FAM-CAM)

ICU Delirium and Cognitive Impairment Study Group: Patient and Family Report: Memories from the ICU

ICU-DIARY.org: Informal network for all health care workers interested in the ICU diary

Nursing Home Toolkit: Promoting Positive Behavioral Health: http://www.nursinghometoolkit.com/

Society of Critical Care Medicine: Clinical practice guidelines for the management of pain, agitation, and delirium in adult patients in ICU important to note that delirium must be resolved before considering a diagnosis of dementia. The persistence of delirium after discharge may interfere with the ability to manage chronic conditions and contribute to poor outcomes (Hain et al, 2012). Further research is needed to determine the reasons for the long-term poor outcomes, whether characteristics of the delirium itself (subtype or duration) influence prognosis, and how the long-term effects might be decreased.

⚡ SAFETY ALERT

Older adults with risk factors for delirium should be screened for delirium upon admission to the hospital, when transitioning from one area of care to another, and before discharge to other care settings or home. In an effort to reduce poor health outcomes, needs should be identified as part of the care coordination process. Individuals with unresolved delirium at discharge should be screened again at 3 months and monitored closely until the delirium has resolved (Lindquist et al, 2011).

◆ PROMOTING HEALTHY AGING: IMPLICATIONS FOR GERONTOLOGICAL NURSING

◆ Assessment

◆ Cognitive Assessment

The cornerstone of evidence-based practice is using the best available evidence to develop the most appropriate interventions for individuals with NCDs. However, before this can occur, it is essential that a comprehensive cognitive assessment

be done to identify reversible conditions that may be the cause of an individual's symptoms. For the older person with cognitive changes, a comprehensive assessment in a memory disorder center with experts in NCD and geriatrics is important (Box 29-7). An important aspect of this is differentiating delirium, dementia, and depression. Older adults should be routinely and regularly assessed for cognitive function in all settings, and nurses must have the skills to recognize cognitive impairment and monitor cognitive functioning. "Assessment of cognitive function is the first and most critical step in a cascade of strategies to prevent, reverse, halt, or minimize cognitive decline" (Braes et al, 2008, p. 42).

Assessing cognitive function can be challenging. Some of the reasons for this include the complexity of cognitive assessment and the existence of several conditions with overlapping symptoms (dementia, depression, delirium). Other reasons include the often atypical presentation of illness in older people and the belief, on the part of health care professionals as well as older people, that alterations in cognitive functioning are part of the "normal" aspects of aging (Chapter 5). Chapter 7 discusses tools that can be used to assess cognitive function and Chapter 23 discusses comprehensive cognitive assessment.

◆ Assessment of Delirium

Prevention of delirium is the first step in caring for vulnerable older adults. An awareness and identification of the risk factors for delirium and a formal assessment of mental status are the first-line interventions for prevention. Nurses play a pivotal role in the identification of delirium, and it is imperative that they

---

BOX 29-7   An Exemplar Program for Comprehensive Dementia Care

About the Center

The Louis and Anne Green Memory and Wellness Center (MWC) is a unique Center of the Christine E. Lynn College of Nursing at Florida Atlantic University in Boca Raton. Grounded in the philosophy of caring espoused by the College, the MWC provides compassionate and innovative programs of care for reflecting best practice, research, and education. The MWC is a state-designated memory disorder clinic and the first adult day center in Florida to receive the designation of "Specialized Alzheimer's Services Center."

Model of Care

Clinical practice at the MWC is illuminated philosophically and operationally by caring science and utilizes a nurse practitioner model designed to provide comprehensive, coordinated care. Nurse practitioners function as the dementia-specific care providers and care managers within a core physician-NP-psychologist-neuropsychologist-social worker team.

Services

Comprehensive memory evaluations are conducted by bilingual interprofessionals within a patient/family-provider partnering framework. Driving evaluations and physical therapy evaluation and treatment are also available. Hearing and honoring the story of the patient and family guide assessment, diagnosis, and ongoing care. Educational programs for caregivers, self-preservation activities such as yoga, caregiver consultations with a certified

care manager, psychotherapy, a caregiver library, and caregiver support groups, including adult children and individuals with early-onset dementia, are offered. Classes are also offered for cognitively healthy individuals in the community who wish to maintain their brain health and there are also a variety of educational programs offered to individuals in the community and care providers.

Adult Day Center

The Adult Day Center provides a wide array of evidence-based therapeutic programs designed to maintain and enhance cognitive and physical function and quality of life. Activities include chair yoga, reminiscence, cognitive stimulation activities, health education (nutrition, exercise, spirituality, mental health/well-being), and creative arts such as painting and drawing, music, cards, puzzles, and board games.

Student Education and Research

Clinical practice experiences for students of the Colleges of Nursing, Medicine, Social Work and other fields are supervised by MWC staff. Continuous engagement in research within the College of Nursing creates the possibility to advance knowledge related to care of individuals with dementia. Current studies include fall prevention for community-residing older adults, patterns of stress in memory center enrollees and their family members, and communication in couples affected by memory problems.

Source: María de los Ángeles Ordóñez, DNP, ARNP/GNP-BC
Director, Louis and Anne Green Memory and Wellness Center
Memory Disorder Clinic Coordinator; Tappen R, Ordonez M, Curtis B: Designing a nurse-managed center grounded in caring: the aesthetics of place and space, *Journal of Art and Aesthetics in Nursing and Health Sciences* 2(1):22, 2014.

accurately report patients' mental status to the medical team so that causative factors can be identified and treated.

Assessment begins with a thorough history and identification of key diagnostic features. Several instruments can be used to assess the presence and severity of delirium. To detect changes, it is very important to determine the person's baseline cognitive status. If the person cannot tell you this, family members or other caregivers who are with the patient can be asked to provide this information. Family members and other caregivers know the person well and will notice subtle changes in behavior. They can give information about whether or not these behaviors. They normal for this person. It is always important to observe the reaction of the individual undergoing a cognitive assessment as the family member or caregiver is responding to the question. In cases where a person is clearly becoming upset, it might be better to ask sensitive questions at another time or discuss the history with the family member or caregiver in another clinical area.

If the patient is alone, the responsible party or the institution transferring the patient can provide this information by phone. It is important to obtain information regarding baseline cognitive function. Do not assume the person's current mental status represents his or her usual state, and do not attribute altered mental status to age alone or assume that dementia is present. All older patients, regardless of their current cognitive function, should have a formal assessment to identify possible delirium when admitted to the hospital.

The Mini-Mental State Exam-2 (MMSE-2) is considered a general test of cognitive status that helps identify mental status impairment. Although the MMSE-2 alone is not adequate for diagnosing delirium, it represents a brief, standardized method to assess mental status and can provide a baseline from which to track changes (Chapter 7). Several delirium-specific assessment instrument are available, such as the Confusion Assessment Method(CAM) (Inouye et al, 1990) recommended by the Hartford Institute for Geriatric Nursing (Box 29-8), and the NEECHAM Confusion Scale (Neelon et al, 1996).

The CAM-ICU is another instrument specifically designed to assess delirium in an intensive care population and has recently been validated for use in critically ill, nonverbal patients who are on mechanical ventilation (Ely et al, 2001; Rigney, 2006). The Family Confusion Assessment Method (FAM-CAM) (Steis et al, 2012) can be used to identify symptoms based on reports from family members (see Box 29-6).

Assessment using the CAM and NEECHAM should be conducted on admission to the hospital, throughout the hospitalization for all patients identified at risk for delirium, and for all patients who exhibit signs and symptoms of delirium or develop additional risk factors (Steis and Fick, 2008). Many acute care settings have made the CAM a part of the electronic medical record.

Once a patient is identified as having delirium, reassessment should be conducted every shift. Documenting specific objective indicators of alterations in mental status rather than using the global, nonspecific term confusion will lead to more appropriate prevention, detection, and management of delirium and its negative consequences. Findings from assessment using a validated instrument are combined with nursing observation,

---

BOX 29-8 The Confusion Assessment Method (CAM) Diagnostic Algorithm*

Feature 1: Acute onset or fluctuating course. This feature is usually obtained from a family member or nurse and is shown by positive responses to the following questions: Is there evidence of an acute change in mental status from the patient's baseline? Did the (abnormal) behavior fluctuate during the day, that is, tend to come and go, or increase and decrease in severity?

Feature 2: Inattention. This feature is shown by a positive response to the following question: Did the patient have difficulty focusing attention, for example, being easily distractible, or having difficulty keeping track of what was being said?

Feature 3: Disorganized thinking. This feature is shown by a positive response to the following question: Was the patient's thinking disorganized or incoherent, such as rambling or irrelevant conversation, unclear or illogical flow of ideas, or unpredictable switching from subject to subject?

Feature 4: Altered level of consciousness. This feature is shown by any answer other than "alert" to the following question: Overall, how would you rate this patient's level of consciousness (alert [normal]), vigilant [hyperalert], lethargic [drowsy, easily aroused], stupor [difficult to arouse], or coma [unarousable])?

*The diagnosis of delirium by CAM requires the presence of features 1 and 2 and either 3 or 4.
From Inouye, S., van Dyck, C., Alessi, C., Balkin, S., Siegal, A. & Horwitz, R. (1990). Clarifying confusion: The confusion assessment method. Annals of Internal Medicine, 113(12), 941-948.

---

chart review, and physiological findings. Delirium often has a fluctuating course and can be difficult to recognize, so assessment must be ongoing and include multiple data sources.

◆ Interventions
◆ Nonpharmacological Approaches

Because the etiology of delirium is multifactorial, interventions that are multicomponent and address more than one risk factor are more likely to be effective (Rosenbloom-Brunton et al, 2010). Interprofessional approaches to prevention of delirium seem to show the most promising results, but continued research is needed to evaluate what type of approach has the most beneficial effect in specific clinical settings. A person-centered approach to care, rather than a disease-focused approach, can yield the best outcomes (Box 29-9).

BOX 29-9 Taking a Person-Centered Approach to Delirium

Mr. M., an 81-year-old male, was admitted to an acute care facility 2 days ago because of a change in his behavior. The admitting diagnoses were dehydration and acute kidney injury. Suddenly one day he was becoming agitated and yelling loudly. The nurse caring for him was busy with an unstable patient in the next bed, so her first response was to medicate him with an antianxiety medication. The clinical practice specialist just happened to be present and recalled the risks for delirium and that nonpharmacological approaches were best. She quickly suggested to the nurse: "Let's move him out of this room to a quieter area." This simple change in environment was effective in reducing Mr. M.'s agitation, and for the next few days before discharge, he remained calm. This exemplar demonstrates the importance of working together to reduce the use of pharmacological interventions in individuals with delirium.

Source: Candice Hickman, MSN, RN, Clinical Practice Specialist.

A well-researched program of delirium prevention in the acute care setting, the Hospital Elder Life Program (HELP) (Inouye et al, 1999), focuses on managing six risk factors for delirium: cognitive impairment, sleep deprivation, immobility, visual impairments, hearing impairments, and dehydration. An interprofessional team of geriatric specialists, including nurses, takes a multifaceted approach to maintain cognitive and physical function for high-risk older adults, maximize independence at discharge, assist with transitions, and prevent unnecessary readmissions. Trained volunteers are also utilized in the HELP program. The program is used in more than 200 hospitals in the United States and internationally.

The Family-HELP program (Box 29-6), an adaptation and extension of the original HELP program, trains family caregivers in selected protocols (e.g., orientation, therapeutic activities, vision and hearing). Initial research demonstrates that active engagement of family caregivers in preventive interventions for delirium is feasible and supports a culture of family-oriented care (Rosenbloom-Brunton et al, 2010).

A recent meta-analysis reported that multicomponent nonpharmacological delirium prevention interventions are effective in reducing delirium incidence and preventing falls, with a trend toward decreasing length of stay and avoiding institutionalization. Fourteen interventional studies were reviewed, and nine of them used the HELP program. Study authors estimate that these interventions can improve quality of life for one million older patients and save the health care system $10 billion annually (Hshieh et al, 2015).

Most of the interventions in the HELP program can be considered quite simple and part of good nursing care. Interventions include the following: offering herbal tea or warm milk instead of sleeping medications, keeping the ward quiet at night by using vibrating beepers instead of paging systems, removing catheters and other devices that hamper movement as soon as possible, encouraging mobilization, assessing and managing pain, and correcting hearing and vision deficits. Fall risk–reduction interventions—such as bed and chair alarms, low beds, reclining chairs, volunteers to sit with restless patients, and keeping routines as normal as possible with consistent caregivers—are other examples of interventions. Box 29-10 presents suggested interventions for delirium.

The use of an intensive care diary may be helpful to patients and family members to make sense of their experience of delirium. The practice of writing a diary was first noted in Denmark and is now being used in a number of other countries, including the United States. Entries into the diary are made by nurses and also by relatives during the patient's stay. The diary is written directly to the patient in everyday language using an empathetic and reflective style and therapeutic communication. It contains daily entries on the current status of the patient and descriptions of situations and surroundings in which the patient might find recognition. The text is often supported by photos. The use of diaries may be a simple and practical intervention that may reduce the level of PTSD-related symptoms for patients and relatives after critical illness (Jones et al, 2012) (see Box 29-6).

BOX 29-10 TIPS FOR BEST PRACTICE
Interventions to Prevent Delirium

- Know baseline mental status, functional abilities, living conditions, medications taken, alcohol use.
- Assess mental status using Mini-Mental State Exam-2 (MMSE-2), Confusion Assessment Method (CAM), or NEECHAM Confusion Scale, and document.
- Correct underlying physiological alterations.
- Compensate for sensory deficits (e.g., hearing aids, glasses, dentures).
- Encourage fluid intake (make sure fluids are accessible).
- Avoid long periods of giving nothing orally.
- Explain all actions with clear and consistent communication.
- Avoid multiple medications, and avoid problematic medications (see Beers Criteria).
- Be vigilant for drug reactions or interactions; consider onset of new symptoms as an adverse reaction to medications.
- Avoid use of sleeping medications; use music, warm milk, or noncaffeinated herbal tea to alleviate discomfort.
- Attempt to find out why behavior is occurring rather than simply medicating for it (e.g., need to toilet, pain, fear, hunger, thirst).
- Avoid excessive bed rest; institute early mobilization.
- Encourage participation in care for activities of daily living (ADLs).
- Minimize the use of catheters, restraints, or immobilizing devices.
- Use least restrictive devices (mitts instead of wrist restraints, reclining geri-chairs with tray instead of vest restraints).
- Hide tubes (stockinette over intravenous [IV] line), or use intermittent fluid administration.
- Activate bed and chair alarms.
- Place the patient near the nursing station for close observation.
- Assess and treat pain.
- Pay attention to environmental noise, light, temperature.
- Normalize the environment (provide familiar items, routines, clocks, calendars).
- Minimize the number of room changes and interfacility transfers.
- Do not place a delirious patient in the room with another delirious patient.
- Have family, volunteer, or paid caregiver stay with the patient.

◆ Pharmacological Approaches

Pharmacological interventions to treat the symptoms of delirium may be necessary if patients are in danger of harming themselves or others, or if nonpharmacological interventions are not effective. However, pharmacological interventions should not replace thoughtful and careful evaluation and management of the underlying causes of delirium. Pharmacological treatment should be one approach in a multicomponent program of prevention and treatment. Research on the pharmacological management of delirium is limited, but with increased understanding of the neuropathogenesis of delirium, drug therapy may become more important.

Antipsychotics (such as haloperidol) are used and found to be effective in certain populations with agitated delirium. The use of dexmedetomidine as a sedative or analgesic may reduce the incidence or duration of delirium, but further research is necessary (Bledowski and Trutia, 20132 Tullmann et al, 2012). Short-acting benzodiazepines are often used to control agitation but may worsen mental status. Psychoactive medications, if used, should be given at the lowest effective dose, monitored closely, and reduced or eliminated as soon as possible so that recovery can be assessed.

BOX 29-11   TIPS FOR BEST PRACTICE

Communicating with a Person Experiencing Delirium

- Know the person's past patterns.
- Look at nonverbal signs, such as tone of voice, facial expressions, and gestures.
- Speak slowly.
- Be calm and patient.
- Face the person and keep eye contact; get to the level of the person rather than standing over him or her.
- Explain all actions.
- Smile.
- Use simple, familiar words.
- Allow adequate time for response.
- Repeat if needed.
- Tell the person what you want him or her to do rather than what you do not want him or her to do.
- Give one-step directions; use gestures and demonstration to augment words.
- Reassure of safety.
- Keep caregivers consistent.
- Assume that communication and behavior are meaningful and an attempt to tell us something or express needs.
- Do not assume that the person is unable to understand or is demented.

The Society of Critical Care Medicine (Barr, 2013) has developed new pain, agitation, and delirium clinical practice guidelines for adult patients in ICU (see Box 29-6). The guidelines place greater emphasis on the use of valid and reliable tools for assessment of pain, agitation/sedation, and delirium in ICU patients; the use of an interprofessional team approach; avoidance of oversedation; encouragement of more active participation in spontaneous awakening and breathing trials; early mobilization programs; pain management; and environmental strategies to preserve sleep-wake cycles.

Caring for individuals with delirium can be a challenging experience. Patients with delirium can be difficult to communicate with, and disturbing behaviors, such as pulling out intravenous (IV) lines or attempting to get out of bed, disrupt medical treatment and compromise safety. It is important for nurses to realize that behavior is an attempt to communicate something and express needs. The patient with delirium feels frightened and out of control. The calmer and more reassuring the nurse is, the safer the patient will feel. Box 29-11 presents some communication strategies that are helpful in caring for people experiencing delirium.

CARE OF INDIVIDUALS WITH MILD AND MAJOR NEUROCOGNITIVE DISORDER

Nurses provide direct care for people with dementia in the community, hospitals, and long-term care facilities. They also work with families and staff, teaching best practice approaches to care and providing education and support. With the rising incidence of dementia, nurses will play an even larger role in the design and implementation of evidence-based practice and provision of education, counseling, and supportive services to individuals with dementia and their caregivers.

The overriding goals in caring for older adults with dementia are to maintain function and prevent excess disability, structure the environment and relationships to maintain stability, compensate for the losses associated with the disease, and create a therapeutic milieu that nurtures the personhood of the individual and maintains quality of life. Box 29-12 presents an overview of general nursing intervention principles in the care of persons with dementia.

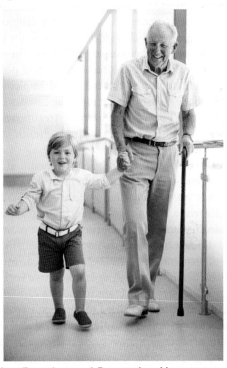

Maintaining Function and Preventing Unnecessary Decline Are Important. (©iStock.com/Squaredpixels)

Nutrition, activities of daily living (ADLs), maintenance of health and function, safety, communication, behavioral changes, caregiver needs and support, and quality of life are the major care concerns for patients, families, and staff caring for individuals with dementia. Five common care concerns for people with major NCD and nursing interventions are discussed in the remainder of this chapter: communication, behavior concerns, ADL care, wandering, and nutrition. Caregiving for persons with dementia is discussed in Chapter 34, and other care

BOX 29-12   General Nursing Interventions in Care of Persons with Dementia

- Address safety.
- Structure daily living to maximize remaining abilities.
- Monitor general health and impact of dementia on management of other medical conditions.
- Support advance care planning and advance directives.
- Educate caregivers in the areas of problem-solving, resource access, long-range planning, emotional support, and respite.

From Evans L, Kurlowicz L: *Complex care needs in older adults with common cognitive disorders,* May 2007, http://hartfordign.org/uploads/File/gnec_state_of_science_papers/gnec_delirium.pdf Accessed October 2014.

concerns such as falls and incontinence are discussed in earlier chapters of this book.

Need for Ongoing Assessment

Assessment of individuals and their caregivers is an especially important nursing role. Beginning at the time of diagnosis and continuing through the course of the disease, individuals and their caregivers require ongoing assessment and monitoring of disease progression and response to therapy. Assessment should occur at least every 6 months to 1 year after diagnosis or any time there is a change in behavior or increase in the rate of decline. Needs change as the disease progresses. The individual should be involved in all discussions to the extent possible. It is essential to evaluate safety awareness and implement safety measures to reduce risks of injury. Ongoing assessment of ability to comprehend benefits and harm of treatment options is essential when making decisions related to health care or obtaining informed consent.

Health care surrogates should be determined, and wishes for palliative and end-of-life care determined. The palliative care movement has yet to reach the majority of individuals with end-stage dementia. Meaningful advance care planning is usually not addressed until far too late in the course of the patient's illness, and it is rare for the grave (and fundamentally terminal) prognosis of dementia to have been discussed. In one 2009 study (Mitchell et al) only 18% of families have ever discussed prognosis with a physician (Sekerak and Stewart, 2014, pages 3, 18). Health care providers need to begin conversations early in the course of dementia with the individual and the family, provide education, explore value and preferences, and facilitate an advance directive (Chapter 35).

Differing Needs in Mild NCD and Those with Early-Onset Dementia

The concerns of individuals and their caregivers in the mild stage and for those with early-onset dementia (EOD) are quite different from those with major NCD. To date, the preponderance of research and intervention programs has been directed toward persons and their families living with major NCD and has focused on preparing caregivers to cope with issues such as behavior problems, incontinence, ADL care, and nursing home placement. Many of these issues are not relevant to those with mild NCD or with early-onset dementia, will not be of interest to them, and can be frightening and misleading as well (Blieszner and Roberto, 2010; Hain et al, 2010).

Areas of concern for caregivers of persons with mild NCD and early-onset dementia center less on personal care needs and more on communication, behavior, and relationships (Box 29-13). Additionally, individuals with mild NCD are aware of their diagnosis and need opportunities to share their feelings and receive support as well. Research must include the voices of those experiencing the health challenge of both mild and moderate NCD (Box 29-14). Interventions that help both the person and his or her caregiver to deal with changing roles, stress, frustration, loss, communication difficulties, and the couple relationship are particularly needed (Hain et al, 2010). Therapeutic programs for both individuals and their

BOX 29-13 RESEARCH HIGHLIGHTS

Interviews were conducted with 10 family caregivers (7 spouses and 3 adult children) of individuals with mild to moderate dementia to explore what matters most to them. Participants were recruited from a Memory and Wellness Center, and the interview took place as part of a free GNP consultation offered at the Center. Questions posed included the following: Can you tell me more about having your loved one diagnosed with mild to moderate dementia? What matters most to you right now? What support and/or information, if any, do you need now? What do you think your future will be like as a caregiver of someone with mild to moderate dementia? What are some of your future hopes and dreams?

Findings reinforced the complexity of the caregiver role, which is plagued with emotional ambiguity as people experience both the rewards and the challenges of caregiving. The participants reported difficulty knowing where to turn for advice and guidance, particularly when related to handling behavior problems. Participants often tried to do it alone and were unaware of the type of resources available, how they worked, or how to access them. They described many stresses but felt guilty for getting angry or frustrated, and they missed the activities in which they used to participate. They were living day to day, afraid of the future, and trying to reorient themselves to a different life and make it as pleasurable as possible for both them and the person with dementia. Their affection and commitment to the loved one made them determined to fight and do their best.

The early stage of dementia may be the most crucial time to intervene and establish a health care provider–patient/family partnership. Support for caregivers should begin at the time of initial diagnosis and continue throughout the disease trajectory because needs vary according to the level of dementia. The study lays the groundwork for further exploration of the efficacy of a GNP consultation as an intervention to determine what matters most to caregivers of persons with mild to moderate dementia, mutual goal setting, and the development of individualized strategies to support caregivers on their journey.

Source: Hain D, Touhy TA, Engström, G: What matters most to caregivers of people with mild to moderate dementia as evidence for transforming care, *Alzheimers Care Today* 11(3):162–171, 2010.

caregivers should be individualized to these varied and changing needs (see Box 29-7).

Person-Centered Care

Irreversible NCDs have no cure, and although new medications offer hope for improved function, the most important treatment for the disease is competent and compassionate person-centered care. Long ago, Mary Opal Wolanin, a gerontological nursing pioneer, suggested that nurses are not as interested in the neurofibrillary tangles in the brain as they are in trying to smooth out the environmental and relational tangles the person and his or her loved ones experience. "Since Alzheimer's affects mind and personality, as well as physical function, there is a great danger that the person can become obscured by the disease, defined by symptoms rather than by her or his unique spirit and continuing sense of self" (Sifton, 2001, p. iv). Person-centered care looks beyond the disease and the tasks we must perform to the person within and our relationship with them. The focus is not on what we need to do to the person but on the person himself or herself and how to enhance well-being and quality of life.

Gerontological nurses know that the person, not the disease, is always the focus of care, and they practice from a belief

BOX 29-14   RESEARCH HIGHLIGHTS

A descriptive phenomenological approach was used to understand the experience of living with early-stage dementia from the person with dementia, the spouse, and the dyad of the person and spouse. Six couples were interviewed individually and as a couple and asked to tell the story of their dementia experience. The themes that emerged from the caregiver narratives indicated that they were trying to do the best they could to ensure that their loved ones receive optimal health care and that life can be as pleasurable as possible. People with dementia are also trying to do their best from the perspective of slowing the disease and not being a burden to their spouse. Similar to other studies, caregivers often do not focus on their own personal needs; instead, they attempt to deal with the psychological roller coaster of living with someone with a neurodegenerative progressive disorder.

Communication difficulties with a loved one can be a major source of stress for caregivers. Individuals with early-stage dementia also experience frustration in trying to communicate effectively and, most importantly, they were quite aware of their own difficulties. Opportunities for both the individual and the caregiver to express frustration and anger over communication difficulties and receive validation of their feelings are important aspects of clinical practice. Effective strategies to maintain and enhance communication and deal effectively with stress can be taught and role-modelled. Of great importance to the individual with dementia was participation in programs that enhance cognition and physical functioning and slow the progression of the disease. Feeling competent and capable in learning new things, participating in stimulating activities, socializing with people who have similar interests, and feeling respected rather than patronized were noted as valuable components of day center programs.

The findings support the importance of living one day at a time by doing the best one can do to promote health and not becoming overwhelmed by what the future may bring. This study provides evidence of how important it is to take a person-centered approach to care and to develop programs that consider the needs of individuals with dementia, their spouse, and the couple dyad throughout the trajectory of the disease. Interventions to enhance couple relationships are important and promote more positive outcomes for the individual with dementia and for the caregiver. Programs and activities aimed at helping the person with early-stage dementia maintain maximum cognitive, physical, and social function for as long as possible are important and are beneficial for both the individual and the caregiver.

Source: Hain D, Touhy TA, Sparks-Compton D, et al: Using narratives of individuals and couples living with early stage dementia to guide practice, *J Nurs Appl Rev Res* 4:82–93, 2014.

that the person with dementia is still a whole person, someone who can think, feel, learn, grow, and be in a relationship (Touhy, 2004). "The person with dementia is not an object, not a vegetable, not an empty body, not a child, but an adult, who, given support, might exercise choices and respond to a respectful approach" (Woods, 1999, p. 35). Person-centered care fosters abilities, supports limitations, ensures safety, enhances quality of life, prevents excess disability, and offers hope. Care for persons with dementia is more than keeping their bodies alive, safe, and clean; performing tasks; and managing behavior—the care must also nourish their souls (Touhy, 2004).

There is a growing body of evidence on the importance of person-centered care and therapeutic work with people with dementia, but the emphasis in the literature and in practice continues to be on the care of the body (bathing, feeding) and the management of aggressive and problematic behavior.

"Despite the emphasis on individualized care and culture change, for many staff, the goal of care hasn't changed: control of behavior is still a priority" (Kolanowski et al, 2010, p. 216).

The emphasis on the decline associated with the disease, the catastrophic behaviors, and the loss of humanness promotes despair, hopelessness, and fear on the part of professional caregivers, patients, and families (Touhy, 2004). Special skills and attitudes are required to nurse the person with dementia, and caring is paramount. It is not an area of nursing that "just anyone can do" (Splete, 2008, p. 11).

COMMUNICATION

The experience of losing cognitive and expressive abilities is both frightening and frustrating. In early stages of NCD people may experience mild difficulty communicating. As the disease progresses, memory, speech, and communication also decline. Older adults experiencing NCD have difficulty expressing their personhood in ways easily understood by others. Identifying receptive and expressive abilities can help the nurse design patient-specific interventions addressing communication challenges. However, the need to communicate and the need to be treated as a person remain despite memory and communication impairments. No group of patients is more in need of supportive relationships with skilled, caring health care providers. People with cognitive and communication impairments "depend on their relationship with and trust of others to provide emotional support, solve problems, and coordinate complex activities" (Buckwalter et al, 1995, p. 15).

Communication with older adults experiencing NCDs requires special skills and patience. Caregivers experience frustration and anxiety when their attempts to communicate with the person who has cognitive limitations are unsuccessful (Williams and Tappen, 2008). NCD affects both receptive and expressive communication components and alters the way people speak. Early in the disease, word finding is difficult (anomia), and remembering the exact facts of a conversation is challenging (Box 29-15).

Individuals with NCD often use nonsensical or "made-up" words such as calling an electric razor a "whisker grinder." Automatic language skills (e.g., hello) are retained for the longest time. The person may wander from the topic of conversation and bring up seemingly unrelated topics. The person may fail to pick up on humor or sarcasm or abstract ideas in conversation.

BOX 29-15   Patient's Descriptions of Communication Difficulties

"I forget words. Sometimes it doesn't mean much and other times it means a great deal. I have learned ways to avoid making mistakes like shaking hands when I don't remember the person's name, joking, looking at their faces for a reaction" (Hain et al, 2014, p. 85).

"There are a range of things you want to say over and over because I think it was a word that was important to say and I'll forget...I hope that what I am saying makes sense" (Hain et al, 2010).

Nonverbal and behavioral responses become especially important as a way of communication as verbal skills become more limited. As the disease progresses, verbal output may become less frequent although the grammar and sounds of the language being spoken remain relatively intact.

Williams and Tappen (2008) remind us that even in the later stages of NCD, the person may understand more than you realize and still needs opportunities for interaction and caring communication, both verbal and nonverbal. Often, health care providers do not communicate with older adults with major NCD, or they limit communication only to task-focused topics.

To effectively communicate with a person experiencing a NCD, it is essential to believe that the person is trying to communicate something that is important. It is critical that nurses recognize various ways a person with dementia may communicate by knowing the person. The best thing we can do is discover what the person is trying to communicate and intervene according to needs. However jumbled it may seem, the person is attempting to tell us something. It is our responsibility as professionals to understand and know how to respond. The person with NCD cannot change his or her communication; we must change ours (Box 29-16).

Nurses can overcome barriers to communication by taking a person-centered approach. A person-centered framework encourages coming to know the person by taking time to find out the individual's story: "Who am I?" In some cases people are unable to disclose a lifetime of memories but taking the time to find out what their background is and making time to be present can contribute to effective communication. A person with NCD, like anyone else, values being recognized as important enough for the nurse to care to listen or pay attention to what is being communicated.

Evidence-Based Communication Strategies

Classic research conducted by Ruth Tappen of Florida Atlantic University (Boca Raton, FL) and colleagues (Tappen et al, 1997, 1999) provided insight into communication strategies that were helpful in creating and maintaining a therapeutic relationship with people with moderate to major NCDs. In these studies,

conversations between 23 participants in the middle and late stages of Alzheimer's disease and a clinical nurse specialist were analyzed to clarify what type of communication techniques were helpful in creating and maintaining a therapeutic relationship. Interviewers were told to "avoid frequent correction of the individual, encourage the individual to engage in conversation, attempt to make the conversation as meaningful as possible, and to assume that any attempt at communication had some meaning to it, however difficult it was to ascertain that meaning" (Tappen et al, 1997, p. 250).

Findings were compared with recommendations in the literature, and specific communication strategies were developed. More than 80% of the participants' responses were relevant in the context of the conversation. The research challenged some of the commonly held beliefs about communication with persons with NCD, for example, avoiding the use of open-ended questions and keeping communication focused only on simple topics, task-oriented topics, and questions that can be answered with yes or no responses.

Findings of this study provided suggestions for specific communication strategies effective in various nursing situations, as well as hope for nurses to establish meaningful relationships that nurture the personhood of people with NCD (Box 29-17). Communication strategies differ depending on the purpose of communication (e.g., performing activities of daily living [ADLs], encouraging expression of feelings). Approaches to communication must be adapted not only to the person's ability to understand but also to the purpose of the interaction. What is appropriate for assessment may be a barrier to conversation that is designed to facilitate expression of concerns and feelings (Williams and Tappen, 2008).

In the past, structured programs of reality orientation (RO) (orienting the person to the day, date, time, year, weather, upcoming holidays) were often used in long-term care facilities and chronic psychiatric units as a way to stimulate interaction and enhance memory. This intervention is still often noted as being of benefit to persons with NCD. However, it has been found that structured RO may place unrealistic expectations on persons with major NCD and may be distressing when they cannot remember these things. Families and professional caregivers can often be heard asking people with NCDs to name relatives, state their birth year, and remember other current facts. One can imagine how upsetting and demoralizing this might be to a person unable to remember.

This does not imply that we should not orient the person to daily activities, time of day, and other important events, but it should be offered without the expectation that the person will remember. Caregivers can provide orienting information as part of general conversation (e.g., "It's quite warm for December 10, but it will be a beautiful day for our lunch date"). Rather than structured RO, a better approach is to go where the person is in his or her own world rather than trying to bring the person's world into yours. For example, if the individual insists that he or she needs to leave the house to meet the school bus, it is more helpful to ask the individual to talk

---

BOX 29-16   TIPS FOR BEST PRACTICE

Communicating Effectively with Individuals with Dementia

Envision a tennis game: The caregiver is like the tennis coach, and whenever the coach plays the ball, he or she seems to be able to put the ball where the person on the other side of the net can return it. The coach also returns the ball in such a way as to keep the rally going; he or she does not return it to score a point or win the match, but rather returns the ball so that the other player is able to reach it and, with encouragement, hit it back over the net again. Similarly, in our communication with people with dementia, our conversation and words must be put into play in such a way such that the person can respond effectively and share thoughts and feelings.

Source: Kitwood T: *Dementia reconsidered: the person comes first,* Bristol, PA, 1999, Open University Press.

BOX 29-17   Four Useful Strategies for Communicating with Individuals Experiencing Cognitive Impairment

Simplification Strategies

Simplification strategies are useful with ADLs:

- Give one-step directions.
- Speak slowly.
- Allow time for response.
- Reduce distractions.
- Interact with one person at a time.
- Give clues and cues as to what you want the person to do. Use gestures or pantomime to demonstrate what it is you want the person to do — for example, put the chair in front of the person, point to it, pat the seat, and say, "Sit here."

Facilitation Strategies

Facilitation strategies are useful in encouraging expression of thoughts and feelings:

- Establish commonalities.
- Share self.
- Allow the person to choose subjects to discuss.
- Speak as if to an equal.
- Use broad openings, such as "How are you today?"
- Employ appropriate use of humor.
- Follow the person's lead.

Comprehension Strategies

Comprehension strategies are useful in assisting with understanding of communication:

- Identify time confusion (in what time frame is the person operating at the moment?).

- Find the theme (what connection is there between apparently disparate topics?). Recognize an important theme, such as fear, loss, or happiness.
- Recognize the hidden meanings (what did the person mean to say?).

Supportive Strategies

Supportive strategies are useful in encouraging continued communication and supporting personhood:

- Introduce yourself, and explain why you are there. Reach out to shake hands, and note the response to touch.
- If the person does not want to talk, go away and return later. Do not push or force.
- Sit closely, and face the person at eye level.
- Limit corrections.
- Use multiple ways of communicating (gestures, touch).
- Search for meaning.
- Know the person's past life history, as well as daily life experiences and events.
- Remember there is a person behind the disease.
- Recognize feelings, and respond.
- Treat the person with respect and dignity.
- Show interest through body posture, facial expression, nodding, and eye contact. Assume a pleasant, relaxed attitude.
- Attend to vision and hearing losses.
- Do not try to bring the person to the present or use reality orientation. Go to where the person is, and enjoy the conversation.
- When leaving, thank the person for his or her time and attention, as well as information.
- Remember that the quality, not the content or quantity, of the interaction is basic to therapeutic communication.

ADLs, Activities of daily living.

about the times he or she did this activity rather than informing the person that his or her children are grown and do not ride the school bus. Validation therapy, developed by Naomi Feil in the 1980s, involves following the person's lead and responding to feelings expressed rather than interrupting to supply factual data. Helping families and caregivers to understand validation therapy can assist in enhancing quality time with their loved ones.

◆ PROMOTING HEALTHY AGING: IMPLICATIONS FOR GERONTOLOGICAL NURSING

Care and communication that respect and value, the dignity, and the worth of every person and use of research-based communication techniques will enhance communication and personhood. "Gerontological nurses who are sensitive to communication and interaction patterns can assist both formal and informal caregivers in using more personal verbal and nonverbal communication strategies that are humanizing and show respect for the person. Similarly, they can monitor and try to change object-oriented communication approaches, which are not only insensitive and dehumanizing but also often lead to diminished self-image and angry, agitated responses on the part of the patient with cognitive impairment" (Buckwalter et al, 1995, p. 15).

BEHAVIOR CONCERNS AND NURSING MODELS OF CARE

Behavior and psychological symptoms of dementia (BPSDs) may present in up to 98% of individuals at some point in the disease trajectory. These symptoms occur in all types of dementia and include anxiety, depression, hallucinations, delusions, aggression, screaming, sleep disturbances, restlessness, agitation, and resistance to care. BPSDs appear to be a consequence of multiple, but sometimes modifiable, interacting factors. These factors are both external and internal and result in part from heightened vulnerability to the environment as cognitive function declines. BPSDs should be viewed as a form of communication that is meaningful (rather than a problem) and is the individual's best attempt to communicate a variety of unmet needs (Kolanowski and Van Haitsma, 2013).

BPSD symptoms cause a great deal of distress to the person and the caregivers and often precipitate institutionalization. Clinically significant BPSDs, if untreated, are associated with faster disease progression than in the absence of such symptoms. For formal caregivers in institutions, caring for older people with BPSD symptoms is positively associated with physical and psychological caregiver burden as well (Kales et al, 2014; Kolanowski et al, 2013; Miyamoto et al, 2010). Family caregivers of individuals with challenging behavioral conditions experience more stress than other caregivers and receive little or no guidance on how to deal with these conditions (Reinhard et al, 2014). In an international study of nursing homes in eight countries, the top two important areas for research were the needs of cognitively impaired residents and the management of challenging behaviors (Morley et al, 2014).

Several nursing models of care are helpful in recognizing and understanding the behavior of individuals with NCDs and can be used to guide practice and assist families and staff in providing care from a more person-centered framework. The *Progressively Lowered Stress Threshold (PLST)* model and the *Need-Driven Dementia-Compromised Behavior (NDDB)* model focus on "the close interplay between person, context, and environment. These models propose that behavior is used to communicate or express, in the best way the person has available, unmet needs (physiological, psychosocial, disturbing environment, uncomfortable social surroundings) and/or difficulty managing stress as the disease progresses" (Evans and Kurlowicz, 2007, p. 7).

The Progressively Lowered Stress Threshold Model

The progressively lowered stress threshold (PLST) model (Hall and Buckwalter, 1987; Hall, 1994) was one of the first models used to plan and evaluate care for people with NCDs in every setting. The PLST model categorizes symptoms of NCD into four groups: (1) cognitive or intellectual losses, (2) affective or personality changes, (3) conative or planning losses that cause a decline in functional abilities, and (4) loss of the stress threshold, causing behaviors such as agitation or catastrophic reactions. Symptoms such as agitation are a result of a progressive loss of the person's ability to cope with demands and stimuli when the person's stress threshold is exceeded. Stressors that may trigger these symptoms are presented in Box 29-18.

Using this model, care is structured to decrease the stressors and provide a safe and predictable environment. Positive outcomes from use of the model include improved sleep; decreased sedative and tranquilizer use; increased food intake and weight; increased socialization; decreased episodes of aggressive, agitated, and disruptive behaviors; increased caregiver satisfaction with care; and increased functional level (DeYoung et al, 2003; Hall and Buckwalter, 1987). Box 29-19 presents the principles of care derived from the PLST model.

Need-Driven Dementia-Compromised Behavior Model

The need-driven, dementia-compromised behavior (NDDB) model (Algase et al, 2003; Kolanowski, 1999; Richards et al, 2000) is a framework for the study and understanding of

---

> ### BOX 29-19 Principles of Care Derived from PLST Model
>
> 1. Maximize functional abilities by supporting all losses in a prosthetic manner.
> 2. Establish a caring relationship, and provide the person with unconditional positive regard.
> 3. Use behaviors indicating anxiety and avoidance to determine appropriate limits of activity and stimuli.
> 4. Teach caregivers to try to find out causes of behavior and to observe and evaluate verbal and nonverbal responses.
> 5. Identify triggers related to discomfort or stress reactions (factors in the environment, caregiver communication).
> 6. Modify the environment to support losses and promote safe function.
> 7. Evaluate care routines and responses on a 24-hour basis, and adjust plan of care accordingly.
> 8. Provide as much control as possible; encourage self-care, offer choices, explain all actions, do not push or force the person to do something.
> 9. Keep the environment stable and predictable.
> 10. Provide ongoing education, support, care, and problem solving for caregivers.
>
> Adapted from Hall GR, Buckwalter KC: Progressively lowered stress threshold: a conceptual model for care of adults with Alzheimer's disease, *Arch Psychiatr Nurs* 1:399–406, 1987.

behavioral symptoms of dementia. All behaviors have meaning and are a form of communication, particularly as verbal communication becomes more limited. The NDDB model proposes that the behavior of persons with dementia carries a message of need that can be addressed appropriately if the person's history and habits, physiological status, and physical and social environment are carefully evaluated (Kolanowski, 1999). Rather than behavior being viewed as disruptive, it is viewed as having meaning and expressing needs. Behavior reflects the interaction of background factors (cognitive changes as a result of dementia, gender, ethnicity, culture, education, personality, responses to stress) and proximal factors (physiological needs such as hunger or pain, mood, physical environment [e.g., light, noise, temperature]) with social environment (e.g., staff stability and mix, presence of others) (Richards et al, 2000).

Optimal care is provided by manipulating the proximal factors that precipitate behavior and by maximizing strengths and minimizing the limitations of the background factors. It is important for caregivers to identify and address the unmet need(s) that arise from both sets of factors rather than ignore the call for help and attempt to control the behavior with the use of sedating drugs (Dettmore et al, 2009). For instance, sleep disruptions are common in people with dementia. If the person is not getting adequate sleep at night, agitated or aggressive behavior during the day may signal the need for more rest. Interventions to modify proximal factors interfering with sleep, such as noise, frequent awakenings during the night, and daytime boredom, can help meet the need for rest and sleep and decrease agitation or aggression.

Despite increased knowledge and awareness that all behavior has meaning, it can be difficult to identify and treat unmet needs when there are environmental stressors such as screaming and pacing that may contribute to caregiver stress (Kovach et al, 2005). Considering the possible poor outcomes related to

---

> ### BOX 29-18 Stressors Triggering BPSD Symptoms (PLST)
>
> Fatigue
> Change of environment, routine, or caregiver
> Misleading stimuli or inappropriate stimulus levels
> Internal or external demands to perform beyond abilities
> Physical stressors such as pain, discomfort, acute illness, and depression

behavior change in persons with major NCD, it is important that nurses have continued education and administrative support to address unmet needs.

PROMOTING HEALTHY AGING: IMPLICATIONS FOR GERONTOLOGICAL NURSING

Assessment

The focus must be on understanding that behavioral expressions communicate distress, and the response is to investigate the possible sources of distress and intervene appropriately. There are many possible reasons for BPSD. After ruling out medical problems (e.g., pneumonia, dehydration, impaction, infection/sepsis, fractures, pain, or depression) as a cause of behavior, continued assessment to identify why distressing symptoms are occurring is important. Conditions such as constipation or urinary tract infections can cause great distress for cognitively impaired individuals and may lead to marked changes in behavior. Pain and discomfort are also common reasons for changes in behavior (striking out, resistance to care) (Cohen-Mansfield, 2013). After careful assessment of other possible causes of pain or discomfort, treatment with a trial of analgesics should be considered.

Understanding what triggers behavior is essential for development of interventions that address the individual's unmet need. Fear, discomfort, unfamiliar surroundings and people, illness, fatigue, depression, need for autonomy and control, caregiver approaches, communication strategies, and environmental stressors are frequent precipitants of behavioral symptoms. "For the individual with late-stage dementia, a good deal of their discomfort comes from non-physiological sources, for example, from difficulty sorting out and negotiating everyday life activities" (Kovach et al, 1999, p. 412).

The need for socialization and support and stimulation to address boredom can also contribute to changes in behavior (Cohen-Mansfield, 2013). Understanding what triggers behavior is important. What may appear as hallucinations or delusions to the caregiver might be misinterpretations by the person of a television program, family photographs, or images reflected in a mirror. "In these cases, it is much safer to turn off the television, remove photographs from the area, or cover a mirror rather than place the patient on an antipsychotic medication" (Hall et al, 2009, pp. 40, 41). Box 29-20 presents precipitating factors for BPSD.

A study exploring sensitivity and specificity of staff nurses to identify behavior changes and the need for further evaluation revealed that verbal symptoms and body part cues (e.g., facial grimacing, tenseness of specific muscle groups, rubbing or guarding specific parts of the body) were the most common behavior changes. However, staff nurses underreported behavior changes in residents with major NCDs and the need for further evaluation. The authors concluded that people with major NCDs have problems communicating their unmet needs, but more importantly the staff is missing the opportunity for early intervention (Kovach et al, 2012).

Putting yourself in the place of the person with NCD and trying to see the world from his or her eyes will help you understand his or her behavior. Box 29-21 presents an example of

---

BOX 29-20 Conditions Precipitating Behavioral Symptoms in Individuals with Dementia

- Communication deficits
- Pain or discomfort
- Acute medical problems
- Sleep disturbances
- Perceptual deficits
- Depression
- Need for social contact
- Hunger, thirst, need to toilet
- Loss of control
- Misinterpretation of the situation or environment
- Crowded conditions
- Changes in environment or people
- Noise, disruption
- Being forced to do something
- Fear
- Loneliness
- Psychotic symptoms
- Fatigue
- Environmental overstimulation or understimulation
- Depersonalized, rushed care
- Restraints
- Psychoactive drugs

BOX 29-21 Understanding Behavior: Seeing Through the Eyes of the Person with Dementia

You are asleep in the chair at home when suddenly you are awakened by a person you have never seen before trying to undress you. Then he or she puts you naked into a hard, cold chair and wheels you down a hallway. Suddenly cold water hits you in the face and the person is touching your private areas. You don't understand why the person is trying to do this to you. You are embarrassed, frightened, cold, and angry. You hit and scream at this person and try to get away.

---

seeing the world from the eyes of the individual with dementia. Questions of what, where, why, when, who, and what now are important components of the assessment of behavior. Box 29-22 presents a framework for asking questions about the possible meanings and messages behind observed behavior. Asking caregivers to play back the situation "as if in a movie" is often helpful in eliciting details and understanding the circumstances associated with the problematic behavior. Except in late-stage NCDs, when verbal communication may be problematic, the perspective of the individual should be elicited to determine what he or she can describe about the situation. It is also important to understand what aspect of the behavior is most problematic or distressing for the individuals and the caregiver and the treatment goal (Kales et al, 2014).

Use of a behavioral log or diary over a 2- to 3-day period to track when the behavior occurs, the circumstances, and the response to interventions is recommended and required in skilled nursing facilities. The Behave-AD, the Cohen-Mansfield Agitation Inventory, and the Neuropsychiatric Inventory for Nursing Homes are examples of reliable instruments that can be used in assessment. Box 29-23 presents examples of some common behaviors and possible strategies.

Interventions
Pharmacological Approaches

All evidence-based guidelines endorse an approach that begins with comprehensive assessment of the behavior and possible causes followed by the use of nonpharmacological interventions as a first line of treatment except in emergency situations when BPSD symptoms

BOX 29-22 Framework for Asking Questions about the Meaning of Behavior

What?

What is being sought? What is happening? Does the behavior have a physical or emotional component or both? What are the person's responses? What would be done if the person was 20 years old instead of 80? What is the behavior saying? What is the emotion being expressed?

Where?

Where is the behavior occurring? What are environmental triggers?

When?

When does the behavior most frequently occur: after activities of daily living (ADLs), family visits, mealtimes?

Who?

Who is involved? Other residents, caregivers, family?

Why?

What happened before? Poor communication? Tasks too complicated? Physical or medical problem? Person being rushed or forced to do something? Has this happened before and why?

What Now?

Approaches and interventions (physical, psychosocial)

Changes needed and by whom?

Who else might know something about the person or the behavior or approaches?

Communicate to all and include in plan of care.

Adapted from Hellen C: Alzheimer's disease: activity focused care, Boston, 1998, Butterworth-Heinemann; Ortigara A. Alzheimer's Care Quarterly 1:91, 2000.

BOX 29-23 Examples of Behavior and Environmental Modification Strategies for Managing BPSD

BEHAVIOR	STRATEGY
Hearing voices	Evaluate hearing or adjust amplification of hearing aids. Assess quality and severity of symptoms. Determine whether they present an actual threat to safety or function. Assess noise around patient's room (e.g., staff talking in hallway).
Aggression	Determine and modify underlying causes of aggression (e.g., pain, caregiver interaction, being forced to do something). Teach caregiver not to confront individual, use distraction, observe facial expression and body posture, leave individual alone if safe, return later for the task (e.g., bathing). Create a calmer, more soothing environment.
Repetitive questioning	Respond with a calm, reassuring voice. Use calm touch for reassurance. Place warm water bottle covered with soft fleece cover on the lap or abdomen (Fitzsimmons et al, 2014). Inform individual of events only as they occur. Structure daily routines. Involve person in meaningful activities.

Adapted from Kales H, Gitlin L, Lyketsos C, et al: Management of neuropsychiatric symptoms of dementia in clinical settings: recommendations from a multidisciplinary expert panel, *J Am Geriatr Soc* 62:762–769, 2014.

could lead to imminent danger or compromise safety (American Geriatrics Society, 2014; Centers for Medicare and Medicaid Services, 2013; Kales et al, 2014). Despite these recommendations, antipsychotic medications to treat BPSD are often given as the first-line response in nursing homes, hospitals, and ambulatory care centers without appropriate determination of whether there is a medical, physical, functional, psychological, psychiatric, social, or environmental cause of the behaviors (Gordon, 2014). Often, these drugs are prescribed in response to frustration and helplessness on the parts of both professionals and loved ones, in addition to inadequate knowledge of BPSD in dementia and nonpharmacological interventions (Kales et al, 2014).

⚡ SAFETY ALERT

Do not use antipsychotics as your first choice to treat behavioral and psychological symptoms of dementia (BPSD). People with dementia often exhibit aggression, resistance to care, and other challenging or disruptive behaviors. In such instances, antipsychotic medications are often prescribed, but they provide limited benefit and can cause serious harm, including stroke and premature death. Use of these drugs should be limited to cases where nonpharmacological measures have failed and patients pose an imminent threat to themselves or others. Identifying and addressing causes of behavior change can make drug treatment unnecessary (American Geriatrics Society, 2014).

Pharmacological approaches may be considered, in addition to nonpharmacological approaches, if there has been a comprehensive assessment of reversible causes of behavior; the person presents a danger to self or others; nonpharmacological interventions have not been effective; and the risk/benefit profiles of the medications have been considered. Staff must document all care planning related to resident behaviors and use and effectiveness of nonpharmacological interventions (Box 29-24). In 2008, the FDA required manufacturers to add a Boxed Warning to conventional antipsychotic drugs to warn about an increased risk of death associated with off-label use of these agents to

BOX 29-24 Investigating Causes of Behavior

- What was the person trying to communicate through the behavior; what were the possible reasons for the person's behavior that led to the initiation of the medication?
- What other approaches and interventions were attempted before the use of the antipsychotic medication?
- Was the family or representative contacted before initiating the medication?
- Were personal needs not being met appropriately or sufficiently, such as hunger, thirst, or constipation?
- Was there fatigue, lack of sleep, or change in sleep patterns that may make the person more likely to misinterpret environmental cues resulting in anxiety, aggression, or confusion?
- Were there environmental factors, for example noise levels that could be causing or contributing to discomfort or misinterpretation of noises such as overhead pagers, alarms, etc. causing delusions or hallucinations?
- Was there a mismatch between the activities or routines selected and the resident's cognitive and other abilities to participate in those activities/routines?

Source: Berkowitz C: Dust off your policies and procedures: CMS releases updates to SOM Appendix PP, *Florida Health Care Association, PULSE,* January 2015.

treat behavioral problems of older people with dementia. Strict federal regulations monitor the use of psychotropic medications in skilled nursing facilities. Antipsychotic medication use in nursing homes may be considered after all possible causes of behavior have been investigated and, if used, should be given at the lowest possible dosage for the shortest period of time, monitored closely for side effects, and subject to gradual dose reduction and re-review (CMS, 2013) (Chapter 9).

In 2012, the Centers for Medicare and Medicaid Services (CMS) launched a nationwide initiative to improve dementia care (Partnership to Improve Dementia Care in Nursing Homes) through individualized approaches, with the goal of reducing the use of unnecessary antipsychotic medications to address behavioral expressions in dementia care. In 2013, data indicated that nursing homes are using less antipsychotic medications and instead seeking person-centered treatments for dementia and other behavioral health care. Use of antipsychotic drugs in now a quality indicator in the 5-Star rating system for nursing homes (Chapter 32).

◆ Nonpharmacological Approaches

Nonpharmacological approaches tend to view behavior as stemming from unmet needs, environmental overload, and interactions of individual, caregiver, and environmental factors. The goals of nonpharmacological treatment are prevention, symptom relief, and reduction of caregiver distress (Kales et al, 2014). These approaches are resident-centered and include interventions such as meaningful activities tailored to the individual's personality and interests, validation therapy, social contact (real or simulated), animal-assisted therapy, exercise, sensory stimulation, art therapy, reminiscence, Montessori-based activities, environmental design (e.g., special care units, homelike environments, gardens, safe walking areas), changes in mealtime and bathing environments, consistent staffing assignments, bright light therapy, aromatherapy, massage, music, relaxation, distraction, nonconfrontational interaction, and pain management (Edgerton and Richie, 2010; Fitzsimmons et al, 2014; Gitlin et al, 2013; Gordon, 2014; Kolanowski et al, 2013).

BOX 29-25   Taking a Person-Centered Approach to BPSD

A retired cardiovascular surgeon with a history of dementia resided in a nursing home and was becoming increasingly agitated. Members of the interprofessional team expressed concerns about his behavior and the request for antipsychotic medications. Ivy, the director of nursing, knew about a new program using iPads for resident-family communication. Taking a person-centered approach, she knew this man was a physician who was now in a medical facility where he was the one receiving care. Upon the recommendation from nursing, the recreational therapist downloaded cardiovascular procedure videos and placed headphones on Dr. A's head. Within a brief time, transformation took place. He became calm and appeared to enjoy the videos. Coming to know the person and recognizing his background led to nonpharmacological approaches to treat BPSD, thus avoiding the use of antipsychotic medication.

Source: Ivy Gordon-Thompson RN, MSN, Director of Nursing, John Knox Village, Pompano Beach, Florida.

Fitzsimmons and colleagues (2014) provide an excellent discussion of sensory and nurturing nonpharmacological interventions for BPSD and discussion of the Simple Pleasures program (Buettner, 1999; Colling and Buettner, 2002). Use of iPads to both prevent and address agitation in individuals with dementia holds interesting possibilities. While further research is needed related to what types of applications and programs are effective, preliminary findings suggest that even individuals with severe cognitive impairment were able to interact with the device and eqisodes of agitation and restlessness were reduced (Ross et al, 2015). Box 29-25 presents an exemplar on use of the iPad to calm agitation behavior.

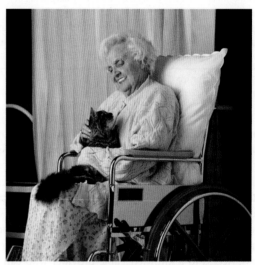

A Nursing Home Resident Enjoying Pet Therapy. (Courtesy Corbis.)

There is a large amount of literature on nonpharmacological interventions, and these approaches are recommended in the culture change movement (Chapter 32). In general, these interventions have shown promise for improving quality of life for persons with dementia despite a lack of rigorous evaluation (Kales et al, 2014). Continued attention must be paid to translating these interventions into real-world practice. Pleasant sensory stimulation and relaxation methods such as bright light therapy, music therapy, Snoezelen (a relaxation technique popular in Europe), and massage have been studied most extensively, and there is good evidence for their effectiveness (Zimmerman et al, 2012). Other therapies with strong support include cognitive training/stimulation; physical exercise, and music (Burgener et al, 2015). Practical guidance for implementing nonpharmacological approaches that emerged from focus groups with direct care providers are presented in Box 29-26.

Gerontological nurse researcher Ann Kolanowski co-led an expert panel that developed an on-line nursing home toolkit: *Promoting Positive Behavioral Health: A Nonpharmacological Toolkit for Senior Living Communities.* The toolkit provides many resources for nurses, other caregivers, and families including behavior assessment tools, clinical decision-making algorithms, and evidence-based approaches to ameliorate or prevent BPSD. CMS also has an on-line training tool specifically for nursing homes that teaches staff how to employ nonpharmacological alternatives in caring for individuals with BPSD: Hand in Hand program (see Box 29-6).

Behavioral health programs must be better integrated with medical care for individuals with dementia. Health care providers and family caregivers can benefit from training in approaches for behavioral concerns. The Alzheimer's Association offers many support groups for families that can assist in relieving stress. Access to a knowledgeable provider who can follow the individual and family throughout the course of the illness is essential and leads to improved outcomes and less distress (Hain et al, 2010). Collaborative care management programs for the treatment of Alzheimer's disease (AD), often led by advanced practice nurses, have been shown to improve quality of care, decrease the incidence of behavioral and psychological symptoms, and decrease caregiver stress (Callahan et al, 2006; Fortinsky et al, 2014; Reuben et al, 2014).

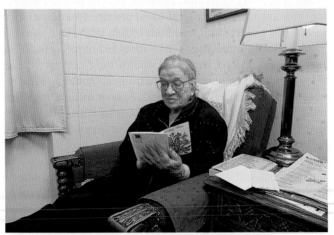

Meaningful Activities Provide Cognitive Stimulation. (From Sorrentino SA, Gorek B: *Mosby's textbook for long-term care assistants,* ed 5, St Louis, MO, 2007, Mosby.)

PROVIDING CARE FOR ACTIVITIES OF DAILY LIVING

The losses associated with dementia interfere with the person's communication patterns and ability to understand and express thoughts and feelings. Perceptual disturbances and misinterpretations of reality contribute to fear and misunderstanding. Often, bathing and the provision of other ADL care, such as dressing, grooming, and toileting, are the cause of much distress for both the person with dementia and the caregiver.

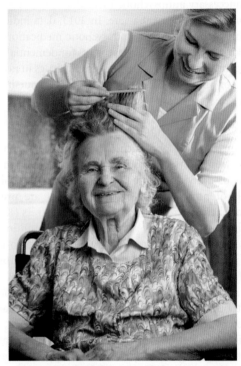

ADL Care Enhances Self-Esteem. (©iStock.com/AlexRaths)

Bathing

Bathing is an essential aspect of everyday life that most people enjoy. However, bathing and care for ADLs can be perceived as a personal attack by persons with dementia who may respond by screaming or striking out. In institutional settings, a rigid focus on tasks or institutional care routines, such as a shower three mornings each week, can contribute to the distress and precipitate distressing behaviors. Being touched or bathed against one's will violates the trust in caregiver relationships and can be considered a major affront (Rader and Barrick, 2000). The behaviors that may be exhibited are not deliberate attacks on caregivers by a violent person, but rather a way to express self in an uncertain situation. The message is, in the words of Rader and Barrick: "Please find another way to keep me clean, because the way you are doing it now is intolerable" (2000, p. 49) (see Box 29-20).

◆ PROMOTING HEALTHY AGING: IMPLICATIONS FOR GERONTOLOGICAL NURSING

◆ Assessment and Interventions

In research conducted in nursing homes, Rader and Barrick (2000) have provided comprehensive guidelines for bathing people with dementia in ways that are pleasurable and decrease distress. Asking the question "What is the easiest, most comfortable, least frightening way for me to clean the person right now?" guides the choice of interventions (Rader and Barrick, 2000, p. 42). *Bathing Without a Battle* is an approach that can be used to create a better bathing experience for people with dementia (Box 29-27).

Another innovative approach being investigated in Sweden is caregiver singing and the use of background music during ADL care in nursing homes. Caregivers play and sing familiar songs during care routines. When compared to usual care practices, this approach enhanced the expression of positive moods and emotions, increased the mutuality of communication, and reduced aggression and resistive care behaviors (Hammar et al, 2011).

WANDERING

Wandering associated with dementia is one of the most difficult management problems encountered in home and institutional settings. One in five people with dementia wander. Wandering is a complex behavior and is not well understood. Wandering is defined as "a syndrome of dementia-related locomotion behavior having a frequent, repetitive, temporally disordered and/or

---

> ### BOX 29-28 Patient Perspectives on Wandering Behavior
>
> *"Wandering and restlessness is one of the by-products of Alzheimer's disease... When the darkness and emptiness fills my mind, it is totally terrifying... Thoughts increasingly haunt me. The only way I can break the cycle is to move"* (Davis, 1989, p. 96).
>
> *"Very often, I wander around looking for something which I know is very pertinent, but then after awhile I forget all about what it was I was looking for. When I'm wandering around, I'm trying to touch base with—anything, actually. If anything appeared I'd probably enjoy it, or look at it or examine it and wonder how it got there. I feel very foolish when I'm wandering around not knowing what I'm doing and I'm not always quite sure how to do any better. It's not easy to figure out what the heck I'm looking for"* (Henderson, 1998).

---

spatially disoriented nature that is manifested in lapping, random and or pacing patterns, some of which is associated with eloping, eloping attempts or getting lost unless accompanied" (Algase et al, 2007, p. 696). Risk factors for wandering include visuospatial impairments, anxiety and depression, poor sleep patterns, unmet needs, and a more socially active and outgoing premorbid lifestyle (Futrell et al, 2014; Lester et al, 2012). Wandering frequency tends to increase as cognitive function decreases (Futrell et al, 2014). There is a need for more research and interventions for this behavior.

Wandering presents safety concerns in all settings. Wandering behavior affects sleeping, eating, safety, and the caregiver's ability to provide care, and it also interferes with the privacy of others. The behavior can lead to falls, elopement (leaving the home or facility), injury, and death (Futrell et al, 2010; Rowe et al, 2010). The stimulus for wandering arises from many internal and external sources. Wandering can be considered a rhythm, intrinsically and extrinsically driven. Box 29-28 presents insight into the behavior of wandering from the perspective of individuals with dementia.

◆ PROMOTING HEALTHY AGING: IMPLICATIONS FOR GERONTOLOGICAL NURSING

◆ Assessment and Interventions

Careful assessment of physical problems that may trigger wandering, such as acute illness, exacerbations of chronic illness, fatigue, medication effects, and constipation, is important. Unmet needs or pain can increase wandering (Futrell et al, 2014). Wandering behaviors can be predicted through careful observation and awareness of the person's patterns. For example, if the person with dementia starts wandering or trying to leave the home in the afternoon every day, meaningful activities such as music, exercise, and refreshments can be provided at this time. Research suggests that wandering may be less likely to occur when the person is involved in social interaction. There are also several instruments to assess risk for wandering, and nurse researcher May Futrell and colleagues (2010, 2014) developed an evidence-based protocol for wandering. There are a number of assistive technology devices and programs that can enhance the

---

> ### BOX 29-27 TIPS FOR BEST PRACTICE
>
> #### *Techniques for Bathing without a Battle*
>
> 1. Rethink the bathing experience.
>   - Make the experience comfortable and pleasurable.
>   - Consider what makes the individual feel good.
>   - Do not be in a hurry.
> 2. Approach techniques such as "let's go get freshened up for the day" and avoiding bathing terminology (e.g. "it's time for your bath") can create a more positive environment.
>   - Tell person it is time to get freshened up and try not to ask "do you want a bath?" because the answer may be no.
> 3. Have the room ready.
>   - Keep the room warm and low-lit.
>   - Hand-held shower head wets one area at a time.
>   - Have a large towel or blanket to preserve dignity and keep person warm.
> 4. Begin bathing least sensitive area first.
>   - Wash legs and feet first, followed by arms, trunk, perineum area, and face last.
> 5. Save washing hair until last or do separately.
> 6. Use distraction techniques.
>   - Consider using music or singing songs that the person likes.
>   - Consider having the person hold a towel or something to provide distraction.
> 7. Consider a towel bath for those who may not respond to the above strategies.
>
> Source: Dougherty J, Long CO: Techniques for bathing without a battle, *Home Healthcare Nurse* 21(1):38–39, 2003.

BOX 29-29   TIPS FOR BEST PRACTICE

Interventions for Wandering or Exiting Behaviors

- Face the person, and make direct eye contact (unless this is interpreted as threatening).
- Gently touch the person's arm, shoulders, back, or waist if he or she does not move away from a door or other exit.
- Call the person by his or her formal name (e.g., Mr. Jones).
- Listen to what the person is communicating verbally and nonverbally; listen to the feelings being expressed.
- Identify the agenda, plan of action, and the emotional needs of the behavior being expressed.
- Respond to the feelings expressed, staying calm.
- Repeat specific words or phrases, or state the need or emotion (e.g., "You need to go home; you're worried about your husband").
- If such repetition fails to distract the person, accompany him or her and continue talking calmly, repeating phrases and the emotion you identify.
- Provide orienting information only if it calms the person. If it increases distress, stop talking about the present situations. Do not "correct" the person or belittle his or her agenda.
- At intervals, redirect the person toward the facility or the home by suggesting, "Let's walk this way now" or "I'm so tired, let's turn around."
- If orientation and redirection fail, continue to walk, allowing the person control but ensuring safety.
- Make sure you have a backup person, but he or she should stay out of eyesight of the person.
- Have someone call for help if you are unable to redirect. Usually the behavior is time limited because of the person's attention span and the security and trust between you and the person.

Adapted from Radar J, Doan J, Schwab M, et al: How to decrease wandering, a form of agenda behavior, *Geriatr Nurs* 6(4):196–199, 1985.

BOX 29-30   TIPS FOR BEST PRACTICE

Recommendations to Avoid Individuals with Dementia Getting Lost

- Do not leave the person with dementia alone in the home.
- Secure the environment so that the person cannot leave by himself or herself while the caregiver is asleep or busy.
- If the person lives in a nursing facility, keep in a supervised area; do frequent checks; use bed, chair, and door alarms and WanderGuard bracelets; identify potential wanderers by special arm bands.
- Disguise doorways by painting pictures (or using posters) such as floral arrangements or bookcases so that they will not be visualized and recognized as a door by the individual with dementia.
- Place locks out of reach, hide keys, and lock windows.
- Consider motion detectors or home security systems that alert when doors are opened.
- Register the person in the Safe Return program of the Alzheimer's Association, and ensure that the person wears the Safe Return jewelry or clothing tags at all times.
- Register with the Silver Alert system if available.
- Let neighbors know that a person with dementia lives in the neighborhood.
- Prepare a search-and-rescue plan in case the person becomes lost.
- Keep copies of up-to-date photos ready for distribution to searchers, police, hospitals, and the media.
- Call the local law enforcement agency and the Safe Return program to report the missing person.
- Conduct a search immediately if the person becomes lost.
- If the person is not found within 6 to 12 hours (or sooner depending on weather conditions), search any wooded areas or fields near where the person was last seen. People with dementia may not seek help or respond to calls and may try to hide from searchers; search in an organized manner with as many searchers as possible.

Adapted from Rowe M: People with dementia who become lost, *Am J Nurs* 103:32–39, 2003.

safety of persons who wander (Chapter 20). Box 29-29 presents other suggested interventions.

Wandering behavior may also result in people with dementia going outside and getting lost, a phenomenon studied by nurse researcher Meredith Rowe (2003). All people with dementia should be considered capable of getting lost. Caregivers must prevent people with dementia from leaving homes or care facilities unaccompanied, register the person in the Alzheimer's Association Safe Return program, and have a plan of action in case the person does become lost. In care facilities, "a risk-management approach needs to include 1) identification of the wanderer; 2) a wandering prevention program; 3) an elopement response plan when patients are missing; and 4) staff mobilization around the problem" (Futrell et al, 2014, p. 22). Rowe also suggests that police must respond rapidly to requests for searches, and the general public should be informed about how to recognize and assist people with dementia who may be lost (Rowe, 2003). Box 29-30 presents specific recommendations from this study.

NUTRITION

Older adults with dementia are particularly at risk for weight loss and inadequate nutrition. Weight loss often becomes a considerable concern in late-stage dementia. Some of the factors predisposing individuals with dementia to nutritional inadequacy include lack of awareness of the need to eat, depression, loss of independence in self-feeding, agnosia, apraxia, vision impairments (deficient contrast sensitivity), wandering, pacing, and behavior disturbances. Weight loss increases risk for infection, pressure wound development and poor wound healing, and hospitalization and is associated with higher mortality and morbidity rates. Nurses, as members of interprofessional teams, play a significant role in assessing nutrition in persons with dementia. Chapter 14 discusses nutritional needs and interventions in depth.

◆ PROMOTING HEALTHY AGING: IMPLICATIONS FOR HEALTHY AGING

◆ Assessment and Interventions

Assessment includes evaluation of nutrition status and identification of eating and feeding problems through observation of meals. The Mini Nutritional Analysis (MNA) is an easy tool to identify those at risk (Chapter 14). Collaborating with a dietitian

BOX 29-31   TIPS FOR BEST PRACTICE

Improving Intake for Individuals with Dementia

- Serve only one dish at a time.
- Provide only one utensil at a time.
- Consider using a "spork" (combination spoon-fork).
- Serve finger foods such as fried chicken, chicken strips, pizza in bite-size pieces, fish sticks, sandwiches.
- Serve soup in a mug.
- Remove any hot items or items that should not be eaten.
- Cut up foods before serving.
- Sit next to the person at his or her level.
- Demonstrate eating motions that the person can imitate.
- Use hand-over-hand feeding technique to guide self-feeding.
- Use verbal cueing and prompting (e.g., take a bite, chew, swallow).
- Use gentle tone of voice, and avoid scolding or demeaning remarks.
- Provide verbal encouragement to participate in eating by talking about food taste and smell.
- Offer small amounts of fluid between bites.
- Help person focus on the meal at hand; turn off background noise, remove clutter from the table.
- Avoid patterned dishes or table coverings.
- Use red plates/glasses/cups; food intake may increase when food is served with high-contrast tableware.
- Use unbreakable dishes that will not slide around.
- Serve smaller, more frequent meals rather than expecting the person to complete a big meal.

Data from Dunne T, Neargarder S, Cipolloni P, Cronin-Golomb A: Visual contrast enhances food and liquid intake in advanced Alzheimer's disease, Clinical Nutrition 23(4):533 538, 2004, Spencer P: How to solve eating problems common to people with Alzheimer's and other dementias. Retrieved June 1, 2015 from https://www.caring.com/articles/alzheimers-eating-problems.

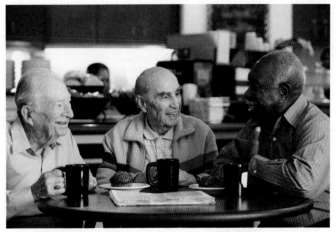

A Pleasurable Dining Experience. (©iStock.com/monkeybusinessimages)

to perform a clinical examination that yields information regarding potential or real nutritional deficits is an excellent way to develop strategies to minimize or improve nutritional status of persons with dementia.

One of the best strategies for managing poor intake is establishing a routine so that the older person does not have to remember time and places for eating. Caregivers should continue to serve foods and fluids that the person likes and has always eaten. Nutrient-dense foods (e.g., peanut butter, protein bars, yogurt) are preferred. Attention to mealtime ambience is important, and the person should be able to take as much time as needed to eat the food. Food should be available 24 hours a day, and the person should be allowed to follow his or her accustomed eating schedule (e.g., late breakfast, early dinner). Other suggestions to enhance food intake for individuals with dementia are presented in Box 29-31.

NURSING ROLES IN THE CARE OF PERSONS WITH DEMENTIA

Caregiving for someone with dementia by family members, or formal caregivers, requires special skills, knowledge of evidence-based practice, and a deep understanding of the person.

Rader and Tornquist (1995) reflect on the knowledge required and provide a view of caregiving roles that is quite useful and understandable for all caregivers. The authors have found that nursing assistants and family caregivers can truly relate to the practical wisdom in these words.

Magician role: To understand what the person is trying to communicate both verbally and nonverbally, we must be a magician who can use our magical abilities to see the world through the eyes, the ears, and the feelings of the person. We know how to use tricks to turn an individual's behavior around or prevent it from occurring and causing distress.

Detective role: The detective looks for clues and cues about what might be causing distress and how it might be changed. We have to investigate and know as much about the person as possible to be a good detective.

Carpenter role: By having a wide variety of tools and selecting the right tools for the job, we build individualized plans of care for each person.

Jester role: Many people with dementia retain their sense of humor and respond well to the appropriate use of humor. This does not mean making fun of but rather sharing laughter and fun. "Those who love their work and do it well employ good doses of humor as part of the care of others, as well as for self-care" (Rader and Barrick, 2000, p. 42). The jester spreads joy, is creative, energizes, and lightens the burdens (Laurenhue, 2001; Rader and Barrick, 2000).

Figure 29-1 presents a nursing situation that one nurse experienced in caring for a patient with dementia who was being admitted to a nursing home. Written from the perspective of the nurse and his knowledge of the patient, the story provides insight into important nursing responses, such as providing person-centered care, implementing therapeutic communication, and establishing meaningful relationships. It is a lovely example of expert gerontological nursing for individuals with dementia and a fitting way to end this chapter.

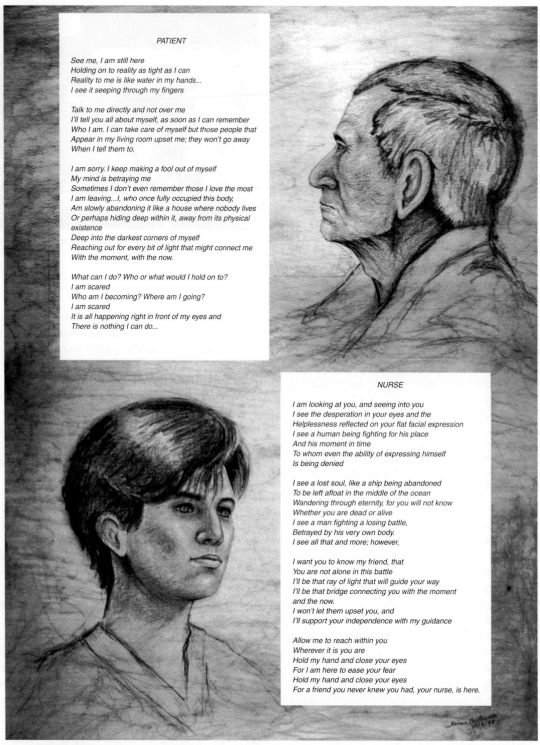

FIGURE 29-1 Nurse and Person. (Copyright ©1998 by Jaime Castaneda, Lake Worth, Fla.)

KEY CONCEPTS

- Nurses must advocate for thorough assessment of any elder who appears to be experiencing cognitive decline and inability to function in important aspects of life. Self-reports or caregiver reports of changes in cognitive function are important indicators for evaluation of cognitive status.

- Delirium results from the interaction of predisposing factors (e.g., vulnerability on the part of the individual due to predisposing conditions such as cognitive impairment, severe illness, and sensory impairment) and precipitating factors/insults (e.g., medications, procedures, restraints, iatrogenic events). Delirium is characterized by an acute onset, fluctuating levels of consciousness, and frequent misperceptions and illusions. It often goes unrecognized and is attributed to age or dementia. People with dementia are more susceptible to delirium. Knowledge of risk factors, preventive measures, and treatment of underlying medical problems is essential to prevent serious consequences.

- Acute illness (e.g., urinary tract infections, respiratory tract infections), medications, and pain are frequently the causes of delirious states in older people. In people with dementia, a change in environment can precipitate delirium.
- In older adults experiencing delirium, a new diagnosis of dementia cannot be made until the delirium is resolved.
- It is essential to view all behavior as meaningful and an expression of needs. The focus must be on understanding that behavioral expressions communicate distress, and the response is to investigate the possible sources of distress and intervene appropriately.
- All evidence-based guidelines endorse an approach that begins with comprehensive assessment of the behavioral and psychological symptoms of dementia and possible causes followed by the use of nonpharmacological interventions as a first line of treatment except in emergency situations when BPSD symptoms could lead to imminent danger or compromise safety.
- Fear, discomfort, unfamiliar surroundings and people, illness, fatigue, depression, need for autonomy and control, caregiver approaches, communication strategies, and environmental stressors are frequent precipitants of behavioral symptoms.
- Individuals with the neurocognitive disorder of dementia respond best to calmness and patience, adaptations of communication techniques, and environments and relationships that enhance function, support limitations, ensure safety, and provide opportunities for a meaningful quality of life. Because individuals with dementia may be unable to express their feelings and needs in ways that are easily understood, the gerontological nurse must always try to understand the world from their perspective.

NURSING STUDY: MAJOR NEUROCOGNITIVE DISORDER: BEHAVIOR

Pat is an 83-year-old retired nurse who was diagnosed with major neurocognitive disorder 3 years ago. Her other diagnoses include hypertension and osteoarthritis. She had a hip replacement 6 years ago and also has pain in her shoulders and knees from the osteoarthritis and some limitation of movement that affects her mobility. She lives with her daughter, who has brought her to the clinic for a medication check.

Her daughter tells you, the nurse, that things have not been going well. The daughter states that Pat has been verbally and physically abusive to her when she tries to bathe and dress her. She hits her and screams "You're hurting me." The daughter says that her mother was a very fastidious person and always wanted to look nice, so she cannot understand why she resists bathing and dressing. The daughter tries to give her mother a shower at least every other day, but the battles have gotten so bad that she has not been able to keep this schedule. The daughter tells you that her mother never took showers, preferring either a tub bath or sponge bathing at the sink. However, the shower is more convenient for the daughter and her mother cannot get in the whirpool tub at her house. She is concerned over her mother's appearance and also deeply hurt that her mother has been so mean to her.

Her mother has been a lovely woman and never acted like this before. She asks you what she can do and if her mother needs some kind of tranquilizer.

Based on the nursing study, develop a nursing care plan using the following procedure*:

- List Pat's comments that provide subjective data.
- List information that provides objective data.
- From these data, identify and state, using an accepted format, two nursing diagnoses you determine are most significant to Pat at this time. List two of Pat's strengths that you have identified from the data.
- Determine and state outcome criteria for each diagnosis. These must reflect some alleviation of the problem identified in the nursing diagnosis and must be stated in concrete and measurable terms.
- Plan and state one or more interventions for each diagnosed concern. Provide specific documentation of the source used to determine the appropriate intervention. Plan at least one intervention that incorporates Pat's existing strengths.
- Evaluate the success of the intervention. Interventions must correlate directly with the stated outcome criteria to measure the outcome success.

*Students are advised to refer to their nursing diagnosis text and identify possible or potential problems.

CRITICAL THINKING QUESTIONS AND ACTIVITIES

1. What internal and external factors could be influencing Pat's behavior?
2. What nursing framework for understanding behavior would be helpful in this situation?
3. Discuss some specific interventions that might be helpful in promoting comfort during bathing for persons with dementia.
4. What type of communication techniques would be helpful in assisting with ADL activities for a person with dementia?
5. How might you help the daughter in understanding and reacting to her mother's behavior?

RESEARCH QUESTIONS

1. What barriers do nurses encounter in recognizing delirium in hospitalized older adults?
2. How does delirium experienced in the hospital affect care outcomes for older people who are discharged home?
3. What are student nurses' feelings about caring for individuals with dementia?
4. What types of programs can be developed to enhance the health of older adults with dementia?
5. What nonpharmacological interventions are most effective in the home setting for individuals with moderate NCD who are resistant to bathing?
6. What are the effects of an interprofessional team approach to dementia care for individuals with BSPD who reside in nursing homes?
7. What type of dining options encourage intake in long-term care facilities?
8. Do educational programs for informal and formal caregivers of older persons with dementia improve understanding and management of behavioral problems?

REFERENCES

Algase DL, Beel-Bates C, Beattie ERA: Wandering in long-term care, *Ann Longterm Care* 11:33–39, 2003.

Algase DL, Moore DH, Vanderweerd C, et al: Mapping the maze of terms and definitions in dementia-related wandering, *Aging Ment Health* 11:686–698, 2007.

American Geriatrics Society: AGS updated Beers Criteria for potentially inappropriate medication use in older adults, *J Am Geriatr Soc* 60(4):616–631, 2012.

American Geriatrics Society: *Choosing wisely: five things physicians and patients should question*, 2014. http://www.american geriatrics.org/health_care_professionals/clinical_practice/clinical_guidelines_recommendations/choosing_wisely2014. Accessed October 2014.

American Psychiatric Association: *Diagnostic and statistical manual of mental disorders*, ed 5, Washington, DC, 2013, American Psychiatric Association.

Balas M, Rice M, Chaperon C, et al: Management of delirium in critically ill older adults, *Crit Care Nurse* 32(4):15–26, 2012.

Barr J: *SCCM releases new pain, agitation and delirium clinical practice guidelines*, 2013. http://www.sccm.org/Communications/Critical-Connections/Archives/Pages/SCCM-Releases-New-Pain,-Agitation-and-Delirium-Clinical-Practice-Guidelines.aspx. Accessed October 2014.

Bienvenu O, Gellar J, Althouse B, et al: Post-traumatic stress disorder symptoms after acute lung injury: a 2-year prospective longitudinal study, *Psychol Med* 43:2657–2671, 2013.

Bledowski J, Trutia A: A review of pharmacologic management and prevention strategies for delirium in the intensive care unit, *The Journal of Lifelong Learning in Psychiatry* XI(4):568–575, 2013.

Braes T, Milisen K, Foremen M: Assessing cognitive function. In Capezuti E, Zwicker D, Mezey M, et al, editors: *Evidence-based geriatric nursing protocols for best practice*, ed 3, New York, 2008, Springer, pp 122-134.

Buckwalter K, Gerdner L, Hall G, et al: Shining through: the humor and individuality of persons with Alzheimer's disease, *J Gerontol Nurs* 21:11–16, 1995.

Buettner LL: Simple pleasures: a multilevel sensorimotor intervention for nursing home residents with dementia, *Am J Alzheimers Dis Other Demen* 14:41–52, 1999.

Burgener S, Jao Y-L, Anderson J, Bossen A: Mechanism of action for nonpharmacological therapies for individuals with dementia: Implications for practice and research, *Res Gerontol Nurs*, Posted May 11, 2015, DOI 10.3928/19404921-20150429-02.

Callahan C, Boustani M, Unversagt F, et al: Effectiveness of collaborative care for older adults with Alzheimer's disease in primary care, *JAMA* 295:2148–2157, 2006.

Centers for Medicare and Medicaid Services: *Center for Clinical Standards and Quality/Survey and Certification Group*, (Memo), May 14, 2013. http://www.cms.gov/Medicare/Provider-Enrollment-and-Certification/SurveyCertification-GenInfo/Downloads/Survey-and-Cert-Letter-13-35.pdf. Accessed May 19, 2015

Cerejeira J, Nogueira V, Luís P, et al: The cholinergic system and inflammation: common pathways in delirium pathophysiology, *J Am Geriatr Soc* 60(4):689–675, 2012.

Cohen-Mansfield J: Nonpharmacologic treatment of behavioral disorders in dementia, *Curr Treat Options Neurol* 15(6):765–785, 2013.

Colling K, Buettner L: Simple pleasures: interventions from the need-driven dementia-compromised behavior model, *J Gerontol Nurs* 28(10):16–20, 2002.

Dahlke S, Phinney A: Caring for hospitalized older adults at risk for delirium: the silent, unspoken piece of nursing practice, *J Gerontol Nurs* 34:41–47, 2008.

Davis R: *My journey into Alzheimer's disease*, Wheaton, IL, 1989, Tyndale House.

Dettmore D, Kolanowski A, Boustani M: Aggression in persons with dementia: use of nursing theory to guide clinical practice, *Geriatric Nursing* 30:8–17, 2009.

DeYoung S, Just G, Harrison R: Decreasing aggressive, agitated, or disruptive behavior: participation in a behavior management unit, *J Gerontol Nurs* 28:22–31, 2003.

Edgerton E, Richie L: Improving physical environments for dementia care: making minimal changes for maximum effect, *Ann Longterm Care* 18:43–45, 2010.

Ely EW, Margolin R, Francis J, et al: Evaluation of delirium in critically ill patients: validation of the Confusion Assessment Method for the intensive care unit (CAM-ICU), *Crit Care Med* 29:1370–1379, 2001.

Evans L, Kurlowicz L: *Complex care needs in older adults with common cognitive disorders, Section A: Assessment and management of dementia*, 2007. http://hartfordign.org/uploads/File/gnec_state_of_science_papers/gnec_delirium.pdf. Accessed November 2014.

Fitzsimmons S, Barba B, Stump M: Sensory and nurturing pharmacological interventions for behavioral and psychological symptoms of dementia, *J Gerontol Nurs* 40(11):9–15, 2014.

Fortinsky R, Delaney C, Harel O, et al: Results and lessons learned from a nurse practitioner-guided dementia care intervention for primary care patients and their family caregivers, *Res Gerontol Nurs* 7(3):126–137, 2014.

Futrell M, Mellilo K, Remington R, et al: Evidence-based practice guideline: wandering, *J Gerontol Nurs* 36:6–16, 2010.

Futrell M, Mellilo K, Remington R, et al: Evidence-based practice guideline: wandering, *J Gerontol Nurs* 40(11):16–23, 2014.

Gitlin L, Mann W, Vogel W, Arthur P, et al: A non-pharmacologic approach to address challenging behaviors of veterans with dementia: description of the tailored activity program—VA randomized trial, *BMC Geriatr* 13:96, 2013.

Gordon M: When should antipsychotics for the management of behavioral and psychological symptoms of dementia be discontinued? *Ann Longterm Care* 22(4), 2014. http://www.annalsoflongtermcare.com/article/antipsychotics-discontinued-management-behavioral-psychological-symptoms-dementia. Accessed October 2014.

Hain D, Tappen R, Diaz S, et al: Cognitive impairment and medication self-management errors in older adults discharged home from a community hospital, *Home Healthc Nurse* 30(4):246–254, 2012.

Hain D, Touhy T, Engstrom G: What matters most to carers of people with mild to moderate dementia as evidence for transforming care, *Alzheimers Care Today* 11:162–171, 2010.

Hall GR: Caring for people with Alzheimer's disease using the conceptual model of progressively lowered stress threshold in the clinical setting, *Nurs Clin North Am* 29:129–141, 1994.

Hall GR, Buckwalter KC: Progressively lowered stress threshold: a conceptual model for care of adults with Alzheimer's disease, *Arch Psychiatr Nurs* 1:399–406, 1987.

Hall G, Gallagher M, Dougherty J: Integrating roles for successful dementia management, *Nurse Pract* 34:35–41, 2009.

Hammar LM, Emami A, Engstrom G, et al: Communicating through caregiver singing during morning care situations in dementia care, *Scand J Caring Sci* 25(1):160–168, 2011.

Henderson C: *Partial view: an Alzheimer's journal*, Dallas, TX, 1998, Southern Methodist Press.

Hshieh T, Yue J, Oh E, Puelle E, et al: Effectiveness of multicomponent nonpharmacological delirium interventions, *JAMA Intern Med.* Published online February 2, 2015. Doi: 10.1001/jamainternmed.2014.7779.

Inouye SK, Bogardus ST Jr, Charpentier PA, et al: A multicomponent intervention to prevent delirium in hospitalized older patients, *N Engl J Med* 340:669–676, 1999.

Inouye SK, van Dyck CH, Alessi CA, et al: Clarifying confusion: the Confusion Assessment: a new method for detection of delirium, *Ann Intern Med* 113:941–948, 1990.

Inouye SK, Westendorp RG, Saczynski JS: Delirium in elderly people, *Lancet* 383:911–922, 2014.

Institute of Medicine: *Envisioning the national health care quality report*, Washington DC, National Academies Press, 2001.

Jones C, Backman C, Griffiths R: Intensive care diaries and relatives' symptoms of posttraumatic stress disorder after critical illness: a pilot study, *Am J Crit Care* 21(3):172–176, 2012.

Kales H, Gitlin L, Lyketsos C, et al: Management of neuropsychiatric symptoms of dementia in clinical settings: recommendations from a multidisciplinary panel, *J Am Geriatr Soc* 62:762–769, 2014.

Kolanowski A: An overview of the need-driven dementia-compromised behavior model, *J Gerontol Nurs* 25:7–9, 1999.

Kolanowski A, Fick D, Frazer C, et al: It's about time: use of nonpharmacological interventions in the nursing home, *J Nurs Scholarsh* 42:214–222, 2010.

Kolanowski A, Resnick B, Beck C, et al: Advances in nonpharmacological interventions, 2011-2012, *Res Gerontol Nurs* 6(1):5–8, 2013.

Kolanowski A, Van Haitsma K: *Promoting positive behavioral health: a non-pharmacologic toolkit for senior living communities*, 2013. http://www.nursinghometoolkit.com. Accessed October 2014.

Kovach C: Assessment and treatment of discomfort for people with late-stage dementia, *J Pain Symptom Manage* 18(6):412–419, 1999.

Kovach C, Noonan P, Schildt A, et al: A model of consequences of need-driven dementia-compromised behavior, *J Nurs Scholar* 37(2):134–140, 2005.

Kovach C, Simpson M, Joosse L, et al: Comparison of the effectiveness of two protocols for treating nursing home residents with advanced dementia, *Res Gerontol Nurs* 5(4):251–263, 2012.

Kuehn B: Delirium often not recognized or treated despite serious long-term consequences, *JAMA* 304:389–390, 2010a.

Kuehn B: Questionable antipsychotic prescribing remains common despite serious risks, *JAMA* 303:1582–1584, 2010b.

Laurenhue K: Each person's journey is unique, *Alzheimers Care Q* 2:79–83, 2001.

Lester P, Garite A, Kohen I: Wandering and elopement in nursing homes, *Ann Longterm Care* 20(3):32–36, 2012.

Lindquist I, Go L, Fleisher J, et al: Improvements in cognition following hospital discharge of community dwelling seniors, *J Gen Intern Med* 26(7):765–770, 2011.

Marcantonio E, Bergmann M, Kiely D, et al: Randomized trial of a delirium abatement program for postacute skilled nursing facilities, *J Am Geriatr Soc* 58:1019–1026, 2010.

Mitchell S, Teno J, Kiely D, et al: The clinical course of advanced dementia, *N Engl J Med* 36(1):1529–1538, 2009.

Miyamoto Y, Tachimori H, Ito H: Formal caregiver burden in dementia: impact of behavioral and psychological symptoms of dementia and activities of daily living, *Geriatr Nurs* 31(4):246–253, 2010.

Morley J, Caplan G, Cesari M, et al: International survey of nursing home research priorities, *J Am Med Dir Assoc* 15(5):309–312, 2014.

Neelon VJ, Champagne MT, Carlson JR, et al: The NEECHAM confusion scale: construction, validation and clinical testing, *Nurs Res* 45:324–330, 1996.

O'Mahony R, Murthy L, Akunne A, et al: Synopsis of the National Institute for Health and Clinical Excellence guideline for prevention of delirium, *Ann Intern Med* 154:746–751, 2011.

Rader J, Barrick A: Ways that work: bathing without a battle, *Alzheimers Care Q* 1:35–49, 2000.

Rader J, Tornquist E: *Individualized dementia care*, New York, 1995, Springer.

Reinhard S, Samis S, Levine C: *Family caregivers providing complex chronic care to people with cognitive and behavioral health conditions*, Insight on the Issues 93, August 2014, AARP Public Policy Institute. http://www.aarp.org/home-family/caregiving/info-2014/family-caregivers-providing-complex-chronic-care-cognitive-behavioral-AARP-ppi-health.html. Accessed October 2014.

Reuben D, Ganz D, Roth C, et al: The effect of nurse practitioner co-management on the care of geriatric conditions, *J Am Geriatr Soc* 61(8):857–867, 2014.

Richards K, Lambert C, Beck C: Deriving interventions for challenging behaviors from the need-driven dementia-compromised behavior model, *Alzheimers Care Q* 1:62–72, 2000.

Rigney T: Delirium in the hospitalized elder and recommendations for practice, *Geriatr Nurs* 27(3):151–157, 2006.

Rosemary, Blieszner R, Roberto K: Care partner responses to the onset of mild cognitive impairment, *Gerontologist* 50:11–22, 2010.

Rosenbloom-Brunton D, Henneman E, Inouye S: Feasibility of family participation in a delirium prevention program for hospitalized older adults, *J Gerontol Nurs* 36:22–33, 2010.

Ross L, Ramirez S, Bhatt A et al: Tables devices (IPad) for control of behavioral symptoms in older adults with dementia, Presented at the American Association for Geriatric Psychiatry (AAGP) 2015 Annual Meeting, March 31, 2015.

Rowe MA: People with dementia who become lost, *Am J Nurs* 103:32–39, 2003.

Rowe MA, Kairalla JA, McCrae CS: Sleep in dementia caregivers and the effect of a nighttime monitoring system, *J Nurs Scholarsh* 42:338–347, 2010.

Sekerak R, Stewart J: Caring for the patient with end-stage dementia, *Annals of Long-Term Care* 22(12):1–17, 2014.

Sifton C: Life is what happens while we are making plans, *Alzheimers Care Q* 2: iv, 2001.

Splete H: Nurses have special strategies for dementia, *Caring Ages* 9:11, 2008.

Steis M, Fick D: Are nurses recognizing delirium? *J Gerontol Nurs* 34:40–48, 2008.

Steis M, Evans L, Hirschman K, et al: Screening for delirium using family caregivers: convergent validity of the Family Confusion Assessment Method and interviewer-rated Confusion Assessment Method, *J Am Geriatr Soc* 60(11): 2121–2126, 2012.

Tappen R, Williams C, Fishman S, et al: Persistence of self in advanced Alzheimer's disease, *Image J Nurs Sch* 31:121–125, 1999.

Tappen R, Williams-Burgess C, Edelstein J, et al: Communicating with individuals with Alzheimer's disease: examination of recommended strategies, *Arch Psychiatr Nurs* 11:249–256, 1997.

Touhy T: Dementia, personhood and nursing: learning from a nursing situation, *Nurs Sci Q* 17:43–49, 2004.

Tullmann D, Mion L, Fletcher K, et al: Delirium prevention, early recognition and treatment. In Capezuti E, Zwicker D, Mezey M, et al, editors: *Evidence-based geriatric nursing: protocols for best practice*, ed 3, New York, 2008, Springer.

Tullmann D, Fletcher K, Foreman M: In Boltz M, Capezuti E, Fulmer T, et al, editors: *Evidence-based geriatric nursing protocols for best practice*, ed 4, New York, 2012, Springer.

Voyer P, Richard S, Doucet L, et al: Examination of the multifactorial model of delirium among long-term care residents with dementia, *Geriatr Nurs* 31:105–114, 2010.

Waszynski C, Petrovic K: Nurses' evaluation of the Confusion Assessment Method: a pilot study, *J Gerontol Nurs* 34:49–56, 2008.

Williams C, Tappen R: Communicating with cognitively impaired persons. In Williams C, editor: *Therapeutic interaction in nursing*, ed 2, Boston, 2008, Jones and Bartlett.

Woods B: Dementia challenges assumptions about what it means to be a person, *Generations* 13:39, 1999.

Zaubler T, Murphy K, Stanton R, et al: Quality improvement and cost savings of the Hospital Elder Life Program in a community hospital, *Psychosomatics* 54(3):219–226, 2013.

Zimmerman S, Anderson W, Brode S, et al: *Comparison of characteristics of nursing homes and other residential long-term care settings for people with dementia* (Comparative Effectiveness Review no. 79, AHRQ publication no. 12[13]-EHC127-EF), Rockville, MD, 2012, Agency for Healthcare Research and Quality.

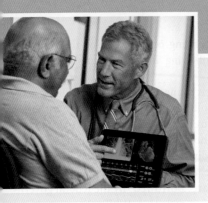

CHAPTER 30

Economics and Health Care in Later Life

Kathleen Jett

http://evolve.elsevier.com/Touhy/TwdHlthAging

A STUDENT SPEAKS

We went on a home visit with our preceptors today. I could hardly stand it. The house was almost bare. The only food he had was left over from the "home-delivered meals" he gets from the local social service organization. The preceptor said that he was doing the best he could with what he had. There were few other community services in his state and he had no family and few friends. I don't know why someone can't help him more!

Evelyn, age 21

AN ELDER SPEAKS

When I was growing up, life was hard. We were so poor we couldn't do much but to hold on tight. When I was lucky I could get work plowing a field for $1 an acre. You work hard and you make do. There were not such things as going to a doctor or hospital; you did the best you could and pray you don't get sick. . . . Then when I turned 65 I got a little check from the government and a red, white, and blue insurance card [Medicare card]. The check isn't much, about $521 a month [SSI], but you know I consider myself blessed and much better off than ever before. And now I don't worry about my health; I will be taken care of, praise the Lord.

Aida at 74 in 1994

LEARNING OBJECTIVES

On completion of this chapter, the reader will be able to:
1. Explain how health care is financed in the United States.
2. Briefly explain the history of Social Security, Supplementary Security Income, and some of the anticipated challenges.
3. Compare the types of health care services available under Medicare.
4. Describe the role of the nurse-advocate in relation to health and economic issues of concern to the older adult.
5. Be able to discuss self-responsibility as conceptualized in the United States.
6. Identify some of the changes in health care delivery instituted through the Affordable Care Act.

ECONOMICS IN LATE LIFE

Social Security

Considered by many to be one of the most successful federal programs in the United States, Social Security was established in 1935 in the depths of the Great Depression (Chapter 1). The primary function was to provide monetary benefits to older retired workers as a means to prevent or minimize their dependency, and therefore financial burden, on younger members of society (National Archives, 2010). It was based on the societal belief that older adults were uniformly poor in relation to younger adults.

Social Security and a number of programs that followed were established as "age-entitlement" programs. This meant that eligible individuals (beneficiaries) could receive monthly monetary benefits simply because of their age and regardless of their actual financial need (Box 30-1). However, the benefits were and are limited to those who have paid taxes on a requisite amount of income (Box 30-2). Nine out of 10 eligible persons in the United States today receive Social Security benefits. In 2014 more than 59 million Americans received almost $863 billion in benefits, including retired workers, dependents (such as minor children of beneficiaries, spouses), persons with disabilities, dependents, and widows or widowers. Social Security is a major source of income for many who are 65 and older, especially those who are unmarried (Figure 30-1). For 22% of those who are married and 47% of those who are unmarried, Social Security makes up 90% of their income. In 2014 the

BOX 30-1   Criteria for Eligibility for Social Security

American citizens or legal residents, at a predetermined age, who are totally and permanently disabled (including blind) or who are married to or an eligible partner of or dependent of someone receiving Social Security are eligible to receive Social Security benefits.

From Social Security Administration: Retirement planner: when to start your benefits, n.d. Available at http://www.socialsecurity.gov/ retire2/applying1.htm Accessed February 2015.

BOX 30-2   Amount of Annual Wages Needed to Receive Social Security Income

In order to receive even the minimal monthly income from Social Security, a person must have worked enough to have earned an adequate number of "credits." In 2014, one credit was equal to an income of $1200 in any one year with a maximum of four credits possible. In order to receive Social Security retirement income, those born after 1929 have to obtain a minimum of 40 credits in a lifetime. Only income from which Social Security taxes are withheld can be used toward a credit (www.ssa.gov). For the current cohort of older adults, this calculation has been most beneficial to white men, who are more likely to have worked the most consistently and at higher salaries than all other groups of workers. It is least beneficial to those who were low wage-earners, who never worked out of the home (e.g., housewives and homemakers), or who took time out of the job market for caregiving and child-rearing activities.

average monthly income from Social Security was $1294 with a maximum of $2642 for those who had reached the "age of full retirement." The benefit is based on a calculation of income during the earning of "credits" (see Box 30-2). The monthly payment increases every year one *delays* receiving the benefit until the age of 70. Depending on the state of the economy of the country, a cost-of-living increase occurs the first of each year.

The program has been managed on what is called a pay-as-you-go system. Payroll taxes on a percentage of one's income are collected from current employees and employers. Social Security funds, although individually deposited, are not reserved for any one individual. No one has an account set aside in his or her name. All funds that are not immediately paid out to beneficiaries are "borrowed" by the federal government for regular operating expenses. While the majority of Social Security taxes collected are reimbursed immediately to current beneficiaries, the government converts the borrowed funds into government bonds and places these in a "trust fund" overseen by the trustees of the fund. Details of the changing status of this fund are provided to the public annually and may be accessed at http://www.ssa.gov/oact/progdata/ funds.html

As long as the amount of contributions from workers exceeds that paid to beneficiaries, the program, as designed, can remain solvent. However, the combination of the increasing number of beneficiaries, the decreasing number of workers (in proportion to the beneficiaries), and the intangible nature of the "trust fund" has resulted in concern that the program will cease to exist in the near future, which is a potentially serious threat to millions who depend entirely on Social Security as the sole source of income. The extent of this threat continues to be hotly debated. While the depth of the concern varies from year to year, a solution has not been found. In an attempt to delay the problem, legislation was passed in 1983 gradually increasing the age when one could

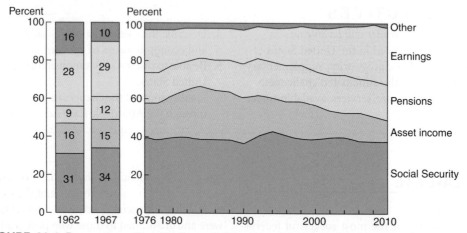

FIGURE 30-1 Percentage Distribution of Sources of Income for Married Couples and Nonmarried Persons Age 65 and Older, 1962–2010. A married couple is age 65 and older if the husband is age 65 and older or if the husband is younger than age 55 and the wife is age 65 and older. The definition of "other" includes, but is not limited to, unemployment compensation, workers' compensation, alimony, child support, and personal contributors. These data refer to the civilian noninstitutionalized population. (From Federal Interagency Forum on Aging-Related Statistics: *Older Americans 2012: key indicators of well-being*, 2012, Washington, DC, 2012, U.S. Government Printing Office. http://www.agingstats.gov/aging-statsdotnet/Main_Site/Data/2012_Documents/Docs/EntireChartbook.pdf Accessed November 12, 2014. With data from Current Population Survey, Annual Social and Economic Supplement, 1977–2011.)

reach "full retirement," and therefore eligible to receive Social Security (Table 30-1).

Supplemental Security Income

Not all older persons living in the United States have income from any source that is adequate to provide even the most basic necessities of life. This is especially true for persons who have spent their lives employed in the agriculture industry, in the food industry, or as domestic workers and have been paid very low wages or on a cash basis. Supplemental Security Income (SSI) was established in 1965 to provide a minimal level of economic support to persons age 65 and older such as Aida (above), those who are blind, or disabled regardless of their earning power in early life or when capable of working. SSI either provides "total support" or supplements a low Social Security benefit (Box 30-3).

Other Late Life Income

Finally, late life income may come from private retirement investments or employer pensions. These monies are held for the beneficiary until such a time when they must begin to "withdraw" some portion of this, at the age determined by the fund. Some private retirement plans offer several choices for receipt of funds. The retiree could elect to take his or her pension in one lump sum or a monthly amount based on his or her own

TABLE 30-1 Full Retirement Age

YEAR OF BIRTH*	FULL (NORMAL) RETIREMENT AGE
1937 or earlier	65
1938	65 and 2 months
1939	65 and 4 months
1940	65 and 6 months
1941	65 and 8 months
1942	65 and 10 months
1943-1954	66
1955	66 and 2 months
1956	66 and 4 months
1957	66 and 6 months
1958	66 and 8 months
1959	66 and 10 months
1960 and later	67

*If you were born on January 1st, you should refer to the previous year. Data from Social Security Administration: *Retirement planner: benefits by year of birth.* http://www.socialsecurity.gov/retire2/agereduction.htm Accessed November 12, 2014.

BOX 30-3 A Monthly Stipend for the Lowest-Income Elders: The SSI Program

In 2015, the Supplementary Security Income program provided for a maximum benefit of $733.00 a month for an eligible individual ($1100 per couple) to provide for basic needs. The determination of the total income the person has already includes the value of "gifts" such as housing. The majority of the recipients are those older than age 65.

From Social Security: SSI federal payment amounts. Available at http://www.ssa.gov/oact/cola/SSIamts.html Accessed February 2015.

BOX 30-4 A Surprising Change of Income

Mrs. Jones lived in a small rural community. Her husband had worked for the same company from the time he was 18 until he died. He had a limited but adequate pension to meet their day-to-day needs, but nothing extra. His Social Security benefit was small due to his lifelong low wages. When Mr. Jones died suddenly, Mrs. Jones was informed that she would no longer receive support from his pension. He had opted for the "no survivor benefit" when he enrolled, meaning that all benefits would cease upon his death.* Because she had never worked outside of the home, Mrs. Jones was dependent solely on her husband's survivor Social Security benefit. She was in danger of losing her home because she could not afford her taxes.

*NOTE: This is no longer legal without the express permission of the potentially surviving spouse.

life expectancy only, or based on the life expectancy of the retiree and spouse or partner. In other words, a person may establish a plan so that he or she receives all or most of the benefit during his or her *expected* lifetime rather than providing for any survivor benefit. Notification of the potential survivor of such a choice is now required, but was not always so in the past. This may still affect some older survivors today (Box 30-4).

ECONOMICS AND HEALTH CARE

Before the industrial revolution of the late 1800s, people in most countries and cultures worked until they were no longer physically able to do so. In many cases the type of work changed as they aged, but the expectation was that the person would continue to contribute to the family or the community until shortly before death. Family members and the community provided care to those who were no longer able to care for themselves (Bohm, 2001). While this is still the case in some countries, as countries industrialized, care of members of the family with diminished capacity became problematic in both social and economic terms. As younger members of the family joined the urban workforce, many elders stayed behind in agricultural areas of the country with less social and caregiving support.

In the early 1900s, almshouses and poor houses emerged to provide care for the frail and ill indigent who did not have family available or able to care for them. Most of these facilities were initially supported by charitable groups, especially religious organizations. Governments eventually became involved when the primary population was the elderly and disabled; they became essentially public nursing institutions. In some places, public monies replaced or supplemented charitable offerings. Local governments were authorized to purchase land and erect facilities through taxes to others. The care of indigent elderly was considered a public responsibility; however, because of the long-held social belief in personal responsibility, those residing in such care facilities were required to contribute any property they owned to help cover the expenses related to their care.

Economic factors are always driving forces in the delivery of health care, regardless of who pays for it and where it is provided. While higher-income countries are struggling to keep up with the escalating costs of technology, persons in low-income countries may not receive even the most rudimentary care. In countries with universal health care, it is supported to a large extent by payroll taxes, which can be significant. The insurance risk is shared among all residents of the country. That is, some level of health care is available to all persons either living in or working in the country. The expectation is that all people can use services while being protected from associated financial hardship. However, at this time there is a very wide variation in who is actually eligible for the "universal health care" within any one country (World Health Organization [WHO], 2014).

With few exceptions health care has always been a purchased service in the United States. It is not considered a universal right. However, the federal government is the major purchaser of health care through its insurance plans (Medicare, Railroad Medicare, Medicaid, and TRICARE) or provided directly through Veterans Services. The major insurance plan available to and used by eligible older adults (≥65 years of age) living in the United States is Medicare (Figure 30-2). For those with very low incomes, they may also be eligible for Medicaid, an insurance plan that is jointly funded by state and federal resources. Although the cost is still beyond the reach of some, many others have been able to purchase insurance in an exchange system within the U.S. health care "Market Place" through the Affordable Care legislation of 2010 (https://www.healthcare.gov/get-covered-a-1-page-guide-to-the-health-insurance-marketplace/).

Changes in Health Care for Older Adults

In 1934 President Franklin D. Roosevelt appointed the Committee on Economic Security (CES) to craft the Social Security system as noted earlier. The original proposal included a universal health insurance plan, but because of much opposition to it, Roosevelt removed it to avoid losing Social Security (Corning, 1969). The American Medical Association opposed any national program of health insurance, believing it to be "socialized medicine," and successfully prevented its implementation (Goodman, 1980). *Fortune* magazine polled the American public in 1942 and found that 76% of those questioned opposed government-financed medical care (Cantril, 1951).

In the early 1960s President Lyndon Johnson recognized that the numbers of older persons, those with serious disabilities, and poor children were increasing significantly and that these vulnerable groups were most often without access to needed health services of any kind. Although opposition continued, Johnson proposed amendments to the Social Security program to address this widespread public health problem. In Senate and House hearings, some legislators described the amendments as steps that would continue to destroy independence and self-reliance and would tax the poor and middle classes to subsidize the health care of the wealthy (Twight, 1997). Nonetheless, legislation was passed in 1965 and 1966 to expand the Social Security system by establishing Medicare (including Medicare for retired railroad workers) and Medicaid.

In a short time after implementation of these plans, millions more people could receive health care and the associated costs escalated rapidly. Prescription drug coverage in the form now known as Medicare Part D was not added until President George W. Bush's administration in 2006. The Affordable Care Act of the Obama administration (2010) contained a number of provisions with the potential to further impact health care services for older adults, especially in the area of coverage for

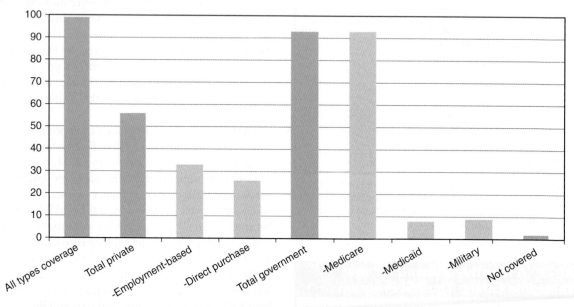

FIGURE 30-2 Percentage of Persons 65 Years of Age and Older by Type of Health Insurance Coverage, 2012. Total private: privately purchased health insurance such as secondary plans; direct purchase: out-of-pocket expenses, especially premiums and co-pays; approximately 99% of all of those at least 65 with approximately 2% having no insurance of any kind. NOTE: A person can be represented in more than one category. (From Administration on Aging: *Health insurance coverage.* http://www.aoa.acl.gov/Aging_Statistics/Profile/2013/15.aspx Accessed November 12, 2014.)

TABLE 30-2 Major Components of the Affordable Care Act that Affect Older Adults

COMPONENT	DESCRIPTION
Primary care	Incentives to providers based on quality and not just quality of care ("evaluation of quality based indicators")
Bundled payments	Payment to hospital for the entire "bundle of care," which will include both the hospital stay and the medical needs for a period of time after discharge
Demonstration projects	Welcoming of creative proposals to improve quality and control cost
Five-star programs	Yearly evaluation and ranking of Medicare Parts C and D
Decreasing out-of-pocket costs for prescription medications	Reduce current size of the donut hole and decrease the co-pay in the donut hole from 100% to 25%; donut hole set to be closed by 2020
No co-pays for those preventive services with most evidence of usefulness*	Increased access to preventive services

*See http://www.medicare.gov/coverage/preventive-visit-and-yearly-wellness-exams.html For "*Is my test covered?*
Adapted from Byman JPW: Financing and organization of health care. In Ham RJ, Sloane PD, Warshaw GA, et al, editors: *Primary care geriatrics: a case-based approach,* ed 6, Philadelphia, 2014, Elsevier, pp 92–101.

BOX 30-5 An Exception to the Late Enrollment Penalties

On April 3, 2014, the U.S. Department of Health and Human Services announced that the Social Security Administration was now able to process requests for Medicare Parts A and B and that the late enrollment penalties, under certain circumstances, would be waived for same-sex partners. This was based on the June 26, 2013, Supreme Court ruling that Medicare is not prevented from recognizing same-sex marriages for the determination of, and entitlement to, benefits.

From U.S. Department of Health and Human Services: *HHS announces important Medicare information for people in same-sex marriages* (Press release), April 3, 2014. http://www.hhs.gov/news/press/2014pres/04/20140403a.html Accessed November 12, 2014.

BOX 30-6 The "Welcome to Medicare" Exam

Must be obtained within 12 months of enrolling in Medicare Part B and must include the following:
Review of medical record
Review of social history related to your health
Education and counseling about preventive services
Health screenings, immunizations, or referrals for other care as needed
Height, weight, and blood pressure measurements
Calculation of body mass index
Simple vision test
Review of risk for depression and level of safety
An offer to discuss advance directives
Written preventive health plan

preventive services (Table 30-2). These provisions are expected to be enacted over a period of years; however, significant changes are possible as opposition continues.

Medicare

Medicare is the insurance plan specifically designed to provide almost universal health care for those who are eligible for Social Security (e.g., older adults, the disabled). It is administered by the Centers for Medicare and Medicaid Services (CMS) and is a part of the Department of Health and Human Services, a special entity created to administer the programs. Medicare is made up of three components: the age-entitlement Medicare A, the purchased Medicare B or the alternative Advantage Plans (Medicare C), and the Prescription Drug Plan (Medicare D).

As soon as a person is 65 (or meets special disability requirements), he or she is automatically enrolled in Medicare A and receives a "red, white, and blue" card indicating coverage. The choices associated with Medicare Parts B, C, and D are selected based on personal preference and availability. Selection and enrollment must take place during a 6-month period beginning 3 months before and ending 3 months after a person's 65th birthday to avoid late enrollment penalties and higher premiums (Medicare, n.d.) (Box 30-5). In 2010 more than 47 million persons received Medicare benefits, almost all of them age 65 or older (U.S. Census Bureau, 2012).

Beginning in 2011, most deductibles and other cost-sharing of many preventive care services (e.g., mammograms) have been removed. Before 2011 there was a free and one-time "Welcome to Medicare" visit (Box 30-6). At this time "wellness

visits" are available at no cost every 12 months after the initial exam (Box 30-7). These are both specifically designed to promote healthy aging. through prevention and early detection (primary and secondary prevention)

Like Social Security, Medicare Part A was designed as a pay-as-you-go system; that is, taxes collected from employers and employees are used for the payment of specific health-related expenses. The funds are not earmarked for any particular taxpayers' future medical expenses. While the federal government

BOX 30-7 Yearly "Wellness" Visit*

Completions of a "Health Risk Assessment"
- A review of your medical and family history, including medications, herbs, and dietary supplements taken
- Developing or updating a list of current providers
- Height, weight, blood pressure, and other routine measurements
- Screening for any cognitive impairment or indications of depression
- Screening for potential functional impairments or safety risks
- Personalized health advice related to assessment, including health risks identified and treatment options
- A screening schedule (like a checklist) for appropriate preventive services

*First one at least 12 months since "Welcome" visit. Cannot include a physical exam of any kind.
See http://www.medicare.gov/coverage/your-medicare-coverage.html to determine coverage, co-pay, and eligibility for screenings.

pays the majority of the health-related costs covered by Medicare Parts B, C, and D, the beneficiaries contribute in the form of premiums and co-pays.

Medicare Part A

Medicare Part A is a hospital insurance plan covering acute care, short-term rehabilitation in a skilled nursing facility or at home and most of the costs associated with hospice care (Box 30-8). Those who have not paid an adequate amount into the U.S. Social Security system (Social Security taxes) may be eligible to purchase Part A coverage for a monthly fee.

Medicare Part B

After January 1, 2007, the premium for Medicare B was based in part on income as reported to the Internal Revenue Service. Medicare B (referred to as *Original Medicare*) provides insurance coverage for many of the services provided on an outpatient basis, such as visits to providers' offices (Box 30-9). An advantage of this Original Part B is choice of the primary care provider and referrals are not usually necessary. Providers who "accept assignment" have agreed to charge only an "allowable fee" that Medicare determines annually. The provider receives 80% of this amount

---

> ### BOX 30-8 Health Services Provided Through Medicare Part A
>
> Designed to partially cover the costs of acute hospitalization semiprivate rooms and any necessary medical services and supplies; care as listed below:
> - a. There is a deductible for days 1 to 60 (each stay) ($1216 in 2014)
> - b. Days 60 to 120 co-pay amounts increase over time
> - d. There is no coverage after 150 days
> - d. Deductibles and co-pays increase every year
> - e. The deductibles and co-pays are either paid out-of-pocket or reimbursed by Medicaid or Medigap policies
>
> Skilled rehabilitative nursing care in a health care facility (only when care by a licensed nurse or physical or occupational therapist is needed):
> - a. Only after a minimum of 72-hour acute care hospital admission *(not observation)*
> - b. The first 20 days are covered at 100%
> - c. Days 21 to 100 with a daily co-pay of more than $100
> - d. No coverage after 100 days
> - e. Coverage ceases the day skilled care is no longer needed
>
> Home health services requiring skilled care (only when care by a licensed nurse or physical or occupational therapist is needed):
> - a. Intermittent skilled care for the purpose of rehabilitation provided in the home
> - b. The person must be ill enough to be considered homebound
> - c. Medicare may pay 80% of the approved amount for durable medical equipment and supplies (e.g., hospital bed)
>
> Hospice care is provided for terminally ill persons expected to live less than 6 months who elect to forgo traditional medical treatment for the terminal illness:
> - a. Co-pay of $5 for Medicare
> - b. Co-pay of 5% for limited respite or pain management stays
> - c. Replaces Medicare Parts A and B for all costs associated with the terminal condition
>
> Inpatient psychiatric care:
> - a. Limited to 190 days in a lifetime
> - b. Partial payment
> - c. Other significant restrictions apply

> ### BOX 30-9 Health Services Provided Through Medicare Part B
>
> Designed to cover some of the costs associated with outpatient or ambulatory services. Deductibles and co-pays are required in most cases:
> 1. Physician, nurse practitioner, or physician assistant medically necessary services
> 2. Limited prescribed supplies
> 3. Medically necessary diagnostic tests
> 4. Physical, occupational, and speech therapy for the purpose of rehabilitation
> 5. Limited durable medical equipment if prescribed by a *physician* and for documented medical necessity
> 6. Outpatient hospital treatment, blood, and ambulatory surgical services
> 7. Some preventive services (many with no co-pay or deductible)
> 8. Diabetic supplies (excluding insulin and other medications) (see Chapter 25)

from Medicare and the patient is responsible for the remaining 20% and any deductible. If the service is provided independently by a nurse practitioner, the reimbursement rate is 85% of the 80%. If a person has a privately funded "secondary" insurance this usually covers the unpaid portion (e.g., the 20%) (see Medigap below) and may include the initial deductible.

A provider who does not accept assignment may charge the patient up to 15% more than the allowable charge. A combination of an increasing number of wealthy elders and fewer primary care providers has spawned a new industry of "boutique" services, including physician practices. For an additional "membership," "convenience," or "surcharge," patients are eligible for a wide range of special services from immediate access to an emergency room to unlimited access to the provider (e.g., via private cell phone).

Medicare Part C

Otherwise referred to as Medicare Advantage Plans (MAPs), Medicare Part C uses a prospective payment system and includes traditional health maintenance organizations (HMOs) and other managed care plans. All traditional services covered by Medicare Part A and Part B must be provided, and additional services, co-pays, and deductibles are predetermined. Medicare Advantage Plans may or may not provide prescription drug benefits; if so, they are referred to as MAP-PDs. Not all MAPs are offered at all locations in the United States. MAP premiums vary in price depending on location and range of services provided; in many cases, there is no premium charged to the member.

MAPs may provide a cost savings to the member, as well as extra benefits in comparison to the Original Medicare Plan. However, special rules must be followed, including the requirement that no care is obtained without a referral from the assigned primary care provider. This person serves as a "gate-keeper" in an effort to ensure that only the highest quality medically necessary care is received. Should a member obtain services without a referral, there is no coverage and all costs are "out-of-pocket."

Medicare C plans are now rated once a year in a 5-star program, on a scale of 0 to 5 with the results available to the public. This information can be used if one wants to change from one program to another at designated times of the year. This is an attempt to hold the Medicare C (Advantage) Plans more accountable for the quality of care they provide (CMS, 2014). The

Affordable Care Act instituted a number of additional options available, especially under Medicare C.

Alternatives to Medicare C. Several new programs have emerged as health care finance is changing in the United States. One of these is the *Private Fee-for-Service Medical Savings Account*. In this plan, the federal government makes monthly payments directly into the person's own private saving account and when health services are obtained the individual pays for them directly. This program comes with high deductibles and the fees charged by the providers are predetermined on a contractual basis between the provider and Medicare. Although no contracted provider can deny services at the agreed rate, noncontracted providers are under no obligation to accept the rate. For information about the range of existing and pending plans see http://www.cms.gov/Medicare/Medicare.html.

Medicare Part D

The Medicare Modernization Act of 2003 established a prescription drug benefit for eligible recipients of Medicare, known as Medicare Part D (Box 30-10). It is an *elective* prescription drug plan (PDP) with associated out-of-pocket premiums and co-payments. All persons with Medicare, except those in MAP-PD programs, are eligible to voluntarily purchase a PDP. However, if one chooses to enroll in a Medicare D program, the same rules and timing related to enrollment and incurring of penalties seen in Medicare B apply. People can change their plans during the "open enrollment" periods each year without penalty or when they have a change of circumstances, such as entering a long-term care facility. Help with the associated costs is available for persons with low incomes. For persons with both Medicare and Medicaid the plan is mandatory, and in most cases the person is arbitrarily assigned to a particular PDP.

As with Medicare C Advantage Plans, the 5-star rating plan is used. Each year the commercial companies that provide Medicare D plans are evaluated and the results are posted on the CMS website (CMS, 2014). Established by the Affordable Care Act, this is an attempt to hold the these commercial plans more accountable for the quality of product they provide, including pricing and patient safety (CMS, 2014).

Nurses, nurse practitioners, physicians, pharmacists, and community volunteers spend hours helping beneficiaries select the insurance plans that best meet their needs and enroll at appropriate times. This sometimes onerous task can be instrumental in promoting healthy aging (Box 30-11).

Supplemental Insurance/Medigap Policies

Because of potentially high deductibles and co-payments, people who have the financial resources often purchase supplemental insurance plans, referred to as Medigap. Some are part of a person's retirement benefit or available to members of organizations such as the American Association of Retired Persons (AARP). While Medicare remains the "primary" insurance, and therefore billed first, the Medigap plans serve as a "secondary insurance"; that is, a monthly premium is paid and, in exchange, many or all of the co-pays and deductibles not covered by the "primary insurance" (i.e., Medicare) are paid. Persons searching for an appropriate plan can be referred to the Medicare website for their state or can request a printed copy of the standard plans (available at www.cms.gov).

Medicaid

Medicaid was established in 1965 as part of the revisions to the Social Security Act at the same time as Medicare. It is a health insurance program jointly funded by federal and state governments using tax dollars. CMS (Centers for Medicare and Medicaid Services) administers the program at the federal level, and a state agency administers it at each state level.

Medicaid covers the costs of health services for low-income children, pregnant women, those who are permanently disabled, and persons age 65 and older who meet the state's eligibility criteria. Eligibility is determined by the state and is based on income and assets, categorical need, and lack of ability to afford any insurance premiums, including those associated with Medicare. The number of persons who can receive Medicaid regardless of their situation is limited in any one state based on fiscal and political decisions.

BOX 30-10   Medicare Prescription Drug Plans (PDPs)

Most PDPs are set up in a similar way with deductibles and co-pays; however, to be a provider in Medicare Part D, the insurance plan must meet the following specific guidelines (2014 figures):

1. Premiums based on the plan (usually dependent on the range of medications covered) plus a payment based on your income (reported to the IRS: e.g., family income $17,000 or less, pay nothing above premium; family income more than $428,000, pay $69.30 above your premium)
2. Annual deductible as low as zero but no greater than $310
3. Co-pay of medications dependent on plan until the "donut hole" is reached ($2850 includes deductible)*
4. Donut hole: Out-of-pocket cost is 47.5% of the 50% required manufacturer discount (down from 100% when it was established with no manufacturer discount)
5. After having spent $4550 in any one year, you receive what is called "catastrophic coverage." This is either 5% for covered drugs or $2.55 for generic covered drugs or $6.35 for covered brand-name drugs

*Note: Under the current plan, the size of the donut hole gets smaller every year. It is scheduled to close in 2020.

Data from Medicare Interactive: Part D: Cost overview. Available at www.medicareinteractive.org a service of the Medicare Rights Center. Accessed September 2014.

BOX 30-11   TIPS FOR BEST PRACTICE

Helping Your Patients Enroll in Medicare Plans that Best Suit Their Needs

When it is time for the person to enroll in Medicare, he or she can be referred to the Medicare website (www.cms.gov). At this website, the person will find not only information about plans available in their areas but also information about the procedures for changing from one plan to another according to personal choice or change in needs. If the person has limited literacy or health literacy, he or she should be referred to their nearest Area Agency on Aging for guidance (for locations, see www.n4a.org).

For elders with low incomes, Medicaid covers all Medicare premiums, co-pays, and deductibles and may provide additional health benefits. Persons who are dually eligible for both Medicare and Medicaid are frequently required to be enrolled in MAP-PD plans. Federal law requires states to provide a certain minimal level of service, and states may add other coverage such as vision care, dentures, prostheses, case management, and other medical or rehabilitative care provided by a licensed health care practitioner. Medicaid pays for the majority of the care provided in nursing homes.

Consistent with the early expectations in the almshouses, if institutional long-term care is needed, the person is expected to be fiscally responsible for his or her own care to the extent possible before depending on the tax support of the community. That is, the person is required to use his or her own assets first to pay for care. When assets are no longer (or ever) available, then Medicaid (funded through taxes) provides a "safety net" to ensure that the poorest disabled and frail adults receive care.

For a person who requires the financial support of Medicaid for a nursing home stay and has a spouse who is able to remain in the community, Congress enacted provisions in 1988 to protect him or her from "spousal impoverishment." Burial funds and only one-half of the combined value of the household goods, including the automobile (up to a limit), are counted as belonging to the patient, are used to determine eligibility, and are not expected to be used to pay for care. On the death of both spouses, it is expected that the amount that Medicaid has spent on the care (and only up to that point) be reimbursed with any remaining funds in the couple's estate.

In the past some people who believed they would soon need nursing home care have transferred funds (sometimes large amounts) to others in order to be eligible for Medicaid to avoid using their own funds to pay for their care. While some transfers are permitted, such as to a spouse or a disabled, dependent child, any other transfer (i.e., to another person or to a trust) is considered Medicaid fraud. When a person applies for Medicaid, a "look-back period" is done to determine if funds have been transferred that would normally be available to the applicant. If transfers were made, Medicaid support will not begin until the costs incurred equal the amount of the transfer. For example, an income-eligible person (monthly income less than the state's determination of institutional Medicaid) who transfers $100,000 and is in a nursing home where the monthly rate is $10,000 would not be eligible for Medicaid for 10 months. This is known as "spend-down." These regulations attempt to ensure that individuals pay what they can for the care they need but still provide a safety net when funds are exhausted.

The majority of the Medicaid funds are used to provide extended long-term nursing home care for older and disabled adults. The federal government has attempted to slow the flow of Medicaid monies to pay for nursing home and other care for the non-poor by a series of laws enacted to require people to pay as much as they can from their own funds. Examples include the following:

- The 1993 Omnibus Budget Reconciliation Act (OBRA) permitted states to recover the costs of nursing home care from a deceased person's estate as noted above.

- The 1996 Health Insurance Portability and Accountability Act (HIPAA) reduced the allowable methods of hiding or transferring monies before needing or entering long-term care.
- The 1997 Balanced Budget Act targeted lawyers and other estate planners, holding them responsible for attempting to circumvent laws that required persons to pay for their own long-term care.

Persons who are near-poor and without assets and with monthly incomes greater than the "low income" limit set by the state are not eligible for assistance with health care expenses under Medicaid. In the absence of the availability of informal caregivers, providing for those who need assistance continues to be a major social and public health problem in the United States (Chapter 32).

Other Means to Finance Health Care

In some parts of the country (and for some persons), alternative plans have been developed to both finance and provide for health needs while aging.

Indian Health Services

The Indian Health Service (IHS) is a federal health program for and with American Indians and Alaskan Natives (http://www.ihs.gov). Services are provided both at the Tribal level and through Urban Indian Health Programs. The provision of health services is complex among this population. Persons who are American Indians and military veterans are eligible for care through Veterans' Services but not through the IHS. If a retired workers they are most likely eligible for Medicare and if low income, they may qualify for Medicaid as well. Traditional IHS care is available to documented members of one of the Indian Nations but is limited to those who have no other source of care. There are a number of programs in development and implementation is intended to promote health among American Indians at all ages, ranging from those who are aging healthfully to those caring for aging and debilitated elders (http://www.ihs.gov/ElderCare).

Program of All-Inclusive Care for the Elderly

The Program of All-inclusive Care for the Elderly (PACE) is a program for Medicaid-eligible seniors providing comprehensive care in community settings. Services vary by site. There is no cost to the participants. For a detailed description, see Chapter 32.

Care for Veterans

The Veterans Health Administration (VHA) system has long held a leadership position in gerontological care. A great deal of the research that guided gerontologists in earlier years was generated through the VA system as were innovations in care. In addition, the majority of geriatric fellowships to train geriatricians have been provided through VA hospitals. The system has been a forerunner of the various continua of care providers now in place. Since early on, this system provided VA-administered nursing homes, home care and community-based programs, respite care, blindness rehabilitation, mental health, and numerous other services in addition to acute hospitals.

In the past, veterans' hospitals and services were available on an as-needed basis for anyone who had served in the uniformed services at any time and for any length of time. It was not necessary for individuals to use their Medicare benefits. However, this system has undergone significant change as the number of veterans has increased. One of the first changes noted included restrictions placed on the use of veterans' hospitals and services. Instead of coverage of any health problem, priorities were set for those health problems that are deemed "service connected" in some way; in other words, the health care problem began when the person was on active duty.

Older and disabled veterans are now expected to obtain and use Medicare for their non–service-connected health problems, with the responsibilities for co-pays and deductibles the same as those for other beneficiaries. An outcry among veterans and veteran groups resulted in the development of a free Medigap policy known as TRICARE for Life (TFL).

TRICARE for Life. TRICARE is provided by the Department of Defense for Medicare-eligible beneficiaries ages 65 and older and their dependents or widows or widowers older than age 65. This plan requires that the person enroll in both Medicare Part A and Part B and pay the premiums for Part B. As a Medigap policy, TFL covers those expenses not covered by Medicare, such as co-pays and costs for prescription medicines. Dependent parents or parents-in-law may be eligible for pharmacy benefits if they turned age 65 on or after April 1, 2001, and are also enrolled in Medicare Part B. For more information about this, see http://www.military.com/benefits/tricare.

Long-Term Care Insurance

Some are electing to purchase additional insurance for their potential future long-term care needs. Ideally, these policies would cover the expenses related to co-pays for long-term care and coverage for what is called custodial care, that is, help with day-to-day needs (as opposed to skilled care). Traditionally, these policies were limited to care in long-term care facilities and provided a flat-rate reimbursement to residents for their costs. However, these policies are becoming more creative and innovative and may, under some circumstances, cover home care costs instead of or in addition to care in long-term care facilities. Many plans are being marketed. To offer assistance to elders, nurses can refer the person to the websites provided by the Administration on Aging (http://longtermcare.gov/) or the American Association for Long-Term Care Insurance (www. aaltci.org).

The purchaser of a long-term care policy is cautioned to read the policy carefully and understand all the details, limitations, and exclusions, such as if the plan covers the amount and type of service that the person would desire if it was needed. They may have a benefit period or a lifetime value. The benefit period may be in days or in dollars spent. Particular concerns are related to dementia because many of the early policies excluded these individuals from home benefits and included very limited institutional benefits. It is advisable to suggest that the persons speak to an independent financial advisor and refer to consumer reports of the particular insurance company and its reliability before applying for a policy.

KEY CONCEPTS

- The Social Security system in the United States provided a guaranteed income for persons who have paid a requisite amount into the system earlier in their lives.
- Both the Social Security and the Medicare insurance programs are based on a "pay-as-you-go" arrangement with funds from current workers used to support current retirees.
- Social Security provides an income to the majority of those retired persons in the United States.

- Medicare is a near-universal health insurance plan for persons who are age 65, blind, permanently disabled, or with end-stage renal disease.
- Medicare is composed of Parts A, B, C, and D. There is no premium for Medicare Part A, hospitalization. There are considerable differences between Parts B and C, which must be selected at the age of eligibility.
- Medicaid provides coverage for the out-of-pocket medical expenses for poor Medicare beneficiaries.

CRITICAL THINKING QUESTIONS AND ACTIVITIES

1. What do elders find most helpful about Medicare? What do they find least helpful?
2. How would elders like to see Medicare changed?
3. What are elders' thoughts and attitudes about managed care?

4. What are the prevalent attitudes of the elderly persons with whom you are acquainted regarding their economic future?
5. Do the older adults you know understand how the changes in the Affordable Care Act affect them?

RESEARCH QUESTIONS

1. Whom do elders most frequently contact when they need legal and economic advice?
2. How many elders feel secure about their economic future?
3. What are the current average out-of-pocket costs for elder health care?

4. How do elders feel about the rationing of health care based on age or survivability?

REFERENCES

Bohm D: Striving for quality in America's nursing homes, *DePaul J Health Care Law* 4:317–366, 2001.

Cantril H: *Public opinion 1935-1946*, Princeton, NJ, 1951, Princeton University Press.

Centers for Medicare and Medicaid Services (CMS): *5-Star plan ratings*, 2014. http://www.cms.gov/Outreach-and-Education/Training/CMSNationalTrainingProgram/Downloads/2013-5-Star-Enrollment-Period-Job-Aid.pdf. Accessed November 25, 2014.

Corning P: *The evolution of Medicare: from idea to law* (Research report no. 29), Washington, DC, 1969, U.S. Department of Health, Education and Welfare, Social Security Administration, Office of Research and Statistics, U.S. Government Printing Office.

Goodman JC: *The regulation of medical care: is the price too high?* (Cato public policy research monograph no. 3), San Francisco, 1980, Cato Institute.

Medicare: *Part B Late enrollment penalty*, n.d. http://www.medicare.gov/your-medicare-costs/part-b-costs/penalty/part-b-late-enrollment-penalty.html. Accessed February 2015.

National Archives: *Social Security marks 75th anniversary August 14*, 2010 Press release. http://www.archives.gov/press/press-releases/2010/nr10-128.html. Accessed 2015.

Twight C: Medicare's origin: the economics and politics of dependency, *Cato J* 16(3):209–338, 1997.

U.S. Census Bureau: *Health & nutrition: Medicare, Medicaid*, 2012. http://www.census.gov/compendia/statab/cats/health_nutrition/medicare_medicaid.html. Accessed September 2014.

World Health Organization (WHO): *What is universal health coverage?* 2014. http://www.who.int/universal_health_coverage/en. Accessed November 25, 2014.

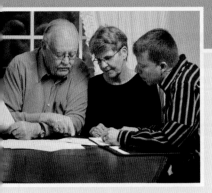

Common Legal and Ethical Issues

Kathleen Jett

AN ELDER SPEAKS

I have had a feeding tube in my stomach for a long time due to cancer. I had been in the hospital recently and even though I disagreed, the social worker was concerned that I could not take care of myself at home. They sent a nurse out to check on me and sure enough, just as she drove up I was pouring my daily beer into my tube. I was so glad she didn't say anything about that, just asked how I was doing!

Henry, age 68

A STUDENT SPEAKS

When I was asked to go on a home visit to Mr. Jones it was obvious that he did not take care of himself. His clothes were dirty and he smelled like urine. But he had no significant health problems and seemed undisturbed by the situation. I really didn't know what to think or do.

Steffen, age 19

LEARNING OBJECTIVES

On completion of this chapter, the reader will be able to:

1. Describe the nurse's responsibility to respect decision-making for those with limited capacity.
2. Differentiate the mechanisms for the protection of those who have limited decision-making capacity and discuss the advantages and disadvantages of each, from least restrictive to most restrictive.
3. Identify the nurse's responsibility for the protection of those with limited capacity.
4. Differentiate between abuse and neglect.
5. Understand the meaning of undue influence and describe how it might be identified.
6. Describe cultural differences in the perception and response to abuse.
7. Identify the ethical conflicts between beneficence and autonomy in self-neglect.
8. Define the nurse's role in the prevention of elder mistreatment.

In the day-to-day practice of caring for older adults, gerontological nurses face questions that are ethical in nature with legal components. In the first section of this chapter, decision-making from a process perspective is considered, specifically when the individual is suspected to have limited decision-making capacity. In the second section, the ethical and legal ramifications of "elder" mistreatment are examined relative to the nurse's role. Although gerontological nurses (unless also attorneys) cannot provide any legal advice, it is imperative that they are able to discuss several key ethical and legal issues frequently encountered in their work.

DECISION-MAKING

Consent is a concept that arises from the ethical principle of *self-determination* or *autonomy*. In the health care setting,

self-determination is documented or expressed through what we refer to as *informed consent*. In most circumstances the consent is implied, such as when the person accepts a medication that is offered or cooperates with a dressing change.

More complex consent is needed under certain circumstances (Box 31-1). In the exception of an emergency, the person must be free from the effect of sedating medications before formal informed consent can be obtained (Zorowitz, 2014). In older adults, it is also important that the nurse ensures that any special needs are addressed (e.g., functional hearing aids, reading glasses) (Box 31-2). Most courts have upheld the requirements of providing information in such a way that an average person could understand it before being asked to make a decision. Consent to participate in research is a more detailed and extensive process because treatments received in such circumstances may not necessarily provide benefit to the participant.

Research with the very frail and those with changing levels of capacity (for any reason) has been difficult and has limited the advancement of science in some areas due to the overriding need to protect the participant.

Informed consent in health care is only possible with the assumption that adults have decision-making *capacity.* Decisional capacity means that a person is able to understand a problem, the risks and benefits of a decision, the alternative options, and the consequences of the decision. Capacity is presumed when the legal age of "adult" is reached, unless adjudicated (decided by a court) to lack such capacity. However, even in the absence of such adjudication, it is sometimes necessary to make professional judgments that influence accepting consent from a particular person.

In Western medicine, an emphasis is placed on autonomous decision-making, and the provider has a responsibility to inform the individual of the decision needed and the individual has the right and responsibility to make his or her decisions whenever possible (Chapter 4). The decision is made within the context of the individual's health values and needs (Box 31-3). In many other belief systems and cultures, decisions, including those related to health care, are shared or delegated responsibilities (see Chapter 4).

In day-to-day gerontological practice with frail elders, it is important to differentiate between legally determined incapacity and day-to-day decision-making. While the person

may still be legally competent, does he or she have the capacity to understand at the level needed for the decision at hand? Deciding which foods to accept is very different from deciding to undergo a surgical procedure. He or she may have no or limited capacity for one type of decision but full capacity for another. A guiding principle is to provide protection to those with questionable capacity and ensure that the person's needs are met and personal rights are protected, all at the same time.

There are a range of modes of protection that can be provided, with the expectation that the least restrictive one is used whenever possible. These options include powers of attorney, conservatorship, and guardianship. It is important that nurses understand the differences and meaning of each.

Advance Care Planning

Gerontological nurses have the responsibility to encourage their patients, neighbors, and family members to discuss their wishes regarding potential incapacity and end-of-life care, otherwise referred to as advance care planning. It is always advisable to legally appoint a surrogate (see following sections) or otherwise formally document one's wishes. The use of living wills is addressed in Chapter 35.

Power of Attorney

A power of attorney (POA) is a person (agent) who has been legally appointed to act on behalf of another in ways that are specifically indicated in a legal document. This may include appointing the person to complete particular transactions or asking the person to assume full responsibility for the assets of another. In some jurisdictions there are two types—a general POA and a durable POA for health care. In both cases the appointment of the POA has been made in advance as a part of "advance care planning" in anticipation of future needs. The agent named as a general POA most often represents the person in matters of business but not those of health care. In many cases, the authority of the general POA is no longer in effect if the person is determined to be incapacitated.

The person appointed as a *durable power of attorney for health care,* referred to as a *health care surrogate,* is responsible for making medical decisions for persons when they are unable to do so for themselves. Whether the surrogate can make end-of-life decisions is determined by state statutes. As soon as the person regains abilities or choses to end the authority of the POA, it is no longer in force unless requested.

This is the least restrictive form of assistance, encompassing decision-making for persons with impaired capacity. All rights and responsibilities afforded by law are retained. An important aspect of this approach is that the person given decision-making rights is someone who has been chosen by the individual rather than appointed by a court.

Health Care Proxy

Most state statutes and cultures provide a "hierarchy" of those who have the authority to act on a person's behalf or when the person has lost (either temporarily or permanently) the capacity to make decisions and has not documented his or her preferences. For example, in the state of Florida this is written into Statute 765.401. All health care facilities have the legal responsibility to follow this "order of decision-maker" (Box 31-4). The decision-making responsibilities proceed down the list until a willing proxy is obtained.

Both surrogates and proxies are expected to use *"substituted judgment"* in making decisions, that is, on the basis of what they believe the person would make if able to do so and not necessarily the surrogate's choice in a similar situation (Zorowitz, 2014) (Box 31-5). As the gerontological nurse works with people who are making decisions about the selection of a surrogate,

---

BOX 31-4   Hierarchy of Appointments of Health Care Proxy by Florida State Statute, from First to Last

Guardian
Spouse
Majority of adult children
Parents
Majority of adult siblings reasonably available for consultation
Adult relative who has exhibited special care and has regular contact
Close friend
Licensed clinical social worker

BOX 31-5   "I Know that is What She Would Want but that is not What I Want"

Mr. and Mrs. Jones had been married for 60 years. She had developed Alzheimer's disease a number of years earlier and reached a point where she did not always know what to do with food in her mouth. She no longer recognized her husband and did not respond in any verbal way. In almost daily distress, her husband intermittently pleaded that a "feeding tube" be placed into her so she could "eat." However, Mrs. Jones had made it very clear to her husband and to all who knew her that she "never wanted artificial nutrition" or to do anything to stop a natural death when she worsened. When Mr. Jones asked for a feeding tube, the only thing we could say was that we were very sorry but her wishes had been made very clearly and that is what we were bound to follow. He would agree that those indeed were her wishes and start to cry.

BOX 31-6   Conservators and Guardians

Conservators
Appointed to manage the finances of the ward and continue in that role until the court appointment is rescinded. Each state is slightly different in how this is handled and defined.

Guardians
Appointed by the court to help the incapacitated person make informed decisions (or makes decisions for the person) about personal and health matters. The guardian is expected to ensure that the ward remains safe and receives adequate and appropriate food, shelter, and personal hygiene. The guardian provides appropriate consent for medical or other professional care as needed and, in some cases, is reflective of the previously expressed wishes of the person.

---

the nurse can encourage persons to carefully consider someone who is willing to uphold their wishes or holds similar values.

Guardians and Conservators

Guardians and conservators are individuals, agencies, or corporations that have been appointed to take care, custody, and control of an incapacitated person and ensure that his or her needs are met and handled responsibly (Box 31-6). Such appointments can only be made at court hearings in which someone demonstrates the elder is incapacitated in some way. In some states it is not required that the elder be present. If the judge agrees that this level of protection is needed, the person is declared incapacitated. Similar to surrogates and proxies, conservators and guardians are expected to use substituted judgment in all decision-making.

In some states limits are set in the appointment of guardianship according to the degree of protection needed. Total dependency means that the person lacks all decision-making capacity and cannot meet even basic needs in any self-sustaining way. Partial dependency means the person may be able to manage certain challenges of life but health or cognitive abilities interfere with more complex decision-making. In the latter situation, a guardian is appointed to protect the person in very specific ways.

There are considerable pros and cons in the use of conservatorships and guardianships, and a major disadvantage is risk for exploitation. The use of these mechanisms of care is the most restrictive, and in most cases the person loses all rights to self-determination and should only be considered in cases of severe impairment, such as for persons with advanced dementia. Nurses working with older adults and their families can encourage the use of advance planning as alternatives that are less restrictive, noting that the definitions and rules vary from state to state.

ELDER MISTREATMENT

Elder mistreatment is a complex phenomenon that includes "elder" abuse and neglect. It is the infliction of actual harm, or a risk for harm, to vulnerable older persons through the action or behavior of others (American Psychological Association

[APA], 2012). It is a universal problem and occurs in all educational, racial, cultural, religious, and socioeconomic groups, in any family configuration and in every setting. It is one of our most unrecognized and underreported social problems today. While there are no reliable statistics available related to the prevalence on a worldwide basis, the World Health Organization estimates that up to 4% to 6% of those older than age 60 have been or will be mistreated (World Health Organization [WHO], 2012). In the United States it is estimated that between 7% and 10% of those 60 and older are mistreated every year, not including financial exploitation (Acierno et al, 2010). However, it is also estimated that only 1 out of 14 cases are ever recognized (National Research Council, 2003). As the population of older adults grows (Chapter 1), so does the expectation that the prevalence of mistreatment will increase as well. The risk is further exacerbated as family caregivers have increasing responsibilities outside of the home (Chapter 34).

In order for mistreatment to occur, the perpetrator and a vulnerable elder must have a trusting relationship of some kind. This may be as simple as a salesperson (financial exploitation) or as complex as a long-time caregiver such as a spouse or a child. Most often "elder mistreatment" is discussed in the context of family caregiving. This may be a lifelong pattern that intensifies in the current situation (Box 31-7). The risk factors for one to become an abuser or be abused are often interconnected (Box 31-8).

Mistreatment at the hands of formal caregivers occurs as well. When a number of different providers are giving care, monitoring becomes especially difficult. Situations of increased potential for formal caregiver abuse include those in which there is inadequate supervision of patient care, poor coordination of services, inadequate staff training, theft and fraud, drug and alcohol abuse by staff, tardiness and absenteeism, unprofessional and criminal conduct, and inadequate record keeping. The nurse should pay particular attention to the person who is alone with a formal caregiver for extended periods of time, with no support from others and no opportunities for respite for the caregiver.

In a study conducted in the year 2000 of 2000 residents of long-term care facilities, 44% reported being abused themselves and 95% reported that they had observed others being abused or neglected (Broyles, 2000). A compilation of survey data in 2008 (see Chapter 31) found 70% of all nursing facilities were found to have at least one "deficiency" relating to the incidence of actual or potential mistreatment; 15% of these resulted in actual harm (U.S. Government Accounting Office, 2008).

BOX 31-7   A Lifelong History of Abuse

A young adult woman was the 24-hour caregiver to her dying grandfather. While he was weak, he could still move about his hospital bed and even get out of it alone from time to time. We noticed that he appeared to regularly make suggestive remarks to his granddaughter and reach toward her. She seemed frightened and always tried to back away. When we were finally able to talk to her alone she quietly said that she was afraid of him; he had sexually assaulted her all of her life. She was assigned by the family to be his caregiver because she was disabled and could not work outside of the home.

BOX 31-8   More Likely to Mistreat and be Mistreated

More Likely to Abuse or Neglect
- Family member
- One with emotional or mental illnesses
- One who is abusing alcohol or other substances
- History of family violence
- Cultural acceptance of interpersonal violence
- Caregiver frustration
- Social isolation
- Impaired impulse control of caregiver

More Likely To Be Abused or Neglected
- Cognitive impairment, especially with aggressive features
- Dependent on abuser
- Physically or mentally frail
- Having abused the caregiver earlier in life
- Women either living alone or in a household with family members
- Having been abused in the past
- Behavior that is considered aggressive, demanding, or unappreciative
- Living in an institutional setting
- Feeling deserving of abuse due to own inadequacies

Adapted from Sehgal SR, Mosqueda L: Mistreatment and neglect. In Ham RJ, Sloane D, Warshaw GA, editors: *Primary care geriatrics: a case-based approach,* ed 6, Philadelphia, 2014, Elsevier, pp 360–364.

In recognition of this escalating social and personal problem, countries have been working hard to understand the issue in their own countries and many have developed proactive programs and policies to identify and provide services to persons at risk (Box 31-9). With the support of the United Nations, creative programs have been implemented in countries across Europe (United Nations Economic Commission for Europe [UNECE], 2013). In the United States there has been an increase in the number of training programs for persons at the

---

BOX 31-9   TIPS FOR BEST PRACTICE

Making a Difference: Opportunities to Reduce Elder Mistreatment

The World Health Organization and the United Nations have exerted a considerable amount of effort to help countries better understand elder mistreatment and develop programs and policies to address this growing problem. To hear concerns from the elder's viewpoint, see the free download *Missing voices: views of older persons on elder abuse* at http://www.who.int/ageing/projects/elder_abuse/missing_voices/en/

Norway has implemented *Vern for Eldre*, which combines municipal and governmental resources to provide an array of services, from hot lines, to calls for help, to actual programs to provide the help needed. In 2013 it was in place in the cities of Oslo, Baerum, and Tronheim.

Adapted from UNECE (United Nations Economic Commission for Europe): Abuse of older persons, Policy Brief # 14, October 2013. Available at http://www.un.org/esa/socdev/ageing/documents/egm/NeglectAbuseandViolenceofOlderWomen/ECE-WG-14.pdf Accessed September 2014.

"front line," such as health professionals and police officers, as well as passage of more stringent laws against mistreatment. Mistreatment of older adults is categorized as either abuse or neglect. However, unlike the case with children, as long as one maintains capacity, nothing can be done without the person's permission.

Abuse

Elder abuse is a violation of human rights and a significant cause of illness, injury, loss of productivity, isolation and despair (WHO, 2014).

Abuse is intentional and may be physical, psychological, medical, financial, or sexual (Box 31-10). It also occurs in the form of discrimination (APA, 2014; National Center on Elder Abuse [NCEA], 2014). Should harm occur, the abuser can be sued for the elder's injuries. If the abuse escalates to a criminal act or if the abuse includes theft of property or money, the perpetrator is subject to criminal prosecution. Many states have reporting statutes that require certain persons, including nurses, who become aware of abuse, neglect, or exploitation to report it to the appropriate authorities. The designated authority can be found in each state's laws (NCEA, 2014).

Most abuse (90%) occurs in the home setting and is committed by adult children or spousal caregivers (NCEA, 2014).

Many factors interfere with the identification of those who are mistreated (Box 31-11). It is further complicated by varying cultural perspectives on abuse (Box 31-12).

Whereas other forms of abuse have external signs, it is more difficult to detect financial exploitation. Care is costly and the person's assets may be gone before it is noticed that charges have been excessive or misappropriated. Changes in banking practices, access to a bank account by an unauthorized person, failure to pay medical or other bills, unexpected changes in a will, or the disappearance of personal items are all evidence of possible financial exploitation. This is the most common form of abuse reported in the United States (New York State Coalition on Elder Abuse, 2011). However, in many Latino families this may not be considered abuse due to the common belief it is appropriate to share funds, even at the expense of one's own needs (NCEA, 2014).

Undue Influence

Undue influence is a means of financial or material exploitation. As described by Quinn (2002, p. 11):

Undue influence is the substitution of one person's will for the true desires of another … Undue influence takes place when one person uses his or her role and power to exploit the trust, dependency or fear of another to gain psychological control over the weaker person's decision-making, usually for financial gain.

Undue influence may occur in an insidious way if the perpetrator isolates the victim from friends and family in some way, such as with the suggestion that he or she is the only one who cares. In other situations the older adult meets a "new friend," who offers to provide "lifelong" care in exchange for the title to property such as one's home. A salesman may make an "offer you just can't refuse" or claims an unneeded repair or replacement.

Undue influence can also occur outside of the caregiving situation; for example, a person provides false affection and even marriage to a lonely person *for the purpose of defrauding the person of assets*. In these cases, intervention is difficult because the victim has developed trust and reliance on the abuser and has entered into the relationship voluntarily. Affection and kindness to the older adult in and of itself is not considered undue influence. It only reaches that point when

---

BOX 31-10   Types of Abuse of Older Adults

Physical abuse: The use of physical force that results in the threat of or the infliction of bodily injury, physical pain, or impairment. It includes, but is not limited to, acts of violence such as striking (with or without an object), pushing, shaking, pinching, and burning. It includes the use of physical restraints, force-feeding, and physical punishment.

Sexual abuse: Nonconsensual sexual contact of any kind, including with those persons unable to give consent. It includes unwanted touching of any kind and sexual assault or battery—such as rape, sodomy, coerced nudity, and forced sexually explicit photographing.

Psychological abuse: The infliction of anguish, pain, or distress through verbal or nonverbal acts, including intimidation or enforced social isolation. This includes verbal assaults, insults, threats, intimidation, humiliation, and harassment. It can include belittling the person in front of others and forced social isolation from family, friends, or usual activities.

Medical abuse: Subjecting a person to unwanted medical treatments or procedures. Examples of this include venipuncture or the insertion of a urinary catheter (also sexual abuse) in those with dementia who refuse the procedure. The use of chemical restraints (e.g., sedatives) for the convenience of care rather than for the protection of the person (**medical neglect:** failure to provide needed medical care).

Financial abuse or material exploitation: The illegal or improper use of another's funds, property, or assets. Exploitation may be accomplished through coercion (undue influence), such as demanding that the person sign checks or other documents, including deeds to property, with the threat of withholding care.

Discrimination: The illegal, cultural or social behavior such as that which is demeaning, belittling, or the withholding of full rights to persons, especially those who are at risk of physical, emotional, or sexual abuse or of financial exploitation as a result of the discrimination.

Abandonment: The desertion of an elder by an individual who had assumed the responsibility of providing care or assistance.

BOX 31-11   Identification of Abuse of Older Adults

Cultural or societal tolerance of violence, especially against women
Shame and embarrassment
Fear of retaliation
Fear of institutionalization
Social isolation
Unacceptability of emotional expression, especially that of fear or distress

Adapted from Sehgal SR, Mosqueda L: Mistreatment and neglect. In Ham RJ, Sloane D, Warshaw GA, et al, editors: *Primary care geriatrics: a case-based approach,* ed 6, Philadelphia, 2014, Elsevier, pp 360–364.

BOX 31-12   Cultural Variations Regarding Abuse and Neglect and Risk for Exploitation

Latino*
- In a study of 198 elders 40% reported abuse of some kind: psychological (25%), financial (16.7%), physical (10.7%), sexual (9%). Only 1.5% had reported it. (Financial not always considered abuse)
- *Machismo:* expectation of men to neglect self on behalf of others if necessary
- *Marianismo:* role expectation of women to tolerate abuse and focus on service of others
- *Vergüenza:* Need to protect the family from shame (above all things)
- *La familia:* emphasis on the family instead of outsiders
- Extreme level of guilt not to provide care to elders at home regardless of the difficulty to do so

Asian/Pacific Islander (in General Terms)*
- Ability to endure violence as a symbol of strength and honor
- Not familiar with the terms of abuse; instead use terms "sacrifice" and "suffering"
- Psychological abuse considered the worst possible type of abuse and the most commonly experienced
- Strong belief in filial duty to care for parents may result in excessive burden on single caregivers due to other obligations such as to financial support oneself
- Defined only within a family setting
- Unacceptability to express emotions

Chinese
- Must be kept in family
- Disrespect most important form of mistreatment
- Cultural disparities in expectations between younger adults and older adults

Asian Indian
- Children leaving the family home may be considered a form of elder abandonment
- Oldest son handles all finances, without question
- As age is venerated, physical abuse very uncommon

Japanese
- 80% report psychological abuse is the worst type of abuse to endure
- Emotional abuse, neglect, physical abuse reported to be perpetrated by daughters-in-law
- Lack of caring for elder is a sign of disrespect and socially unacceptable
- Suffering is expected to be done in a stoic manner
- Fatalism to suffering, should it occur
- Self-blame
- Those who expose a family "shame" may be considered a traitor and be sanctioned

Korean
- Financial exploitation as defined in the United States not considered a form of abuse
- High tolerance for neglect
- Placing in nursing home shameful and a form of abuse

Vietnamese
- Family problems to be kept at home; cannot be disclosed to outsiders
- Neglect brings shame to family
- Psychological "silent treatment" most serious and reported

*May or may not be applicable to any one subcultural group. It is always recommended for the nurse to find the correct language used and not to make assumptions; these are general variations; the subgroups of Korean and others are more specific. See following references for guidance in addressing issues with culture groups.

From National Center on Elder Abuse: *Research briefs,* 2014. http://ncea.aoa.gov/Library/Review/Brief/index.aspx Accessed October 2014. See also *Mistreatment of Lesbian, Gay, Bisexual and Transgender (LGBT) Elders* at same site.

---

the relationship leads to persuasion or coercion that limits the person's ability to make independent or informed choices. These situations are being examined more carefully in the courts, and some states are activating legal protections against undue influence (Quinn, 2002; Quinn and Tomita, 2003). Quinn has developed guidelines for nurses attempting to identify signs of undue influence (Box 31-13).

Impact of Elder Abuse

The abuse of elders has effects that are far more reaching than is usually discussed. Posttraumatic stress syndrome and lowered self-efficacy even after the termination of the abusive situation may never be resolved (Comijs et al, 1999). Those subjected to even minimal abuse have been found to have a 300% higher risk for death than those who have never been abused (Dong et al,

---

BOX 31-13   Signs of Undue Influence

- Actions inconsistent with his or her life history. Actions run counter to the person's previous lifelong values and beliefs.
- Makes sudden changes with regard to financial management. Examples include cashing in insurance policies or changing titles on bank accounts or real estate property.
- Elder changes his or her will and previous disposition of assets.
- Elder is taken to practitioners different from those he or she has always trusted. Examples include bankers, stockbrokers, attorneys, physicians, and realtors.
- Elder is systematically isolated from or is continually monitored when with others who care about him or her.
- Someone unexpectedly moves into the person's home, or the elder is moved into someone's home under the guise of providing better care.
- Someone attempts to get income checks directed differently from the usual arrangement.
- Documents are suddenly signed frequently as the elder nears death.

- A history of mistrust exists in the elder's family, especially with financial affairs, and the elder places unusual trust in newfound acquaintances.
- Statements of the elder and the alleged abuser vary concerning the elder's affairs or disposition of assets.
- A power imbalance exists between the parties in matters of finances or health.
- The stronger person unduly benefits by the transaction.
- The elder is never left alone with anyone. No one is allowed to speak to the elder without the alleged abuser having a way of finding out about it.
- Unusual patterns arise in the elder's finances. For instance, numerous checks are written out to "cash," always in round numbers, and often in large amounts.
- The elder reports meeting a "wonderful new friend who makes me feel young again." The elder then becomes suspicious of family and begins to avoid family gatherings.
- The elder is pressed into a transaction without being given time to reflect or contact trusted advisors.

Adapted from Quinn M: Undue influence and elder abuse: recognition and intervention strategies, *Geriatr Nurs* 23:11–16, 2002.

2011). In addition, older adults who have been victims of violence have more health problems than other older adults, including increased bone or joint problems, digestive problems, depression or anxiety, chronic pain, hypertension, and cardiovascular disease (Dyer et al, 2000).

Neglect

Neglect is a form of mistreatment resulting from the *failure* of action by a caregiver or through one's own behavior or choices. Neglect of self and neglect by caretakers are often difficult to define because they are intertwined with energy, lifestyle, and resources. Nurses are particularly challenged by issues of self-neglect when the ethical principle of beneficence (do good) counters that of autonomy (self-determination) (Zorowitz, 2014). In either case, the needs of the individual may not become known until there is a medical crisis when the person's unmet needs become visible to others.

Neglect by a Caregiver

Neglect by a caregiver requires a socially (formally or informally) recognized role and responsibility of a person to provide care to a vulnerable other. Neglect is most often passive mistreatment, such as an act of omission. It is not only the failure to provide the goods and services—such as food, medication, medical treatment, and personal care—necessary for the well-being of the frail elder, but also the failure or inability to recognize your responsibility to provide such goods and services. Neglect is active when care is withheld deliberately and for malicious reasons (Quinn and Tomita, 2003). In some cases this level of neglect would be considered abuse as well. Neglect by caregivers occurs for many reasons (Box 31-14).

Self-Neglect

Self-neglect is a behavior in which people fail to meet their own basic needs in the manner in which the average person would in similar circumstances. It generally manifests itself as a refusal to, or failure to, provide themselves with adequate safety, food, water, clothing, shelter, personal hygiene, or health care. It may be due to diminished capacity, but it also may be the result of a long-standing lifestyle, homelessness, or alcoholism or other substance abuse. It is important for the nurse to remember that there are many mentally competent people who understand the consequences of their decisions and make conscious and voluntary decisions to engage in acts that threaten their health or safety as a matter of personal choice. There are both ethical and legal questions as to how much health care professionals can and should intervene in these situations.

PROMOTING HEALTHY AGING: IMPLICATIONS FOR GERONTOLOGICAL NURSING

Nurses are expected to provide safety and security to the persons under their care to the extent possible. When caring for vulnerable elders, it also may mean wrestling with difficult and problematic legal and ethical issues. This may include questioning the person's decision-making capacity related to a request by another health care provider for an informed consent (see Box 31-2). It may involve contacting protective services when there is evidence of potential abuse or even working for an abuse hotline or international program for the protection of older adults (see www.who.org).

Clues to Potential Incapacity

As noted, unless adjudicated (declared by the courts) otherwise, all adults have a presumed capacity to control their lives, including what happens to their bodies; that is, they have the autonomous legal and ethical right to determine whether or not to receive treatment. It is always necessary to determine whether the appearance of incapacity is truly one of impairment or whether it is simply the manifestation of choices that are inconsistent with the preferences, expectations, or values of the health care system or the nurse, caregiver, surrogate, or proxy (Torke et al, 2010).

Lack of capacity is *not* a question of preference or a question of the person's values or choices, but the ability to understand the problem at hand, the choice made, and its consequences. The nurse is expected to work toward preserving the individual's integrity, independence, dignity, and assets to the extent possible.

What is the Nurse's Responsibility Regarding Issues of Capacity?

In many settings where gerontological nurses provide care to elders, ethical and legal questions of capacity and decision-making authority can occur quickly. While working in a nursing facility, the author regularly heard from previously distant or uninvolved relatives of elders who were still able to make all but the most complex decision. The presumed relative would insist that he or she was the person's "power of attorney" and therefore had the right to override an individual's decisions or would insist on access to the person's medical and health information. In such a situation, several nursing actions are expected, including asking the elder's opinion on the situation (Box 31-15).

If the facility is provided with authentic documentation that a person is actually the resident's guardian, then indeed all

---

BOX 31-14 Examples of Causes of Neglect by Caregivers

Caregiver personal stress and exhaustion
Multiple role demands
Caregiver incompetence
Unawareness of importance of the neglected care
Financial burden of caregiving limiting resources available
Caregivers' own frailty and advanced age
Unawareness of community resources available for support and respite

---

BOX 31-15 Dealing with Potential Questions of the Right to Decision-Making

1. Clarify the issues at hand and the conflicts that are present.
2. Discuss the situation with the elder/patient/resident of a long-term care facility.
3. Participate in the gross assessment of the elder's capacity and the situations to which this may apply.
4. Clarify the type of POA that is held, including obtaining a copy of the document for the patient's record (via the help of facility attorney).
5. Document where clearly visible (to staff only) to whom and what health information can be released.

requests and instructions must be followed. However, as an advocate, the nurse still has a responsibility to protect the patient from neglect or exploitation from all sources, including guardians, surrogates, or proxies. Nurses who are consulted about legal issues should not attempt to provide legal advice but, instead, should refer the person to an elder law attorney, preferably one who is certified by the National Elder Law Foundation (www.nelf.org). The nurse who is interested can also access this site for more detailed information related to elder law. The state or local bar association is an additional source of information.

◆ Elder Mistreatment

When working with frail and vulnerable elders, nurses must always be vigilant and sensitive to the signs and symptoms of mistreatment. In addition to the obvious indicators of physical abuse (e.g., unexplained bruises), the nurse looks for more subtle signs (Box 31-16). For the person who is clearly competent

---

BOX 31-16   Signs of Mistreatment

The first signs that further evaluation may be necessary are if the histories given by the (usually cognitively intact) elder and the caregiver are inconsistent or the caregiver refuses to leave the elder alone with the nurse. While it is always important to ask the elder if he or she is a recipient of abuse/shame/suffering/family disharmony/moral cruelty, one cannot assume that this will be acknowledged. While there is more than one category of abuse and abuse combined with neglect, the specific signs would include:

Physical Abuse
- Unexplained bruising or lacerations in unusual areas in various stages of healing
- Fractures inconsistent with functional ability

Sexual Abuse
- Bruises or scratches in the genital or breast area
- Fear or an unusual amount of anxiety related to either routine or necessary exam of the anogenital area
- Torn undergarments or presence of blood

Medical Abuse
- Caregiver repeatedly requesting procedures that are not recommended and not desired by elder

Medical Neglect
- Unusual delay between the beginning of a health problem and when help is sought
- Repeated missed appointments without reasonable explanations

Psychological Abuse
- Caregiver does all of the talking in a situation, even though the elder is capable
- Caregiver appears angry, frustrated, or indifferent while the elder appears hesitant or frightened
- Caregiver or the care recipient aggressive toward one another or the nurse

Neglect by Self or Caregiver
- Weight loss
- Uncharacteristically neglected grooming
- Evidence of malnutrition and dehydration
- Fecal/urine smell
- Inappropriate clothing to the situation or weather
- Insect infestation

---

and refuses assessment, this cannot be done. For a person with unmet needs or other signs of abuse or neglect, as well as questionable capacity, intervention is required.

A full and specialized assessment includes the immediate determination of the person's safety. Further assessment of mistreatment involves a number of very sensitive components and tools developed by experts in the field that may be very useful (Box 31-17). Assessment of mistreatment in the cross-cultural setting is especially difficult; however, helpful guidelines can be found at The National Center on Elder Abuse through the Administration on Aging (http://www.ncea.aoa.gov/Library/Review/Brief/index.aspx). Because of the sensitive nature of such an assessment, specialized training is recommended for all gerontological nurses.

◆ Mandatory Reporting

In most states and U.S. jurisdictions, licensed nurses are "mandatory reporters," that is, persons who are required to report suspicions of abuse to the state, usually to a group called Adult Protective Services (APS) (National Adult Protective Services Association [NAPSA], 2014). The standard for reporting is one of reasonable belief; that is, the nurse must have a reasonable belief that a vulnerable person either has been or is likely to be abused, neglected, or exploited.

Usually these reports are anonymous. If the nurse believes the elder to be in immediate danger, the police are notified. How the nurse accomplishes this varies with the work setting. In hospitals and nursing homes, suspicions of abuse are often reported first internally to the facility social worker. In the home care setting, the report is made to the nursing supervisor. It would be very unusual for the nurse not to approach this subject through his or her employer. However, the nurse who is a neighbor, friend, or privately paid caregiver may be under obligation to make the report directly. In the nursing home or licensed assisted living facility, the nurse has the additional resource of calling the state long-term care ombudsman for help.

In each state, ombudsmen are either volunteers or paid staff members who are responsible for acting as advocates for vulnerable elders in institutions (www.ltcombudsman.org). All reports, either to the state ombudsman or to APS, will be investigated. A unique aspect of elder abuse compared with child abuse is that the physically frail (and even abused or neglected) but mentally competent adult can, and often does, refuse intervention. These adults cannot be removed from harmful situations without their permission, much to the frustration of the nurse and other health care providers.

BOX 31-17   RESOURCES FOR BEST PRACTICE
Assessment of Mistreatment

See elder mistreatment assessment information at
   http://consultgerirn.org/
   http://www.cdc.gov/violenceprevention/elderabuse/index.html
   www.ncea.aoa.gov
   http://www.who.int/ageing/projects/elder_abuse/en/

Prevention of Abuse

In the ideal situation, gerontological nurses are alert to potential mistreatment of vulnerable elders and take steps to prevent the occurrence of abuse or neglect. In some situations, the abuse may have been preventable, and in others, it is less likely. If the mistreatment is the result of psychopathological conditions, especially if the situation is long-standing, the nurse probably cannot prevent the abuse. However, nurses can make sure that the potential victims know how to get help if it is needed and are aware of the resources that are available to them; in addition, nurses can provide support and encouragement that it is possible for elders to remove themselves from these dangerous situations. The nurse can also work with the elder, caregiver, and community support groups to increase the social network of at-risk elders (e.g., promote more community activities and involve elders in the lives of their neighbors).

If the abusive behavior is learned or a response to stress, the situation may be subject to change. Learned abuse, theoretically, can be unlearned and may respond to a close working relationship with a mentoring professional who can demonstrate positive problem solving and new ways of managing difficult situations.

If the abuse is triggered by the stress of caregiving, nurses can be very proactive and help all involved take action to lessen the stress. This may include finding respite services, changing the situation entirely (giving permission to the caregiver to relinquish the role), referring to support groups for expression of frustrations and peer support, teaching people how to use crisis hotlines, and providing access to professional consultation, victim support groups, or victim volunteer companions; most importantly, thoughtful and compassionate care is imperative for both the victim and the perpetrator (Centers for Disease Control and Prevention [CDC], 2014). See Box 31-18 for tips on the prevention of elder mistreatment.

Finally, for elders who become incapacitated, legal protection at some level may be necessary. Gerontological nurses can become familiar with the laws that specifically affect older adults in their state. This can be done by selecting continuing education programs to update knowledge in the field of elder law and protection. Nurses are in a position to assist elders and family members seek legal representation when necessary and to help them find solutions that may solve potential caregiving problems in the least restrictive manner possible. Although initiating these interventions is usually the responsibility of the social worker and enacted by lawyers and judges, the nurse should understand the basic concepts and the types of legal protection for elders and other incapacitated persons.

BOX 31-18 TIPS FOR BEST PRACTICE

Prevention of Elder Mistreatment

- Make professionals aware of potentially abusive situations.
- Help families develop and nurture informal support systems.
- Link families with support groups.
- Teach families stress management techniques.
- Arrange comprehensive care resources.
- Provide counseling for troubled families.
- Encourage the use of respite care and day care.
- Obtain necessary home health care services.
- Inform families of resources for meals and transportation.
- Encourage caregivers to pursue their individual interests.

Advocacy

An advocate is one who maintains or promotes a cause; defends, pleads, or acts on behalf of another; and fights for someone who cannot fight.

Topics for advocacy can include protection of specific rights (e.g., promoting the least restrictive residential alternative), finding the best nursing home, or testifying at the judicial appointment of a conservator. Other areas of advocacy include the rights of medical patients, the right to have the in-home supportive services needed to assist with care, and the right to access government programs that support caregiving and prevent abuse (e.g., Area Agencies for Aging, veterans' programs). Nurse-advocates function in various arenas: with their own and other disciplines within their own agencies, with other agencies, with physicians, with families, with neighbors and community representatives, with professional organizations, with legislators, and with courts.

Nurses act as advocates when they support people as autonomous free agents who have the right to make decisions and to be involved in all conversations about their health care needs. In a health care setting, advocacy is acting for or on behalf of another in terms of pleading for and supporting the best interests of that other person with respect to choice, provision, and refusal of health care as appropriate. However, situations occur in the care of older adults when the elder either is not strong enough or does not have the mental capacity to exert measures to protect his or her own interests. When this occurs, the nurse's role is to ensure not only that the person is protected but also that his or her voice, when he or she can or could express himself or herself, is not lost.

▉ KEY CONCEPTS

- Informed consent is based on the ethical principle of autonomy, which requires the capacity to understand a situation, the choices that are available, and the consequences of a decision.
- In the health care setting, an individual may be legally competent but have diminished or varying levels of capacity to make health-related decisions.
- Varying levels of protection are available to protect persons with diminished capacity and to ensure that his or her voice is still heard.
- Elder mistreatment is an umbrella term that covers abuse, neglect, exploitation, and abandonment.
- The nurse has a legal responsibility in most states to report suspected mistreatment of frail or disabled elders.

NURSING STUDY: WHEN CAN YOU INTERVENE?

Mrs. Henry, 87 years old, is admitted to the medical/surgical floor of a community hospital with a fractured right orbit and ruptured eye globe. Her husband attends to her with care and concern, trying to anticipate her needs. He is active and appears much younger than his stated age of 85. The emergency department report states the cause of the injury as "fall at home." Although Mrs. Henry is alert and oriented, she appears very thin, frail, and withdrawn. Her husband also voices concern that she seems confused at times. When the gerontological clinical nurse specialist arrives to do a basic intake, she reports to the nurses that she is concerned that Mrs. Henry has been abused. Her husband answers all the questions posed to his wife, and, as he does so, Mrs. Henry seems to withdraw even further from both him and the staff. Mr. Henry does not leave his wife's side for hours. Finally he leaves for a quick cup of coffee, and the nurse

who had been providing care quickly goes into the room and asks Mrs. Henry what happened. She begins to cry and says that her husband hit her. She is immediately offered shelter and protection. She declines, saying that she has nowhere else to go but back home and that she will be okay. The husband returns to find the nurse talking to his wife privately and immediately gathers up her things, and they leave the hospital against medical advice.

- Identify the risk factors for elder abuse in this situation.
- Provide the subjective data suggesting abuse.
- Provide the objective data suggesting abuse in this situation.
- Describe the nurse's legal responsibility to Mrs. Henry at this time.
- Describe the next step the nurse can take on the departure of a patient who reports abuse but declines intervention.

CRITICAL THINKING QUESTIONS AND ACTIVITIES

1. After reading this chapter, discuss with a classmate why you believe some elders feel that they have no options but to endure abuse of any kind.

2. If you were the nurse making home visits to the man and his granddaughter described in Box 17-7, what would you do? What if this were your neighbor?

3. Why might Mrs. Henry believe she has no options?

RESEARCH QUESTIONS

1. What are your responsibilities for reporting elder abuse in your state?

2. What resources are available to frail elders in your community who are attempting to escape from abuse?

REFERENCES

Acierno R, Hernandez MA, Amstadter AB, et al: Prevalence and correlates of emotional, physical, sexual, and financial abuse and potential neglect in the United States: the national elder mistreatment study, *Am J Public Health* 100(2):292–297, 2010.

American Psychological Association (APA): *Elder abuse and neglect: in search of solutions,* 2012. http://www.apa.org/pi/aging/resources/guides/elder-abuse.aspx?item=1. Accessed September 2014.

Broyles, K: *The silenced voice speaks out: a study of abuse and neglect of nursing home residents* (Report from the Atlanta Long Term Care Ombudsman Program and Atlanta Legal Aid Society to the National Citizens Coalition for Nursing Home Reform), Atlanta, GA, 2000, Authors.

Centers for Disease Control (CDC): *Elder abuse: prevention strategies,* 2014. http://www.cdc.gov/violenceprevention/elderabuse/prevention.html. Accessed October 2014.

Comijs HC, Penninx BW, Knipscheer KP, et al: Psychological distress in victims of elder mistreatment: the effects of social support and coping, *J Gerontol B Psychol Sci Soc Sci* 54(4):240–245, 1999.

Dong X, Simon MA, Beck T, et al: Elder abuse and mortality: the role of psychological and social wellbeing, *Gerontology* 57(6):549–558, 2011.

Dyer CB, Pavlik VN, Murphy KP, et al: The high prevalence of depression and dementia in elder abuse or neglect, *J Am Geriatr Soc* 48:205–208, 2000.

National Adult Protective Services Association (NAPSA): *About NAPSA,* 2014. http://www.napsa-now.org/about-napsa/. Accessed November 25, 2014.

National Center on Elder Abuse (NCEA): *Statistics and data,* 2014. http://ncea.aoa.gov/Library/Data/index.aspx. Accessed November 2014.

National Research Council: *Elder mistreatment: abuse, neglect and exploitation in an aging America,* Washington, DC, 2003, National Academies Press.

New York State Coalition on Elder Abuse: *Under the radar: New York State Elder Abuse Prevalence Study,* Lifespan of Greater Rochester, Inc, Weill Cornell Medical Center of Cornell University, & New York City Department for the Aging, 2011.

Quinn M: Undue influence and elder abuse: recognition and intervention strategies, *Geriatr Nurs* 23:11–16, 2002.

Quinn M, Tomita SK: *Elder abuse and neglect: causes, diagnoses and intervention strategies,* ed 3, New York, 2003, Springer.

Torke AM, Moloney R, Siegler M, et al: Physicians' view on the importance of patient preferences in surrogate decision-making, *J Am Geriatr Soc* 58(3):533–538, 2010.

United Nations Economic Commission for Europe (UNECE): *Abuse of older persons* (Policy brief no. 14), October 2013. http://www.unece.org/fileadmin/DAM/pau/age/Policy_briefs/ECE-WG-14.pdf. Accessed November 25, 2014.

U.S. Government Accounting Office: *Nursing homes: federal monitoring surveys demonstrate continued understatement of serious care problems and CMS oversight weaknesses* (Publication GAO–08-517), 2008.

World Health Organization (WHO): *World elder abuse awareness day, 2012.* http://www.un.org/en/events/elderabuse. Accessed October 2014.

Zorowitz RA: Ethics. In Ham RJ, Sloane D, Warshaw GA, et al, editors: *Primary care geriatrics: a case-based approach,* ed 6, Philadelphia, 2014, Elsevier, pp 77–91.

CHAPTER 32

Long-Term Care

Theris A. Touhy

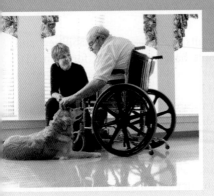

http://evolve.elsevier.com/Touhy/TwdHlthAging

A STUDENT SPEAKS

I feel so depressed when I see all the older people in nursing homes. I don't know how families can put loved ones into a nursing home and I have promised my parents that I will never do that to them.

John, age 25

AN ELDER SPEAKS

This nursing home is my home now. We are all like a family, and I will die here. The girls that help me during the day, we treat one another like family members. We have some days when we are grumpy, some days we are happy, and we don't hold our feelings back, just like you would do with your own family at home.

Helen, age 88

LEARNING OBJECTIVES

On completion of this chapter, the reader will be able to:

1. Define long-term care and describe the long-term care system.
2. Describe factors influencing the provision of long-term care.
3. Identify differences between the focus of acute and long-term care.
4. Discuss long-term care as a component of the health care system in the United States and in other countries.
5. Describe several long-term care options for older adults including continuing care retirement communities, residential care facilities, skilled nursing facilities, and community-based programs such as PACE and adult day health.
6. Assist older adults and their families in making an informed choice when relocation to a more protected setting becomes necessary.
7. Discuss interventions to improve care for older adults in skilled nursing facilities including quality improvement, culture change, and transitional care.

The term long-term care (LTC) is often only associated with nursing homes and with care of older people but long-term care describes a variety of services, including medical and nonmedical care, provided on an ongoing basis to people of all ages who have a chronic illness or physical, cognitive, or developmental disabilities. Long-term care can be provided informally or formally in a range of environments, from an individual's home to the home of a friend or relative, an adult day health center, independent and assisted living facilities, continuing care retirement communities, skilled nursing facilities, and hospice (Applebaum et al, 2013).

Long-term services and supports (LTSS) consist predominantly of assistance or supervision with activities of daily living (ADLs), such as bathing, dressing, toileting, or eating, or with instrumental activities of daily living (IADLs), such as shopping or cleaning. Older adults receive the majority of long-term services and supports on a yearly basis (56%), but children and younger adults also receive this type of care. Children younger than age 18 are a small percentage of the total population (4%)

requiring LTSS but can have substantial needs that will last a lifetime (United States Senate, 2013).

Most people with LTC needs live in their own home with family, friends, and volunteers (as well as hired personnel) providing most of the care. However, the bulk of long-term care throughout the developed world is informal unpaid care provided by family members. More than 80% of individuals needing long-term care support and services receive help informally from friends and relatives (Frank, 2012) (Chapter 34). The nature of family caregiving is changing as more individuals are discharged early from acute settings with increasingly complex medical care needs to be met in the home (United States Senate, 2013).

FUTURE PROJECTIONS

The number of older people needing long-term services and supports is dramatically increasing year after year, and the challenge of ensuring the quality and financial stability of care provision is one faced by governments in both the developed and the developing world (Mor et al, 2014). Worldwide, the number of people older than age 80, those most likely to need long-term care services, will increase by 233% between 2008 and 2040 (Applebaum et al, 2013). In the coming years, most families will have a member with a need for long-term care services and supports. However, with shrinking family sizes, there will be fewer potential caregivers and reliance on formal care services can be expected to expand (Frank, 2012) (Chapter 34). Of baby boomers, 70% can expect to use some form of long-term care and 33% will spend at least 3 months in a nursing home before they die. A fivefold increase in spending on LTC is projected by 2045 in the United States (Frank, 2012).

A recent report on long-term services and supports states: "We lack a national solution to providing quality long-term services and supports that are equitable and affordable for all in need of such services. Our nation faces an unprecedented public policy challenge of how to transform our system of long-term services and supports (LTSS) to promote independence among older adults and people with disabilities and provide support for family members who help them" (Reinhard et al, 2014). While progress has been made, it is not adequate to meet the needs of aging baby boomers and beyond.

COSTS OF LONG-TERM CARE

In the United States, LTC is expensive and becoming more expensive; costs have outpaced inflation since 2003 (Table 32-1). LTC coverage in the United States is overly reliant on institutional care and primarily financed by individuals or Medicaid (Markkanen et al, 2012). Low- and moderate-income older people will be most affected by increased costs (e.g., those having to spend their personal savings or rely on unpaid family members for care) (Kaiser Family Foundation, 2013). Only people in the wealthiest 10% to 20% of older adult households have savings that could absorb the risks of high LTSS spending (Frank, 2012; Reinhard et al, 2014). Finding a way to pay for long-term care is a growing concern for people of all

TABLE 32-1   Costs of U.S. Long-Term Care Services and Support Programs

SERVICE	COST
Homemaker services	National median hourly rate: $19
Home health aide	National median hourly rate: $20
Adult day health	National median daily rate: $65
Assisted living facility	National median monthly rate: $3500 Annual cost: $42,000
Nursing home care	National median daily rate (semiprivate room): $212 Annual cost: $90,000
Costs of LTC services and support programs at home	Estimated to be $1800/month

Data from Genworth 2014 Cost of Care Survey: https://www.genworth.com/corporate/about-genworth/industry-expertise/cost-of-care.html. Accessed September 2014.

ages, especially older adults, persons with disabilities, and their families. Most people have not planned for their LTC needs and are not knowledgeable about existing resources (Harris-Kojetin et al, 2013).

The total U.S. long-term care spending is currently financed through a mixture of Medicaid, Medicare, out-of-pocket spending, private long-term care insurance, and appropriations from the Older Americans Act (Chapter 30). It is important to remember that the majority of long-term care services are not paid for at all. They are provided by unpaid caregivers, primarily family members and friends of those needing services. Without family caregivers, the present level of long-term care could not be sustained (Chapter 34).

Medicaid

Medicaid is the primary payer for long-term care services and supports for people who have low incomes and who deplete their personal savings to pay for medical and long-term care. Without affordable private-insurance options or public insurance alternatives, such as a national long-term care insurance system or expanded coverage for Medicare beneficiaries, there will be continued reliance on the Medicaid program. Medicaid accounts for more than 62% of national long-term care spending in the United States. Of this amount, about 55% is for institutional care and 45% is for home and community-based services. In most areas of the country, the supply and use of nursing homes is greater than those of other long-term care service options (Harris-Kojetin et al, 2013).

At present, more Medicaid spending is directed toward institutional care but national and state initiatives are directed toward changing the bias from institutional care to more home and community-based services (HCBS) that are usually less expensive and reflective of the desires of people to "age in place." Despite recent improvements, under federal law, Medicaid initiatives for HCBS must not increase Medicaid spending. As a result, states are forced to limit eligibility for these services and impose other requirements to keep costs down. Many states cap enrollment in HCBS and many have waiting lists for services (Markkanen et al, 2012; United States Senate, 2013). Where you live really matters because there are large differences across the states in how well they are doing in expanding and funding LTSS (Reinhard et al, 2014) (Figure 32-1).

The Patient Protection and Affordable Care Act (ACA) establishes new home and community-based service options, demonstration projects, and incentives to states to institute improvements as part of several changes to Medicaid (Okrent, 2012). The success of community-based programs depends on the ability of states and the federal government to build consumer-friendly, coordinated programs while maintaining costs that will be affordable for taxpayers and effective in meeting needs. Several states, including Minnesota and Washington, are developing innovative LTSS systems that include easy-to-access information, care coordination, nursing home preadmission and transition services, and a wide selection of home and community-based and managed care options (United States Senate, 2013).

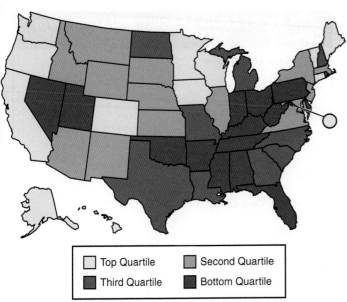

FIGURE 32-1 State Ranking on Overall LTSS System Performance, 2014. (From AARP: Raising expectations, 2014. http://www.longtermscorecard.org/ Accessed November 14, 2014.)

Legend:
- Top Quartile
- Second Quartile
- Third Quartile
- Bottom Quartile

Medicare

Medicare is not designed to provide coverage for long-term care services. Medicare covers acute and post-acute medical care for people 65 years of age and older and for younger populations who qualify for Social Security because of disability. Many people think that Medicare covers long-term care; however, in reality, it provides limited coverage for nursing home stays and home health care (Chapter 30). Medicare does not cover the costs of care in chronic, custodial, and long-term care units. If the older person was admitted to the nursing home because of a dementia diagnosis and the need for assistance with ADLs and maintenance of safety, Medicare would not cover the cost of care unless there was some skilled need.

Private Long-Term Care Insurance

Long-term care insurance pays for approximately 7% of national long-term care spending. Relatively few people have purchased this type of insurance (Okrent, 2012). Barriers to the purchase of long-term care insurance include the inability of many people to afford coverage, the belief that LTC is covered by their general policies or by Medicare, and the reluctance of private insurers to write policies for those in poor health (the individuals most likely to require LTC services) (Freundlich, 2014). Some new and more cost-effective options for LTC insurance are emerging, as well as proposed reforms to encourage more individuals to obtain coverage, such as the Partnership for Long-Term Care program (United States Senate, 2013).

Out-of-Pocket Spending

For those who do not qualify for Medicare or Medicaid benefits, the costs of long-term care are paid out-of-pocket.

Out-of-pocket spending accounts for about 22% of national spending for long-term care (Okrent, 2012). LTC is the largest expenditure for older adults in the United States (Markkanen et al, 2012).

LTC AND THE U.S. HEALTH CARE SYSTEM

The U.S. health care system has been focused on delivering acute care needs and addressing time-limited and specific illnesses or injuries as they occur in episodes, driven by restrictions of Medicare, Medicaid, and private insurance. Such a system does not address the increasingly complex and long-term needs of people with chronic conditions who need acute and long-term services and support systems. Traditionally, health care has been made up of two sectors: acute care and ambulatory care. Each setting has been viewed as an independent entity with little coordination or recognition of LTC as an integral part of the continuum of care.

Today, the total spectrum of care has been expanded to include long-term and post-acute care services (LTPAC), which includes nursing homes, assisted living facilities, home care, and hospice (Golden and Shier, 2012-2013) (Figure 32-2). However, in the United States today, the LTC system is complex and fragmented, isolated from other service providers, and poorly funded; it also is confusing and difficult for the individual and the caregiver to access and negotiate.

Access to services is dependent of funding governed by a mix of federal, state, and local rules and procedures. Separate agencies have unique eligibility rules, intake, and assessment processes. When individuals need long-term care, they and their families must find and arrange for services on their own, sometimes on short notice when the need arises from a medical event or change in the individual's functional capacity.

There is no comprehensive approach to care coordination. As a result, services and supports may not be provided in the most appropriate setting by the most appropriate provider, the

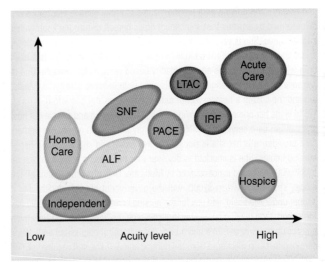

FIGURE 32-2 LTPAC Spectrum of Care. (From John F. Derr, RPh; JD and Associates Enterprises, Inc.)

individual's needs and preferences may not be met, and their caregivers may experience substantial stress trying to arrange for or provide care. This fragmented, provider- and setting-centered approach (as opposed to a person-centered approach) results in unmet needs, risk for injuries, and adverse outcomes (Nazir et al, 2014; United States Senate, 2013). There is also a critical shortage of well-prepared health care professionals and direct care staff to provide LTC, putting the individual who needs LTC at further risk of poor outcomes (Chapter 2).

Health care professionals who have not had experience in the long-term care system are often unaware of the many differences between the systems. Unless they have experienced the problems in their own families, they may be unaware of the challenges associated with obtaining quality care for individuals with long-term needs (Box 32-1). It is important for health care professionals, especially nurses, to understand the total spectrum of care and the differences between acute and long-term care (Boxes 32-2 and 32-3). "Without addressing the obstacles discussed above, we will continue to move forward with a partial view of older adults—one seen through an acute and medical lens, rather than seeing a person with a story, a family system, and a community" (Golden and Shier, 2012-2013, p. 11).

GLOBAL APPROACHES TO LTC

Most countries are facing increasing challenges surrounding long-term care for the growing numbers of older people. Many of these developed countries have been preparing for big increases in their older populations and the associated growth in the need for long-term care services for many years (Polivka, 2012; Zhan, 2013). Every developed country in the world, except for the United States and the United Kingdom, has some

---

BOX 32-2 Focus of Acute and Long-Term Care

Acute Care Orientation
- Illness
- High technology
- Short term
- Episodic
- One-dimensional
- Professional
- Medical model
- Cure

Long-Term Care Orientation
- Function
- High touch
- Extended
- Interdisciplinary model
- Ongoing
- Multidimensional
- Paraprofessional and family
- Care

Adapted from Ouslander J, Osterweil D, Morley J: *Medical care in the nursing home*, New York, 1997, McGraw-Hill.

BOX 32-3 Goals of Long-Term Care

1. Provide a safe and supportive environment for chronically ill and functionally dependent people.
2. Restore and maintain highest practicable level of functional independence.
3. Preserve individual autonomy.
4. Maximize quality of life, well-being, and satisfaction with care.
5. Provide comfort and dignity at the end of life for residents and their families.
6. Provide coordinated interdisciplinary care to subacutely ill residents who plan to return to home or a less restrictive level of care.
7. Stabilize and delay progression, when possible, of chronic medical conditions.
8. Prevent acute medical and iatrogenic illnesses, and identify and treat them rapidly when they do occur.
9. Create a homelike environment that respects the dignity of each resident.

Adapted from Ouslander J, Osterweil D, Morley J: *Medical care in the nursing home*, New York, 1997, McGraw-Hill.

BOX 32-1 One Woman's Story

Myra is an 86-year-old woman who lives in her own condominium apartment in Florida. Her diagnoses include osteoarthritis and hypertension. She is a widow with no children or close relatives. She has about $80,000 in savings and is very careful living on a limited income monthly budget. Her hands are so deformed by arthritis that she cannot dress herself or turn the knob on her kitchen stove. She is very alert but is having increasing difficulty living alone. Friends and neighbors have been helping as much as they can. She has been on a waiting list for home and community-based services for a month. Due to her savings, she is not eligible for assistance with in-home care under Medicaid and the cost of a homemaker or aide is more than she can afford.

She visits her primary care provider for her annual exam and asks about how she can get care services so that she can stay in her own home. Her primary care provider tells her she is not safe to live alone and she is given a list of nursing homes. She is shocked to discover that the nursing home can cost up to $90,000 yearly and is not covered by Medicare. Only after she spends all the money she has, down to $2000, will the government step in, declare her a pauper under Medicaid, and pay for the nursing home bill. Medicare would pay for a short-term nursing home stay (full coverage for 20 days and partial coverage for up to 80 days if she had a prior 3-day hospital admission) and skilled care needs. Upon discharge from the nursing home, if she still required skilled care, she could receive part-time home health care (RN supervision, therapy, home health aide a couple of hours per day for personal care).

---

system for universal long-term care. The United States and the United Kingdom (excluding Scotland) are the only developed countries that still operate a means-tested system (Medicaid in the United States). Most governments have established collectively financed systems for personal and nursing home care cost. It may be social insurance (e.g., Germany, Japan, Korea), a personal care benefit (e.g., paying informal caregivers in cash or in-kind for services) (e.g., France, Italy, Australia), or fully integrated social care (e.g., Sweden, Norway) (Box 32-4).

On average, countries spend about 1.5% of their Gross National Product on public long-term care programs—much less than they spend on health care. There is a lot of variation, with the United States spending about 1%, well below the average. The Netherlands and Sweden spend far more (3.5% and

Roger is an 87-year-old widowed man who lives alone in the home he has owned for more than 40 years. He fell and broke his hip and received care in the hospital in his local municipality. All of his care in the hospital, including rehabilitation, was covered by the government. When he was ready for discharge, a care plan meeting with Roger, his family/significant others, the district nurse in his municipality, social worker, and therapists was held to evaluate how much care he will need following discharge. He will not be discharged until the plan is decided. If Roger is able to return home safely, he will receive personal care up to several times a day (getting up, dressing, grooming, toileting, meals, going to bed) at no charge to him. Services are supported through taxes and administered through the local municipalities.

If his family wants to provide some of this care, they can receive a stipend equivalent to the salary of the paid caregivers. Care plan meetings are held with the team to determine the type of services he needs, as well as the frequency; however, he can receive home assistance until his function improves and he is able to live safely at home. If he continues to need extensive care at home (24 hours/day) that is more expensive than nursing home care, he will be evaluated for nursing home care. If he needs to go to a nursing home, he must go to a home in his area. Individuals with the greatest need have priority and sometimes there is a waiting period before admission. He may pay a small fee for the nursing home depending on his income level but probably not more than $150 to $200 per month. The remaining costs are covered through the government benefits. The district nurse will continue to coordinate his care and evaluate his status while he is in the nursing home.

Source: Personal communication, Gabriella Engstrom RN, PhD.

BOX 32-5   U.S. Senate Commission on LTC: Selected Recommendations

- Strengthen LTSS financing through private options for financial protection (long-term care insurance, tax preference for long-term care policies, protection for catastrophic long-term care costs).
- Strengthen LTSS financing through social insurance (comprehensive Medicare benefit for LTSS through increase in Medicare payroll tax and creation of Part A premium).
- Eliminate the 3-day hospital stay requirement for SNF coverage.
- Reconsider the requirement for home health services under Medicare that the individual be "homebound."
- Create a more responsive, integrated, person-centered and fiscally responsible LTSS delivery system that ensures people can access quality services in settings they choose.
- Promote active involvement of individuals and family caregivers in making care decisions and ensuring delivery of care in the least restrictive setting consistent with their preferences.
- Integrate LTSS with medical and health-related care including effective management of transitions. Establish a single point of contact for LTSS on the care team (personal navigator, care coordinator).
- Develop a standardized assessment tool that can produce a single care plan across care settings.
- Enhance options and improve focus on quality across settings, with particular attention to home and community-based care.
- Create livable communities and more opportunities to "age-in-place" (e.g., Villages, NORC) (Chapter 20).
- Develop a national strategy to support family caregivers.
- Create meaningful career ladders for direct care workers to improve access to career advancement opportunities and improved compensation.

Source: United States Senate, Commission on Long-Term Care: *Report to the Congress*, Sept 13, 2013. http://www.gpo.gov/fdsys/pkg/GPO-LTCCOMMISSION/content-detail.html Accessed September 2014.

3.6%, respectively). Private long-term care insurance barely exists in most countries (Colombo et al, 2011; Gleckman, 2011; Markkanen et al, 2012).

All nations need to take steps to prepare for the growing numbers of older people by creating sustainable financing systems, developing better ways to support informal caregivers, and focusing efforts on prevention and chronic care management. By sharing best practices, nations can learn from each other in designing systems of care that support the health and well-being of their citizens (Applebaum et al, 2013). As the United States looks to improving the LTC system, there is a slow shift away from a solely acute medical model and more emphasis on managing chronic disease and long-term care and prevention while lowering costs and preserving quality (Belli, 2013). The United States Senate Commission on Long-Term Care *Report to the Congress* (2013) provides a comprehensive look at the existing system and offers many excellent best practice recommendations for improvement. A few are presented in Box 32-5.

◆ **PROMOTING HEALTHY AGING: IMPLICATIONS FOR GERONTOLOGICAL NURSING**

We know we can do better providing care to those with long-term needs even in times of fiscal restraint through creative planning and utilization of best practices. Gerontological nurse educators, researchers, and providers must be knowledgeable about the full spectrum of LTPAC so that they can assist individuals and their caregivers to obtain the most appropriate care to enhance health and well-being. Nurses must also "advocate

for improved financing and delivery of LTC services to reach the goal of quality, equitable, seamless, and affordable person-centered LTC for all in need of such services" (Markkanen et al, 2012, p. 20).

FORMAL LONG-TERM CARE SERVICE PROVIDERS

The following section describes some of the types of facilities and programs providing long-term care services in the United States. Services available and characteristics of the individuals served are discussed. It is important for nurses in all practice settings to be knowledgeable about the range of services so that they can assist older adults and their families in making decisions when the need for long-term care arises. Nurses who practice in acute care need to know the characteristics of the setting from which the patient is admitted, and to which they will be discharged, in order to create appropriate discharge plans and effective transitions of care. Most nurses work in one setting and are not familiar with the requirements of other settings or the needs of individuals in these settings. As a result, there are often significant misunderstandings and criticisms of care in different settings across the continuum. We can no longer work in our individual "silos" and not be concerned with what happens after the patient is out of our particular institution.

Community Care

Program for All-Inclusive Care for the Elderly

This program is a Medicaid and Medicare program that provides community services to people age 55 or older who would otherwise need a nursing home level of care. Participants must meet the criteria for nursing home admission, prefer to remain in the community, and be eligible for Medicare and Medicaid. While all Program for All-inclusive Care for the Elderly (PACE) participants must be certified to need nursing home care to enroll in the program, only about 7% of participants reside in a nursing home. If participants need nursing home care, the program pays for that care. If the individual has Medicaid, he or she will not have to pay a monthly premium for the long-term care portion of the PACE benefit. If the individual does not qualify for Medicaid but has Medicare, there will be a monthly premium to cover the long-term care portion of the PACE benefit and a premium for Part D Medicare drugs. However, there is never a deductible or co-payment for any drug, service, or care approved by the PACE team.

PACE provides a comprehensive continuum of primary care, acute care, home care, adult day health care, nursing home care, and specialty care by an interdisciplinary team. PACE is a capitated system in which the team is provided with a monthly sum to provide all care to the enrollees, including medications, eyeglasses, and transportation to care, as well as urgent and preventive care. PACE is now recognized as a permanent provider under Medicare and a state option under Medicaid. In 2014, there were 104 PACE programs operational in 31 states. PACE has been approved by the U.S. Department of Health and Human Services (USDHHS) Substance Abuse and Mental Health Services Administration (SAMHSA) as an evidence-based model of care. Models such as PACE are innovative care delivery models, and continued development of such models is important as the population ages (National PACE Association, 2014) (Box 32-6).

Adult Day Services

Adult day services (ADSs) are community-based group programs designed to provide social and some health services to adults who need supervised care in a safe setting during the day. They also offer caregivers respite from the responsibilities of caregiving, and most provide educational programs, support groups, and individual counseling for caregivers. There are approximately 5685 adult day programs across the United States—a 35% increase since 2002. Adult day centers are serving populations with higher levels of physical disability and chronic disease, and the number of older people receiving adult day services has increased 63% over the past 12 years (National Adult Day Services Association, 2014).

ADSs are increasingly being utilized to provide community-based care for conditions like Alzheimer's disease and for transitional care and short-term rehabilitation following hospitalization. Nearly half of all participants have some level of dementia. Staff ratios in ADS are one direct care worker to six clients. Almost 80% of centers have professional nursing staff, 50% have a social worker, and 60% offer case management services. Most also offer transportation services.

Some ADSs are private pay, and others are funded through Medicaid home and community-based waiver programs, state and local funding, and the Veterans Administration (Table 32-1). The Patient Protection and Affordable Care Act provides additional funding to states for home and community-based care. Pilot programs have been implemented through Medicare and are being evaluated. ADSs hold the potential to meet the need for cost-efficient and high-quality long-term care services, and continued expansion and funding are expected. Adult day services are an important part of the LTPAC continuum and a cost-effective alternative or supplement to home care or institutional care. Athough further research is needed on patient and caregiver outcomes of ADS, findings suggest that they improve health-related quality of life for participants and improve caregiver well-being. Local area agencies on aging are good sources of information about adult day services and other community-based options (National Adult Day Services Association, 2014).

Continuing Care Retirement Communities

Life care communities, also known as continuing care retirement communities (CCRCs), provide the full range of residential options, from single-family homes to skilled nursing facilities all in one location. Most of these communities provide access to these levels of care for a community member's entire remaining lifetime, and for the right price, the range of services may be guaranteed. Having all levels of care in one location allows community members to make the transition between levels without life-disrupting moves. For married couples in which one spouse needs more care than the other, life care communities allow them to live nearby in a different part of the same community. This industry is maturing, and there are almost 1900 CCRCs in the United States (Maag, 2012). More than 80% of CCRCs are managed by not-for-profit organizations. Entrance fees can range from as low as $20,000 for a non-purchase (rental) agreement to buy-in fees among the most expensive CCRCs of up to $500,000. The average monthly cost of living in a not-for-profit CCRC is $2672. It is important to remember that in most CCRCs, the residence purchased usually belongs to the community after the death of the owner.

Residential Care/Assisted Living

Residential care/assisted living (RC/AL) is a long-term care option that provides housing and services for close to 1 million older adults in the United States and is the fastest growing housing option for older adults (Beeber et al, 2014). A recent survey reported that almost half of older adults would move to an assisted living community if they could no longer care for themselves (Maag, 2012). RC/AL is known by more than 30 different names across the country, including adult congregate facilities, foster care homes, personal care homes, homes for the elderly, domiciliary care homes, board and care homes, rest homes, family care homes, retirement homes, and assisted living facilities.

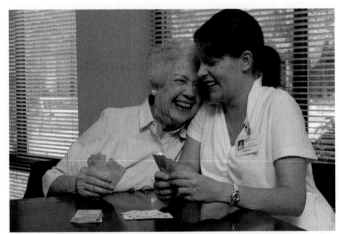

Providing nursing services in assisted living facilities promotes physical and psychosocial health. (From Potter PA: *Basic nursing: essentials for practice*, ed 7, St Louis, MO, 2010, Mosby.)

RC/AL is viewed as more cost effective than nursing homes while providing more privacy and a homelike environment. Medicare does not cover the cost of care in these types of facilities. Eighty-six percent of individuals in RC/AL pay for their care from their personal resources, but there is some assistance for low-income individuals through Medicaid and state programs of waivers. Private and long-term care insurance may also cover some costs (Assisted Living Federation of America, 2013). The rates charged and the services those rates include vary considerably, as do regulations and licensing.

Assisted living. A popular type of RC/AL is assisted living facilities (ALFs), also called *board and care homes* or *adult congregate living facilities*. Assisted living is a residential long-term care choice for older adults who need more than an independent living environment but do not need the 24 hours/day skilled nursing care and the constant monitoring of a nursing home. There are 51,367 assisted living facilities in the United States. Box 32-7 presents information about the typical assisted living resident. Assisted living settings may be a shared room or a single-occupancy unit with a private bath, kitchenette, and communal meals. They all provide some support services.

BOX 32-7   Profile of a Resident in an Assisted Living Facility

- 86.9 years old
- Female (74%)
- Needs help with 2-3 activities of daily living
- 87% need help with meal preparation
- 81% need help managing medications
- 45% to 67% have Alzheimer's disease or other dementia types of diagnoses
- Length of stay: 22 months
- 59% move to a nursing facility
- 33% die while a resident of an assisted living facility

Assisted living is more expensive than independent living and less costly than skilled nursing home care, but it is not inexpensive (Table 32-1). Costs vary by geographical region, size of the unit, and relative luxury. Most ALFs offer two or three meals per day, light weekly housekeeping, and laundry services, as well as optional social activities. Each added service increases the cost of the setting but also allows for individuals with resources to remain in the setting longer, as functional abilities decline. Consumers are advised to inquire as to exactly what services will be provided and by whom if an ALF resident becomes more frail and needs more intensive care.

Many seniors and their families prefer ALFs to nursing homes because they cost less, are more homelike, and offer more opportunities for control, independence, and privacy. However, many residents of ALFs have chronic care needs and over time may require more care than the facility is able to provide. Services (e.g., home health, hospice, homemakers) can be brought into the facility, but some question whether this adequately substitutes for 24-hour supervision by registered nurses (RNs). Not all states require a nurse in assisted living facilities, but between 47% and 70% of these settings employ an RN or licensed practical nurse (LPN)/licensed vocational nurse (LVN). RNs may oversee care at a single site or oversee care to multiple settings. LPN/LVNs may coordinate clinical care as a health supervisor or manager. In the ALF, there is no organized team of providers such as that found in nursing homes (i.e., nurses, social workers, rehabilitation therapists, pharmacists).

With the growing numbers of older adults with dementia residing in ALFs, many are establishing dementia-specific units. It is important to investigate services available, as well as staff training when making decisions as to the most appropriate placement for older adults with dementia. Continued research is needed on best care practices and outcomes of care for people with dementia in both ALFs and nursing homes. The Alzheimer's Association has issued a set of dementia care practices for ALFs and nursing homes (Alzheimer's Association, 2009).

The Joint Commission and the Commission for Accreditation of Rehabilitation Facilities have published standards for accreditation of ALFs, but many are advocating for more comprehensive federal and state standards and regulations. The nonmedical nature of ALFs is a primary factor in keeping costs more reasonable than those in nursing facilities, but costs are still high for those without adequate funds. Appropriate standards of care must be developed, and care outcomes monitored to ensure that residents are receiving quality care in this setting, which is almost devoid of professional nursing. Further research is needed on care outcomes of residents in ALFs and the role of unlicensed assistive personnel, as well as RNs, in these facilities (Kaskie et al, 2015).

Advanced practice gerontological nurses are well suited to the role of primary care provider in ALFs, and many have assumed this role. The American Assisted Living Nurses Association has established a certification mechanism for nurses working in these facilities and has also developed a *Scope and Standards of Assisted Living Nursing Practice for Registered Nurses*. The Assisted Living Federation of America and the National Center for Assisted Living provide a consumer guide for choosing an assisted living residence (see Box 32-6).

Skilled Nursing Facilities (Nursing Homes)

Nursing homes are the settings for the delivery of around-the-clock care for those needing specialized care that cannot be provided elsewhere. Nursing homes are a complex health care setting that is a mix of hospital, rehabilitation facility, hospice, and dementia-specific units, and they are a final home for many elders. When used appropriately, nursing homes fill an important need for families and elders.

Characteristics of Nursing Homes

The settings called *nursing homes* or *nursing facilities* most often include up to two levels of care: a *skilled nursing care* (also called *subacute care*) facility is required to have licensed professionals with a focus on the management of complex medical needs; and a *chronic care* (also called *long-term* or *custodial*) facility is required to have 24-hour personal assistance that is supervised and augmented by professional and licensed nurses. Often, both kinds of services are provided in one facility. There are approximately 15,700 certified nursing homes in the United States, and 1.3 million older adults reside in nursing homes (Harris-Kojetin et al, 2013). Nursing home residents represent the most frail of all older adults. Their needs for 24-hour care could not be met in the home or residential care setting or may have exceeded what the family was able to provide.

The majority of nursing homes are for-profit organizations, and nursing home chains own over half of all nursing homes (Harrington et al, 2012). The number of nursing home beds is decreasing in the United States as a result of the increased use of residential care facilities and more reimbursement by Medicaid programs for community-based care alternatives. However, in most areas of the country, the supply and use of nursing homes is still greater than those of other long-term care service options (Harris-Kojetin et al, 2013) (see Table 32-1).

Subacute Care (Short-Term)

Subacute care is more intensive than traditional nursing home care and several times more costly, but far less costly than care in a hospital. Skilled nursing facilities are the most frequent site of postacute care in the United States. The expectation is that the patient will be discharged home or to a less intensive setting. Length of stay is usually no more than 1 to 3 months. In addition

to skilled nursing care, rehabilitation services are an essential component of subacute units. Length of stay is usually less than 1 month and is largely reimbursed by Medicare. Patients in subacute units are usually younger and less likely to be cognitively impaired than those in traditional nursing home care. Generally, higher levels of professional staffing are found in the subacute setting than those in the traditional nursing home setting because of the acuity of the patient's condition (Chapter 2).

Chronic Care (Long-Term)

Nursing homes also care for patients who may not need the intense care provided in subacute units but still need ongoing 24-hour care. This may include individuals with severe strokes, dementia, or Parkinson's disease, and those receiving hospice care. Residents of long-term facilities are predominantly women, 80 years or older, widowed, and dependent in ADLs and instrumental activities of daily living (IADLs). About 50% of residents in nursing homes are cognitively impaired, and nursing homes are increasingly caring for people at the end of life. Twenty-three percent of Americans die in nursing homes, and this figure is expected to increase to 40% by 2040 (Agency for Healthcare Quality and Research, 2011; Teno et al, 2013). While the percentage of older people living in nursing homes at any given time is low (4% to 5%), those who live to age 85 will have a 1 in 2 chance of spending some time in a nursing home. This could be for subacute care, ongoing long-term care, or end-of-life care.

Interprofessional Team Model in Subacute and Long-Term Care

An interprofessional team, working with the resident and family, assesses, plans, and implements care in nursing homes and all facilities that provide rehabilitation and restorative programs (Box 32-8). Rehabilitation and restorative care is increasingly important in light of shortened hospital stays that may occur before conditions are stabilized and the older adult is not ready to function independently. The opportunity to work collaboratively with a team is one of the most exciting aspects of practice in long-term care facilities.

Professional Nursing in Long-Term Care

There are a wide range of opportunities for professional nursing in nursing homes (Chapter 2). The American Health Care

---

BOX 32-8   Interprofessional Teams in Nursing Homes

Patient
Family/significant others
Nurse
Primary care provider: physician, nurse practitioner
Physical, occupational, speech therapists
Social worker
Dietitian
Discharge planner/case manager
Psychologist
Prosthetist and orthotist
Audiologist

Association (2010) predicts a 41% increase in the need for RNs in long-term care between 2000 and 2020. The setting "provides abundant opportunities for transformative learning and practice in areas that are core to 21st century nursing: managing chronic illness and palliative care in ways that are patient-centered and evidence-based, working with interdisciplinary teams, supervising unlicensed caregivers, and developing systems for quality improvement" (Cartwright, 2010, p. 243). Professional nursing practice in this setting is different from acute care in terms of competencies, focus, and goals of care. Nursing education programs and facility orientation and training programs must prepare nurses to practice competently in this important and growing care setting (Box 32-9).

Nursing homes are often blamed for all of the societal problems associated with the aging of our population. Daily, millions of dedicated caregivers in nursing homes are providing competent and compassionate care to very sick older people against great odds, such as a lack of support, inadequate salaries and staff, inadequate funding, and a lack of respect. It is time for their stories to be told, and it is time to recognize their needs for adequate and well-trained staff to do this very important work. Although there are continued challenges and opportunities to improve care in nursing homes (and care in all settings for older adults) and in the fabric of the long-term care system, many nursing homes provide an environment that truly represents the best of caring and quality of life.

We agree with Eliopoulos (2010), who states: "The many positive aspects of nursing in long-term care facilities are often overshadowed by an uncomplimentary image of care in this setting, influenced by a history laden with scandals and the media's readiness to highlight the abuses and substandard conditions demonstrated by a small minority. This negative image is compounded by reimbursement policies that significantly limit the ability to provide high-quality care" (p. 365).

More RN direct-care time per resident in nursing facilities is associated with fewer pressure ulcers, fewer hospitalizations, fewer urinary tract infections, less weight loss, fewer catheterizations, and less deterioration in the ability to perform ADLs (Horn et al, 2005). Total nursing staffing and RN staffing levels are predictors of nursing home quality and are negatively associated with total deficiencies, quality of care deficiencies, and serious deficiencies that may cause harm or jeopardy to nursing homes residents (Horn et al, 2005; Kim et al, 2009; Spillsbury et al, 2011). The use of nurse practitioners in nursing homes is also associated with improved patient outcomes and satisfaction (Chapter 2).

Despite the evidence of improved outcomes associated with professional nurse presence in nursing homes, federal requirements require only one RN in the nursing facility for 8 hours a day, a figure quite shocking considering the ratio of RNs to patients in acute care, even in the face of shortages in this setting. Federal regulations require adequate staffing to meet the needs of the residents, and most nursing homes go beyond this minimal RN staffing, particularly in subacute units. However, the federal government has not acted to mandate increases in minimum RN staffing requirements. Many groups dealing with issues of the aging, as well as the ANA, have supported the

BOX 32-9   RESEARCH HIGHLIGHTS

Comparing Long-Term Care Nursing Work with Intensive Care Unit Nursing Work

A pilot study (Leppa, 2004) was conducted to explore the nature of nursing work in LTC nursing home environments (subacute, Medicare, dementia units) and to compare it with the nature of nursing work in ICU environments, using the Leatt Measure of Nursing Technology (Leatt and Schneck, 1981). This instrument operationalizes and measures the nature of nursing work in terms of uncertainty (percentage of patients with more than one diagnosis and with complex nursing problems and how much nursing intuition or judgment is required in providing care); variability (percentage of patients with similar health problems in the unit and the variety of nursing techniques used); and instability (percentage of patients requiring frequent observation and care or specialized monitoring and potential emergency situations).

Findings suggest that the nature of work in LTC and ICU environments is comparable in terms of work uncertainty, variability, and instability. Long-term care nursing scores for uncertainty and variability in nursing work were as high as ICU scores. The LTC respondents emphasized the complexity of the medical and psychosocial needs of their patients and families as one theme in the nature of their work. In LTC, nurses must attend to the needs of both individual patients and the wider community. They must grasp how other patients, family members, and nursing staff are affected by the care provided, especially in the dementia units. Respondents discussed the fragility of their patients, the importance of knowing their patterns, and the need for astute observational skills to detect subtle alterations that could indicate a change in physiology.

ICU care and LTC require different nursing skills, judgment, and knowledge, but the results of this study suggest that the work of nurses in LTC is as complex and demanding as ICU nursing work and that there are many similarities in terms of uncertainty and nursing judgment, patient variability, and instability. LTC nursing work is performed on multiple levels (individual, family, patient groups, and patient–nursing assistant groups) across the continuum of care (rehabilitation, subacute, custodial, and palliative) and presents a wide variety of opportunities for student learning and professional nursing practice. "The ICU work environment is a biomedically intensive environment and the LTC nursing environment is a nursing intensive environment...highly autonomous and centered on nursing care" (Leppa, 2004, p. 32).

Further study is needed to explore the breadth of nursing work in LTC from the perspective of LTC nurses and patients. A better understanding of the complexities of this type of nursing work may help attract more students and nurses to this specialty. LTC nursing work is challenging and highly autonomous, requires specialized knowledge and skills, and should be seen as different, not as "less than" because it does not involve as much medical technology.

ICU, Intensive care unit; *LTC,* long-term care.
Data from Leppa CJ: The nature of long-term care nursing work, *J Gerontol Nurs* 30:26–33, 2004.

critical need for adequate staffing in nursing homes. An expert panel on nursing home care convened by the John A. Hartford Institute for Geriatric Nursing (Harrington et al, 2000) provided comprehensive recommendations for improved RN staffing and increased gerontological nursing education requirements for all staff (Box 32-10). Continued research on new models of care delivery and the appropriate mix of all levels of nursing staff in subacute and long-term units is needed to improve outcomes.

Nursing Assistants

Although it is important to promote professional nursing care for all elders, nursing assistants provide the majority of direct

---

BOX 32-10   Expert Panel Recommendations: Professional Nursing in Nursing Homes

Bachelor of science in nursing (BSN) degree for directors of nursing
Increased staffing ratios for RNs, LPNs, and nursing assistants
Most nursing homes should have a full-time CNS or GNP on staff

Source: Harrington C, Kovner C, Mezey M, et al: Experts recommend minimum staffing standards for nursing facilities in the United States, *Gerontologist* 40(1):5–16, 2000.

---

care in nursing homes and significantly contribute to the quality of life for residents. Research results support the deep commitment and passion that nursing assistants bring to their jobs as they "struggle to find and maintain a balance between the task-oriented needs of residents (e.g., bathing, toileting, feeding) and develop relationships and building community" (Carpenter and Thompson, 2008, p. 31). The significance and importance of close personal relationships between nursing assistants and residents, often described as "like family," is emerging as a central dimension of quality of care and positive outcomes (Bowers et al, 2000, 2003; Bradshaw et al, 2012; Carpenter and Thompson, 2008; Ersek et al, 2000; Fisher and Wallhagen, 2008; Sikma, 2006; Touhy et al, 2005). The commitment and dedication of nursing home staff must be honored and supported. They have much to teach us about aging, nursing, and caring. Box 32-11 presents a description of caring themes expressed by nursing home caregivers.

BOX 32-11   How We Care: Voices of Nursing Home Staff

Responding to What Matters
Taking time to do the little things, competence, cleanliness, meeting basic needs, safe administration of medications, kindness and consideration

Caring as a Way of Expressing Spiritual Commitment
Spiritual beliefs lead staff to long-term care and continue to motivate and guide the special care they give to residents; they reflect a spiritual commitment to caring for residents as expressed in the golden rule: "Do unto others as you would like done to you."

Devotion Inspired by Love for Others
Deep connection between staff and residents described as being like family, caring for residents as you would for your own mother or father, sharing of good and bad times, going out on a limb to be an advocate, listening, and staying with residents when others had given up

Commitment to Creating a Home Environment
Nursing home is the resident's home, staff are guests in the home; the importance of cleanliness, privacy, good food, and feeling part of a family

Coming to Know and Respect Person as Person
Treating residents, families, and one another with respect and dignity, being recognized for the person you are, intimate knowing of likes and dislikes, individualized care

Adapted from Touhy T, Strews W, Brown C: Expressions of caring as lived by nursing home staff, residents, and families, *Int J Human Caring* 9:31, 2005.

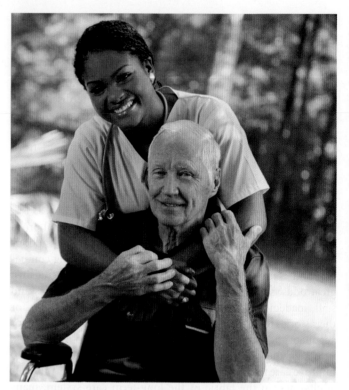

Caring relationships between staff and residents in long-term care enhance quality of care. (©iStock.com/Pamela Moore)

Critical shortages of nursing assistants exist now in residential care facilities, skilled care, and home care, and these shortages will worsen in the future. Recruitment, retention, and high turnover rates are a problem in nursing homes. Several recent studies have investigated the relationship of factors such as turnover, work satisfaction, staffing, and power relations to quality of care and positive outcomes in nursing homes. Results support the importance of developing a culture of respect in which the work of nursing assistants is understood and valued at all levels of the organization. An important nursing role in long-term care is the supervision and education of nursing assistants to enable them to competently perform in their role as an essential member of the care team.

One of the most important components of the culture change movement (discussed later) is the creation of models of care that value and honor the important work of nursing assistants. Culture change must be equally concerned about the needs of residents and the well-being of staff (Thomas and Johansson, 2003). "An organization that learns to give love, respect, dignity, tenderness, and tolerance to all members of the staff will soon find these same virtues being practiced by the staff" (Thomas and Johansson, 2003, p. 3).

Until health care professionals and our society make a real commitment to providing adequate wages, individual supports (e.g., health insurance, education, career ladders), and an appreciation of their significant contribution to quality of nursing home care, these neglected workers cannot be expected to have the energy or incentive to extend themselves to the elders in their care (Kash et al, 2007). Care of the frail elderly and seriously ill persons is labor intensive, is costly, and requires specialized knowledge. Reasonable workloads, enhanced education and training, and adequate reimbursement are essential.

Resident Bill of Rights

Regulations have also been created to protect the rights of the residents of nursing homes. Residents in long-term care facilities have rights under both federal and state laws. The staff of the facility must inform residents of these rights and protect and promote their rights. The rights to which the residents are entitled should be conspicuously posted in the facility (Box 32-12). Also, the Long-Term Care Ombudsman Program is a nationwide effort to support the rights of both the residents and the facilities. In most states, the program provides trained volunteers to investigate rights and quality complaints or conflicts. All reporting is anonymous. Each facility is required to post the name and contact information of the ombudsman assigned to the facility.

QUALITY OF CARE IN SKILLED NURSING FACILITIES

Nursing homes are one of the most highly regulated industries in the United States. The Omnibus Budget Reconciliation Act (OBRA) of 1987 and the frequent revisions and updates are designed to improve the quality of resident care and have had a positive impact. Some of the requirements of OBRA and subsequent legislation include the following: comprehensive resident assessments (Minimum Data Set [MDS]) (Chapter 7), increased training requirements for nursing assistants, elimination of the use of medications and restraints for the

purpose of discipline or convenience, higher staffing requirements for nursing and social work staff, standards for nursing home administrators, and quality assurance activities. The Affordable Care Act (ACA) provided additional legislation to support quality and performance improvement in nursing homes. The Quality Assurance Performance Improvement (QAPI) requires all nursing homes participating in Medicare or Medicaid programs to implement a QAPI program to assess quality of care provided to residents and to improve outcomes (see Box 32-6). CMS has activities under way with regard to pay-for-performance based on quality indicators for both the nursing home and the home health settings. Box 32-13 presents quality measures.

Nursing homes were the first to publish on-line quality information, which is now available for hospitals and other health care organizations. In 2007 CMS instituted the skilled nursing facility scorecard, known as Nursing Home Compare, which provides a 5-star rating system for ranking all licensed facilities. Nursing Home Compare helps professionals, consumers and their families, and caregivers to compare nursing homes (www.medicare.gov/NHCompare). This rating system is based on the nursing home's most recent health inspection (highest weight), staffing, and quality measures.

In 2015 an additional quality measure for use of antipsychotic medication in short-stay and long-stay residents who do not have a diagnosis of schizophrenia, Huntington's disease, or Tourette syndrome was added to the 5-star rating system. This change supports the national goal of reducing inappropriate prescribing of antipsychotics in long-term care by 30% by the end of calendar year 2016. Additionally, algorithms to more

---

BOX 32-12   Bill of Rights for Long-Term Care Residents

- The right to voice grievances and have them remedied
- The right to information about health conditions and treatments and to participate in one's own care to the greatest extent possible
- The right to choose one's own health care providers and to speak privately with one's health care providers
- The right to consent to or refuse all aspects of care and treatments
- The right to manage one's own finances, if capable, or to choose one's own financial advisor
- The right to be transferred or discharged only for appropriate reasons
- The right to be free from all forms of abuse
- The right to be free from all forms of restraint to the extent compatible with safety
- The right to privacy and confidentiality concerning one's person, personal information, and medical information
- The right to be treated with dignity, consideration, and respect in keeping with one's individuality
- The right to immediate visitation and access at any time for family, health care providers, and legal advisors; the right to reasonable visitation and access for others

Note: This list of rights is a sampling of federal and several states' lists of rights of residents or participants in long-term care. Nurses should check the rules of their own state for specific rights in law for that state.

BOX 32-13   Quality Measures for Nursing Homes

Percent of Short-Stay Residents

Self-report moderate to severe pain
Have pressure ulcers that are new or worsened
Assessed and appropriately given seasonal influenza and pneumococcal vaccines
Have newly received antipsychotic medications

Percent of Long-Term Residents

Experienced one or more falls with major injury
Self-report moderate to severe pain
Have pressure ulcers (those at high risk)
Assessed and appropriately given seasonal influenza and pneumococcal vaccines
Have lost control of their bowels or bladder (those at low risk)
Have a catheter inserted and left in their bladder
Physically restrained
Help with activities of daily living has increased
Lost too much weight
Have depressive symptoms
Receive an antipsychotic medication

Source: Centers for Medicare and Medicaid Services: *Quality measures,* 2014. http://www.cms.gov/Medicare/Quality-Initiatives-Patient-Assessment-Instruments/NursingHomeQualityInits/NHQIQuality Measures.html Accessed December 1, 2014.

accurately reflect staffing levels were adjusted (Annals of Long-Term Care, 2015). Quality of care in skilled nursing homes is improving. In skilled nursing facilities nationwide, the average performance has improved in 12 of the 15 reported clinical outcome quality measures over the past 5 years and the percentage of facilities receiving an overall rating of 4 or 5 stars has increased to 43% of facilities (American Health Care Association, 2013). Advanced practice nurses, either on-site or in consultation, are linked to improved quality of care in nursing homes (Dyck et al, 2014).

Advancing Excellence in America's Nursing Homes

Another quality improvement initiative is the Advancing Excellence in America's Nursing Homes. This is an ongoing, voluntary campaign to help nursing homes achieve measurable improvement in the quality of care and quality of life for residents and staff. The campaign works with CMS to identify national goals for improvement and publish free downloadable quality improvement (QI) resources. There have been significant improvements nationally in some of the CMS quality measures since the campaign began. Restraint use has shown the greatest improvement, but the presence of pain and pressure ulcers has also shown improvement (Bakerjian and Zisberg, 2013).

Improving Quality of Transitional Care in Nursing Homes

Transitional care is discussed in depth in Chapter 2, but some further information related to improving the quality of transitional care in nursing homes is presented in this section. Most current models of transitional care focus on care transitions from hospital to home, but increasing attention is being directed to other types of transitions such as hospital to nursing home and nursing home, to hospital. Providing a seamless continuum of care through improved coordination of acute care, post-acute care, and long-term care services and including better management of transitions between care settings are essential in health care today to address both cost and quality issues.

One of four individuals admitted to post-acute care in skilled nursing facilities was rehospitalized within 30 days and up to 67% of these readmissions may have been either preventable, futile, or directly related to diagnoses that could have been treated in the nursing homes. The cost of these avoidable admissions has been estimated as high as $4 billion annually. In addition to cost, hospitalization of nursing home residents potentially causes harm, both mentally and physically, to the resident and increases stress for the family/significant others. Hospital admission also puts the individual at risk for iatrogenic adverse events and medical errors (Mor et al, 2014; Ouslander et al, 2010). Penalties are already imposed on hospitals for avoidable readmissions, and it is expected that these penalties will also be instituted for skilled nursing facilities with high rates of preventable hospital readmissions starting in 2017 (Medicare News Digest, 2013).

QAPI program improvement requirements under the Affordable Care Act include attention to improving transitional care processes and effectively managing acute changes in an individual's condition while in the nursing home. Components

of transitional care models and best practices in transitional care are presented in Chapter 2. Interventions to Reduce Acute Care Transfers (INTERACT) is an exemplar program for reducing the frequency of transfers to the acute hospital from nursing homes. INTERACT is a quality improvement program with communication tools, care paths or clinical tools, and advance care planning tools to assist nursing homes in identifying and managing acute changes in condition without hospital transfer when safe and feasible (interact2.net). Other successful interventions include the use of nurse practitioners working in collaborative teams with physicians, standardized admission assessments, palliative care consultations for residents with recurrent hospitalizations, and interprofessional case conferences (Toles et al, 2013).

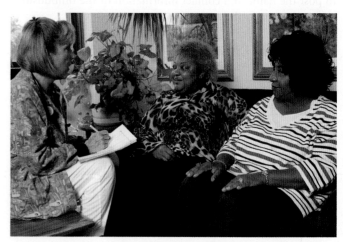

Working with the patient and the caregiver to provide education to enhance self-care abilities and to facilitate linkages to resources is important for the consideration of promoting safe discharges and transitions to home and other care settings. (From Potter PA: *Basic nursing: essentials for practice*, ed 7, St Louis, MO, 2010, Mosby.)

Many health care reform measures such as accountable care organizations, medical (health) homes, bundled payments for an episode of care, and penalties for unnecessary readmissions have led to efforts to improve communication and coordination between hospitals and nursing homes. Many health systems are forming partnerships (often called continuing care networks or CCNs) with skilled nursing facilities offering sub-acute care services. These continuing care networks are intended to improve patient outcomes, decrease unnecessary hospital readmissions, and increase cost-effectiveness. Several Medicare demonstration projects are ongoing as well.

Choosing a Quality Nursing Home

While the national rating system for nursing homes is helpful for evaluating quality, CMS advises consumers to use additional sources of information because the rating system should not substitute for visiting nursing homes since it is a "snap shot" of the care in individual nursing homes (Nazir et al, 2014). The most appropriate method of choosing a nursing home is to personally visit the facility, meet with the director of nursing, observe care routines, discuss the potential resident's needs, and use a format such as the one presented in Box 32-14 to ask questions. CMS provides a nursing home checklist on its website, and the National Citizens' Coalition for Nursing Home Reform also provides resources for choosing a nursing home and understanding quality measures (see Box 32-6). Nurse researchers Marilyn Rantz and Mary Zywgart-Stauffacher (2009) published a book, *How to Find the Best Eldercare*, based on their research.

Nurses play an important role in helping individuals and their family/significant others understand the discharge process and their post hospital needs, particularly if discharge to a skilled nursing facility is planned. CMS recommends that an evaluation of discharge needs to be performed at least 48 hours before discharge, but ideally, discharge planning should begin on admission (Nazir et al, 2014). Patient and family education should include the role of skilled nursing facilities in rehabilitation, role of members of the interprofessional team, interpretation of five-star ratings, and other information on how to choose a facility.

The Culture Change Movement

Across the United States, as well as internationally, the movement to transform nursing homes from the typical medical model into "homes" that nurture quality of life for older people and support and empower frontline caregivers is changing the face of long-term care. Begun by the Pioneer Network, a national not-for-profit organization that serves the culture change movement, many facilities are changing from a rigid institutional approach to one that is person centered. CMS has endorsed culture change and has also released a self-study tool for nursing homes to assess their own progress toward culture change. The Affordable Care Act includes a national demonstration project on culture change to develop best practices and the development of resources and funding to undertake culture change.

Culture change is the "process of moving from a traditional nursing home model—characterized as a system unintentionally designed to foster dependence by keeping residents, as one observer put it, 'well cared for, safe, and powerless'—to a regenerative model that increases residents' autonomy and sense of control" (Brawley, 2007, p. 9). The ultimate vision of culture change is to improve the lives of residents and staff by centering facility's philosophies, organizational structures, environmental designs, and care around practices that support residents' needs and preferences (Hartmann et al, 2013). Older people in need of long-term care want to live in a homelike setting that does not look and function like a hospital. They want a setting that allows them to make decisions they are used to making for themselves, such as when to get up, take a bath, eat, or go to bed.

BOX 32-14   Selecting a Nursing Home

Central Focus
- Residents and families are the central focus of the facility.

Interaction
- Staff members are attentive and caring.
- Staff members listen to what residents say.
- Staff members and residents smile at one another.
- There is a prompt response to resident and family needs.
- Meaningful activities are provided on all shifts to meet individual preferences.
- Residents engage in activities with enjoyment.
- Staff members talk to cognitively impaired residents; cognitively impaired residents are involved in activities designed to meet their needs.
- Staff members do not talk down to residents, talk as if they are not present, ignore yelling or calling out.
- Families are involved in care decisions and daily life in facility.

Milieu
- Calm, active, friendly
- Presence of community, volunteers, children, plants, animals

Environment
- No odor, clean, and well maintained
- Rooms personalized
- Private areas
- Protected outside areas
- Equipment in good repair

Individualized Care
- Restorative programs for ambulation, ADLs
- Residents well dressed and groomed
- Resident and family councils
- Pleasant mealtimes, good food, residents have choices
- Adequate staff to serve meals and assist residents
- Flexible meal schedules, food available 24 hours per day
- Ethnic food preferences available

Staff
- Well trained, high level of professional skill
- Professional in appearance and demeanor
- RNs involved in care decisions and care delivery
- Active staff development programs
- Physicians and advanced practice nurses involved in care planning and staff training
- Adequate staff (more than the minimum required) on each shift
- Low staff turnover

Safety
- Safe walking areas indoors and outdoors
- Monitoring of residents at risk for injury
- Restraint-appropriate care, adequate safety equipment and training on its use

ADLs, Activities of daily living; *RNs,* registered nurses.
Adapted from Rantz MJ, Mehr DR, Popejoy L, et al: Nursing home care quality: a multidimensional theoretical model, *J Nurs Care Qual* 12:30–46, 1998.

They want caregivers who know them and understand and respect their individuality and their preferences. Box 32-15 presents some of the differences between an institution-centered culture and a person-centered culture.

While further research is needed, some results suggest that person-centered care is associated with improved organizational performance, including higher resident and staff satisfaction, better workforce performance, and higher occupancy rates (Alliance for Quality Nursing Home Care and American Health Care Association, 2011; Hartmann et al, 2013). Examples of philosophies and programs of culture change are the Eden Alternative (companion animals, indoor plants, frequent visits by children, involvement with the community), the Green House Project (small homes designed for 10 to 12 residents), and the Wellspring Model. The Eden Alternative is best known for the addition of animals, plants, and children to nursing homes. However, cats and dogs are not the heart of culture change. Truly transforming a nursing home starts at the top and requires involvement of all levels of staff and changes in values, attitudes, structures, and management practices. The principles central to culture change are presented in Box 32-16.

Nurses should take a leadership role in the culture change movement. Box 32-17 presents nursing home cultural change competencies for nurses. The culture change movement is

growing rapidly, and ongoing research is needed to demonstrate costs, benefits, and outcomes (Hartmann et al, 2013; Mueller et al, 2013). Additionally, strategic and cost-efficient methods of assisting nursing homes to implement culture change are needed and will require strong nursing leadership (Eliopoulos, 2013).

◆ PROMOTING HEALTHY AGING: IMPLICATIONS FOR GERONTOLOGICAL NURSING

Nurses play a key role in improving quality of care in nursing homes through evidence-based practice and leadership in quality improvement initiatives. Nursing research has contributed significantly to the evidence-based interventions to improve quality of care in the nursing home. Further research needs to be directed to other LTPAC settings. For

---

BOX 32-16   Principles of Culture Change

- Care and activities are directed by the residents.
- The environment and care practices support a homelike atmosphere.
- Relationships among staff and residents are supported and fostered.
- Increased attention to respect of staff and the value of caring are promoted.
- Staff is empowered to respond to the residents' needs and desires.
- The organizational hierarchy is flattened to support collaborative decision-making for staff.
- Comprehensive and continuous quality improvement underscores all activities and decisions to sustain a person-directed organizational culture.

Adapted from Mueller C, Burger S, Rader J, et al: Nurse competencies for person-directed care in nursing homes, *Geriatr Nurs* 34: 101–104, 2013.

BOX 32-17   Nursing Home Culture Change Competencies for Nurses

Models, teaches, and utilizes effective communication skills such as active listening, giving meaningful feedback, communicating ideas clearly, addressing emotional behaviors, resolving conflict, and understanding the role of diversity in communication.

Creates systems and adapts daily routines and "person-directed" care practices to accommodate resident preferences.

Views self as part of team, not always the leader.

Evaluates the degree to which person-directed care practices exist in the care team and identifies and addresses barriers to person-directed care.

Views the care setting as the residents' home and works to create attributes of home.

Creates a system to maintain consistency of caregivers for residents.

Exhibits leadership characteristics/abilities to promote resident-directed care.

Role models person-directed care.

Problem solves complex medical/psychosocial situations related to resident choice and risk.

Facilitates team members, including residents and families, in shared problem solving, decision-making, and planning.

Source: Mueller C, Burger S, Rader J, et al: Nurse competencies for person-directed care in nursing homes, *Geriatr Nurs* 34:101–104, 2013.

BOX 32-15   Institution-Centered versus Person-Centered Culture

Institution-Centered Culture

- Schedules and routines are designed by the institution and staff, and residents must comply.
- Focus is on tasks that need to be accomplished.
- Rotation of staff among units occurs.
- Decision-making is centralized with little involvement of staff or residents and families.
- There is a hospital environment.
- Structured activities are provided to all residents.
- There is little opportunity for socialization.
- Organization exists for employees rather than residents.
- There is little respect for privacy or individual routines.

Person-Centered Culture

- Emphasis is on relationships between staff and residents.
- Individualized plans of care are based on residents' needs, usual patterns, and desires.
- Staff members have consistent assignments and know the residents' preferences and uniqueness.
- Decision-making is as close to that of the resident as possible.
- Staff members are involved in decisions and plans of care.
- Environment is homelike.
- Meaningful activities and opportunities for socialization are available around the clock.
- There is a sense of community and belonging—"like family."
- There is involvement of the community—children, pets, plants, outings.

Adapted from The Pioneer Network. Available at www.pioneernetwork.net. Accessed August 8, 2008.

many, nursing in long-term care offers the opportunity to practice the full scope of nursing, establish long-term relationships with patients and families, and make a significant difference in patient outcomes. While medical management is important, the need for expert nursing is the most essential service provided.

More and more nursing graduates will practice in LTPAC settings, and education must prepare them for these roles. Health care reform initiatives also offer many new roles for nurses skilled in care across the continuum. Nurses are increasingly recognized as important to improved health outcomes for the individual with long-term care needs.

KEY CONCEPTS

- Long-term care describes a variety of services, including medical and nonmedical care (assistance with ADLs and IADLs), provided on an ongoing basis to people of all ages who have a chronic illness or physical, cognitive, or developmental disabilities.
- Long-term care can be provided informally or formally in a range of environments, from an individual's home to the home of a friend or relative, an adult day health center, independent and assisted living facilities, continuing care retirement communities, skilled nursing facilities, and hospice.
- The total spectrum of health care in the United States care has been expanded to include LTPAC services which include nursing homes, assisted living facilities, home care, and hospice.
- The bulk of long-term care throughout the developed world is informal unpaid care provided by family members. Without family caregivers, the present level of long-term care could not be sustained.
- The number of older people needing long-term services and support is dramatically increasing year after year, and the

challenge of ensuring the quality and financial stability of care provision is one faced by governments in both the developed and the developing world.
- LTC coverage in the U.S. is expensive, fragmented, overly reliant on institutional care, and primarily financed by individuals or their caregivers or by Medicaid.
- Nursing homes are the settings for the delivery of around-the-clock care for those needing specialized care that cannot be provided elsewhere. Nursing homes are a complex health care setting that is a mix of hospital, rehabilitation facility, hospice, and dementia-specific units, and they are a final home for many elders.
- Quality of care in skilled nursing homes is improving. In skilled nursing facilities nationwide, the average performance has improved. Professional nurse staffing results in improved outcomes.
- Culture change in nursing homes is a growing movement to develop models of person-centered care and improve outcomes and quality of life.

NURSING STUDY: TRANSITIONS ACROSS THE CONTINUUM

Ray is 85 years old and was recently admitted to the hospital from his own home following a fall with resultant fracture of the right hip. He was brought to the hospital by paramedics after a neighbor checked on him because they had not heard any sounds from his apartment. He had been lying on the floor for 8 hours unable to call for help. He lives alone in a one-bedroom condominium. His wife of 50 years died 4 years ago. His three adult children and their families live out of state but keep in close contact with their father and visit several times a year. The last time they saw their father was 4 months before his hospitalization.

Before the hip fracture, Ray was fairly capable of taking care of himself but since the death of his wife, his memory and mood have declined. He is hard of hearing in both ears but often refuses to wear his hearing aids, claiming that they distort all sounds and are a bother. He only occasionally left his apartment and had lost a great deal of weight. His neighbors reported that he was falling frequently and there were repeated calls to 911 for assistance. He had several "fender-benders" and had limited his driving to shopping and church. His children were becoming increasingly worried about him living alone. He refused to consider moving to live nearer or with his children or to an assisted living facility. He did not want to be a bother to his children. His home is full of family pictures, pictures from his worldwide travels with his wife, memorabilia from his days as a police officer, and antique furniture. He has a little dog who gives him great enjoyment.

Following a surgical repair of his fractured hip, he experienced delirium and his mental status declined. He received physical therapy but had difficulty following the orders for partial weight bearing on the affected leg. He became incontinent

and required an adult brief. He also developed a necrotic pressure ulcer on his right heel. The hospital case manager recommended to the family that he be transferred to a skilled nursing facility for further rehabilitation, treatment of the pressure ulcer, and possible long-term care placement. It was felt that he could not return safely to his home because of his mental status and functional decline. His finances were limited, so a home that accepted both Medicare and Medicaid was recommended.

Even though the family had promised their father that they would never put him in a nursing home and felt terrible, they agreed with the decision and felt relieved that he would not be living alone. Worried that he would be upset, they decided not to tell him that he would not be going home. They decided to sell his apartment to provide some money for his nursing home care. The children divided the furniture and memorabilia between them and sold the remaining household items. They chose not to tell him that they had done this and when he asked, they said: "When you get better, then you can go home." Ray's mental status continued to decline. He was unable to walk independently, experienced weight loss and sleep problems, and became more withdrawn.

Based on the case study, develop a nursing care plan using the following procedure*:
- List Ray's and the family comments that provide subjective data.
- List information that provides objective data.
- From these data, identify and state, using an accepted format, two nursing diagnoses you determine are most significant to Ray at this time. List two of Ray's strengths that you have identified from the data.

Continued

- Determine and state outcome criteria for each diagnosis. These must reflect some alleviation of the problem identified in the nursing diagnosis and must be stated in concrete and measurable terms.
- Plan and state one or more interventions for each diagnosed problem. Provide specific documentation of the source used to determine the

appropriate intervention. Plan at least one intervention that incorporates Ray's strengths.
- Evaluate the success of the interventions. Interventions must correlate directly with the stated outcome criteria to measure the outcome success.

*Students are advised to refer to their nursing diagnosis text and identify possible or potential problems.

CRITICAL THINKING QUESTIONS AND ACTIVITIES

1. If you were in the role of a hospital case manager, how might you have helped this family with the discharge decision?
2. Would Ray be appropriate for an assisted living facility upon discharge from the hospital? Why or why not? What services would need to be in place for him to be discharged to an assisted living facility? How would he pay for these services?
3. Would Ray be appropriate for discharge home following hospitalization? What would home health provide under Medicare? What other services might he need? How would he pay for these services?
4. What type of interventions might you have implemented to enhance Ray's adjustment to the nursing home?
5. What are some of the obstacles that families of older people face when their loved one needs a great deal of care? Do you

think that families should provide the care rather than placing loved ones with 24-hour care needs in nursing homes? If this was your family, what challenges might present in providing 24-hour care for a loved one?
6. Would you be willing to pay more taxes or be required to purchase long-term care insurance to pay for long-term care? Do you think individuals should be responsible for paying for their own long-term care needs?
7. Would you consider nursing practice in long-term care? Why or why not? What can education programs do to more adequately prepare students for practice in LTC and encourage them to consider working in these settings?

RESEARCH QUESTIONS

1. What are the experiences of older people seeking care assistance to remain in their own homes?
2. What are the differences in the characteristics of residents of ALFs and nursing homes?
3. How do outcomes of care differ for older people living in ALFs and nursing homes?
4. What are the best practice approaches to the provision of long-term care for older people?

5. How do younger and older people in different countries feel about increased taxes for government support of long-term care?
6. Are younger people preparing for their future long-term care needs?
7. What is the relationship between a culture change model and care outcomes in nursing homes?
8. How does the role of the professional nurse differ between acute and long-term care?

REFERENCES

Agency for Healthcare Research and Quality: *Comparison of characteristics of nursing homes and other residential long-term care settings for people with dementia,* 2011. http://effectivehealthcare.ahrq.gov/index.cfm/search-for-guides-reviews-and-reports/?pageaction=displayproduct&productid=832. Accessed September 2014.

Alliance for Quality Nursing Home Care and American Health Care Association: *2011 Annual quality report: a comprehensive report on the quality of care in America's nursing homes and rehabilitation facilities,* 2011. http://www.ahcancal.org/quality_improvement/Documents/2011QualityReport.pdf. Accessed September 2014.

Alzheimer's Association: *Dementia care practice: recommendations for assisted living residences and nursing homes,* 2009. http://www.alz.org/national/documents/brochure_DCPRphases1n2.pdf. Accessed September 2014.

American Health Care Association: *U.S. long-term care workforce at a glance,* 2010. http://www.ahcancal.org/research_data/staffing/Documents/WorkforceAtAGlance.pdf. Accessed September 2014.

American Health Care Association: *2013 Quality report, Washington, DC,* 2013, American Healthcare Association. http://www.ahcancal.org/qualityreport/Documents/AHCA_2013QR_ONLINE.pdf. Accessed September 2014.

Annals of Long-Term Care: *Prepping for Nursing Home Compare 3.0: what are the changes and how will they affect practice?* http://www.annalsoflongtermcare.com/content/prepping-nursing-home-compare-30-what-are-changes-and-how-will-they-affect-practice. Accessed February 2015.

Applebaum R, Bardo A, Robbins E: International approaches to long-term services and supports, *Generations* 37(1):59–65, 2013.

Assisted Living Federation of America: *Assisted living,* 2013. http://www.alfa.org/alfa/Assisted_Living_Information.asp. Accessed September 2014.

Bakerjian D, Zisberg A: Applying the Advancing Excellence in America's Nursing

Homes Circle of Success to improving and sustaining quality, *Geriatr Nurs* 34: 402–411, 2013.

Beeber A, Cohen L, Zimmerman S, et al: Differences in assisted living staff perceptions, experience, and attitudes, *J Gerontol Nurs* 40(1):41–49, 2014.

Belli D: *Can Japan serve as a model for U.S. health and long-term care systems? San Francisco*, 2013, American Society on Aging. http://www.asaging.org/blog/can-japan-serve-model-us-health-and-long-term-care-systems. Accessed November 2014.

Bowers BJ, Esmond S, Jacobson N: The relationship between staffing and quality in long-term care facilities: exploring the views of nurse aides, *J Nurs Care Qual* 14:55–64, 2000.

Bowers BJ, Esmond S, Jacobson N: Turnover reinterpreted: CNAs talk about why they leave, *J Gerontol Nurs* 29(3):36-43, 2003.

Bradshaw S, Playford D, Riazi A: Living well in care homes: a systematic review of qualitative studies, *Age Ageing* 41:429-440, 2012.

Brawley E: What culture change is and why an aging nation cares, *Aging Today* 28: 9–10, 2007.

Cartwright J: Opportunities for practice and educational transformations through unlikely partnerships, *J Nurs Educ* 49(5):243–244, 2010.

Colombo F, Llena-Nozel A, Mercia J, et al: *Help wanted? Providing and paying for long-term care*, Paris, 2011, OECD Publishing.

Carpenter J, Thompson SA: CNAs' experiences in the nursing home: "It's in my soul," *J Gerontol Nurs* 34:25–32, 2008.

Dyck M, Schwinderhammer T, Butcher H: Quality improvement in nursing homes, *J Gerontol Nurs* 40(7):21–31, 2014.

Eliopoulos C: *Gerontological nursing*, Philadelphia, 2010, Wolters Kluwer/Lippincott Williams & Wilkins.

Eliopoulos C: Let's open our eyes to the barriers to culture change, *Ann Longterm Care* 21(12):44–45, 2013.

Ersek M, Kraybill B, Hansberry J: Assessing the educational needs and concerns of nursing home staff regarding end-of-life care, *J Gerontol Nurs* 26:16–26, 2000.

Fisher L, Wallhagen M: Day-to-day care. The interplay of CNAs' views of residents and nursing home environments, *J Gerontol Nurs* 34:26–33, 2008.

Frank R: Long-term care financing in the United States: sources and institutions, *Appl Econ Perspect Policy* 34(2):333–345, 2012.

Freundlich N: *Long-term care: what are the issues? (Robert Wood Johnson Foundation issue brief)*, Health Policy Snapshot, 2014. http://www.rwjf.org/en/research-publications/find-rwjf-research/2014/02/long-term-care—what-are-the-issues-.html. Accessed September 2014.

Gleckman H: *Long-term care in the U.S. and the rest of the world*, 2011. http://howardgleckman.com/2011/06/long-term-care-in-the-u-s-and-the-rest-of-the-world. Accessed September 2014.

Golden R, Shier G: What does "care transitions" really mean? *Generations* 36(4): 6–12, 2012–2013.

Harrington C, Kovner C, Mezey M, et al: Experts recommend minimum staffing standards for nursing facilities in the United States, *Gerontologist* 40(1):5–16, 2000.

Harrington C, Olney B, Carrillo H, et al: Nurse staffing and deficiencies in the largest for-profit chains and chains owned by private equity companies, *Health Services Research* 47(1, Part 1): 106–128, 2012.

Harris-Kojetin L, Sengupta M, Park-Lee E, et al: *Long-term care services in the United States*: 2013 overview, Hyattsville, MD, 2013, National Center for Health Statistics.

Hartmann C, Snow A, Allen R, et al: A conceptual model for culture change evaluation in nursing homes, *Geriatr Nurs* 34: 388–394, 2013.

Horn S, Buerhas P, Bergstrom N, et al: RN staffing time and outcomes of long-stay nursing home residents, *Am J Nurs* 105(11):58–70, 2005.

Kaiser Family Foundation: *Five key facts about the delivery and financing of long-term services and supports*, 2013. http://kff.org/medicaid/fact-sheet/five-key-facts-about-the-delivery-and-financing-of-long-term-services-and-supports. Accessed September 2014.

Kash B, Castle N, Phillips C: Nursing home spending, staffing and turnover, *Health Care Manage Rev* 43:253–262, 2007.

Kaskie B, Nattinger M, Potter A: Policies to protect persons with dementia in assisted living: Déjà vu all over again? *The Gerontologist* 55(2):199-209, 2015.

Kim H, Kovner C, Harrington C, et al: A panel data analysis of the relationships of nursing home staffing levels and standards of regulatory deficiencies, *J Gerontol B Psychol Sci Soc Sci* 64:269–278, 2009.

Leatt P, Schneck R: Nursing subunit technology: a replication, *Adm Sci Q* 26:225–236, 1981.

Maag S: *CCRCs today: the real deal about retirement communities*, Leading Age, Jan 17, 2012: http://www.leadingage.org/How_to_Respond_to_Media_Inquiries.aspx. Accessed December 1, 2014.

Markkanen P, Abdallah L, Lee J, et al: Long-term care in the United States and Finland: policy and lessons to be learned, *J Gerontol Nurs* 38(12):16–21, 2012.

Medicare News Digest: *Skilled nursing facilities could face readmission penalties*, 2013. http://www.medicarenewsdigest.com/Pages/ExternalArticle.aspx?featured=d47c5396-5643-6f71-bd80-ff0000115b4a. Accessed September 2014.

Mor V, Intrator I, Feng Z, et al: The revolving door of hospitalization from skilled nursing facilities, *Health Aff* 29(1):57–64, 2010.

Mor V, Leone T, Maresso A: *Regulating long-term care: an international comparison*. Cambridge, UK, 2014, Cambridge University Press.

Mueller C, Burger S, Rader J, et al: Nurse competencies for person-directed care in nursing homes, *Geriatr Nurs* 34:101–104, 2013.

National Adult Day Services Association: *About adult day services*, 2014. http://nadsa.org/learn-more/about-adult-day-services. Accessed September 2014.

National PACE Association: *What is PACE?* 2014. http://www.npaonline.org/website/article.asp?id=12&title=Who,_What_and_Where_Is_PACE. Accessed September 2014.

Nazir A, Little M, Arling G: More than just location: helping patients and families select an appropriate skilled nursing facility, *Ann Longterm Care* 22(11), 2014. http://www.annalsoflongtermcare.com/article/more-just-location-helping-patients-and-families-select-appropriate-skilled-nursing-facility. Accessed September 2014.

Okrent D: Long-term care. In *Covering health issues*, ed 6, Chapter 9, Washington, DC, 2012, Alliance for Health Reform. http://www.allhealth.org/sourcebookcontent.asp?CHID=125. Accessed September 2014.

Ouslander J, Lamb G, Perloe M, et al: Potentially avoidable hospitalizations of nursing home residents: frequency, causes, and costs, *J Am Geriatr Soc* 58:627–635, 2010.

Polivka L: The challenge of long-term care, *Next Avenue*, May 21, 2012. http://www.nextavenue.org/article/2012-02/challenge-long-term-care. Accessed September 2014.

Rantz M, Zwygart-Stauffacher M: *How to find the best elder care*, Minneapolis, MN, 2009, Fairview Press.

Reinhard S, Kasner E, Houser A, et al: *Raising expectations, 2014: a state scorecard on long-term services and supports for older adults, people with physical disabilities, and family caregivers,* AARP, Commonwealth Fund, SCAN Foundation, 2014. http://www.longtermscorecard.org. Accessed September 2014.

Sikma S: Staff perceptions of caring: the importance of a supportive environment, *J Gerontol Nurs* 32:22–29, 2006.

Spillsbury K, Hewitt C, Stirk L, et al: The relationship between nurse staffing and quality of care in nursing homes: a systematic review, *Int J Nurs Studies* 48(5):732–750, 2011.

Teno J, Gozato P, Bynum J, et al: Change in end-of-life care Medicare beneficiaries, *JAMA* 309(5):470–477, 2013.

Thomas WH, Johansson C: Elderhood in Eden, *Top Geriatr Rehabil* 19:282–290, 2003.

Toles M, Young H, Ouslander J: Improving care transitions in nursing homes, *Generations*, Jan 31, 2013. http://asaging.org/blog/improving-care-transitions-nursing-homes. Accessed September 2014.

Touhy T, Strews W, Brown C: Expressions of caring as lived by nursing home staff, residents, and families, *Int J Human Caring* 9: 31, 2005.

United States Senate, Commission on Long-Term Care: *Report to the Congress,* September 13, 2013. http://www.gpo.gov/fdsys/pkg/GPO-LTCCOMMISSION/content-detail.html. Accessed September 2014.

Zhan H: Population aging and long-term care in China, *Generations* 37(1):53–57, 2013.

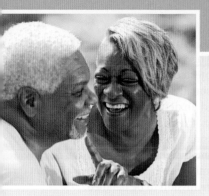

CHAPTER **33**

Intimacy and Sexuality

Theris A. Touhy

http://evolve.elsevier.com/Touhy/TwdHlthAging

A STUDENT SPEAKS

I'm sorry but I cannot imagine my grandparents having sexual intercourse or being interested in information about sexual health. I never thought much about sexuality and older people but, I must say, I do hope that I will have a fulfilling sexual life when I am old.

Jennifer, age 21

AN ELDER SPEAKS

These early morning hours are terribly lonely ... that's when I have such a longing for someone who loves me to be there just to touch and hold me ... and to talk to.

Sister Marilyn Schwab
From Schwab M: A gift freely given: the personal journal of Sister Marilyn Schwab, Mt Angel, Ore.,
1986, Benedictine Sisters.

LEARNING OBJECTIVES

On completion of this chapter, the reader will be able to:

1. Discuss touch and intimacy as integral components of sexuality.
2. Discuss the physiological, social, and psychological factors that affect sexual function as people age.
3. Identify the effects of illness on sexual function and adaptations to enhance sexual health.
4. Describe the various approaches to sexuality assessment that may reduce nurse-client anxiety in discussing a sensitive area.
5. Discuss challenges related to intimacy and sexuality for individuals with dementia and those residing in long-term care facilities.
6. Discuss the rising incidence of HIV/AIDS and sexually transmitted illnesses among older individuals and interventions to promote safe practices.
7. Develop a plan of care for an elder to promote sexual health.

TOUCH

Touch is the first of our senses to develop and provides us with our most fundamental means of contact with the external world (Gallace and Spence, 2010). It is the oldest, most important, and most neglected of our senses. Touch is 10 times stronger than verbal or emotional contact. All other senses have an organ on which to focus, but touch is everywhere. Touch is unique because it frequently combines with other senses. An individual can survive without one or more of the other senses, but no one can survive and live in any degree of comfort without touch.

In the absence of touching or being touched, people of all ages can become sick and become touch starved. "Touch is experienced physically as a sensation, as well as affectively as emotion and behavior (Mammarella et al, 2012). The interaction of

touch affects the autonomic, reticular, and limbic systems, and thus profoundly affects the emotional drives" (Kim and Buschmann, 2004, p. 35).

The human yearning for physical contact is embedded in our language in such figurative terms as "keep in touch," "handle with care," and "rubbed the wrong way." We will focus on touch as an overt expression of closeness, intimacy, and sexuality. We believe an individual must recognize the power of touch and its intimacy to fully comprehend sexuality. Touch and intimacy are integral parts of sexuality, just as sexuality is expressed through intimacy and touch. Together, touch and intimacy can offer the older adult a sense of well-being. Throughout life, touch provides emotional and sensual knowledge about other individuals—an unending source of information, pleasure, and pain.

445

Response to Touch

The Touch Model proposed by Hollinger and Buschmann (1993) suggests that attitudes toward touch and acceptance of touch affect the behaviors of both caregivers and patients. Two types of touch occur during the nurse-patient relationship: procedural and nonprocedural. Procedural touch (task-oriented or instrumental touch) is physical contact that occurs when a particular task is being performed. Nonprocedural touch (expressive physical touch) does not require a task but is affective and supportive in nature, such as holding a patient's hand.

Everyone has definite feelings, opinions, and comfort with touch based on his or her own life experience. "Individuals learn the boundaries of tactual communication culturally" (Kim and Buschmann, 2004, p. 37). Cultural and religious norms determine the appropriateness and acceptability of touch. For example, touch of any kind between members of the opposite sex outside of the family is strictly forbidden in traditional Muslims. The nurse should ask the person's permission before touching and not assume that a person likes or wants to be touched (Rheaume and Mitty, 2008) (Chapter 4).

Of all health care professionals, nurses have the most frequent opportunities to provide gentle, reassuring, renewing touch. Therapeutic, caring touch by the nurse is a potent healing intervention. It is important that touching be done with respect regarding the person's comfort and with the nurse's intention of providing a comforting and healing modality within the nurse-patient relationship.

Touch Zones

Hall (1969) identifies different categories of touching—expanding or contracting zones around which every individual extends the sensory experience of touching, smelling, hearing, and seeing. The categories of touching include the intimate, vulnerable, consent, and social zones (Figure 33-1). Providing care in the zone of intimacy, which is identified as generally the area within an arm's length of the individual's body and is the

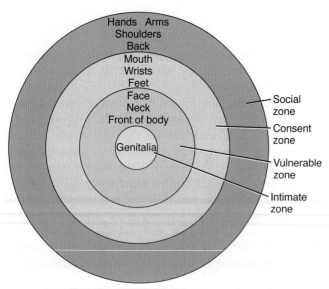

FIGURE 33-1 Zones of Intimacy or Sexuality.

space used for comforting, protecting, and lovemaking, is part of the nurse's function. The vulnerable zone is highly sexually charged and will be protected. The most intimate area, the genitalia, is the most personally protected area of the body and causes the most stress and anxiety when approached, touched, or viewed by the caregiver. The consent zone requires the nurse to seek out or ask permission to touch or initiate procedures to these areas. The social zone includes the areas of the body that are the least sensitive or embarrassing to be touched and that do not necessarily require permission to be handled.

Illness, confinement, and dependency seen in institutionalization are stresses on the intimate zone of touch. Just as caregivers enter a room without knocking, so they often intrude into the intimate circle of touch without asking. A person's need for privacy and personal space is strongly related to acceptance and response to touch. If the need for privacy and distance is great, touch should be used judiciously. The parameters of the intimate zone of touch are examined in this chapter to emphasize the importance of understanding behavior that might occur when the nurse enters this arena.

Touch Deprivation

Montagu (1986) noted that "tactile hunger" becomes more powerful in later life when other sensuous experiences are diminished and direct sexual expression is often no longer possible or available. Furthermore, Montagu believes the cause of illness may be greatly influenced by the quality of tactile support received. Do older people suffer touch deprivation? Many elders may if they are separated from caring others. Older men, in particular, may find it hard to reach out to others for comforting and caring touch. The previous lifestyles of these men often discouraged touch, except in the intimacy of sexual contact, which may no longer be available to them (Montagu, 1986).

Older women are allowed considerably more freedom to touch, although they may lack the opportunity. Studies have shown that older women have reduced access to nonsexual intimacy, such as greeting someone with a hug or kiss or playing or cuddling with a grandchild (Waite et al, 2009). Since older women are more often widowed, reduced access to these other forms of nonsexual intimacy can further deprive them of warm and loving contact.

In the cases of the isolated or institutionalized older person, higher death rates are more related to the quality of human relationships than they are to the degree of cleanliness, nutrition, and physical disabilities on which we focus. Sansone and Schmitt (2000) noted that older people in nursing homes experience touch every day as they are bathed, dressed, toileted, fed, and positioned. The type of touch they desire is not task-oriented touch but "gentle, patient, conscious touch of another person that says to them, 'I'm here, I care, you are important to me.' It's the kind of touch that goes beyond routine and bonds one human being with another" (p. 304).

Adaptation to Touch Deprivation

An outstanding feature of touch according to Ackerman (1995) is that it does not have to be performed by a person or

Hadfield J: The health of grandparents raising grandchildren, *J Gerontol Nurs* 40(4):32–42, 2014.

Hooyman N, Kiyak H: *Social gerontology: a multidisciplinary perspective*, ed 9, Boston, 2011, Allyn & Bacon.

Institute of Medicine: *Retooling for an aging America: building the healthcare workforce*, 2008. http://www.iom.edu/Reports/2008/Retooling-for-an-Aging-America-Building-the-Health-Care-Workforce.aspx. Accessed May 2014.

Jablonski R, Vance D, Beattie E: The invisible elderly: lesbian, gay, bisexual, and transgender older adults, *J Gerontol Nurs* 39(11):46–52, 2013.

Jackson L, Howe N, Tobias P: *The global aging preparedness index*, ed 2, Washington, DC, 2013, Center for Strategic and International Studies. http://csis.org/publication/global-aging-preparedness-index-second-edition. Accessed December 1, 2014.

Keyes K, Pratt C, Galea S, et al: The burden of loss: unexpected death of a loved one and psychiatric disorders across the life course in a national study, *Am J Psychiatry* 171:864–871, 2014.

Korporaal M, van Groenou M, Tilburg T: Health problems and marital satisfaction among older couples, *J Aging Health* 25:1279–1298, 2013.

Kwock T, Wong B, Ip I, et al: Telephone-delivered psychoeducational intervention for Hong Kong Chinese dementia caregivers: a single-blinded randomized controlled trial, *Clin Int Aging* 8:1191–1197, 2013.

Legacy Project: *Grandparents today*, 2014. http://www.tcpnow.com/guides/gptoday.html. Accessed May 2014.

Lindemann E: Symptomatology and management of acute grief, *Am J Psychiatry* 101:141–160, 1944.

Livingston G, Barber J, Rapaport P, et al: Clinical effectiveness of a manual based coping strategy programme (START, STrAtegies for Relatives) in promoting the mental health of careers of family members with dementia: pragmatic randomized controlled trial, *BMJ* 347:6276, 2013. http://dx.doi.org/10.1136/bmj.f6276. Accessed May 2014.

Livingston G, Parker K: *Since the start of the great recession, more children raised by grandparents*, 2010. http://www.pewsocialtrends.org/2010/09/09/since-the-start-of-the-great-recession-more-children-raised-by-grandparents. Accessed May 2014.

Lowenthal MF, Haven C: Interaction and adaptation: intimacy as a critical variable, *Am Sociol Rev* 33:20–30, 1968.

Lund M: Caregiver, take care, *Geriatr Nurs* 26:152–153, 2005.

Lusardi A, Mitchell O: *Financial literacy and planning: implications for retirement wellbeing* (National Bureau of Economic Research [NBER] working paper no. 17078), 2011. http://www.nber.org/papers/w17078. Accessed May 2014.

Mast M: To use or not to use: a literature review of factors that influence family caregivers' use of support services, *J Gerontol Nurs* 39(1):20–28, 2013.

McNamara T, Williamson J: What can other countries teach us about retirement? *Generations* 37(1):33–37, 2013.

Meiner S: *Gerontological nursing*, ed 4, St. Louis, MO, 2011, Mosby.

Messecar D: Family caregiving. In Boltz M, Capezuti E, Fulmer T, et al, editors: *Evidence-based geriatric nursing protocols for best practice*, ed 4, New York, 2012, Springer, pp 469–499.

MetLife: *Report on American grandparents*, New York, 2011, MetLife Mature Market Institute.

Minton M, Barron C: Spousal bereavement assessment: review of bereavement-specific measures, *J Gerontol Nurs* 34:34–48, 2008.

Musil C, Gordon N, Warner C, et al: Grandmothers and caregiving to grandchildren: continuity, change, and outcomes over 24 months, *Gerontologist* 51(1):86–100, 2011.

National Institute on Aging, National Institutes of Health: *Why population aging matters: a global perspective*, 2007. http://www.nia.nih.gov/sites/default/files/WPAM.pdf. Accessed May 2014.

Newell R, Dowd O, Netinho S, et al: Stress among caregivers of chronically ill older adults: implications for nursing practice, *J Gerontol Nurs* 38(9):18–29, 2012.

Ostwald S: Who is caring for the caregiver? Promoting spousal caregiver's health, *Fam Community Health* 32:S5–S14, 2009.

Polivka L: A future out of reach? The growing risk in the U.S. retirement security system, *Generations* 36(2):12–17, 2012.

Robinson B: Validation of a Caregiver Strain Index, *J Gerontol* 38:344–348, 1983.

Ryan A, Taggart L, Truesdale-Kennedy M, et al: Issues in caregiving for older people with intellectual disabilities and their ageing family carers: a review and commentary, *Int J Older People Nurs* 9(3):217–226, 2014.

Schulz R, Beach SR: Caregiving as a risk factor for mortality: the caregiver health effects study, *JAMA* 262:2215–2219, 1999.

Schumacher K, Beck CA, Marren JM: Family caregivers: caring for older adults, working with their families, *Am J Nurs* 106:40–49, 2006.

Services and Advocacy for Gay, Lesbian, Bisexual, and Transgender Elders (SAGE) and Movement Advancement Project: *Improving the lives of LGBT older adults*, 2010. http://www.lgbtmap.org/policy-and-issue-analysis/improving-the-lives-of-lgbt-older-adults. Accessed May 2014.

Shahly V, Chatterji S, Gruber M, et al: Cross-national differences in the prevalence and correlates of burden among older family caregivers in the World Health Organization World Mental Health Surveys, *Psychol Med* 43(4):865–879, 2013.

Silverstein M, Angelli J: Older parents' expectations of moving closer to their children, *J Gerontol B Psychol Sci Soc Sci* 53:S153–S163, 1998.

Smith G, Palmieri P, Hancock G, et al: Custodial grandmothers' psychological distress, dysfunctional parenting, and grandchildren's adjustment, *Int J Aging Hum Dev* 67:327–357, 2008.

Sorrell J: Moving beyond caregiver burden, *J Psychosoc Nurs Ment Health Serv* 52(3):15–18, 2014.

Stanford P, Usita P: Retirement: who is at risk? *Generations* 26:45, 2002.

Taggart L, Truesdale-Kennedy M, Ryan A, et al: Examining the support needs of ageing family carers in developing future plans for a relative with an intellectual disability, *J Intellect Disabil* 18(3):217–234, 2012.

Thompson M: Millions expect to outlive their retirement savings, *CNN Money*, Feb 9, 2013. http://money.cnn.com/2013/02/19/retirement/retirement-savings-report. Accessed May 2014.

Touhy TA: Nurturing hope and spirituality in the nursing home, *Holist Nurs Pract* 15:45–56, 2001.

U.S. Census Bureau: *American families and living arrangements*, 2013. www.census.gov/hhes/families. Accessed May 2014.

Van Etten D, Gautam R: Custodial grandparents raising grandchildren: lack of legal relationship is a barrier for services, *J Gerontol Nurs* 38(6):18–22, 2012.

van Groenou M, Hoogendijk E, van Tilburg T: Continued and new personal relationships in later life: differential effects of health, *J Aging Health* 25:274–295, 2013.

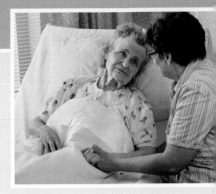

Loss, Death, and Palliative Care

Kathleen Jett

http://evolve.elsevier.com/Touhy/TwdHlthAging

A STUDENT SPEAKS

When I started nursing school I was so afraid that I would have to take care of someone who was dying—or maybe even died! Then I found out that to share the time before death with a person is a special privilege.

Ana, age 20

AN ELDER SPEAKS

When we were in our 60s, my friends and I met over cards, went on trips, and experienced all of the joys of retirement. We didn't have much time to worry about aches and pains. In our 70s we had less time to play because we were busy visiting one another in the hospital or in nursing homes. In our 80s we met frequently again, but it was usually at our friends' funerals, leaving little time for cards or travel. Now that I am in my 90s, hardly any of my friends are still alive; you know it gets kind of lonely, so you just have to make new younger friends!

Theresa, age 93

LEARNING OBJECTIVES

On completion of this chapter, the reader will be able to:

1. Compare and contrast the needs of elders in response to varying types of losses.
2. Differentiate different types of grief and the needs of the griever.
3. Discuss the attributes that are needed by the nurse to provide the highest quality of care to those experiencing loss or death.
4. Discuss the benefits and limitations of the available conceptual frameworks for dying and grieving.
5. Identify aspects of palliative care in which there is a special need to work within the cultural boundaries.
6. Develop interventions that will enhance coping and the reestablishment of equilibrium within the family.
7. Differentiate a living will from DNR orders and explain the roles and responsibilities of the nurse as they relate to each of them.

LOSS, GRIEF, AND BEREAVEMENT

Loss, dying, and death are universal, incontestable events of the human experience. With age, the number of losses increases. Some of these are associated with normal changes, such as the loss of joint flexibility (Chapter 26), and others are related to changes in everyday life and transitions, such as moving and retirement (Chapter 34). Other losses include the loss of loved ones through death or the anticipation of one's own approaching death. Some deaths are considered normative and expected, such as that of older parents, while the death of adult children or grandchildren is always nonnormative and unexpected.

Loss of any kind has the potential to trigger grief and mourning. The terms *grief* and *mourning* and a third term, *bereavement*, are often used interchangeably. It has been suggested that bereavement can be used to refer to the fact that a loss has occurred (Zisook and Shear, 2009). Grief is the response to a loss, and mourning is the outward expression of loss. Mourning is a socially and culturally prescribed behavior following, and around the time of, a loss, especially from death. In many traditions, wearing black is part of mourning behavior. Although there are well-defined rituals in response to loss through death, no guidelines exist for many other losses, such as independent functional ability, the long-time companionship of a pet, or self-concept following a mastectomy.

In later life one loss and its accompanying grief is often superimposed on others. No sooner has the individual begun to grieve for one when another occurs. When the losses accumulate in quick succession, the griever may become incapacitated

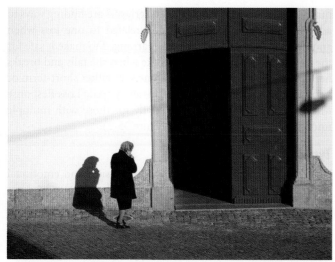

Expressions of Mourning. Funeral on Friday. (©JB55, https://www.flickr.com/photos/jb55/)

and require careful and skilled support and guidance. This phenomenon can lead to a continual state of grieving, known as *bereavement overload*.

This chapter addresses grief as a response to loss, palliative care, and some of the ethical and legal issues surrounding end-of-life decision-making. The purpose of this chapter is to provide gerontological nurses the basic information needed to promote effective grieving and good and appropriate deaths. Loss is considered broadly to include anything that has meaning to the person.

GRIEF WORK

Researchers have tried for years to understand the grieving process *(grief work)*, resulting in a number of models and theories to explain and predict the human response. Pioneer thanatologist (one who studies the dying process) Elisabeth Kübler-Ross is best known for describing what became known as the stages of dying (1969). Other early theorists included Rando (1995), Corr (2000), and the early work of Doka (1989). Each of these authors described successful grieving as movement through predictable stages, phases, or tasks until one eventually was able to "let go" of that which was lost (Hall, 2011). These early

models have strongly influenced how nurses, physicians, other health care professionals, and society in general have thought about grieving and dying.

Newer approaches have described grief work as more of a circular process in which a continued attachment to that which has been lost, at some level, is "normal" (Hall, 2011). Although the theories are intended to describe physical death and related grief, we propose that these same models can serve as a framework for understanding other types of meaningful losses in the lives of older adults.

The Loss Response Model

The Loss Response Model (LRM) is influenced by the systems' work of nurse theorist Dr. Betty Newman (Alward, 2010) and the writing of nurse Barbara Giacquinta (1977), psychiatrist Avery Weisman (1979), and thanatological scholars Doka (2002) and Neimeyer and Sands (2011) (Jett and Jett, 2014). It can be used to improve the understanding of grieving and to assist nurses in caring and comforting those who have experienced, or are experiencing, a loss. A framework is provided from which nursing interventions can be easily developed.

In the Loss Response Model, griever(s) are viewed as part of a system that is striving to maintain equilibrium or stability (Figure 35-1). However, the *impact* of the loss (or the anticipation of it) results in *disequilibrium* or instability within the system. The system is in chaos, the grievers are emotionally and functionally compromised *(functional disruption)*, and it is difficult for them to accomplish their usual activities of daily living (Chapter 7). Common, simple activities, such as dressing, that normally take a few minutes may take much longer. Deciding which clothing to wear may seem too complex a task. Even as the tasks are accomplished, the person may complain of feeling distracted, restless, "at loose ends," and numb (Richardson et al, 2013). Men who complained of numbness have been found to have higher cortisol levels (i.e., indicators of physiologically prolonged stress) than comparative women (Richardson et al, 2013).

Nurses can make a significant contribution to the family in fostering even momentary stability by knowing what questions to ask at the time of death, such as the following: Does the person have a living will or has he or she made personal wishes known for this time? What cultural or familial rituals are important right now? Is there anyone who should be called at this time? Would a spiritual advisor be a support for you right now?

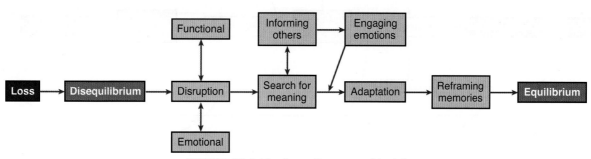

FIGURE 35-1 The Loss Response Model.

Have funeral arrangements already been made? If not, who can help you with this? Parallel questions can be used in the situations of other types of loss.

As the system attempts to stabilize and grievers attempt to make sense of the chaos and integrate the loss into their lives, they *search for meaning*, asking such questions as the following: Why did this happen to us (me)? How will we survive the loss? In reacting to the loss of a child or a grandchild, thoughts of "why wasn't it me?" are common. Searching for meaning is difficult, and as it is done, *others are informed of the loss*. Each time the story is repeated, *emotions are engaged* in ways that are consistent with the griever's culture and personality. While acute grief may be triggered at each telling, the intensity of the sorrow becomes less and the duration shorter. Movement toward a new equilibrium progresses as the person incorporates the loss.

As roles and situations change, *adaptation* is necessary. In the language of the LRM, adaptation is a process in which the system changes in order to survive. For example, when a person is no longer able to do a task due to loss of ability, someone else must step in to perform it; when the elder patriarch dies, it may be a cultural expectation that the eldest son assumes his father's roles and responsibilities.

Finally, if the system is to survive, it must redefine itself. This is accomplished not by forgetting or ignoring the loss but by *reframing memories*. In the case of a death, family portraits and reunions will still be possible, just different from how they were before, and new memories can and will be made. Similarly, if celebrations had always been at the home of the elder (eliciting the sights, smells, and memories of childhood), the elder's move to a nursing home will prevent this custom. Adaptation leads to the development of new memories when the celebrations are held at the home of another, such as that of a child. The system can return to a new but different steady state. The nurse serves as a role model who displays the behavioral qualities of responsiveness, authenticity, commitment, and competence, that is, caring.

However, grieving is not linear, especially in later life. At any point in the movement toward stabilization, new disturbances may lead to renewed instability. The grievers are finding ways to adapt to the functional disruption related to one loss when another occurs. A home has been rearranged to make it safe for the person who has suffered a stroke when she falls and breaks her hip, necessitating a nursing home stay, either short-term or permanent, due to the combined losses. A cyclic Loss Response Model is most appropriate, especially for those with multiple underlying chronic conditions (Figure 35-2).

Types of Grief

Grieving takes enormous amounts of physical and emotional energy. It is the hardest thing anyone can do and may be especially hard for those who are accumulating losses, as one does with aging, or face multiple losses at the same time, such as following a catastrophic event. The most common types of grief are anticipatory, acute, shadow (a type of chronic grief), and complicated. Another type, disenfranchised or unspeakable grief, may be occurring and hidden for one reason or another, but nonetheless can be quite significant.

Anticipatory Grief

Anticipatory grief is the response to a real or perceived loss before it occurs—a dress rehearsal, so to speak. One grieves in preparation for a potential loss, such as the loss of belongings (e.g., selling a home), moving (e.g., into a nursing home), knowing that a body part or function is going to change (e.g., amputation), or in anticipation of the death of a loved one. Behaviors that may signal anticipatory grief include preoccupation with the particular loss, unusually detailed planning, or a sudden change in attitude toward the thing or person to be lost. Some feel more in control of the situation because anticipatory grief facilitates planning and preparation for death by saying goodbyes or preparing for burials if that is accepted in the person's culture. In other cases anticipatory grief leads to declines in spousal health even before the death (Vable et al, 2014).

If the loss is certain but the timing is either uncertain or not occurring as expected, anticipatory grieving may be particularly difficult, not because the loss is desired, but in

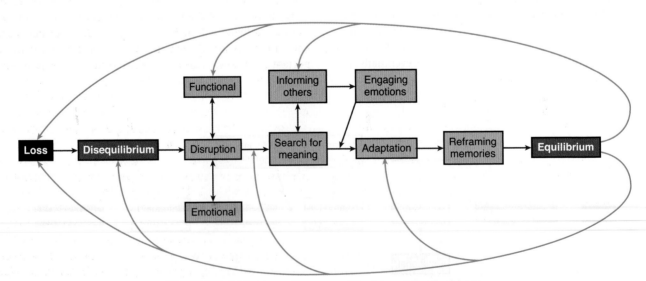

FIGURE 35-2 The Loss Response Model and Cyclical Loss.

response to the emotional ups and downs of the waiting, with the system staying in a state of disequilibrium. Glaser and Strauss (1968) describe this as an *interruption in sentimental order;* no one knows quite how to behave. Family and friends, and nurses as professional grievers, usually deal much more easily with known losses at a known time or in a set manner (Glaser and Strauss, 1968).

Anticipatory grief can also result in the phenomenon of premature detachment from an individual who is dying or detachment of the dying person from others. Pattison (1977) calls the latter *sociological death* and the former *psychological death.* In either case, the person who is dying is no longer involved in day-to-day activities of living and essentially suffers a premature death.

Acute Grief

Acute grief is a crisis. It has a definite syndrome of somatic, functional, and emotional symptoms of distress that occur in waves lasting varying lengths of time during the period of impact. Symptoms may occur every time others are informed of the loss or acknowledged by the self or others in the form of condolences. Preoccupation with the loss is a phenomenon similar to daydreaming and is accompanied by a sense of unreality. Depending on the situation, feelings of self-blame or guilt may be present and manifest themselves as hostility or anger toward friends and family. The intense stress of acute grief may lead to significant declines in physical health and the manifestation of depressive symptoms (Utz et al, 2012). The older adult who is acutely grieving may say things like "If only I had forced him/her to see the doctor sooner!"

Acute grief will be the most intense in the months immediately after the loss and lessen over time. Acute grief is experienced at a national or global level after catastrophic events, such as the 2001 attack on the World Trade Center in New York City or the Ebola Outbreak in 2014.

Shadow Grief

Grieving takes time, but over the months, the intense pain of the acute period of impact lessens as memories are reframed. But the old memories never go away completely. There are often moments of intermittent sadness referred to as *shadow grief* (Horacek, 1991). It may temporarily inhibit some function but is considered a normal response. While most often discussed in the context of perinatal death, a type of shadow death can occur at any age. It may be triggered by anniversary dates (birthdays, holidays, anniversaries) or by sensory stimuli, such as the smell of perfume, a color, or a sound (Carr et al, 2014) (Box 35-1).

People deal with this in many different ways. Each year, hundreds of people visit the Vietnam War Memorial in Washington, DC, to remember and leave items that connect them to those who have died. Similarly, individuals make pilgrimages to the Wailing Wall in Jerusalem, praying and placing prayer papers in the crevices of the wall. In Mexico, the annual holiday called "Day of the Dead" is a time when people visit the graves of their family members, leave food, grieve anew, and feel a renewed sense of connection with those who have died before them.

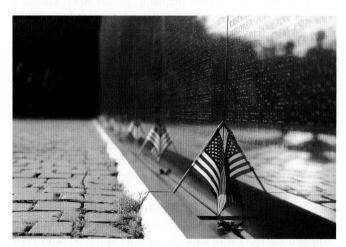

Remembering Those Lost. U.S. flags at the Vietnam Veterans Memorial Wall in Washington, DC. (©Austin Kirk, https://www.flickr.com/photos/aukirk/)

Complicated Grief

Shadow grief is a type of chronic grief that is considered healthy and restorative. Yet for others, the shadows are debilitating. Those who are survivors of major tragedies, war, rape, abuse, and other horrific events are also grieving; the "shadows" are often debilitating and now recognized as posttraumatic stress. This is a form of complicated grief.

Complicated grief also comes in the form of acute grief that does not significantly lessen over the months and even years after the loss. Obstacles of one form or another interfere with the evolution toward the *reestablishment of equilibrium;* stability is elusive. The memories resist being reframed. Issues of guilt, anger, and ambivalence toward the person who has died are factors that will impede the grieving process until these issues are resolved. Reactions are exaggerated and memories are experienced as if they are fresh, over and over again.

Signs of possible complicated grief include excessive yearning and longing, decreased interest in everyday activities, and insomnia that lingers for an extended period of time or surfaces months or years later (Shear et al, 2013). It may trigger a new major depressive episode or cause one to reappear (Goldstein and Morrison, 2014). If the depression is manifested in cognitive difficulties, it may be misinterpreted as dementia, especially in the very frail (Chapter 28). Complicated grief requires the professional intervention of a grief counselor, a psychiatric nurse practitioner, or a psychologist who is skilled in helping grieving elders (Corless, 2006).

Disenfranchised Grief

The person whose loss cannot be openly acknowledged or publicly mourned experiences what is called *disenfranchised* or *unspeakable grief*. The grief is stigmatizing, socially disallowed, or unsupported (Doka, 2002). The death is one that is socially condoned, such as that associated with capital punishment, or when a survivor does not have a socially recognized right to be perceived as a person in bereavement. The relationship is not recognized, the loss is not sanctioned, the griever is not recognized, and public mourning is not acceptable (Doka, 2002; Hall, 2011). Disenfranchised grief frequently occurs when same-sex partnerships or marriages are not acknowledged by the family of the deceased or in secret relationships (e.g., extramarital), in which the griever cannot tell others of the meaning or depth of the attachment. It may follow the death of an estranged family member, death caused by suicide, death due to acquired immunodeficiency syndrome (AIDS), or by families of death row inmates (Beck and Jones, 2007-2008; Jones and Beck, 2007-2008).

The person in late life can experience disenfranchised grief when family or friends do not understand the full meaning of the loss, for example, of a person's retirement, the death of a pet, or gradual losses caused by chronic conditions. Families coping with a member who has Alzheimer's disease may also experience disenfranchised grief when others perceive the death as a "blessing" and fail to support the griever or caregiver who has struggled for years with anticipatory grief and now must cope with the actual death.

Factors Affecting Coping with Loss

To cope effectively with loss is to have the ability to move from a state of chaos, i.e., disequilibrium, and instability to one of stability and equilibrium. It is to find meaning in the loss and be able to find a way to reframe memories. Many factors affect the ability to cope with loss and grief (Box 35-2).

Psychiatrist Avery Weisman described those who are more likely to effectively deal with loss as "good copers"—individuals or families who have successfully navigated through crises in the past (Box 35-3) (1979, pp. 42-43). In other words, they can acknowledge the loss and try to make sense of it. They can maintain composure when necessary, can generally use good judgment, and can remain optimistic and appropriately hopeful without denying the loss. Good copers seek guidance when it is needed.

On the contrary, those who cope less effectively have few, if any, of these abilities. They tend to be more rigid, pessimistic, and demanding. They are more likely to be dogmatic and expect perfection in themselves and others. Ineffective copers are more likely to live alone, socialize little, and have few close friends or have an ineffective support network. They may have a history of mental illness or have guilt, anger, or ambivalence toward the person who has died or that which has been lost. The person is more likely have unresolved past conflicts or be facing the loss at the same time as secondary life stressors. In some cases they will have fewer opportunities as a result of the loss (Chapter 30). They are the elders who are most in need of the expert interventions of grief counselors and skilled, sensitive gerontological nurses.

BOX 35-2 Factors Influencing the Grieving Process

Physical
Number of concurrent medical conditions
Use of sedatives (delays but does not lessen grief)
Nutritional state: if inadequate, reduces the ability to cope or meet demands of daily living; inadequate rest can lead more quickly to mental and physical exhaustion
Exercise: if inadequate, limits emotional outlet; may increase aggressive feelings, tension, and anxiety

Emotional
Unique nature and meaning of loss
Individual coping behavior, personality, and mental health
Individual level of maturity and intelligence
Previous experience with loss or death
Social, cultural, ethnic, religious, or philosophic background
Sex-role conditioning
Immediate circumstances surrounding loss
Timeliness of the loss
Perception of preventability (sudden vs. expected)
Perceived importance of the loss or relationship to that which is lost
Number, type, and quality of secondary losses
Presence of concurrent stresses or crises

Social
Individual support systems and the acceptance of assistance of its members
Individual sociocultural, ethnic, religious, or philosophic background
Educational, economic, and occupational status
Ritual

Modified from Beare PG, Myers JL: *Adult health nursing*, ed 3, St Louis, MO, 1998, Mosby.

BOX 35-3 Identifying Those with Better Coping Skills

- Avoid avoidance.
- Confront realities, and take appropriate action.
- Focus on solutions.
- Redefine problems.
- Consider alternatives.
- Have good communication with others.
- Seek and use constructive help.
- Accept support when offered.
- Can keep up their morale.

From Weisman A: *Coping with cancer,* New York, 1979, McGraw-Hill, pp 42–43.

◆ PROMOTING HEALTHY AGING WHILE GRIEVING: IMPLICATIONS FOR GERONTOLOGICAL NURSING

Loss, grief, and death are parts of the lives of all and occur with increasing frequency with aging. The goal of the gerontological nurse is not to prevent grief but to support those who are coping with grief and facilitate the return of stability to the system each time a new loss occurs. Although the acute emotions associated with the impact of the loss will usually abate, any long-term detrimental effects can be ameliorated. While promoting healthy aging, the nurse works with grieving elders as part of the normal workday; this is both a privilege and a responsibility. It is one of the few areas in nursing in which small actions can make a large difference in the quality of life for the persons to whom we provide care.

◆ Assessment

The goal of the grief assessment is to differentiate those who are likely to cope effectively from those who are less likely so that appropriate interventions can be planned (Box 35-4). A grief assessment is based on knowledge of the grieving process and

"coming to know" the grievers. Data are obtained through observation in the context of culture (Goldstein et al, 2004).

A grief assessment is based on listening to the expression of spiritual or existential concerns and needs and the relationship to that which has been or will be lost. How many other stressful or demanding events or circumstances are going on in the griever's life? How meaningful is the loss? Answers to these questions will help determine the potential intensity of support needed and the risk for complicated grieving.

The nurse determines what stress management techniques are normally used and if they have been helpful (e.g., talking it out) or detrimental (e.g., substance abuse) in the past. Are usual support systems available? Was the griever's identity closely tied to that which is lost, such as a lifelong athlete who is faced with never walking again? If the loss is of a partner, how was the relationship? The loss of an abusive or controlling partner may liberate the survivor, who may feel guilty for not feeling the grief that others expect (Box 35-5). For many older women who depended on their spouses financially, death may leave them impoverished, significantly complicating their grief. A survivor may be suddenly homeless after the loss of a domestic partner in jurisdictions in which such relationships are unrecognized. Knowing more about the loss and its effect on the elder's life will enable the nurse to construct and implement appropriate and caring interventions.

BOX 35-4   Assessment of the Dying Patient and Family

Patient

Age
Gender
Coping styles and abilities
Social, cultural, ethnic background
Previous experience with illness, pain, deterioration, loss, grief
Mental health
Lifestyle
Fulfillment of life goals
Amount of unfinished business
The nature of the illness (death trajectory, problems particular to the illness, treatment, amount of pain)
Time passed since diagnosis
Response to illness
Knowledge about the illness or disease
Acceptance or rejection of the diagnosis
Amount of striving for dependence or independence
Feelings and fears about illness
Location of the patient (home, hospital, nursing home)
Family rules, norms, values, and past experiences that might inhibit grief or interfere with a therapeutic relationship

Family

Developmental stage of the family
Existing subsystems
Geographic proximity of support network
Degree of flexibility or rigidity
Type of communication
Rules, norms, expectations
Values, beliefs
Quality of emotional relationships
Dependence, interdependence, freedom of each member
Closeness or disengaged from the dying member
Established extrafamilial interactions
Strengths and vulnerabilities of the family
Style of leadership and decision-making
Unusual methods of problem solving, crisis resolution
Family resources (personal, financial, community)
Current problems identified by the family
Quality of communication with the caregivers
Immediate and long-range anticipated needs

From Hess PA: Loss, grief, and dying. In Beare P, Myers J: *Adult health nursing*, ed 3, St Louis, MO, 1998, Mosby.

◆ Interventions

Weisman (1979) described the work of health care professionals as "countercoping." Although he was speaking of working with people with cancer, it is equally applicable to working with people who are grieving other losses. "Countercoping is like counterpoint in music, which blends melodies together into a basic harmony. The patient copes; the therapist [nurse] countercopes; together they work out a better fit" (Weisman, 1979, p. 109).

Like good copers, good gerontological nurses must be flexible, practical, resourceful, and abundantly optimistic. Nurses introduce themselves, establish rapport, learn the cultural rules regarding the situation, and explain their roles (e.g., nurse practitioner, charge nurse, staff nurse) and the time they will be available. The nurse fosters the griever's movement from disequilibrium and instability to a new, albeit modified, steady state (Box 35-6).

BOX 35-5   "Now I can buy that blouse I have been wanting!"

Sam and Hannah had been married more than 50 years. During that time Hannah's children often encouraged her to leave Sam since he was consistently psychologically abusive and controlling. In the last couple of years of his life, these qualities intensified so that she was forbidden to purchase only the necessities of life, even with her own money. He died after a prolonged illness, but even before the elaborate funeral expected in her culture, she exclaimed (to those closest to her), "Now I can buy that blouse I have been wanting, and maybe a new couch, too!"

BOX 35-6   TIPS FOR BEST PRACTICE

Helping Grievers Move through the Impact of Loss to the Reestablishment of New Memories

Functional Disruption
- Provide functional assistance

Searching for Meaning
- Provide reliable sources of information (e.g., websites)
- Inform appropriate providers of the person's need for information and make sure they receive it
- Active listening

Engaging Emotions
- "Give permission" to express emotions
- Offer physical presence
- Offer to locate usual sources of support during times of crisis (e.g., minister, tribal elder)
- Active listening

Informing Others
- Offer physical presence
- Active listening

Adaptation
- Identify meaningful events influenced by the loss
- Help find new ways of replacing that which has been lost
- Offer discussions of how the loss has affected life
- Active listening

Reframing Memories
- Offer to discuss mechanisms to develop new memories without denying connection with that or with whom has been lost
- Encourage reminiscence
- Facilitate opportunities for culturally based and desired bereavement rituals
- Assure grievers that stability will return
- Active listening

Impact and Functional Disruption

If it is the time of *impact* (e.g., just after a new serious diagnosis, at the death of a family member, at the time of a move to a care facility), nurses can provide a safe environment ensuring that basic needs, such as meals and rest, are met. At all times, active listening is preferable to giving advice. When listening, the nurse soon discovers that it is not the actual loss that is of utmost concern but, rather, the fear associated with the loss. If the nurse listens carefully to both the stated and the implied expressions, statements such as the following may be heard: "How will I go on?" "What will I do now?" "What will become of me?" "I don't know what to do." "How could he (she) do this to me?" Because the nurse knows that there will be some resolution, such comments may seem exaggerated or melodramatic, but to the one who is grieving, there seems to be no end to the pain. The person who is actively grieving cannot yet look ahead or know that the despair and other feelings will resolve. The nurse can soften the despair by fostering *reasonable and appropriate hope*, such as, "You will make it through one moment at a time, and I will be here to help."

Nurses observe for *functional disruption* and offer support and direction. When the death is imminent or at the time of death, the nurse may have to ask difficult questions, such as the following: Are there any cultural or family rituals that are important at this time? Does the person have a living will? Who is the proxy? Have funeral arrangements been made? Who needs to be notified; does this include a spiritual advisor? The nurse helps the family establish priorities and determine how to accomplish them and encourages the family to delay what they can. The nurse can either complete the task (e.g., tell them that you are going to wash the dishes; do not ask) or find a friend or other family member who is less affected and able to step in to minimize the functional disruption.

Searching for Meaning, Engaging Emotions, and Informing Others

As grievers search for meaning, the nurse facilitates coping with loss by helping elders get the information they feel they need, consider alternatives, and find ways to make their grief manageable. In this way clarification is supported (Weisman, 1979).

Sometimes families are looking for information about a disease or trying to understand how to find the best hospital for a treatment or the best nursing home for a long-term stay (Chapter 32). The nurse assists in obtaining the information whenever possible. With the availability of Internet search engines and devices such as touch screens and tablets, this is often straightforward even as simply as providing key search terms. While paying attention to health literacy, many sources provide reliable information in a range of languages. Active listening often helps grievers make sense of the loss and find meaning in it as they experience a change in their reality. Often this means helping the person contact a health care provider, an elder in their culture, or a spiritual leader.

The expressions of emotion, be they moments of panic, hysteria, or silence, may make grief less frightening. In some cultures catharsis is expected, and in others it is the nurse who gives the griever the "permission" needed to emote. Sometimes it is a spiritual search and help is in the form of finding a resource or a place of peace, such as the chapel. Often, what is needed most is someone to listen to the existential and unanswerable questions, the "whys" and "hows," without giving answers. At other times it may be appropriate to be directive, such as suggesting that "This is not a good time to make any major decisions" (Weisman, 1979).

Sometimes nurses feel a need to help *inform others* for the grievers, thinking that this is an expression of caring. While it appears to be, it is more therapeutic for grievers or designated cultural spokespersons to talk to others about the losses, and nurses should refrain from intervening in this way. Instead, the nurse can offer to find a phone number or just offer to "be there" when the news is being shared. In this way, the nurse provides support when the griever's emotions engage and at the same time shows respect for the person's and family's cultural roles.

Adaptation

As the person or family moves toward equilibrium after the impact of a loss, be it a death, a move to a nursing home, or other change, the nurse can help the person reorganize this new life. The nurse talks with the elder about what was most valued about that which has been lost, determines what habits and rituals were comforting related to this, and finds ways to incorporate these in a new way to the new environment (Box 35-7). For example, if the person always had a cup of tea before bed but now does not have access to a kitchen, "cup of tea at bedtime" can become part of the individualized plan of care.

Memories Reframed and the Return to Equilibrium and a New Steady State

For the system to return to equilibrium and a new steady state, however fleeting, new memories are needed. Reminiscence is often helpful in creating these. The nurse collaborates with grievers by encouraging them to share stories with others and repeat them as often as needed (Weisman, 1979). Listening to the story, endlessly repeated, is difficult to do and it is likely to change with each retelling, but this means that memories are being reframed as a new steady state is approached. Reminiscence allows the reality of the loss to filter slowly into the unconscious mind. It helps the griever acknowledge that the loss is indeed real and that life can go on, even though the future may be experienced in a different way. At the time when new memories are being developed, drawing out anecdotes and vignettes of his or her life before the loss will allow the person to be seen from a different perspective. The nurse serves as a role model who displays the behavioral qualities of responsiveness, authenticity, commitment, and competence, that is, caring.

DYING AND DEATH

Before the 1900s, most women and men died at home. Women died during childbirth, and men died of unknown causes. During times of war, most men died in battle or from battle-associated injuries. The life expectancy at birth in 1900 was 46.3 years for men and 48.3 years for women (United States). Now both men and women live well into their 70s and beyond (see Chapter 1). While most people prefer to die at home, they most often die in acute care hospitals with wide variation in prevalence by country of residence. In a study of 16 million deaths in developed countries, 54% occurred in hospitals, ranging from 78% in Japan to 20% in China. The older the person is, the more likely he or she is to die in a residential care facility (Broad et al, 2013). In an English study, the vast majority of persons died in acute care facilities, with the exception of the most cognitively impaired persons, who were more likely to die in care homes (Perrels et al, 2014).

Dying is both a challenging life experience and a private one. How people deal with their own dying is often a reflection of the way they responded to earlier losses and stressors. Most people probably die as they have lived, that is, the manner in which one faces dying is an expression of personality, circumstances, illness, and culture.

Although not all older adults have had fulfilling lives or have a sense of completion, transcendence, or self-actualization (Chapter 36), their deaths at the age or after that of their parents is considered normative. If dying occurs after a particularly prolonged or painful illness, it is sometimes rationalized as a relief, at least in part. The deaths of the older community members at the time of catastrophic events, such as the Indian Ocean tsunami of 2004, are never considered an acceptable loss of human potential. A major question arises when considering dying and death in late life. When is a person with multiple chronic or repeated acute or progressive health problems considered to be "dying"? Both treatable chronic conditions and those associated with an irreversible terminal condition often occur at the same time, more so as we age (Goldstein and Morrison, 2014).

While the signs and symptoms attributed to terminal conditions may appear obvious, they can easily be confused with frailty and exacerbations of chronic diseases. However, the nurse can look for signs of an approaching death when the person begins using "coded communication," such as saying good-bye instead of the usual goodnight, giving away cherished possessions as gifts, urgently contacting friends and relatives with whom the person has not communicated with for a long time, and having direct or symbolic premonitions that death is near.

Anxiety, depression, restlessness, and agitation are behaviors that are frequently categorized as manifestations of confusion or dementia but may also be responses to the inability to express feelings of foreboding and a sense of life escaping one's grasp. Ensuring that the person remains comfortable, whether the condition is chronic, acute, or terminal, is the work of the nurse and other members of the caring team. Many people have said that death is not the problem; it is the dying that takes the work. This is true for all involved: the person who is dying, the loved ones, the professional caregivers such as the nurses, and the nursing assistants in care facilities, who are too often invisible grievers.

The Family

Today's older adults are usually members of both multigenerational and more complex family constellations, consisting of ex-spouses and partners, step-grandchildren, and fictive kin (those considered family as a result of affective bonds). Although members may be geographically distant, in many cases some degree of filial ties may exist (Chapter 34). When an elder becomes seriously or terminally ill and cannot uphold his or her role or obligation, the family balance or dynamics are significantly altered (*functional disruption*). For example, new arrangements are needed when an elder who has been providing

---

BOX 35-7   **TIPS FOR BEST PRACTICE**

Helping the Person Adapt to the Loss of a Former Ritual

The grandmother who had always hosted her eldest daughter's birthday party can still do that even if she is now a resident in a long-term care facility. The nurse can help the resident reserve a private space within the facility, send out invitations, and have the birthday party as always but now reframe it as catered by the facility in the elder's new "home."

childcare or help with meal preparation is no longer able to do so. This change may cause considerable familial distress, as will the need for elder care when day-to-day help seems impossible due to the work demands and schedules of adult children, grandchildren, nieces, and nephews. Even the elder who is single and relies on friends and neighbors finds a change in the relationships. Depending on the role the individual has in the family/friend constellation, while changes may not occur at the time of diagnosis, they will as any associated frailty advances (Chapter 21). Roles and traits of the person who is now considered to be dying may create adjustment difficulties in the soon-to-be survivors, whether they are partners, spouses, adult children, or grandchildren. Adult children often begin to see their own mortality through the death of their parents as a new family is established.

The idea that family members can remain involved with the dying person may be a source of constant conflict as they anticipate and plan for life without the dying family member. This change requires enormous energy by family members who are already burdened with their own anticipatory grief, daily living, and, in many cases, raising their own children and possibly grandchildren. A number of tasks may facilitate healthy adaptation to the loss of a family member.

Family members have to separate their own identities from that of the patient and learn to tolerate the reality that another family member will die while they live on. The ability of the family to support, love, and provide intimacy may lead to exhaustion, impatience, anger, and a sense of futility if the dying is prolonged. Family members may be at different points in grief than the patient or each other, which can hinder communication when it is needed the most. As the illness worsens, physical disability increases, and the patient's needs intensify, so may the family members' feelings of helplessness and frustration.

Responding to the effects of grief requires acknowledging feelings that surface before and after the death. Coming to terms with the reality of the impending loss means that family members often go through a period of self-reflection. Because people are "supposed to" die in old age according to social norms, the grief responses may not be exceptionally intense and this can lead to either guilt or relief for the person who is suffering.

The family may feel extremely pressured to provide very personal care during the final days of a relative's life. They may feel caught between experiencing the present and remembering the person as he or she was, between pushing for more interventions with the potential to extend the dying or letting life take its natural course. Nurses often hear families lament that they "can't give up on them," even if this runs counter to the elder's wishes (Chapter 31).

Despite the family's grief and pain, they must give the patient permission to die; let the loved one know that it is all right to let go and leave them. This gesture is the last act of love and dignity that the family can offer. Occasionally, no family is available to say, "It's okay to let go." The task then falls to the nurse who has developed a meaningful relationship with the person through care.

◆ PROMOTING A GOOD DEATH: IMPLICATIONS FOR GERONTOLOGICAL NURSING

The needs of the dying are like threads in a piece of cloth. Each thread is individual but necessary to the integrity and completeness of the fabric. If one thread is pulled, it touches the other threads, affecting the fabric's appearance, the thread placement, and the stability of the piece. When one need is unmet, it will affect all others because they are all interwoven. Separating the physical, psychological, and spiritual needs of the dying in late life in order to identify specific interventions and approaches is difficult because of their interconnection. There are several ways to approach an understanding of the needs of persons who are dying and the responsibilities of the nurse in the promotion of a healthy death (Figure 35-3).

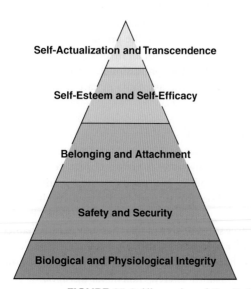

Self-Actualization and Transcendence	To share and come to terms with the unavoidable future To perceive meaning in death
Self-Esteem and Self-Efficacy	To maintain respect in the face of increasing weakness To maintain independence to the extent possible To feel like a normal person, a part of life right to the end To preserve personal identity
Belonging and Attachment	To talk To be listened to with understanding To be loved and to share love To be with a caring person when dying
Safety and Security	To be given the opportunity to voice hidden fears To trust those who care for him or her To feel that he or she is being told the truth To be secure
Biological and Physiological Integrity	To obtain relief from physical symptoms To conserve energy To be free from pain

FIGURE 35-3 Hierarchy of the Dying Person's Needs, Based on Maslow.

The 6 C's Approach

Psychiatrist Avery Weisman (1979) identified six needs of the dying: care, control, composure, communication, continuity, and closure (the 6 C's). The importance of each to the person is influenced by his or her personality, culture, experiences, religious and philosophical beliefs, orientation, the prior degree of life involvement, and perhaps gender. Weisman's approach can provide a framework for the nurse in the development of interventions when caring for those who are dying.

Care

The dying person should have the best care possible; this means freedom from pain, conservation of energy, expert management of symptoms, and support at all times. Common symptoms include dyspnea, fatigue, pain, and those that are more specific to the cause of terminal condition. In aging they accompany the symptoms the person has due to concurrent chronic disease. It is never acceptable for the person's *symptoms* to remain either untreated or undertreated.

The chronic pain that often accompanies dying is not going to stop and usually requires a regimen of narcotic and adjuvant drug therapy administered around the clock and on time, not just as requested by the patient (Chapter 27). Providing adequate relief must be done without concern of addiction or overall effect on respiratory status; relief of pain is paramount.

Pain goes beyond the physical to that which is spiritual and psychological, induced by depression, anxiety, fear, and other unresolved emotional concerns that are just as strong and just as real. When emotional needs are not met, the total pain experience is exacerbated or intensified. Medication alone cannot relieve this pain. Instead, empathetic listening and allowing those who are dying to verbalize what is on their minds are important interventions that must be based on the energy and stamina that are available at any one time. If tears and sadness are present, silence and touch, if acceptable, are worth more than words can convey. Gentleness, closeness, and sitting near the person may be appropriate. The counsel of the person's spiritual advisor may be needed.

Diversional activity can sometimes ease pain: a backrub to relieve tension, a foot massage, radio or television, or exposure to art and music. If hearing is impaired, headphones are very useful. If vision is impaired, talking books or a volunteer reader can be found. In many instances, psychological pain can be relieved if the person feels safe and has someone close by to converse, to listen, and to be with.

Dying requires much energy to cope with the physical assault of illness on the body and the spiritual and emotional unrest that dying initiates. Care means helping the person conserve energy. How much can the individual do without becoming physically and emotionally taxed? What activities of daily living are most important for the person to do independently? How much energy is needed for the patient to talk with those who are the most important without becoming exhausted? Only the person who is dying can answer these questions, and the nurse can advocate for the person to be given the opportunity to do so. By meeting the needs for freedom from pain and conservation of energy, the nurse has already begun to ensure that the person receives optimal care in order to maximize the quality of life to the extent possible for the time that remains.

Control

As death gets closer, people often feel that they have less and less control over their lives and bodies. The person is in the process of losing everything he or she has ever known or would ever know. The potential loss of identity, independence, and control over bodily functions can lead to threatened self-esteem. The person may begin to feel ashamed, humiliated, and like a "burden." Control is the need to remain in a collaborative role relating to one's own living and dying and as active a participant in the care as desired. The nurse can help the person meet these needs by taking every opportunity to return the control to the person and, in doing so, bolster self-esteem. Essential to the facilitating of self-esteem is the premise that the values of the patient must figure significantly in the decisions that will affect the course of dying. Whenever possible, the nurse can have the person decide when to groom, eat, wake, and sleep, and so on. The nurse never has the right to determine the activities of the individual, especially relating to visitors and how time is spent.

Composure

Dying is an emotional activity—for the dying and for those around them. The need for composure is that which enables the person to modulate emotional extremes within cultural norms as is appropriate. This is not to avoid the sadness; this is to have moments of relief.

Communication

The need for communication is broad, from the need for information to make decisions, to the need to share information. Although the type and content of communication that is acceptable to the person vary, the nurse has a responsibility to ensure that the person has an opportunity for the communication he or she desires.

Communication includes auditory, visual, and tactile stimulation to appropriately nurture and foster quality of life while dying. Verbal and nonverbal communication is necessary to convey positive messages. Hand-holding, placing an arm around the shoulder, or sitting on the edge of the bed as culturally appropriate conveys to the person that the nurse or caregiver is available to listen.

In a classic study of terminal illness in the hospital, Glaser and Strauss (1963) identified four types of communication: *closed awareness, suspected awareness, mutual pretense,* and *open awareness*. Each of these influenced the work on the hospital unit. Closed awareness is described as "keeping the secret." Hospital staff and the family and friends know that the patient is dying, but the patient does not know it or keeps the secret as well. Generally, caregivers invent a fictitious future for the patient to believe in (e.g., next year we are going on the cruise we always wanted), in hopes that it will boost the patient's morale. Although this happens less today with the legislation related to patients' rights, it still occurs. In suspected awareness, the patient suspects that he or she is going to die. Hints are bandied back and forth, and a contest ensues for control of the information. Mutual pretense is a situation of "let's pretend." Everyone knows the death is approaching, but the patient, family, friends, nurses, and physicians do not talk about it—real feelings are kept hidden, and too often, so are questions. Open awareness acknowledges the reality of approaching death. The patient may ask, "Will I die?" and "How and when will I die?" "What is it going to be like?" The patient becomes resigned to dying, and the family grieves with the patient rather than for the patient. The nurse can encourage open awareness whenever possible while respecting the patient's cultural patterns and behaviors. It is essential to note that what is said and to whom is culturally determined. Talking about dying or death may be considered taboo, and speaking to the wrong person may be very inappropriate (Coolen, 2012).

Continuity

The need for continuity is fulfilled by preserving as normal a life as possible while dying; by transcending the present, continuity helps to maintain self-esteem. Often a dying patient can feel shut off from the rest of the world at a time when he or she is still capable of being involved and active in some way. Providing stimuli such as photographs and mementos, enabling the individual to stay at home, or enabling individuality or other culturally appropriate experiences in the institutional setting engenders continuity and self-esteem. Self-esteem and dignity complement each other. Dignity involves the individual's ability to maintain a consistent self-concept.

Loneliness may be the result of a loss of continuity with one's life and a diminution of one's concept of self and results in spiritual or existential distress. The nurse may ask about the person's life and those things most valued and work with the family and the patient or resident on a plan to remain engaged in as many of the activities and past roles as long as possible. A father who watches a certain ballgame with his son every Sunday can continue to do this regardless of the need to be in a hospital, a nursing home, or an inpatient hospice unit. If the person is bed-bound at home, it may be more practical to have the bed in a central area rather than in a distant room. Treating the person as an intelligent adult says, "I care" and "You're not alone" and "You are important." Others prefer some time alone and have valued solitude (Box 35-8). This too can be respected as a way of enhancing the continuity of a long life. The nurse can find out the personal preferences and values of the person and work toward honoring these.

Closure

The need for closure is the need for the opportunity for reconciliation, transcendence, and self-actualization (Chapter 36) (Maslow, 1943). Reminiscence is one way of putting life in order, to evaluate the pluses and minuses of life, and to think about the legacies left behind. It is a means of resolving conflicts, giving up possessions, and making final good-byes. Learning to say "good-bye" today leaves open the possibility of many more "hellos." Pain and other symptoms that are not well cared for may interfere with this reconciliation, making appropriate interventions by the nurse especially important.

BOX 35-8   Meditation Coping

Mrs. Herbert was a spry 76-year-old white woman. She was the sole caregiver of her husband with mid-stage Alzheimer's disease. The hospital had arranged for her husband to share a room with her while her diagnostic tests were completed and her symptoms stabilized before she went home. She had just been diagnosed with metastatic breast cancer, with a terminal diagnosis. The nurses thought that she was becoming increasingly irritable and agitated after her initial calmness. As an advanced practice nurse on an oncology unit, I was called to assess Mrs. Herbert and recommend a treatment plan. We talked for a while—about her life, her plans for the future, and her usual coping mechanisms. She explained that she had everything under control and had already made arrangements for home care in the process of planning for the eventual long-term care needs of her husband. As she started to cry, she said, "It's just so hard with my life disrupted here. Every morning for years I have meditated for 30 minutes. My husband respects my need for quiet, and afterward I think I can do anything! I have not been able to meditate since I have been here; the nurses and staff are always coming in my room or calling on the room's intercom—I can't find any moments of peace!" The nurses and I worked out a plan with Mrs. Herbert. Every morning between 6:00 and 6:30 AM, she would not be disturbed. A "Do Not Disturb" sign would be placed on the intercom at the nurses' station and on her door. A noticeable change was seen in just a few days; Mrs. Herbert was calmer and coping well again. She was most appreciative to "have my life back again."

Kathleen Jett

For some, closure means coming to terms with their spiritual selves, with the Great Spirit, Jesus, God, Allah, or Buddha—of that which has meaning to the person. If the patient has existential or spiritual needs, arranging for pastoral care may be offered but should never be done without the person's permission. The nurse can foster transcendence by providing patients with the time and privacy for self-reflection and an opportunity to talk about whatever they need to talk about, especially about the meanings of their lives and the meanings of their deaths.

Spirituality

In 2009, a group of experts in palliative care gathered to come to a consensus on the spiritual dimension care at the end of life (National Consensus Project, 2009). This meeting was driven in part by discovery that while addressing the spiritual needs of persons who are dying had long been an expectation of providers of hospice and palliative care, they were not often met. In 2013 the *Palliative Care Guidelines* were updated to stress the responsibility of health care professionals to assess spiritual and existential needs at all times during the dying process and when needs were identified, ensure that they were addressed. The *Guidelines* emphasized the importance of the interdisciplinary team, including the chaplain or other spiritual advisor. The nurse is reminded of the importance of attending to spiritual and cultural rituals that are important to the patient and family as a means of comfort and support (Herman, 2013).

The spiritual dimension of persons who are dying deals with the transcendental or existential relationship between the dying person and another—between the person and his or her god or the person and significant others. Signs of spiritual distress while dying include expressions of hopelessness, meaninglessness, guilt, and despair, all of which can emerge indirectly through anxiety, depression, or anger. At the specific direction of the patient, interventions may involve calling the patient's choice of a religious leader; sharing spiritual readings that are consistent with the patient's beliefs; reciting meditative poems and playing music of the person's choice; obtaining religious articles such as amulets, a Bible, or a rosary; or praying. The nurse is strongly cautioned that these interventions must be consistent with the culture and express wishes of the patient and may not at any time be suggested based the nurse's belief system.

Hope

Hope is a fluid concept that changes as dying comes closer. At the beginning, the person hopes for a cure. When a prognosis is given, the hope may change to "as much time as possible." As death approaches, the hope may be for a good death, one that is symptom free (Box 35-9).

Hope is expectancy of fulfillment, an anticipation, or relief from something. Hope is based on the belief of the possible, the support of meaningful others, a sense of well-being, overall coping ability, and a purpose in life. Hope empowers, generates courage, motivates action and achievement, and can counter physiological, spiritual, and emotional dysfunction. Hope involves faith and trust.

It can be classified as desirable or expectational (Pattison, 1977). Expectational hope sounds like "I hope to get better" or "I hope my children get here in time." If this hope is a reflection of expectations that are not realistic, they can increase stress for the person and caregiver. However, this hope can be modified without being lost. In desirable hope, the wishes are something that would be appreciated if it were to occur without the fixed expectation that it will, will not, or must occur. The nurse can respond to the comment "I hope I get better" from someone who is rapidly declining with "That would be really great; in the meantime, there is so much we can do."

Nurses seldom recognize the small things they do, routinely and unconsciously, to impart hope. The act of helping with grooming conveys a quiet belief that the person matters. Pain relief and comfort measures reinforce the recognition of an individual's needs and reinforce the value of the person.

Promoting Equilibrium for the Family

The nurse is often present and supporting the family at the moment of death and in the moments preceding it. Regardless of the age of the survivors, they, too, have needs and nurses have a responsibility to care for them. This may be in the form of the interventions that promote equilibrium to a system now in chaos. Nursing interventions that promote health at the time of loss include actions that empower the family to cope with the death in a manner consistent with their traditions. In a small ethnography, Herbert and colleagues (2007) found that family caregivers most needed prognostic information and were unlikely to ask for this. Hearing from the provider what the death would "look like" was a key ingredient the families found missing.

PALLIATIVE CARE

According to the World Health Organization, palliative care is "an approach to care which improves the quality of life of patients and their families facing life-threatening illness, through the prevention, assessment and treatment of pain and other physical, psychological and spiritual problems" (World Health Organization, 2010). Providing such care is part of day-to-day practice of gerontological nurses who routinely care for elders having life-limiting conditions, such as Alzheimer's disease or Parkinson's disease (Chapter 23). The primary goal of palliative care is to prevent or to minimize suffering. It is often provided through interdisciplinary formal systems to help people understand their options and make health-related decisions that are consistent with their values and to facilitate seamless transitions when movement from one care setting is necessary.

Most importantly, palliative care is offered simultaneously with life-prolonging or stabilizing care for those living with chronic conditions (Figure 35-4). When working with older adults and their families, the focus is very often on amelioration

---

BOX 35-9   Indicators of an Appropriate and Good Death

- Care needed is received, and it is timely and expert.
- One is able to control one's life and environment to the extent that is desired and possible and in a way that is culturally consistent with one's past life.
- One is able to maintain composure when necessary and to the extent desired.
- One is able to initiate and maintain communication with significant others for as long as possible.
- Life continues as normal as possible while dying with the added tasks that may be needed to deal with and adjust to the inevitable death.
- One can maintain desirable hope at all times.
- One is able to reach a sense of closure in a way that is culturally consistent with one's practices and life patterns.

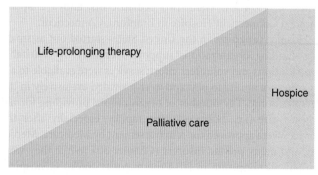

FIGURE 35-4 Palliative care is offered simultaneously with life-prolonging and curative therapies for persons living with serious, complex, and advanced illness. (From Ham RJ, Sloane PD, Warshaw GA, et al, editors: *Primary care geriatrics*, ed 6, Philadelphia, 2014, Elsevier.)

of cognitive and functional limitations and support to the caregiver(s) who are coping with multiple issues simultaneously.

Purely palliative care may be elected when previously curative treatments are no longer effective, such as with end-stage cancer, AIDS, or end-stage heart disease. It may also be appropriate when an individual with multiple comorbid conditions or a health care proxy makes the decision to forego any aggressive treatment of chronic or new health problems. It must be noted that the provision of palliative care does not means that any simple curative treatments to transient new problems are automatically withheld, such as the treatment of a urinary tract infection or other infection when the terminal illness is heart disease, cancer, or chronic obstructive pulmonary disease (COPD).

Whereas initially palliative care was provided primarily by specialized organizations, today it is provided regardless of setting and by anyone sharing these goals and skills. This may be in the ambulatory care clinic when the focus of the care of the person with neurodegenerative disorders is comfort (Chapter 23) or in specialized beds in an acute care or long-term care facility.

Providing Palliative Care through Hospice Services

The model for the modern day hospice is based on the medieval concept of hospitality in which a community assists the traveler at dangerous points along a journey. The dying are also travelers along the continuum of life and wellness, in a community consisting of friends and family, as well as health care providers. However, for many years, providing comfort to those approaching death was lacking. In 1952 Englishwoman Dame Cicely Saunders, a nurse, social worker, physician, and writer, began working at St. Joseph's Hospice in London. The goal of her work and study was to reduce pain. In 1967 she established Saint Christopher's Hospice, also in London, based on the principles of teaching, clinical research, and the provision of expert and holistic pain and symptom relief (St. Christopher's, 2014). Inspired by the work of Dame Saunders, Dr. Florence Wald, the Dean of the College of Nursing at Yale, and physician Dr. Elisabeth Kübler-Ross championed the hospice concept in the United States. In 1974 Dr. Wald, two pediatricians, and a chaplain founded Connecticut Hospice in Branford, Connecticut.

Hospice programs in the United States started out as small, free-standing organizations supported entirely by charitable contributions and volunteer effort; services were available to all, regardless of ability to pay, and were provided exclusively in the person's home. The number of organizations providing formal hospice care (i.e., hospices) grew rapidly, especially after the services were approved for reimbursement by Medicare, Medicaid, and many private insurers (Chapter 30). While they were initially all nonprofit, in 2014 the majority (66%) of hospices were for-profit corporations (National Hospice and Palliative Care Organization [NHPCO], 2014). The variations in origins and styles reflect the particular needs of the community, the style of leadership, funding sources, political forces, and available resources for health and social services in the community in which they were established or continue to exist. While the care provided is palliative, it is within the specific context of a signed agreement between the individual and the organization in which the person has elected to receive care-only therapy for an identified diagnosis. Hospice services are limited to those for whom two physicians have agreed that the person has a prognosis of 6 months or less.

At a minimum, services include medical, nursing, nursing assistant, chaplain, social work, and volunteer support. Potential services may also include massage, music, art, pet therapy, and other nonpharmacological interventions to promote comfort and quality of life. Hospices provide care not only to the dying but also to their families and friends through support groups and other bereavement services before and after the deaths.

The majority of hospice care is provided in people's homes to support an identified informal caregiver. The home becomes the primary center of care, and it is provided by family members or friends, who are taught basic care, including diet, exercise, and medication management with intermittent visits from the hospice staff. Volunteers, as members of the team, are a unique aspect of care; chores are performed, and friendship and companionship are provided to the patient and family.

Many hospices today have free-standing care centers where a patient may go to provide caregivers with short periods of respite or when intense symptom management is more than is possible at home. Those hospices without centers may have agreements with skilled nursing homes or acute care hospitals where the same symptom management can be achieved. Once stabilized, the person returns home.

The unprecedented contribution of hospice continues to be the provision of comfort for those who are dying and of support for those close to them. Through both pharmacological and nonpharmacological means, control of pain and other symptoms can often be accomplished without denying the patient's full alertness and the ability to communicate to others. The crux of accomplishing this end is the anticipation of symptoms and intervention by the caregiver before problems occur. Both hospice and other palliative care programs support and guide the family in patient care and ensure safe passage (e.g., for the patient, that he or she will not die alone; and that the family will not be abandoned).

Nursing practice in hospice incorporates the expression of the mind-body continuum. Nursing is considered the cornerstone of hospice care. The nurse provides much of the direct care and functions in a variety of roles: as staff nurse giving direct care, as coordinator implementing the plan of the interdisciplinary team, as executive officer responsible for research and educational activities, and as advocate for the patient and hospice in the clinical and political arena.

DECISION-MAKING AT THE END OF LIFE

Who makes end-of-life decisions has been the subject of research, debate, and federal legislation in the United States. Although people have always had opinions about their wishes, in the past these were made in the context of the prevailing principle of paternalism, that is, reliance on physicians to make the decisions they would make for their own children. This perspective has been replaced by presumed autonomy in the health care setting based on a Euro-American or Western perspective (Spoelhof and Elliott, 2012) (Chapters 4 and 31). Persons from many other culture groups place less emphasis on the individual and more, if not all, on identified cultural or familial decision-makers (Mazanec and Panke, 2010).

Decision-making about life-prolonging measures when death is inevitable is a legal, ethical, medical, and professional issue faced by gerontological nurses in their daily work. Yet the lines between living and dying are quite blurred, especially for the medically frail, or for an older adult with a multitude of chronic conditions. Considerable ethical conflicts arise from the technological advances available in some parts of the world or when there is ambivalence of whether death is to be fought or allowed to proceed naturally. Nonetheless, the nurse is obligated to know legal restrictions related to decision-making and then work with the elder and family on how these are consistent with their cultural patterns and rituals related to the end of life. For example, Hispanic elders are more likely to defer decision-making to other members of the family based on the belief that they know and will act on their wishes (Coolen, 2012).

Living Wills

Since the passage of the Patient Self-Determination Act (PSDA) in 1991 in the United States, any agency that is reimbursed by Medicare for services is required to provide all patients with information about their rights to make their own health care decisions, accept or refuse treatment, and complete an advance directive of some kind, especially living wills (Chapter 31). In the outpatient setting, providers (e.g., physicians, nurse practitioners, and physician assistants) are encouraged, but not obligated to provide this information.

The Patient Self-Determination Act (PSDA) recognized a living will (LW) as an advance directive (AD) that is specifically related to a situation in which a person is facing a terminal illness and unable to speak for herself or himself. It is a morally and, in some jurisdictions, legally binding document in which adults could express their wishes regarding end-of-life decisions for some future time when they were unable to do so for themselves. LWs may be as limited as decisions regarding the use of resuscitation or as detailed as decisions about dialysis, antibiotics, tube feedings, and so on (Box 35-10). The LW includes the appointment of a proxy to uphold patients' wishes when they are no longer able to do so. As the proxy is selected by the individual, the legal assumption is that a designated person has more authority than the next-of-kin.

An LW can be revoked only by the individual, either verbally or in writing. The person may also indicate revocation by tearing, burning, or destroying the document, preferably in front of witnesses. Directives may also be amended; formal language is not necessary, and one can add items in writing or cross out unwanted passages, but only the creator of the document may do so. If the person becomes incompetent, revocation is no longer possible, and the last statement of wishes stands. Nurses should know the details of AD and LW requirements in the state, country, or other jurisdiction in which they practice. The nurse should also be familiar with the LW form or forms available in the organization in which he or she is employed. The exact format and signature requirements (e.g., notary) for advance directives including living wills vary from state to state.

Barriers to Completing Advance Directives

While neither the concept of advance planning nor the PSDA is new, the number of persons with completed directives, including LWs, remains very low. Those more likely (21%) to have completed them are older, have more comorbidities, or are widowed. A contributing factor for people to complete living wills is involvement of the health care provider (Van Scoy et al, 2014). However, for multiple reasons, too often this does not occur (Spoelhof and Elliott, 2012).

British community nurses reported lack of resources, lack of public awareness, and difficulties talking about death as barriers to implementing advance care planning (Seymour et al, 2010). The majority (84%) of participants in a study designed to increase the number of persons who completed advance planning felt that it was irrelevant to their personal needs. In another study of a multiethnic, multilingual inpatient population, 369 patients were asked if their physicians had discussed advance care decision-making with them. Only 41% reported conversations, and the finding was across various education, age, ethnic, and language groups (Kulkarni et al, 2011).

In some cultures there are appointed spokespersons and decision-makers, which is in direct conflict with the Western model and regulations related to the PSDA (Box 35-11). Interpreters, used to assist the health care professional with explanations to their non–English-speaking patients, may not facilitate a clear translation of an AD because of cultural beliefs surrounding death or anticipation of poor health, such as the belief of many in the Haitian culture that speaking of death is taboo and may cause it to occur more quickly (Coolen, 2012).

To clarify documentation of end-of-life decisions even further, the POLST® (Physicians Orders for Life-Sustaining Treatment) document was created. The document is signed by the physician and the patient and can be used between care settings (POLST, 2012). The POLST is not an advance directive; it is a physician order to health care facilities.

BOX 35-10   TIPS FOR BEST PRACTICE

A living will is not the same as a do-not-resuscitate (DNR) order or a do-not-hospitalize (DNH) order, which are medical directives to health care professionals and are not personal advance directives. Neither the DNR order nor the DNH order should be written without a discussion of the implications with the patient and/or proxy. The nurse is often the one to facilitate this order in either case.

BOX 35-11   Cultural Barriers to the Completions of Advance Directives, Including Living Wills

Distrust of the health care system (especially in groups who have experienced violence or discrimination in the United States or their country of origin)
Cultural pattern of *Collectivism*: Family rather than individual is "decision-maker"
Preference for physician, as expert, to make the decision
Taboo to talk about death or dying
Influence of faith and spirituality: Illness as a test of faith
Belief that life is a gift from God that must be protected
Death as a part of the cycle of life and must not be disturbed
Dying away from home may lead to a disturbance of the spirits
Cannot die at home as the spirit will linger

From Coolen PR: Cultural relevance in end-of-life care, *EthnoMed*, May 1, 2012. https://ethnomed.org/clinical/end-of-life/cultural-relevance-in-end-of-life-care Accessed October 2014.

◆ PROMOTING HEALTHY AGING: IMPLICATIONS FOR GERONTOLOGICAL NURSING

Although nurses cannot provide legal information, they do serve as resource persons ready to discuss many of the questions people have about end-of-life decision-making, especially how these affect their care (Box 35-12). The nurse must consider the factors previously discussed and must ensure that patients are informed of their rights related to the PSDA in a culturally sensitive manner. The nurse may be responsible to inquire about the presence of an existing advance directive, to offer and explain the option, and to ensure that any existing directive still reflects the person's wishes. The nurse is also responsible for ensuring that existing or newly created advance directives are available in the appropriate locations in the medical record.

The nurse can help the elder to understand interventions (e.g., cardiopulmonary resuscitation [CPR], intubations, and artificial nutrition) and their consequences. The nurse can explain that choosing no further intervention is not "giving up"

BOX 35-12   RESOURCES FOR BEST PRACTICE

National Hospice and Palliative Care Organization: www.nhpco.org
Hospice and Palliative Care Nurses Association: www.hpna.org
   Includes: Core Competencies, Statements on the Scope and Standards of Hospice and Palliative Care for Nurses at all levels, Certification in Palliative Care Nursing
National Academy of Elder Law Attorneys: www.naela.org
Resources for information about living wills, including downloadable documents:
   Information and forms for living wills and other advance directives: www.fivewishes.com
   Extensive information on advance care planning: www.caringinfo.org
POLST: Physician Orders for Life-Sustaining Treatment Paradigm: http://www.polst.org/

but is an active decision to allow a natural death to occur. Personal bias cannot be injected into the discussion (e.g., religious affiliation or otherwise) under any circumstances. The nurse is an impartial advocate for the patient regardless of decision or setting, but it is particularly important in the long-term care environment (Herbert et al, 2011). There, the nurse advocates for the self-determination of all patients to the best possible extent, even those with limited cognitive function.

The nurse acts as a patient advocate by bringing decision-makers, elders, and health providers together to discuss the difficult issues addressed in executing a directive or simply to discuss the elder's wishes. The nurse may also be the one who obtains the appropriate AD or LW form for the elder who is well or ill.

No one can think of all possible contingencies that might require decisions regarding life-limiting conditions. The use of values' assessments may help clarify what the elder holds important in his or her life and how this relates to his or her desires for health care and quality of life. Does the elder want measures to be taken to prolong life at all costs, or does he or she wish for a natural death? What are the boundaries in which suffering can be minimized? Are there any persons the elder feels comfortable with who can act as a proxy and will ensure that the elder's wishes will be carried out? Answers to these questions are helpful in the promotion of an appropriate and good death. Before a directive is completed, the family and support persons should discuss whether those who are to be involved are comfortable with the decisions and will adhere to the directive. For elders without family, the nurse may become a sounding board, but he or she must take care to not influence the outcome and may never serve as a proxy in a patient's living will.

Approaching Death

In 1991, the U.S. Supreme Court reviewed the case of *Cruzan v. State of Missouri* and confirmed a person's right to refuse unwanted treatment. No distinction was made between withholding and withdrawing the treatment. Later, case law characterized tube feeding and intravenous feeding as medical treatments (also referred to as *artificial sustenance*) and therefore these could be refused as well. Nonetheless, questions remained. These "rights" have not always been granted, and questions have been raised regarding the relationship between patients' wishes and the responsibilities and activities of health care providers. The questions have become more and more complex as states and countries wrestle with questions of physician-assisted suicide, euthanasia, terminal sedation, and double effect.

Physician-Assisted Suicide

The potential for a person's ultimate control of his or her dying has risen to state and Supreme Court levels in the United States and to equivalent levels in other countries. In 1994 and again in 1997, voters in Oregon passed legislation legalizing a person's right to end his or her life in very specific circumstances (Box 35-13). The voters in Washington State passed similar legislation in 2008 with identical restrictions (Death with Dignity National Center, 2014). Vermont's right to die legislation

BOX 35-13 Rules Governing Physician-Assisted Suicide*

Competent adult

Free of depression

Prognosis of <6 months to live

Two requests, both verbal and in writing, repeated 15 days apart

Two witnesses to the request; one must not be an heir, related, or employed by the health care facility caring for the patient

Has been informed of alternatives

Has received counseling to ensure that the person is fully informed regarding the risks of such actions

Neither physicians nor nurses are permitted to administer the product that will result in death

*Oregon and Washington states.

BOX 35-14 TIPS FOR BEST PRACTICE

Safe Conduct

The responsibility of the nurse is to provide what is referred to as "safe conduct," helping the dying and their families navigate through unknown waters to a good and appropriate death (i.e., one that a person would choose if choosing was possible). A good and appropriate death is one in which one's needs are met for as long as possible, and life is never without meaning.

was passed in 2013. In 2009 the Montana courts ruled that there was nothing in the state law prohibiting physician-assisted suicide, but no definitive laws have been passed (Death with Dignity National Center, 2014). As of this writing physician-assisted suicide is being discussed at all levels in the state of New Mexico. It is legal in Belgium, The Netherlands, Luxemburg, and Switzerland. In many other states and countries, persons' involvement is subject to criminal prosecution. The numbers of people who have chosen this route to end their suffering have been few. At the same time, the number of referrals to palliative care programs and hospice services has increased.

Palliative Sedation

In 1997, the U.S. Supreme Court declared that while universal physician-assisted suicide was illegal, pharmacological sedation for the relief of refractory symptoms (e.g., pain, nausea and vomiting, dyspnea), by whatever means necessary, was acceptable. This has been referred to as *terminal sedation* but is more accurately called *palliative sedation.* The intent of the sedation is to provide comfort but to go no further. This is based on the concept of *double effect*—that is, if the sedation provides comforts even if it is possible that death is hastened, it is considered neither assisted suicide nor euthanasia and is acceptable. While replete with ethical questions, the *intention* must be to relieve the suffering with treatment and to that extent only (Seale et al, 2014). Active euthanasia, wherein the goal is death instead of relief, remains illegal everywhere in the United States but is legal in Luxemburg (Steck et al, 2013), The Netherlands (Seale et al, 2014), and Belgium (Chambaere et al, 2010; Roelands et al, 2014).

◆ PROMOTING HEALTHY DYING WHILE AGING: IMPLICATIONS FOR GERONTOLOGICAL NURSING

Nurses are professional grievers, in caring for those who are frail and in any setting; we are repeatedly exposed to the death of our patients. Some consider the death of a patient as a failure—they have "lost" the person they cared for. However, when it is a good death, it can be viewed as a professional success because the nurse provided safe conduct for the dying elder and gently cared for the survivors (Box 35-14). We can use the reminders of our own mortality as motivation to live the best we can with the time we have. Nurses can seek support and support each other. As grievers, we too may need to tell the story of the dying person to those professionals around us, in either formal or informal support groups; and we need to listen to our colleagues' stories.

Caring for older adults requires knowledge of the grieving and dying processes, as well as skills in providing relief of symptoms or palliative care (Table 35-1). However, it is also acknowledged that working daily with the grieving or dying is an art. The development of the art necessitates inner strength. The nurse needs to have spiritual strength—strength from within. This does not mean that the nurse must have a specific religious orientation or affiliation but, rather, that he or she has a positive belief in self, a connection to others, and a belief that life has meaning. The effective nurse has developed a personal philosophy of life and of death. Although this may change over time and cannot be assumed to be held by anyone else, one's beliefs about life and death will help the nurse through difficult times. Emotional maturity allows the nurse to deal with disappointment and postponement of immediate wants or desires. Maturity means that the nurse can reach out for help for self when needed. Finally, to provide comfort to grieving persons, nurses must be comfortable with their own lives or at least be able to set aside their own sadness and grief while working with that of others (Box 35-15).

It is always important to remember that some nurses are unable to care for the dying because of their own unresolved conflicts and should not be expected to function in these roles. This may be a temporary situation associated with events in the nurse's life or something deeper, such as a traumatic experience in the death of a loved one. The nurse should recognize his or her limitations and should defer care to another nurse when appropriate. In doing so, the nurse gives the most compassionate care possible.

TABLE 35-1   Best Nursing Practice: Signs and Symptoms of Approaching Death

PHYSICAL	RATIONALE	INTERVENTION
Coolness	Diminished peripheral circulation to increase circulation to vital organs	Socks, light cotton blankets or warm blankets if needed; *do not use electric blanket*
Increased sleeping	Conservation of energy	Respect need for increased rest; inquire as to their wishes regarding timing of companionship
Disorientation	Metabolic changes	Identify self by name before speaking to patient; speak softly, clearly, and truthfully
Fecal and/or urinary incontinence	Increased muscle relaxation	Change bedding as needed; use bed pads; *avoid indwelling catheter*s
Noisy respirations	Poor circulation of body fluids, immobilization, and the inability to expectorate	Elevate the head with pillows, or raise the head of the bed, or both; gently turn the head to the side to drain
Restlessness	Metabolic changes and relative cerebral anoxia	Calm the patient by speech and action; reduce light; gently rub back, stroke arms, or read aloud; play soothing music; *do not use restraints*
Decreased intake of food and fluids	Body conservation of energy for function	Provide nutrition within limits expressed by patient or in advance directive; semisolid liquids easiest to swallow; protect mouth and lips from discomfort of dryness
Decreased urine output	Decreased fluid intake and decreased circulation to kidney	None
Altered breathing pattern	Metabolic and oxygen changes	Elevate the head of bed; speak gently to patient
EMOTIONAL OR SPIRITUAL	**PRESUMED RATIONALE**	**INTERVENTION**
Withdrawal	Prepares the patient for release and detachment and letting go	Continue communicating in a normal manner using a normal voice tone; identify self by name; give permission to die
Vision-like experiences of dead friends or family; religious vision	Preparation for transition	Accept the reality of the experience for the person; reassure him or her that the feeling is normal
Restlessness	Tension, fear, unfinished business	Listen to patient express his or her fears, sadness, and anger; facilitate completion of business if possible
Unusual communication	Signals readiness to let go	Say what needs to be said to the dying patient; kiss, hug, cry with him or her as appropriate

BOX 35-15   Nursing Skills Needed for the Practice of Palliative/End-of-Life Care

- Have ability to talk to patients and families about dying.
- Be knowledgeable about symptom control and pain-control techniques.
- Have ability to provide comfort-oriented nursing interventions.
- Recognize physical changes that precede imminent death.
- Deal with own feelings.
- Deal with angry patients and families.
- Be knowledgeable and deal with the ethical issues in administering end-of-life palliative therapies.
- Be knowledgeable, and inform patients about ADs.
- Be knowledgeable of the legal issues in administering end-of-life palliative care.
- Be adaptable and sensitive to religious and cultural perspectives.

Modified from White KR, Coyne PJ, Patel UB: Are nurses adequately prepared for end-of-life care? *J Nurs Scholarsh* 33:147–151, 2001., Sigma Theta Tau International.

KEY CONCEPTS

- Grief is a physical, emotional, and spiritual/existential response to loss.
- The Loss Response Model can be used to guide the development of nursing interventions designed to optimize the quality of life for those who are grieving and those who are dying.
- Persons who are at risk for complicated grieving should receive specialized and skilled supportive care.
- The individual's response to loss and grief is similar to how he or she has dealt with other stressors in life.
- An individual is living until he or she has died; the nurse works with the elder and significant others to maintain as high a quality of life as possible before, during, and after the loss or death.
- Hope is fluid and empowering; it can be appropriately supported during any aspect of the process of loss, grief, and mourning. Hope generates courage and resilience.

- Palliative care is that which focuses on comfort rather than cure.
- Hospice is a specific interprofessional approach to the provision of palliative care.
- Palliative care can be provided regardless of setting.
- Advance directives and living wills provide persons the opportunity to express their end-of-life wishes and appoint a proxy to act on those wishes, when they are unable to do so for themselves.
- Physician-assisted suicide is now legal or permitted in several states and countries. As a result of the law, the care of the dying has improved.
- Double effect is the accepted practice that permits the provision of as much medication as needed to relieve suffering, even if the amount has the potential to hasten death. It occurs in the context of palliative sedation.

NURSING STUDY: COPING WITH DYING

Jesse was simply unable to believe that his wife was dying. The physician told Jesse that Jeanette was in the early stages of multiple myeloma, and that she might die in less than a year or she might have remissions and live another decade. Jesse and his wife had worked hard all their lives and raised two sons. Now they were both retired and financially secure and thought the best years of their lives were ahead of them. However, both Jesse and Jeanette were the type who approached a problem head-on. They gathered all the relevant material they could find about multiple myeloma and assiduously studied it. Jeanette said that she did not want to mention her problem to others because she thought that she was unable to deal with "their piteous cancer looks." She also stressed that she expected to have long remissions and to live at least 10 more years. So why trouble friends and family? As a result of her decision, Jesse was unable to share his fear and grief because he had promised to respect Jeanette's wishes in that regard. She began a series of chemotherapeutic drugs, and friends began to notice her leth-

argy. They began to worry about her, but she insisted, "I'm just fine." Six months passed with a steady downward course in Jeanette's condition. Her sons began to suspect she had a malignancy, and one son, Rob, asked outright, "Are you hiding a serious illness from us?" She denied it, but Rob also noticed that Jesse was withdrawing into himself and that he was drinking more than usual. Rob knew something was wrong but was at a loss. When Rob went to the family physician for his annual checkup, the office nurse said, "Oh, Rob, how is your mother doing?"

- Considering the situation and the current regulations about the protection of patient privacy, how would you respond to the son's next question if you were the nurse?
- As a nurse, how could you promote communication within this family to help them move toward open awareness?
- What is your priority in attending to the needs of Jesse? Of Jeanette? Of their children?

CRITICAL THINKING QUESTIONS AND ACTIVITIES

1. Explore your responses to being given a terminal diagnosis. What coping mechanisms work for you?
2. With which level of awareness approach would you be most comfortable? As a nurse? As a patient?
3. If you believe that you are able, discuss your grief process when you dealt with the loss of someone special in your life.
4. Practice with a partner several methods that you will use to introduce the topic of dying with a client who is critically ill and is not expected to live.

5. Describe how you would deal with a dying person and his or her family when these family members are especially protective of each other.
6. Discuss and strategize how you would bring up the topic of advance directives.
7. Explore with family and friends their thoughts on completing an advance directive.

RESEARCH QUESTIONS

1. What advance directive is legally recognized in your state?
2. What is the American Nurses Association viewpoint on nurses' involvement in assisted suicide?

3. Select a culture other than your own and explore loss, grief, and morning rituals. How often are they used?

REFERENCES

Alward PD: Betty Newman's system model. In Parker ME, Smith MC, editors: *Nursing theories and nursing practice*, ed 3, Philadelphia, 2010, FA Davis, pp 182–201.

Beck E, Jones SJ: Children of the condemned: grieving the loss of a father on death row, *Omega (Westport)* 56(2): 191–215, 2007–2008.

Broad JB, Gott M, Kim H, et al: Where do people die? An international comparison of the percentage of deaths occurring in hospital and residential care setting in 45 populations, using published and available statistics, *Int J Public Health* 58(2):257–267, 2013.

Carr D, Sonnega J, Nesse RM, et al: Do special occasions trigger psychological distress among older bereaved spouses? An empirical assessment of clinical wisdom, *J Gerontol B Psychol Sci Soc Sci* 69(1): 113–122, 2014.

Chambaere K, Bilsen J, Cohn J, et al: Physician-assisted deaths under the euthanasia law in Belgium: a population-based survey, *CMAJ* 182(9):895–901, 2010.

Coolen PR: *Cultural relevance in end-of-life care*, 2012. https://ethnomed.org/clinical/end-of-life/cultural-relevance-in-end-of-life-care. Accessed October 2014.

Corless IB: Bereavement. In Ferrell BR, Coyle N, editors: *Textbook of palliative nursing*, ed 2, New York, 2006, Oxford University Press, pp 531–544.

Corr CA, Nabe CM, Corr DM: *Death and dying, life and living*, ed 3, Stamford City, CT, 2000, Wadsworth.

Death with Dignity National Center: *Death with dignity acts*, 2014. http://www.deathwithdignity.org/acts. Accessed October 2014.

Doka KJ: Disenfranchised grief. In Doka KJ, editor: *Disenfranchised grief: recognizing hidden sorrow*, Lexington, MA, 1989, Lexington Books.

Doka, KJ: *Disenfranchised grief: new directions, challenges, and strategies for practice*, Champaign, IL, 2002, Research Press.

Giacquinta B: Helping families face the crisis of cancer, *Am J Nurs* 77:1585–1588, 1977.

Glaser B, Strauss A: *Awareness of dying*, Chicago, 1965, AVC.

Glaser BG, Strauss AL: *Time for dying*, Chicago, 1968, Aldine.

Goldstein C, Anapolsky E, Park J, et al: Research guiding practice related to cultural issues at end of life care, *Geriatr Nurs* 25:58–59, 2004.

Goldstein NB, Morrison BS: Palliative care. In Ham RJ, Sloane PD, Warshaw GA, et al, editors: *Primary care geriatrics: a case-based approach*, ed 6, Philadelphia, 2014, Elsevier, pp 164–174.

Hall C: *Beyond Kübler-Ross: recent developments in our understanding of grief and bereavement, InPsych 2011*. http://www.psychology.org.au/publications/inpsych/2011. Accessed October 2014.

Herman C: *National Consensus Project updates: palliative care guidelines*, Aging Today Online, Sept 26, 2013. http://www.nationalconsensusproject.org/guidelines_download2.aspx. Accessed October 2014.

Herbert K, Moore H, Rooney J: The nurse advocate in end-of-life care, *Oschsner J* 11(4):325–329, 2011.

Herbert RS, Schultz R, Copeland V, et al: What questions do family caregivers want to discuss with health care providers in order to prepare for the death of a loved one? An ethnographic study of caregivers of patients at end of life, *J Palliat Med* 11:476–483, 2007.

Horacek BJ: Toward a more viable model of grieving and consequences for older persons, *Death Studies* 15:459–472, 1991.

Jett KJ, Jett SW: *The loss response model*, unpublished manuscript, 2014.

Jones SJ, Beck E: Disenfranchised grief and nonfinite loss as experienced by the families of death row inmates, *Omega (Westport)* 54(4):281–299, 2007–2008.

Kübler-Ross E: *On death and dying*, New York, 1969, Macmillan.

Kulkarni SP, Karliner LS, Auerbach AD, et al: Physician use of advance care planning discussions in diverse hospitalized population, *J Immigr Minor Health* 13(3): 620–624, 2011.

Maslow AH: A theory of human motivation, *Psychol Rev* 50:370–396, 1943.

Mazanec P, Panke JT: Cultural considerations in palliative care. In Ferrell BR, Coyle N: *Oxford textbook of palliative nursing*, ed 3, New York, 2010, Oxford University Press, pp 701–713.

National Consensus Project: *Clinical practice guidelines for quality palliative care*, ed 2, 2009. http://www.nationalconsensusproject.org. Accessed October 2014.

National Hospice and Palliative Care Organization (NHPCO): *NHPCO Facts and figures: hospice care in America*, 2014. http://www.nhpco.org/sites/default/files/public/Statistics_Research/2014_Facts_Figures.pdf. Accessed November 2014.

Neimeyer RA, Sands DC: Meaning reconstruction in bereavement: from principles to practice. In Neimeyer RA, Harris DL, Winokuer HR, et al, editors: *Grief and bereavement in contemporary society: bridging research and practice*, New York, 2011, Routledge.

Pattison EM: The experience of dying. In Pattison EM, editor, *The experience of dying*, Englewood Cliffs, NJ, 1977, Prentice-Hall.

Perrels AJ, Fleming J, Zhao J, et al: Place of death and end-of-life transitions experienced by very old people with differing cognitive status: retrospective analysis of a prospective population-based cohort aged 85 and over, *Palliat Med* 28(3): 220–233, 2014.

POLST: *What is POLST®?* 2012. http://www.polst.org. Accessed October 2014.

Rando TA: Grief and mourning: accommodating to loss. In Wass H, Neimyer RA, editors: *Dying—facing the facts, Philadelphia*, 1995, Taylor & Francis, pp 211–241.

Richardson VE, Bennett KM, Carr D, et al: How does bereavement get under the skin? The effects of late-life spousal loss on cortisol levels, *J Gerontol B Psychol Sci Soc Sci*, Dec 19, 2013. [Epub ahead of print]. http://www.ncbi.nlm.nih.gov/pubmed/24259378.

Roelands M, Van den Block L, Geurts S, et al: Attitudes of Belgian students of medicine, philosophy and law towards euthanasia and the conditions for its acceptance, *Death Studies* Sept 25, 2014. [Epub ahead of print].

Seale C, Raus K, Bruinsma S, et al: The language of sedation in end-of life care: the ethical reasoning of care providers in three countries. *Health (London)*, Nov 10, 2014. [Epub ahead of print].

Seymour J, Almack K, Kennedy S: Implementing advance care planning: a qualitative study of community nurses' views and experiences, *BMC Palliat Care* 9:4, 2010. doi: 10.1186/1472-684X-9-4.

Shear MK, Ghesquiere A, Glickman K: Bereavement and complicated grief, *Curr Psychiatry Rep* 15(11):406, 2013.

Spoelhof GD, Elliott B: Implementing advance directives in office practice, *Am Fam Physician* 85(5):461–466, 2012.

St. Christopher's: *Dame Cicely Saunders—her life and her work*, 2014. http://www.stchristophers.org.uk/about/damecicelysaunders. Accessed October 2014.

Steck N, Egger M, Maessen M, et al: Euthanasia and assisted suicide in selected European countries and the US states: a systematic literature review, *Med Care* 51(10):936–944, 2013.

Utz RL, Caserta M, Lund D: Grief, depressive symptoms, and physical health among recently bereaved spouses, *Gerontologist* 52(4):460–471, 2012.

Vable AM, Subramanian SV, Rist PM, et al: Does the "widowhood effect" precede spousal bereavement? Results from a nationally representative sample, *Am J Geriatr Psychiatry* S1064–781 (14):00145–6, May 14, 2014. [Epub ahead of print].

Van Scoy LJ, Howrylak J, Nguyen A, et al: Family structure, experience with end-of-life decision making, and who asked about advanced directives, *J Palliat Med* 17(10):1099–1106, 2014.

Weisman A: *Coping with cancer*, New York, 1979, McGraw-Hill.

World Health Organization: *WHO definition of palliative care*, 2010. http://www.who.int/cancer/palliative/definition/en. Accessed October 2014.

Zisook S, Shear K: Grief and bereavement: what psychiatrists need to know, *World Psychiatry* 8(2):67–74, 2009.

36 | CHAPTER

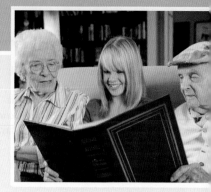

Self-Actualization, Spirituality, and Transcendence

Priscilla Ebersole* and Theris A. Touhy

http://evolve.elsevier.com/Touhy/TwdHlthAging

A STUDENT SPEAKS

Well, I always went to church with my parents when I was a child, but it was really boring. Now, I sometimes go with my grandmother to make her happy. I see how important it is to her, and I wonder if it will be important to me when I get really old. I'm just too busy right now.

Lori, age 22

AN ELDER SPEAKS

This is a real problem! I have three children and don't want them to squabble over my things when I'm gone. I would like it if they would each choose something special that would remind them of me, but every time I bring it up they cut me off and won't talk about it. I know there will be a big fight over the piano!

Mabel, age 74

LEARNING OBJECTIVES

On completion of this chapter, the reader will be able to:

1. Provide a comprehensive definition of self-actualization and identify several qualities of self-actualized elders.
2. Discuss the nursing role in relation to the self-actualization of elders.
3. Describe several examples of transcendence as experienced by older people.
4. Specify various types of creative self-expression and describe their positive impact on health, illness, and quality of life among older adults.
5. Understand the meaning of spirituality in the lives of older people and discuss nursing interventions to facilitate spiritual well-being.
6. Define the concept of legacy and name several types of legacies and what the nurse can do to facilitate their expression.

Self-actualization, spirituality, and *transcendence* are vague, ambiguous terms that mean whatever the theorist thinks. These expressions also serve as umbrella terms for other conditions and situations that are addressed throughout this chapter. These terms overlap a great deal, but we have attempted to tease out the meanings for the reader, knowing that the perception of the reader will cast a particular interpretation that we may not have thought or intended. These conditions are ineffable, within the awareness of the individual but often inexpressible. Why, if these concepts are so obscure, do we include them as the final chapter in a text for nurses working with elders? Because these concepts are the life tasks of aging, seldom fully approached earlier. Concerns of the young are to become established as adults; middle-aged persons are overwhelmed with the requirements of success and survival.

Older people are more in touch with their inner psychological life than at any other point in the life cycle (Cohen, 2006). Ferreting out the reason for being and the meaning of life is the concern of elders. "As people age, confronting mortality is part of it, but as things change, they begin to recognize who they are and who they aren't, the strengths they have and haven't. They begin to think about the value and meaning of life. Tending to look more inwards rather than outwards often happens when we are 45 to 50, but there's a screaming need for it when we reach 85 or 90" (Bernstein, 2009; www.agingwellmag.com/news/septstory1.shtml).

*Special thanks to Dr. Priscilla Ebersole, the original author of this chapter, for her foundational and very wise contributions.

An understanding of the developmental phases in the second half of life assists in understanding the journey toward self-actualization (Box 36-1).

Nurses will likely see numerous older people who are apparently not seeking any of these esoteric states of existence and have never tried to cultivate their deepest inner nature. We live in a mechanistic, scientifically based culture in which cultivation of immeasurable states of being has not been necessarily regarded or regarded at all. The dramatic increase in the population of older people has been considered a problem to be solved in an era of dwindling resources rather than a resource to enrich society. Attempting to sort, dissect, and classify everything is a hazard of our society.

Despite all the human efforts for the past millennia, we have not been able to completely grasp or dissect the human soul. I have many times approached this subject incorrectly by asking individuals what it is like to be old. Now that I am old, what it is like seems too concrete. What is the meaning of this stage of life? Every nurse must ask this question of his or her older clients, friends, and parents. Do not ask on your way out the door. For many people, this notion will take some pondering. For some, it will open the door of their later lives just a crack. Others will be enlightened and will teach you a great deal.

SELF-ACTUALIZATION

Self-actualization is the highest expression of one's individual potential and implies inner motivation that has been freed to express the most unique self or the "authentic person" (Maslow, 1959, p. 3). The crux of self-actualization is defining life in such a way as to allow room for continual discovery of self. A critical consideration in developing self-actualization is an underlying sense of mastery and a sense of coherence in the life situation. This effort depends to a large extent on individual attributes, as well as self-esteem. In this unit, we hope to expose the nurse to the myriad evidences of self-actualization in old age and suggest ways in which the nurse can assist older people in seeking their own unique way of living, growing, and making meaning. The focus is on nursing actions that may encourage elders to seek new possibilities within themselves.

Characteristics of the Self-Actualized

In old age, threats to self-esteem are strong if value is measured only by attainment, containment, power, and influence. Ethics, values, humor, courage, altruism, and integrity flourish in people who continue to grow toward self-actualization. Numerous other attributions can be mentioned. We focus only on those qualities that seem most pertinent to the older people whom health care professionals are serving (Box 36-2).

Courage

Courage is the quality of mind or spirit that enables a person to conquer fear and despair in the face of difficulty, danger, pain, or uncertainty. An older man with diabetes, amputations, and failing vision sits in his room at the retirement home, looking out the window for hours each day, for weeks, months, and years. Yet he retains his positive spirit and love of life. This is courage. An older lady crippled with arthritis attends her ailing spouse, who no longer recognizes her. This is courage. When asking older people how they keep going day by day, various answers are given. No one has ever said to me, "It is because I am courageous." Older people need to be told. A gold star can be given to people who have lived and survived the long battle of living many years filled with both joy and pain. Memorials are made for people who die in battle, but few monuments are raised to those who courageously wake every morning with no great purpose or challenge to push them out of bed.

Tara Cortes, Executive Director of the Hartford Institute for Geriatric Nursing, shares the following quote from a 91-year-old gentleman: "It's a decision I make every morning when I wake up. I have a choice; I can spend the day in bed recounting

---

BOX 36-1 Developmental Phases in the Second Half of Life

Midlife reevaluation: Early 40s to late 50s and characterized by seriously confronting the sense of one's own mortality and thinking about time remaining instead of time gone by. A catalyst for uncovering unrealized creative sides of ourselves.

Liberation: Mid-50s to mid-70s and characterized by a sense of personal freedom to speak one's mind and do what needs to be done. With retirement comes a new experience of personal liberation and having time to experiment with something different.

Summing-up: Late 60s to the 80s and beyond and characterized by the desire to find larger meaning in the story of one's life and to deal with unresolved conflicts and unfinished business. Motivation to give the wisdom accrued throughout life, share lessons and fortunes through autobiography and personal storytelling, philanthropy, community activism, and volunteerism.

Encore: Any time from the late 70s to the end of life and characterized by the desire to restate and reaffirm major themes in one's life and explore new variations on those themes or further attend to unfinished business or unresolved conflicts and a desire to live well until the end.

From Cohen G: Research on creativity and aging: the positive impact of the arts on health and illness, *Generations* 30(1):7–15, 2006.

BOX 36-2 Traits of Self-Actualized People

- Time competent: The person uses past and future to live more fully in the present.
- Inner directed: The person's source of direction depends on internal forces more than on others.
- Flexible: The person can react situationally, without unreasonable restrictions.
- Sensitive to self: The person is responsive to his or her own feelings.
- Spontaneous: The person is able and willing to be himself or herself.
- Values self: The person accepts and demonstrates strengths as a person.
- Accepts self: The person approves of self, in spite of weaknesses or deficiencies.
- Positively views others: The person sees both the bad and the good in others as essentially good and constructive.
- Positively views life: The person sees the opposites of life as meaningfully related.
- Acceptance of aggressiveness: The person is able to accept own feelings of anger and aggressiveness.
- Capable of intimate contact: The person is able to develop warm interpersonal relationships with others.

the difficulty I have with parts of my body that no longer work, or get out of bed and be thankful for the ones that do. Each day is a gift, and as long as my eyes open, I'll focus on the new day and all the happy memories I've stored away just for this time in my life" (Cortes, 2013). The capacity of the spirit to find meaning in existence is often remarkable. Nurses may ask, "What sustains you in your present situation?"

Altruism

A high degree of helping behaviors is present in many older people. The very old will remember the Great Depression and the altruism that kept people physically and spiritually alive. Neighbor helped neighbor long before the government came to the rescue. Apparently, a sense of meaning in life is strongly tied to survival and is derived from the conviction of, in some way, being needed by others. Many nurses are in the field because of altruistic motives and can understand the importance of assisting others. This idea might be discussed with the elder.

Volunteering often involves new role development and endeavors that expand one's awareness. When volunteer services are considered as a means of personal enrichment and an expression of altruism, it is important for the elder to augment some latent interest areas and launch into pursuits perhaps unavailable earlier because of time constraints or other commitments. Nurses may question elders about latent interests and talents that they may want to cultivate.

Humor

Metcalf (1993) explains humor: it originates in the Latin root *humour,* meaning fluid and flexible, able to flow around and wear away obstacles. In the same way that water sustains our life and well-being, humor sustains our mental well-being. Cousins (1979) and many other researchers have recognized the importance of humor in recovery from illness. The physiological effects of humor stimulate production of catecholamines and hormones and increase pain tolerance by releasing endorphins.

Elders often initiate humor, and, in our seriousness, we may overlook the dry wit or, worse, perceive it as confusion. Older people are not a humorless group and frequently laugh at themselves. Objections to jokes about old age seem to emanate from the young far more than the old. Perhaps the old, from the vantage point of a lifetime, can more clearly see human predicaments. Ego transcendence (Peck, 1955) allows one to step back and view the self and situation without the intensity and despair of the egocentric individual.

Continuous Moral Development

The moral development of mankind, on an individual and collective basis, has been of interest to philosophers and religious leaders throughout history. The driving forces of morality are love (Plato) and intellect (Aristotle).

Kohlberg's refinements of his original theories have focused on the evidence, derived from autobiographies, that in maturity, transformations of moral outlook take place. Kohlberg posited old age as a seventh stage of moral development that goes beyond reasoning and reaches awareness of one's relative participation in universal morality. This stage of moral development involves identification with a more enduring moral perspective than that of one's own life span (Kohlberg and Power, 1981). This effort involves moral expansion and the exemplary impact of the fully developing elder on the following generations, born and unborn. We have come to believe that these exemplary lives may be the most important function of elders as we decry the honor and recognition given to individuals who seem to have little integrity or reliability. Each individual carries a mass of motivations and desires. Some people are stunted, and some will flourish. Youngsters must have models of honorable, truthful, and honest elders if we hope to cultivate these qualities in society and human experience.

Self-Renewal

Self-renewal is an ongoing process that ideally continues through adult life as one becomes self-actualized (Hudson, 1999). According to Hudson, self-renewal involves the following:

- Commitment to beliefs
- Connecting to the world
- Times of solitude
- Episodic breaks from responsibility
- Contact with the natural world
- Creative self-expression
- Adaptation to changes
- Learning from down times

Collective Self-Actualization

The collective power of self-actualized older people has already brought about many changes in society. Power is a term describing the capacity of an individual or group to accomplish something, to take command, to exert authority, and to influence. The self-actualized older person is powerful and confident. Power is the gateway to resources and recognition.

The age-equality movement, older citizens returning to school, and the revolution of older people in movements such as the Gray Panthers have produced major changes in the status and recognition of older people. Gray Panthers recognize that issues of aging are not narrow or exclusive but, rather, are representative of human rights for people of all ages. Maggie Kuhn (1979), founder of the Gray Panthers, died in 1995 at the age of 89, but her beliefs and followers survive. Kuhn perceived that the issues confronting older people are not those of self-interest. As "elders of the tribe," the old should seek "survival of the tribe" (Kuhn, 1979, p. 3).

WISDOM

Wisdom is an ancient concept that has historically been associated with the elders of a society. Wisdom represents the pinnacle of human development and can be compared to Maslow's self-actualization or Erickson's ego integrity. In many cultures, older people are respected for their years of experience and are awarded the role of wise elder in political, judicial, cultural, and religious systems.

Over the last 2 decades, there has been renewed interest in the concept of wisdom and the capacity of the aging brain to develop unique capacities (Ardelt, 1997, 2000, 2003, 2004; Baltes 1991; Baltes and Smith, 2003, 2008). Many skills improve with age but are not identified on standard cognitive screens, and certain testing conditions have exaggerated age-related declines in cognitive performance (Chapter 5). The bulk of research has focused on cognitive declines and strategies to help older people find ways to overcome cognitive failings. Because of this emphasis, research on cognitive capacities in aging and possible ways to stimulate wisdom has been limited.

Moving beyond Piaget's formal operational stage of cognitive development, adult development theories propose a more advanced cognitive stage, the postformal operational stage. In this stage, individuals develop the skills to view problems from multiple perspectives, utilize reflection, and communicate thoughtfully in complex and emotionally challenging situations (Parisi et al, 2009). Recent neuroimaging research has suggested that changes in the brain, once seen only as compensation for declining skills, are now thought to indicate development of new capacities (Chapter 5).

Characteristics of Wisdom

One does not become wise simply because one grows old. Nor is wisdom achieved simply because of an accumulation of life experiences. Most agree that the achievement of wisdom is a developmental process that requires the ability to "integrate experiences across time and utilize these experiences in a reflective manner" (Parisi et al, 2009, p. 867). Maturity, integrity, generativity, the ability to overcome negative personality characteristics such as neuroticism or self-centeredness, superior judgment skills in difficult life situations, the ability to cope with difficult challenges in life, and a strong sense of the ultimate meaning and purpose of life are also associated with wisdom (Ardelt, 2004) (Box 36-3). Wisdom is a major contributor to successful aging (Reichstadt et al, 2010). The renewed emphasis on wisdom and other cognitive capabilities that can develop with age provides a view of aging that reflects the history of many cultures and provides a much more hopeful view of both aging and human development.

Paths to growing older and wiser can be fostered throughout life. Viewing older people as resources for younger people, our society places the reason for and the immense value of aging at the center of focus. This is in contrast to the view of aging as inevitable decline, personal diminishment, disengagement from life, and a drain on society. Nursing too must turn to the wise leaders who came before us as we chart our course for the future (Chapter 2). Priscilla Ebersole, one of the geriatric nursing pioneers and co-author of this chapter, shares her reflections on wisdom from the perspective of her 86 years (Box 36-4).

With the prospect of longer and healthier lives, older people are looking for more meaningful and challenging ways to foster continued growth and contribute to society. Programs such as Foster Grandparents, the Experience Corps, and the Sage-ing Guild are examples of this new view.

BOX 36-3   Dimensions of Wisdom

- Cognitive: Knowledge and acceptance of the positive and negative aspects of human nature, the limits of knowledge, and of life's unpredictability and uncertainties; a desire to know the truth and comprehend the significance and deeper meaning of experiences, phenomena, and events
- Reflective: Being able to perceive phenomena and events from multiple perspectives; self-awareness, self-examination, self-insight; absence of subjectivity and projections (e.g., the tendency to blame other people or circumstances for one's own situation, decisions, or feelings)
- Affective: Sympathetic and compassionate love for others; positive emotions and behaviors toward others

From Ardelt M: Wisdom as expert knowledge system: a critical review of a contemporary operationalization of an ancient concept, *Hum Dev* 47:257–285, 2004.

BOX 36-4   Reflections on Wisdom: Priscilla Ebersole, Geriatric Nursing Pioneer

In thinking about wisdom, I wonder what it is and if we ever achieve anything near that in one lifetime. I now have more questions about life than I have answers.

Where are we in the process of human evolution? We seem to be consumed with speed and technical wonders. What about the extrasensory perceptions and amazing coincidences that seemingly arise randomly? Are we still primitives?

Dying: Doesn't it present more questions? I have become immunized as so many I love have preceded me, but it would be wonderful to know how much time I have—or would it?

How can one develop true compassion? I have flashes of it, but find I still have many judgmental feelings about many persons and events. Is this not practical?

How can I learn more from others? I am rather trapped in my own skin and imperfections.

Is it true that our hormones really affect us so much? Yes, undoubtedly I have become much more aggressive with the almost total loss of estrogen. Do I care?

Is the search for prolongevity a worthy goal? Only when one is healthy and has something to offer the world. But, really, what is healthy? Only function? Mind health?

Does history really teach us anything? Though we seem to repeat so much of it yet pondering it and our roots remains significant for me. And what about the universe, both macro and micro of which we really still know so little? Pondering and wondering, I will never know even a bit of all I wish.

Yet becoming old is *becoming* as life seems to hold many lifetimes in one. There are so many challenges and circumstances that change one's perspective and beliefs. One begins to feel a part of and connected to every living thing. The youth and elders in one's lifetime are so significant in one's philosophy. Grandchildren and great grandchildren open new vistas of thought and opportunities to redo some of the faltering actions of parenthood.

It seems one important goal is to learn to enjoy life in spite of all the bumps one experiences along the way. One of my granddaughters said she loves to see how much I enjoy life and her ability to see that in me is something I will always treasure. That is a gift I hope to leave with her and others whom I contact. I think I have learned to really enjoy this precious gift of life. Catherine, my friend who died at 106, taught me more about aging than any experience in my life. She still giggled like a school girl as she told me of some amusing event in her life.

CREATIVITY

Creativity is a bridge between the growing self and the transcending of self. Creativity may be the transit mechanism between self-actualization (the reaching of one's highest potential) and the step beyond, to transcend the limitations of ego. "Creativity has always been at the heart of our experience as human beings ... this need for creativity never ends" (Perlstein, 2006, p. 5). American culture has neglected to recognize the innate creativity in elders, who are too often viewed as debilitated, in need of medical attention, and the focus of societal problems. Promoting health in aging is more than targeting problems and developing interventions for health promotion and disease prevention. Aging encompasses potential and problems. A focus on creativity and aging and the positive impact of the arts on health, illness, and quality of life is gaining importance in our understanding of health and well-being among older adults.

The National Center for Creative Aging, established in 2001, is dedicated to fostering the relationship between creative expression and quality of life for older people. The *Beautiful Minds: Finding Your Lifelong Potential* campaign is an initiative from the Center that focuses on raising awareness of people who are keeping their minds beautiful and the actions people can take to maintain the brain. Research suggests that there are four dimensions to brain health: the nourished mind, the socially connected mind, the mentally active mind, and the physically active mind. These dimensions stress the importance of healthy diet, social engagement, cognitive stimulation, and physical activity to brain health.

Products of creativity are less important than creative attitudes. Curiosity, inquisitiveness, wonderment, puzzlement, and craving for understanding are creative attitudes. Much of the natural creative imagination of childhood is subdued by enculturation. In aging, some people seem able to break free of excessive enculturation and again express their free spirit when practical matters no longer demand their sole attention.

Creativity is often considered in terms of the arts, literature, and music. A truly self-actualized person may express creativity in any activity. Breaking through the habitual or traditional mode into authentic expression of self is creativity, whether it is through cooking, cleaning, planting, poetry, art, or teaching. Creative expression does not necessarily mean that the older person has to create a work of art. Subtler ways of expressing creativity are present even in the frailest of older people. Consider Dr. Ebersole's description of Catherine at 100 years old and living in a nursing home (Box 36-5).

Creative Arts for Older Adults

Maximizing the use of self in the later years in unique ways might be termed creative self-actualization. Many individuals will need the stimulus of an interested person to uncover latent interests and talents. Other people will need encouragement to try new avenues of self-expression—some will be fitting for them and others not. Several ideas are presented here for nurses working with older people who may need an introduction to creative use of leisure time.

BOX 36-5   Another View of Creativity: Catherine

Catherine was self-actualized and creative to the best possible extent. Her physical constraints were enormous: She had no material assets, her range of activity was limited to her small cubicle in a skilled nursing facility, and her body was frail. However, her spirit was strong, and she knew and used her potential. Catherine's creativity was expressed at each meal when she rearranged, mixed, and added to her food. She carefully chopped a pickle and sprinkled it on her cottage cheese and added a little honey to her applesauce. Each meal was a small adventure. Several friends would visit regularly and bring Catherine small items she enjoyed. They could always count on being entertained with creatively embroidered tales of the past. The gifts they brought were always used in extraordinary ways. A scarf might be tied around her head. Powder, perfume, books, and other things would be bartered for favors from staff members or given as gifts. Her radio brought news of the day interspersed with classical music. Catherine created a milieu in which she enjoyed life and maintained her self-esteem. That she was self-actualized was never in doubt. Her artistry overflowed in myriad small gestures.

Wikstrom suggests that art and aesthetics "help individuals know themselves, become more alive to human conditions, provide a new way of looking at themselves and the world, and offer opportunities for participation in new visual and auditory experiences" (2004, p. 30). Each person has a private, symbolic, feeling world that can be brought out by certain expressive activities.

Creative arts and expression offer great value to people with dementia and hold tremendous promise to improve quality of life. Programs of dance, storytelling (Chapter 6), music, poetry, and art should be included in activities for individuals with dementia. Killick (1997, 2000, 2008) has done beautiful work with poetry writing for persons who have dementia, and he has said that "people with dementia can often find a real solace and satisfaction and a creativity in speaking in this way and having it recognized as being of value because they're so used to being put down" (Killick, 2005).

At the Louis and Anne Green Memory and Wellness Center in the Christine E. Lynn College of Nursing at Florida Atlantic University, the "Artful Memories" program provides opportunities for individuals with mild to moderate dementia to learn techniques of artistic creation and expression in artistic media in a supportive and nonjudgmental environment (Chapter 29) (Figure 36-1). Works created are on display at the Center and in

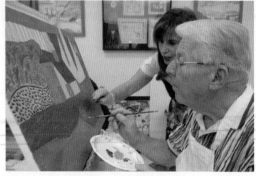

FIGURE 36-1 Artful Memories Program. (Courtesy of the Louis and Anne Green Memory and Wellness Center of the Christine E. Lynn College of Nursing at Florida Atlantic University.)

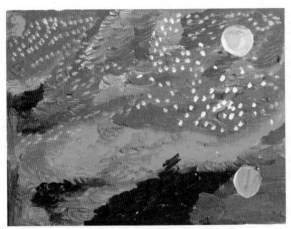

FIGURE 36-2 Artwork created by Frances Hope Goldstein in the Florida Atlantic University (FAU) Louis and Anne Green Memory and Wellness Center "Artful Memories" program.

art museums and have been made into calendars as well (Figure 36-2). Participants have derived a great deal of pleasure, pride, stimulation, and camaraderie from the time spent creating art. More ideas for developing creative activities are presented in Box 36-6.

RECREATION

Recreation is akin to creation. The wisdom of regularly scheduled periods of recreation and recuperation following creative acts can be traced to early Jewish writings and the creation story. If God needed time to rest and recuperate, we certainly do. Inherent in creative acts is time for renewal, time for re-creation. Burnout and boredom are companions of monotony and shorten the perceived life span by emptiness and vanished time. A change of scene or companions may be exhilarating. The opportunity to be outside or look at beautiful scenery is also renewing. Many long-term care facilities are providing opportunities for gardening and enjoying nature. Retreats from routine to periods of recreation are important, as are retreats following intensive efforts. Resources that can enhance recreational activities and programs are presented in Box 36-7.

BRINGING YOUNG AND OLD TOGETHER

Larson (2006) suggests that intergenerational programs can "help older and younger people look beyond their generational stereotypes and know each other (body, mind, and spirit)" (p. 39). Intergenerational programs can be those in which older people assist younger people (tutoring, mentoring, childcare, foster grandparent programs); those in which younger people assist older people (social visits, meal assistance); and those in which younger and older people serve together. Benefits of intergenerational programs for younger people include increased self-esteem and self-worth, improved behavior, increased involvement and success in school work, and a sense of historical and personal continuity. For older people, contact with younger

BOX 36-6 Ideas for Developing Creative Abilities

Art

Using oil pastels, create a drawing that represents self, or select three colors you like and three colors you dislike, using all six colors to create a self-portrait.

Draw a representation of your world.

Create a collage or mobile out of an assortment of materials and pictures that can represent subjects, such as the self, part of self you like or dislike, or the family.

In small groups, use clay to create an art piece or a statement.

Music

Play a variety of music; focus discussion on imagery and any feelings that the music evokes.

Discuss or have clients bring in music that elicits feelings of sadness, happiness, and so on.

Show a picture (can be cut from a magazine), and ask members to see if they can imagine the sounds that might go with the picture.

Express self or group through dance and movement to select music.

Movement

Create a movement to fit the way you are feeling while introducing self to group.

Have members stand and initiate a slow, swaying motion (good exercise with which to end the group session).

Have members mirror each other's movements, such as hands or the entire body, creating a duet.

Imagery

Use guided fantasies and imagery to facilitate stress reduction and relaxation, awareness, the power of one's own healing capability, and self-expression through symbols and symbolisms.

Writing

Encourage journals or diaries; set a group time available to write and share ideas.

In small groups, create a group poem.

Read selected poems or stories as a group, and then share reactions and feelings from the readings.

Create a book to be distributed to the group consisting of a collection of members' writings.

people can promote life satisfaction, decrease isolation, help develop new skills and insights, promote fulfillment, establish new and meaningful relationships, and provide a sense of meaning and purpose (Larson, 2006). Examples of such programs include the Elders Share the Arts, Roots and Branches Theatre Company, and the Liz Lerman Dance Exchange.

Recognizing the developmental significance of contact between the generations, some long-term care facilities have included children in their milieu in various ways:

- *As residents* (children with profound developmental disabilities or severe neurological disabilities): Elders rock, stroke, and cuddle these children, providing stimulation for both.
- *As a service to employees* (day care centers for children of employees): Elders sometimes assist in the care and special programs for the children, such as reading stories or teaching basic skills (tying shoes, telling time).

BOX 36-7 Resources to Enhance Recreational Activities/Programs

- Local florists may present a flower show or provide a flower-arranging activity.
- Police/fire departments may give safety presentations.
- Local religious leaders may lead readings and discussions of religious/philosophical works.
- Craft suppliers may give demonstrations.
- Local pharmacists may give talks on medication use.
- Nurses or nursing students may give talks on health and well-being in aging.
- Clothing stores can sponsor fashion shows.
- Bakeries may give demonstrations of pastry decoration.
- Beauty supply houses may give makeup demonstrations.
- Travel agencies may present slide shows.
- Librarians may institute great book discussions or other activities.
- Students from community colleges may provide numerous educational events and activities.
- Garden clubs or horticultural groups may provide gardening classes.
- Collectors' clubs may talk about collecting stamps, antiques, coins, or memorabilia.
- Historical societies may give tours to historic places of interest.
- Whenever possible, events should be planned as field trips to the sites of the locals involved because trips add elements of additional interest, stimulation, and involvement in the community at large.

- *In adopt-a-grandparent programs:* One child affiliates with a resident with periodic visits, cards, and inclusion of the grandparent in some special family events.

Nurses in the community may want to explore potential intergenerational experiences that may be of interest to their older clients. Area Agencies on Aging can provide information on intergenerational programs that are available in the community. Although we recommend intergenerational contact when desired by the older person, certain pitfalls must be considered. Not all older people will enjoy contact with children. Contacts with the very young, energetic child must be brief, or else the elder is likely to be exhausted, and the benefits will decrease. In intergenerational programs, young people need consistent supervision, support, and training in the developmental aspects of old age. Similarly, elders will also benefit from education and support in understanding developmental tasks of children, as well as effective methods of intergenerational communication.

◆ PROMOTING HEALTHY AGING: IMPLICATIONS FOR GERONTOLOGICAL NURSING

In this unit, we have considered what aging can be and that the last years can truly actualize the most unique capacities of older people. Our functions as nurses who value self-actualization are (1) to continually spur our clients to ask "What is possible and suitable for me?" and (2) to assist them in finding appropriate resources and, when needed, assist in implementing activities toward self-actualization. The nature of self-actualization is self-determination and direction. Nurses are ancillary to the process but may be needed to stir the beginnings of the search. In doing so, we may move forward with our own search.

Self-actualization implies that one actualizes the potential of self through various mechanisms. We have mentioned only a few of these mechanisms in a somewhat cursory manner, knowing that these individually instituted actions have a force of their own and that once activated go far beyond the professionals' involvement. Activities such as yoga, focused meditation, the discipline of karate, and other forms of centered concentration are segued into spirituality and transcendence.

SPIRITUALITY

Spirituality is a rather indescribable need that drives individuals throughout life to seek meaning and purpose in their existence. Spirituality is difficult to define, though many people have tried. We can observe the body and we can imagine the mind in operation and measure intelligence, but there is no computed tomography (CT) scan of the spirit (Bell and Troxel, 2001). Understanding spirituality is far more elusive than learning about the pathology associated with disease and illness.

Spirituality has been defined as a "quality of a person derived from the social and cultural environment that involves faith, a search for meaning, a sense of connection with others, and a transcendence of self, resulting in a sense of inner peace and well-being" (Delgado, 2007, p. 230). The spiritual aspect of people's lives transcends the physical and psychosocial to reach the deepest individual capacity for love, hope, and meaning. Erickson's concept of ego integrity and Maslow's concept of self-actualization seem closely related to development of a spiritual self.

Aging as a biological process has been studied extensively. Less attention has been paid to the study of aging as a spiritual process. As people age and move closer to death, spirituality may become more important. Declining physical health, loss of loved ones, and a realization that life's end may be near often challenge older people to reflect on the meaning of their lives. Spiritual belief and practices often play a central role in helping older adults cope with life challenges and are a source of strength in the lives of older adults (Hodge et al, 2010). Nursing studies of spirituality and aging indicate that spirituality increases in importance and is a source of hope, aids in adaptation to illnesses, and has a positive influence on quality of life in chronically ill older adults (Cherry et al, 2013; Edlund, 2014; Lowry and Conco, 2002; O'Brien, 2003; Touhy, 2001a,b; Touhy et al, 2005). The ultimate goal for promoting spirituality is to support and enhance quality of life.

Spirituality must be considered a significant factor in understanding healthy aging. Rowe and Kahn's (1998) model of successful aging includes active engagement in life, minimal risk and disability, and high cognitive and physical function. Crowther and colleagues (2002) maintain that spirituality must be the fourth element of the model and is interrelated with all of the others (Edlund, 2014). Spirituality may be particularly important to healthy aging in "historically disadvantaged populations who display remarkable strength despite adversities in their lives" (Hooyman and Kiyak, 2005, p. 213). Spiritual well-being may be considered the ability to experience and integrate meaning and purpose in life through connectedness with self, others, art, music, literature, nature, or a power greater than oneself (Gaskamp et al, 2006).

Spirituality and Religion

Distinguishing between religion and spirituality is a concern for many health professionals. Religious beliefs and participation in religious obligations and rites are often the avenues of spiritual expression, but they are not necessarily interchangeable. "Religion can be described as a social institution that unites people in a faith in God, a higher power, and in common rituals and worshipful acts. A god, divinity, and/or soul is always included in the concept" (Strang and Strang, 2002, p. 858). Each religion involves a particular set of beliefs. Spirituality is a broader concept than religion and encompasses a person's values or beliefs, search for meaning, and relationships with a higher power, with nature, and with other people. The concept of spirituality is found in all cultures and societies.

For some people, particularly older people, formalized religion helps them feel fulfilled. The majority of older adults describe themselves as both spiritual and religious (Hodge et al, 2010). Gerontologists appreciate the significance of religion and spirituality in promoting the well-being of elders. "Although aging changes can affect the body and the mind, there is no evidence that the spirit succumbs to the aging process, even in the presence of debilitating physical and emotional illness" (Heriot, 1992, p. 23).

For some older people, particularly those who are frail or cognitively impaired, meeting spiritual needs may be a greater challenge than for healthier elders (Powers and Watson, 2011). Functional decline and dependence can threaten the sense of identity and connection with others and the world, thus causing a loss of spirit (Leetun, 1996; Touhy 2001a). The spiritual aspect transcends the physical and psychosocial to reach the deepest individual capacity for love, hope, and meaning. The spiritual person can rise above that which is humanly expected in a situation. For example, a dying elder in great pain who was being cared for by Dr. Ebersole said: "This is so hard for you." That he was able to see beyond himself at that time was difficult to believe.

◆ PROMOTING HEALTHY AGING: IMPLICATIONS FOR GERONTOLOGICAL NURSING

◆ Assessment

Assessment of spirituality is as important as assessment of physical, emotional, and social dimensions (Edlund, 2014). A spiritual history opens the door to a conversation about the role of spirituality and religion in a person's life. People often need permission to talk about these issues. Without a signal from the nurse, patients may feel that such topics are not welcome. Patients welcome a discussion of spiritual matters and want health professionals to consider their spiritual needs.

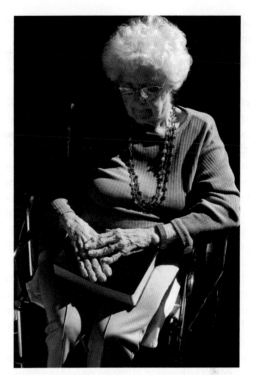

Prayer. (©iStock.com/Lisa Thornberg)

The older person may have a pressing need to talk about philosophy and spiritual development. Private time for prayer, meditation, and reflection may be needed.

Nurses may neglect to explore this issue with elders because religion and spirituality may not seem the high priority. The client should be assured that religious longings and rituals are important and that opportunities will be made available as desired. Nurses need to be knowledgeable and respectful about the rites and rituals of varying religions, cultural beliefs, and values (Chapter 4). Religious and spiritual resources, such as pastoral visits, should be available in all settings where older people reside. It is important to avoid imposing one's own beliefs and to respect the person's privacy on matters of spirituality and religion (Touhy and Zerwekh, 2006).

Spiritual care entails assisting individuals to find a sense of meaning and reconciliation with others and with a transcendent reality, while encouraging them to strengthen their spiritual life as they choose. Nurses may not lead individuals to soul growth and acceptance when facing illness and disability but may have the privilege of accompanying them on the journey. If spiritual growth is the primary focus of the older person, clergy will be best suited to work with the person. Reflection, feedback, comfort, and affirmation are all a part of being with the elder, providing the supports that release energy for spiritual seeking.

An emphasis on spirituality in nursing is not new; nursing has encompassed the spiritual from its origin. The science of nursing was not seen as separate from the art and spirit of the discipline. Florence Nightingale's view of nursing was derived from her spiritual philosophy, and she considered nursing a spiritual experience, "intrinsic to human nature, our deepest and most potent resource for healing" (Macrae, 1995, p. 8). Many nursing theories address spirituality, including those of Neuman, Parse, and Watson (Martsolf and Mickley, 1998). Nursing and medicine are beginning to reclaim some of the essential healing values from their roots.

The essence of being spiritual is being whole or holistic, and attention to the spiritual needs of patients is a critical dimension of holistic nursing care. Yet surveys with practicing nurses suggest that most have had little, if any, education in spiritual care. Many nurses view spiritual nursing responses in religious terms and may feel that spirituality is a religious matter better left to clergy and religious leaders. Heriot (1992) suggested that nurses need to understand care of the human spirit both within and outside the context of religion. Goldberg (1998) asserted that the connection in the nurse-patient relationship is central to spiritual care but that most nurses are "carrying out spiritual interventions at an unconscious level" (p. 840). She called for education and research to help nurses become more aware of the importance of connection and use of self in relationships as ways of bringing the elements of spiritual care into conscious awareness.

An evidence-based guideline for promoting spirituality in the older adult (Gaskamp et al, 2006) provides a framework for spiritual assessment and interventions. The guideline identifies older adults who may be at risk for spiritual distress and who might be most likely to benefit from use of the guideline (Box 36-8). Spiritual distress or spiritual pain is "an individual's perception of hurt or suffering associated with that part of his or her person that seeks to transcend the realm of the material. Spiritual distress is manifested by a deep sense of hurt stemming from feelings of loss or separation from one's God or deity, a sense of personal inadequacy or sinfulness before God and man, or a pervasive condition of loneliness" (Gaskamp et al, 2006, p. 9).

The person experiencing spiritual distress is unable to experience the meaning of hope, connectedness, and transcendence. Spiritual distress may be manifested by anger, guilt, blame, hatred, expressions of alienation, turning away from family and friends, inability to derive pleasure, and inability to participate in religious activities that have previously provided comfort.

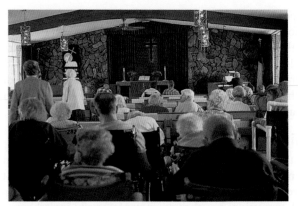

Residents Attend a Religious Service at a Nursing Center. (From Sorrentino SA, Gorek B: *Mosby's textbook for long-term care assistants,* ed 5, St Louis, MO, 2007, Mosby.)

Spiritual Assessment Tools

There are formal spiritual assessments, but open-ended questions can also be used to begin dialogue about spiritual concerns (Box 36-9). Simply listening to patients as they express their fears, hopes, and beliefs is important. Spiritual assessments are intended to elicit information about the core spiritual needs and how the nurse and other members of the health care team can respond to them. These include the Faith, Importance/Influence, Community and Address (FICA) Spiritual History (Puchalski and Romer, 2000), and the Brief Assessment of Spiritual Resources and Concerns (Koenig and Brooks, 2002; Meyer, 2003) (Box 36-10). The Joint Commission requires spiritual assessments in hospitals, nursing homes, home care organizations, and many other health care settings providing services to older adults. The process of

---

BOX 36-8   Identifying Elders at Risk for Spiritual Distress

- Individuals experiencing events or conditions that affect the ability to participate in spiritual rituals
- Diagnosis and treatment of a life-threatening, chronic, or terminal illness
- Expressions of interpersonal or emotional suffering, loss of hope, lack of meaning, need to find meaning in suffering
- Evidence of depression
- Cognitive impairment
- Verbalized questioning or loss of faith
- Loss of interpersonal support

Data from Gaskamp C, Sutter R, Meraviglia M, et al: Evidence-based guideline: promoting spirituality in the older adult, *J Gerontol Nurs* 32:8–13, 2006.

BOX 36-9   Questions to Begin Dialogue about Spiritual Concerns

- Tell me more about your life.
- What has been most meaningful in your life?
- To whom do you turn when you need help?
- What brings you joy and comfort?
- What are you most proud of?
- How have you found strength throughout your life?
- What are you hopeful about?
- Is spiritual peace important to you? What would help you achieve it?
- Is your religion or God significant in your life? Can you describe how?
- Is prayer or meditation helpful?
- What spiritual or religious practices bring you comfort?
- Are there religious books or materials that you want nearby?
- What are you afraid of right now?
- What do you wish you could still do?
- What are your concerns at this time for the future?
- What matters most to you right now?

Adapted from Touhy T, Zerwekh J: Spiritual caring. In Zerwekh J: *Nursing care at the end of life: palliative care for patients and families,* Philadelphia, 2006, FA Davis; Hospice of the Florida Suncoast, 2001.

BOX 36-10 Brief Assessment of Spiritual Resources and Concerns

Instructions: Use the following questions as an interview guide with the older adult (or caregiver if the older adult is unable to communicate).

- Does your religion/spirituality provide comfort or serve as a cause of stress? (Ask to explain in what ways spirituality is a comfort or stressor.).
- Do you have any religious or spiritual beliefs that might conflict with health care or affect health care decisions? (Ask to identify any conflicts.)
- Do you belong to a supportive church, congregation, or faith community? (Ask how the faith community is supportive.)
- Do you have any practices or rituals that help you express your spiritual or religious beliefs? (Ask to identify or describe practices.)
- Do you have any spiritual needs you would like someone to address? (Ask what those needs are and if referral to a spiritual professional is desired.)
- How can we (health care providers) help you with your spiritual needs or concerns?

From Gaskamp C, Sutter R, Meraviglia M, et al: Evidence-based guideline: promoting spirituality in the older adult, *J Gerontol Nurs* 32:10, 2006. Adapted from Meyer CL: How effectively are nurse educators preparing students to provide spiritual care? *Nurse Educ* 28(4):185–190, 2003; Koenig HG, Brooks RG: Religion, health and aging: implications for practice and public policy, *Public Policy Aging Rep* 12:13–19, 2002.

BOX 36-11 RESEARCH HIGHLIGHTS

The study investigated the associations among hope, meaning in life, self-transcendence, and nurse-patient interaction in a sample of 202 cognitively intact Finnish nursing home residents. Residents completed the Herth Hope Index, the Purpose in Life Test, the Self-Transcendence Scale, and the Nurse-Patient Interaction Scale. Statistical analysis revealed a significant direct relationship of nurse-patient interaction on hope, meaning in life, and self-transcendence. Findings suggest that nurse-patient interaction in the nursing home setting may be a critical resource to health and well-being of residents. The researchers recommended that nursing home caregivers should be given more time for interacting with their patients and education should be provided to assist in developing and appreciating the caring interaction skills that provide hope, meaning, and self-transcendence.

Sources: Hagan G: Nurse-patient interaction is a resource for hope, meaning in life and self-transcendence in nursing home patients, *Scand J Caring Sci* 28:74–88, 2014.

BOX 36-12 Spiritual Nursing Responses

- Relief of physical discomfort, which permits focus on the spiritual
- Creating a peaceful environment
- Comforting touch, which fosters nurse-patient connection
- Authentic presence
- Attentive listening
- Knowing the patient as a person
- Listening to life stories
- Sharing fears and listening to self-doubts or guilt
- Fostering forgiveness and reconciliation
- Validating the person's life and ensuring persons they will be remembered
- Sharing caring words and love
- Encouraging family support and presence
- Fostering connections to that which is held sacred by the person
- Praying with and for the patient
- Respecting religious traditions and providing for access to religious objects and rituals
- Referring the person to a spiritual counselor

Sources: Gaskamp C, Sutter R, Meraviglia M, et al: *J Gerontol Nurs* 32:8, 2006; Touhy T, Brown C, Smith C: Spiritual caring: end of life in a nursing home, *J Gerontol Nurs* 31:27–35, 2005.

---

spiritual assessment is more complex than completing a standardized form and must be done within the context of the nurse-patient relationship.

For older people with cognitive impairment, information about the importance of spirituality and religious beliefs can be obtained from family members. Nurses often see cognitive impairments as obstacles or excuses to providing spiritual care to people with dementia. Nurturing mind, body, and spirit is part of holistic nursing, and nurses must provide opportunities to all elders, no matter how impaired, to live life with meaning, purpose, and hope (Touhy, 2001b).

◆ Interventions

The caring relationship between nurses and persons nursed is the heart of nursing that touches and supports the spirit and enhances health and well-being (Haugan, 2014) (Box 36-11). Knowing persons in their complexity, responding to that which matters most to them, identifying and nurturing connections, listening with one's being, using presence and silence, and fostering connections to that which is held sacred by the person are spiritual nursing responses that arise from within the caring, connected relationship (Touhy et al, 2005). Suggestions for spiritual care interventions are presented in Box 36-12.

Know that caring for an aging body is the least of the work with older people. "Limiting care to the physical needs denies elders the opportunity to live out their life with meaning, purpose, and hope" (Touhy, 2001a, p. 45). Recognizing the primacy of the spirit is essential. Some very spiritual individuals are unable to articulate their knowing. Therefore, do not negate that aspect of an individual's experience because it is not expressed verbally. Realizing that biopsychosocial aspects of aging are all shards of the spirit will integrate every aspect of your work in gerontological nursing.

Nurturing the Spirit of the Nurse

"Because spiritual care occurs over time and within the context of relationship, probably the most effective tool at the nurse's disposal is the use of self" (Soeken and Carson, 1987, p. 607). Thinking about what gives your own life meaning and value helps in developing your spiritual self and assists you in being able to offer spiritual support to patients. Examples of activities include finding quiet time for meditation and reflection; keeping your own faith traditions; being with nature; appreciating the arts; spending time with those you love; and journaling (Touhy and Zerwekh, 2006). Giving your patient the best spiritual care stems from taking care of your own spiritual needs first. Find ways to nourish your own spirit. Nurses often do not take the time to do so and become dispirited. This is especially true for nurses who work with dying patients and experience grief and loss repeatedly. Having someone to talk to about feelings is important. Practicing compassion for oneself is essential to authentic practice of compassion for others (Touhy and Zerwekh, 2006) (Box 36-13).

Faith Community Nursing

Faith community nursing (FCN) is a specialty practice for professional nursing with established scope and standards of practice. The focus of faith community nursing is "the protection, promotion and optimization of health and abilities, prevention of illness and injury, and responding to suffering in the context of values, beliefs and practices of a faith community" (American Nurses Association [ANA], 2005, p. 1). FCN was originally known as *parish nursing,* but the name was changed to faith community nursing to reflect the broader scope of the practice and the full range of faiths (Dyess and Chase, 2010).

In a literature review of the current state of research for FCN, Dyess et al. (2010) noted that FCN began 20 years ago and is widely implemented today in many faith communities in the United States and in multiple countries around the world. These authors suggest that FCN can assist in bridging the gaps in care in the current health care system, contribute to a reduction in acute health care costs, promote health and disease prevention, and integrate faith with health care to promote positive health outcomes. Models of care such as those implemented in FCN may be particularly relevant to meeting the health maintenance needs and spiritual needs of older people with chronic illness living in the community.

Nurses who are involved in religious organizations can also be advocates for increasing the attention given to the health needs of older people. Nurses may even spearhead particular services to older people, such as peer counseling, health screening activities, day care, home visitation programs, and respite for families. Many religious organizations reach out to homebound elders in their community by offering visits from clergy or church members, involvement in prayer circles, and other activities to maintain connection with their faith community. Communities nationwide have organized interfaith volunteer services to provide in-home services for isolated frail elders. Many of these efforts have been organized and supported by the Robert Wood Johnson Foundation, and the national Faith Based Initiative also provides support for faith-based programs.

TRANSCENDENCE

Transcendence is the high-level emotional response to religious and spiritual life and finds expression in numerous rituals and modes of cosmic consciousness. Rituals provide a means of connecting with everyone through the ages who has observed similar rituals. These modes of thinking and feeling are sometimes unfamiliar to individuals who are immersed in the necessary materialistic concerns of young adulthood, yet moments do occur throughout life when one is deeply aware of being part of a larger scheme. Although some of the material in this chapter may be obscure, it is the springboard for learning to appreciate the full life cycle. The privilege of briefly walking alongside an elder on the last great journey can be truly inspiring.

Transcending is roused by the desire to go beyond the self as delimited by the material and the concrete aspects of living, to expand self-boundaries and life perspectives. "Transcendence involves detachment and separation from life as it has been lived to experience a reality beyond oneself and beyond what can be seen or felt" (Touhy and Zerwekh, 2006, p. 229). Creative thought and actions are vehicles of both self-actualization and self-transcendence, the bridge to universal expression and existence. Self-transcendence is generally expressed in five modes: creative work, religious beliefs, children, identification with nature, and mystical experiences (Reed, 1991). This section of the chapter deals with various mechanisms by which one transcends the purely physical limitations of existence.

Some people may use asceticism, self-denial, and rigorous rituals to reach the peaks of human experience; many others find more prosaic approaches just as effective. The thesis of Maslow's writings is that mystic, sacred, and transcendent experiences frequently arise from the ordinary elements of one's life (Maslow, 1970). Gardening, reading, holding an infant, dealing with loss, and numerous other normal events have elements of mystery.

With each death of a loved one, throughout life, one is reborn to a slightly altered state. When deaths of significant others abound in the later years, elders must be given the opportunity to express how they personally have been altered by the loss. We can speculate that with each personal loss, one moves slightly closer to the universal and away from the individual until, toward the end, one feels an affiliation with all living things—animal, plant, and mineral. Some older people have achieved a state of existence that transcends the limits of the failing body.

Gerotranscendence

The theory of gerotranscendence (Tornstam, 1994, 1996, 2005) (Chapter 3) theorizes that human aging brings about a general potential for gerotranscendence, a shift in perspective from the material world to the cosmic and, concurrent with that, an

---

BOX 36-13   Personal Spirituality Questions for Reflection for Nurses

- What do I believe in?
- How do I find purpose and meaning in my life?
- How do I take care of my physical, emotional, and spiritual needs?
- What are my hopes and dreams?
- Whom do I love, and who loves me?
- How am I with others?
- What would I change about my relationships?
- Am I willing to heal relationships that trouble me?

Source: Touhy T, Zerwekh J: Spiritual caring. In Zerwekh J: *Nursing care at the end of life: palliative care for patients and families,* Philadelphia, 2006, FA Davis.

increasing life satisfaction. Gerotranscendence is thought to be a gradual and ongoing shift that is generated by the normal processes of living, sometimes hastened by serious personal disruptions. An understanding of transcendence and the unique characteristics of this transformation as one ages is important to the continued growth and development of older people. Indices of gerotranscendence are summarized in Box 36-14.

Achieving Transcendence

Time Transcendence

Life as experienced ordinarily involves the chronological passage of time. Some types of conscious experience alter our time perception, but the unconscious destroys time. Therefore the release of the unconscious transcends the limitations of time that conscious life experience generally imposes on us. If we conquer time, we conquer annihilation and the dimensions of time that lie within the mind. Recognizing the importance of time perception, particularly in old age, is a fertile field to explore more fully. Influences on time perception include age, imminent death, level of activity, emotional state, outlook on the future, and the value attached to time. Conclusions from studies of older people generally support the view that elders perceive time as passing quickly and favor the past over the present or the future.

Peak Experiences

A peak experience is when one momentarily transcends the self through love, wisdom, insight, worship, commitment, or creativity. These experiences are the extraordinary events in one's life that clearly demonstrate self-actualization and personal authenticity. Peak experience is the time when restrictive boundaries seem to vanish, and one feels more aware, more complete, more ecstatic, or more concerned for others. Peak experiences include many modes of transcending one's ordinary limitations. Spiritual and paranormal experiences, creative acts, courage, and humor may all produce peak experiences. Keeping oneself open to transcendence involves finding the places in which such experiences can break through: soul-stirring concerts, sunrises, sunsets, or raging storms on mountaintops (Kimble, 1993). Each individual seeks states of being in which he or she feels part of a larger whole.

Meditation

Many types and rituals of meditation have flourished in Western societies in the past 2 decades. Some methods of meditation have been used for thousands of years in Eastern cultures. Whatever the method, the goal is to quiet the mind and center oneself. When the mind slows, the body relaxes and less oxygen and nutrients are needed. Mindfulness meditation can decrease pain, improve sleep, and enhance well-being and quality of life. Meditation may also improve cognitive function (Newberg et al, 2010). Other benefits of meditation are presented in Box 36-15.

Effective meditation requires approximately 20 minutes of focusing on a sound, a thought, or an image. Practicing two or more times daily will bring calmness, better health, and higher energy levels in its wake. Although meditation can be accomplished in any setting, a place with few distractions is helpful. People who meditate with consistency often begin to be aware of a transcendent state of being. Nurses may introduce the values of meditation to older adults and serve as guides in the beginnings of such activities. Chanting psalms, reciting poetry by rote, praying, saying the rosary, practicing yoga, and playing a musical instrument are all mechanisms of release and renewal that may bring one into higher states of awareness.

Hope as a Transcendent Mechanism

Hope is the belief in the future and the expectation of fulfillment. Hope is the anchor that sustains life in the most difficult times and in the face of doubts and ennui. Some level of hope must be maintained to survive and to die in peace. Hope embodies desires and expectations and the limitless possibilities of humans in all times and places—present, past, and future. For many elders, hope is a major means of coping, and those who lose hope lose the capacity and desire for survival.

O'Connor (1996) enumerates the critical aspects of hope: (1) the presence of an inner human energy, (2) positive expectations for the future, (3) motivation for action, and (4) formulations of meaningful, realistic goals. O'Connor further states that a person without hope has no goals or expectations for the future. All practicing nurses have observed how a small goal or hope for the future can sustain an elder. The grandson's graduation from college, the daughter's return from her travels, or even a birthday may keep an elder alive until the event is safely fulfilled.

BOX 36-14 Characteristics of Individuals with a High Degree of Gerotranscendence

- Have high degrees of life satisfaction
- Engage in self-controlled social activity
- Experience satisfaction with self-selected social activities
- Social activities not essential to their well-being
- Midlife patterns and ideals no longer prime motivators
- Demonstrate complex and active coping patterns
- Have greater need for solitary philosophizing
- May appear withdrawn when engaged in inner development
- Have accelerated development of gerotranscendence fomented by life crises
- Feel shifts in perception of reality

BOX 36-15 Benefits of Meditation

- Increased measured intelligence
- Increased short-term and long-term recall
- Decreased anxiety, depression, and irritability
- Greater perceived self-actualization (realization of potential)
- Better mind-body coordination
- Increased perceptual awareness
- Normalization of blood pressure
- Relief from insomnia
- Normalization of weight

Central to the instillation of hope is the caring relationship between nurses and patients. Nursing responses that instill hope foster harmony, healing, and wholeness. Caring relationships characterized by unconditional positive regard, encouragement, and competence help patients feel loved and cared about, thus inspiring hope. A patient's hope for cure may change to a hope for freedom from pain, day-to-day experiences to enjoy precious moments of life, time to accomplish life goals before life is over, sharing love with family and friends, relief of suffering, death with dignity, and eternal life. Nurses may foster hope by doing the following:

1. Presenting honestly the limits of human knowledge
2. Controlling symptoms and providing comfort
3. Encouraging patient and family to become involved in positive experiences that transcend the current situation
4. Determining significant aspects of the individual's life
5. Fostering spiritual processes and finding meaning
6. Exploring beliefs and values of the elder
7. Promoting connection and reconciliation
8. Providing opportunities for prayer, meditation, scripture reading, clergy visits, and religious rituals, if meaningful for the elder

Other hope-promoting experiences are presented in Box 36-16.

Transcendence in Illness

Serious illnesses influence how one perceives the meaning of life. A distinct shift in goals, relationships, and values often occurs among people who have survived life-threatening

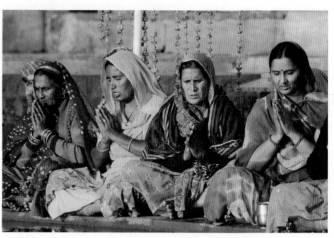

Prayer Is an Important Spiritual Practice in Many Cultures.
(©iStock.com/kaetana_istock)

episodes. A heightened awareness of beauty and of caring relationships may occur, but a long period of emotional "splinting" may be necessary while recovering from the psychic wound of body betrayal. Newman (1994) contends that disease can be a manifestation of health as one confronts the crisis and, as it reveals, the special meanings.

Steeves and Kahn (1987) found from their work in hospice care that certain conditions facilitate the search for meaning in illness, noting the following:

- Suffering must be bearable and not all-consuming if one is to find meaning in the experience.
- A person must have access to and be capable of perceiving objects in the environment. Even a small window on the world may be sufficient to match the limited energy one has to attend.
- One must have time that is free of interruption and a place of solitude to experience meaning.
- Clean, comfortable surroundings and freedom from constant responsibility and decision-making free the soul to search for meaning.
- An open, accepting atmosphere in which to discuss meanings with others is important.

Accompanying someone in his or her grief and quest for meaning in painful events is a privilege nurses are often given. This spiritual intimacy means being willing to suffer with another, and both the nurse and the client will reap the benefits. One of the great rewards of working with older clients is observing and participating as they turn suffering into a spiritual event.

Sister Rosemary Donley (1991) defines the nursing role in the spiritual search of suffering individuals as compassionate accompaniment, meaning entering into another's reality and quietly, attentively sharing the experience. "Nurses need to be with people who suffer, to give meaning to the reality of suffering and, in so far as possible, to remove suffering and its causes. Here lies the spiritual dimensions of health care" (Donley, 1991, p. 180). The challenge is to find meaning and some purpose in the affliction that, unchallenged, entwines and chokes identity.

BOX 36-16 Hope-Promoting Activities

- Feel the warmth of the sun.
- Share experiences children are having.
- See the crystal blue of the sky.
- Enjoy a garden or fresh flowers.
- Savor the richness of black coffee at breakfast.
- Feel the tartness of grapefruit to wake up the taste buds.
- Watch the activities of an animal in a tree outside the window.
- Benefit from each encounter with another person.
- Write messages to grandchildren, nieces, or nephews.
- Study a favorite painting.
- Listen to a symphony.
- Build highlights into each day such as meals, visits, Bible reading.
- Keep a journal.
- Write letters.
- Make a tape recording of your life story.
- Have hope objects or symbols nearby.
- Share hope stories.
- Focus on abilities, strengths, and past accomplishments.
- Encourage decision-making about daily activities; foster a sense of control.
- Extend caring and love to others.
- Appreciate expressions of caring concern.
- Renew loving relationships.

Adapted from Jevne R: Enhancing hope in the chronically ill, *Humane Med* 9:121–130, 1993; Miller, J: *Coping with chronic illness: overcoming powerlessness*, Philadelphia, 1983, FA Davis; Touhy T, Zerwekh J: Spiritual caring. In Zerwekh J: *Nursing care at the end of life: palliative care for patients and families*, Philadelphia, 2006, FA Davis.

LEGACIES

A legacy is one's tangible and intangible assets that are transferred to another and may be treasured as a symbol of immortality. The purpose of legacies is to supersede death. Courage, wisdom, and insights that we perceive in our elders become part of their legacy. The desire for meaning and immortality seems to be the basic motivation for leaving a legacy. Extending one's authentic self to others can be an important activity in the last years. Throughout life, shared experiences provide satisfaction, but in the last years this exchange allows one to gain a clearer perspective on how his or her movement on earth has had impact.

Older people must be encouraged to identify that which they would like to leave and who they wish the recipients to be. This process has interpersonal significance and prepares one to leave the world with a sense of meaning. A legacy can provide a transcendent feeling of continuation and tangible or intangible ties with survivors.

Legacies are manifold and may range from memories that will live on in the minds of others to bequeathed fortunes. Box 36-17 is a partial list of legacies. The list is as diverse as individual contributions to humanity. Legacies are generative and are identified and shared best as one approaches the end of life. This activity reinforces integrity.

Certain questions allow the older person to consider a legacy if he or she is ready to do so. For example:

- What is the meaning to you of your life experience right now?
- Have you ever thought of writing an autobiography?
- If you were able to leave something to the younger generation, what would it be?
- Have you ever thought of the impact your generation has had on the world?
- What has been most meaningful in your life?

BOX 36-17 Examples of Legacies

- Oral histories
- Autobiographies
- Written or video histories
- Shared memories
- Taught skills
- Works of art and music
- Publications
- Human organ donations
- Endowments
- Objects of significance
- Tangible or intangible assets
- Personal characteristics, such as courage or integrity
- Bestowed talents
- Traditions and myths perpetuated
- Philanthropic causes
- Progeny children and grandchildren
- Methods of coping
- Unique thought: Darwin, Einstein, Freud, Nightingale, and others

- What possessions have special meaning for you? Who else is interested in them?
- Do you see some of your genetic traits emerging in your grandchildren?

Types of Legacies

Autobiographies and Life Histories

Oral histories are an approach to immortality. As long as one's story is told, one remains alive in the minds of others. Doers leave their products and live through them. Powerful figures are remembered in fame and infamy. The quiet, unobtrusive person survives in the memory of intimates and in family anecdotes. Everyone has a life story.

Autobiographies and recorded memoirs can serve a transcendent purpose for people who are alone—and for many who are not. Nurses can encourage older people to write, talk, or express in other ways the meaning of their lives. The human experience and the poignant anecdotes bind people together and validate the uniqueness of each brief journey in this level of awareness and the assurance that one will not be forgotten. Dying patients can express and order their memories through audiotapes, CDs, videotapes, or DVDs, which are then bequeathed to families if the older person desires.

Sharing one's personal story creates bonds of empathy, illustrates a point, conveys some of the deep wisdom that we all have, and connects us with our deepest human consciousness. "It is only when people who have loved and cared for us reach the end of life that we see the full gift we have received from them. By leaving us their reminiscences, their spirits can continue in our lives as a living memorial" (Grudzen and Soltys, 2000, p. 8). See Chapter 6 for additional discussion of storytelling, reminiscence, and life review.

Creation of Self through Journaling

Through the personal journal, one can, in thoughtful reflection, discover meaning and patterns in daily events. The self becomes a coherent story with successive revisions as old events are reread and perceived in new contexts. The journals of elders provide rich descriptions of the interior lives of the authors. May Sarton (1984) and Florida Scott-Maxwell (1968) are two of the best-known authors. The study of these journals and of the journals of less-known and less articulate elders assists nurses in understanding the inner experience of older people and, perhaps, their own.

Collective Legacies

Each person is a link in the chain of generations (Erikson, 1963) and as such may identify with generational accomplishments. An older woman may think of herself as a significant part of a generation that survived the Great Depression. A middle-aged man may identify with the generation that walked on the moon. The years of youthful idealism are impressed in one's memory by the political or ideological climate of the time. This time is the stage when one searches for a fit in the larger society.

The importance of collective legacies to nurses lies in how they use this knowledge. For instance, the nurse may ask, "Who were the great people of your time?" "Which ones were important to you?" "What events of your generation changed the world?" "What were the most important events you experienced?" Mentioning certain historical events or asking about individual reactions is sometimes helpful.

Childless individuals are becoming more prevalent with each passing generation, and they must find a way to outlive the self through a legacy. Many people choose a social legacy. Florence Nightingale would be one such person, with the grand legacy she left to nurses.

Legacies Expressed through Other People

One's legacy can be expressed in many ways—through the development of others in a teaching or learning situation or through mentorship, patronage, shared talents, organ donations, and genetic transmission. Some creative works and research are legacies left to successive generations for continued modification and growth. In other words, one's legacy may be a product of his or her own brought to fruition through someone else who may also become an intermediary to later developments. Thus people and generations are tied in sequential progress. Some examples may illustrate this type of legacy:

- An older man cried as he talked of his grandson's talent as a violinist. Both the man and his grandson shared their love for the violin, and the grandfather believed that he had genetically and personally contributed to his grandson's development as an accomplished musician.
- A professor emeritus spoke of visiting her son in a distant state and hearing him expound ideas that had been partially developed by the professor and her father before her.
- People who amass a fortune and allocate certain funds for endowment of artists, scientific projects, and intellectual exploration are counting on others to complete their legacy.

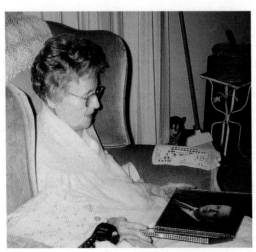

Widow Reflecting on Her Deceased Husband's Legacy.
(From Black JM, Hawks JH: *Medical-surgical nursing: clinical management for positive outcomes*, ed 7, St Louis, MO, 2005, Saunders.)

Living Legacies

Many older people wish to donate their bodies to science or donate body parts for transplant. This mechanism is a means to transcend death. Parts of the body keep another person alive, or, in the case of certain diseases, the deceased body may provide important information leading to preventive or restorative techniques in the future. Donation of body parts in old age may not be encouraged because they are often less viable than those from younger people. Nonetheless, older bodies are welcome for use as cadavers. The Dementia Brain Bank Research Program has been operated by the Alzheimer's Research Center for more than 30 years. The Brain Bank has collected more than 2500 brains obtained from individuals enrolled in the autopsy program who suffered from some form of dementia. It is one of the world's largest collections of brain tissue, which contributes to research on the neurochemistry, physiology, and diagnosis of dementing illnesses. People who are interested in providing such a legacy should be encouraged to call the nearest university biomedical center or brain bank registry and obtain more information. The nurse then has a postmortem obligation to the client to assist in carrying out his or her wishes.

Property and Assets

Wealth may be viewed as a means toward power more often than transcendence; therefore some older people are often reluctant to disperse material goods before their death. Some elders use the future legacy as a means to exert power and control over offspring. One man said, "So long as I have that bankroll, they've got to treat me with respect" (Lustbader, 1996). The power to exert influence, to punish, and to reward is often bound up in an anticipated estate distribution.

Estates can be planned in certain ways that are decidedly advantageous for the planner, as well as the recipient, in terms of control and avoidance of lengthy probate proceedings and taxation. Because the laws are complex and ever-changing, using the services of an estate planner would be advisable. The nurse's responsibility regarding wills may be limited to advising older people to obtain legal counsel while they are healthy and competent and plan how they would like to distribute their worldly goods.

Personal Possessions

Possessions carry more meaning as time passes; individuals change, but the possession remains much the same. A possession is a way of symbolically hanging on to individuals who are gone or times that are past. For some people, keeping personal possessions is a means of hanging on to the self that is changing with time. Cherished possessions passed on through several generations may have achieved meaning through the close family member to whom they belonged. One's personally significant items become highly charged with memories and meaning, and transferring them to friends and kin can be a tender experience. Personal possessions should never be dispersed without the individual's knowledge. Because of the uncertainty of late life lucidity, these issues should be discussed early with older individuals.

People who are approaching death must be given the opportunity to distribute their important belongings appropriately to those whom they believe will also cherish them. Nurses may encourage elders to plan the distribution of their significant items carefully. Deciding when and how best these possessions should be given is often difficult. Some people choose to distribute possessions before dying. In these cases, nurses often need to help family members accept these gifts, appreciating the meaning and recognizing the significance.

◆ PROMOTING HEALTHY AGING: IMPLICATIONS FOR GERONTOLOGICAL NURSING

"The responsibility of the nurse is not to make people well, or to prevent their getting sick, but to assist people to recognize the power that is within them to move to higher levels of consciousness" (Newman, 1994, p. xv). In this chapter, we have examined methods of expanding one's limited existence by developing the authentic self, transcendent self, and spiritual self and several mechanisms used to establish immortality through a legacy. These areas often become major issues in the latter part of life, and the nurse will find it a revealing, absorbing, and challenging task to be a part of this effort. An important point is that some people may avoid any such interest or concern, particularly when angry, in pain, or denying their own mortality. Nurses need not push the individual to accomplish this task but should be available to assist the person and family members.

The basic mysteries of life elude scientific researchers, yet they are the essence of existence with meaning. Remembering, feeling, dreaming, worshipping, and grasping one's connection to the universe are the realities of the human spirit.

Being old is not the centrality of the self—spirit is. Spirit synthesizes the total personality and provides integration, energizing force, and immortality. Nurses who care for older people have a great privilege in being able to accompany them on the final journey of their lives. It calls for a nurse who is willing to enter into meaningful spirit-sharing relationships. Such relationships have the potential to enhance inner harmony and healing. There may be no greater goal in caring for elders than helping a person see a life well lived and meaningful to themselves and others, thus providing hope that life's journey was not in vain. Taking advantage of these opportunities will enrich our nursing, our inner selves, and the spiritual well-being of the elders whom we nurse. As gerontological nursing scholar Sarah Gueldner (2007) so eloquently stated:

"We must help each older adult to continue to experience and express the passions that, over a lifetime, have become who they are. Older adults should continue to make their unique and precious contributions to society, and we must not fail to take note of it in even the frailest and quietest of individuals. We must give them voice and time on the center stage of life and help them connect with each other and with society in a way that fosters appreciation of the traits, talents, and memories that still define their being" (p. 4).

The authors of this book hope that you find as much joy and fulfillment in your nursing with older people as we have.

▎ KEY CONCEPTS

- Self-actualization is a process of developing one's most authentic self. Maslow thought of self-actualization as the pinnacle of human development.
- Self-actualized individuals embody qualities of courage, humor, high moral development, and seeking to learn more about themselves and others.
- Opportunities for pursuing interests will assist individuals in developing latent talents, expressing their creativity, and rising beyond daily concerns.
- Groups working toward societal humanitarian advancement may accomplish collective actualization.
- Creativity emanates from people who are self-actualized and may be expressed in everyday activities, as well as the arts, music, theater, and literature.
- Transcending the material and physical limitations of existence through ritual and spiritual means is an especially important aspect of aging.
- Gerotranscendence is a theory proposed by Tornstam that implies a natural shift in concerns that occurs in the aging

process. Elders are thought to spend more time in reflection, to spend less on materialistic concerns, and to find more satisfaction in life. This effort is an attempt to define aging not by the standards of young and middle adulthood but as having distinctive characteristics of its own.
- Illnesses that occur have the potential for altering one's fundamental beliefs and hopes. Nurses must give elders the opportunity to discuss the meanings of an illness. Some people find that these experiences bring new insights; others are angry. Empathic nurses will provide a sounding board while the elder makes sense of an illness within a satisfactory framework.
- Nurses need not neglect discussing spirituality with elders. Elders will respond only if it has significance for them.
- Spiritual nursing interventions emanate from the caring relationship between the older person and the nurse. The most important tool at the nurse's disposal is the use of self.

NURSING STUDY: SELF-ACTUALIZATION, SPIRITUALITY, AND TRANSCENDENCE

Melba had no children but had numerous nieces and nephews, though she did not feel particularly close to any of them. She had been a nursing instructor at a community college and had enjoyed her students but had not developed a sustained relationship with any of them after they had completed her courses. At her level of nursing education, the opportunity for mentorship was lacking, though she had occasionally taken students under her wing and arranged special experiences that they particularly desired. Because she had taught several courses each year, Melba never really developed a strong affiliation to a specialty but considered herself a pediatric nurse. She had not made any major contributions to the field in terms of research or publications; a few reviews, continuing education workshops, and some nursing newsletters had really been the extent of her work outside of that which was required. Melba's husband died in 1988, and she had felt very much alone since that time, especially after her retirement 3 years ago. Before her husband's death, Melba had been too busy to think about the ultimate meaning of all her years of teaching and wifely activities. With time on her hands, she began to wonder what it all meant. Had she done anything meaningful? Had she really made a difference in anything or in anyone's life? Was anyone going to remember her in any special way? So many questions were making her morose. She had never been a religious person, though her husband had been a devout Catholic. He had believed that God had a purpose for him in life, and though he was not always able to understand what it might be, he seemed to have a sense of satisfaction. She began to wonder if she should go to church—would that make her feel less depressed?

One Sunday morning, Melba had decided to attend her neighborhood Catholic church, but on her way out she slipped on the icy walkway and sustained bilateral Colles' fractures. After a brief emergency room visit for assessment, immobilization of the wrists, and medications, Melba was sent back home with an order for home health and social service assessment on the following day. Of course, she had extreme difficulty managing the most basic self-care while keeping her wrists immobilized and was very dejected. When the home health nurse arrived the next morning, to Melba's amazement, it was a former student who had graduated 4 years previously. Melba was more chagrined than pleased and greeted her with, "Oh, I hate to have you see me so helpless. I've been feeling so useless, and, now with these wrists, I am totally useless." If you were the home health nurse, how would you begin working with Melba, knowing that you would be limited to just a few visits?

Based on the nursing study, develop a nursing care plan using the following procedure*:

* List Melba's comments that provide subjective data.
* List information that provides objective data.
* From these data, identify and state, using an accepted format, two nursing diagnoses you determine are most significant to Melba at this time. List two of Melba's strengths that you have identified from the data.
* Determine and state the outcome criteria for each diagnosis. These must reflect some alleviation of the problem identified in the nursing diagnosis and must be stated in concrete and measurable terms.
* Plan and state one or more interventions for each diagnosed problem. Provide specific documentation of the sources used to determine the appropriate intervention. Plan at least one intervention that incorporates Melba's existing strengths.
* Evaluate the success of the intervention. Interventions must correlate directly with the stated outcome criteria to measure the outcome success.

*Students are advised to refer to their nursing diagnosis text and identify possible or potential problems.

CRITICAL THINKING QUESTIONS AND ACTIVITIES

1. Discuss the meanings and the thoughts triggered by the student's and elder's viewpoints as expressed at the beginning of the chapter. How do they vary from your own experience?
2. How do nursing students learn about spirituality and spiritual nursing interventions?
3. What activities might be helpful in developing your own sense of spirituality?
4. How do cultural beliefs and traditions affect one's concept of spirituality?
5. How can nurses enhance spiritual care, self-actualization, and transcendence of self among elders?

RESEARCH QUESTIONS

1. What aspects of intergenerational programs are enjoyed by younger and older individuals?
2. Who makes wills and when do they make them?
3. What are the motivating differences between gifts given during life and those given after one's death?
4. What is the perspective of older people related to spiritual assessment and interventions by nurses?
5. How do nurses describe the spiritual interventions they use with older people?
6. How do nurses recognize aspects of gerotranscendence?

REFERENCES

American Nurses Association: *Faith community nursing: scope and standards of practice*, Silver Spring, MD, 2005, American Nurses Association.

Ardelt M: Wisdom and life satisfaction in old age, *J Gerontol B Psychol Sci Soc Sci* 52:15–27, 1997.

Ardelt M: Antecedents and effects of wisdom in old age: a longitudinal perspective on aging well, *Res Aging* 22:360–394, 2000.

Ardelt M: Empirical assessment of a three-dimensional wisdom scale, *Res Aging* 25(3):275–324, 2003.

Ardelt M: Wisdom as expert knowledge system: a critical review of a contemporary operationalization of an ancient concept, *Hum Dev* 47:257–285, 2004.

Baltes P: The many faces of human ageing: toward a psychological culture of old age, *Psychol Med* 21:837–854, 1991.

other living thing. Some sustenance or peace for the old may be gained from the self-contained stimulation of a rocking chair or slowly stroking an animal's fur or wearing something that provides sensory stimulation. Music, perceived through the skin as well as the ears, may be another source of touch stimulation that is self-induced. Skin touched by the vibrations of music is enveloped and caressed. Music and dancing seem to be two important mechanisms of enjoyment of older people (Chapter 36). In later years, older adults often return to dancing after decades of ignoring the pleasurable activity. Perhaps this desire is a response to the need for more touch.

Therapeutic Touch

Touch is a powerful healer and a therapeutic tool that nurses can use to satisfy "touch hunger" of older people. Nursing has recognized the importance of touch and has the social sanctions to touch the body in the intimate and personal care of a person, an opportunity too often not fully used for the betterment of the older person's adaptation to environment and location in time and space. Touch can serve as a means of providing sensory stimulation, reducing anxiety, relieving physical and psychological pain, and comforting the dying, as well as sexual expression.

Kreiger's experiments with therapeutic touch (1975) demonstrate physiological and psychological improvement in patients who are exposed to consistent "doses" of touch. "Hands-on healing and energy-based interventions have been found in cultures throughout history, dating back at least 5000 years" (Wang and Hermann, 2006, p. 34). "Laying on of the hands" and the power of touch to heal had largely disappeared with the scientific revolution. The phenomenon has reemerged as healing touch and therapeutic touch movements. A growing body of research supports the healing power of touch, and *Energy Field, Disturbed* is an approved nursing diagnosis (Wang and Hermann, 2006).

Many nurses have learned how to perform therapeutic and healing touch and use these modalities in their practice with people of all ages. Positive outcomes of interventions utilizing touch in nursing homes, particularly with people with dementia and agitated behaviors, have been reported (Box 33-1). Further research on the use of touch with older people is needed. Touch is a powerful tool to promote comfort and well-being when working with elders.

INTIMACY

Although intimacy is often thought of in the context of sexual performance, it encompasses more than sexuality and includes five major relational components: commitment, affective intimacy, cognitive intimacy, physical intimacy, and interdependence (Youngkin, 2004). "Intimacy is from a Greek word meaning 'closest to; inner lining of blood vessels'" (Steinke, 2005, p. 40). It is a warm, meaningful feeling of joy. Intimacy includes the need for close friendships; relationships with family, friends, and formal caregivers; spiritual connections; knowing that one matters in someone else's life; and the ability

BOX 33-1 RESEARCH HIGHLIGHTS

Effects of Slow-Stroke Back Massage and Hand Massage on Relaxation in Older People

Massage is a traditional nursing intervention and a part of early nursing history. Yet few studies have examined the benefits of massage for older people. The authors conducted a review of the psychological and physiological effects of slow-stroke back massage and hand massage with older people. A total of 21 studies were reviewed, and the most common protocols were 3-minute slow-stroke back massage and 10-minute hand massage. Overall, statistically significant improvements in physiological and psychological indicators provide support for the use of slow-stroke back massage and hand massage with older people in clinical practice across settings. Outcomes of these forms of massage included reduction of anxiety, increase in relaxation, and reduction in verbal aggression and aggressive behaviors in individuals with dementia.

Nurses can be educated in the knowledge and skill needed to administer these techniques into practice and educate caregivers on their use. Slow-stroke back massage and hand massage for relaxation may be an effective alternative to pharmacological therapy in reducing stress and improving quality of life for older people.

Data from Harris M, Richards K: The physiological and psychological effects of slow-stroke back massage and hand massage on relaxation in older people, *J Clin Nurs* 19:917–926, 2010.

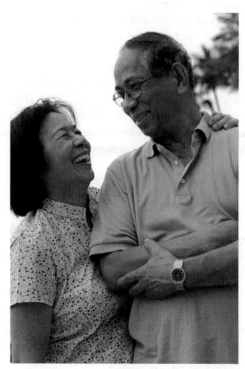

Older couples enjoy love and companionship. (©iStock.com/DanielBendjy)

to form satisfying social relationships with others (Steinke, 2005; Syme, 2014).

Youngkin (2004) points out that older people may be concerned about changes in sexual intimacy, but "social relationships with people important in their lives, the ability to

interact intellectually with people who share similar interests, the supportive love that grows between human beings (whether romantic or platonic), and physical nonsexual intimacy are equally—and in many instances more—important than the physical intimacy of direct sexual relations. All of these facets of intimate life are integrally woven into the fabric of aging, along with other influences that can make life rewarding" (p. 46). Intimacy needs change over time, but the need for intimacy and satisfying social relationships remains an important component of healthy aging.

SEXUALITY

Sexuality is a state of physical, emotional, mental, and social well-being in relation to sexuality; it is not merely the absence of disease, dysfunction, or infirmity. It is a central aspect of being human and encompasses sex, gender identities and roles, sexual orientation, eroticism, pleasure, intimacy, and reproduction (World Health Organization, 2014). As a major aspect of intimacy, sexuality includes the physical act of intercourse, as well as many other types of intimate activity. It includes components such as sexual desire, activity, attitudes, body image, gender-role activity, and sexual self-esteem (Syme, 2014; Zeiss and Kasl-Godley, 2001). Sexuality provides the opportunity to express passion, affection, admiration, and loyalty. It can also enhance personal growth and communication. Sexuality also allows a general affirmation of life (especially joy) and a continuing opportunity to search for new growth and experience.

Sexuality, similar to food and water, is a basic human need, yet it goes beyond the biological realm to include psychological, social, and moral dimensions (Waite et al, 2009) (Figure 33-2). The constant interaction among these spheres of sexuality works to produce harmony. The linkage of the four dimensions

composes the holistic quality of an individual's sexuality. "Historically, sexuality has been perceived more narrowly in a biomedical context, with emphasis placed on the sexual response cycle, hetero-normative behaviors (e.g., penile-vaginal intercourse), and heterosexist and ageist assumptions" (Syme, 2014, p. 36). A holistic view better reflects the philosophy of healthy aging for all individuals. Box 33-2 presents *Healthy People 2020* goals related to sexual health.

The social sphere of sexuality is the sum of cultural factors that influence the individual's thoughts and actions related to interpersonal relationships, as well as sexuality related to ideas and learned behavior. Television, radio, literature, and the more traditional sources of family, school, and religious teachings combine to influence social sexuality. The belief of that which constitutes masculine and feminine is deeply rooted in the individual's exposure to cultural factors (Chapter 4).

The psychological domain of sexuality reflects a person's attitudes, feelings toward self and others, and learning from experiences. Beginning with birth, the individual is bombarded with cues and signals of how a person should act and think about the use of "dirty words" or body parts. Conversation is self-censored in the presence of or in discussion with certain people. The moral aspect of sexuality, the "I should" or "I shouldn't," makes a difference that is based in religious and cultural beliefs or in a pragmatic or humanistic outlook.

The final dimension, biological sexuality, is reflected in physiological responses to sexual stimulation, reproduction, puberty, and growth and development. Because of the interrelatedness, these dimensions affect each other directly or indirectly whenever an aspect of sexuality is out of harmony.

Sexuality is a vital aspect to consider in the care of the older person regardless of the setting. Sexuality exists throughout life in one form or another in everyone. All older people have a need to express sexual feelings, whether the individuals are healthy and active or whether they are frail. Sexuality is linked with the person's personality and identity and has a significant role in promoting better life adaptation (Bach et al, 2013; Steinke, 2013). Sex and intimacy cannot be ignored since adults are living longer and healthier lives and engaging in a variety of intimate and sexual behaviors (Syme, 2014).

Acceptance and Companionship

Sexuality validates the lifelong need to share intimacy and have that offering appreciated. Sexuality is love, warmth, sharing, and touching between people, not just the physical act of coitus.

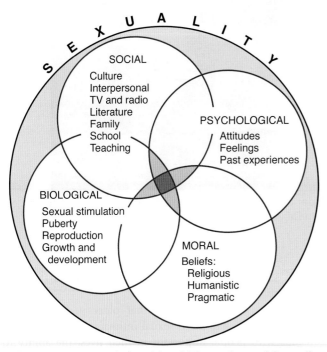

FIGURE 33-2 Interrelationship of Dimensions of Sexuality.

> **BOX 33-2   HEALTHY PEOPLE 2020**
> - Improve the health, safety, and well-being of lesbian, gay, bisexual, and transgender (LGBT) individuals.
> - Promote healthy sexual behaviors, strengthen community capacity, and increase access to quality services to prevent sexually transmitted diseases (STDs) and their complications.
> - Prevent human immunodeficiency virus (HIV) infection and its related illness and death.

Data from U.S. Department of Health and Human Services, Office of Disease Prevention and Health Promotion: Healthy People 2020, 2012. http://www.healthypeople.gov/2020.

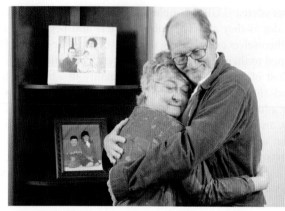

Love and affection are important to older persons. (From Sorrentino SA, Gorek B: *Mosby's textbook for long-term care assistants,* ed 5, St Louis, MO, 2007, Mosby.)

Margot Benary-Isbert, in her book *The Vintage Years* (1968), expresses the essence of sexuality most eloquently (p. 200):

> *Let us not forget old married couples who once shared healthy and happy days as they now share the unavoidable limitations of old age and grow even closer together in love and patience. When they exchange a smile, a glance, one can guess that they still think each other beautiful and loveable.*

SEXUAL HEALTH

The World Health Organization defines sexual health as a state of physical, emotional, mental, and social well-being related to sexuality (2014). Sexual health is a realistic phenomenon that includes four components: personal and social behaviors in agreement with individual gender identity; comfort with a range of sexual role behaviors and engagement in effective interpersonal relations with both sexes in a loving relationship or long-term commitment; response to erotic stimulation that produces positive and pleasurable sexual activity; and the ability to make mature judgments about sexual behavior that is culturally and socially acceptable. "Sexual health, as with physical health, is not simply the absence of sexual dysfunction or disease, but, rather a state of sexual well-being that includes a positive approach to a sexual relationship and anticipation of a pleasurable experience without fear, shame, or coercion" (Rheaume and Mitty, 2008, p. 342).

These interpretations address the multifaceted nature of the biological, psychosocial, cultural, and spiritual components of sexuality and imply that sexual behavior is the capacity to enhance self and others. Sexual health is individually defined and wholesome if it leads to intimacy (not necessarily coitus) and enriches the involved parties.

Factors Influencing Sexual Health
Expectations
Older adults are becoming increasingly open in their attitudes and beliefs about sexuality (Syme, 2014). However, a large number of cultural, biological, psychosocial, and environmental factors can influence the sexual behavior of older adults.

The older person may be confronted with barriers to the expression of his or her sexuality by reflected attitudes, health, culture, economics, opportunity, and historic trends. Factors affecting a person's attitudes on intimacy and sexuality include family dynamics and upbringing and cultural and religious beliefs (Chapter 4).

Older people often internalize the broad cultural proscriptions of sexual behavior in late life that hinder the continuance of sexual expression. There remains a prevailing assumption that as we age, we become sexually undesirable, incapable of sex, or asexual (DiNapoli et al, 2013). Health care professionals are not immune to these stereotypes and may assume sexual issues are of lesser concern to older adults and neglect to address this important aspect of healthy aging. Much sexual behavior stems from incorporating other people's reactions. Older people do not feel old until they are faced with the fact that others around them consider them old. Similarly, older adults do not feel asexual until they are continually treated as such.

An often quoted statement by Alex Comfort (1974) sums it up nicely: "In our experiences, old folks stop having sex for the same reasons they stop riding a bicycle—general infirmity, thinking it looks ridiculous, no bicycle." Box 33-3 presents some of the myths about sexuality in older women that may be held by older people themselves and by society in general.

Activity Levels

For both heterosexual and homosexual individuals, research supports that liberal and positive attitudes toward sexuality, greater sexual knowledge, satisfaction with a long-term relationship or a current intimate relationship, good social networks, psychological well-being, and a sense of self-worth are associated with greater sexual interest, activity, and satisfaction. Both early studies of sexual behavior in older adults and more recent ones indicate that most elders continue to be interested in sex, engage in a variety of sexual and intimate behaviors, and find their sexual lives satisfying (Lindau et al, 2007; Lindau and Gavrilova, 2010).

Determinants of sexual activity and functioning include the interaction of each partner's sexual capacity, physical health, motivation, conduct, and attitudes, as well as the quality of the

---

BOX 33-3 Sexuality and Aging Women: Common Myths

- Masturbation is an immature activity of youngsters and adolescents, not older women.
- Sexual prowess and desire wane during the climacteric, and menopause is the death of a woman's sexuality.
- Hysterectomy creates a physical disability that results in the inability to function sexually.
- Sex has no role in the lives of older people, except as perversion or remembrance of times past.
- Sexual expression in old age is taboo.
- Older people are too old and frail to engage in sex.
- The young are considered lusty and virile; elders are considered lecherous.
- Sex is unimportant or over in the lives of the older individuals.
- Older women do not wish to discuss their sexuality with professionals.

dyadic relationship (Waite et al, 2009). Having a sexual partner, frequent intercourse, good health, low level of stress, and an absence of financial worries enhanced a happy sexual relationship (Fisher, 2010). Patterns of sexual activity in earlier years are a major predictor of sexual activity in later life, and individuals with higher levels of sexual activity in middle age show less decline with advanced age (Kennedy et al, 2010).

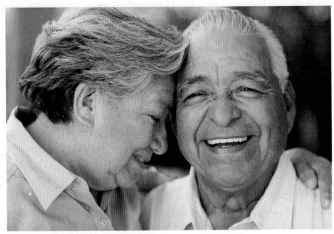

Sexuality is an important need in late life and affects pleasure, adaptation, and a general feeling of well-being. (©iStock.com/Aldo Murillo)

Sexual activity is closely tied to overall health, and individuals with better health are more likely to be sexually active. The most common reason for sexual inactivity among heterosexual couples is the male partner's health. Men are more sexually active than women, most likely because women live longer and may not have a partner. Women, especially those not in a relationship, were more likely than men to report lack of interest in sex (Lindau et al, 2007; Lindau and Gavrilova, 2010).

Cohort and Cultural Influences

The era in which a person was born influences attitudes about sexuality. Women in their 80s today may have been strongly influenced by the prudish Victorian atmosphere of their youth and may have experienced difficult marital adjustments and serious sexual problems early in their marriages. Sexuality was not openly expressed or discussed, and this was a time when "pleasurable sex was for men only; women engaged in sexual activity to satisfy their husbands and to make babies" (Rheaume and Mitty, 2008, p. 344). These kinds of experiences shape beliefs and knowledge about sexual expression, as well as comfort with sexuality, particularly for older women. It is important to come to know and understand the older person within his or her social and cultural background and not make judgments based on one's own belief system.

The next generation of older people (baby boomers) has experienced other influences, including more liberal attitudes toward sexuality, the women's movement, a higher number of divorced adults, the human immunodeficiency virus (HIV) epidemic, and increased numbers of lesbian, gay, bisexual, and

transgendered (LGBT) couples, that will affect their views and attitudes as they age. The baby boomers and beyond, as they find themselves experiencing sexuality beyond the age they had assigned to their elders, may alter current perceptions.

Most of what is known about sexuality in aging has been gained through research with well-educated, healthy, white older adults. Further research is needed among culturally, socially, and ethnically diverse older people; those with chronic illness; and LGBT older people. Suzman (2009) suggests the importance of early life experiences in understanding aging and sexual patterns, an area missing when studies focus on experiences after age 65 only.

Biological Changes with Age

Acknowledgment and understanding of the age changes that influence sexual physiology, anatomy, and the stages of sexual response may partially explain alteration in sexual behavior to accommodate these changes and facilitate continued pleasurable sex. Characteristic physiological changes during the sexual response cycle do occur with aging, but these vary among individuals depending on general health factors. The changes occur abruptly in women starting with menopause but more gradually in men, a phenomenon called *andropause* (Kennedy et al, 2010). The "use it or lose it" phenomenon applies here: the more sexually active the person is, the fewer changes he or she is likely to experience in the pattern of sexual response. Changes in the appearance of the body (wrinkles, sagging skin) may also affect the older person's security about his or her sexual attractiveness (Arena and Wallace, 2008). Table 33-1 summarizes physical changes in the sexual response cycle.

Older people who do not understand the physical changes that affect sexual activity become concerned that their sex life is approaching its natural conclusion with the onset of menopause or, for men, when they discover a change in the firmness of their erection or the decreased need for ejaculation with each orgasm or when the refractory period is extended between episodes of intercourse. A major nursing role is to provide information about these changes, as well as appropriate assessment and counseling within the context of the individual's needs.

SEXUAL DYSFUNCTION

Sexual dysfunction is defined as impairment in normal sexual functioning and can have many causes, both physical and psychological. Sexual disorders in older people have not been well studied, but generally, the following four categories are described: hypoactive sexual desire disorder; sexual arousal disorder; orgasmic disorder; and sexual pain disorders (Arena and Wallace, 2008).

Male Dysfunction

Erectile dysfunction (ED) is the most prevalent sexual problem in men. ED is defined as the inability to achieve and sustain an erection sufficient for satisfactory sexual intercourse in at least 50% or more attempts. When discussing ED with older men, it is important to provide education about normal age-related changes as well. Older men require more physical penile

TABLE 33-1   Physical Changes in Sexual Responses in Old Age

FEMALE	MALE
Excitation Phase	
Diminished or delayed lubrication (1 to 3 minutes may be required for adequate amounts to appear)	Less intense and slower erection (but can be maintained longer without ejaculation)
Diminished flattening and separation of labia majora	Increased difficulty regaining an erection if lost
Disappearance of elevation of labia majora	Less vasocongestion of scrotal sac
Decreased vasocongestion of labia minora	Less pronounced elevation and congestion of testicles
Decreased elastic expansion of vagina (depth and breadth)	
Breasts not as engorged	
Sex flush absent	
Plateau Phase	
Slower and less prominent uterine elevation or tenting	Decreased muscle tension
Nipple erection and sexual flush less often	No color change at coronal edge of penis
Decreased capacity for vasocongestion	Slower penile erection pattern
Decreased areolar engorgement	Delayed or diminished erectile and testicular elevation
Labial color change less evident	
Less intense swelling or orgasmic platform	
Less sexual flush	
Decreased secretions of Bartholin's glands	
Orgasmic Phase	
Fewer number and less intense orgasmic contractions	Decreased or absent secretory activity (lubrication) by Cowper's gland before ejaculation
Rectal sphincter contraction with severe tension only	Fewer penile contractions
	Fewer rectal sphincter contractions
	Decreased force of ejaculation (approximately 50%) with decreased amount of semen (if ejaculation is long, seepage of semen occurs)
Resolution Phase	
Observably slower loss of nipple erection	Vasocongestion of nipples and scrotum slowly subsides
Vasocongestion of clitoris and orgasmic platform	Very rapid loss of erection and descent of testicles shortly after ejaculation
	Refractory time extended (time required before another erection ranges from several to 24 hours, occasionally longer)

Adapted from Kennedy G, Martinez M, Garo N: Sex and mental health in old age, *Prim Psychiatry* 17:21–30, 2010.

stimulation and a longer time to achieve erection, and the duration of orgasm may be shorter and less intense (Rheaume and Mitty, 2008).

An erection is governed by the interaction among the hormonal, vascular, and nervous systems. A problem in any of these systems can cause ED. Of course, multiple causes exist for this problem in older men. Nearly one-third of ED is a complication of diabetes. Alcoholism, medications, depression, and prostate cancer and treatment are also causes of ED in older men. The new nerve-saving microsurgical techniques used for prostatectomies often spare erectile function. Anxiety and relationship issues are additional causes of ED, and, as Rheaume and Mitty (2008) note, some men may have widower's syndrome (difficulty achieving erection because they harbor guilt about pursuing a sexual relationship after the death of their spouse). Testosterone levels have little to do with ED but can have a major effect on libido (sexual desire).

The use of phosphodiesterase inhibitors such as sildenafil (Viagra), vardenafil (Levitra), and tadalafil (Cialis) has revolutionized treatment for ED regardless of cause. Some have commented that this can be called "the Viagratization of the older population." Contraindications to the use of these medications include use of nitrate therapy, heart failure with low blood pressure, certain antihypertensive regimens, and other medications and cardiovascular conditions (Chapter 9).

Before the availability of these medications, intracavernosal injections with the drugs papaverine and phentolamine, vasoactive agents that reduce resistance of arteriolar and cavernosal smooth muscle tissue of the penis, were used. Penile implants of the semirigid, adjustable-malleable, or hinged and inflatable types are available when impotence does not respond to other treatments or is irreversible. The hinged and inflatable types, which are inserted in the testicular area, are the most popular. Another alternative is the vacuum pump device, which works by creating a vacuum that draws blood into the penis, causing an erection. Vacuum pumps are available in manual and battery-operated versions and may be covered by Medicare if deemed medically necessary.

Female Dysfunction

Female dysfunction is considered "persistent impediment to a person's normal pattern of sexual interest, response, or both" (Kaiser, 2000, p. 1174). Female sexual function can be influenced by factors such as culture, ethnicity, emotional state, age,

and previous sexual experiences, as well as age-related changes in sexual response. Frequency of intimacy depends more on the age, health, and sexual function of the partner or the availability of a partner, rather than on their own sexual capacity. Postmenopausal changes in the urinary or genital tract as a result of lower estrogen levels can make sexual activity less pleasurable (Rheaume and Mitty, 2008). Dyspareunia, resulting from vaginal dryness and thinning of the vaginal tissue, occurs in one-third of women older than age 65. In many instances, using water-soluble lubricants such as K-Y Jelly, Astroglide, Slip, and HR lubricating jelly during foreplay or intercourse can resolve the difficulty. Topical low-dose estrogen creams, rings, or pills that are introduced into the vagina may also help to plump tissues and restore lubrication, with less absorption than oral hormones (Kennedy et al, 2010; Rheaume and Mitty, 2008).

Women can experience arousal disorders resulting from drugs such as anticholinergics, antidepressants, and chemotherapeutic agents and from lack of lubrication from radiation, surgery, and stress. Orgasmic disorders also may result from drugs used to treat depression. Unlike ED, studies of vascular insufficiency are less clear in women with sexual dysfunction. Prolapse of the uterus, rectoceles, and cystoceles can be surgically repaired to facilitate continued sexual activity. Urinary incontinence (UI) is another condition that may affect sexual activity for both men and women. Appropriate assessment and treatment are important because many causes of UI are treatable (Chapter 16).

ALTERNATIVE SEXUAL LIFESTYLES: LESBIAN, GAY, BISEXUAL, AND TRANSGENDER

Discrimination in health and social systems affects gays, lesbians, bisexuals, and transgender individuals of all ages. Older individuals may be even more at risk for discrimination as a result of lifelong experiences with marginalization and oppression. They may have been shunned by family or friends, religious organizations, and the medical community; ridiculed or physically attacked; or labeled as sinners, perverts, or criminals. It was not until 1973 that homosexuality was removed from the *Diagnostic and Statistical Manual of Mental Disorders* (Institute of Medicine, 2011; Jablonski et al, 2013; Lim et al, 2014). Gay and lesbian older people face the "double stigma" of being both old and homosexual, with lesbians facing the triple threat of being women, old, and having a different sexual orientation (Agronin, 2004; Jablonski et al, 2013).

As a result of lifelong discrimination and negative experiences with health care agencies and personnel, LGBT older adults are much less likely than their heterosexual peers to access needed health and social services or identify themselves as gay or lesbian to health care providers (SAGE and MAP, 2010). As a result, they are at greater risk for poorer health than their heterosexual counterparts. Gay and bisexual men may have more chronic conditions and suffer greater psychological distress, and even the more affluent and educated may be uninsured (Lim et al, 2014; Wallace et al, 2011). Among LGBT individuals, transgender older adults have the most difficulty accessing health care and are more likely to experience financial barriers, receive inferior care, and be denied health care (Jablonski et al, 2013).

Although recently published reports (American Society on Aging and MetLife, 2010; Fredriksen-Goldsen et al, 2011; Institute of Medicine, 2011; SAGE and MAP, 2010) have added to the body of knowledge about aging LGBT individuals, there is still a lack of knowledge, as well as research. Research has been conducted primarily with middle class white gay men and lesbians in urban areas. Even less is known about bisexual and transgender older people.

The United States Department of Health and Human Services (HHS) has recommendations to address LGBT health care issues including collection of health data through federally funded surveys, guidance to states regarding access to federal welfare programs for LGBT families and protection of same-sex partner's assets when his or her family uses Medicaid for long-term care, and expanded outreach regarding the range of HHS funding opportunities for organizations that serve the LGBT community (U.S. Department of Health and Human Services, 2014).

◆ PROMOTING HEALTHY AGING: IMPLICATIONS FOR GERONTOLOGICAL NURSING

◆ Assessment

Health care providers may assume that their LGBT patients are heterosexual and neglect to obtain a sexual history, discuss sexuality, or be aware of their particular medical needs. Providers receive little education and training in the needs of this population and may lack sensitivity when caring for older LGBT individuals (Jablonski et al, 2013; Lim et al, 2014). Sensitivity is of utmost importance when attempting to obtain a health history. Using open-ended questions such as "Who is most important to you?" or "Do you have a significant other?" is much better than asking "Are you married?" This form of the question allows the nurse to look beyond the rigid category of family.

If the patient identifies as transgender, it is important to ask how the patient wishes to be addressed. Asking individuals if they consider themselves as primarily heterosexual, homosexual, or bisexual is also better. This question conveys recognition of sexual variety. Euphemisms are frequently used for a life partner (e.g., roommate, close friend). An older lesbian woman in a health care situation may refer to herself indirectly by saying "people like us." Nurses need to become more aware of these nuances and try to understand the fear of discovery that is apparent in the older gay man and lesbian woman. These elders are of a generation in which they were, and may still be, closeted because of the homophobic experiences they had throughout their younger years.

◆ Interventions

Better support and care services for LGBT individuals by care providers should include working through homophobic attitudes and discomfort discussing sexuality, learning about special issues facing LGBT individuals, and becoming aware of resources in the community specific to this population. When

caring for transgender older adults, it is important to use discretion and sensitivity when obtaining medical and surgical histories and performing physical examinations (Jablonski et al, 2013).

Facilities or agencies in the community need to be assessed from the perspective of the client, patient, or resident who may be gay, lesbian, bisexual, or transgender. It is important that service providers create programs that are inclusive and culturally appropriate for all individuals (Chapter 4). Only about 15% of the Area Agencies on Aging offer services tailored to the needs of LGBT older adults (Jablonski et al, 2013). The National Center for Transgender Equality (2011) recommends revising federal Medicaid regulations to explicitly prohibit discrimination based on gender identity and sexual orientation in home- and community-based services (National Center for Transgender Equality, 2011).

Programs to increase awareness of the needs of LGBT elders and reduce discrimination are necessary especially in light of the anticipated increase in older LGBT individuals. Chapter 34 provides further discussion of relationship and family issues of elder LGBT individuals and suggestions for resources.

INTIMACY AND CHRONIC ILLNESS

Chronic illnesses and their related treatments may bring many challenges to intimacy and sexual activity. Physical capacity may be affected by illness and psychological factors (anxiety, depression) affect sexual activity (Steinke, 2013). Often, patients and their partners are given little or no information about the effect of illnesses on sexual activity or strategies to continue sexual activity within functional limitations. Individuals want and need information on sexual functioning, and health care professionals need to become more knowledgeable and more actively involved in sexual counseling.

Nurse researcher Dr. Elaine Steinke (2013) provides specific information and sexual counseling strategies for individuals with cardiovascular and pulmonary diseases and cancer. Sexual counseling recommendations for health care professionals working with individuals with cardiovascular disease can be found in a consensus statement from the American Heart Association and the European Society of Cardiology Council on Cardiovascular Nursing and Allied Professions (Steinke et al, 2013).

Table 33-2 presents suggestions for individuals with chronic illness. Timing of intercourse (mornings or when energy level is

TABLE 33-2	**Chronic Illness and Sexual Function: Effects and Interventions**	
CONDITION	**EFFECTS/PROBLEMS**	**INTERVENTIONS**
Arthritis	Pain, fatigue, limited motion Steroid therapy may decrease sexual interest or desire	Advise patient to perform sexual activity at time of day when less fatigued and most relaxed Suggest use of analgesics and other pain-relief methods before sexual activity Encourage use of relaxation techniques before sexual activity, such as a warm bath or shower, application of hot packs to affected joints Advise patient to maintain optimal health through a balance of good nutrition, proper rest, and activity Suggest that he or she experiment with different positions, use pillows for comfort and support Recommend use of a vibrator if massage ability is limited Suggest use of water-soluble jelly for vaginal lubrication
Cardiovascular disease	Most men have no change in physical effects on sexual function; one-fourth may not return to pre–heart attack function; one-fourth may not resume sexual activity Women do not experience sexual dysfunction after heart attack Fear of another heart attack or death during sex Shortness of breath	Encourage counseling on realistic restrictions that may be necessary **Post–myocardial infarction (MI):** Those able to engage in mild to moderate physical activity without symptoms can generally resume sexual activity; those with a complicated MI may need to resume sexual activity gradually over a longer period of time Avoid large meals several hours before sex Avoid anal sex Instruct patient and spouse on alternative positions to avoid strain and allow for unrestricted breathing Stop and rest if chest pain is experienced, take nitroglycerin if prescribed, and seek emergency treatment for sustained chest pain **Post-CABG or pacemaker or ICD insertion:** Avoid strain or direct pressure on device/incision Individuals with poorly controlled arrhythmias should not engage in sexual activity until the condition is well managed Instruct individual that ICD could fire with sex, although uncommon; a change in device setting may be needed

Continued

TABLE 33-2   Chronic Illness and Sexual Function: Effects and Interventions—cont'd

CONDITION	EFFECTS/PROBLEMS	INTERVENTIONS
Cerebrovascular accident (stroke)	Depression May or may not have sexual activity changes Often erectile disorders occur Change in role and function of partners Decreased physical endurance, fatigue Mobility and sensory deficits Perceptual and visual deficits Communication deficits Cognitive and behavioral deficits Fear of relapse or sudden death	Encourage counseling Instruct patient to use alternative positions Suggest use of a vibrator if massage ability is limited Suggest use of pillows for positioning and support Suggest use of water-soluble jelly for lubrication Suggest alternate forms of sexual expression acceptable to the individuals
Chronic obstructive pulmonary disease (COPD)	No direct impairment of sexual activity, although affected by coughing, exertional dyspnea, positions, and activity intolerance Medications may lead to erectile difficulties	Encourage patient to plan sexual activity when energy is highest Instruct patient to use alternative positions; use ample pillows for support and elevate the upper body, or use a sitting up-right position; avoid any pressure on the chest Advise patient to plan sexual activity at time medications are most effective Suggest use of oxygen before, during, or after sex, depending on when it provides the most benefit Teach partner to observe for breathing difficulty and allow time for change of positions and time to catch breath when needed
Diabetes	Sexual desire and interest unaffected Neuropathy and/or vascular damage may interfere with erectile ability; about 50% to 75% of men have erectile disorders; a small portion have retrograde ejaculation Some men regain function if diagnosis of diabetes is well accepted, if diabetes is well controlled, or both Women have less sexual desire and vaginal lubrication Decrease in orgasms/absence of orgasm can occur; less frequent sexual activity; local genital infections	Recommend possible candidates for penile prosthesis Suggest use of alternative forms of sexual expression Recommend immediate treatment of genital infections
Cancers		
Breast	No direct physical affect; there is a strong psychological effect: loss of sexual desire, body-image change, depression/reaction of partner	Refer to support groups, sex therapists, counselors Encourage open expression of sexual concerns
Prostate	Incontinence can occur following surgery Erectile dysfunction Psychological effects Use of nerve-sparing surgery causes less dysfunction	Kegel exercises and routine toileting Use of phosphodiesterase inhibitors Provide information related to sexual functioning/continence
Most other cancers	Men and women may lose sexual desire temporarily Men may have erectile dysfunction; dry ejaculation; retrograde ejaculation Women may have vaginal dryness, dyspareunia Both men and women may experience anxiety, depression, pain, nausea from chemo-therapy, radiation, hormone therapy, and nerve damage from pelvic surgery	New sexual positions may be helpful; explore alternative sexual activities

CABG, Coronary artery bypass graft; *ICD,* implantable cardioverter-defibrillator.

Data from Steinke EE: Sexuality and chronic illness, *J Gerontol Nurs* 39(11):18–27, 2013.

highest), oral or anal sex, masturbation, appropriate pain relief, and different sexual positions are all strategies that may assist in continued sexual activity. There is no consensus on what kind of position the individual should assume for sexual activity, but a lesser amount of energy is expended with the person on the bottom during use of the missionary position. Alternative positions may require less energy and may be more comfortable depending on the situation (Figure 33-3) (Kennedy et al, 2010; Steinke, 2013; Steinke et al, 2013).

For individuals with cardiac conditions, manual stimulation (masturbation) may be an alternative that can be used early in the recovery period to maintain sexual function if the practice is not objectionable to the patient. Studies show that masturbation is less taxing on the heart and makes less oxygen demand. Although self-stimulation is steeped in myth and fear, masturbation is a common and healthy practice in late life. Individuals without partners or those whose spouses are ill or incapacitated find that masturbation is helpful. As children, today's older population was discouraged from practicing this pleasurable activity with stories of the evils of fondling a person's own genitals.

Attitudes have changed over the years and the National Social Life, Health, and Aging project (NSHAP) study reported that more than 50% of male participants and 25% of female participants acknowledged masturbating, regardless of whether or not they had a sexual partner (Lindau et al, 2007). Masturbation provides an avenue for resolution of sexual tensions, keeps sexual desire alive, maintains lubrication and muscle tone of the vagina, provides mild physical exercise, and preserves sexual function in individuals who have no other outlet for sexual activity and gratification of their sexual need.

One couple, who had long sustained a satisfactory sexual relationship, was unable to imagine engaging in the alternative modes of sexual expression (cunnilingus, mutual masturbation, and repositioning) that were suggested when the wife developed severe osteoarthritis. The old gentleman brought the worn and dog-eared illustrative pamphlet back to the nurse in the health clinic. "She just won't go for it, nurse!" In such cases, the most well-meant advice may not be useful. To resolve such incompatible needs, the nurse may best counsel the most sexually active and liberal partner in ways to achieve orgasm while still remaining sexually comforting for the other partner.

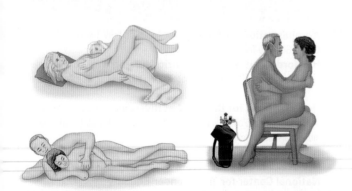

FIGURE 33-3 Adaptations of Sexual Positions for Individuals with Chronic Illness.

INTIMACY AND SEXUALITY IN LONG-TERM CARE FACILITIES

Research is needed on sexuality in residential care facilities and nursing homes, but surveys suggest that a significant number of older people living in these settings might choose to be sexually active if they had privacy and a sexual partner (Messinger-Rapport et al, 2003). Intimacy and sexuality among residents includes the opportunity to have not only coitus but also other forms of intimate expressions, such as hugging, kissing, hand holding, and masturbation. Wallace (2003) commented that the sexual needs of older adults in long-term care facilities should be addressed with the same priority as nutrition, hydration, and other well-accepted needs. The institutionalized older person has the same rights as noninstitutionalized elders to engage in or refrain from sexual activity.

Attitudes about intimacy and sexuality among long-term care staff and, often, family members may reflect general societal attitudes that older people do not have sexual needs or that sexual activity is inappropriate. Families may have difficulty understanding that their older relative may want to have a new relationship. Nursing home staff generally have limited knowledge of late-life sexuality and may view residents' sexual acts as problems rather than as expressions of the need for love and intimacy (DiNapoli et al, 2013). Reactions may include disapproval, discomfort, and embarrassment, and caregivers may explicitly or implicitly discourage or deny intimacy needs.

Privacy is a major issue in nursing homes that can prevent fulfillment of intimacy and sexual needs. Suggestions for providing privacy and an atmosphere accepting of sexual activity include the availability of a private room, not interrupting when doors are closed and sexual activity is taking place, allowing residents to have sexually explicit materials in their rooms, and providing adaptive equipment, such as side rails or trapezes and double beds. In one facility where one of the authors (T.T.) worked, the staff would assist one of the female residents to be freshly showered, perfumed, and in a lovely nightgown when she and her partner wanted to have sexual relations.

Interventions

Staff, family, and resident education programs to promote awareness, provide education on sexuality and intimacy in later life, involve residents in discussions of sexuality, and discuss interventions to respond to residents' needs are important in long-term care settings. Staff education should include the opportunity to discuss personal feelings about sexuality, changes associated with aging, the impact of diseases and medications on sexual function, sexual expression among same-sex residents, as well as role-playing and skill training in sexual assessment and intervention (DiNapoli et al, 2013). Rheaume and Mitty (2008) suggest the use of *The Sexual Dysfunction Trivia Game* (Skinner, 2000) and the *Staff Attitudes about Intimacy and Dementia (SAID)* (Kamel and Hajjar, 2003) in staff education programs and policy development.

INTIMACY, SEXUALITY, AND DEMENTIA

Intimacy and sexuality remain important in the lives of persons with dementia and their partners throughout the illness. Intimacy and sexuality may "serve as a nonverbal form of communication and intimacy when other cognitive skills and functions have declined" (Agronin, 2004, p. 13). Yet sexual behavior between life partners when one has dementia is not often addressed and individuals with dementia may be viewed as asexual. Nurses need to have an awareness of the sexual needs of the individual with dementia and their partner and be comfortable discussing this area with both. Robinson and Davis (2013) suggest asking the question: "How has dementia affected your sexual relationship?" (Robinson and Davis, 2013, p. 35).

As dementia progresses, particularly in persons living in long-term care facilities, intimacy and sexuality issues may present challenges, especially regarding the impaired person's ability to consent to sexual activity, and require accurate assessment and documentation. Inappropriate sexual behavior (exposing oneself, masturbating in public, or making inappropriate sexual advances or sexual comments) may also occur in long-term care settings. These behaviors are most distressing to staff and to other residents. Sexual inappropriateness (sexual disinhibition) is one of the least understood aspects of dementia. Individuals with subtypes of dementia that include frontal lobe impairment (Pick's disease and alcoholic dementia) may exhibit more sexually inappropriate behavior (Balasubramaniam et al, 2013).

These kinds of behavior may be triggered by unmet intimacy needs or may be symptoms of an underlying physical problem, such as a urinary tract or vaginal infection. The lack of privacy in nursing homes may lead to sexually inappropriate behavior in public areas. Social cues such as explicit television shows may also precipitate behaviors. Bodily contact, such as in bathing residents, may be misinterpreted as a sexual act or romantic advance.

"A resident with dementia might be mistaking another person for his or her spouse and begin exhibiting unwelcome intimate behavior toward that person. On the other hand, sexual expression between residents could indicate development of a new relationship, as beautifully depicted in the 2007 movie with Julie Christie, Away from Her. Former Supreme Court Justice Sandra Day O'Connor poignantly described the relationship between her husband, who had Alzheimer's disease, and another resident in a residential care setting" (www.usatoday.com/news/nation/2007-11-12-court_N.htm) (Rheaume and Mitty, 2008, p. 348).

Rheaume and Mitty (2008) suggest that an interdisciplinary sexual assessment to determine the underlying need that the person is expressing and how it might be addressed is important. Encouraging family and friends to touch, hug, kiss, and hold hands when visiting may help to meet touch and intimacy needs and decrease inappropriate sexual behavior. Also, allowing the person to stroke a pet or hold a stuffed animal may be helpful. Behavioral and nonpharmacological interventions are first-line treatment. Aggressive or violent behavior may require limit setting, working with the resident and family, providing for sexual expression in a nonharmful manner, and pharmacological treatment if indicated (Messinger-Rapport et al, 2003). Staff will need opportunities for discussion and assistance with interventions.

Sexuality among nursing home residents with dementia is a sensitive topic, and there are no national guidelines for determining sexual consent capacity among individuals with severe dementia (DiNapoli et al, 2013). Determination of a cognitively impaired person's ability to consent to participation in a sexual activity involves concepts of voluntary participation, mental competence, and an understanding of the risks and benefits. The Hebrew Home in Riverdale, New York, initiated model sexual policies in 1995. The recently updated policies are valuable resources on intimacy, sexuality, and sexual behavior for older people with dementia (2014) (Box 33-4).

HIV/AIDS AND OLDER ADULTS

An increasingly significant trend in the global HIV epidemic is the growing number of people aged 50 years and older who are living with HIV. This trend is occurring in both developed and developing countries. For the first time since the start of the HIV epidemic, 10% of the adult population living with HIV in low- and middle-income countries is aged 50 years or older. In China, the proportion of people 50 years and older living with HIV/AIDS increased from 16.5% in 2007 to 42.7% in 2011. In Zambia, persons 50 years and older with HIV infections account for 20.4% of all HIV infections (Heckman, 2014; UNAIDS Report, 2013).

In the United States, nearly 37% of people with HIV in the United States are older than age 50. Predictions are that this figure could rise to 50% by 2015 and to 70% by 2020 (Figure 33-4) (HIVAge.org, 2014). The racial/ethnic disparities in HIV/AIDS among older people parallel trends among all age groups with higher rates among African Americans and Hispanics/Latinos. Fourteen percent of gay or bisexual men are HIV positive (Jablonski et al, 2013). Women older than

---

BOX 33-4 RESOURCES FOR BEST PRACTICE

- **Administration on Aging:** Older Adults and HIV Toolkit
- **CDC:** Guide to Taking a Sexual History
- **Hartford Institute for Geriatric Nursing**: Wallace, M: Issues regarding sexuality, Protocol: Sexuality in the Older Adult: See Assessment Series for video illustrating use of PLISSIT model
- **Hebrew Home for the Aged at Riverdale**: The Center for Older Adult Sexuality: Policy and guidelines for sexual expression among individuals with dementia in long-term care
- **HIVAge.org:** resources, research
- **HIV Wisdom for Older Women**
- **National Center for Transgender Equality**
- **National Institute on Aging**: Sexuality in later life, Sexuality and older people

The Aging of the HIV Epidemic in the US
CDC Surveillance Data

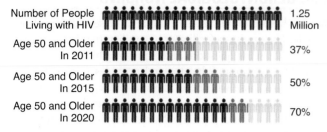

Number of People Living with HIV		1.25 Million
Age 50 and Older In 2011		37%
Age 50 and Older In 2015		50%
Age 50 and Older In 2020		70%

FIGURE 33-4 HIV and Older Adults. Data estimations are based on CDC surveillance data. (From http://hiv-age.org. Used with permission from S.E. Karpiak, PhD.)

age 60 make up one of the fastest-growing risk groups and 70% of older HIV-positive women are African American or Hispanic/Latina (Greene et al, 2013). Most got the virus from sex with infected partners (CDC, 2013; HIV Wisdom for Older Women, 2010).

While rates of HIV/AIDS have remained relatively stable in younger age groups, the number of older people infected with the virus is growing. The largest increase in HIV diagnoses from 2008 to 2010 was among people ages 65 and older (Baron-Faust, 2013; CDC, 2013). The incidence is expected to continue to increase as more individuals become infected later in life, and those who were infected in early adulthood live longer as a result of advances in disease treatment.

The compromised immune system of an older individual makes him or her even more susceptible to HIV or AIDS than a younger person. Older women who are sexually active are at high risk for HIV/AIDS (and other sexually transmitted infections) from an infected partner, resulting, in part, from normal age changes of the vaginal tissue—a thinner, drier, friable vaginal lining that makes viral entry more efficient. (CDC, 2013; UNAIDS, 2013). Studies show that sexually active older men and women do not routinely use condoms, thus increasing their risk of sexually transmitted diseases. Recently widowed or divorced individuals may not understand the need for practicing safe sex because they do not worry about an unwanted pregnancy and may not understand the risk of sexually transmitted diseases (Johnson, 2013). Box 33-5 presents some other risk factors.

Assessment

Physicians, nurse practitioners, and other health professionals need to increase their knowledge of HIV in older adults and become comfortable taking a complete sexual history and talking about sex with all older adults. A thorough sex and drug use/assessment screening should be conducted with attention to HIV risk factors (Johnson, 2013). The idea that elders are not sexually active limits health care providers' objectivity to recognize HIV/AIDS as a possible diagnosis.

AIDS in older adults has been called the "Great Imitator" because many of the symptoms, such as fatigue, weakness, weight loss, and anorexia, are common to other disease conditions and may be attributed to normal aging. Additionally, older people may blame possible symptoms on aging or be reluctant to seek testing or share symptoms due to the stigma they associate with the disease (National Institute on Aging, 2009). Older adults living with HIV/AIDS are thought to experience a "double stigma" of being both old and HIV/AIDS positive (National Resource Center on LGBT Aging, 2011).

Most U.S. guidelines recommend HIV testing among high-risk groups regardless of age, but routine screening recommendations differ and some have a cut-off age of 65 years. The Joint Academy of HIV Medicine, the American Geriatrics Society, and the AIDS Community Research Initiative of America recommend routine opt-out screening, regardless of age (Greene et al, 2013). Medicare covers annual screenings for HIV for those who are at increased risk and those who ask for the test. Also covered is annual screening for those who are at increased risk for sexually transmitted infections (STIs). A home HIV test system is made by the Home Access Health Corporation and is the only system approved by the FDA. It is available at retail pharmacies (National Institute on Aging, 2009).

Interventions

Lack of awareness about HIV in older people results in older people diagnosed with HIV infection late in the course of their disease, meaning a late start to treatment, possibly more damage to their immune system, and poorer prognoses than younger individuals (CDC, 2013; UNAIDS, 2013). HIV-infected adults may also be at increased risk of geriatric syndromes that complicate their treatment and face higher rates of cardiovascular disease, diabetes, hypertension, and cancer (HIVAge.org, 2014). Some research has reported more cognitive deficits in individuals with HIV, and this may be due to the systemic inflammation that also promotes neuroinflammation (Jablonski et al, 2013).

Antiretroviral therapy (ART) can be more complicated if there are chronic illnesses, comorbidities, and polypharmacy (Kazer, 2012). Long-term effects of antiretroviral therapy are also not well studied. However, there is no evidence that response to therapy is different in older people than in younger individuals and some data suggest that older individuals may be more adherent to ART. Presently, guidelines for care of adults

60 to 80 years of age with HIV are somewhat limited because this population has not been studied in clinical trials or pharmacokinetic trials (Greene et al, 2013). Box 33-6 presents a disease-stage summary of care.

Misinformation about HIV is more common in older adults and they may know less about the disease than younger individuals (Kazer et al, 2013; UNAIDS, 2013). Educational materials and programs aimed at older adults need to be developed. They should include information about what HIV/AIDS is and how it is (and is not) transmitted, risk-reduction counseling, symptoms of which to be aware, and the treatments that are available.

Jane Fowler, director of the National HIV Wisdom for Older Women program (WOW), suggests that HIV/AIDS educational campaigns and programs are not targeted to older individuals and asks, "How often does a wrinkled face appear on a prevention poster?" (HIV Wisdom for Older Women, 2010). The National Institute on Aging provides an HIV/AIDS toolkit with resources designed specifically for education of older people (see Box 33-4).

BOX 33-6 Disease-Stage Summary of Care (HIV/AIDS) in Advanced Age

Early-Stage Care
- Discuss sexual history.
- Perform routine screening for HIV.
- HIV symptoms are often atypical in older adults.
- If HIV positive, antiretroviral therapy should be started in all older patients regardless of CD4 T-lymphocyte count.
- No specific guidelines exist for choosing antiretroviral drugs in HIV-positive older adults.
- Choice of ART depends on factors such as pill burden, dosing frequency, comorbid disease, drug interactions, and local drug availability.
- Provide education on HIV transmission reduction strategies and adherence to drug therapy.

Chronic-Stage Care
- HIV-associated non-AIDS conditions are more likely to impact mortality than HIV.
- Management of comorbidities should be prioritized (cardiovascular, hepatic, renal, bone, central nervous system).
- Modifiable lifestyle risk factors, focusing on health maintenance and prevention, should be addressed.
- Risk for polypharmacy and drug interactions should be considered.
- Risk for social isolation should be considered since social support can influence health outcomes.

Advanced-Stage Care
- Provide ongoing discussions of end-of-life preferences, choice of living environment, and safety.
- Prognosis is an increasingly important component of decision-making related to screening, adding medications, and considering invasive treatments.
- Palliative care is an important consideration in older HIV-positive patients.
- Best models of care are not well-defined but will require integration of HIV, primary care, and geriatric expertise.

Adapted from Greene M, Justice AC, Lampiris HW, et al: Management of human immunodeficiency virus infection in advanced age, *JAMA* 309(13):1397–1405, 2013.

◆ PROMOTING HEALTHY AGING: IMPLICATIONS FOR GERONTOLOGICAL NURSING

Nurses have multiple roles in the area of sexuality and older people. The nurse is a facilitator of a milieu that is conducive to the person asking questions and expressing his or her sexuality. The nurse is also an educator and provides information and guidance to those who need it. Some older people remain or want to remain sexually active, whereas others do not see this as an important part of their life. Nurses should open the door to discussions of sexual concerns in a nonjudgmental manner, helping those who want to continue to be sexually active, and making it clear that stopping sex is an acceptable option for others.

Assessment

Sexuality and intimacy are crucial to healthy aging, and the way these are expressed among older adults is changing, particularly with the aging of the baby boomers and upcoming generations. When promoting healthy aging, nurses must consider increasingly open attitudes toward sexuality, dating and developing new relationships, the challenges of facilitating intimacy in residential settings, and the importance of promoting sexual health and safe sex practices (Syme, 2014). Being aware of one's own feelings about sexuality and attitudes toward intimacy and sexuality in older people of all sexual preferences is important. Only after confronting one's own attitudes, values, and beliefs can the nurse provide support without being judgmental.

Anticipation of problems in older individuals' sexual experiences can ward off anxiety, misconceptions, and an arbitrary cessation of sexual pleasure. Validation of the normalcy of sexual activity and a discussion of the physiological changes that occur either with age or as a result of illness are important. Adaptations that will promote sexual function for individuals with chronic illness should be provided. Screening for HIV/AIDS and other sexually transmitted diseases and education about safe sexual practices are also important (Box 33-7) (Johnson, 2013).

BOX 33-7 TIPS FOR BEST PRACTICE

Screening for Sexually Transmitted Infections among Older Adults

- Adults who are sexually active should talk to their health care provider about STI testing.
- All adults should be tested at least once for HIV.
- All sexually active older women with risk factors such as new or multiple sex partners or who live in communities with a high burden of disease should be screened annually for chlamydia and gonorrhea.
- Screening is recommended at least once a year for syphilis, chlamydia, gonorrhea, and HIV for all sexually active gay men, bisexual men, and other men who have sex with men.

From Johnson B: Sexually transmitted infections and older adults, *J Gerontol Nurs* 39(11):53–60, 2013.

In addition, the myth that elders do not engage in sexual activity must be put to rest. After age 50, only 38% of U.S. men and 22% of U.S. women report discussing sexual activity with their health care provider and only about one-fourth of U.S. adults, without obvious risk for HIV acquisition, are screened for HIV (Greene et al, 2013). When questions about sexual issues are asked or when the older adult is examined, the nurse needs to be particularly cognizant of the era and culture in which the individual has lived to understand the factors affecting conduct. Box 33-8 provides other suggestions for assessment, from the perspective of the older adult. The CDC provides a guide to taking a sexual history (see Box 33-4).

Currently, there are no instruments that could be used in clinical practice or research to assess the sexual health of the older population. Nurse researcher Meredith Kazer and colleagues (2013) report on the preliminary development of the Geriatric Sexuality Inventory and note that having a self-report instrument to replace open-ended questions may be an effective strategy to decrease the discomfort of health care providers and older adults in discussing sexuality.

A medication review is essential because many medications affect sexual functioning. Often, medications are prescribed to both older men and women without attention to the sexual side effects. If medications that affect sexual function are necessary, adjustment of doses, use of alternative agents, and prescription of antidotes to reverse the sexual side effects are important (Box 33-9).

The PLISSIT Model (Annon, 1976) is a helpful guide for discussion of sexuality (Box 33-10). Youngkin (2004) provides suggestions for use of the PLISSIT Model with older people:

- **Permission:** Obtain permission from the client to initiate sexual discussion. Allow the person to discuss concerns related to sexual issues, and gather information about what might have changed in the person's life to affect sexual needs and response. Questions such as the following can be used: "What concerns or questions do you have about fulfilling your sexual needs?" or "In this era of HIV and other sexually transmitted infections, I ask all my patients about sexual practices and concerns. Are there any questions I can answer for you?"

BOX 33-8 TIPS FOR BEST PRACTICE
Guidelines for Health Care Providers in Talking to Older Adults about Sexual Health

Health Care Providers Should Spend Time with Older Adults
- Be available to discuss the subject.
- Give us your full attention.
- Allow time to ask questions.
- Take time to answer questions.
- Health care providers should use clear and easy-to-understand words.
- Use plain, everyday language.
- Explain medical terms in plain English.
- Give explanations or answers to questions in simple terms.

Health Care Providers Should Help Older Adults Feel Comfortable Talking about Sex
- Help us to break the ice.
- Make us feel comfortable in asking questions.
- Offer permission to express feelings and needs.
- Do not be afraid or embarrassed to discuss sexuality problems.

Health Care Providers Should be Open-Minded and Talk Openly
- Do not assume there are no concerns.
- Be open.
- Ask direct questions about sexual activity and attitudes.
- Discuss sexual concerns freely.
- Answer questions honestly.
- Just talk about it.
- Do not evade sexual concerns.
- Be willing to discuss sexual problems.
- Probe sexual concerns if elder wishes.

Health Care Providers Should Listen
- Be prepared to listen.
- Listen so that we feel you are interested in our problems.
- Let us talk.

Health Care Providers Should Treat Older Adults with a Respectful and Nonjudgmental Attitude
- See us as individuals with sexual needs.
- Accept us for what we are: gay, straight, bisexual.
- Be nonjudgmental.
- Show genuine concern and respect.

Health Care Providers Should Encourage Discussion
- Make opportunities for one-to-one discussion.
- Provide privacy.
- Promote candid discussion.
- Provide discussion groups to ask questions.
- Develop support groups.

Health Care Providers Can Give Advice or Suggestions
- Provide information.
- Offer to find solutions and alternatives to given situations.
- Provide explicit pamphlets; explain sexual positions, lubrication.
- Discuss old taboos.
- Give suggestions of ways to help solve sexual problems.

Health Care Providers Need to Understand that Sex is Not Just for the Young
- Try to eliminate the idea that sex and love are just for younger people.
- Acknowledge that sexual impulses are healthy and do not disappear as individuals age.
- Treat older adults as normal sexual beings and not as asexual elderly people.
- Recognize that sex can improve—can become even better when one is older.

From Kazer MW, Grossman S, Kerins G, et al: Validity and reliability of the Geriatric Sexuality Inventory, *J Gerontol Nurs* 39(11):38–45, 2013.

BOX 33-9   Medications that May Affect Sexual Health

Antihypertensive agents
Medications for prostate diseases
Cholesterol medications
Antidepressant agents
Other medications that affect mood
Anticholinergic agents
Pain medications (narcotics)
Osteoporosis medications
Oral hypoglycemic agents
Insulin
Chemotherapy for cancer

BOX 33-10   PLISSIT Model

P—Permission from the client to initiate sexual discussion
LI—Providing the **Limited Information** needed to function sexually
SS—Giving **Specific Suggestions** for the individual to proceed with sexual relations
IT—Providing **Intensive Therapy** surrounding the issues of sexuality for the clients (may mean referral to specialist)

Compiled from Annon J: The PLISSIT model: a proposed conceptual scheme for behavioral treatment of sexual problems, *J Sex Educ Ther* 2:1–15, 1976; Wallace M: Best practices in nursing care to older adults: sexuality, *Dermatol Nurs* 15:570–571, 2003; Youngkin EQ: The myths and truths of mature intimacy, *Adv Nurse Pract* 12:45–48, 2004.

- **Limited Information:** Provide the limited information to function sexually (Wallace, 2003). Offer teaching about the normal age-associated changes that affect sexual performance or how illness may affect sexuality. Encourage the person to learn more about the concern from books and other sources.
- **Specific Suggestions:** Offer suggestions for dealing with problems such as lubricants for atrophic vaginitis; use of condoms to prevent sexually transmitted infections; proper use of ED medications; how to communicate sexual and other needs; ways to increase comfort with coitus or ways to be intimate without coital relations.
- **Intensive Therapy:** Refer as appropriate for complex problems that require specialist intervention.

◆ Interventions

Interventions will vary depending on the needs identified from the assessment data. Following a comprehensive assessment, interventions may center on the following categories: (1) education regarding age-associated change in sexual function; (2) compensation for age-associated changes and effects of chronic illness; (3) effective management of acute and chronic illness affecting sexual function; (4) provision of education on HIV and STIs and reduction of risk factors; (5) removal of barriers associated with fulfilling sexual needs; and (6) special interventions to promote sexual health in cognitively impaired older adults (Arena and Wallace, 2008) (see Box 33-4).

KEY CONCEPTS

- Touch provides sensory stimulation, reduces anxiety, and provides pain relief, comfort, and sexual expression.
- The absence of touch, a powerful sense, threatens survival.
- Sexuality is love, sharing, trust, and warmth, as well as physical acts. Sexuality provides an individual with self-identity and affirmation of life.
- Sexual activity continues in aging, though adaptations are needed for the age-related changes of the male and female genital systems.
- Generally speaking, medications, ill health, and lack of a partner affect sexual activity.
- Further research is needed to promote knowledge and understanding of the sexual health of LGBT older adults.
- AIDS awareness and the practice of safe sex among older adults are still lacking. Health professionals, too, do not consider older adults at risk for AIDS, even though the incidence of AIDS in the older population is rapidly increasing.
- The major role of the nurse in enhancing the sexual health of older adults in the community or in long-term care settings is education and counseling about sexual function; adaptations for age-related changes and chronic conditions; prevention of HIV/AIDS and STDs in sexually active older adults; and the maintenance of sexuality for the older adult's health, well-being, and pleasure.

NURSING STUDY: SEXUALITY IN LATE LIFE

George was a 70-year-old man who had been widowed for 6 years. He lived alone in a lovely home in the hills of San Francisco. His many friends tried to introduce him to a lady who would be attractive to him, but they were unaware of his real concerns. Although George was attracted to young, energetic women, often barely older than his daughters, he was justifiably cautious regarding their sincere attraction to him because he had a considerable estate. In addition, his sexual desire was waning and his capacity for sexual performance was unpredictable. One thing George expressed fairly frequently was, "I don't like demands made on me." To further complicate the picture, George had begun to take medication to reduce his benign prostatic hypertrophy (BPH) that had become increasingly troublesome. The medication further reduced his sexual desire. In addition, George's sleep pattern was disturbed by the need to arise three or four times each night to void. George came to the clinic for follow-up evaluation of his BPH, and, while talking with the nurse, he began crying uncontrollably, much to his embarrassment and the nurse's surprise because George had always seemed to be a rather solid and stoic fellow who was reluctant to discuss feelings.

Based on the case study, develop a nursing care plan using the following procedure*:
- List George's comments that provide subjective data.
- List information that provides objective data.
- From these data, identify and state, using an accepted format, two nursing diagnoses you determine are most significant to George at this time. List two of George's strengths that you have identified from the data.

- Determine and state outcome criteria for each diagnosis. These criteria must reflect some alleviation of the problem identified in the nursing diagnosis and must be stated in concrete and measurable terms.
- Plan and state one or more interventions for each diagnosed problem. Provide specific documentation of the sources used to determine the appropriate intervention. Plan at least one intervention that incorporates George's existing strengths.
- Evaluate the success of the intervention. Interventions must correlate directly with the stated outcome criteria to measure the outcome success.

*Students are advised to refer to their nursing diagnosis text and identify possible or potential problems.

CRITICAL THINKING QUESTIONS AND ACTIVITIES

1. How would you begin discussing sexuality with George?
2. What are the factors that may be underlying George's sexual distress?
3. With a partner, role-play and demonstrate your interpersonal interaction with George in this situation.
4. What resources or recommendations would you suggest for George?

RESEARCH QUESTIONS

1. What do women find are the most troubling changes in their sexuality as they grow older?
2. What do men find are the most troubling changes in their sexuality as they grow older?
3. What are the differences in sexual feelings and expression in the 60-year-old, the 70-year-old, the 80-year-old, and the 90-year-old individual?
4. What are the chronic disorders that most affect sexual performance of men and women, and how are individuals affected?
5. How many individuals older than age 60 have ever been given the opportunity to provide a thorough sexual history?
6. What community and health resources are available to meet the needs of LGBT older adults?
7. What is the knowledge level about HIV/AIDS for people older than age 65?

REFERENCES

Ackerman D: *A natural history of the senses*, New York, 1995, Vantage Books.

Agronin M: Sexuality and aging: an introduction, *CNS Longterm Care* 12–13, 2004.

American Society on Aging and MetLife: *Still out, still aging*, 2010. https://www.metlife.com/assets/cao/mmi/publications/studies/2010/mmi-still-out-still-aging.pdf. Accessed November 2014.

Annon J: The PLISSIT model: a proposed conceptual scheme for behavioral treatment of sexual problems, *J Sex Educ Ther* 2:1–15, 1976.

Arena J, Wallace M: Issues regarding sexuality. In Capezuti E, Swicker D, Mezey M, et al, editors: *Evidence-based geriatric nursing protocols for best practice*, ed 3, New York, 2008, Springer, pp 629–648.

Bach L, Mortimer J, Vandeweerd C, et al: The association of physical and mental health with sexual activity in older adults in a retirement community, *J Sex Med* 10(11):2671–2678, 2013.

Balasubramaniam M, Clark L, Jensen T, et al: Medroxyprogesterone acetate treatment for sexually inappropriate behavior in a patient with frontotemporal dementia, *Ann Longterm Care* 21(11):30–36, 2013.

Baron-Faust R: *HIV/AIDS in older adults: rising, and unchecked*, 2013. http://www.rheumatologynetwork.com/articles/hivaids-older-adults-rising-and-unchecked. Accessed May 2014.

Benary-Isbert M: *The vintage years*, New York, 1968, Abingdon Press.

Centers for Disease Control and Prevention: *HIV among older Americans*, 2013. http://www.cdc.gov/hiv/risk/age/olderamericans. Accessed May 2014.

Comfort A: Sexuality in old age, *J Am Geriatr Soc* 22:440–442, 1974.

DiNapoli E, Breland G, Allen R: Staff knowledge and perceptions of sexuality and dementia of older adults in nursing homes, *J Aging Health* 25:1087–1105, 2013.

Fisher L: *Sex, romance and relationships: AARP survey of midlife and older adults*, May 2010. http://assets.aarp.org/rgcenter/general/srr_09.pdf. Document1Accessed August 2014.

Fredriksen-Goldsen K, Hyun-Jun K, Emlet C, et al: *The aging and health report: disparities and resilience among lesbian, gay, bisexual, and transgender older adults*, 2011. http://www.lgbtagingcenter.org/resources/resource.cfm?r=419. Accessed May 2014.

Gallace A, Spence C: The science of interpersonal touch: an overview, *Neurosci Biobehav Rev* 34:246–259, 2010.

Greene M, Justice A, Lampiris H, et al: Management of human immunodeficiency virus infection in advanced age, *JAMA* 309(13):1387–1405, 2013.

Hall ET: *The hidden dimensions*, Garden City, New York, 1969, Doubleday.

Hebrew Home at Riverdale: *The Center for Older Adult Sexuality, Policies and Procedures concerning sexual expression at the Hebrew Home at Riverdale*. http://www.hebrewhome.org/uploads/ckeditor/files/sexualexpressionpolicy.pdf. Accessed February 13, 2015.

Heckman T: *Introduction to current issues on HIV/AIDS in older adults*, 2014. http://www.apa.org/pi/aids/resources/exchange/2014/01/introduction.aspx. Accessed May 2014.

HIVAge.org: *Geriatric syndromes are common among HIV-infected adults*, Apr 4, 2014. http://hiv-age.org/2014/04/geriatric-syndromes-common-among-older-hiv-infected-adults. Accessed May 2014.

HIV Wisdom for Older Women: *Things you should know about HIV and older women*,

2010. http://www.hivwisdom.org/facts.html. Accessed May 2014.

Hollinger LM, Buschmann MT: Factors influencing the perception of touch by elderly nursing home residents and their health caregivers, *Int J Nurs Stud* 30:445–461, 1993.

Institute of Medicine: *The health of lesbian, gay, bisexual, and transgender people: building a better foundation for better understanding*, 2011. http://www.iom.edu/Reports/2011/The-Health-of-Lesbian-Gay-Bisexual-and-Transgender-People.aspx. Accessed May 2014.

Jablonski R, Vance D, Beattie E: The invisible elderly: lesbian, gay, bisexual, and transgender older adults, *J Gerontol Nurs* 39(11):46–52, 2013.

Johnson B: Sexually transmitted infections and older adults, *J Gerontol Nurs* 39(11): 53–60, 2013.

Kaiser FE: Sexual dysfunction in men; sexual dysfunction in women. In Beers MH, Berkow R, editors: *The Merck manual of geriatrics*, ed 3, Whitehouse Station, NJ, 2000, Merck.

Kamel H, Hajjar R: Sexuality in the nursing home, part 2: managing abnormal behavior—legal and ethical issues, *J Am Med Dir Assoc* 4:203–206, 2003.

Kazer M: Issues regarding sexuality. In Boltz M, Capezuti E, Fulmer T, et al, editors: *Evidence-based geriatric nursing protocols for best practice*, ed 4, New York, 2012, Springer, pp 500–515.

Kazer M, Grossman S, Kerins G, et al: Validity and reliability of the Geriatric Sexual Inventory, *J Gerontol Nurs* 39(11):40–45, 2013.

Kennedy G, Martinez M, Garo N: Sex and mental health in old age, *Prim Psychiatry* 17: 22–30, 2010.

Kim EJ, Buschmann MBT: Touch-stress model and Alzheimer's disease: using touch intervention to alleviate patients' stress, *J Gerontol Nurs* 30:33–39, 2004.

Kreiger D: Therapeutic touch: the imprimatur of nursing, *Am J Nurs* 75:784–787, 1975.

Lim F, Brown D, Justin K, et al: Addressing health care disparities in the lesbian, gay, bisexual, and transgender population, *Am J Nurs* 114(6):24–34, 2014.

Lindau S, Gavrilova N: Sex, health, and years of sexually active life gained due to good health: evidence from two US populations based cross sectional surveys of ageing, *BMJ* 340:c810, 2010. http://www.bmj.com/content/340/bmj.c810. Accessed May 2014.

Lindau S, Schumm L, Laumann E, et al: A study of sexuality and health among older adults in the United States, *N Engl J Med* 357:762–774, 2007.

Mammarella N, Fairfield B, Di Domenico A: When touch matters: an affective tactile intervention for older adults, *Geriatr Gerontol Int* 17(4):722–724, 2012.

Messinger-Rapport BJ, Sandhu SK, Hujer ME: Sex and sexuality: is it over after 60? *Clin Geriatr* 11:45–53, 2003.

Montagu A: *Touching: the human significance of the skin*, ed 3, New York, 1986, Harper & Row.

National Center for Transgender Equality: *Improving the lives of transgender older adults*, 2011. http://transequality.org/Issues/seniors.html. Accessed May 2014.

National Institute on Aging: *HIV, AIDS, and older people*, 2009. http://www.nia.nih.gov/health/publication/hiv-aids-and-older-people. Accessed May 2014.

National Resource Center on LGBT Aging: *HIV/AIDS and older adults: fact versus fiction*, 2011. http://www.lgbtagingcenter.org/resources/resource.cfm?r=322. Accessed May 2014.

Rheaume C, Mitty E: Sexuality and intimacy in older adults, *Geriatr Nurs* 29:342–349, 2008.

Robinson K, Davis S: Influence of cognitive decline on sexuality in individuals with dementia and their caregivers, *J Gerontol Nurs* 39(11):31–36. 2013.

Sansone P, Schmitt L: Providing tender touch massage to elderly nursing home residents: a demonstration project, *Geriatr Nurs* 21:303–308, 2000.

Services and Advocacy for Gay, Lesbian, Bisexual, and Transgender Elders (SAGE) and Movement Advancement Project (MAP): *Improving the lives of LGBT older adults*, 2010. http://www.lgbtmap.org/policy-and-issue-analysis/improving-the-lives-of-lgbt-older-adults. Accessed May 2014.

Skinner KD: Creating a game for sexuality and aging: the sexual dysfunction trivia game, *J Contin Educ Nurs* 31:185–189, 2000.

Steinke E: Intimacy needs and chronic illness, *J Gerontol Nurs* 31:40–50, 2005.

Steinke E: Sexuality and chronic illness, *J Gerontol Nurs* 39(11):18–27, 2013.

Steinke E, Jaarsma T, Barnason S, et al: Sexual counseling for individuals with cardiovascular disease and their partners: a consensus statement from the American Heart Association and the ESC Council on Cardiovascular Nursing and Allied Professions (CCNAP), *Circulation* 128:2075–2096, 2013. https://circ.ahajournals.org/content/early/2013/07/29/CIR.0b013e31829c2e53. Accessed May 2014.

Suzman R: The National Social Life, Health, and Aging Project: An introduction, *J Gerontol B Psychol Sci Soc Sci* 64:i5–i11, 2009.

Syme M: The evolving concept of older adult sexual behavior and its benefits, *Generations* 38(1):35–41, 2014.

United National (UNAIDS): *HIV and aging*, 2013. http://www.unaids.org/sites/default/files/media_asset/20131101_JC2563_hiv-and-aging_en_0.pdf. Accessed February 2015.

U.S. Department of Health and Human Services: *LGBT health and well-being*, 2014. http://www.hhs.gov/lgbt. Accessed May 2014.

Waite L, Laumann E, Das A, et al: Sexuality: measures of partnerships, practices, attitudes, and problems in the National Social Life, Health and Aging Study, *J Gerontol B Psychol Sci Soc Sci* 64 (Suppl 1):i56–i66, 2009.

Wallace M: Best practices in nursing care to older adults: sexuality, *Dermatol Nurs* 15:570–571, 2003.

Wallace SP, Cochran SD, Durazo EM, et al: *The health of aging lesbian, gay and bisexual adults in California*. Los Angeles, CA, 2011, UCLA Center for Health Policy Research. http://www.ncbi.nlm.nih.gov/pmc/articles/PMC3698220/. Accessed February 13, 2015.

Wang K, Hermann C: Pilot study to test the effectiveness of healing touch on agitation in people with dementia, *Geriatr Nurs* 27:34–40, 2006.

World Health Organization: *Sexual and reproductive health: defining sexual health*, 2014. http://www.who.int/reproductive-health/topics/sexual_health/sh_definitions/en. Accessed August 2014.

Youngkin EQ: The myths and truths of mature intimacy, *Adv Nurse Pract* 12:45–48, 2004.

Zeiss A, Kasl-Godley J: Sexuality in older adults' relationships, *Generations* 25:18, 2001.

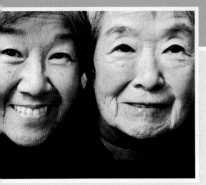

Relationships, Roles, and Transitions

Theris A. Touhy

http://evolve.elsevier.com/Touhy/TwdHlthAging

A STUDENT SPEAKS

I'm really worried about retirement! That is ridiculous at my age, but I keep reading and hearing about Social Security and Medicare running out of money for the baby boom generation. Those are my parents! What about me?

Joseph, age 30

AN ELDER SPEAKS

I thought when my children left home that my most important job was done. But they came home again and again, and then my mother-in-law came to live with us. Finally, the kids were really on their own and married, so now I take care of the grandchildren while they both work to make ends meet. I just pray daily that my husband will remain healthy. I don't think I could deal with one more thing.

Esther, age 64

LEARNING OBJECTIVES

On completion of this chapter, the reader will be able to:

1. Explain the issues involved in adapting to transitions and role changes in later life.
2. Discuss changes in family structure and functions in society today.
3. Examine family relationships in later life.
4. Identify the range of caregiving situations and the potential challenges and opportunities of each.
5. Discuss nursing responses with older adults experiencing caregiver roles or other transitions.

This chapter examines the various relationships, roles, and transitions that characteristically play a part in later life. Important roles include those of spouse, partner, parent, grandparent, great-grandparent, sibling, friend, and caregiver. The role functions of these relationships shift as societal norms and economics change. Even more changes are expected as the first wave of baby boomers enters young-old age. The major concerns of this group are maintaining health and independence, having adequate health care coverage, ensuring the preservation of Social Security, and meeting caregiving demands. This major change in the aging landscape is only one of the massive social changes that have altered the patterns of work, family, and kinship structure in recent decades.

Concepts of family structure and function—the transitions of retirement, widowhood, widowerhood, and caregiving—are examined. Nursing interventions to support older adults in maintaining fulfilling roles and relationships and adapting to transitions are discussed.

LATER LIFE TRANSITIONS

Role transitions that occur in late life include retirement, grandparenthood, widowhood, and becoming a caregiver or recipient of care. These transitions may occur predictably or may be imposed by unanticipated events. Retirement is an example of a predictable event that can and should be planned long in advance, although for some, it can occur unexpectedly as a result of illness, disability, or being terminated from a job. To the degree that an event is perceived as expected and occurring at the right time, a role transition may be comfortable and even welcomed. Those persons who must retire "too early" or are widowed "too soon" will have more difficulty adapting than those who are at an age when these events are expected.

The speed and intensity of a major change may make the difference between a transitional crisis and a gradual and comfortable adaptation. Most difficult are the transitions that incorporate losses rather than gains in status, influence, and

opportunity. The move from independence to dependence and becoming a care recipient is particularly difficult. Conditions that influence the outcome of transitions include personal meanings, expectations, level of knowledge, preplanning, and emotional and physical reserves. Cohort, cultural, and gender differences are inherent in all of life's major transitions. Those transitions that make use of past skills and adaptations may be less stressful. The ideal outcome is when gains in satisfaction and new roles offset losses.

Retirement

Issues of work and retirement for older adults are a cultural universal topic because every culture has mechanisms for retiring their elders. While retirement patterns differ across the world, in industrialized nations, as well as in many developing nations, the expectation is that older workers will cease full-time career job employment and be entitled to economic support (McNamara and Williamson, 2013). However, whether that support will be adequate, or even available, is a growing concern worldwide.

In the United States and many European countries and Australia, the problems are emerging as the generation born after World War II moves into retirement. Developing countries face similar issues with the growth of the older population combined with decreasing birth rates. Governments may not be able to afford retirement systems to replace the tradition of children caring for aging parents. Most countries are not ready to meet what is projected to be one of the defining challenges of the twenty-first century (Jackson et al, 2013).

Retirement, as we formerly knew it, has changed. The transitions are blurring, and the numerous patterns and styles of retiring have produced more varied experiences in retirement. Retirement is no longer just a few years of rest from the rigors of work before death. It is a developmental stage that may occupy 30 or more years of one's life and involve many stages. Some individuals will be retired longer than they worked.

Retirees are living longer, and declining birth rates mean there will be fewer workers to support them. Countries are scaling down retirement benefits and raising the age to start collecting them. Individuals can expect to work longer before retirement and many plan to continue to work after they retire. Some do so because of economic need, whereas others have a desire to remain involved and productive.

The Great Recession and the declining economy have contributed to a rising level of economic risk facing retirees. More than half of the world's working population claims they are not preparing adequately for a comfortable retirement, and nearly 20% are saving nothing at all (Thompson, 2013). Single senior households, mostly women, are at even greater financial vulnerability and 36% are at serious financial risk (Polivka, 2012). Obviously, health and financial status affect decisions and abilities to work or engage in new work opportunities. The baby boomers increasingly face the prospect of working longer, and 33% of this generation do not own assets and have little in savings or projected retirement income beyond Social Security. The majority of baby boomers plan to work after 65 or not retire at all (Hooyman and Kiyak, 2011).

With growing concerns about unemployment across the globe, opportunities for work may be limited and strategies to increase older adults' employability are important. They have been initiated in many countries in the European Union (McNamara and Williamson, 2013). Individuals will be seeking new career paths later in life and look to employers to help them. Continuing education, workplace design, and part-time employment opportunities for older workers will be needed, and rising retirement ages will require reconsideration of early retirement provisions (National Institute on Aging, National Institutes of Health, 2007).

Special Considerations in Retirement

In the United States, retirement security depends on the "three-legged stool" of Social Security pensions, savings, and investments (Stanford and Usita, 2002). Older people with disabilities, those who have lacked access to education or held low-paying jobs with no benefits, and those not eligible for Social Security are at increased economic risk during retirement years. Non-white older persons, women—especially widows and those divorced or never married—immigrants, and gay and lesbian men and women often face greater challenges related to adequate income and benefits in retirement. Unmarried women, particularly African Americans, face the most negative prospects for retirement now and for at least the next 20 years (Hooyman and Kiyak, 2011).

Inadequate coverage for women in retirement is common because their work histories have been sporadic and diverse. Women often retire earlier than anticipated because of family needs. Whereas most men have always worked outside the home, it is only within the past 30 years that this has been the expectation of women. Therefore large cohort differences exist. Traditionally, the variability of women's work histories, interrupted careers, the residuals of sexist pension policies, Social Security inequities, and low-paying jobs created hazards for adequacy of income in retirement. The scene is gradually changing in many respects, but the gender bias remains (Chapter 30).

Barriers to equal treatment for LGBT couples include job discrimination, unequal treatment under Social Security, pension plans, and 401(k) plans. LGBT couples are not eligible for Social Security survivor benefits, and unmarried partners cannot claim pension plan rights after the death of the pension plan participant. These policies definitely place LGBT elders at a disadvantage in retirement planning.

Retirement Planning

Current research suggests that retirement has positive effects on life satisfaction and health, although this may vary depending on the individual's circumstances. Decisions to retire are often based on financial resources; attitudes toward work, family roles, and responsibilities; the nature of the job; access to health insurance; chronological age; health; and self-perceptions of ability to adjust to retirement. Retirement planning is advisable during early adulthood and essential in middle age. However, people differ in their focus on the past, present, and future and their realistic ability to "put away something" for future needs. One-third of adults in their 50s have failed to develop any kind of retirement savings plan (Lusardi and Mitchell, 2011).

Retirement preparation programs are usually aimed at employees with high levels of education and occupational status,

those with private pension coverage, and government employees. Thus the people most in need of planning assistance may be those least likely to have any available, let alone the resources for an adequate retirement. Individuals who are retiring in poor health, minorities, women, those in lower socioeconomic levels, and those with the least education may experience greater concerns in retirement and may need specialized counseling and targeted education efforts (Lusardi and Mitchell, 2011).

◆ PROMOTING HEALTHY AGING: IMPLICATIONS FOR GERONTOLOGICAL NURSING

Successful retirement adjustment depends on socialization needs, energy levels, health, adequate income, variety of interests, amount of self-esteem derived from work, presence of intimate relationships, social support, and general adaptability (Box 34-1). Nurses may have the opportunity to work with people in different phases of retirement or participate in retirement education and counseling programs (Box 34-2).

Talking with clients older than age 50 about retirement plans, providing anticipatory guidance about the transition to retirement, identifying those who may be at risk for lowered income and health concerns, and referring to appropriate resources for retirement planning and support are important nursing interventions. Additionally, the period of preretirement and retirement may be an opportune time to enhance the focus on health promotion and illness/injury prevention. (Chapter 1).

It is important to build on the strengths of the individual's life experiences and coping skills and to provide appropriate

counseling and support to assist individuals to continue to grow and develop in meaningful ways during the transition from the work role. In ideal situations, retirement offers the opportunity to pursue interests that may have been neglected while fulfilling other obligations. However, for too many individuals, retirement presents challenges that affect both health and well-being, and nurses must be advocates for policies and conditions that allow all older people to maintain quality of life in retirement.

◆ Death of a Spouse or Life Partner

Losing a spouse or other life partner after a long, close, and satisfying relationship is the most difficult adjustment one can face, aside from the loss of a child. This loss is a stage in the life course that can be anticipated but seldom is considered. Spousal bereavement in later life is a high probability for women and, while less common among men, still a significant event. Nearly 73% of women 85 years and older are widowed compared with 35% of men (United States Census Bureau, 2013).

The death of a life partner is essentially a loss of self. The mourning is as much for oneself as for the individual who has died. A core part of oneself has died with the partner, and even with satisfactory grief resolution, that aspect of self will never return. Even those widows and widowers who reorganize their lives and invest in family, friends, and activities often find that many years later they still miss their "other half" profoundly.

With the loss of the intimate partner, several changes occur simultaneously in almost every domain of life and have a significant impact on well-being: physical, psychological, social, practical, and economic. Individuals who have been self-confident and resilient seem to fare best (Bennett and Soulsby, 2012). The transitional phase of grief, if handled appropriately, leads to the confirmation of a new identity, the end of one stage of life, and the beginning of another.

Gender differences on widowhood are found in the literature. Bereaved husbands may be more socially and emotionally vulnerable. Suicide risk is highest among men older than 80 years of age who have experienced the death of a spouse (Chapter 28). Widowers adapt more slowly than widows to the loss of a spouse and often remarry quickly. Loneliness and the need to be cared for are factors influencing widowers to pursue new partners. Having associations with family and friends, being members of a church community, and continuing to work or engage in activities can all be helpful in the adjustment period following the death of a wife. Common bereavement reactions of widowers are listed in Box 34-3 and should be discussed with male clients.

BOX 34-1 Predictors of Retirement Satisfaction

- Good health
- Functional abilities
- Adequate income
- Suitable living environment
- Strong social support system characterized by reciprocal relationships
- Decision to retire involved choice, autonomy, adequate preparation, higher-status job before retirement
- Retirement activities that offer an opportunity to feel useful, learn, grow, and enjoy oneself
- Positive outlook, sense of mastery, resilience, resourcefulness
- Good marital or partner relationship
- Sharing similar interests to spouse/significant other

Data from Hooyman N, Kiyak H: *Social gerontology: a multidisciplinary perspective*, ed 9, Boston, 2011, Allyn & Bacon.

BOX 34-2 Phases of Retirement

Remote: Future anticipation with little real planning
Near: Preparation and fantasizing regarding retirement
Honeymoon: Euphoria and testing of the fantasies
Disenchantment: Letdown, boredom, sometimes depression
Reorientation: Developing a realistic and satisfactory lifestyle
Stability: Personal investment in meaningful activities
Termination: Loss of role resulting from illness or return to work

---

BOX 34-3 Common Widower Bereavement Reactions

- Search for the lost mate
- Neglect of self
- Inability to share grief
- Loss of social contacts
- Struggle to view women as other than wife
- Erosion of self-confidence and sexuality
- Protracted grief period

◆ PROMOTING HEALTHY AGING: IMPLICATIONS FOR GERONTOLOGICAL NURSING

◆ Assessment

Nurses working with bereaved individuals will need to review Lindemann's classic grief studies to understand the initial somatic responses of the bereaved (Lindemann, 1944) (Chapter 35). There is an elevated risk of morbidity and mortality, particularly in the early bereavement period (DiGiacomo et al, 2013). The likelihood of a heart attack or stroke doubles in the critical 30-day period after a partner's death. The risk seems likely to be the result of adverse physiological responses associated with acute grief (Carey et al, 2014). The bereavement period is also associated with an elevated risk of multiple psychiatric disorders, particularly if the death was unexpected (Keyes et al, 2014) (Chapter 28). This is an important time for nurses to assess the health status of the individual and provide interventions to assist in coping. However, the risks of effects of spousal bereavement and increasing age on health, particularly chronic issues, remain elevated even among those long past the event (10+ years), so ongoing surveillance and assessment are indicated (Das, 2013).

Feelings of the bereaved one are not orderly or progressive; they are conflicted, ambivalent, suicidal, full of rage, and often suspicious. Bereaved individuals may exhibit personality disorganization that would be considered mentally aberrant or frankly psychotic under other circumstances. Some people handle grief with less apparent decompensation. Grief reactions must be accepted as personally valid and useful evidences of healing. deVries (2001) discusses the signs of ongoing bonds and connections with the deceased (e.g., dreaming of the deceased, ongoing daily communication, "checking in") that persist long after death and counsels professionals to reexamine the idea that there is a timetable for "resolution" of grief. Maintaining bonds with the deceased is considered normal and healthy (Bennett and Soulsby, 2012). There are several tools that can be used to assess aspects of the bereavement process including coping, grief symptomatology, personal growth, continuing bonds, and health risk assessment (Minton and Barron, 2008).

◆ Interventions

Nurses will interact with bereaved older people in many settings. Knowing the stages of transition to a new role as a widow or widower will be useful in determining interventions, although each individual is unique in this respect. Individuals respond to losses in ways that reflect the nature and meaning of the relationships, as well as the unique characteristics of the bereaved. Patterns of adjustment are presented in Box 34-4. With adequate support, reintegration can be expected in 2 to 4 years. People with few familial or social supports may need professional help to get through the early months of grief in a way that will facilitate recovery.

To support the grieving person, it is necessary to extend one's own self to reconnect the bereaved person with a world of warmth and caring. No one nurse or family member can accomplish this task alone. Hundreds of small, caring gestures build strength and confidence in the grieving person's ability and willingness to survive. Additional information about dying, death, and grief can be found in Chapter 35.

BOX 34-4 Patterns of Adjustment to Widowhood

Stage 1: Reactionary (First Few Weeks)
Early responses of disbelief, anger, indecision, detachment, and inability to communicate in a logical, sustained manner are common. Searching for the mate, visions, hallucinations, and depersonalization may be experienced.
Intervention: Support, validate, be available, listen to individual talk about mate, reduce expectations.

Stage 2: Withdrawal (First Few Months)
Depression, apathy, physiological vulnerability; movement and cognition are slowed; insomnia, unpredictable waves of grief, sighing, and anorexia occur.
Intervention: Protect individual against suicide, monitor health status, and involve in support groups.

Stage 3: Recuperation (Second 6 Months)
Periods of depression are interspersed with characteristic capability. Feelings of personal control begin to return.
Intervention: Support accustomed lifestyle patterns that sustain and assist individual to explore new possibilities.

Stage 4: Exploration (Second Year)
Individual begins new ventures, testing suitability of new roles; anniversaries, holidays, birthdays, and date of death may be especially difficult.
Intervention: Prepare individual for unexpected reactions during anniversaries. Encourage and support new trial roles.

Stage 5: Integration (Fifth Year)
Individual will feel fully integrated into new and satisfying roles if grief has been resolved in a healthy manner.
Intervention: Assist individual to recognize and share own pattern of growth through the trauma of loss.

RELATIONSHIPS IN LATER LIFE

The classic study of Lowenthal and Haven (1968) has been reviewed in detail and elaborated many times since its inception. The importance of caring relationships and the presence of a confidante as a buffer against "age-linked social losses" are demonstrated in the study. Maintaining a stable intimate relationship was more closely associated with good mental health and high morale than was a high level of activity or elevated role status. Individuals seem able to manage stresses if some relationships are close and sustaining.

Increasingly evident is that a caring person may be a significant survival resource. Frequently nurses become the caring other in an older person's life, especially among elders living in nursing homes (Touhy, 2001). Social bonding increases health status through as yet undetermined physiological pathways, though studies in psychoneuroimmunology are giving us clues. Social support is related to psychological and physical well-being, and participation in meaningful social activities is also a modifying factor that may offset the risk of dementia.

Friendships

Friends are often a significant source of support in late life. The number of friends may decline, but the majority of older adults have at least one close friend with whom they maintain close contact, share confidences, and can turn to in an emergency.

The social network may narrow as one ages with intimate personal relationships being maintained and the more instrumental relationships discontinued (van Groenou et al, 2013). Research supports the value of friendship for older people across the globe in promoting health and well-being (Blieszner, 2014).

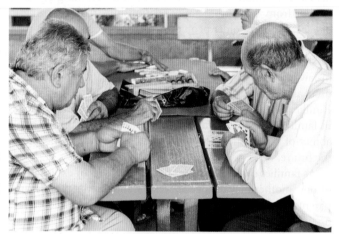

Friends play an important role in the lives of older adults. (By Michal Osmenda from Brussels, Belgium [CC BY 2.0 (http://creativecommons.org/licenses/by/2.0)], via Wikimedia Commons.)

Friendships are often sustaining in the face of overwhelming circumstances. Friends provide the critical elements of satisfactory living that families may not, providing commitment and affection without judgment. Personality characteristics between friends are compatible because the relationships are chosen and caring is shared without obligation. Trust, demonstrations of caring, and mutual problem solving are important aspects of the friendships. Friends may share a lifelong perspective or may bring a totally new intergenerational viewpoint into one's life. Late-life friendships often develop out of changing situations, such as relocation to retirement or assisted living communities, widowhood, and involvement in volunteer pursuits. As desires and pursuits change, some friendships evolve that the person never would have considered in his or her youth.

Considering the obvious importance of friendship, it seems to be a neglected area of exploration and a seldom considered resource for professionals working with older people. Because close friendships have such influence on the sense of well-being of elders, anything done to sustain them or assist in building new friendships and social networks will be helpful. Internet access and social media offer new opportunities to interact with friends or even to form new friendships (Blieszner, 2014). Generally, women tend to have more sustaining friendships than do men, and this factor contributes to resilience, a characteristic linked to successful aging (Hooyman and Kiyak, 2011) (Chapter 28).

Nurses may include questions about the individual's friendship and their importance and availability in their assessment of older adults. While friendships do provide much support, they are also a further source of grief in old age. The loss of friends through death occurs often and nurses must appreciate the nature of this loss. Encouraging intergenerational friendships and linking older adults to resources for social participation and meaningful activities are important interventions.

FAMILIES

Changing Family Structure

The idea of family evokes strong impressions of whatever an individual believes the typical family should be. Because everyone comes from a family, these impressions have powerful symbolic meanings. However, in today's world, the definition of family is in a state of flux. As recently as 100 years ago, the norm was the extended family made up of parents, their grown children, and the children's children, often living together and sharing resources, strengths, and challenges. As cities grew and adult children moved in pursuit of work, parents did not always come along, and the nuclear family evolved. The norm in the United States became two parents and their two children (nuclear family), or at least that was the norm in what has been considered mainstream America. This pattern was not as common among ethnically diverse families where the extended family is often the norm. However, families are changing, and today only about 19% of U.S. households are composed of nuclear families (United States Census Bureau, 2013).

Changing family patterns pose significant challenges for the future of long-term care because 80% to 90% of all long-term care services and supports are provided by spouses, adult children, and other informal caregivers. Baby boomers are more likely to live alone than previous generations, and single-person households are increasing (Blanchard, 2014). Other countries are also experiencing changes in family composition, and even values, as the numbers of older citizens increase and the younger members of society become more mobile and move away from their home (Batiashvili and Gerzmava, 2013). In China, the extended family is disappearing and the country has enacted a new law mandating that family members must attend to the spiritual needs of older family members and visit them frequently if they live apart. Nearly half of the country's seniors live apart from their children (Atlantic Cities, 2013).

A decrease in fertility rates has reduced family size, and American families are smaller today than ever before. The average number of children per family declined from 1.3 in 1970 to 0.9 in 2013 (U.S. Census Bureau, 2013). The high divorce and remarriage rate results in households of blended families of children from previous marriages and the new marriage. The new modern family includes single-parent families, blended families, gay and lesbian families, domestic partnerships, and childless families. Fewer families altogether are common. Older people without families, either by choice or by circumstance, have created their own "families" through communal living with siblings, friends, or others. Indeed, it is not unusual for childless persons residing in long-term care facilities to refer to the staff as their new "family."

Multigenerational Families

In the United States, multigenerational families have grown by approximately 60% since 1990 and 1 in 6 Americans live in a multigenerational ("multigen") household (Generations United, 2014; Hooyman and Kiyak, 2011). Multigenerational families are more common among other cultures, but the growth of multigenerational households in the United States has accelerated during the economic downturn. This growing trend is expected

to continue and has benefits for older family members, as well as younger ones (Generations United, 2011). "Multigen" remodeling or new home building to accommodate intergenerational families is an increasing trend. Box 34-5 presents tips when planning to add an older person to the household.

BOX 34-5   TIPS FOR BEST PRACTICE

Adding an Older Person to the Household

Questions to Ask

- What are the needs of the new member and of the family?
- Where will space be allotted for the new member?
- How will the new member be included in existing family patterns?
- How will responsibilities be shared?
- What resources in the community will assist in the adjustment phase?
- Is the environment safe for the new member?
- How will family life change with the added member, and how does the family feel about it?
- What are the differences in socialization and sleeping patterns?
- What are the older person's strong needs and expectations?
- What are the older person's skills and talents?

Modifications that May Need to be Made

- Arrange semiprivate living quarters if possible.
- Regularly schedule visits to other relatives to give each family time for respite and privacy.
- Arrange adult day health programs and senior activities for the older person to help keep contact with members of his or her own generation. Consider how the older person will feel about giving up familiar surroundings and friends.

Potential Areas of Conflict

- Space: especially if someone has given up his or her space to the older relative.
- Possessions: older people may want to move possessions into the house; others may not find them attractive or may insist on replacing them with new things.
- Entertaining: times when old and young feel the need or desire to exclude the other from social events.
- Responsibilities and chores: the older person may feel useless if he or she does nothing and may feel in the way if he or she does something.
- Expenses: increased cost of home maintenance, food, clothing, and recreation may not be shared appropriately.
- Vacations: whether to go together or alone; young persons may feel uneasy not taking the older person out and may feel resentful if they must.
- Childrearing: disagreement over childrearing policies.
- Childcare: grandparental babysitting may be welcomed by family and resented by older person, or, if not allowed, older person may feel lack of trust in capability.

Ways to Decrease Areas of Conflict

- Respect privacy.
- Discuss space allocations.
- Discuss the older person's furnishings before move.
- Make it clear in advance when social events include everyone or exclude someone.
- Make clear decisions about household tasks; all should have responsibility geared to ability.
- Have the older person pay a share of expenses and maintain a separate phone to reduce strain and increase feelings of independence.

Family Relationships

Family members, however they are defined, form the nucleus of relationships for the majority of older adults and their support system if they become dependent. A long-standing myth in society is that families are alienated from their older family members and abandon their care to institutions. Nothing could be further from the truth. Family relationships remain strong in old age, and most older people have frequent contact with their families. Most older adults possess a large intergenerational web of significant people, including sons, daughters, stepchildren, in-laws, nieces, nephews, grandchildren, and great-grandchildren, as well as partners and former partners of their offspring. Families provide the majority of care for older adults. Changes in family structure will have a significant impact on the availability of family members to provide care for older people in the future.

As families change, the roles of the members or expectations of one another may change as well. Grandparents may assume parental roles for their grandchildren if their children are unable to care for them; or grandparents and older aunts and uncles may assume temporary caregiving roles while the children, nieces, and nephews work. Adult children of any age may provide limited or extensive caregiving to their own parents or aging relatives who may become ill or impaired. A spouse, sibling, or grandchild may become a caregiver as well.

Close-knit families are more aware of the needs of their members and work to resolve problems and find ways to meet the needs of members, even if they are not always successful. Emotionally distant families are less available in times of need and have greater potential for conflict. If the family has never

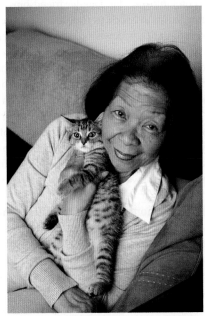

Pets are a part of the family and are particularly beneficial to older adults. They provide companionship, comfort, and caring. (©iStock.com/michellegibson)

been close and supportive, it will not magically become so when members grow older. Resentments long buried may crop up and produce friction or psychological pain. Long-submerged conflicts and feelings may return if the needs of one family member exceed those of the others.

In coming to know the older adult, the gerontological nurse comes to know the family as well, learning of their special gifts and their life challenges. The nurse works with the elder within the unique culture of his or her family of origin, present family, and support networks, including friends.

Types of Families
Traditional Couples

The marital or partnered relationship in the United States is a critical source of support for older people, and nearly 55% of the population age 65 and older is married and lives with a spouse. Although this relationship is often the most binding if it extends into late life, the chance of a couple going through old age together is exceedingly slim. Women older than age 65 are three times as likely as men of the same age to be widowed. Men who survive their spouse into old age ordinarily have multiple opportunities to remarry if they wish. Even among the oldest-old, the majority of men are married. A woman is less likely to have an opportunity for remarriage in late life.

Often, older couples live together but do not marry because of economic and inheritance reasons. In late marriages or remarriage, developing an intimate, sharing relationship between individuals who have had 75 or 80 years of separate experiences often brings conflicting ideologies into the new relationship and can be an enormous challenge. Older people who remarry usually choose someone they have previously known and with whom they share similar backgrounds and interests.

The needs, tasks, and expectations of couples in late life differ from those in earlier years. Some couples have been married more than 60 or 70 years. These years together may have been filled with love and companionship or abuse and resentment, or anything in between. However, in general, marital status (or the presence of a long-time partner) is positively related to health, life satisfaction, and well-being (Korporaal et al, 2013). For all couples, the normal physical and sociological circumstances in late life present challenges. Some of the issues that strain many of these relationships include (1) the deteriorating health of one or both partners; (2) limitations in income; (3) conflicts with children or other relatives; (4) incompatible sexual needs; (5) mismatched needs for activity and socialization.

Divorce. In the past, divorce was considered a stigmatizing event. Today, however, it is so common that a person is inclined to forget the ostracizing effects of divorce from 60 years ago. The divorce rate among people 50 years of age and older has doubled in the past 20 years. Older couples are becoming less likely to stay in an unsatisfactory marriage, and with the aging of the baby boomers, divorce rates will continue to rise. Health care professionals must avoid making assumptions and be alert to the possibility of marital dissatisfaction

in old age. Nurses should ask, "How would you describe your marriage?"

Long-term relationships are varied and complex, with many factors forming the glue that holds them together. Marital breakdown may be more devastating in old age because it is often unanticipated and may occur concurrently with other significant losses. Nurses and other health care professionals must be concerned with supporting a client's decision to seek a divorce and with assisting him or her in seeking counseling in the transition. Divorce will initiate a grieving process similar to the death of a spouse, and a severe disruption in coping capacity may occur until the individual adjusts to a new life. The grief may be more difficult to cope with because no socially sanctioned patterns have been established. In addition, tax and fiscal policies favor married couples, and many divorced elderly women are at a serious economic disadvantage in retirement.

Nontraditional Couples

As the variations in families grow, so do the types of coupled relationships. Among the types of couples we see today are lesbian, gay, bisexual, and transgender (LGBT) couples. Although the number of LGBT people of any age has remained elusive given the reluctance many have about disclosing their status, an estimated 1.75 to 4 million Americans more than 60 years of age are LGBT with projections that this figure is likely to double by 2030 (Administration on Aging, 2014; Jablonski et al, 2013).

Most LGBT adults older than age 60 are single because the ability to legally marry is a recent occurrence. Many have been part of a live-in couple at some time during their life, but as they age, they are more likely to live alone. Gay and bisexual men older than age 50 are twice as likely to live alone as heterosexual men of the same age, while older lesbian and bisexual women are about one-third more likely to live alone. Approximately one-third of the lesbians "come out" after age 50. Many lesbians married, raised children, divorced, and led double lives.

In the case of transgender people, medical providers for many years required candidates for sex reassignment surgery to divorce their spouses, move to a new place, and construct a false personal history consistent with their new gender expression. These practices resulted in transgender people losing even more of their social and personal support systems than might otherwise have been the case (SAGE and MAP, 2010).

It is important to recognize that there are considerable differences in the experiences of younger LGBT individuals when compared with those who are older. Older LGBT individuals did not have the benefit of antidiscrimination laws and support for same-sex partners and are more likely to have kept their relationships hidden than those who grew up in the modern day gay liberation movement. Transgender and bisexual individuals are less likely to "be out" (American Society on Aging and MetLife, 2010).

Some LGBT individuals may have developed social networks of friends, members of their family of origin, and the

larger community, but many lack support. Because many LGBT couples may have no or fewer children, they will have fewer caregivers as they age. The continued legal and policy barriers faced by LGBT elders contribute to the challenges for those in domestic partnerships as they age. Organizations that serve LGBT elders in the community need to enhance outreach and support mechanisms to enable them to maintain independence and age safely and in good health. Box 34-6 presents resources for LGBT elders.

Increasing numbers of same-sex couples are choosing to have families, and this will call for greater understanding of these "new" types of families, young and old. The majority of research has involved gay and lesbian couples, and much less is known about bisexual and transgender relationships. Much more knowledge of cohort, cultural, and generational differences among age groups is needed to understand the dramatic changes in the lives of LGBT individuals in family lifestyles.

Elders and Their Adult Children

In adulthood, relationships between the generations become increasingly important for most people. Older parents enjoy being told about the various activities and successes of their offspring, and these adult children begin to see aspects of themselves that have developed from their parents. At times, the relationships may become strained because the younger adults

are more concerned with their own spouses, partners, and children. The parents are no longer central to their lives, though offspring may be central to the lives of their parents. The most difficult situations occur when the elder parents are openly critical or judgmental about the lives of their offspring. In the best of situations, adult children shift to the role of friend, companion, and confidant to the elder, a concept known as filial maturity.

By and large, elders and their children have relationships that are reciprocal in nature and characterized by affection and mutual support. These relationships are both the most important and potentially the most conflicted. Family resources are shared from birth and usually in some way until and after death. These resources may be tangible, such as money, belongings, and housing. Intangible resources may include advice, support, guidance, and day-to-day assistance with life. Elders provide a family history perspective, models for growing old, assistance with grandchildren, a sense of continuity, and a philosophy of aging.

Most older people see their children on a regular basis, and even children who do not live close to their older parents maintain close connections, so *"intimacy at a distance"* can occur (Hooyman and Kiyak, 2011; Silverstein and Angelli, 1998). Approximately 50% of older people have daily contact with their adult children; nearly 80% see an adult child at least once a week; and more than 75% talk on the phone at least weekly with an adult child (Hooyman and Kiyak, 2011).

Never-Married Older Adults

Approximately 5% of women and 4% of men today have never married. Older people who have lived alone most of their lives often develop supportive networks with siblings, friends, and neighbors. Never-married older adults may demonstrate resilience to the challenges of aging as a result of their independence and may not feel lonely or isolated. Furthermore, they may have had longer lifetime employment and may enjoy greater financial security as they age. Single older adults will increase in the future because being single is increasingly more common in younger years.

Grandparents

The role of grandparenting, and increasingly great-grandparenthood, is experienced by most older adults. The numbers of grandparents are at record highs and still growing at more than twice the overall population growth rate. There were an estimated 65 million grandmothers and grandfathers in 2010. By 2020, they are projected to reach 80 million, at which time they will be nearly one-in-three adults (MetLife, 2011). Sixty-eight percent of individuals born in 2000 will have four grandparents alive when they reach 18; and 76% will have at least one grandparent at 30 years of age (Hooyman and Kiyak, 2011). Great-grandparenthood will become more common in the future in light of projections of a healthier aging.

As the term implies, the "grands" are a step beyond parents in their concerns, exposure, and responsibility. The majority of grandparents derive great emotional satisfaction from their grandchildren. Historically, the emphasis has been on the progressive aging of the grandparent as it affects the relationship with the grandchild, but little has been said about the effects of

---

BOX 34-6   RESOURCES FOR BEST PRACTICE

Administration on Aging: National Resource Center on LGBT Aging

Agency for Healthcare Research and Quality: Family caregiving guideline

Alzheimer's Association: EssentiALZ—Care training resources, e-learning workshops, DVDs, online care training for dementia care and certification for professionals

Caregiver Action Network: Resources, education

Caregiving Resource Center

Family Caregiver Alliance

Hartford Institute for Geriatric Nursing: Family Caregiving Standard of Practice Protocol

Lavender Health: Site maintained by a team of nurses; educational resources and PPT presentations on LGBT health issues and best practices for LGBT communities

Lesbian and Gay Aging Issues Network (LGAIN): A constituent group of the American Society on Aging that works to raise awareness about the concerns of LGBT elders and the unique barriers they encounter in gaining access to housing, health care, long-term care, and other needed services

National Alliance for Caregiving: International resources and best practices in caregiving

National Resource Center on LGBT Aging: Technical assistance resource center aimed at improving the quality of services and supports offered to lesbian, gay, bisexual, and transgender (LGBT) older adults

Services and Advocacy for Gay, Lesbian, Bisexual, and Transgender Elders (SAGE)

The Centers for Disease Control and Prevention (CDC): Caregiving for adults

The Grandmother Project: U.S. nonprofit organization working to strengthen the leadership role of grandmothers in improving health for women and children in Laos, Senegal, Mali, Uzbekistan, and Albania

U.S. Administration on Aging: National Family Caregiver Support Program

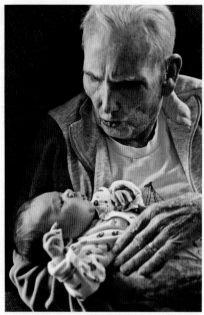

The author's grandson and his maternal great-grandfather. (Photo courtesy Ben Aronoff, Fogline Studios.)

the growth and maturation of the grandchild on the relationship. Many young adults who have had close contact with their grandparents report that this relationship was very meaningful in their lives. Growing numbers of adult grandchildren are assisting in caregiving for grandparents.

The age, vitality, and proximity of both grandchild and grandparent produce a kaleidoscope of possible activities and interactions as both progress through their aging processes. Approximately 80% of grandparents see a grandchild at least monthly, and nearly 50% do so weekly. Geographic distance does not significantly affect the quality of the relationship between grandparents and their grandchildren. The Internet is increasingly being used by distant grandparents as a way of staying involved in their grandchildren's lives and forging close bonds (Hooyman and Kiyak, 2011) (Chapter 5).

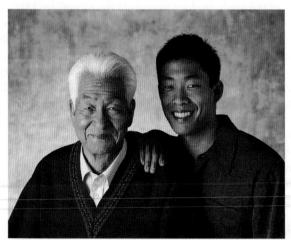

Grandparenting is an important role for elders. (Copyright ©Getty Images.)

Younger grandparents typically live closer to their grandchildren and are more involved in childcare and recreational activities (Box 34-7). Older grandparents with sufficient incomes may provide more financial assistance and other types of instrumental help. The need for support for adult children and grandchildren has the potential to increase during current economic conditions and may pose significant financial concerns for older people (Goyer, 2010). Grandparent-headed households are one of the fastest growing U.S. family groups, and this phenomenon is taking place in other countries as well (Hadfield, 2014). Approximately 2.5 million grandparents are responsible for raising their grandchildren (Legacy Project, 2014). This phenomenon is discussed later in the chapter.

Siblings

Late-life sibling relationships are poorly understood and have been neglected by researchers. As individuals age, they often have more contact with siblings than they did in the years when family and work demands were more pressing. About 80% of older people have at least one sibling, and they are often strong sources of support in the lives of never-married older persons, widowed persons, and those without children. For many elders, these relationships become increasingly important because they have a long history of memories and are of the same generation and similar backgrounds.

Sibling relationships become particularly important when they are part of the support system, especially among single or widowed elders living alone. The strongest of sibling bonds is thought to be the relationship between sisters. When blessed with survival, these relationships remain important into late old age. Service providers should inquire about sibling relationships of past and present significance.

The loss of siblings has a profound effect in terms of awareness of one's own mortality, particularly when those of the same gender die. When an elder reaches the age of the sibling who died, the reaction can be quite disruptive. Not only is grieving activated, but also rehearsal for one's own death may occur. In some cases in which an elder sibling survives younger ones, there may be not only a deep grief but also pangs of guilt: "Why them and not me?" (Chapter 35).

Fictive Kin

Fictive kin are nonblood kin who serve as "genuine fake families," as expressed by Virginia Satir. These nonrelatives become surrogate family and take on some of the instrumental and

---

BOX 34-7   A Grandmother as Seen by an 8-Year-Old Child

"A grandmother is a woman who has no children of her own. That is why she loves other people's children."

"Grandmothers have nothing to do. They are just there: when they take us for a walk they go slowly, like caterpillars along beautiful leaves. They never say, 'Come on, faster, hurry up!'"

"Everyone should try to have a grandmother, especially those who don't have a TV."

From *Ageing in Focus*, March 2006.

affectional attributes of family. Fictive kin are important in the lives of many elders, especially those with no close or satisfying family relationships and those living alone or in institutions. Fictive kin includes both friends and, often, paid caregivers. Primary care providers, such as nursing assistants, nurses, or case managers, often become fictive kin. Professionals who work with older people need to recognize the instrumental and emotional support, as well as the mutually satisfying relationships, that occur between friends, neighbors, and other fictive kin who assist older adults who are dependent.

CAREGIVING

Rosalyn Carter said: "There are four kinds of people in the world: those who have been caregivers, those who are currently caregivers, those who will be caregivers, and those who will need caregivers" (Alzheimer's Reading Room, 2013).

Gerontological nurses are most likely to encounter elders with their family and friends in situations relating to caregiving of some kind. Family members and other unpaid caregivers provide the majority of care for older adults in the United States. In both the United States and other countries, women provide the majority of caregiving (Columbo et al, 2011). The most common caregiver arrangement is that of an adult female child providing care to an older female parent (Messecar, 2012).

Among individuals older than 70 years of age who require care, whites are more likely to receive help from spouses; Hispanics are more likely to receive help from their adult children; and African Americans are the most likely to receive help from a nonfamily member (Messecar, 2012). However, family caregiving has become a normative experience (similar to marriage, working, or retirement) for many of America's families and cuts across racial, ethnic, and social class distinctions. Box 34-8 presents some statistics on caregiving.

Caregiving is considered a major public health issue across the globe, and attention to the physical and mental health of caregivers is receiving increased attention. The aging of the population, the absence of clear signs of a reduction of disability among older adults, the developing looseness of family ties, and the growing female labor market participation are challenging long-term care services worldwide. Initiatives supporting older family caregivers are especially needed in low and lower middle income countries (Columbo et al, 2011; Shahly et al, 2013).

Current trends suggest that the use of paid, formal care by older persons in the community has been decreasing, while their sole reliance on family caregivers has been increasing (Family Caregiver Alliance, 2012). The need for family caregivers will increase substantially, but the number of family caregivers who are available to provide care is decreasing substantially as well. In the United States, informal care provided by caregivers is universally recognized as the foundation of the long-term care system.

Informal caregivers basically provide free services to care recipients (Mast, 2013). These services are valued at $375 billion per year—more than that spent by the U.S. government on Medicare (Sorrell, 2014). Without family caregivers, the present level of long-term care could not be sustained. Additionally,

BOX 34-8   Facts about Caregiving

- 65.7 million caregivers make up 29% of the U.S. adult population (31% of households) providing care to someone who is ill, disabled, or aged.
- Family caregivers are children (41.3%), spouses (38.4%), and other family and friends (20.4%).
- The average duration of a caregiver's role is 4.6 years.
- On average, caregivers spend 20.4 hours/week providing care.
- 43.5 million adult family caregivers care for someone who has Alzheimer's disease or other dementia. They provide care an average of 1 to 4 years more than caregivers of individuals with other illnesses.
- 66% of caregivers are female and their average age is 48. Older caregivers are more likely to care for a spouse or partner; their average age is 63 years and one-third of them are in poor health.
- The number of male caregivers is smaller but increasing, and continued research is needed to address their unique needs. Among spousal caregivers 75 years and older, both sexes provide equal amounts of care.
- 14% of gay men are full-time caregivers.
- 1.4 million children 8 to 18 years of age provide care for an adult relative, and 73% are caring for a parent or grandparent.
- Rates of caregiving vary by ethnicity; approximately 72% are white; 13% are African American; 12% Hispanic; and 2% Asian American.
- African American caregivers are more likely to be younger and unmarried; have less formal education and fewer financial resources; and to be sandwiched between caring for an older person and a younger person younger than age 18 or caring for more than one older person. They are more likely to live with the care recipient and provide more hours of care and are more likely to report unmet needs in terms of support and access to services.
- 70% of working caregivers suffer work-related difficulties due to their caregiving roles.
- Caregiving can have serious negative effects on mental and physical health. Approximately 40% to 70% of caregivers have clinically significant symptoms of depression.
- Caregiving can also present financial burdens, and women who are family caregivers are 2.5 times more likely than noncaregivers to live in poverty.

Data from Family Caregiver Alliance: *Selected caregiver statistics,* 2012. https://caregiver.org/selected-caregiver-statistics Accessed May 2014.

there is a growing shortage of all levels of health care workers for long-term care services. The Institute of Medicine report (2008) states that "unless action is taken immediately, the health care workforce will lack the capacity (in both size and ability) to meet the needs of older patients in the future" (p. 23).

Some suggest that the conception of caregiving is different among the baby boomer generation. While they recognize their responsibility to care for ill family members, they view themselves as partners in the organization of care and want to negotiate and set limits to the amount and kind of care they wish to undertake. "This will require the existence of alternative resources to family care and policy and practice that no longer takes family caregiving for granted" (Guberman et al, 2012). Baby boomer caregivers and upcoming generations will expect more support and formal assistance from national and local agencies in a coordinated long-term care network (Family Caregiver Alliance, 2012; Mast, 2013) (Chapter 32).

Impact of Caregiving

Although caregiving is a means to "give back" to a loved one and can be a source of joy in the giving, it is also stressful. "Caregiving

is a very complex issue, and assuming a caregiving role is a time of transition that requires a restructuring of one's goals, behaviors, and responsibilities. It requires taking on something new, but it is also about loss—of what was and what could have been" (Lund, 2005, p. 152). Caregivers are considered to be "*the hidden patient*" (Schulz and Beach, 1999, p. 2216).

Family caregiving has been associated with increased levels of depression and anxiety, poorer self-reported physical health, compromised immune function, higher rates of insomnia, increased alcohol use, and increased mortality (Newell et al, 2012; Mast, 2013; Sorrell, 2014). Caregiver burden is defined as the negative psychological, economic, and physical effects of caring for a person who is impaired. Whereas not all caregivers experience stress and caregiver burden, the circumstances that are more likely to cause problems with caregiving include competing role responsibilities (e.g., work, home), advanced age of the caregiver, high-intensity caregiving needs, insufficient resources, financial difficulty, poor self-reported health, living in the same household with the care recipient, dementia of the care recipient, length of time caregiving, and prior relational conflicts between the caregiver and care recipient. Caregivers of persons with dementia experience even greater emotional and physical stress than other caregivers (Ching-Tzu et al, 2014; Livingston et al, 2013). Unrelieved caregiver stress increases the potential for abuse and neglect (Newell et al, 2012) (Chapter 31). Boxes 34-9 and 34-10 present further information on caregiver stress.

The positive benefits of caregiving have been given more attention in recent years, but further research is needed to help understand what factors influence how caregivers perceive the experience. Positive benefits of caregiving may include enhanced self-esteem and well-being, personal growth and satisfaction, and finding or making meaning through caregiving (Sorrell, 2014). Caregiving is perceived as rewarding if the caregiver feels needed and useful, has a close and reciprocal relationship with the care recipient, and has an adequate support network (Mast, 2013).

BOX 34-9 Caregiver Needs

- Finding time for myself
- Keeping the person I care for safe
- Balancing work and family responsibilities
- Managing emotional and physical stress
- Finding easy and satisfying activities to do with the care recipient
- Learning how to talk to physicians
- Making end-of-life decisions
- Moving or lifting the care recipient; bathing and dressing
- Managing incontinence or toileting problems
- Managing the challenging behaviors of the care recipient
- Negotiating health care and home and community-based services
- Managing complex medication schedules or high-tech medical equipment
- Choosing a home health agency, assisted living, or skilled nursing facility
- Finding non-English educational material

From Curry L, Walker C, Hogstel MO: Geriatric Nursing 27:166, 2006; Family Caregiver Alliance: Caregiver assessment: principles, guidelines and strategies for change, Report from a National Consensus Development Conference (Vol. 1), San Francisco, 2006, The Alliance.

BOX 34-10 TIPS FOR BEST PRACTICE
Reducing Caregiver Stress

- Educate yourself about the disease or medical condition.
- Contact the appropriate disease-related organization to learn about resources and education and support groups to help you adapt to the challenges you encounter.
- Find a health care professional who understands the disease.
- Consult with other experts to help plan for the future (legal, financial).
- Tap your social resources for assistance.
- Take time for relaxation and exercise.
- Use community resources.
- Maintain your sense of humor.
- Explore religious beliefs and spiritual values.
- Participate in pleasant, nurturing activities such as reading a good book, taking a warm bath.
- Seek supportive counseling when you need it.
- Identify and acknowledge your feelings; you have a right to ALL of them.
- Set realistic goals.
- Attend to your own health care needs.

From U.S. Department of Health and Human Services Administration on Aging, National Family Caregiver Support Program Resources: *Taking care of yourself*, 2014. http://www.acl.gov/NewsRoom/Publications/Index.aspx Accessed May 2014.

Patricia Archbold and colleagues studied caregiving as a role and examined how the relationships between the caregiver and care recipient (mutuality) and the preparation of the caregiver for the tasks and stresses of caregiving (preparedness) influence reactions to caregiving (Archbold et al, 1990). Most caregivers are not prepared for the many responsibilities they face and receive no formal instruction in caregiving activities. Lack of preparedness can greatly increase the caregiver's stress (Messecar, 2012). Figure 34-1 presents a caregiver preparedness scale that nurses can use to determine caregiver needs. Caregivers who have a positive relationship with the care recipient (mutuality) and are prepared for caregiving experience less stress and find caregiving more meaningful (Ching-Tzu et al, 2013). Further research is needed to understand the complexities of the caregiving and care-receiving role and provide a theory base for nursing interventions.

Spousal Caregiving

Eighty percent of persons who live with spouses with disabilities provide care for them. An older spousal caregiver may have significant health problems that are neglected in deference to the greater needs of the incapacitated partner. The disabled spouse may need physical care that is beyond the capabilities of the spousal caregiver. Spousal caregivers provide more intensive, time-consuming care than other family caregivers, as much as 56 hours of care per week on average. They are also less likely to receive assistance from other family members.

Older spouses are at greater risk for negative consequences and often take on greater burdens than they can reasonably handle and wait longer for outside help, using formal services as a last resort. Spousal caregivers are more prone to loneliness and depression and have a 63% greater chance of dying

YOUR PREPARATION FOR CAREGIVING

We know that people may feel well prepared for some aspects of giving care to another person, and not as well prepared for other aspects. We would like to know how well prepared you think you are to do each of the following, even if you are not doing that type of care now.

	Not at all prepared	Not too well prepared	Somewhat well prepared	Pretty well prepared	Very well prepared
1. How well prepared do you think you are to take care of your family member's physical needs?	0	1	2	3	4
2. How well prepared do you think you are to take care of his or her emotional needs?	0	1	2	3	4
3. How well prepared do you think you are to find out about and set up services for him or her?	0	1	2	3	4
4. How well prepared do you think you are for the stress of caregiving?	0	1	2	3	4
5. How well prepared do you think you are to make caregiving activities pleasant for both you and your family member?	0	1	2	3	4
6. How well prepared do you think you are to respond to and handle emergencies that involve him or her?	0	1	2	3	4
7. How well prepared do you think you are to get the help and information you need from the health care system?	0	1	2	3	4
8. Overall, how well prepared do you think you are to care for your family member?	0	1	2	3	4

9. Is there anything specific you would like to be better prepared for? _____

_____

_____

_____

_____

MEAN SCORE of the number of items answered: _____

FIGURE 34-1 Caregiver Preparedness Scale. (From Archbold PG, Stewart BJ, Greenlick MR, et al: Mutuality and preparedness as predictors of caregiver role strain, *Res Nurs Health* 13:375–385, 1990. Reprinted with permission from John Wiley & Sons.)

than people of the same age who are not caring for spouses (Ostwald, 2009). More wives than husbands provide care, but this is expected to change as the life expectancy for men increases.

Older spouses caring for disabled partners also face many role changes. Older women may need to learn to drive, manage money, or make decisions by themselves. Male caregivers may need to learn how to cook, shop, do laundry, and provide personal care to their wives. Spousal caregivers also deal with the added responsibilities of caregiving while at the same time dealing with the anticipated loss of their spouse. Nurses should be alert to situations in which health care personnel may be able to provide supports and resources that make it possible for an individual to assume new responsibilities without being totally overwhelmed. Adult day programs, respite care services, or periodic assistance from a home health aide or homemaker may make it possible for the couple to continue to live together. It is important to pay attention to the physical and mental health needs of the caregiver, as well as the care recipient.

Caring for Individuals with Dementia

More than 70% of individuals with dementia live at home, and family and friends provide nearly 75% of their care. There are 15 million people providing care for a loved one with dementia. These caregivers provide more hours of help than caregivers of other older people and nearly 60% rate the emotional stress of caregiving as high or very high. More than one-third report symptoms of depression. Factors that

increase the stress of caregiving include grief over the multiple losses that occur, the physical demands and duration of caregiving (up to 20 years), and resource availability. Demands are intensified if the care recipient demonstrates behavioral disturbances and impairments in activities of daily living (ADLs) and instrumental activities of daily living (IADLs) (Alzheimer's Association, 2013).

The number of individuals with Alzheimer's disease and other dementias will escalate rapidly in coming years. By 2050, the number of people age 65 and older with Alzheimer's disease may nearly triple. The rising numbers of individuals with dementia, issues related to caregiving, and health care costs of dementia are public health concerns across the globe. Chapter 29 discusses dementia in depth.

Aging Parents Caring for Developmentally Disabled Children

Although we tend to think of caregivers as middle-aged adults caring for elders, an unknown number of elders are caring for their middle-aged children who are physically and mentally disabled. In the past century, developmentally disabled children usually died before reaching adulthood; now, with improved care, they are surviving. For the first time in history, individuals with developmental disabilities are outliving their parents. Planning for their future is an area posing challenges for older people and for service providers internationally (Ryan et al, 2014; Taggart et al, 2012).

With increased survival, adults with developmental disabilities are also at risk for developing chronic illness and will need more care and services. For example, individuals with Down syndrome are more likely to develop dementia. Often, the burden of caring for a developmentally disabled child has been carried by parents for their entire adult life and will end only with the death of the parent or the adult child. Parental caregivers who are aging face changes in their financial resources and health that affect their continued caregiving ability. A majority of these caregivers worry how their child will receive care if they develop a debilitating illness or die.

In the United States, the Planned Lifetime Assistance Network (PLAN), available in some states through the National Alliance for the Mentally Ill, provides lifetime assistance to individuals with disabilities whose parents or other family members are deceased or can no longer provide for their care. The Alzheimer's Association and other aging organizations offer education and support programs for both parents and their developmentally disabled adult children in some communities. There is a continued need for the development of both in-home and community options for developmentally disabled adults who are aging (Ryan et al, 2014; Taggart et al, 2012).

Grandparents Raising Grandchildren

Around the world, an increasing number of grandparents are raising grandchildren in households without a biological parent. More than 2.5 million grandparents are providing primary care (custodial grandparents) for grandchildren in the United States and grandparent-headed households are one of the fastest-growing U.S. family groups (Hadfield, 2014). In the United

States, 1 out of every 10 children lives with a grandparent, and 41% of those children are being raised primarily by that grandparent. More than two-thirds of grandparent primary caregivers are younger than 60 years of age, and 62% are female. Nearly one in five are living below the poverty line (Hadfield, 2014; Livingston and Parker, 2010). The phenomenon of grandparents serving as primary caregivers is more common among African Americans and Hispanics than whites, but the increase in grandparent primary caregiving across the past decade has been much more pronounced among whites (a 19% increase) (Hadfield, 2014; Livingston and Parker, 2010).

The reasons grandparents take a child into the home without his or her parents vary among countries, groups, and individuals. Many grandparents have become, by default, the primary caregivers of grandchildren because the parents are unable to provide the care needed as a result of child abuse, teen pregnancy, imprisonment, joblessness, military deployment, drug and alcohol addictions, illness, death, and other social problems.

In China, grandparent caring is increasing as a result of the number of parents relocating far from home for job opportunities. In Africa and other developing countries, grandparents and other relatives are caring for millions of children orphaned due to the HIV/AIDS epidemic (Hadfield, 2014). Grandparents in these developing countries face great challenges in providing basic subsistence for their grandchildren, and often for themselves.

Research is lacking related to the effect of grandparent caregiving on health status, but existing literature suggests that there are economic, health, and social challenges inherent in this role. Single non-white women caring for their grandchildren appear to be the highest risk group for depression (Hadfield, 2014). Often, crisis situations precipitate the decision, and time for preparation is not available. In many cases, grandparents assume care so that their grandchildren's care is not taken over by the public care system (del Bene, 2010). The unexpected career of caregiving for grandchildren and the "off timing" of this family role transition contribute to the challenges faced (Musil et al, 2011).

As with other types of caregiving, there are both blessings and burdens and caregivers' experiences will be unique (Hadfield, 2014). However, for many grandparents the challenges may include limited income and financial support through the welfare system, lack of informal support systems, loss of leisure activities in retirement, and shame or guilt related to their children's inability to parent. Physical and mental stressors appear to be greater when grandparents are raising a chronically ill or special-needs child or a child with behavioral problems, or experiencing chronic illness themselves (del Bene, 2010; Hooyman and Kiyak, 2011).

Interventions

Routine screening and monitoring of the psychological distress of primary care grandparents and offering support, advice, and referral to reduce stressors are important. Health care institutions, schools, and churches are potential sites where grandparents could access needed information and support (Van Etten and Gautam, 2012). Education and training programs and

support groups are valuable resources that should be available in communities. Nurses can be instrumental in developing and conducting these types of interventions. The National Family Caregiver Support Program (NFCSP), under the Older Americans Act program, provides support services, education and training, counseling, and respite care. Nurses can refer the grandparents to their local area agency on aging to inquire about available resources. Box 34-6 presents resources for grandparents.

Further research is needed to determine the type of interventions most beneficial (Smith et al, 2008). The experiences of children who have been raised by a grandparent, as well as the experiences of grandfathers raising grandchildren, also need to be investigated. Suggestions for nursing interventions with older adults providing primary care to their grandchildren are presented in Box 34-11.

Long-Distance Caregiving

Because of the increasing mobility of today's global society, more children move away for education or employment and do not return home. When the parent needs help, it must be provided "long distance." This is perhaps one of the most difficult situations, and it presents unique challenges. The usual impulse is to want to move the elder into the family's home or to a more accessible location for the family, but this may not be best for an elder or for the family. Issues that need to be considered in long-distance caregiving include identifying a local person who will be available quickly in emergency situations; identifying reliable individuals or services that will provide daily monitoring if necessary; identifying acceptable facilities for assisted living or nursing home care if that becomes necessary; determining which family member is most likely to be free to travel to the elder if needed; and being sure that legalities regarding advance directives, a will, and power of attorney (for health care and financial) have been established.

A profession and industry have emerged to assist the geographically distant family member to ensure that an older relative will receive care. This profession is made up of geriatric care managers, some of whom are nurses or social workers. A care manager can be hired to do everything a family member would do if able, from being available in an emergency, to helping with estate planning, to making arrangements for a move to a nursing home. These services are available primarily to those who are able to pay for them because they are not covered by private insurance, Medicare, or any public agencies. Although these services are expensive, they may be far less expensive than alternative living arrangements or institutional placement.

Similar services may be available for persons with very low incomes by asking the local Area Agency on Aging about local "Community Care for the Elderly" programs. When incomes are too high to qualify for Medicaid and too low to pay for private care managers, the persons and their families must do the best they can. Long-distance care then depends on the goodness of neighbors, local friends, and apartment managers and frequent trips by the long-distance caregiver to the elder.

◆ PROMOTING HEALTHY AGING: IMPLICATIONS FOR GERONTOLOGICAL NURSING

◆ Assessment

◆ Family Assessment

A comprehensive assessment of the elder includes assessment of the family. Often, nurses see families in times of crisis when an older family member needs care. It is important for the nurse to be aware of his or her vision of what a "family" should be and what a "family" should do. Our values should not enter into assessment and intervention with clients. Meiner (2011, p. 113) reminds us that we should not "label families as 'dysfunctional.' It is necessary to identify the strengths within each family and to build on those strengths while recognizing the family's limitations in providing support and caregiving." Thus, the nurse's role is to teach, monitor, and strengthen the family system so as to maintain health and wellness of the entire family structure.

◆ Caregiver Assessment

Family members who assume the caregiving role experience both stressors and benefits. The stresses, the expectations of future needs and problems, and the positive aspects of the caregiving situation should be explored. Caregiver assessment includes how the family member can help the care recipient and how the health care team can help the person providing care. Several validated caregiver assessment instruments are available, including the Preparedness for Caregiving Scale (see Figure 34-1) (Archbold et al, 1990), the Caregiver Strain Index developed by Robinson (1983), and the Modified Caregiver Strain Index (Figure 34-2).

◆ Interventions

In designing interventions to support caregiving, a partnership model, combining the "nurse's professional expertise with the caregiver's knowledge of the family member, is recommended" (Schumacher et al, 2006, p. 47). Given the range of caregiving situations and the uniqueness of each, interventions must be tailored to individual needs (Messecar, 2012). "There is no single, easily implemented and consistently effective method for eliminating the stresses and/or strain of being a caregiver" (Messecar, 2012, p. 479). Interventions include risk assessment, education about caregiving and stress, needed care skills, caregiver

---

BOX 34-11 TIPS FOR BEST PRACTICE

Interventions with Grandparent Caregivers

- Early identification of at-risk grandparents
- Comprehensive assessment of physical, psychosocial, and environmental factors affecting those in the caregiving role for grandchildren
- Anticipatory guidance and counseling about child growth and development and other child-raising issues
- Referral to resources for support, counseling, and financial assistance
- Advocacy for policies supportive of grandparents who have assumed a caregiving role

Directions: Here is a list of things that other caregivers have found to be difficult. Please put a checkmark in the columns that apply to you. We have included some examples that are common caregiver experiences to help you think about each item. Your situation may be slightly different, but the item could still apply.

	Yes, On a Regular Basis = 2	Yes, Sometimes = 1	No = 0
My sleep is disturbed (For example: the person I care for is in and out of bed or wanders around at night)	_____	_____	_____
Caregiving is inconvenient (For example: helping takes so much time or it's a long drive over to help)	_____	_____	_____
Caregiving is a physical strain (For example: lifting in or out of a chair; effort or concentration is required)	_____	_____	_____
Caregiving is confining (For example: helping restricts free time or I cannot go visiting)	_____	_____	_____
There have been family adjustments (For example: helping has disrupted my routine; there is no privacy)	_____	_____	_____
There have been changes in personal plans (For example: I had to turn down a job; I could not go on vacation)	_____	_____	_____
There have been other demands on my time (For example: other family members need me)	_____	_____	_____
There have been emotional adjustments (For example: severe arguments about caregiving)	_____	_____	_____
Some behavior is upsetting (For example: incontinence; the person cared for has trouble remembering things; or the person I care for accuses people of taking things)	_____	_____	_____
It is upsetting to find the person I care for has changed so much from his/her former self (For example: he/she is a different person than he/she used to be)	_____	_____	_____
There have been work adjustments (For example: I have to take time off for caregiving duties)	_____	_____	_____
Caregiving is a financial strain	_____	_____	_____
I feel completely overwhelmed (For example: I worry about the person I care for; I have concerns about how I will manage)	_____	_____	_____

[Sum responses for "Yes, on a regular basis" (2 pts each) and "yes, sometimes" (1 pt each)]

Total Score =

FIGURE 34-2 Modified Caregiver Strain Index. (From Thornton M, Travis SS: Analysis of the reliability of the Modified Caregiver Strain Index, *J Gerontol B Psychol Sci Soc Sci* 58(2):S129, 2003. Copyright ©The Gerontological Society of America. Reproduced by permission of the publisher.)

health and home safety, support groups, linkages to ongoing support, counseling, resource identification, relief/respite from daily care demands, and stress management.

Education provided by nurses to help prepare the caregiver for the caregiving role, particularly at the time of discharge from the hospital or nursing home, can help to prevent role strain and lessen burden (Sorrell, 2014). With many caregivers trying to balance caregiving responsibilities while working, educational programs offered in the workplace can be beneficial for both the caregiver and the employer (Box 34-12) (Curry et al, 2006). When the nurse works with a family from a different culture that may have rituals and routines unfamiliar to him or her, the nurse needs to be particularly careful to respect these differences. The nurse can work with the family to make the best use of their strengths, whatever they may be. Each family member can be valued for what he or she brings to the situation. Service providers need to enhance cultural competence and design programs that are culturally acceptable (Chapter 4).

Linking caregivers to community resources, such as respite care, adult day programs, and financial support resources, is important. Respite care allows the caregiver to take a break from caregiving for various periods of time. Respite care may be provided in institutions, in the home, or in other community settings. Nurses should be aware of respite care resources in their communities, and the local Area Agency on Aging can provide information on respite care and other caregiver services. These interventions, when available, can alleviate much of the stress of caregiving but are utilized infrequently or very late in the course of caregiving in the United States (Mast, 2013). Many countries in Europe offer generous respite care services as part of the long-term care system. *Healthy People 2020* objectives for long-term services and supports are presented in Box 34-13. Box 34-14 presents nursing interventions for caregivers.

Tailored multicomponent interventions designed to match a specific target population seem to have the most positive outcomes on caregiver burden and stress—for example, groups designed to assist caregivers caring for individuals with early-stage dementia or those with Parkinson's disease. Programs that work collaboratively with care recipients and their families and are more intensive and modified to the caregiver's needs are also more successful. Effective programs should include training on needed skills (managing difficult behaviors, personal care problems), finding and using resources, handling emotional and physical responses to care, self-care for the caregiver, individual consultation and therapy, and ongoing assistance and support (Alzheimer's Association, 2014; Messecar, 2012; Sorrell, 2014). Box 34-15 presents results from a telephone-delivered intervention for dementia caregivers in China.

Interventions with caregivers must always consider the great variability in family structures, resources, traditions, and history. The range of adaptations is enormous, and the goal is always to restore the balance of the system to the greatest extent possible and support caregivers in their caring. The family can be visualized as a mobile structure with many parts, and when one part is touched, each part shifts to regain the balance. The intrusion of professionals in a family system will temporarily unbalance the system and may provide an opportunity to restore the balance in a

---

BOX 34-12   Topics for Workplace Caregiver Assistance Programs

- Normal and healthy aging
- Communicating effectively with older adults
- Medication use
- Caring for the caregiver
- Specific health information
- Community resources
- Supplemental services
- Housing and long-term care options
- Medicare, Medigap, and other insurance (e.g., long-term care)
- Support groups
- End-of-life and legal information (e.g., advance directives)

From Curry LC, Walker C, Hogstel MO: Educational needs of employed family caregivers of older adults: evaluation of a workplace project, *Geriatr Nurs* 27:166–173, 2006.

 BOX 34-13   HEALTHY PEOPLE 2020

Long-Term Services and Supports

- Reduce the proportion of unpaid caregivers of older adults who report an unmet need for caregiver support services.
- Reduce the proportion of noninstitutionalized older adults with disabilities who have an unmet need for long-term services and supports.

Data from U.S. Department of Health and Human Services, Office of Disease Prevention and Health Promotion: Healthy People 2020, 2012. http://www.healthypeople.gov/2020.

---

healthier manner, sometimes by adding an element or increasing the weight of one or decreasing the weight of another. Further research is needed to provide the foundation for nursing interventions with family caregivers, particularly among racially and ethnically diverse families and nontraditional families. Resources for caregiving are presented in Box 34-6.

BOX 34-14   TIPS FOR BEST PRACTICE

Nursing Actions to Create and Sustain a Partnership with Caregivers

- Surveillance and ongoing monitoring
- Coaching: helping caregivers apply knowledge and develop skills
- Teaching: providing information and instruction
- Providing accurate and complete information about services; determine with the family referrals for services based on needs and preferences of caregiver and care recipient; mutually determine with the family services that are affordable, acceptable, and logistically feasible
- Fostering partnerships: fostering communication and collaboration between the caregiver and the care recipient and between them and the nurse
- Providing psychosocial support: attending to psychosocial well-being; help the caregiver and family identify effective coping strategies
- Coordinating: orchestrating the work of other health care team members and the activities of the caregiver

Data from Eilers J, Heermann JA, Wilson ME, et al: Independent nursing actions in cooperative care, *Oncol Nurs Forum* 32:849–855, 2005; Mast M: To use or not to use: a literature review of factors that influence family caregivers' use of support services, *J Gerontol Nurs* 39(1):20–28, 2013; Schumacher K, Beck CA, Marren JM: Family caregivers: caring for older adults, working with their families, *Am J Nurs* 106:40–49, 2006.

BOX 34-15   RESEARCH HIGHLIGHTS

This single-blinded randomized controlled trial investigated the effectiveness of a 12-week telephone-delivered psychoeducational intervention in alleviating caregiver burden and enhancing caregiver self-efficacy among caregivers of individuals with dementia in China. The focus of the intervention was to provide emotional support; direct caregivers to appropriate resources; encourage them to attend to their own physical, emotional, and social needs; and provide education on strategies to cope with ongoing concerns.

Participants in the telephone-delivered psychoeducational program demonstrated significant reductions in caregiver burden and improvements in self-efficacy compared with the control group. A telephone-based intervention offers flexibility for caregivers who may not have time to travel to a face-to-face program (Kwock et al, 2013). Dementia is still seen as a stigma in Chinese society, and the authors note that a telephone intervention may be more acceptable than joining a group.

From Kwock T, Wong B, Ip I, et al: Telephone-delivered psychoeducational intervention for Hong Kong Chinese dementia caregivers: a single-blinded randomized controlled trial, *Clin Int Aging* 8:1191–1197, 2013.

KEY CONCEPTS

- Roles define individual and societal expectations of function.
- The ability to successfully negotiate transitions and develop new and gratifying roles depends on personal and environmental supports, timing, clarity of expectations, personality, and degree of change required.
- Numerous patterns of retirement exist, and therefore retirement per se cannot be viewed categorically.
- Preretirement planning and postretirement follow-up significantly affect positive adaptation to the transition.
- Elders and their family members carry a long history. Current family dynamics must be understood within the context of family history.
- Loss of a spouse/life partner is the role change that has the greatest potential for life disruption, and nursing support can make a significant positive difference in the transition.

- Widowers are a neglected group in the literature and in the service arena. These men are particularly vulnerable to physical and mental stress.
- Family members and other unpaid caregivers provide 80% of care for older adults in the United States.
- Grandparents are increasingly assuming primary caregiving roles with grandchildren.
- Caregiving activities are one of the most major social issues of our time, as well as a significant global public health problem.
- Nursing interventions with caregivers include risk assessment, education about caregiving and stress, needed care skills, caregiver health and home safety, support groups, linkages to ongoing support, counseling, resource identification, relief/respite from daily care demands, and stress management.

NURSING STUDY: RETIREMENT

Sandy was a professor at a small, private college in a metropolitan area. Although she had taught nursing for 25 years and loved her work, it had been a demanding year, and she was very tired. A rumor had recently circulated that the college was in trouble financially. Some of the most affluent alumni could no longer be counted on for gifts and endowments because the football coach had not produced a winning team for several years. Because the tuition was becoming exorbitant, the college had recently lost some students to one of the three state college campuses within driving distance of the city. The trustees of the college, in a move to cut expenses, offered an incentive to professors who were willing to retire early; an extra year of service credit was presented for every 6 years worked. Sandy was only 55 years old but thought that the 4 years of extra credit would bring her near the minimum retirement age for Social Security (an error, of course, because her age did not change with her service credit). Rather impulsively, Sandy decided to accept the offer after telling colleagues, "Well, you know how I love to travel. Why wait until I'm too old to enjoy retirement? Why don't you think about the offer, too? This is a once-in-a-lifetime opportunity." Near the end of the academic year, the celebrations began: recognition, plaques, expressions of gratitude from students, and envy from her associates. The send-off was wonderful. In the summer, Sandy withdrew her savings and booked a cruise to the Greek islands. The journey was lovely, and she enjoyed every moment. Sandy began to feel depressed when she got off the ship but knew it was only because the elegant cruise was over. However, as fall came around, Sandy began to feel more depressed. Most of her friends were teachers, and they were all back at work. Sandy briefly thought of going to Pittsburgh to visit her sister but decided against the idea because she and her sister had really

never been very compatible. Then Sandy was hit with some of the realities of early retirement: she was unable to withdraw any of her considerable tax-deferred savings before she was 59{1/2} years of age without significant penalty, her health insurance coverage was considerably less comprehensive after retirement, her colleagues were all busy, and she was very bored. Then the real blow fell. The college, in desperation, had dipped into the retirement funds to remain solvent, and the retirees' pensions were now at risk. Sandy's sister, who was a nurse, called to announce that she wanted to come and stay a few days while she attended a conference in the city. When she arrived, Sandy overwhelmed her with the litany of woes. If you were Sandy's sister, what would you do?

Based on the nursing study, develop a nursing care plan using the following procedure*:

- List Sandy's comments that provide subjective data.
- List information that provides objective data.
- From these data, identify and state, using an accepted format, two nursing diagnoses you determine are most significant to Sandy at this time. List two of Sandy's strengths that you have identified from the data.
- Determine and state outcome criteria for each diagnosis. These criteria must reflect some alleviation of the problem identified in the nursing diagnosis and must be stated in concrete and measurable terms.
- Plan and state one or more interventions for each diagnosed problem. Provide specific documentation of the source used to determine the appropriate intervention. Plan at least one intervention that incorporates Sandy's existing strengths.
- Evaluate the success of the intervention. Interventions must correlate directly with the stated outcome criteria to measure the outcome success.

*Students are advised to refer to their nursing diagnosis text and identify possible or potential problems.

CRITICAL THINKING QUESTIONS AND ACTIVITIES

1. Identify several important family and social roles that elder members of your family fulfill.
2. What are the factors to consider in role transitions, and how can transitions be made smoother?
3. What factors must be considered in the decision to retire?
4. Discuss the differences you would expect in adaptation to retirement between an individual who retired because of ill health and one who retired because he or she desired to do so.
5. How do you think retirement differs for men and women?
6. Describe what you think would be an ideal retirement.
7. Discuss how you think an individual can prepare for widowhood.
8. Discuss the meanings and the thoughts triggered by the young person's and elder's viewpoints expressed at the beginning of the chapter. How do these vary from your own experience?

RESEARCH QUESTIONS

1. What are the challenges associated with older people working longer?
2. What are the patterns of adaptation of widowers? How do the patterns differ for young-old and old-old?
3. Who divorces in later life and for what reasons?
4. What are the differences between grandparenting and great-grandparenting?
5. Are there differences in the experience of primary grandparent caregivers based on ethnicity, race, and culture?
6. How do adults who were raised by grandparents view this experience?
7. Do interventions to improve the physical health of caregivers relate to less reported stress and improved health outcomes?
8. What are the reactions of elders to the care given by their offspring?
9. How do upcoming generations view caregiving responsibilities?

REFERENCES

Administration on Aging: *Diversity,* 2014. http://www.aoa.gov/AoA_programs/Tools_Resources/diversity.aspx. Accessed May 2014.

Alzheimer's Association: *Alzheimer's facts and figures,* 2014. http://www.alz.org/alzheimers_disease_facts_and_figures.asp#quickFacts. Accessed May 2014.

Alzheimer's Reading Room: *Quote of the day,* 2013. http://www.alzheimersreadingroom.com/2009/11/quote-of-day-caregivers.html. Accessed May 2014.

American Society on Aging and MetLife: *Still out, still aging,* 2010. https://www.metlife.com/assets/cao/mmi/publications/studies/2010/mmi-still-out-still-aging.pdf. Accessed November 18, 2014.

Archbold PG, Stewart BJ, Greenlick MR, et al: Mutuality and preparedness as predictors of caregiver role strain, *Res Nurs Health* 13:375–384, 1990.

Atlantic Cities: *The wake-up call in China: "Visit your parents" law,* 2013. http://www.theatlanticcities.com/politics/2013/07/wake-call-chinas-visit-your-parents-law/6377. Accessed May 2014.

Batiashvili G, Gerzmava O: Administration on Aging, Global comparison of formal and informal caregiving, *Eur Sci J* 2:89–97, 2013.

Bennett K, Soulsby L: Well-being in bereavement, *Illn Crises Loss* 20(4):321–337, 2012.

Blanchard J: Aging in community: the communitarian alternative to aging in place alone, *Generations* 37(4), 2013–2014. http://asaging.org/blog/aging-community-communitarian-alternative-aging-place-alone. Accessed May 2014.

Blieszner R: The worth of friendships: can friends keep us happy and healthy? *Generations* 38(1):24–30, 2014.

Carey I, Shah S, DeWilde S, et al: Increased risk of acute cardiovascular events after partner bereavement, *JAMA* 174(4):598–605, 2014.

Ching-Tzu Y, Hsin-Yun L, Yea-Ing L: Dyadic relational resources and role strain in family caregivers of persons living with dementia at home: a cross-sectional survey, *Int J Nurs Studies* 51(4):593–602, 2014.

Columbo F, Llena-Nozal A, Mercier J, et al: *Help wanted? Providing and paying for LTC,* OECD Health Policy Studies, OECD Publishing, 2011. http://dx.doi.org/10.1787/9789264097759-en. Accessed May 18, 2015

Curry LC, Walker C, Hogstel MO: Educational needs of employed family caregivers of older adults: evaluation of a workplace project, *Geriatr Nurs* 27:166–173, 2006.

Das A: Spousal loss and health in late life: moving beyond emotional trauma, *J Aging Health* 25:221–242, 2013.

del Bene S: African American grandmothers raising grandchildren: a phenomenologi-cal perspective of marginalized women, *J Gerontol Nurs* 36:32–40, 2010.

deVries B: Grief: intimacy's reflection, *Generations* 25:75–80, 2001.

DiGiacomo M, Lewis J, Nolan M, et al: Health transitions in recently widowed women: a mixed methods study, *BMC Health Serv Res* 13:143, 2013.

Family Caregiver Alliance, National Center on Caregiving: *Selected caregiver statistics,* 2012. https://caregiver.org/selected-caregiver-statistics. Accessed May 2014.

Generations United: *Family matters: multigenerational families in a volatile economy,* 2011. http://www.gu.org/RESOURCES/Publications/FamilyMattersMultigenerationalFamilies.aspx. Accessed December 1, 2014.

Generations United: *What is a multigenerational household?* 2014. http://www2.gu.org/OURWORK/Multigenerational/MultigenerationalHouseholdInformation.aspx. Accessed May 2014.

Goyer A: *Grandparents increasingly fill need as caregivers,* 2010, AARP. http://www.aarp.org/relationships/grandparenting/info-12-2010/more_grandparents_raising_grandchildren.html. Accessed August 2014.

Guberman N, Lavoie JP, Blein L, et al: Baby boom caregivers: care in the age of individualization, *Gerontologist* 52(2):210–218, 2012.